About the Authors

Frances Sienkiewicz Sizer

M.S., R.D.N., F.A.N.D., attended Florida State University where, in 1980, she received her B.S., and in 1982 her M.S., in nutrition. She is certified as a charter Fellow of the Academy of Nutrition and Dietetics. She is a founding member and vice president of Nutrition and Health Associates, an information and resource center in Tallahassee, Florida, that maintains an ongoing bibliographic database tracking research in more than 1,000 topic areas of nutrition. Her textbooks include *Life Choices: Health Concepts and Strategies*; *Making Life Choices*; *The Fitness Triad: Motivation, Training, and Nutrition*; and others. She also authored *Nutrition Interactive*, an instructional college-level nutrition CD-ROM that pioneered the animation of nutrition concepts in college classrooms. She has consulted with an advisory board of professors from around the nation with a focus on innovations in nutrition education. She has lectured at universities and at national and regional conferences and supports local hunger and homelessness relief organizations in her community.

Eleanor Noss Whitney

Ph.D., received her B.A. in biology from Radcliffe College in 1960 and her Ph.D. in biology from Washington University, St. Louis, in 1970. Formerly on the faculty at Florida State University and a dietitian registered with the Academy of Nutrition and Dietetics, she now devotes her time to research, writing, and consulting in nutrition, health, and environmental issues. Her earlier publications include articles in *Science*, *Genetics*, and other journals. Her textbooks include *Understanding Nutrition*, *Understanding Normal and Clinical Nutrition*, *Nutrition and Diet Therapy*, and *Essential Life Choices* for college students and *Making Life Choices* for high school students. Her most intense interests presently include energy conservation, solar energy uses, alternatively fueled vehicles, and ecosystem restoration. She is an activist who volunteers full-time for the Citizens Climate Lobby.

Brief Contents

The five **Dietary Reference Intake** tables are on pages A, B, and C at the back of the book in this edition, relocated there from the front cover in previous editions.

Contents

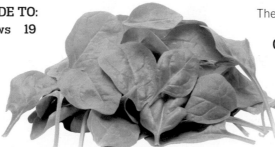

Norman Chan/Shutterstock.com

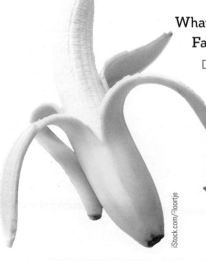

iStock.com/Floortje

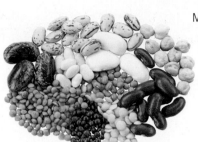

CHAPTER 7
The Vitamins   218

Evgeny Karandaev/Shutterstock.com

CHAPTER 8
Water and Minerals   270

CHAPTER 9
Energy Balance and Healthy Body Weight   317

George Nazmi Bebawi/Shutterstock.com

Tim UR/Shutterstock.com

CHAPTER **15**

Hunger and the Future of Food   567

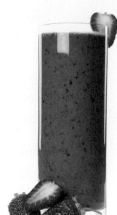

Olyina/Shutterstock.com

Dietary Reference Intakes and Other Standards
(at the back of the book)

Preface

A billboard in Louisiana reads, "Come as you are. Leave different," meaning that once you've seen, smelled, tasted, and listened to Louisiana, you'll never be the same. This book extends the same invitation to its readers: come to nutrition science as you are, with all of the knowledge and enthusiasm you possess, with all of your unanswered questions and misconceptions, and with the habits and preferences that now dictate what you eat.

But leave different. Take with you from this study a more complete understanding of nutrition science. Take a greater ability to discern between nutrition truth and fiction, to ask sophisticated questions, and to find the answers. Finally, take with you a better sense of how to feed yourself in ways that not only please you and soothe your spirit but nourish your body as well.

For more than four decades, *Nutrition: Concepts and Controversies* has been a cornerstone of nutrition classes across North America, serving the needs of students and professors. In keeping with our tradition, in this, our 15th edition, we continue exploring the ever-changing frontier of nutrition science, confronting its mysteries through its scientific roots. We maintain our sense of personal connection with instructors and learners alike, writing for them in the clear, informal style that has become our trademark.

Pedagogical Features

Throughout these chapters, features tickle the reader's interest and inform. For both verbal and visual learners, our logical presentation and our lively figures keep interest high and understanding at a peak. The photos that adorn many of our pages add pleasure to reading.

Many tried-and-true features return in this edition: Each chapter begins with What Do You Think? questions to pique interest. What Did You Decide? at the chapter's end asks readers to draw conclusions. A list of Learning Objectives (LO) offers a preview of the chapter's major goals, and the LO reappear under section headings to make clear the main take-away messages. Do the Math margin features challenge readers to solve nutrition problems, with examples provided. Think Fitness reminders alert readers to links among nutrition, fitness, and health. Food Feature sections act as bridges between theory and practice; they are practical applications of the chapter concepts. The consumer sections, entitled A Consumer's Guide To . . ., lead readers through an often bewildering marketplace with scientific clarity, preparing them to move ahead with sound marketplace

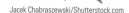
Jacek Chabraszewski/Shutterstock.com

decisions. Each Consumer's Guide ends with review questions to improve recall of the main points.

By popular demand, we have retained our Snapshots of vitamins and minerals, which now reflect the 2015 Daily Values. These concentrated capsules of information depict food sources of vitamins and minerals, present DRI values, and offer the chief functions of each nutrient along with deficiency and toxicity symptoms.

New or major terms are defined in the margins of chapter pages or in nearby tables, and they also appear in the Glossary at the end of the book. Terms defined in margins are printed in **blue** boldface type; terms in tables are in **black**. Readers who wish to locate any term can quickly do so by consulting the Index, which lists the page numbers of definitions in boldface type. Each chapter closes with the indispensible Self Check that provides study questions, with answers in Appendix G to provide immediate feedback to the learner.

Controversies

The Controversies of this book's title invite you to explore beyond the safe boundaries of established nutrition knowledge. These optional readings, which appear at the end of each chapter, delve into current research themes and ongoing debates among nutrition scientists. These fast-changing topics capture interest and demonstrate how scientific investigations both build nutrition knowledge and challenge it.

Chapter Contents

Chapter 1 begins the text with a personal challenge to students. It asks the question so many people ask of nutrition educators—"Why should people care about nutrition?" We answer with a lesson in the ways in which nutritious foods affect diseases and present a continuum of diseases from purely genetic in origin to those almost totally preventable by nutrition. After presenting some beginning facts about the genes, nutrients, bioactive food components, and nature of foods, the chapter goes on to present the *Healthy People* goals for the nation. It concludes with a discussion of scientific research and quackery.

Chapter 2 brings together the concepts of nutrient standards, such as the Dietary Reference Intakes, and diet planning using the Dietary Guidelines for Americans 2015–2020. Chapter 3 presents a thorough, but brief, introduction to the workings of the human body from the genes to the organs, with major emphasis on the digestive system and its microbiota. Chapters 4 through 6 are devoted to the energy-yielding nutrients: carbohydrates, lipids, and protein. Controversy 4 has renewed its focus on theories and fables surrounding the health effects of added sugars in the diet. Controversy 5 considers the scientific underpinnings of lipid guidelines.

Chapters 7 and 8 present the vitamins, minerals, and water. Chapter 9 relates energy balance to body composition, obesity, and underweight and provides guidance on lifelong weight maintenance. Chapter 10 presents the relationships among physical activity, athletic performance, and nutrition, with some guidance about products marketed to athletes. Chapter 11 applies the essence of the first 10 chapters to chronic disease development and prevention.

Chapter 12 delivers urgently important concepts of food safety and ends with practical pointers for applying them in real-life situations. It also addresses the usefulness and safety of food additives, including artificial sweeteners and artificial fats. Chapters 13 and 14 emphasize the importance of nutrition through the life span, with issues surrounding childhood obesity in Controversy 13. Chapter 14 includes nutrition advice for feeding preschoolers, schoolchildren, teens, and the elderly.

Chapter 15 devotes attention to hunger and malnutrition, both in the United States and throughout the world. It also touches on the vast network of problems that threaten the future food supply, and explores potential paths to solutions.

Our Message to You

Our purpose in writing this text, as always, is to enhance our readers' understanding of nutrition science. We also hope the information on this book's pages will reach beyond the classroom into our readers' lives. Take the information you find inside this book home with you. Use it in your life: nourish yourself, educate your loved ones, and nurture others to be healthy. Stay up with the news, too—for despite all the conflicting messages, inflated claims, and even quackery that abound in the marketplace, true nutrition knowledge progresses with a genuine scientific spirit, and important new truths are constantly unfolding.

New to This Edition

Every section of each chapter of this text reflects the changes in nutrition science occurring since the last edition. The changes range from subtle shifts of emphasis to entirely new sections that demand our attention. Appendix F supplies current references; older references may be viewed in previous editions, available from the publisher.

Inside Front Cover Pages
- The DRI tables, previously located on the inside front cover pages, have joined other standards at the back of the book, pages A through C.

Chapter 1
- Updated leading causes of death figure.
- Updated midcourse review of HP2020.
- Defined term *macronutrients* and *micronutrients*.
- Defined term *meta-analysis*.

- Controversy definitions and descriptions follow Academy of Nutrition and Dietetics,
- Definition of Terms List (2017).
- Updated NDTR credentials.

Chapter 2
- Updated U.S. diet compared with ideals figure.
- Defined term *nutritional equivalents*.
- Major revision to diet planning section and tables.
- Expanded and clarified Food Lists for Weight Management coverage.
- New food label comparison figure.
- Improved phytochemical tables.
- Moved Table C2–3 to instructors' materials.

Chapter 3
- Reorganized chapter for greater focus on digestive tract and functions. Moved other body systems to instructors' materials.
- Revamped figure of pH values.
- Reorganized figure of small intestinal lining.
- Introduced and defined term *microbiome*.
- Reorganize table of foods and intestinal gas.
- Major reorganization, update, and streamlining of the alcohol Controversy.

Chapter 4
- New explanation of energy nutrients percentages in relation to total calorie intake.
- New figure of percentages of energy nutrients.
- Moved figure of fiber composition to instructors' materials.
- New figure of strategies to increase fiber intake.
- Shortened glycemic index coverage.
- Major diabetes coverage moved to Chapter 11.
- New section on diabetes and hypoglycemia, explaining failure of blood glucose control.
- New section on sugar alcohols.
- New sugar alcohol table.
- Controversy is streamlined and updated.

Chapter 5
- Defined term *shortening*.
- Defined term *inflammation*.
- Updated and improved coverage of EPA and DHA.
- Moved figure of fish oil supplement label to instructors' materials.
- New bar graph figure of lipids in grain foods.
- Updated Controversy.

Chapter 6
- Added bone broth discussion to Consumer's Guide.
- Removed adult bone loss from protein excess.
- New figure comparing energy and protein in Greek-style yogurt and a commercial highprotein shake.
- Condensed and combined tables in Controversy section.
- New sample 2,000-calorie menu for a day of vegetarian meals.

Chapter 7
- Fully updated each vitamin section.
- Converted photos to figures, as follows: Vitamin E in Oils; Vitamin K for newborns; Folate and neural tube defects.
- Moved table of Vitamin D in disease to instructors' materials.
- New Consumer's Guide on food processing and vitamins.
- New figure of the effect of folic acid fortification on neural tube defect prevalence in selected countries of the world.
- Updated Controversy section; addressed current supplement contamination concerns.
- New figure of how to read a food label.

Chapter 8
- Reorganized, updated water section.
- Reorganized sodium sections.
- Replaced figure of sodium sources.
- New figure of sodium on a food label.
- Created new figures from photos as follows: Osmosis (eggplant); goiter; iodized salt label; nonheme iron absorption; zinc deficiency.
- New figure of average daily sodium intakes in U.S. adults.
- New photo of calcium sources.
- Moved section on tracking calcium to instructors' materials.
- Updated Controversy.

Chapter 9
- New obesity maps reflecting newer analytical methods.
- Defined clinical term *adiposity-based chronic disease*.
- Added sleep function of ghrelin.
- Refined section on microbiome and obesity.
- Addressed efficacy of artificial sweeteners.
- Added discussion of genetic alterations in obesity.
- New summary figure of factors in obesity development.
- Added sleeve gastrectomy to surgical options.
- New explanation of intermittent fasting.
- Defined term *exergaming*.
- Addressed cultural differences in dietary energy density.
- Updated terminology associated with female athlete triad.
- New table of harms from anorexia nervosa.

Chapter 10
- Reorganized several major sections.
- Addressed energy availability and energy need concepts.
- Addressed gastrointestinal effects of ultraendurance events.
- New carbohydrate and protein recommendations from the Academy of Nutrition and Dietetics (AND).
- New figure of anemia in female athletes.
- New hydration schedule from AND.
- Applied guidelines for nutrient timing from the International Society of Sports Nutrition.
- New discussion of beetroot and dietary nitrite among ergogenic aids.

Chapter 11
- Complete chapter reorganization to focus on nutrition and chronic diseases.
- Removed discussion of infectious disease.
- New table of chronic disease risk factors.
- New table of adult blood pressure standards.
- New major section on diabetes; new table of misconceptions about diabetes.
- Introduced term *precision medicine*.
- Addressed consumer privacy in genetic testing.

Chapter 12
- Defined terms *pathogen, intoxication, and endemic*.
- Added term *toxin-mediated infections*.
- New section on the FDA Food Safety Modernization Act, with definition.
- Expanded coverage of package dating.
- Defined FDA's new Produce Safety Rule.
- Moved kitchen test table to new Food Feature.
- Restructured thermometer and safe temperature figures for clarity.
- New Food Feature: *Handling Real-Life Challenges to Food Safety*.
- New figure on selective breeding.
- Defined *gene editing* and CRISPR technology.
- Described and added new figure of genetically engineered salmon.
- Added consumer concerns about glyphosate to summary table.

Chapter 13
- Deleted the infant mortality figure.
- Replaced the spina bifida figure.
- Added a new table of seafood advice for pregnant and lactating women.
- Replaced the sketched figure of facial characteristics of FAS with photo of FAS child.
- Reorganized table of supplements for breastfed infants.
- Added a discussion and definition of responsive feeding.
- Added hunger and satiety signals to the table of infant development.
- New table of parental strategies against childhood obesity.
- New adequate sleep section and table.

Chapter 14
- Updated MyPlate figure.
- Updated and improved allergy section.
- Condensed and updated PMS coverage.
- New section on weight loss and overweight in aging.
- Restructured, updated vitamin D section.
- Addressed the Mediterranean Eating Pattern in Alzheimer's disease development.
- New figure of controllable factors associated with dementia in aging.
- New figure of caffeine sources.

Chapter 15
- New figure of trends in prevalence of food insecurity.
- Updated hunger sections.
- Several new figures.

Appendix Changes:
- Deleted the Table of Food Composition.
- Previous Appendix I, Chemical Structures, is now Appendix A.

Ancillary Materials

Students and instructors alike will appreciate the innovative teaching and learning materials that accompany this text.

MindTap: A new approach to highly personalized online learning. Beyond an eBook, homework solution, digital supplement, or premium website, MindTap is a digital learning platform that works alongside your campus LMS to deliver course curriculum across the range of electronic devices in your life. MindTap is built on an "app" model allowing enhanced digital collaboration and delivery of engaging content across a spectrum of Cengage and non-Cengage resources.

Instructor Companion Site: Everything you need for your course in one place! This collection of book-specific lecture and class tools is available online via www.cengage.com/login. Access and download PowerPoint presentations, images, instructors' manual, videos, and more.

Test Bank with Cognero: Cengage Learning Testing Powered by Cognero is a flexible online system that allows you to:
- Author, edit, and manage test bank content from multiple Cengage Learning solutions.
- Create multiple test versions in an instant.
- Deliver tests from your LMS, your classroom, or wherever you want.

Diet & Wellness Plus: Diet & Wellness Plus helps you understand how nutrition relates to your personal health goals. Track your diet and activity, generate reports, and analyze the nutritional value of the food you eat. Diet & Wellness Plus includes over 75,000 foods as well as custom food and recipe features. The new Behavior Change Planner helps you identify risks in your life and guides you through the key steps to make positive changes. Diet & Wellness Plus is also available as an app that can be accessed from the app dock in MindTap.

Global Nutrition Watch: Bring currency to the classroom with Global Nutrition Watch from Cengage Learning. This user-friendly website provides convenient access to thousands of trusted sources, including academic journals, newspapers, videos, and podcasts, for you to use for research projects or classroom discussion. Global Nutrition Watch is updated daily to offer the most current news about topics related to nutrition.

Acknowledgments

Our thanks to our partners Linda Kelly DeBruyne and Sharon Rolfes for decades of support. Thank you, David Warren Cox for generating our orderly endnote lists.

We are also grateful to the nutrition professionals who updated sections of this edition.

- Linda DeBruyne, M.S., R.D.N. (Chapters 11 and 13). Linda received her master's degree in nutrition from Florida State University and is a founding member of Nutrition and Health Associates. She also coauthors the college nutrition texts *Nutrition and Diet Therapy* and *Nutrition for Health and Health Care*.
- Shannon Dooies Gower-Winter, M.S., R.D.N./L.D.N. (Chapter 7). Shannon graduated from Florida State University with her master's degree in nutrition. She has taught nutrition at Florida State University and lectured on topics related to childhood nutrition throughout the state. She has conducted research in the area of nutritional neuroscience, where her work focused on various roles of zinc in the brain. Her research has been presented at regional and national scientific conferences, and she has coauthored multiple articles in peer-reviewed journals.

Our special thanks to our publishing team—Miriam Myers, Lori Hazzard, and Carol Samet—for their superb work and dedication to excellence.

We would also like to thank **MPS North America LLC** for their work on the student and instructor ancillaries for the 15th edition, which includes the test bank, instructors' manual, and PowerLecture.

Reviewers of Recent Editions

As always, we are grateful for the instructors who took the time to comment on this revision. Your suggestions were invaluable in strengthening the book and suggesting new lines of thought. We hope you will continue to provide your comments and suggestions.

Samuel Adeyeye, *Georgia Southern University*
Katherine Alaimo, *Michigan State University*
Linda Armstrong, *Normandale Community College*
Tammy Lee Christensen, *Hostos Community College (CUNY)*
Dorinda M. Cosimano, *Kean University*
Katie Ferraro, *Santa Rosa Junior College*
Shoshana Freedman, *Glendale Community College*
Keith R. Hench, Ph.D., *Kirkwood Community College*
Rachel K. Johnson, *University of Vermont*
Lauren Lavretsky, *University of Texas at El Paso*
David Lightsey, *M.S., Bakersfield College*
Cheryl McAfee, RDN, LD, *Prince George's Community College*
Letty Moreno-Brown, *El Paso Community College/University of Texas, El Paso*
Molly Ranney, *Finger Lakes Community College*
Victoria Rethmeier, *Southeast Community College*
Laura Rokosz, *EGGLROCK Nutrition, LLC*
Laurie Runk, *Coastline Community College*
Christie Shubert, *University of North Florida*
Taylor C. Wallace, *George Mason University*

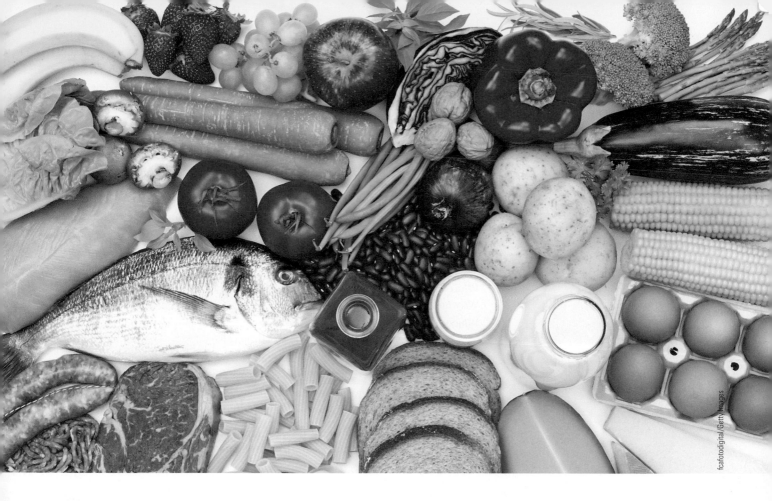

1 Food Choices and Human Health

Learning Objectives

After reading this chapter, you should be able to accomplish the following:

LO 1.1 Describe the ways in which food choices impact a person's health.

LO 1.2 List the seven major categories of nutrition and weight-related objectives included in the publication *Healthy People 2020*.

LO 1.3 Name the six classes of nutrients.

LO 1.4 Give examples of the challenges and solutions to choosing a health-promoting diet.

LO 1.5 Describe the science of nutrition.

LO 1.6 Describe the characteristics of the six stages of behavior change.

LO 1.7 Explain how the concept of nutrient density can facilitate diet planning.

LO 1.8 Evaluate the authenticity of any given nutrition information source.

What do you think?

Can your diet make a real difference between getting **sick** or staying **healthy**?

Are **supplements** more powerful than food for ensuring good nutrition?

What makes your favorite foods your **favorites**?

Are **news and media nutrition reports** informative or confusing?

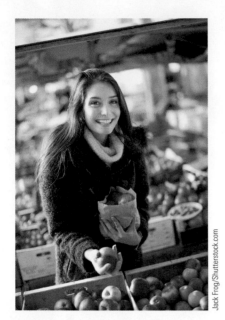

When you choose foods with nutrition in mind, you can enhance your own well-being.

If you care about your body, and if you have strong feelings about **food**, then you have much to gain from learning about **nutrition**—the science of how food nourishes the body. Nutrition is a fascinating, much-talked-about subject. Each day, newspapers, Internet websites, radio, and television present stories of new findings on nutrition and heart health or nutrition and cancer prevention, and at the same time, advertisements and commercials bombard us with multicolored pictures of tempting foods—pizza, burgers, cakes, and chips. If you are like most people, when you eat you sometimes wonder, "Is this food good for me?" or you berate yourself, "I probably shouldn't be eating this."

When you study nutrition, you learn which foods serve you best, and you can work out ways of choosing foods, planning meals, and designing your **diet** wisely. Knowing the facts can enhance your health and your enjoyment of eating while relieving your feelings of guilt or worry that you aren't eating well.

This chapter addresses these "why," "what," and "how" questions about nutrition:

- *Why* care about nutrition? Why be concerned about the **nutrients** in your foods? Why not just take supplements?
- *What* are the nutrients in foods, and what roles do they play in the body? What are the differences between vitamins and minerals?
- *What* constitutes a nutritious diet? How can you choose foods wisely, for nutrition's sake? What factors motivate your choices?
- *How* do we know what we know about nutrition? How does nutrition science work, and how can a person keep up with changing information?

Controversy 1 concludes the chapter by offering ways to distinguish between trustworthy sources of nutrition information and those that are less reliable.

A Lifetime of Nourishment

LO 1.1   Describe the ways in which food choices impact a person's health.

If you live for 65 years or longer, you will have consumed more than 70,000 meals, and your remarkable body will have disposed of 50 tons of food. The foods you choose exert cumulative effects on your body.[1]* As you age, you will see and feel those effects—if you know what to look for.

Your body renews its structures continuously. Each day, it builds a little muscle, bone, skin, and blood, replacing old tissues with new. It may also add a little fat if you consume excess food energy (calories) or subtract a little if you consume less than you require. Some of the food you eat today becomes part of "you" tomorrow.

The best food for you, then, is the kind that supports the growth and maintenance of strong muscles, sound bones, healthy skin, and sufficient blood to cleanse and nourish all parts of your body. This means you need food that provides not only the right amount of energy but also sufficient nutrients—that is, enough water, carbohydrates, fats, protein, vitamins, and minerals. If the foods you eat provide too little or too much of any nutrient today, your health may suffer just a little today. If the foods you eat provide too little or too much of one or more nutrients every day for years, then in later life you may suffer severe disease effects.

A well-chosen diet supplies enough energy and enough of each nutrient to prevent **malnutrition**. Malnutrition includes deficiencies, imbalances, and excesses of nutrients, alone or in combination, any of which can take a toll on health over time.

KEY POINTS

- The nutrients in food support growth, maintenance, and repair of the body.
- Deficiencies, excesses, and imbalances of energy and nutrients bring on the diseases of malnutrition.

food scientifically, materials, usually of plant or animal origin, that contain essential nutrients, such as carbohydrates, fats, proteins, vitamins, or minerals, and that are ingested and assimilated by an organism to produce energy, stimulate growth, and maintain life; socially, a more limited number of such materials defined as acceptable by a culture.

nutrition the study of the nutrients in foods and in the body; sometimes also the study of human behaviors related to food.

diet the foods (including beverages) a person usually eats and drinks.

nutrients components of food that are indispensable to the body's functioning. They provide energy, serve as building material, help maintain or repair body parts, and support growth. The nutrients include water, carbohydrate, fat, protein, vitamins, and minerals.

malnutrition any condition caused by excess or deficient food energy or nutrient intake or by an imbalance of nutrients. Nutrient or energy deficiencies are forms of undernutrition; nutrient or energy excesses are forms of overnutrition.

*Reference notes are in Appendix F.

Table 1–1

Leading Causes of Death in the United States

Chronic diseases cause the great majority of deaths among U.S. adults and account for more than 85 percent of U.S. health-care costs.

	Percentage of Total Deaths
1. **Heart disease**	23.5
2. **Cancers**	22.5
3. Chronic lung disease	5.7
4. **Strokes**	5.0
5. Accidents	5.0
6. Alzheimer's disease	3.3
7. **Diabetes mellitus**	2.9
8. Pneumonia and influenza	2.2
9. Kidney disease	1.8
10. Suicide	1.6

Note: The diseases highlighted in bold have relationships with diet.

Sources: National Center for Chronic Disease Prevention and Health Promotion, Chronic disease prevention and health promotion, www.cdc.gov/chronicdisease, 2017, updated regularly; J. Q. Xu and coauthors, Deaths: Final data for 2013, National Vital Statistics Reports 64 (Hyattsville, MD: National Center for Health Statistics, 2016).

The Diet–Health Connection

Your choice of diet profoundly affects your health, both today and in the future. Among the common lifestyle habits that profoundly affect development of these diseases, only two are more influential than food habits: smoking and using other forms of tobacco and drinking alcohol in excess. Of the leading causes of death listed in Table 1–1, four—heart disease, cancers, strokes, and diabetes—are directly related to nutrition, and another—accidents—is related to drinking alcohol.

Many older people suffer from debilitating conditions that could have been largely prevented had they applied the nutrition principles known today. The **chronic diseases**—heart disease, diabetes, some kinds of cancer, dental disease, and adult bone loss—all have a connection to poor diet. These diseases cannot be prevented by a good diet alone; they are to some extent determined by a person's genetic constitution, activities, and lifestyle. Within the range set by your genetic inheritance, however, the likelihood of developing these diseases is strongly influenced by your daily choices.

KEY POINT

- Nutrition profoundly affects health.

Genetics, Nutrition, and Individuality

Figure 1–1 demonstrates that genetics and nutrition affect different diseases to varying degrees. The **anemia** caused by sickle-cell disease, for example, is purely hereditary and thus appears at the left of Figure 1–1 as a genetic condition largely unrelated to nutrition. Nothing a person eats affects the person's chances of contracting this anemia, although nutrition therapy may help ease its course. At the other end of the spectrum, iron-deficiency anemia most often results from undernutrition. Diseases and conditions of poor health appear all along this continuum, from almost entirely genetically based

chronic diseases degenerative conditions or illnesses that progress slowly are long in duration, and lack an immediate cure. Chronic diseases limit functioning, productivity, and the quality and length of life. Examples include heart disease, cancer, and diabetes.

anemia a blood condition in which red blood cells, the body's oxygen carriers, are inadequate or impaired and so cannot meet the oxygen demands of the body.

Figure 1–1

Nutrition and Disease

Not all diseases are equally influenced by diet. Some, such as sickle-cell anemia, are almost purely genetic. Some, such as diabetes, may be inherited (or the tendency to develop them may be inherited in the genes) but may be influenced by diet. Some, such as vitamin-deficiency diseases, are purely dietary.

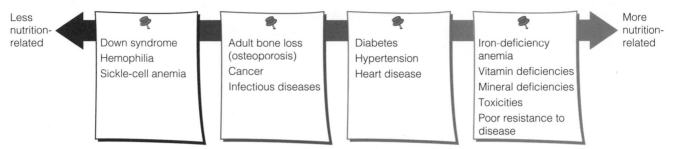

Less nutrition-related

Down syndrome
Hemophilia
Sickle-cell anemia

Adult bone loss (osteoporosis)
Cancer
Infectious diseases

Diabetes
Hypertension
Heart disease

Iron-deficiency anemia
Vitamin deficiencies
Mineral deficiencies
Toxicities
Poor resistance to disease

More nutrition-related

genome (GEE-nome) the full complement of genetic information in the chromosomes of a cell. In human beings, the genome consists of about 35,000 genes and supporting materials. The study of genomes is *genomics*. Also defined in Controversy 11.

genes units of a cell's inheritance; sections of the larger genetic molecule DNA (deoxyribonucleic acid). Each gene directs the making of one or more of the body's proteins.

DNA an abbreviation for deoxyribonucleic (dee-OX-ee-RYE-bow-nu-CLAY-ick) acid, the thread-like molecule that encodes genetic information in its structure; DNA strands coil up densely to form the chromosomes (Chapter 3 provides more details).

to purely nutritional in origin; the more nutrition-related a disease or health condition is, the more successfully sound nutrition can prevent it.

Furthermore, some diseases, such as heart disease and cancer, are not one disease but many. Two people may both have heart disease but not the same form; one person's cancer may be nutrition-related, but another's may not be. Individual people differ genetically from each other in thousands of subtle ways, so no simple statement can be made about the extent to which diet can help any one person avoid such diseases or slow their progress.

The identification of the human **genome** establishes the entire sequence of the **genes** in human **DNA**. This work has, in essence, revealed the body's instructions for making all of the working parts of a human being. The human genome is 99.9 percent the same in all people; all of the normal variations such as differences in hair color, as well as variations that result in diseases such as sickle-cell anemia, lie in the 0.1 percent of the genome that varies. Nutrition scientists are working industriously to apply this

THINK FITNESS — Why Be Physically Active?

Why should people bother to be physically active? A person's daily food choices can powerfully affect health, but the combination of nutrition and physical activity is more powerful still. People who combine regular physical activity with a nutritious diet can expect to receive at least some of these benefits:

- Reduced risks of cardiovascular diseases, diabetes, certain cancers, hypertension, and other diseases.
- Increased endurance, strength, and flexibility.
- More cheerful outlook and less likelihood of depression.
- Improved mental functioning.
- Feeling of vigor.

- Feeling of belonging—the companionship of sports.
- Stronger self-image.
- Reduced body fat and increased lean tissue.
- A more youthful appearance, healthy skin, and improved muscle tone.
- Greater bone density and lessened risk of adult bone loss in later life.
- Increased independence in the elderly.
- Sound, beneficial sleep.
- Faster wound healing.
- Reduced menstrual symptoms.
- Improved resistance to infection.

If even half of these benefits were yours for the asking, wouldn't you step up to claim them? In truth, they are yours to claim, at the price of including physical activity in your day. Chapter 10 explores the topics of fitness and physical activity.

start now! Ready to make a change? Go to this book's website at www.cengage.com, access MindTap, and open the Diet & Wellness Plus program. Track your physical activities—all of them—for three days. After you have recorded your activities, see how much time you spent exercising at a moderate to vigorous level. Should you increase the intensity level and amount of your activity?

new wealth of knowledge to benefit human health. Later chapters expand on the emerging story of nutrition and the genes.

- Diet influences long-term health within the range set by genetic inheritance.
- Nutrition exerts little influence on some diseases but strongly affects others.

Other Lifestyle Choices

Besides food choices, other lifestyle choices affect people's health. Tobacco use and alcohol and other substance abuse can destroy health. Physical activity, sleep, emotional stress, and other environmental factors can also modify the severity of some diseases. Physical activity is so closely linked with nutrition in supporting health that most chapters of this book offer a feature called Think Fitness, such as the previous one.

- Life choices, such as being physically active or using tobacco or alcohol, can improve or damage health.

The Nation's Nutrition Objectives

LO 1.2   List the seven major categories of nutrition and weight-related objectives included in the publication *Healthy People 2020*.

The U.S. Department of Health and Human Services has set specific 10-year objectives to guide national health promotion efforts.[2] The vision of its *Healthy People 2020* is a society in which all people live long, healthy lives. Table 1–2 (p. 6) provides a quick scan of the nutrition and weight-related objectives set for this decade. The inclusion of nutrition and food-safety objectives shows that public health officials consider these areas to be top national priorities.

In 2015, the nation's health report was mixed: more adults reported spending the recommended amount of leisure time in physical activity; at the same time, most people's diets still lacked vegetables, and obesity rates were creeping higher.[3] To fully meet the *Healthy People* nutrition goals, our nation must change its eating habits.

The next section shifts focus to the nutrients at the core of nutrition science. As your course of study progresses, the individual nutrients will become like old friends, revealing more and more about themselves as you move through the chapters.

- Each decade, the U.S. Department of Health and Human Services sets health and nutrition objectives for the nation.

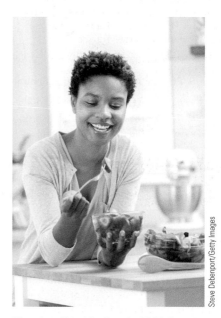

The aim of Healthy People 2020 *is to help people live long, healthy lives.*

The Human Body and Its Food

LO 1.3   Name the six classes of nutrients.

As your body moves and works each day, it must use **energy**. The energy that fuels the body's work comes indirectly from the sun by way of plants. Plants capture and store the sun's energy in their tissues as they grow. When you eat plant-derived foods such as fruit, grains, or vegetables, you obtain and use the solar energy they have stored. Plant-eating animals obtain their energy in the same way, so when you eat animal tissues, you are eating compounds containing energy that came originally from the sun.

The body requires six kinds of nutrients—families of molecules indispensable to its functioning—and foods deliver these. Table 1–3 (p. 6) lists the six classes of nutrients. Four of these six are **organic**; that is, the nutrients contain the element carbon derived from living things.

energy the capacity to do work. The energy in food is chemical energy; it can be converted to mechanical, electrical, thermal, or other forms of energy in the body. Food energy is measured in calories, defined on page 8.

organic carbon containing. Four of the six classes of nutrients are organic: carbohydrate, fat, protein, and vitamins. Organic compounds include only those made by living things and do not include compounds such as carbon dioxide, diamonds, and a few carbon salts.

Table 1–2

Healthy People 2020, Selected Nutrition and Body Weight Objectives

Many other Objectives for the Nation are available at www.healthypeople.gov.

1. Chronic Diseases

- Reduce the proportion of adults with osteoporosis.
- Reduce the death rates from cancer, diabetes, heart disease, and stroke.
- Reduce the annual number of new cases of diabetes.

2. Food Safety

- Reduce outbreaks of certain infections transmitted through food.
- Reduce severe allergic reactions to food among adults with diagnosed food allergy.

3. Maternal, Infant, and Child Health

- Reduce the number of low-birthweight infants and preterm births.
- Increase the proportion of infants who are breastfed.
- Reduce the occurrence of fetal alcohol syndrome (FAS).
- Reduce iron deficiency among children, adolescents, women of childbearing age, and pregnant women.
- Reduce blood lead levels in lead-exposed children.
- Increase the number of schools offering breakfast.

4. Food and Nutrient Consumption

- Increase vegetables, fruit, and whole grains in the diets of those aged 2 years and older, and reduce solid fats and added sugars.

5. Eating Disorders

- Reduce the proportion of adolescents who engage in disordered eating behaviors in an attempt to control their weight.

6. Physical Activity and Weight Control

- Increase the proportion of children, adolescents, and adults who are at a healthy weight.
- Reduce the proportions of children, adolescents, and adults who are obese.
- Reduce the proportion of people who engage in no leisure-time physical activity.
- Increase the proportion of schools that require daily physical education for all students.

7. Food Security

- Eliminate very low food security among children in U.S. households.

Source: www.healthypeople.gov.

Table 1–3

Elements in the Six Classes of Nutrients

The nutrients that contain carbon are organic.

	Carbon	Oxygen	Hydrogen	Nitrogen	Minerals
Carbohydrate	✓	✓	✓		
Fat	✓	✓	✓		
Protein	✓	✓	✓	✓	b
Vitamins	✓	✓	✓	✓[a]	h
Minerals					✓
Water		✓	✓		✓

[a]*All of the B vitamins contain nitrogen; amine means nitrogen.*
[b]*Protein and some vitamins contain the mineral sulfur; vitamin B_{12} contains the mineral cobalt.*

Meet the Nutrients

The human body and foods are made of the same materials, arranged in different ways (see Figure 1–2). When considering quantities of foods and nutrients, scientists often measure them in **grams** or fractions of grams, units of weight.

The Energy-Yielding Nutrients   Of the four organic nutrients, three are **energy-yielding nutrients**, meaning that the body can use the energy they contain. These are carbohydrate, fat, and protein, often referred to as the **macronutrients**, and they contribute to the calories you consume. Among them, protein stands out for doing double duty: it can yield energy, but it also provides materials that form structures and working parts of body tissues. (Alcohol yields energy, too—see Table 1–4 comments.)

Vitamins and Minerals   The fourth and fifth classes of nutrients are the vitamins and the minerals, sometimes referred to as **micronutrients** because they are present in tiny amounts in living tissues. These provide no energy to the body. A few minerals serve as parts of body structures (calcium and phosphorus, for example, are major constituents of bone), but all vitamins and minerals act as regulators. As regulators, the vitamins and minerals assist in all body processes: digesting food; moving muscles; disposing of wastes; growing new tissues; healing wounds; obtaining energy from carbohydrate, fat, and protein; and participating in every other process necessary to maintain life. Later chapters are devoted to these six classes of nutrients.

Water   Although last on the list, water is foremost in quantity among the six classes of nutrients in the body. The body constantly loses water, mainly through sweat, breath, and urine, and that water must constantly be replaced. Without sufficient water, the body's cells cannot function.

The Concept of Essential Nutrients   When you eat food, then, you are providing your body with energy and nutrients. Furthermore, some of the nutrients are **essential nutrients**, meaning that if you do not ingest them, you will develop deficiencies; the body cannot make these nutrients for itself. Essential nutrients are found in all six classes of nutrients. Water is an essential nutrient; so is a form of carbohydrate; so are some lipids, some parts of protein, all of the vitamins, and the minerals important in human nutrition.

Figure 1–2
Components of Food and the Human Body

Foods and the human body are made of the same materials.

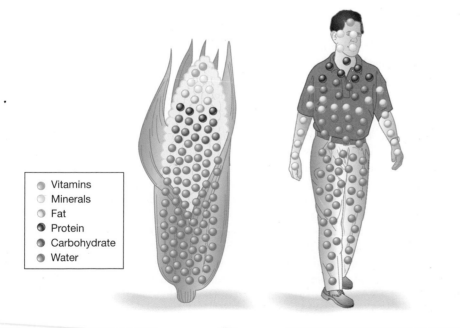

- Vitamins
- Minerals
- Fat
- Protein
- Carbohydrate
- Water

Table 1–4
Energy-Yielding Nutrients

The energy a person consumes in a day's meals comes from these three energy-yielding nutrients; alcohol, if consumed, also contributes energy at a rate of about 7 calories per gram (see note).

Energy Nutrient	Energy
Carbohydrate	4 cal/g
Fat (lipid)	9 cal/g
Protein	4 cal/g

Note: Alcohol is not classed as a nutrient because it interferes with growth, maintenance, and repair of body tissues.

grams (g) metric units of weight. About 28 grams equal an ounce. A *milligram* is one-thousandth of a gram. A *microgram* is one-millionth of a gram.

energy-yielding nutrients the nutrients the body can use for energy: carbohydrate, fat (also called *lipids*), and protein. These also may supply building blocks for body structures.

macronutrients another name for the energy-yielding nutrients: carbohydrate, fat, and protein.

micronutrients nutrients required in very small amounts: the vitamins and minerals.

essential nutrients the nutrients the body cannot make for itself (or cannot make fast enough) from other raw materials; nutrients that must be obtained from food to prevent deficiencies.

You may wonder why **fiber**, famous for its beneficial health effects, is not listed among the essential nutrients. The reason is that most fiber passes through the body unabsorbed, and omitting it from the diet does not reliably cause a specific deficiency disease. Even so, in research, health benefits often follow eating a fiber-rich diet (Chapter 4 has details).[4]

Calorie Values Food scientists measure food energy in kilocalories, units of heat. This book uses the common word **calories** to mean the same thing. It behooves the person who wishes to control food energy intake and body fatness to learn the calorie values of the energy nutrients, listed in Table 1–4. The most energy-rich of the nutrients is fat, which contains 9 calories in each gram. Carbohydrate and protein each contain only 4 calories in a gram. Weight, measure, and other conversion factors needed for the study of nutrition appear in Appendix C at the back of the book.

Scientists have worked out ways to measure the energy and nutrient contents of foods. They have also calculated the amounts of energy and nutrients various types of people need—by gender, age, life stage, and activity. Thus, after studying human nutrient requirements (in Chapter 2), you will be able to state with some accuracy just what your own body needs—this much water, that much carbohydrate, so much vitamin C, and so forth. So why not simply take pills or **dietary supplements** in place of food? Because, as it turns out, food offers more than just the six basic nutrients.

KEY POINTS

- The energy-yielding nutrients are carbohydrates, fats (lipids), and protein.
- The regulator nutrients are vitamins and minerals.
- Foremost among the nutrients in food is water.
- Essential nutrients in the diet prevent deficiencies.
- Food energy is measured in calories; nutrient quantities are often measured in grams.

Can I Live on Just Supplements?

Nutrition science can state what nutrients human beings need to survive—at least for a time. Scientists are becoming skilled at making **elemental diets**—life-saving liquid diets of precise chemical composition for hospital patients and others who cannot eat ordinary food. These formulas, administered for days or weeks, support not only continued life but also recovery from nutrient deficiencies, infections, and wounds. Formulas can also stave off weight loss in the elderly or anyone in whom eating is impaired.[5]

Formula diets are essential to help sick people to survive, but they do not enable people to thrive over long periods. Even in hospitals, elemental diet formulas do not support optimal growth and health and may even lead to medical complications. Although serious problems are rare and can be detected and corrected, they show that the composition of these diets is not yet perfect for all people in all settings.

Lately, marketers have taken these liquid supplement formulas out of the medical setting and have advertised them heavily to healthy people of all ages as "meal replacers" or "insurance" against malnutrition. The truth is that real food is superior to such supplements. Most healthy people who eat a nutritious diet need no dietary supplements at all.

Food Is Best Even if a person's basic nutrient needs are perfectly understood and met, concoctions of nutrients still lack something that foods provide. Hospitalized clients who are fed nutrient mixtures through a vein often improve dramatically when they can finally eat food. Something in real food is important to health—but what is it? What does food offer that cannot be provided through a needle or a tube? Science has some partial explanations, some physical and some psychological.

In the digestive tract, the stomach and intestine are dynamic, living organs, changing constantly in response to the foods they receive—even to just the sight, aroma, and taste of food. When a person is fed through a vein, the digestive organs, like unused muscles, weaken and grow smaller. Medical wisdom now dictates that a person should be fed through a vein for as short a time as possible and that real food taken by mouth

fiber a collective term for various indigestible plant materials, many of which bear links with human health. See also Chapter 4.

calories units of energy. In nutrition science, the unit used to measure the energy in foods is a kilocalorie (also called *kcalorie* or *Calorie*): it is the amount of heat energy necessary to raise the temperature of a kilogram (a liter) of water 1 degree Celsius. This book follows the common practice of using the lowercase term *calorie* (abbreviated *cal*) to mean the same thing.

dietary supplements pills, liquids, or powders that contain purified nutrients or other ingredients (see Controversy 7).

elemental diets diets composed of purified ingredients of known chemical composition; intended to supply, to the greatest extent possible, all essential nutrients to people who cannot eat foods.

Chapter 1 Food Choices and Human Health

should be reintroduced as early as possible. The digestive organs also release hormones in response to food, and these send messages to the brain that bring the eater a feeling of satisfaction: "There, that was good. Now I'm full." Eating offers both physical and emotional comfort.

Complex Interactions   Foods are chemically complex. In addition to their nutrients, foods contain **phytochemicals**, compounds that confer color, taste, and other characteristics to foods. Some may be **bioactive** food components that interact with metabolic processes in the body and may affect disease risks. Even an ordinary baked potato contains hundreds of different compounds. Nutrients and other food components interact with each other in the body and operate best in harmony with one another. In view of all this, it is not surprising that food gives us more than just nutrients. If it were otherwise, *that* would be surprising.

KEY POINTS

- Nutritious food is superior to supplements for maintaining optimal health.
- Most healthy people who eat a nutritious diet do not need supplements at all.

The Challenge of Choosing Foods

LO 1.4   Give examples of the challenges and solutions to choosing a health-promoting diet.

Well-planned meals convey pleasure and are nutritious, too, fitting your tastes, personality, family and cultural traditions, lifestyle, and budget. Given the astounding numbers and varieties available, consumers can easily lose track of what individual foods contain and how to put them together into a health-promoting diet. A few definitions and basic guidelines can help.

The Abundance of Foods to Choose From

A list of the foods available 100 years ago would be relatively short. It would consist mostly of **whole foods**—foods that have been around for a long time, such as vegetables, fruit, meats, milk, and grains (Table 1–5 defines food types, p. 10; terms in tables are in black bold type, margin definitions are in blue). These foods have been called basic, unprocessed, natural, or farm foods. By any name, these foods form the basis of a nutritious diet. On a given day, however, well over 80 percent of our population consumes too few servings of fruit and vegetables each day.[6] And when people do choose to eat a vegetable, the one they most often choose is potatoes, usually prepared as French fries. Such choices, repeated over time, make development of chronic diseases more likely.

The number and types of foods supplied by the food industry today is astounding, as Figure 1–3 (p. 10) illustrates. Tens of thousands of foods now line the market shelves—many are processed mixtures of the basic ones, and some are constructed entirely from highly processed ingredients.[7] Ironically, this abundance often makes it more difficult, rather than easier, to plan a nutritious diet.

The food-related terms defined in Table 1–5 reveal that all types of food—including **fast foods, processed foods**, and **ultra-processed foods**—offer various constituents to the eater, some more health-promoting than others.[8] You may also hear about **functional foods**, a marketing term coined to identify those foods containing substances, natural or added, that might lend protection against chronic diseases. The trouble with trying to single out the most health-promoting foods is that almost every naturally occurring food—even chocolate—is functional in some way with regard to human health.[9]

The extent to which foods support good health depends on the calories, nutrients, and phytochemicals they contain. In short, to select well among foods, you need to know more than their names; you need to know the foods' inner qualities. Even more

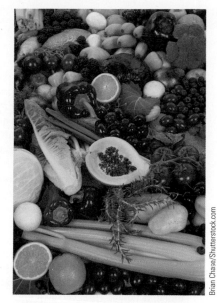

Some foods offer phytochemicals in addition to the six classes of nutrients.

phytochemicals bioactive compounds in plant-derived foods (*phyto*, pronounced FYE-toe, means "plant").

bioactive having chemical or physical properties that affect the functions of the body tissues. See Controversy 2.

Table 1–5

Glossary of Food Types

- **enriched foods** and **fortified foods** foods to which nutrients have been added. If the starting material is a whole, basic food such as milk or whole grain, the result may be highly nutritious. If the starting material is a concentrated form of sugar or fat, the result is less nutritious.
- **fast foods** restaurant foods that are available within minutes after customers order them—traditionally, hamburgers, French fries, and milkshakes; more recently, salads and other vegetable dishes as well. These foods may or may not meet people's nutrient needs, depending on the selections provided and on the energy allowances and nutrient needs of the eaters.
- **functional foods** whole or modified foods that contain bioactive food components believed to provide health benefits, such as reduced disease risks, beyond the benefits that their nutrients confer. However, all nutritious foods can support health in some ways; Controversy 2 provides details.
- **medical foods** foods specially manufactured for use by people with medical disorders and administered on the advice of a physician.
- **natural foods** a term that has no legal definition but is often used to imply wholesomeness.

- **organic foods** understood to mean foods grown without synthetic pesticides or fertilizers. In chemistry, however, all foods are made mostly of organic (carbon-containing) compounds.
- **processed foods** foods subjected to any process, such as milling, alteration of texture, addition of additives, cooking, or others. Depending on the starting material and the process, a processed food may or may not be nutritious.
- **staple foods** foods used frequently or daily—for example, rice (in East and Southeast Asia) or potatoes (in Ireland). Many of these foods are sufficiently nutritious to provide a foundation for a healthful diet.
- **ultra-processed foods** a term used to describe highly palatable food products of manufacturing made with industrial ingredients and additives, such as sugars, refined starches, fats, salt, and imitation flavors and colors, with little or no whole food added. Examples: sugary refined breakfast cereals, candies, cookies, fried chicken nuggets, potato "tots," ready-to-heat meals, snack chips and cakes, and soft drinks.
- **whole foods** milk and milk products; meats and similar foods such as fish and poultry; vegetables, including dried beans and peas; fruit; and grains. These foods are generally considered to form the basis of a nutritious diet. Also called *basic foods*.

important, you need to know how to combine foods into nutritious diets. Foods are not nutritious by themselves; each is of value only insofar as it contributes to a nutritious diet. A key to wise diet planning is to make sure that the foods you eat daily, your **staple foods**, are especially nutritious.

KEY POINT

- Foods that form the basis of a nutritious diet are whole foods, such as ordinary milk and milk products; meats, fish, and poultry; vegetables and dried peas and beans; fruit; and grains.

Figure 1–3

Grocery Options Then and Now

All foods once looked like this ...

... but now many foods look like this.

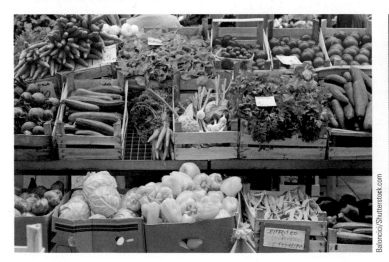

Baloncici/Shutterstock.com

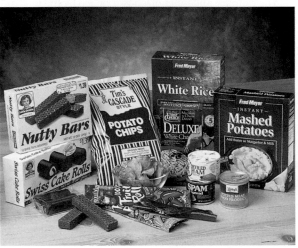

© Polara Studios, Inc.

Chapter 1 Food Choices and Human Health

How, Exactly, Can I Recognize a Nutritious Diet?

A nutritious diet is really an **eating pattern**, a habitual way of choosing foods, with five characteristics. First is **adequacy**: the foods provide enough of each essential nutrient, fiber, and energy. Second is **balance**: the choices do not overemphasize one nutrient or food type at the expense of another. Third is **calorie control**: the foods provide the amount of energy you need to maintain appropriate weight—not more, not less. Fourth is **moderation**: the foods do not provide excess fat, salt, sugar, or other unwanted constituents. Fifth is **variety**: the foods chosen differ from one day to the next. In addition, to maintain a steady supply of nutrients, meals should occur with regular timing throughout the day. To recap, then, a nutritious diet is an eating pattern that follows the A, B, C, M, V principles: Adequacy, Balance, Calorie control, Moderation, and Variety.

Adequacy   Any nutrient could be used to demonstrate the importance of dietary adequacy. Iron provides a familiar example. It is an essential nutrient: you lose some every day, so you have to keep replacing it, and you can get it into your body only by eating foods that contain it.[†] If you eat too few iron-containing foods, you can develop iron-deficiency anemia. With anemia, you may feel weak, tired, cold, sad, and unenthusiastic; you may have frequent headaches; and you can do very little muscular work without disabling fatigue. Some foods are rich in iron; others are notoriously poor. If you add iron-rich foods to your diet, you soon feel more energetic. Meat, fish, poultry, and **legumes** are rich in iron, and an easy way to obtain the needed iron is to include these foods in your diet regularly.

Balance   To appreciate the importance of dietary balance, consider a second essential nutrient, calcium. A diet lacking calcium causes poor bone development during the growing years and increases a person's susceptibility to disabling bone loss in adult life. Most foods that are rich in iron are poor in calcium. Calcium's richest food sources are milk and milk products, which happen to be extraordinarily poor iron sources. Clearly, to obtain enough of both iron and calcium, people have to balance their food choices among the types of foods that provide both nutrients. Balancing the whole diet to provide enough of every one of the 40-odd nutrients the body needs for health requires considerable juggling, however. As you will see in Chapter 2, food group plans ease this task by clustering rich sources of nutrients into food groups that will help you to achieve both dietary adequacy and balance within an eating pattern that meets your needs.

Calorie Control   Energy intakes should not exceed or fall short of energy needs. Named *calorie control*, this characteristic ensures that energy intakes from food balance energy expenditures required for body functions and physical activity. Eating such a diet helps control body fat content and weight. The many strategies that promote this goal appear in Chapter 9.

Moderation   Intakes of certain food constituents such as saturated fats, added sugars, and salt should be limited for health's sake. Some people take this to mean that they must never indulge in a delicious beefsteak or hot-fudge sundae, but they are misinformed: moderation, not total abstinence, is the key.[10] A steady diet of steak and ice cream might be harmful, but once a week as part of an otherwise healthful eating pattern, these foods may have little impact; as once-a-month treats, these foods would have practically no effect at all. Moderation also means that limits are necessary, even for desirable food constituents. For example, a certain amount of fiber in foods contributes to the health of the digestive system, but too much fiber leads to nutrient losses.

eating pattern the combination of foods and beverages that constitute an individual's complete dietary intake over time; a person's usual diet.

adequacy the dietary characteristic of providing all of the essential nutrients, fiber, and energy in amounts sufficient to maintain health and body weight.

balance the dietary characteristic of providing foods of a number of types in proportion to each other, such that foods rich in some nutrients do not crowd out the diet foods that are rich in other nutrients.

calorie control the dietary characteristic of controlling energy intake; a feature of a sound diet plan.

moderation the dietary characteristic of providing constituents within set limits, not to excess.

variety the dietary characteristic of providing a wide selection of foods—the opposite of monotony.

legumes (leg-GOOMS, LEG-yooms) beans, peas, and lentils, valued as inexpensive food sources of protein, vitamins, minerals, and fiber that contribute little fat to the diet. Also defined in Chapter 6.

[†]A person can also take supplements of iron, but as later discussions demonstrate, eating iron-rich foods is preferable.

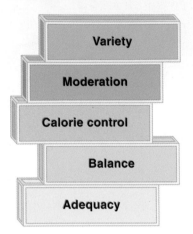

Variety

Moderation

Calorie control

Balance

Adequacy

Variety   As for variety, nutrition scientists agree that people should not eat the same foods, even highly nutritious ones, day after day, for a number of reasons. First, a varied diet is more likely to be adequate in nutrients. Second, some less-well-known nutrients and phytochemicals could be important to health, and some foods may be better sources of these than others. Third, a monotonous diet may deliver large amounts of toxins or contaminants. Such undesirable compounds in one food are diluted by all the other foods eaten with it and are diluted still further if the food is not eaten again for several days. Finally, variety adds interest—trying new foods can be a source of pleasure.

Variety applies to nutritious foods consumed within the context of all of the other dietary principles just discussed. Relying solely on the principle of variety to dictate food choices could easily result in a low-nutrient, high-calorie eating pattern with a variety of nutrient-poor snack foods and sweets. If you establish the habit of using all of the principles just described, you will find that choosing a healthful diet becomes as automatic as brushing your teeth or falling asleep. Establishing the A, B, C, M, V habit (summed up in Figure 1–4) may take some effort, but the payoff in terms of improved health is overwhelming. Table 1–6 takes an honest look at some common excuses for *not* eating well.

KEY POINT

- A well-planned diet is adequate, balanced, moderate in energy, and moderate in unwanted constituents and offers a variety of nutritious foods.

Why People Choose Foods

Eating is an intentional act. Each day, people choose from the available foods, prepare the foods, and decide where to eat, which customs to follow, and with whom to dine. Many factors influence food-related choices.

Cultural and Social Meanings Attached to Food   Like wearing traditional clothing or speaking a native language, enjoying traditional **cuisines** and **foodways** can be a celebration of your own or a friend's heritage. Sharing **ethnic foods** can be symbolic: people offering foods are expressing a willingness to share cherished values with others. People accepting those foods are symbolically accepting not only the person doing the offering but also the person's culture. Developing **cultural competence** is particularly important for professionals who help others to achieve a nutritious diet.[11]

Cultural traditions regarding food are not inflexible; they keep evolving as people move about, learn about new foods, and teach each other. Today, some people are ceasing to be **omnivorous** and are becoming **vegetarians**. Vegetarians often choose this lifestyle because they honor the lives of animals or because they have discovered the health and other advantages associated with eating patterns rich in beans,

---

Table 1–6

What's Today's Excuse for Not Eating Well?

If you find yourself saying, "I know I should eat well, but I'm too busy" (or too fond of fast food, or have too little money, or a dozen other excuses), take note:

- *No time to cook.* Everyone is busy. Convenience packages of fresh or frozen vegetables, jars of pasta sauce, and prepared meats and salads make nutritious meals in little time.
- *Not a high priority.* Priorities change drastically and instantly when illness strikes—better to spend a little effort now nourishing your body's defenses than to spend enormous resources later fighting illnesses.

- *Crave fast food and sweets.* Occasional fast-food meals and sweets in moderation are acceptable in a nutritious diet.
- *Too little money.* Eating right may cost a little more than eating poorly, but the cost of coping with a chronic illness is unimaginably high.
- *Take vitamins instead.* Vitamin pills or even advertised "nutritional drinks" cannot make up for consistently poor food choices.

Sources: D. P. Reidlinger, T. A. Sanders, and L. M. Goff, How expensive is a cardioprotective diet? Analysis from the CRESSIDA study, Public Health Nutrition (2017), epub ahead of print, doi: 10.1017/S1368980016003529; M. M. Abdullah, J. P. Jones, and P. J. Jones, Economic benefits of the Mediterranean-style diet consumption in Canada and the United States, Food and Nutrition Research (2015), epub, doi: 10.3402/fnr.v59.27541; M. Rao and coauthors, Do healthier foods and diet patterns cost more than less healthy options? A systematic review and meta-analysis, BMJ Open 3 (2013): e004277.

whole grains, fruit, nuts, and vegetables. Controversy 6 explores the strengths and weaknesses of both vegetarians' and meat eaters' diets.

Factors that Drive Food Choices Taste prevails as the number-one factor driving people's food choices, with price following closely behind.[12] Consumers also value convenience so highly that they are willing to spend almost half of their food budgets on meals prepared outside the home. Fewer people are learning the skills needed to prepare nutritious meals at home.[13] Instead, they frequently eat out, bring home ready-to-eat meals, or have food delivered. When they do cook, they want to prepare meals in 15 to 20 minutes, using only a few ingredients. Such convenience incurs a cost in terms of nutrition, however: eating away from home reduces intakes of fruit, vegetables, milk, and whole grains. It also increases intakes of calories, saturated fat, sodium, and added sugars. Convenience doesn't have to mean that nutrition flies out the window, however. This chapter's Food Feature (p. 20) explores the trade-offs of time, money, and nutrition that many busy people face today.

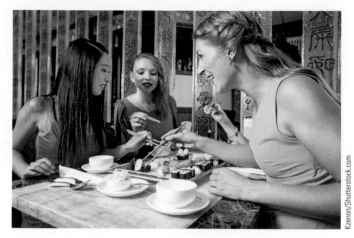

Sharing traditional food is a way of sharing culture.

Many other factors—psychological, physical, social, and philosophical—also influence people's food choices. College students, for instance, often choose to eat at restaurants to socialize, to get out, to save time, or to date; they are not always conscious of their bodies' needs for nutritious food. A list of other factors follows:

- *Advertising.* The media have persuaded you to consume these foods.
- *Availability.* They are present in the environment and accessible to you.
- *Cost.* They are within your financial means.[14]
- *Emotional comfort.* They can make you feel better for a while.
- *Habit.* They are familiar; you always eat them.
- *Nutrition and health benefits.* You think they are good for you.
- *Personal preference and genetic inheritance.* You like the way these foods taste.
- *Positive or negative associations. Positive:* They are eaten by people you admire, or they indicate status, or they remind you of fun. *Negative:* They were forced on you, or you became ill while eating them.
- *Region of the country.* They are foods favored in your area.
- *Social norms.* Your companions are eating them, or they are offered and you feel you cannot refuse them.[15]
- *Values or beliefs.* They fit your religious tradition, square with your political views, or honor the environmental ethic.
- *Weight.* You think they will help control body weight.

One other factor affects food choices:

- *Nutrition and health benefits.* You think they are good for you.[16]

The next section addresses one of the "how" questions posed earlier in this chapter: How do we know what we know about nutrition?

cuisines styles of cooking.

foodways the sum of a culture's habits, customs, beliefs, and preferences concerning food.

ethnic foods foods associated with particular cultural subgroups within a population.

cultural competence having an awareness and acceptance of one's own and others' cultures and abilities, leading to effective interactions with all kinds of people.

omnivorous people who eat foods of both plant and animal origin, including animal flesh.

vegetarians people who exclude from their diets animal flesh and possibly other animal products such as milk, cheese, and eggs.

KEY POINTS
- Cultural traditions and social values often revolve around foodways.
- Many factors other than nutrition drive food choices.

The Science of Nutrition

LO 1.5   Describe the science of nutrition.

Understanding nutrition depends upon a firm base of scientific knowledge. This section describes the nature of such knowledge.

Figure 1–5

The Scientific Method

Research scientists follow the scientific method. Note that most research projects result in new questions, not final answers. Thus, research continues in a somewhat cyclical manner.

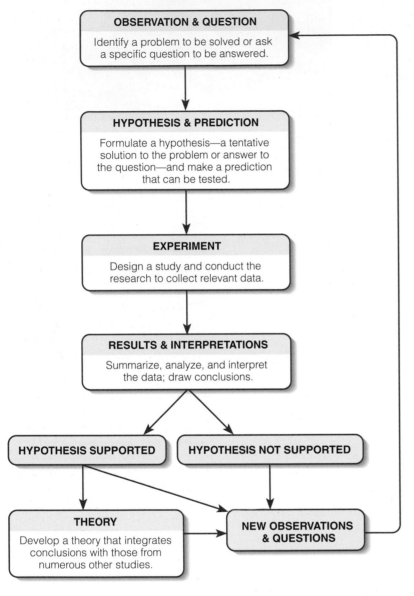

OBSERVATION & QUESTION

Identify a problem to be solved or ask a specific question to be answered.

HYPOTHESIS & PREDICTION

Formulate a hypothesis—a tentative solution to the problem or answer to the question—and make a prediction that can be tested.

EXPERIMENT

Design a study and conduct the research to collect relevant data.

RESULTS & INTERPRETATIONS

Summarize, analyze, and interpret the data; draw conclusions.

HYPOTHESIS SUPPORTED

HYPOTHESIS NOT SUPPORTED

THEORY

Develop a theory that integrates conclusions with those from numerous other studies.

NEW OBSERVATIONS & QUESTIONS

Unlike sciences such as astronomy and physics, nutrition is a relatively young science. Most nutrition research has been conducted since 1900. The first vitamin was identified in 1897, and the first protein structure was not fully described until the mid-1940s. Because nutrition science is an active, changing, growing body of knowledge, new findings often seem to contradict one another or are subject to conflicting interpretations. Bewildered consumers complain in frustration, "Those scientists don't know anything. If they don't know what's true, how am I supposed to know?"

Yet experimenters have confirmed many nutrition facts with great certainty through repeated testing. To understand why apparent contradictions exist, we need to look first at what scientists do.

The Scientific Approach

In truth, it is a scientist's business not to know. Scientists obtain facts by systematically asking honest, objective questions—that's their job. Following the scientific method (outlined in Figure 1–5), researchers attempt to answer scientific questions. They design and conduct various experiments to test for possible answers (see Figure 1–6, and Table 1–7 on p. 16). When they have ruled out some possibilities and found evidence for others, they submit their findings not to the news media but to boards of reviewers composed of other scientists who try to pick apart the findings and often call for further evidence before approving publication. Finally, the work is published in scientific journals where still more scientists can read it. Then the news reporters read it and write about it, and the public can read about it, too. In time, other scientists replicate the experiments and report their own findings, which either support or refute earlier conclusions.

KEY POINTS

- Nutrition is a young and fast-growing science.
- Scientists ask questions and then design research experiments to test possible answers.
- Researchers follow the scientific method and apply it to various research study designs.

Scientific Challenge

An important truth in science is that one experiment does not "prove" or "disprove" anything. When a finding has stood up to rigorous repeated testing in several kinds of experiments performed by several different researchers it is finally considered confirmed. Even then, strictly speaking, science consists not of facts that are set in stone but of *theories* that can always be challenged and revised. Some findings, though, such as the theory that the earth revolves about the sun, are so well supported by observations and experimental findings that they are generally accepted as facts. What we "know" in nutrition is confirmed in the same way—through years of replicating study findings. This slow path of repeated studies stands in sharp contrast to the media's desire for today's latest news.[17]

Figure 1–6

Examples of Research Design

The type of study chosen for research depends upon what sort of information the researchers require. Studies of individuals (**case studies**) yield observations that may lead to possible avenues of research. A study of a man who ate gumdrops and became a famous dancer might suggest that an experiment be done to see if gumdrops contain dance-enhancing power.

Studies of whole populations (**epidemiological studies**) provide another sort of information. Such a study can reveal a **correlation**. For example, an epidemiological study might find no worldwide correlation of gumdrop eating with fancy footwork but, unexpectedly, might reveal a correlation with tooth decay.

Studies in which researchers actively intervene to alter people's eating habits (**intervention studies**) go a step further. In such a study, one set of subjects (the **experimental group**) receives a treatment, and another set (the **control group**) goes untreated or receives a **placebo** or sham treatment. If the study is a **blind experiment**, the subjects do not know who among the members receives the treatment and who receives the sham. If the two groups experience different effects, then the treatment's effect can be pinpointed. For example, an intervention study might show that withholding gumdrops, together with other candies and confections, reduced the incidence of tooth decay in an experimental population compared to that in a control population.

Laboratory studies can pinpoint the mechanisms by which nutrition acts. What is it about gumdrops that contributes to tooth decay: their size, shape, temperature, color, ingredients? Feeding various forms of gumdrops to rats might yield the information that sugar, in a gummy carrier, promotes tooth decay. In the laboratory, using animals or plants or cells, scientists can inoculate with diseases, induce deficiencies, and experiment with variations on treatments to obtain in-depth knowledge of the process under study. Intervention studies and laboratory experiments are among the most powerful tools in nutrition research because they show the effects of treatments.

Case Study

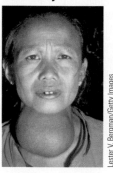

Lester V. Bergman/Getty Images

"This person eats too little of nutrient X and has illness Y."

Epidemiological Study

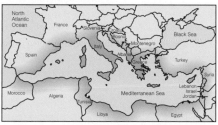

"This country's food supply contains more nutrient X, and these people suffer less illness Y."

Intervention Study

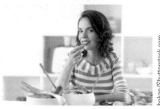

bokan/Shutterstock.com

"Let's add foods containing nutrient X to some people's food supply and compare their rates of illness Y with the rates of others who don't receive the nutrient."

Laboratory Study

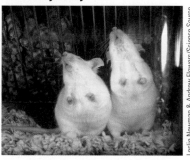

Leslie Newman & Andrew Flowers/Science Source

"Now let's see if a nutrient X deficiency causes illness Y by inducing a deficiency in these rats."

To repeat: the only source of valid nutrition information is slow, painstaking, well-designed, unbiased, repeatable scientific research. We believe a nutrition fact to be true because it has been supported, time and again, in experiments designed to rule out all other possibilities.[18] For example, we know that eyesight depends partly on vitamin A because:

- In case studies, individuals with blindness report having consumed a steady diet devoid of vitamin A; and

- In epidemiological studies, populations with diets lacking in vitamin A are observed to suffer high rates of blindness; and

- In intervention studies (**controlled clinical trials**), vitamin A–rich foods provided to groups of people with vitamin A deficiency reduce their blindness rates dramatically; and

Table 1–7

Research Design Terms

- **blind experiment** an experiment in which the subjects do not know whether they are members of the experimental group or the control group. In a *double-blind experiment*, neither the subjects nor the researchers know to which group the members belong until the end of the experiment.
- **case study** a study of a single individual. When in clinical settings, researchers can observe treatments and their apparent effects. To prove that a treatment has produced an effect requires simultaneous observation of an untreated similar subject (a *case control*).
- **control group** a group of individuals who are similar in all possible respects to the group being treated in an experiment but who receive a sham treatment instead of the real one. Also called *control subjects*.
- **controlled clinical trial** an experiment in which one group of subjects (the **experimental group**) receives a treatment and a comparable group (the **control group**) receives an imitation treatment and outcomes for the two are compared. Ideally, neither subjects nor researchers know who receives the treatment and who gets the placebo (a double-blind study).
- **meta-analysis** a computer-driven statistical summary of evidence gathered from multiple previous studies.

- **correlation** the simultaneous change of two factors, such as the increase of weight with increasing height (a *direct* or *positive* correlation) or the decrease of cancer incidence with increasing fiber intake (an *inverse* or *negative* correlation). A correlation between two factors suggests that one may cause the other but does not rule out the possibility that both may be caused by chance or by a third factor.
- **epidemiological studies** studies of populations; often used in nutrition to search for correlations between dietary habits and disease incidence; a first step in seeking nutrition-related causes of diseases.
- **experimental group** the people or animals participating in an experiment who receive the treatment under investigation. Also called *experimental subjects*.
- **intervention studies** studies of populations in which observation is accompanied by experimental manipulation of some population members—for example, a study in which half of the subjects (the *experimental subjects*) follow diet advice to reduce fat intakes, while the other half (the *control subjects*) do not, and both groups' heart health is monitored.
- **laboratory studies** studies that are performed under tightly controlled conditions and are designed to pinpoint causes and effects. Such studies often use animals as subjects.
- **placebo** a sham treatment often used in scientific studies; an inert, harmless medication. The *placebo effect* is the healing effect that the act of treatment, rather than the treatment itself, often has.

- In laboratory studies, animals deprived of vitamin A and only that vitamin begin to go blind; when it is restored soon enough in the diet, their eyesight returns; and
- Further laboratory studies elucidate the molecular mechanisms for vitamin A activity in eye tissues; and
- Replication of these studies yields the same results.
- Later, a **meta-anlysis** of previous studies also detects the effect.

Now we can say with certainty, "Eyesight depends upon sufficient vitamin A."

KEY POINTS

- Single studies must be replicated before their findings can be considered valid.
- A theory is strengthened when results from follow-up studies with a variety of research designs support it.

Can I Trust the Media for Nutrition Information?

The news media are hungry for new findings, and reporters often latch onto hypotheses from scientific laboratories before they have been fully tested. Also, a reporter who lacks a strong understanding of science may misunderstand or misreport complex scientific principles.[19] To tell the truth, sometimes scientists get excited about their findings, too, and leak them to the press before they have been through a rigorous review by the scientists' peers. As a result, the public is often exposed to late-breaking nutrition news stories before the findings are fully confirmed. Then, when a hypothesis being tested fails to hold up to a later challenge, consumers feel betrayed by what is simply the normal course of science at work.

Real scientists are trend watchers. They evaluate the methods used in each study, assess each study in light of the evidence gleaned from other studies, and modify little by little their picture of what may be true. As evidence accumulates, the scientists become more and more confident about their ability to make recommendations that apply to people's health and lives.

Sometimes media sensationalism overrates the importance of even true, replicated findings. For example, the media eagerly report that oat products lower blood cholesterol, a lipid indicative of heart disease risk. Although the reports are true, they often fail to mention that eating a nutritious diet that is low in certain fats is still the major step toward lowering blood cholesterol. They also may skip over important questions: How much oatmeal must a person eat to produce the desired effect? Do little oat bran pills or powders meet the need? Do oat bran cookies? If so, how many cookies? For oatmeal, it takes a bowl and a half daily to affect blood lipids. A few pills or cookies do not provide nearly so much bran and certainly cannot undo damage from an ill-chosen diet.

Today, the cholesterol-lowering effect of oats is well established. The whole process of discovery, challenge, and vindication took almost 10 years of research. Some other lines of research have taken much longer. In science, a single finding almost never makes a crucial difference to our knowledge, but like each individual frame in a movie, it contributes a little to the big picture. Many such frames are needed to tell the whole story. The Consumer's Guide section (p. 19) offers some tips for evaluating news stories about nutrition.

KEY POINT

- News media often sensationalize single-study findings and so may not be trustworthy sources.

National Nutrition Research

As you study nutrition, you are likely to hear of findings based on ongoing nationwide nutrition and health research projects. A national food and nutrient intake survey, called *What We Eat in America*, reveals what we know about the population's food and supplement intakes. It is conducted as part of a larger research effort, the **National Health and Nutrition Examination Surveys (NHANES)**, which also conducts physical examinations and measurements and laboratory tests.[20] Boiled down to its essence, NHANES involves:

- Asking people what they have eaten and
- Recording measures of their health status.

Past NHANES results have provided important data for developing growth charts for children, guiding food fortification efforts, developing national guidelines for reducing chronic diseases, and many other beneficial programs. Some agencies involved with these efforts are listed in Table 1–8.

KEY POINT

- National nutrition research projects, such as NHANES, provide data on U.S. food consumption and nutrient status.

Table 1–8
Nutrition Research and Policy Agencies

These agencies are actively engaged in nutrition policy development, research, and monitoring:

- Centers for Disease Control and Prevention (CDC)
- U.S. Department of Agriculture (USDA)
- U.S. Department of Health and Human Services (DHHS)
- U.S. Food and Drug Administration (FDA)

Changing Behaviors

LO 1.6   Describe the characteristics of the six stages of behavior change.

Nutrition knowledge is of little value if it only helps people to make A's on tests. The value comes when people use it to improve their diets. To act on knowledge, people must change their behaviors, and although this may sound simple enough, behavior change often takes substantial effort.

National Health and Nutrition Examination Surveys (NHANES) a program of studies designed to assess the health and nutritional status of adults and children in the United States by way of interviews and physical examinations.

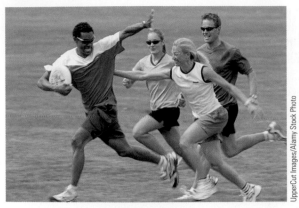
Many people need to change their daily routines to include physical activity.

The Process of Change

Psychologists often describe the six stages of behavior change, offered in Table 1–9. Knowing where you stand in relation to these stages may help you move along the path toward achieving your goals. When offering diet help to others, keep in mind that their stages of change can influence their reaction to your message.

Taking Stock and Setting Goals

Once aware of a problem, you can plan to make a change. Some problems, such as *never* consuming a vegetable, are easy to spot. More subtle dietary problems, such as failing to meet your need for calcium, may be hidden but can exert serious repercussions on health. Tracking food intakes over several days' time and then comparing intakes to standards (see Chapter 2) can reveal all sorts of interesting tidbits about strengths and weaknesses of your eating pattern.

Once a weakness is identified, setting small, achievable goals to correct it becomes the next step to making improvements. The most successful goals are set for specific behaviors, not overall outcomes. For example, if losing 10 pounds is the desired outcome, goals should be set in terms of food intakes and physical activity to help achieve weight loss. After goals are set and changes are under way, a means of tracking progress increases the likelihood of success.

Start Now

As you progress through this text, you may want to change some of your own habits. To help you, little reminders entitled "Start Now" close each chapter's Think Fitness section with an invitation to visit this book's website (p. 21). There, you can take inventory of your current behaviors, set goals, track progress, and practice new behaviors until they become as comfortable and familiar as the old ones were.

KEY POINTS

- Behavior change follows a multistep pattern.
- Setting goals and monitoring progress facilitate behavior change.

Table 1–9

The Stages of Behavior Change

Stage	Characteristics	Actions
Precontemplation	Not considering a change; have no intention of changing; see no problems with current behavior.	Collect information about health effects of current behavior and potential benefits of change.
Contemplation	Admit that change may be needed; weigh pros and cons of changing and not changing.	Commit to making a change and set a date to start.
Preparation	Preparing to change a specific behavior, taking initial steps, and setting some goals.	Write an action plan, spelling out specific parts of the change. Set small-step goals; tell others about the plan.
Action	Committing time and energy to making a change; following a plan set for a specific behavior change.	Perform the new behavior. Manage emotional and physical reactions to the change.
Maintenance	Striving to integrate the new behavior into daily life and striving to make it permanent.	Persevere through lapses. Teach others and help them achieve their own goals. (This stage can last for years.)
Adoption/Moving On	The former behavior is gone, and the new behavior is routine.	After months or a year of maintenance without lapses, move on to other goals.

A CONSUMER'S GUIDE TO . . .

Reading Nutrition News

At a coffee shop, Nick, a health-conscious consumer, sets his cup down on the Lifestyle section of the newspaper. He glances at the headline—"Eating Fat OK for Heart Health!"—and jumps to a wrong conclusion: "Do you mean to say that I could have been eating burgers and butter all this time? I can't keep up! As soon as I change my diet, the scientists change their story." Nick's frustration is understandable. Like many others, he feels betrayed when, after working for years to make diet changes for his health's sake, headlines seem to turn dietary advice upside down. He shouldn't blame science, however.

Tricks and Traps

The trouble started when Nick was "hooked" by a catchy headline. Media headlines often seem to reverse current scientific thought because new "breakthrough" studies are exciting; they grab readers' attention and make them want to buy a newspaper, book, or magazine. (By the way, you can read the true story behind changing lipid intake guidelines in Controversy 5.) Even if Nick had read the entire newspaper article, he could have still been led astray by phrases like "Now we know" or "The truth is." Journalists use such phrases to imply finality, the last word. In contrast, scientists use tentative language, such as "may" or "might," because they know that the conclusions from one study will be challenged, refined, and even refuted by others that follow.

Markers of Authentic Reporting

To approach nutrition news with a trained eye, look for these signs of a scientific approach:

- When an article describes a scientific study, that study should have been published in a peer-reviewed journal, such as the *American Journal of Clinical Nutrition* (see Figure 1–7). An unpublished study may or may not be valid; readers have no way of knowing because the study lacks scrutiny by other experts (the authors' peers).

- The news item should describe the researchers' methods. In truth, few popular reports provide these details. For example, it matters whether the study participants numbered 8 or 80,000 or whether researchers personally observed participants' behaviors or relied on self-reports given over the telephone.

- The report should define the study subjects—were they single cells, animals, or human beings? If they were human beings, the more you have in common with them (age and gender, for example), the more applicable the findings may be for you.

- Valid reports also present new findings in the context of previous research. Some reporters in popular media regularly follow developments in a research area and thus acquire the background knowledge needed to report meaningfully. They strive for adequacy, balance, and completeness, and they cover such things as cost of a treatment, potential harms and benefits, strength of evidence, and who might stand to gain from potential sales relating to the finding.*

- For a helpful *scientific* overview of current topics in nutrition, look for review articles written by experts. They regularly appear in scholarly journals such as *Nutrition Reviews*.

The most credible sources of scientific nutrition information are scientific journals. Controversy 1, which follows this chapter, addresses other sources of nutrition information and misinformation.

* An organization that promotes valid health-care reporting is HealthNewsReview.org, available at www.healthnewsreview.org/.

Figure 1–7

Peer-Reviewed Journals

For the whole story on a nutrition topic, read articles from peer-reviewed journals such as these. A review journal examines all available evidence on major topics. Other journals report details of the methods, results, and conclusions of single studies.

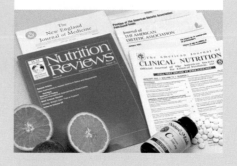

Moving Ahead

Develop a critical eye, and let scientific principles guide you as you read nutrition news. When a headline touts a shocking new "answer" to a nutrition question, approach it with caution. It may indeed be a carefully researched report that respects the gradual nature of scientific discovery and refinement, but more often it is a sensational news flash intended to grab your attention.

Review Questions†

1. To keep up with nutrition science, consumers should _____.

   a. seek out the health and fitness sections of newspapers and magazines and read them with a trained eye

   b. read studies published in peer-reviewed journals, such as the

(continued)

† Answers to Consumer's Guide review questions are in Appendix G.

American Journal of Clinical Nutrition

c. look for review articles published in peer-reviewed journals, such as *Nutrition Reviews*

d. all of the above

2. To answer nutrition questions _____.

   a. rely on articles that include phrases such as "Now we know"

   or "The answer is," which appear to provide conclusive answers to nutrition questions

   b. look to science for answers, with the expectation that scientists will continually revise their understandings

   c. realize that problems in nutrition are probably too complex for consumers to understand

   d. a and c

3. Scholarly review journals such as *Nutrition Reviews* _____.

   a. are behind the times when it comes to nutrition news

   b. discuss all available research findings on a topic in nutrition

   c. are filled with medical jargon

   d. are intended for use by practitioners only, not students

---

FOOD FEATURE

Nutrient Density: How to Get Enough Nutrients without Too Many Calories

LO 1.7 Explain how the concept of nutrient density can facilitate diet planning.

In the United States, only a tiny percentage of adults manage to choose an eating pattern that achieves both adequacy and calorie control. The foods that can help in doing so are foods richly endowed with nutrients relative to their energy contents; that is, they are foods with high **nutrient density**.[21] Figure 1–8 is a simple depiction of this concept. Consider calcium sources, for example. Ice cream and fat-free milk both supply calcium, but a cup of rich ice cream contributes more than 350 calories, whereas a cup of fat-free milk has only 85—and almost double the calcium. Most people cannot, for their health's sake, afford to choose foods without regard to their energy contents. Those who do very often exceed calorie allowances while leaving nutrient needs unmet.

Among foods that often rank high in nutrient density are the vegetables, particularly the nonstarchy vegetables such as dark leafy greens (cooked and raw), red bell peppers, broccoli, carrots, mushrooms, and tomatoes.[22] These inexpensive foods take time to prepare, but time invested in this way pays off in

nutrient density a measure of nutrients provided per calorie of food. A *nutrient-dense food* provides needed nutrients with relatively few calories.

Figure 1–8

A Way to Judge which Foods Are Most Nutritious

These two breakfasts provide about 500 calories each, but they differ greatly in the nutrients they provide per calorie. Note that the sausage in the larger breakfast is lower-calorie turkey sausage, not the high-calorie pork variety. Making small changes like this at each meal can add up to large calorie savings, making room in the diet for more servings of nutritious foods and even some treats.

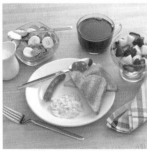

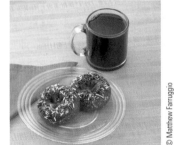

© Matthew Farruggio

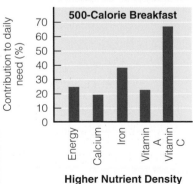

Higher Nutrient Density

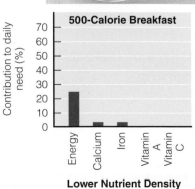

Lower Nutrient Density

(continued)

nutritional health. Twenty minutes spent peeling and slicing vegetables for a salad is a better investment in nutrition than 20 minutes spent fixing a fancy, high-fat, high-sugar dessert. Besides, the dessert ingredients often cost more money and strain the calorie budget, too.

Time, however, is a concern to many people. Today's working families, college students, and active people of all ages may have little time to devote to food preparation. Busy cooks should seek out convenience foods that are nutrient-dense, such as bags of ready-to-serve salads, ready-to-cook fresh vegetables, refrigerated prepared low-fat meats and poultry, canned beans, and frozen vege-

tables. A tip for lower-cost convenience is to double the amount of whole vegetables for a recipe; wash, peel, and chop them; and then refrigerate or freeze the extra to use on another day. Dried fruit and dry-roasted nuts require only that they be kept on hand and make a tasty, nutritious topper for salads and other foods. To round out a meal, fat-free milk or yogurt is both nutritious and convenient. Other convenience selections, such as most potpies, many frozen pizzas, ramen noodles, and "pocket"-style pastry sandwiches, are less nutritious overall because they contain too few vegetables and too many calories, making them low in nutrient density. The Food Features of

later chapters offer many more tips for choosing convenient and nutritious foods.

All of this discussion leads to a principle that is central to achieving nutritional health: no particular foods must be included or excluded in the diet. Instead, your eating pattern—the way you combine foods into meals and the way you arrange meals to follow one another over days and weeks—determines how well you are nourishing yourself.[23] Nutrition is a science, not an art, but it can be used artfully to create a pleasing, nourishing diet. The rest of this book is dedicated to helping you make informed choices and combine them artfully to meet all the body's nutrition needs.

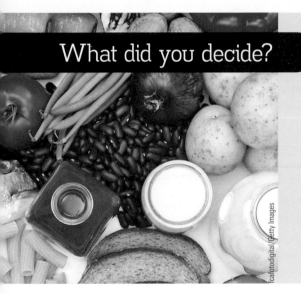

What did you decide?

Can your diet make a real difference between getting **sick** or staying **healthy**?

Are **supplements** more powerful than food for ensuring good nutrition?

What makes your favorite foods your **favorites**?

Are **news and media nutrition reports** informative or confusing?

What's online?

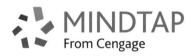

MINDTAP
From Cengage

Visit www.Cengage.com to access MindTap, a complete digital course that includes Diet & Wellness Plus, interactive quizzes, videos, and more.

Self Check

1. (LO 1.1) Both heart disease and cancer are due to genetic causes, and diet cannot influence whether they occur.
   T F

2. (LO 1.1) Some conditions, such as _____, are almost entirely nutrition related.
   a. cancer
   b. Down syndrome
   c. iron-deficiency anemia
   d. sickle-cell anemia

3. (LO 1.2) The nutrition objectives for the nation, as part of *Healthy People 2020*,
   a. envision a society in which all people live long, healthy lives.
   b. track and identify cancers as a major killer of people in the United States.
   c. set U.S. nutrition- and weight-related goals, one decade at a time.
   d. a and c.

4. (LO 1.2) According to a national health report,
   a. most people's diets lacked enough fruit, vegetables, and whole grains.
   b. fewer adults reported being sufficiently physically active.
   c. the number of overweight people was declining.
   d. the nation had fully met the previous *Healthy People* objectives.

5. (LO 1.3) Energy-yielding nutrients include all of the following except _____.
   a. vitamins   c. fat
   b. carbohydrates   d. protein

6. (LO 1.3) Organic nutrients include all of the following except _____.
   a. minerals   c. carbohydrates
   b. fat   d. protein

7. (LO 1.3) Both carbohydrates and protein have 4 calories per gram.
   T F

8. (LO 1.4) One of the characteristics of a nutritious diet is that the diet provides no constituent in excess. This principle of diet planning is called _____.
   a. adequacy   c. moderation
   b. balance   d. variety

9. (LO 1.4) Which of the following is an example of a processed food?
   a. carrots   c. nuts
   b. bread   d. watermelon

10. (LO 1.4) People most often choose foods for the nutrients they provide.
    T F

11. (LO 1.5) Studies of populations in which observation is accompanied by experimental manipulation of some population members are referred to as _____.
    a. case studies
    b. intervention studies
    c. laboratory studies
    d. epidemiological studies

12. (LO 1.5) An important national food and nutrient intake survey, called *What We Eat in America*, is part of _____.
    a. NHANES
    b. FDA
    c. USDA
    d. none of the above

13. (LO 1.6) Behavior change is a process that takes place in stages.
    T F

14. (LO 1.6) A person who is setting goals in preparation for a behavior change is in a stage called *precontemplation*.
    T F

15. (LO 1.7) A slice of peach pie supplies 357 calories with 48 units of vitamin A; one large peach provides 42 calories and 53 units of vitamin A. This is an example of _____.
    a. calorie control
    b. nutrient density
    c. variety
    d. essential nutrients

16. (LO 1.7) A person who wishes to meet nutrient needs while not overconsuming calories is wise to master
    a. the concept of nutrient density.
    b. the concept of carbohydrate reduction.
    c. the concept of nutrients per dollar.
    d. French cooking.

17. (LO 1.8) "Red flags" that can help to identify nutrition quackery include
    a. enticingly quick and simple answers to complex problems.
    b. efforts to cast suspicion on the regular food supply.
    c. solid support and praise from users.
    d. all of the above.

18. (LO 1.8) In this nation, stringent controls make it difficult to obtain a bogus nutrition credential.
    T F

Answers to these Self Check questions are in Appendix G.

Sorting Imposters from Real Nutrition Experts

LO 1.8   Evaluate the authenticity of any given nutrition information source.

From the time of snake oil salesmen in horse-drawn wagons to today's Internet sales schemes, nutrition **quackery** has been a problem that often escapes government regulation and enforcement. To avoid being sitting ducks for quacks, consumers themselves must distinguish between authentic, useful nutrition products or services and a vast array of faulty advice and outright scams.

Each year, consumers spend a deluge of dollars on nutrition-related services and products from both legitimate and fraudulent businesses. Each year, nutrition and other health **fraud** diverts tens of *billions* of consumer dollars from legitimate health care.

More than Money at Stake

When scam products are garden tools or stain removers, hoodwinked consumers may lose a few dollars and some pride. When the products are ineffective, untested, or even hazardous "dietary supplements" or "medical devices," consumers stand to lose the very thing they are seeking: good health. When a sick person wastes time with

quack treatments, serious problems can advance while proper treatment is delayed. And ill-advised "dietary supplements" have inflicted dire outcomes, even liver failure, on previously well people who took them in hopes of *improving* their health.

Information Sources

When questions about nutrition arise, most people consult the Internet, a popular book or magazine, or television for the answer.[1]* Sometimes these sources provide sound, scientific, trustworthy information. More often, though, **infomercials**, **advertorials**, and **urban legends** (defined in Table C1–1) pretend to inform but in fact aim primarily to sell products by making fantastic promises of health or weight loss with minimal effort and at bargain prices.

How can people learn to distinguish valid nutrition information from misinformation? Some quackery is easy to identify—like the claims of the salesman in Figure C1–1—whereas other types are more subtle. Between the extremes of accurate scientific data and intentional

* Reference notes are in Appendix F

Table C1–1
Quackery Terms

- **advertorials** lengthy advertisements in newspapers and magazines that read like feature articles but are written for the purpose of touting the virtues of products and may or may not be accurate.
- **anecdotal evidence** information based on interesting and entertaining, but not scientific, personal stories.
- **critical thinking** the mental activity of rationally and skillfully analyzing, synthesizing, and evaluating information.
- **fraud** or **quackery** the promotion, for financial gain, of devices, treatments, services, plans, or products (including diets and supplements) claimed to improve health, well-being, or appearance without proof of safety or effectiveness. (The word *quackery* comes from the term *quacksalver*, meaning a person who quacks loudly about a miracle product—a lotion or a salve.)
- **infomercials** feature-length television commercials that follow the format of regular programs but are intended to convince viewers to buy products and not to educate or entertain them.
- **urban legends** stories, usually false, that may travel rapidly throughout the world via the Internet, gaining the appearance of validity solely on the basis of repetition.

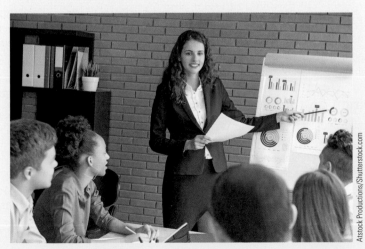

Who speaks on nutrition?

quackery lies an abundance of nutrition misinformation.† An instructor at a gym, a physician, a health-food store clerk, an author of books, or an advocate for a "cleansing diet" product or weight-loss gadget may sincerely believe that the recommended nutrition regimen is beneficial. But what qualifies these people to give nutrition advice? Would following

† Reliable information on quackery is available. Search for the National Council Against Health Fraud or the Food and Drug Administration on the Internet, or call (888) INFO-FDA.

Too good to be true
Enticingly quick and simple answers to complex problems. Says what most people want to hear. Sounds magical.

Suspicions about food supply
Urges distrust of current medical approaches and suspicions about regular foods. Touts "alternatives" that are often inferior or even dangerous, but are kept on the market in the name of "freedom of choice." May use the term "natural" to imply safety.

Testimonials
Support and praise by people who "felt healed," "felt younger," "lost weight," and the like as a result of using the product or treatment. One person is not a statistically significant sample.

Fake credentials
Uses title "doctor," "university," or the like but has created or bought the title—it is not legitimate.

Unpublished studies
Claims to cite "scientific" studies but not studies published in reliable journals.

A **SCIENTIFIC BREAKTHROUGH!** FEEL **STRONGER**, **LOSE** WEIGHT. **IMPROVE** YOUR MEMORY ALL WITH THE HELP OF **VITE-O-MITE!** OH, SURE, YOU MAY HAVE HEARD THAT **VITE-O-MITE** IS NOT ALL THAT WE SAY IT IS, BUT THAT'S WHAT THE FDA WANTS YOU TO THINK! **OUR DOCTORS** AND SCIENTISTS SAY IT'S THE ULTIMATE VITAMIN SUPPLEMENT. SAY "NO!" TO THE WEAKENED VITAMINS IN TODAY'S FOODS! **VITE-O-MITE** INCLUDES **POTENT SECRET INGREDIENTS** THAT YOU CANNOT GET FROM ANY OTHER PRODUCT! ORDER ONE BOTTLE RIGHT NOW AND WE'LL SEND YOU ANOTHER ONE FOR FREE!

Logic without proof
The claim seems to be based on sound reasoning but hasn't been scientifically tested and shown to hold up.

Persecution claims
Claims of persecution by the medical establishment or a fake government conspiracy or claims that physicians "want to keep you ill so that you will continue to pay for office visits."

Authority not cited
Studies cited sound valid but are not referenced, so that it is impossible to check and see if they were conducted scientifically.

Motive: personal gain
Those making the claim stand to make a profit if it is believed.

Advertisement
Claims are made by an advertiser who is paid to promote sales of the product or procedure. (Look for the word "Advertisement" in tiny print somewhere on the page.)

Latest innovation/time-tested
Fake scientific jargon is meant to inspire awe. Claims of being "ancient remedies" are meant to inspire trust.

their advice be helpful or harmful? To sift meaningful nutrition information from rubbish, you must learn to identify both.

Chapter 1 explained that valid nutrition information arises from scientific research and does not rely on **anecdotal evidence** or testimonials. Table C1–2 lists some sources of such authentic nutrition information.

Identifying nutrition misinformation requires more than simply gathering accurate information, though. It also requires you to develop skills in **critical thinking**. Critical thinking allows a person who has gathered information to:

- Understand how concepts are related.
- Evaluate the pros and cons of an argument.
- Detect inconsistencies and errors in thinking.
- Solve problems.
- Judge the relevance of new information.

This book's Controversy sections are dedicated to helping you to develop your critical thinking skills.

Nutrition on the Net

If you have a question, the World Wide Web on the Internet has an answer. The "Net" offers convenient access to reliable reports of scientific research published in refereed journals, but it also delivers an abundance of incomplete, misleading, or inaccurate informa-tion. Simply put: anyone can publish anything on the Internet. For example, popular self-governed Internet "ency-clopedia" websites allow anyone to post information or change others' postings on all topics. Information on the sites may be correct, but it may not be—readers must evaluate it for themselves. Table C1–3 provides some clues to judg-ing the reliability of nutrition information websites.

Personal Internet sites, known as "weblogs" or "blogs," contain the authors' personal opinions and are often not reviewed by experts before post-ing. In addition, e-mail messages often circulate hoaxes and scare stories. Be suspicious when:

Credible Sources of Nutrition Information

Government agencies, volunteer associations, consumer groups, and professional organizations provide consumers with reliable health and nutrition information. Credible sources of nutrition information include:

- Nutrition and food science departments at a university or community college
- Local agencies such as the health department or County Cooperative Extension Service
- Government resources such as:

Centers for Disease Control and Prevention (CDC)	www.cdc.gov
Department of Agriculture (USDA)	www.usda.gov
Department of Health and Human Services (DHHS)	www.hhs.gov
Dietary Guidelines for Americans	fnic.nal.usda.gov /dietary-guidance
Food and Drug Administration (FDA)	www.fda.gov
Health Canada	www.hc-sc.gc.ca/index-eng.php
Healthy People	www.healthypeople.gov
Let's Move!	www.letsmove.gov
MyPlate	www.choosemyplate.gov
National Institutes of Health	www.nih.gov
Physical Activity Guidelines for Americans	www.health.gov/paguidelines

- Volunteer health agencies such as:

American Cancer Society	www.cancer.org
American Diabetes Association	www.diabetes.org
American Heart Association	www.heart.org/HEARTORG

- Reputable consumer groups such as:

American Council on Science and Health	www.acsh.org
International Food Information Council	www.foodinsight.org

- Professional health organizations such as:

Academy of Nutrition and Dietetics	www.eatright.org
American Medical Association	www.ama-assn.org
Dietitians of Canada	www.dietitians.ca

- Journals such as:

American Journal of Clinical Nutrition	ajcn.nutrition.org
Journal of the Academy of Nutrition and Dietetics	www.andjrnl.org
New England Journal of Medicine	www.nejm.org
Nutrition Reviews	www.ilsi.org

- Someone other than the sender or some authority you know wrote the contents.
- A phrase like "Forward this to everyone you know" appears anywhere in the piece.
- The piece states, "This is not a hoax"; chances are it is.
- The information seems shocking or something that you've never heard from legitimate sources.
- The language is overly emphatic or sprinkled with capitalized words or exclamation marks.
- No references are offered or, if present, prove to be of questionable validity when examined.
- Websites such as www.quackwatch.org or www.urbanlegends.com have debunked the message.

In contrast, one of the most trustworthy Internet sites for scientific

Is This Site Reliable?

To judge whether an Internet site offers reliable nutrition information, answer the following questions.

Who? Who is responsible for the site? Is it staffed by qualified professionals? Look for the authors' names and credentials. Have experts reviewed the content for accuracy?

When? When was the site last updated? Because nutrition is an ever-changing science, sites need to be dated and updated frequently.

Where? Where is the information coming from? The three letters following the dot in a Web address identify the site's affiliation. Addresses ending in "gov" (government), "edu" (educational institute), and "org" (organization) generally provide reliable information; "com" (commercial) sites represent businesses and, depending on their qualifications and integrity, may or may not offer dependable information. Many reliable sites provide links to other sites to facilitate your quest for knowledge, but this provision alone does not guarantee a reputable intention. Be aware that any site can link to any other site without permission.

Why? Why is the site giving you this information? Is the site providing a public service or selling a product? Many commercial sites provide accurate information, but some do not. When money is the prime motivation, be aware that the information may be biased.

What? What is the message, and is it in line with other reliable sources? Information that contradicts common knowledge should be questioned.

investigation is the National Library of Medicine's PubMed website, which provides free access to over 10 million abstracts (short descriptions) of research papers published in scientific journals around the world.[2] Many abstracts provide links to full articles posted on other sites. The site is easy to use and offers instructions for beginners. Figure C1–2 introduces this resource.

Who Are the True Nutrition Experts?

Most people turn to their physicians for dietary advice, but physicians vary in their knowledge of nutrition. Physicians have extensive training in human biochemistry and physiology, the bedrocks of nutrition science, but typical medical schools in the United States do not require students to take a comprehensive nutrition course, such as the class taken by students reading this text.[3]

An exceptional physician has a specialty area in clinical nutrition and is highly qualified to advise on nutrition. Membership in the Academy of Nutrition and Dietetics or the Society for Clinical Nutrition, whose journals are cited many times throughout this text, can be a clue to a physician's nutrition knowledge.

Fortunately, a credential that indicates a qualified nutrition expert is easy to spot—you can confidently call on a **registered dietitian nutritionist (RDN)**. To become an RDN, a person must earn a bachelor's or master's of science degree from an **accredited** college or university based on course work that typically includes biochemistry, chemistry, human anatomy and physiology, microbiology, and food and nutrition sciences, along with food service systems management, business, statistics, economics, computer science, sociology, and counseling or education courses. Then the person must complete an accredited and supervised practice program and, finally, pass a national examination administered by the Academy of Nutrition and Dietetics. Once credentialed, the expert must maintain **registration** by participating in required continuing education activities.

Additionally, some states require that **nutritionists** and **dietitians** obtain a **license to practice**. Meeting state-established criteria in addition to **registration** with the **Academy of Nutrition and Dietetics** certifies that an expert is the genuine article. Table C1–4 defines nutrition specialists along with other relevant terms.

RDNs are easy to find in most communities because they perform a multitude of duties in a variety of settings (see Table C1–5). They work in food service operations, pharmaceutical companies, sports nutrition programs, corporate wellness programs, the food industry, home health agencies, long-term care institutions, private practice, community and public health settings, cooperative extension offices,[§] research centers, universities, hospitals, health maintenance organizations (HMO), and other facilities. In hospitals, they may offer **medical nutrition therapy** as part of patient care, or they may run the food service operation, or they may specialize as **certified diabetes educators (CDE)** to help people with diabetes manage the disease. **Public health nutritionists** take leadership roles in government agencies as expert consultants and advocates or in direct service delivery. A **certified specialist in sports dietetics (CSSD)** counsels people who must perform physically for sports, emergency response, military defense, and the like.[4] The roles are so diverse that many pages would be required to cover them thoroughly.

[§] Cooperative extension agencies are associated with land grant colleges and universities and may be found in the telephone book's government listings or on the Internet.

Figure C1–2

PubMed (www.ncbi.nlm.nih.gov/pubmed): Internet Resource for Scientific Nutrition References

The U.S. National Library of Medicine's PubMed website offers tutorials to help teach beginners to use the search system effectively. Often, simply visiting the site, typing a query in the search box, and clicking *Search* will yield satisfactory results.

For example, to find research concerning calcium and bone health, typing in "calcium bone" nets almost 3,000 results. To refine the search, try setting limits on dates, types of articles, languages, and other criteria to obtain a more manageable number of abstracts to peruse.

Type search terms here   Refine the search by setting limits   Use "help" resources to answer questions

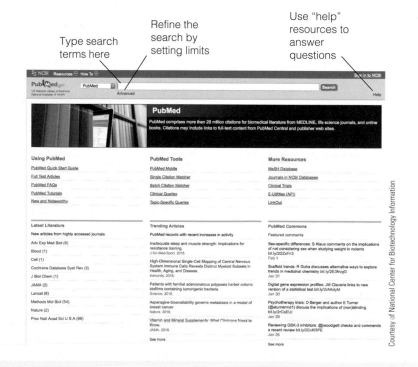

Courtesy of National Center for Biotechnology Information

- **Academy of Nutrition and Dietetics (AND)** the professional organization of dietitians in the United States (formerly the American Dietetic Association). The Canadian equivalent is the Dietitians of Canada (DC), which operates similarly.
- **accredited** approved; in the case of medical centers or universities, certified by an agency recognized by the U.S. Department of Education.
- **certified diabetes educator (CDE)** a health-care professional who has completed an intensive professional training program and examination to earn a certificate attesting to the attainment of knowledge and skill in educating people with diabetes to help them manage their disease through medical and lifestyle means. Professional certifications in many other practice areas also exist.
- **certified specialist in sports dietetics (CSSD)** a Registered Dietitian Nutritionist with special credentials and expertise to deliver safe, effective, evidence-based nutrition assessments and guidance for health and performance to athletes and other physically active people.
- **nutrition and dietetics technician, registered (NDTR)** a dietetics professional who has completed an academic degree from an accredited college or university and an approved dietetic technician program. This professional has also passed a national examination and maintains registration through continuing professional education.
- **dietitian** a person trained in the science of nutrition and dietetics. See also *Registered Dietitian Nutritionist.*
- **diploma mill** an organization that awards meaningless degrees without requiring students to meet educational standards. Diploma mills are not the same as diploma forgers (providing fake diplomas and certificates bearing the names of real, respected institutions). Although visually indistinguishable from authentic diplomas, forgeries can be unveiled by checking directly with the institution.
- **Fellow of the Academy of Nutrition and Dietetics (FAND)** members of the academy who are recognized for their outstanding service and integrity in the dietetics profession.
- **license to practice** permission under state or federal law, granted on meeting specified criteria, to use a certain title (such as *dietitian*) and to offer certain services. Licensed dietitians may use the initials LD after their names.
- **medical nutrition therapy** nutrition services used in the treatment of injury, illness, or other conditions; includes assessment of nutrition status and dietary intake and corrective applications of diet, counseling, and other nutrition services.
- **nutritionist** someone who studies or advises others on nutrition, and who may or may not have an academic degree in the nutrition. In states with responsible legislation, the term applies only to people who have master of science (MS) or doctor of philosophy (PhD) degrees from properly accredited institutions.
- **public health nutritionist** a dietitian or other person with an advanced degree in nutrition who specializes in public health nutrition.
- **registered dietitian nutritionist (RDN)** food and nutrition experts who have earned at least a bachelor's degree from an accredited college or university with a program approved by the Academy of Nutrition and Dietetics. The dietitian must also serve in an approved internship or coordinated program, pass the registration examination, and maintain professional competency through continuing education. Many states also require licensing of practicing dietitians. Also called *registered dietitian (RD)*.
- **registration** listing with a professional organization that requires specific course work, experience, and passing of an examination.

In some facilities, a dietetic technician assists a registered dietitian nutritionist in administrative and clinical responsibilities. A dietetic technician has been educated in nutrition and trained to perform practical tasks in patient care, food service, and other areas of dietetics.[5] Upon passing a national examination, the technician earns the title **nutrition and dietetics technician, registered (NDTR).**

Detecting Fake Credentials

In contrast to RDNs and other credentialed nutrition professionals, thousands of people possess fake nutrition degrees and claim to be nutrition counselors, nutritionists, or "dietists." These and other such titles may sound meaningful, but most of these people lack the established credentials of Academy of Nutrition and Dietetics–sanctioned dietitians. If you look closely, you can see signs that their expertise is fake.

Educational Background

A fake nutrition expert may display a degree from a six-week course of study; such a degree is simply not the same as the extensive requirements for legitimate nutrition credentials. In some cases, schools posing as legitimate institutions are actually **diploma mills**—fraudulent businesses that sell certificates of competency to anyone who pays the fees, from under a thousand dollars for a bachelor's degree to several thousand for a doctorate. To obtain these "degrees," a candidate need not read any books or pass any examinations, and the only written work is a signature on a check. Here are a few red flags to identify these scams:

- A degree is awarded in a very short time—sometimes just a few days.
- A degree can be based entirely on work or life experience.
- An institution provides only an e-mail address, with vague information on physical location.
- It provides sample styles of certificates and diplomas for choosing.
- It offers a choice of graduation dates to appear on a diploma.

Selling degrees is big business; networks of many bogus institutions are often owned by a single entity. In 2011, more than 2,600 such diploma and accreditation mills were identified, and 2,000 more were under investigation.

Accreditation and Licensure

Lack of proper accreditation is the identifying sign of a fake educational institution. To guard educational quality, an accrediting agency recognized by the U.S. Department of Education certifies those schools that meet the criteria defining a complete and accurate schooling, but in the case of nutrition, quack accrediting agencies cloud the picture. Fake nutrition

Professional Responsibilities of Registered Dietitian Nutritionists

Registered Dietitian Nutritionists perform varied and important roles in the workforce. This table lists just a few responsibilities of just a few specialties.

Specialty	Sample Responsibilities
Education	■ Write curricula to deliver to students nutrition knowledge that is appropriate for their goals and that meets criteria of accrediting agencies and professional groups. ■ Teach and evaluate student progress; research, write, and publish.
Food Service Management	■ Plan and direct an institution's food service system, from kitchen to delivery. ■ Plan and manage budgets; develop products; market services.
Health and Wellness	■ Design and implement research-based programs for individuals or populations to improve nutrition, health, and physical fitness.
Hospital Health Care/Clinical Care	■ Design and implement disease prevention services. ■ Order therapeutic diets independently. ■ Coordinate patient care with other health-care professionals. ■ Assess client nutrient status and requirements. ■ Provide client care and diet plan counseling.
Laboratory Research	■ Design, execute, and interpret food and nutrition research. ■ Write and publish research articles in peer-reviewed journals and lay publications. ■ Provide science-based guidance to nutrition practitioners. ■ Write and manage grants.
Public Health Nutrition	■ Influence nutrition policy, regulations, and legislation. ■ Plan, coordinate, administer, and evaluate food assistance programs. ■ Consult with agencies; plan and manage budgets.
Sports Team Nutrition	■ Provide individual and group/team nutrition counseling and education to enhance the performance of competitive and recreational athletes, on-site and during travel. ■ Perform assessments of body composition. ■ Track and document performance and other outcomes. ■ Manage budgets, dining facilities, and personnel.

Sources: Academy Quality Management Committee, Academy of Nutrition and Dietetics: Revised 2017 Scope of Practice for the Registered Dietitian Nutritionist, *Journal of the Academy of Nutrition and Dietetics* 118 (2018): 141–165.

degrees are available from schools "accredited" by more than 30 phony accrediting agencies.**

** To find out whether an online school is accredited, write the Distance Education and Training Council, Accrediting Commission, 1601 Eighteenth Street, NW, Washington, D.C. 20009; call 202-234-5100; or visit their website (www.detc.org).

To find out whether a school is properly accredited for a dietetics degree, visit the U.S. Department of Education's Database of Accredited Postsecondary Institutions and Programs at https://ope.ed.gov/accreditation. You can also write the Academy of Nutrition and Dietetics, Division of Education and Research, 120 South Riverside Plaza, Suite 2000, Chicago, Illinois 60606–6995; call 800-877-1600; or visit their website (www.eatright.org).

The American Council on Education publishes Accredited Institutions of Postsecondary Education Programs, a directory of accredited institutions, professionally accredited programs, and candidates for accreditation that is available at many libraries. For additional information, write the American Council on Education, One Dupont Circle NW, Suite 800, Washington, D.C. 20036; call 202-939-9382; or visit their website (www.acenet.edu).

State laws do not necessarily help consumers distinguish experts from fakes; some states allow anyone to use the title *dietitian* or *nutritionist*. But other states have responded to the need by allowing only RDNs or people with certain graduate degrees and state licenses to call themselves dietitians. Licensing provides a way to identify people who have met minimum standards of education and experience.

A Failed Attempt to Fail

To dramatize the ease with which anyone can obtain a fake nutrition degree, one writer paid $82 to enroll in a nutrition diploma mill that billed itself as a correspondence school. She made every attempt to fail, intentionally giving all wrong answers to the examination questions. Even so, she received a "nutritionist" certificate at the end of the course, together with a letter from the "school" officials explaining that they were sure she must have misread the test.

Would You Trust a Nutritionist Who Eats Dog Food?

In a similar stunt, Mr. Eddie Diekman was named a "professional member" of an association of nutrition "experts" (see Figure C1–3). For his efforts, Eddie received a diploma suitable for framing and displaying. Eddie is a cocker spaniel. His owner, Connie B. Diekman, then president of the American Dietetic Association, paid Eddie's tuition to

Figure C1–3

A "Professional Member" of a Fake Association

Eddie displays his professional credentials.

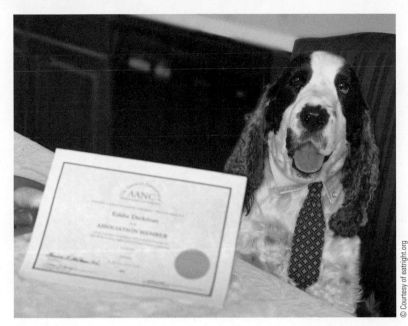

© Courtesy of eatright.org

prove that he could be awarded the title "nutritionist" merely by sending in his name.

Staying Ahead of the Scammers

In summary, to stay one step ahead of the nutrition quacks, check a provider's qualifications. First, look for the degrees and credentials listed after the person's name (such as MD, RDN, MS, PhD, or LD). Then, find out what you can about the reputations of institutions that are affiliated with the provider. If the person objects, or if your findings raise suspicions, look for someone better qualified to offer nutrition advice. Your health is your most precious asset, and protecting it is well worth the time and effort it takes to do so.

Critical Thinking

1. Describe how you would respond to the following situation:

    A friend has started taking ginseng, a supplement that claims to help with weight loss. You are thinking of trying ginseng, but you want to learn more about the herb and its effects before deciding. What research would you do, and what questions would you ask your friend to determine if ginseng is a legitimate weight loss product?

2. Recognizing a nutrition authority that you can consult for reliable nutrition information can be difficult because it is so easy to acquire questionable nutrition credentials. Read the education and experience of the "nutrition experts" described as follows and put them in order, beginning with the person with the strongest and most trustworthy nutrition expertise and ending with the person with the weakest and least trustworthy nutrition expertise:

    1. A nutrition and dietetics technician, registered (NDTR) working in a clinic

    2. A highly successful athlete/coach who has a small business as a nutrition counselor and sells a line of nutrition supplements

    3. An individual who has completed 30 hours of nutrition training through the American Association of Nutrition Counseling

    4. A Registered Dietitian Nutritionist (RDN) associated with a hospital

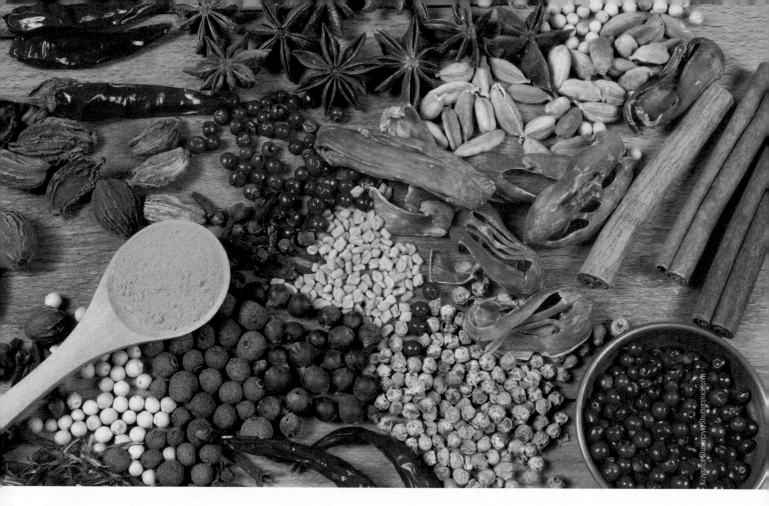

2 Nutrition Tools—Standards and Guidelines

Learning Objectives

After completing this chapter, you should be able to accomplish the following:

LO 2.1 State the significance of Dietary Reference Intakes (DRI) and Daily Values as nutrient standards.

LO 2.2 Define the role of the Dietary Guidelines as part of the overall U.S. dietary guidance system.

LO 2.3 Describe how the USDA Eating Patterns support the planning of a nutritious diet.

LO 2.4 Given a specified number of calories, create a healthful diet plan using the USDA Eating Patterns.

LO 2.5 Describe the information that appears on food labels.

LO 2.6 Compare one day's nutrient-dense meals with meals not planned for nutrient density.

LO 2.7 Summarize the potential health effects of phytochemicals from both food sources and supplements.

How can you tell **how much of each nutrient** you need to consume daily?

Are the health claims on food labels **accurate and reliable**?

Can we trust the **government's dietary recommendations**?

Can certain "**superfoods**" boost your health with more than just nutrients?

E ating well is easy in theory—just choose foods that supply appropriate amounts of the essential nutrients, fiber, phytochemicals, and energy without excess intakes of fat, sugar, and salt, and be sure to get enough physical activity to help balance the foods you eat. In practice, eating well proves harder to do. Many people are overweight, or are undernourished, or suffer from nutrient excesses or deficiencies that impair their health—that is, they are malnourished. You may not think that this statement applies to you, but you may already have less than optimal nutrient intakes without knowing it. Accumulated over years, the effects of your habits can seriously impair the quality of your life.

Putting it positively, you can enjoy the best possible vim, vigor, and vitality throughout your life if you learn now to nourish yourself optimally. To learn how, you first need some general guidelines and the answers to several basic questions. How much of each nutrient and how many calories should you consume? Which types of foods supply which nutrients? How much of each type of food do you have to eat to get enough? And how can you eat all these foods without gaining excess weight? This chapter begins by identifying some ideals for nutrient and energy intakes and ends by showing how to achieve them.

Nutrient Recommendations

LO 2.1 State the significance of Dietary Reference Intakes (DRI) and Daily Values as nutrient standards.

Nutrient recommendations are sets of standards against which people's nutrient and energy intakes can be measured. Nutrition experts use the recommendations to assess intakes and to offer advice on amounts to consume. Individuals may use them to decide how much of a nutrient they need and how much is too much.

Two Sets of Standards

Two sets of standards are important for students of nutrition: one for people's nutrient intakes and one for food labels. The first set are the **Dietary Reference Intakes (DRI)**. A committee of nutrition experts from the United States and Canada develops, publishes, and updates the DRI.* The DRI committee has set recommended intakes and limits for all of the vitamins and minerals, as well as for carbohydrates, fiber, lipids, protein, water, and energy.

The other standards, the **Daily Values**, are familiar to anyone who has read a food label. Nutrient standards—the DRI and Daily Values—are used and referred to so often that they

Dietary Reference Intakes (DRI) a set of five lists of values for measuring the nutrient intakes of healthy people in the United States and Canada. The lists are Estimated Average Requirements (EAR), Recommended Dietary Allowances (RDA), Adequate Intakes (AI), Tolerable Upper Intake Levels (UL), and Acceptable Macronutrient Distribution Ranges (AMDR).

Daily Values nutrient standards used on food labels and on grocery store and restaurant signs.

---

* This is a committee of the Food and Nutrition Board of the National Academy of Sciences' Institute of Medicine.

Figure 2–1

Alphabet Soup?

Don't let the "alphabet soup" of nutrient intake standards confuse you. Their names make sense when you learn their purposes.

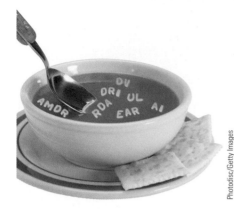

Photodisc/Getty Images

Recommended Dietary Allowances (RDA) nutrient intake goals for individuals; the average daily nutrient intake level that meets the needs of nearly all (97 to 98 percent) healthy people in a particular life stage and gender group.

Adequate Intakes (AI) nutrient intake goals for individuals set when scientific data are insufficient to allow establishment of an RDA value and assumed to be adequate for healthy people.

Tolerable Upper Intake Levels (UL) the highest average daily nutrient intake levels that are likely to pose no risk of toxicity to almost all healthy individuals of a particular life stage and gender group.

Estimated Average Requirements (EAR) nutrient values used in nutrition research and policy making and the basis upon which RDA values are set; the average daily nutrient intake estimated to meet the requirement of half of the healthy individuals in a particular life stage and gender group.

Acceptable Macronutrient Distribution Ranges (AMDR) values for carbohydrate, fat, and protein expressed as percentages of total daily caloric intake; ranges of intakes set for the energy-yielding nutrients that are sufficient to provide adequate total energy and nutrients while minimizing the risk of chronic diseases.

are printed in full on the very last group of pages of this book, pp. A, B, and C. Nutritionists refer to these values by their acronyms, and this book does, too (see Figure 2–1).

KEY POINTS

- The Dietary Reference Intakes are U.S. and Canadian nutrient intake standards.
- The Daily Values are U.S. standards used on food labels.

The DRI Lists and Purposes

For each nutrient, the DRI establish a number of values, each serving a different purpose. The values that most people find useful are those that set goals for nutrient intakes (RDA, AI, and AMDR, described next) and those that describe nutrient safety (UL, addressed later). In total, the DRI include five sets of values:

1. **Recommended Dietary Allowances (RDA)**—adequacy
2. **Adequate Intakes (AI)**—adequacy
3. **Tolerable Upper Intake Levels (UL)**—safety
4. **Estimated Average Requirements (EAR)**—research and policy
5. **Acceptable Macronutrient Distribution Ranges (AMDR)**—healthful ranges for energy-yielding nutrients

RDA and AI—Recommended Nutrient Intakes A great advantage of the DRI values lies in their applicability to the diets of individuals.[†] People may adopt the RDA and AI as their own nutrient intake goals. The AI values are not the scientific equivalent of the RDA, however.

The RDA form the indisputable bedrock of the DRI recommended intakes because they derive from solid experimental evidence and reliable observations—they are expected to meet the needs of almost all healthy people. AI values, in contrast, are based as far as possible not only on the available scientific evidence but also on some educated guesswork. Whenever the DRI committee members find insufficient evidence to generate an RDA, they establish an AI value instead. This book refers to the RDA and AI values collectively as the DRI.

EAR—Nutrition Research and Policy The EAR, also set by the DRI committee, establish the average nutrient requirements for given life stages and gender groups that researchers and nutrition policy makers use in their work. Public health officials may also use them to assess the prevalence of inadequate intakes in populations and make recommendations. The EAR values form the scientific basis upon which the RDA values are set (a later section explains how).

UL—Safety Beyond a certain point, it is unwise to consume large amounts of any nutrient, so the DRI committee sets the UL to identify potentially toxic levels of nutrient intake. Usual intakes of a nutrient below its UL pose a low risk of causing illness; chronic intakes above the UL pose increasing risks. The UL are indispensable to consumers who take supplements or consume foods and beverages to which vitamins or minerals have been added—a group that includes almost everyone. Public health officials also rely on UL values to set safe upper limits for nutrients added to our food and water supplies.

The DRI numbers for nutrients do not mark a rigid line dividing safe and hazardous intakes (as Figure 2–2 illustrates). Instead, nutrient needs fall within a range, and a danger zone exists both below and above that range. People's tolerances for high doses of nutrients vary, so caution is in order when nutrient intakes approach the UL values (listed at the back of the book, p. C).

Some nutrients lack UL values. The absence of a UL for a nutrient does not imply that it is safe to consume it in any amount, however. It means only that insufficient data exist to establish a value.

[†] Reference notes are in Appendix F.

Figure 2-2

The Naïve View versus the Accurate View of Optimal Nutrient Intakes

A common but naïve belief is that consuming *less* than the DRI amount of a nutrient is dangerous, but that consuming any amount more is safe. The accurate view, shown on the right, is that DRI values fall within a safety range, with the UL marking tolerable upper levels.

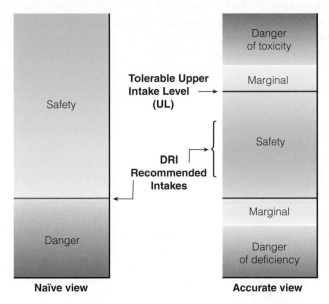

Naïve view   **Accurate view**

AMDR—Calorie Percentage Ranges   The DRI committee also sets healthy ranges of intake for carbohydrate, fat, and protein known as Acceptable Macronutrient Distribution Ranges. Each of these three energy-yielding nutrients contributes to the day's total calorie intake, and their contributions can be expressed as a percentage of the total. According to the committee, a diet that provides adequate energy in the following proportions can provide adequate nutrients while minimizing the risk of chronic diseases:

- 45 to 65 percent of calories from carbohydrate.
- 20 to 35 percent of calories from fat.
- 10 to 35 percent of calories from protein.

The chapters on the energy-yielding nutrients revisit these ranges.

Fortunately, you don't have to calculate these percentages for yourself when planning nutritious meals. The sample calculation in the margin shows how the math is done, but policy makers have translated these guidelines into a pattern of food groups that relieves the meal planner of this task. (See "Dietary Guidelines for Americans," beginning on page 36.).[2]

KEY POINTS

- The DRI include nutrient intake goals for individuals, standards for researchers and public policy makers, and tolerable upper limits.
- RDA, AI, EAR, and UL are all DRI standards, along with AMDR ranges for energy-yielding nutrients.

Understanding the DRI

Nutrient recommendations have been much misunderstood. One young woman posed this question: "Do you mean that some bureaucrat says that I need exactly the same amount of vitamin D as everyone else? Do they really think that 'one size fits all'?" In fact, the opposite is true.

Do the Math

Calculate the percentage of calories from an energy nutrient in a day's meals by using this general formula:

(A nutrient's calorie amount ÷ total calories) × 100

Calculate the percentage of calories from protein in a day's meals:

A day's meals provide 50 grams of protein and 1,754 total calories.

1. Convert the protein *grams* to protein *calories* (protein provides 4 calories per gram):

    50 g protein × 4 cal per g = ____ cal from protein

2. Using this answer, apply the general formula:

    (protein calorie amount ÷ total calories) × 100

    (___ ÷ 1,754) × 100 = ___ percent calories from protein.

Follow the same procedure when considering carbohydrate (4 cal per g) and fat (9 cal per g).

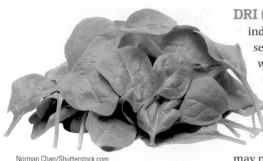

DRI for Population Groups The DRI committee acknowledges differences among individuals and takes them into account when setting nutrient values. It has made separate recommendations for specific groups of people—men, women, pregnant women, lactating women, infants, and children—and for specific age ranges. Children aged 4 to 8 years, for example, have their own DRI. Each individual can look up the recommendations for his or her own age and gender group. Within each age and gender group, the committee advises adjusting nutrient intakes in special circumstances that may increase or decrease nutrient needs, such as illness or smoking. Later chapters provide details about who may need to adjust intakes of which nutrients.

For almost all healthy people, a diet that consistently provides the RDA or AI amount for a specific nutrient is very likely to be adequate in that nutrient. To make your diet nutritionally adequate, aim for nutrient intakes that, over time, average 100 percent of your DRI.

Other Characteristics of the DRI The following facts will help put the DRI into perspective:

- The values reflect daily intakes to be achieved on average, over time. They assume that intakes will vary from day to day and are set high enough to ensure that the body's nutrient stores will meet nutrient needs during periods of inadequate intakes lasting several days to several months, depending on the nutrient.
- The values are based on available scientific research to the greatest extent possible and are updated to reflect current scientific knowledge.
- The values are based on the concepts of probability and risk. The DRI are associated with a low probability of deficiency for people of a given life stage and gender group, and they pose almost no risk of toxicity for that group.
- The values are intended to ensure optimal intakes, not minimum requirements. They include a generous safety margin and meet the needs of virtually all healthy people in a specific age and gender group.
- The values are set in reference to certain indicators of nutrient adequacy, such as blood nutrient concentrations, normal growth, or reduction of certain chronic diseases or other disorders, rather than prevention of deficiency symptoms alone.

The DRI Apply to Healthy People Only The DRI are designed for health maintenance and disease prevention in healthy people, not for the restoration of health or repletion of nutrients in those with deficiencies. Under the stress of serious illness or malnutrition, a person may require a much higher intake of certain nutrients or may not be able to handle even the DRI amount. Therapeutic diets take into account the increased nutrient needs imposed by certain medical conditions, such as recovery from surgery, burns, fractures, illnesses, malnutrition, or addictions.

KEY POINTS

- The DRI set separate recommendations for specific groups of people at different ages.
- The DRI intake recommendations (RDA and AI) are up-to-date, optimal, and safe nutrient intakes for healthy people in the United States and Canada.

How the Committee Establishes DRI Values— An RDA Example

A theoretical discussion will help to explain how the DRI committee goes about setting DRI values. Suppose we are the DRI committee members with the task of setting an RDA for nutrient X (an essential nutrient).[‡] Ideally, our first step will be to find out how much of that nutrient various healthy individuals need. To do so, we review studies of deficiency states, nutrient stores and their depletion, and the factors influencing them.

balance study a laboratory study in which a subject is fed a controlled diet and the intake and excretion of a nutrient are measured. Balance studies are valid only for nutrients such as calcium (chemical elements) that do not change while they are in the body.

[‡]This discussion describes how an RDA value is set. To set an AI value, the committee would use some educated guesswork, as well as scientific research results, to determine an approximate amount of the nutrient most likely to support health.

Chapter 2 Nutrition Tools—Standards and Guidelines

We then select the most valid data for use in our work. Serious science goes into setting all of the five nutrient standards that comprise the DRI, but setting the RDA demands the most rigorous science and tolerates the least guesswork.

Determining Individual Requirements

One experiment we would review or conduct is a **balance study**. In this type of study, scientists measure the body's intake and excretion of a nutrient to find out how much intake is required to balance excretion. For each individual subject, we can determine a **requirement** to achieve balance for nutrient X. With an intake below the requirement, a person will slip into negative balance or experience declining stores that could, over time, lead to deficiency of the nutrient.

We find that different individuals, even of the same age and gender, have different requirements. Mr. A needs 40 units of the nutrient each day to maintain balance; Mr. B needs 35; Mr. C needs 57. If we look at enough individuals, we find that their requirements are distributed, as shown in Figure 2–3—with most requirements near the midpoint (here, 45) and only a few at the extremes.

Accounting for the Needs of the Population   To set the value, we have to decide what intake to recommend for everybody. Should we set it at the mean (45 units in Figure 2–3)? This is the Estimated Average Requirement for nutrient X, mentioned earlier as valuable to scientists and policy makers but not appropriate as an individual's nutrient goal. The EAR value is probably close to everyone's minimum need, assuming the distribution shown in Figure 2–3. (Actually, the data for most nutrients indicate a distribution that is much less symmetrical.) But if people took us literally and consumed exactly this amount of nutrient X each day, half the population would begin to develop nutrient deficiencies and, in time, even observable symptoms of deficiency diseases. Mr. C (at 57 units) would be one of those people.

Perhaps we should set the recommendation for nutrient X at or above the extreme—say, at 70 units a day—so that everyone will be covered. (Actually, we didn't study everyone, and some individual we didn't happen to test might have an even higher requirement.) This might be a good idea in theory, but what about a person like Mr. B who requires only 35 units a day? The recommendation would be twice his requirement, and to follow it, he might spend money needlessly on foods containing nutrient X to the exclusion of foods containing other vital nutrients.

The Decision   The decision we finally make is to set the value high enough so that 97 to 98 percent of the population will be covered but not so high as to be excessive (Figure 2–4 illustrates such a value). In this example, a reasonable choice might be 63 units a day. Moving the value farther toward the extreme would pick up a few additional people, but it would inflate the recommendation for most people, including Mr. A and Mr. B. The committee makes judgments of this kind when setting the DRI for many nutrients. Relatively few healthy people have requirements that are not covered by the DRI.

KEY POINT

- The DRI are based on scientific data and generously cover the needs of virtually all healthy people in the United States and Canada.

Setting Energy Requirements

In contrast to the recommendations for nutrients, the value set for energy, the **Estimated Energy Requirement (EER)**, is not generous; instead, it is set at a level predicted to maintain body weight for an individual of a particular age, gender, height, weight, and physical activity level consistent with good health. The energy DRI values reflect a balancing act: enough food energy is critical to support health and life, but too much energy causes unhealthy weight gain. Because even small amounts of excess energy consumed day after day cause unneeded weight gain and increase chronic disease risks, the DRI committee did not set a Tolerable Upper Intake Level for energy.

Figure 2–3

Individuality of Nutrient Requirements

Each square represents a person. A, B, and C are Mr. A, Mr. B, and Mr. C. Each has a different requirement.

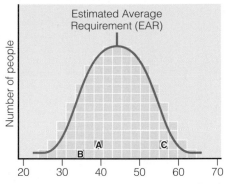

Figure 2–4

Nutrient Recommended Intake: Example

Intake recommendations for most vitamins and minerals are set so that they will meet the requirements of nearly all people.

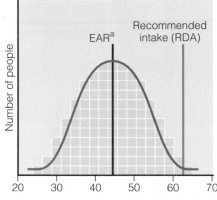

aEstimated Average Requirement

requirement the amount of a nutrient that will just prevent the development of specific deficiency signs; distinguished from the DRI value, which is a generous allowance with a margin of safety.

Estimated Energy Requirement (EER) the average dietary energy intake predicted to maintain energy balance in a healthy adult of a certain age, gender, weight, height, and level of physical activity consistent with good health.

- Estimated Energy Requirements are predicted to maintain body weight and to discourage unhealthy weight gain.

Why Are Daily Values Used on Labels?

On learning about the Daily Values, many people ask why yet another set of nutrient standards is needed for food labels—why not use the DRI? The reason they are not used is that DRI values for a nutrient vary, sometimes widely, to address the different nutrient needs of different population groups. Food labels, in contrast, must list a single value for each nutrient that may be used by anyone who picks up a package of food and reads the label.[3]

The Daily Values reflect the highest level of nutrient need among all population groups, from children of age 4 years through aging adults; for example, the Daily Value for iron is 18 milligrams (mg), an amount that far exceeds a man's RDA of 8 mg (but that meets a young woman's high need precisely). Thus, the Daily Values are ideal for allowing general comparisons among *foods*, but they cannot serve as nutrient intake goals for individuals. The recently updated Daily Values are listed in the back of the book, p. Y.

- The Daily Values are standards used solely on food labels to enable consumers to compare the nutrient values of foods.

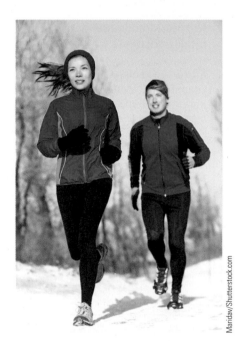

The Dietary Guidelines recommend physical activity to help balance calorie intakes to achieve and sustain a healthy body weight.

Dietary Guidelines for Americans

LO 2.2   Define the role of the Dietary Guidelines as part of the overall U.S. dietary guidance system.

> **Appendix B** offers World Health Organization (WHO) guidelines.

Many countries set dietary guidelines to answer the question, "What should I eat to stay healthy?" In this country, the U.S. Department of Agriculture publishes its *Dietary Guidelines for Americans* as part of a national nutrition guidance system. Although the DRI values set nutrient intake goals, the *Dietary Guidelines for Americans* offer food-based strategies for achieving them. If everyone followed their advice, people's energy intakes and most of their nutrient needs would fall into place.[4][§] Table 2–1 lists the 2015–2020 Dietary Guidelines and their key recommendations.

The Guidelines Promote Health   People who follow the Dietary Guidelines—that is, those who do not overconsume calories, who take in enough of a variety of nutrient-dense foods and beverages, and who make physical activity a habit—often enjoy the best possible health. Only a few people in this country fit this description, however. Instead, about half of American adults suffer from one or more *preventable* chronic diseases related to poor diets and sedentary lifestyles.

How Does the U.S. Diet Compare with the Guidelines?   The Dietary Guidelines committee reviewed nationwide survey results reflecting current nutrient intakes, along with biochemical assessments and other forms of evidence. The results are clear: important needed nutrients are undersupplied by the current U.S. diet, while other, less healthful nutrients are oversupplied (see Table 2–2).[5] Figure 2–5 (p. 38) shows that, typically, people take in far too few nutritious foods from most food groups when compared with the ideals of the Dietary Guidelines for Americans (discussed fully in the next section). They also take in too many calories and too much red and processed meat, refined grain, added sugar, sodium, and saturated fat.

[§] The USDA Eating Patterns may not meet the DRI for vitamin D or potassium.

Table 2–1

Dietary Guidelines for Americans 2015–2020: Guidelines and Recommendations

The Dietary Guidelines and key recommendations should be applied in their entirety to people 2 years of age and older; they are interconnected and each component can affect the others.

Dietary Guidelines	Key Recommendations
1. *Follow a healthy eating pattern across the life span.* All food and beverage choices matter. Choose a healthy eating pattern at an appropriate calorie level to help achieve and maintain a healthy body weight, support nutrient adequacy, and reduce the risk of chronic disease.	**Consume a healthy eating pattern that accounts for all foods and beverages within an appropriate calorie level.** *A healthy eating pattern includes:* ■ A variety of vegetables from all of the subgroups—dark green, red and orange, legumes (beans and peas), starchy, and other. ■ Fruit, especially whole fruit. ■ Grains, at least half of which are whole grains. ■ Fat-free or low-fat dairy, including milk, yogurt, cheese, and/or fortified soy beverages. ■ A variety of protein foods, including seafood, lean meats and poultry, eggs, legumes (beans and peas), and nuts, seeds, and soy products. ■ Oils.
2. *Focus on variety, nutrient density, and amount.* To meet nutrient needs within calorie limits, choose a variety of nutrient-dense foods across and within all food groups in recommended amounts.	
3. *Limit calories from added sugars and saturated fats and reduce sodium intake.* Consume an eating pattern low in added sugars, saturated fats, and sodium. Cut back on foods and beverages higher in these components to amounts that fit within healthy eating patterns.	*A healthy eating pattern limits:* ■ Saturated fats and *trans* fats, added sugars, and sodium. ■ Consume less than 10 percent of calories per day from added sugars. ■ Consume less than 10 percent of calories per day from saturated fats. ■ Consume less than 2,300 milligrams per day of sodium.
4. *Shift to healthier food and beverage choices.* Choose nutrient-dense foods and beverages across and within all food groups in place of less healthy choices. Consider cultural and personal preferences to make these shifts easier to accomplish and maintain.	■ If alcohol is consumed, it should be consumed in moderation—up to one drink per day for women and up to two drinks per day for men—and only by adults of legal drinking age.
5. *Support healthy eating patterns for all.* Everyone has a role in helping to create and support healthy eating patterns in multiple settings nationwide, from home to school to work to communities.	**Meet the *Physical Activity Guidelines for Americans.***

Source: U.S. Department of Health and Human Services and U.S. Department of Agriculture, 2015–2020 Dietary Guidelines for Americans, 8th edition (2015), available at http://health.gov/dietaryguidelines/2015/guidelines/.

Table 2–2

Shortfall Nutrients and Overconsumed Nutrients

These nutrients are chronically under- or overconsumed in relation to their DRI recommendations, indicating a need for change in U.S. eating habits. Added sugars, not listed, are also overconsumed, but no DRI standard exists for added sugars.

Shortfall nutrients: Chronically undersupplied in U.S. diets

■ Vitamin A	■ Calcium
■ Vitamin C	■ Iron (for some girls and women; see Chapter 8)
■ Vitamin D	■ Magnesium
■ Vitamin E	■ Fiber
■ Folate	■ Potassium

Overconsumed nutrients: Chronically oversupplied in U.S. diets

■ Saturated fat	■ Sodium

Source: U.S. Department of Agriculture and U.S. Department of Health and Human Services, Scientific Report of the 2015 Dietary Guidelines Advisory Committee (2015), D-1:89, available at www.health.gov.

Figure 2-5

How Does the Typical U.S. Diet Stack Up?

The average U.S. diet needs improvements—more whole grains, fewer refined grains, more vegetables and fruit, and more milk—to meet intake goals. In addition, most Americans greatly exceed recommendations for added sugars, saturated fats, and sodium.

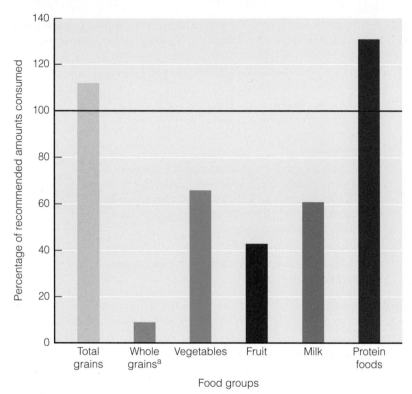

aHalf of the grains you eat should be whole grains.

Source: USDA Economic Research Service, *2015.*

Note that the Dietary Guidelines for Americans do not require that you give up your favorite foods or eat strange, unappealing foods. They advocate achieving a healthy dietary pattern through wise food and beverage choices and not by way of supplements except when medically necessary. With a little planning and a few adjustments, almost anyone's diet can contribute to health instead of disease. Part of the plan must also be to exercise optimally to help achieve and sustain a healthy body weight, and this chapter's Think Fitness box (p. 39) offers some guidelines, while Chapter 10 provides details.

Our Two Cents' Worth If the experts who develop the Dietary Guidelines for Americans were to ask us, our focus would fall on this recommendation: choose carefully, but enjoy your food. The joys of eating are physically beneficial to the body because they trigger health-promoting changes in the nervous, hormonal, and immune systems. When the food is nutritious as well as enjoyable, then the eater obtains all the nutrients needed to support proper body functioning, as well as for the healthy skin, glossy hair, and natural attractiveness that accompany robust health. Remember to enjoy your food.

KEY POINTS

- The Dietary Guidelines for Americans address problems of undernutrition and overnutrition.
- They recommend following a healthful eating pattern and being physically active.
- Key nutrients of concern are lacking in many U.S. diets; others are oversupplied.

THINK FITNESS — Recommendations for Daily Physical Activity

The USDA's Physical Activity Guidelines for Americans suggest that to maintain good health, adults should engage in at least 2½ hours of moderate physical activity each week.[6] A brisk walk at a pace of about 100 steps per minute (1,000 steps over 10 minutes) constitutes "moderate" activity. In addition:

- Physical activity can be intermittent, a few minutes here and there, throughout the week.

- Resistance activity (such as weight-lifting) can be a valuable part of the exercise total for the week.

- Small increases in moderate activity bring health benefits. There is no threshold that must be exceeded before benefits begin.

For weight control or additional health benefits, more than the minimum amount of physical activity is required. Details can be found in later chapters.

start now! Ready to make a change? Set a goal of 30 minutes per day of physical activity (walking, jogging, biking, weight training, etc.), and then track your actual activity for five days. You can do this with a pencil and paper, or use the Track Activity feature of Diet & Wellness Plus, available in MindTap at www.Cengage.com.

Diet Planning Using the USDA Eating Patterns

LO 2.3   Describe how the the USDA Eating Patterns support the planning of a nutritious diet.

Diet planning connects nutrition theory with the food on the table. To help people achieve the goals of the Dietary Guidelines for Americans, the USDA employs a **food group plan** known as the USDA Eating Patterns.** Figure 2–6 (pp. 40–41) displays the food groups used in this plan. By using the plan wisely and by learning about the energy-yielding nutrients, vitamins, and minerals in various foods (as you will in coming chapters), you can achieve the goals of a nutritious diet first mentioned in Chapter 1: adequacy, balance, calorie control, moderation, and variety.

> Phytochemicals and their potential biological actions are explained in **Controversy 2**.

If you design your diet around this plan, it is assumed that you will obtain adequate and balanced amounts of the two dozen or so essential nutrients and hundreds of potentially beneficial phytochemicals because all of these compounds are distributed among the same foods. It can also help you to limit calories and potentially harmful food constituents.

The Food Groups and Subgroups

Figure 2–6 defines the major food groups and their subgroups. The USDA specifies portions of various foods within each group (left column of Figure 2–6) that are **nutritional equivalents** and thus can be treated interchangeably in diet planning. It also lists the key nutrients provided by foods within each group, information worth noting and remembering. The foods in each group are well-known contributors of the key nutrients listed, but you can count on these foods to supply many other nutrients as well. Note also that the figure sorts foods within each group by **nutrient density**.

Vegetable Subgroups and Protein Food Subgroups   Not every vegetable supplies every key nutrient attributed to the Vegetables group, so the vegetables are sorted into subgroups by their nutrient contents. All vegetables provide valuable fiber and the mineral potassium, but many from the "red and orange vegetables" subgroup are known for their vitamin A content; those from the "dark green vegetables" provide a wealth of folate; "starchy vegetables" provide abundant carbohydrate; and "legumes" supply substantial iron and protein.

food group plan a diet-planning tool that sorts foods into groups based on their nutrient content and then specifies that people should eat certain minimum numbers of servings of foods from each group.

nutritional equivalents the portion sizes of various foods needed to deliver similar amounts of any of the nutrients that characterize a particular food group. For example, in the vegetable group, 1 cup cooked kale and 2 cups raw kale are nutritional equivalents because both contain similar amounts of the mineral iron.

nutrient density a measure of nutrients provided per calorie of food. A *nutrient dense food* provides vitamins, minerals, and other nutrients with little or no solid fats, added sugars, refined starches, or sodium.

**USDA Eating Patterns may also be called USDA Food Patterns.

Figure 2–6
USDA Food Groups and Subgroups

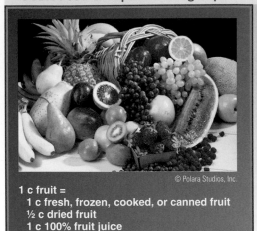

1 c fruit =
1 c fresh, frozen, cooked, or canned fruit
½ c dried fruit
1 c 100% fruit juice

Fruit contributes folate, vitamin A, vitamin C, potassium, and fiber.

Consume a variety of fruit, and choose whole or cut-up fruit more often than fruit juice.

Apples, apricots, avocados, bananas, blueberries, cantaloupe, cherries, grapefruit, grapes, guava, honeydew, kiwi, mango, nectarines, oranges, papaya, peaches, pears, pineapples, plums, raspberries, strawberries, tangerines, watermelon; dried fruit (dates, figs, prunes, raisins); 100% fruit juices

Limit fruit that contains solid fats and/or added sugars:
Canned or frozen fruit in syrup; juices, punches, ades, and fruit drinks with added sugars; fried plantains

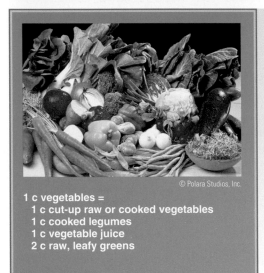

1 c vegetables =
1 c cut-up raw or cooked vegetables
1 c cooked legumes
1 c vegetable juice
2 c raw, leafy greens

Vegetables contribute folate, vitamin A, vitamin C, vitamin K, vitamin E, magnesium, potassium, and fiber.

Consume a variety of vegetables each day, and choose from all five subgroups several times a week.

Vegetable subgroups:
Dark green vegetables: Broccoli and leafy greens such as arugula, beet greens, bok choy, collard greens, kale, mustard greens, romaine lettuce, spinach, turnip greens, watercress

Red and orange vegetables: Carrots, carrot juice, pumpkin, red bell peppers, sweet potatoes, tomatoes, tomato juice, vegetable juice, winter squash (acorn, butternut)

Legumes: Black beans, black-eyed peas, garbanzo beans (chickpeas), kidney beans, lentils, navy beans, pinto beans, split peas, white beans, soybeans and soy products such as tofu

Starchy vegetables: Cassava, corn, green peas, hominy, lima beans, potatoes

Other vegetables: Artichokes, asparagus, bamboo shoots, bean sprouts, beets, brussels sprouts, cabbages, cactus, cauliflower, celery, cucumbers, eggplant, green beans, green bell peppers, iceberg lettuce, mushrooms, okra, onions, seaweed, snow peas, zucchini

Limit vegetables that contain solid fats and/or added sugars:
Baked beans, candied sweet potatoes, coleslaw, french fries, potato salad, refried beans, scalloped potatoes, tempura vegetables

1 oz grains =
1 slice bread
½ c cooked rice, pasta, or cereal
1 oz dry pasta or rice
1 c ready-to-eat cereal flakes
3 c popped popcorn

Grains contribute folate, niacin, riboflavin, thiamin, iron, magnesium, selenium, and fiber.

Make most (at least half) of the grain selections whole grains.

Grain subgroups:
Whole grains: amaranth, barley, brown rice, buckwheat, bulgur, cornmeal, millet, oats, quinoa, rye, wheat, and wild rice and whole-grain products such as breads, cereals, crackers, and pastas; popcorn

Enriched refined products: bagels, breads, cereals, pastas (couscous, macaroni, spaghetti), pretzels, white rice, rolls, tortillas

Limit grains that contain solid fats and/or added sugars:
Biscuits, cakes, cookies, cornbread, crackers, croissants, doughnuts, fried rice, granola, muffins, pastries, pies, presweetened cereals, taco shells

Figure 2–6

USDA Food Groups and Subgroups *(continued)*

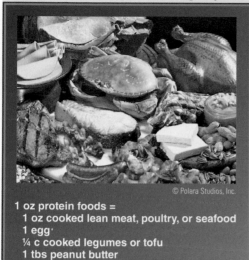

© Polara Studios, Inc.

1 oz protein foods =
1 oz cooked lean meat, poultry, or seafood
1 egg·
¼ c cooked legumes or tofu
1 tbs peanut butter
½ oz nuts or seeds

Protein foods contribute protein, essential fatty acids, niacin, thiamin, vitamin B$_6$, vitamin B$_{12}$, iron, magnesium, potassium, and zinc.

Choose a variety of protein foods from the three subgroups, including seafood in place of meat or poultry twice a week.

Protein food subgroups:
Seafood: Fish (catfish, cod, flounder, haddock, halibut, herring, mackerel, pollock, salmon, sardines, sea bass, snapper, trout, tuna), shellfish (clams, crab, lobster, mussels, oysters, scallops, shrimp)

Meats, poultry, and eggs: Lean or low-fat meats (fat-trimmed beef, game, ham, lamb, pork, veal), poultry (no skin), eggs

Nuts, seeds, and soy products: Unsalted nuts (almonds, cashews, filberts, pecans, pistachios, walnuts), seeds (flaxseeds, pumpkin seeds, sesame seeds, sunflower seeds), legumes, soy products (textured vegetable protein, tofu, tempeh), peanut butter, peanuts

Limit protein foods that contain solid fats and/or added sugars:
Bacon; baked beans; fried meat, seafood, poultry, eggs, or tofu; refried beans; ground beef; hot dogs; luncheon meats; marbled steaks; poultry with skin; sausages; spare ribs

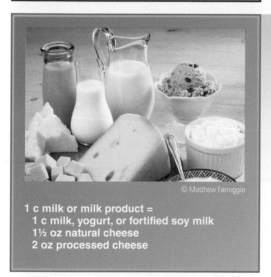

© Matthew Farruggio

1 c milk or milk product =
1 c milk, yogurt, or fortified soy milk
1½ oz natural cheese
2 oz processed cheese

Milk and milk products^a contribute protein, riboflavin, vitamin B$_{12}$, calcium, potassium, and, when fortified, vitamin A and vitamin D.

Make fat-free or low-fat choices. Choose other calcium-rich foods if you don't consume milk.

Fat-free or 1% low-fat milk and fat-free or 1% low-fat milk products such as buttermilk, cheeses, cottage cheese, yogurt; fat-free fortified soy milk

Limit milk products that contain solid fats and/or added sugars:
2% reduced-fat milk and whole milk; 2% reduced-fat and whole-milk products such as cheeses, cottage cheese, and yogurt; flavored milk with added sugars such as chocolate milk, custard, frozen yogurt, ice cream, milkshakes, pudding, sherbet; fortified soy milk

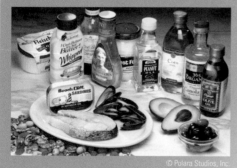

© Polara Studios, Inc.

1 tsp oil =
1 tsp vegetable oil
1 tsp soft margarine
1 tbs low-fat mayonnaise
2 tbs light salad dressing

Oils are not a food group, but are featured here because they contribute vitamin E and essential fatty acids.

Use oils instead of solid fats, when possible.

Liquid vegetable oils such as canola, corn, flaxseed, nut, olive, peanut, safflower, sesame, soybean, sunflower oils; mayonnaise, oil-based salad dressing, soft *trans* fat-free margarine; unsaturated oils that occur naturally in foods such as avocados, fatty fish, nuts, olives, seeds (flaxseeds, sesame seeds), shellfish

Limit solid fats:
Animal fats, butter, shortening, stick margarine.

^{a} This text refers to "Milk and Milk Products" to indicate the foods of this group that are recommended for meeting nutrient needs (see Table 2–1); the USDA uses the broader term "Dairy Products."

The Protein Foods group falls into subgroups, too. All protein foods dependably supply iron and protein, but their fats vary widely. "Meats" tend to be higher in saturated fats that should be limited. "Seafood" and "nuts, seeds, and soy products" tend to be low in saturated fats while providing essential fats that the body requires.

Grain Subgroups and Other Foods Among the grains, the foods of the "Whole Grain" subgroup supply fiber and a wide variety of nutrients. Refined grains lack many of these beneficial compounds but provide abundant energy. The Dietary Guidelines suggest that at least half of the grains in a day's meals be whole grains or that at least three servings of whole-grain foods be included in the diet each day. (Grain serving sizes in 1-ounce equivalents are listed in Figure 2–6.)

Spices, herbs, coffee, and tea provide few, if any, nutrients but can add flavor and pleasure to meals. Some, such as tea and spices, are particularly rich in potentially beneficial phytochemicals—see this chapter's Controversy section.

Variety among and within Food Groups Varying food choices, both among the food groups and within each group, helps ensure adequate nutrient intakes and also protects against consuming large amounts of toxins or contaminants from any one food. Achieving variety may require some effort, but knowing which foods fall into which food groups eases the task.

KEY POINTS

- The USDA Eating Patterns divide foods into food groups based on key nutrient contents.
- People who consume the specified amounts of foods from each group and subgroup achieve dietary adequacy, balance, and variety.

Choosing Nutrient-Dense Foods

To help people control calories and achieve and sustain a healthy body weight, the Dietary Guidelines instruct consumers to base their diets on the most nutrient-dense foods from each group. Unprocessed or lightly processed foods are generally best because many processes strip foods of beneficial nutrients and fiber and others add salt, sugar, or solid fat. Highly processed foods often have low nutrient density, and so must be minimized to meet the Dietary Guidelines.[7] Figure 2–7 displays some low-nutrient density foods and beverages that present mostly solid fats, added sugars, and alcohol to the diet.

Uncooked (raw) oil is worth notice in this regard. Oil is pure, calorie-rich fat and is therefore low in nutrient density, but a small amount of raw oil from sources such as avocados, olives, nuts, and fish, or even raw vegetable oil, provides vitamin E and essential lipids that other foods lack. High temperatures used in frying destroy these nutrients, however, so the recommendation specifies *raw* oil.

> Nutrient density was explained in **Chapter 1**, page 20.

Solid Fats, Added Sugars, and Alcohol Reduce Nutrient Density **Solid fats** deliver saturated fat and *trans* fat, terms that will become familiar after reading Chapter 5. Sugars in all their forms (described in Chapter 4) deliver carbohydrate calories. Figure 2–8 demonstrates how solid fats and added sugars add **empty calories** to foods, reducing their nutrient density. Solid fats include:

- Naturally occurring fats, such as milk fat and meat fats.
- Added fats, such as butter, cream cheese, hard margarine, lard, sour cream, and shortening.

Added sugars include:

- All caloric sweeteners, such as brown sugar, candy, honey, jelly, molasses, soft drinks, sugar, and syrups.

The USDA suggests that intakes of solid fats and added sugars should be limited.

Alcoholic beverages are a top contributor of empty calories to the diets of many U.S. adults, but they provide few nutrients.[8] People who drink alcohol should monitor and

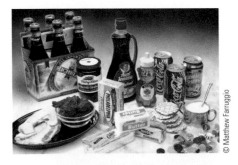

Figure 2–7

Some Sources of Solid Fats, Added Sugars, and Alcohol

Limit intakes of foods and beverages like these.

© Matthew Farruggio

solid fats fats that are high in saturated fat and usually not liquid at room temperature. Some common solid fats include butter, beef fat, chicken fat, pork fat, stick margarine, coconut oil, palm oil, and shortening.

empty calories calories provided by added sugars and solid fats with few or no other nutrients. Other empty calorie sources include alcohol, and highly refined starches, such as corn starch or potato starch, often found in ultra-processed foods.

Chapter 2 Nutrition Tools—Standards and Guidelines

Figure 2–8

How Solid Fats and Added Sugars Add Empty Calories to Nutrient-Dense Foods

The purple bars show the calorie counts of the most nutrient-dense forms of selected foods; the green bars show how many empty calories are contributed by sugars and fats.

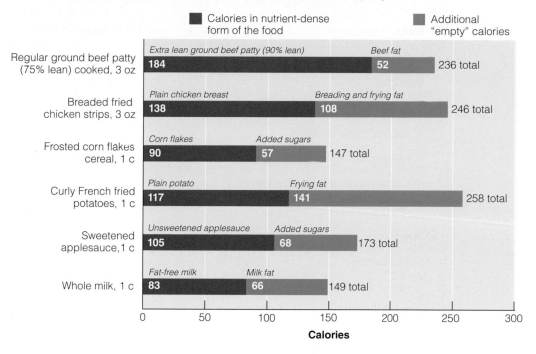

■ Calories in nutrient-dense form of the food   ■ Additional "empty" calories

Regular ground beef patty (75% lean) cooked, 3 oz
Extra lean ground beef patty (90% lean) **184** | *Beef fat* **52** | 236 total

Breaded fried chicken strips, 3 oz
Plain chicken breast **138** | *Breading and frying fat* **108** | 246 total

Frosted corn flakes cereal, 1 c
Corn flakes **90** | *Added sugars* **57** | 147 total

Curly French fried potatoes, 1 c
Plain potato **117** | *Frying fat* **141** | 258 total

Sweetened applesauce, 1 c
Unsweetened applesauce **105** | *Added sugars* **68** | 173 total

Whole milk, 1 c
Fat-free milk **83** | *Milk fat* **66** | 149 total

Calories: 0   50   100   150   200   250   300

moderate their intakes, not to exceed one drink a day for women and two for men. People in many circumstances should never drink alcohol (see Controversy 3).

KEY POINTS

- Following the USDA Eating Patterns requires choosing nutrient-dense foods most often.
- Solid fats, added sugars, and alcohol should be limited.

Diet Planning

LO 2.4   Given a specified number of calories, create a healthful diet plan using the USDA Eating Patterns.

The USDA Eating Patterns specify the amounts of foods needed from each food group to create a healthful diet for a given number of calories. In this chapter, we explore this system using a 2,000-calorie diet as an example (see Table 2–3, p. 44). Of course, people's energy needs vary widely with age, gender, and activity level, so to find your own pattern (or anyone else's), you first must obtain an approximation of how many calories are needed per day, and then select an appropriate eating pattern. Here's how:

- Start by flipping to Appendix H at the back of the book (gold bars on its page margins help distinguish it).
- Once there, study Table H–1 to decide how active you are, a critical variable for determining calorie need.
- Then, turn to Table H–2. Look at the top line and find yourself among the people described there. Look at the column of numbers below and find your estimated energy need.
- Armed with your calorie need, turn to Appendix E (purple bars), and choose an eating pattern that appeals to you—Healthy U.S.-style,

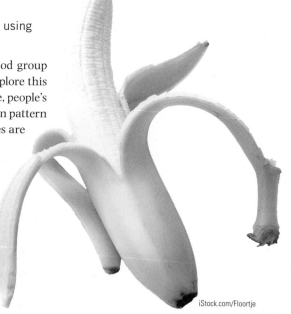

iStock.com/Floortje

Table 2–3

Healthy U.S.-Style Eating Pattern at the 2,000-Calorie Level

Notice that the recommended amounts of food from each major food group are needed *per day;* amounts from the subgroups are needed *per week.*

Food Group[a]	Daily Amounts[b]
Fruit	**2 c/day**
Vegetables	**2½ c/day**
Dark-green vegetables	1½ c/week
Red and orange vegetables	5½ c/week
Legumes (beans and peas)	1½ c/week
Starchy vegetables	5 c/week
Other vegetables	4 c/week
Grains	**6 oz/day**
Whole grains	3 oz
Refined grains	3 oz
Milk and Milk Products	**3 c/day**
Protein Foods	**5½ oz/day**
Seafood	8 oz/week
Meats, poultry, eggs	26 oz/week
Nuts seeds, soy products	5 oz/week
Oils	**27 g/day**
Limit on calories for other uses[c]	270 cal/day

[a] *All foods are assumed to be in nutrient-dense forms, lean or low-fat and prepared without added fats, sugars, refined starches, or salt.*

[b] *Food group amounts are in cup-equivalents (c-eq) or ounce-equivalents (oz-eq); these equivalents are listed under the food photos of Figure 2–6, (pp. 40–41). Oils are shown in grams (g).*

[c] *If all food choices are in nutrient-dense forms, a few calories remain unmet by the Eating Pattern ("limit on calories for other uses.") Calories up to the specified limit can be used for added sugars, added refined starches, solid fats, alcohol, or to eat more than the recommended amount of food in a food group.*

Source: U.S. Department of Health and Human Services and U.S. Department of Agriculture, 2015–2020 Dietary Guidelines for Americans, 8th edition (2015), available at https://health.gov/dietaryguidelines/2015/guidelines/appendix-3/.

DASH, Healthy Vegetarian, or Healthy Mediterranean-style. All are equally effective. Find your calorie level on the top of your chosen pattern, and follow the column to find out how much of each food group will meet your needs. Use these numbers as we do in Table 2–3.

For vegetables and protein foods, notice in Table 2–3 that the daily intakes should be divided among all the subgroups over a week's time. The weekly amounts are listed under the daily goal. It is not necessary to eat foods from every subgroup each day. With judicious selections, the diet can supply all the needed nutrients and provide some luxury items as well (termed "calories for other uses" on the table).

Now the diet planner can begin to translate the USDA Eating Patterns into foods on the plate by assigning each of the food groups to meals and snacks, as shown in Table 2–4. Then the plan can be filled in with real foods to create a menu. For example,

Table 2–4

A Sample Day's Plan, 2,000 Calories

This diet plan is one of many possibilities for our day's meals. Figure 2–16, Monday's Meals (p. 57), illustrates the completed diet plan.

Food Group	Recommended Amounts	Breakfast	Lunch	Snack	Dinner	Snack
Fruit	2 c	½ c		½ c	1 c	
Vegetables	2½ c		1 c		2 c	
Grains	6 oz	1 oz	2 oz	½ oz	2 oz	½ oz
Protein Foods	5½ oz		2 oz		3½ oz	
Milk	3 c	1 c		1 c		1 c
Oils	6 tsp		2 tsp		4 tsp	

the breakfast in Table 2–4 calls for 1 ounce of grains, 1 cup of milk, and ½ cup of fruit. Here's one possibility for this meal:

    1 cup ready-to-eat cereal = 1 ounce grains

    1 cup fat-free milk = 1 cup milk

    1 medium banana = 1/2 cup fruit

Our completed diet plan is shown in Figure 2–16 (p. 57) in the Food Feature of this chapter. We chose healthy U.S.-style foods, but many other choices are possible, so long as they adhere to the principles of the Dietary Guidelines for Americans.

Note that our plan meets nutrient needs with calories to spare—enough for some extra servings of nutritious foods, or one small treat, such as a 6-ounce serving of plain frozen yogurt or a 12-ounce sugar-sweetened soda. Alternatively, the diet planner endeavoring to lose weight can choose to skip such additions to create the desired calorie deficit.

KEY POINT

- The USDA Eating Patterns provide templates for diet planning at various calorie levels.

MyPlate Educational Tool

For consumers with Internet access, the USDA's MyPlate online suite of educational tools eases the use of the USDA Eating Patterns.[9] Figure 2–9 displays its logo. Computer-savvy consumers will find an abundance of MyPlate support materials and diet assessment tools on the website (www.choosemyplate.gov). Those without computer access can meet the same diet-planning goals by following this chapter's principles and working with pencil and paper, as illustrated later.

KEY POINT

- The concepts of the USDA Eating Patterns are demonstrated in the MyPlate online educational tools.

Flexibility of the USDA Eating Patterns

The USDA Eating Patterns can be pleasingly flexible. For example, users can substitute fat-free yogurt for fat-free milk because both supply the key nutrients for the Milk and Milk Products group. Legumes, an extraordinarily nutrient-rich food, provide many of the nutrients that characterize the Protein Foods group, but they also constitute a

Figure 2–9

USDA MyPlate

Note that vegetables and fruit occupy half the plate and that the grains portion is slightly larger than the portion of protein foods. A diet that follows the USDA Eating Patterns reflects these ideals.

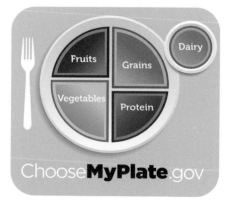

Source: United States Department of Agriculture

Figure 2–10

A Sampling of Ethnic Food Choices

	Grains	Vegetables	Fruit	Protein Foods	Milk
Asian 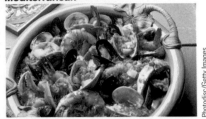	Rice, wheat or rice noodles, millet, wheat or rice wrappers and crepes	Baby corn, bamboo shoots, bok choy, green onions, leafy greens (such as amaranth), mung bean sprouts, snow peas, mushrooms, water chestnuts, kelp	Carambola, guava, kumquat, loquat, lychee, melons, mandarin orange, persimmon	Soybeans and soy products such as miso and tofu, duck and other poultry, eggs, fish, octopus, pork, sea urchin, squid and other seafood, cashews, peanuts	Soy milk
Mediterranean 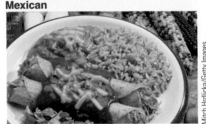	Pita bread, pastas, rice, couscous, polenta, bulgur, focaccia, Italian bread	Artichokes, eggplant, tomatoes, peppers, cucumbers, fennel, grape leaves, leafy greens, leeks, onions	Berries, dates, figs, grapes, lemons, olives, oranges, pomegranates	Fish and other seafood, gyros, lamb, chicken, pork, sausage, lentils, fava beans, tree nuts (almonds, walnuts)	Ricotta, provolone, Parmesan, feta, mozzarella, and goat cheeses; yogurt and yogurt beverages
Mexican	Hominy, masa (corn flour dough), rice, tortillas (corn or flour)	Bell peppers, cactus, cassava, chayote, chili peppers, corn, jicama, onions, summer squash, tomatoes, winter squash, yams	Avocado, banana, guava, lime, mango, orange, papaya, plantain	Beans, refried beans, beef, chicken, chorizo, eggs, fish, goat, pork	Cheese, custard, milk in beverages

Brent Hofacker/Shutterstock.com

Photodisc/Getty Images

Mitch Hrdlicka/Getty Images

Vegetable subgroup, so legumes in a meal can count as a serving of either meat or vegetables. Consumers can adapt the plan to mixed dishes such as casseroles and to national and cultural foods as well, as Figure 2–10 illustrates.

Vegetarians can use adaptations of the USDA Eating Patterns in making sound food choices, too. The food group that includes the meats also includes nuts, seeds, and products made from soybeans. The Vegetable group includes legumes, counted as protein foods for vegetarians. In the food group that includes milk, soy milk and pea milk (beverages made from legumes) can fill the same nutrient needs, provided that they are fortified with calcium, riboflavin, vitamin A, vitamin D, and vitamin B_{12}. Therefore, for all sorts of careful diet planners, the USDA Eating Patterns provide road maps for all sorts of healthful diets.

See **Appendix E** for vegetarian and Mediterranean eating patterns, and **Controversy 6** for vegetarian diet planning.

KEY POINT

- People with a wide variety of eating styles can use the USDA Eating Patterns to plan pleasing, nutritious diets.

Food Lists for Weight Management

A special set of lists to help people manage their calorie intakes are the Food Lists for Diabetes and Weight Management. The lists were originally developed for use not only by people with diabetes but also make a valuable tool for anyone concerned about calories. These lists are shown in Table 2–5. Notice that they emphasize two characteristics of foods: their portion sizes and their calorie amounts.

Table 2–5

Estimating Calories with Food Lists for Diabetes and Weight Management

These calorie values are estimates for average portions of foods within various categories. Appendix D provides details about the calorie values and energy nutrient contents of individual foods on these lists.

Food Lists	Average Calories
Starch	**80**
1 slice bread	
½ c cooked cereals, most grains, legumes, and starchy vegetables	
⅓ c pasta or rice	
1 oz low-fat crackers	
Sweets[a]	**70**
1 tbs sugar	
1 tbs syrup	
1 frozen juice bar	
Fruit	**60**
Milk and Milk Substitutes	
1 c fat-free, low-fat milk (0–1%)	**100**
⅔ c (6 oz) fat-free yogurt (plain or Greek)	**100**
1 c reduced-fat milk (2%)	**120**
1 c whole milk	**160**
Nonstarchy Vegetables	**25**
Proteins[b]	
1 oz lean	**45**
1 oz medium-fat	**75**
1 oz high-fat	**100**
Fats	**45**
1 tsp oil or solid fat	
1 tbs salad dressing	
Alcohol (½ ounce ethanol without mixers; details in Controversy 3)	**100**

[a]Sweets, desserts, baked goods, and beverages vary widely in calorie contents; see Appendix D for details.
[b]Plant-based proteins vary in calorie contents.

Source: Adapted from American Diabetes Association and Academy of Nutrition and Dietetics, Choose Your Foods: Food Lists for Diabetes (2014), available from www.diabetes.org (catalog no. 310X14) or www.eatright.org (ISBN: 978-0-8809-387-4).

Of course, individual foods vary from the examples shown in the table, but these averages are useful. (Appendix D provides details on individual foods.)[††] A dieter who has memorized the average values of Table 2–5 may survey any plate of food and quickly calculate, "Let's see: I've got two breads here, one fruit, one vegetable, one protein food . . . yes, this meal will give me about 320 calories—just what I'm shooting for."

[††]These lists were formerly known as the Exchange Lists.

Controlling Portion Sizes at Home and Away

"May I take your order, please?" Put on the spot when eating out, a diner must quickly choose from a large, visually exciting menu. No one brings a scale to a restaurant to weigh portions, and physical cues used at home, such as measuring cups are at home. Restaurant portions have no standards. When ordering "a burger," for example, the sandwich may arrive resembling a 2-ounce kids' sandwich or a ¾-pound behemoth. Even at home, portion sizes can be mystifying—how much spaghetti is enough?

How Big Is Your Bagel?

When college students are asked to bring "medium-sized" foods to class, they reliably bring bagels weighing from 2 to 5 ounces, muffins from 2 to 8 ounces, baked potatoes from 4 to 9 ounces, and so forth. Knowledge of appropriate daily amounts of food is crucial to controlling calorie intakes, but consumers need help to estimate portion sizes, whether preparing meals at home or choosing from restaurant menus.

Practice with Weights and Measures

At home, practice measuring foods. To estimate the size of food portions, remember these common objects:

- 3 ounces of meat = the size of the palm of a woman's hand or a deck of cards

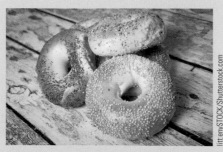

How much does your bagel weigh?

litt emySTOCK/Shutterstock.com

- 1 medium potato or piece of fruit = the size of a tennis ball
- 1½ ounces cheese = the size of a 9-volt battery
- 1 ounce lunch meat or cheese = 1 slice
- 1 cup cooked pasta = the size of a baseball
- 1 pat (1 tsp) butter or margarine = a slice from a quarter-pound stick of butter about as thick as 150 pages of this book (pressed together).
- Most ice cream scoops hold ¼ cup = a lump about the size of a golf ball. (Test the size of your scoop—fill it with water and pour the water into a measuring cup. Now you have a handy device to measure portions at home—use the scoop to serve mashed potatoes, pasta, vegetables, rice, and cereals.)

Among volumetric measures, 1 "cup" refers to an 8-ounce measuring cup (not a teacup or drinking glass) filled to level (not heaped up, or shaken, or pressed down). Tablespoons and teaspoons refer to measuring spoons (not flatware), filled to level (not rounded or heaping). For dry foods, cheeses, and other foods measured by weight, "ounces" signify weight and cannot be equated to volume. An ounce of cereal (such as Rice Krispies) may fill a whole cup but an ounce of granola fills only a quarter cup.

Buy New Bowls

Take a moment to consider the size of your plates, bowls, utensils, and other tableware. Tableware seems to function as a sort of visual gauge for sizing up food portions. In research, people eating from large containers often eat more per sitting than those eating from smaller ones (details in Chapter 9). Thus, if your dinnerware looks more like serving platters than plates, try using luncheon-sized plates instead. The same holds true for bowls and spoons; if yours are giant-sized, invest in smaller ones.

Colossal Cuisine in Restaurants

Figure 2–11 shows that, over the past decades, consumers have doubled the percentage of their food budgets spent on foods eaten away from home. Two other trends occurred during the same period: food portions grew larger and therefore higher in calories (see Figure 2–12), and people's body weights increased to higher, less healthy levels.

Figure 9–13 of Chapter 9 illustrates calorie information on a restaurant menu.

Large chain restaurants, including fast-food restaurants, post calorie information on menus and menu boards for each standard food item.

Figure 2–11

Dining Out Trends, United States

People today are spending a greater proportion of their total food budgets on restaurant meals and other foods eaten away from home.

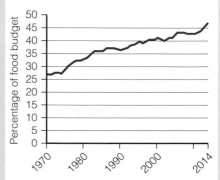

Source: Economic Research Service, U.S. Department of Agriculture, Food Expenditures, 2017, available at www.ers.usda.gov/data-products/food-expenditures .aspx.

Figure 2–12

A Shift toward Colossal Cuisine

The portion sizes of many foods have increased dramatically over past decades, and so have people's body sizes. Fast foods, steaks, candy bars, baked potatoes, pasta servings, and even popcorn servings are much larger today than those typically consumed in the past.

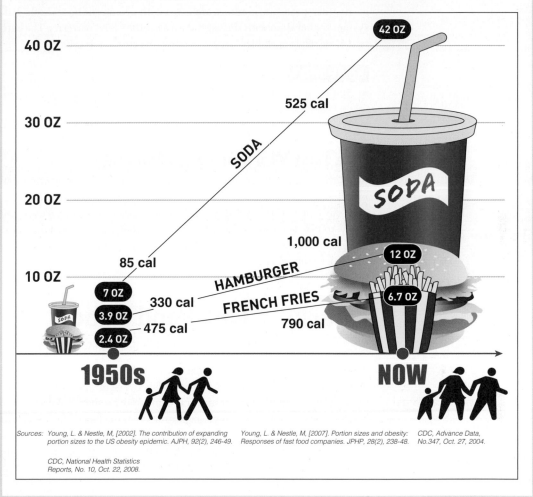

Sources: Young, L. & Nestle, M, [2002]. The contribution of expanding portion sizes to the US obesity epidemic. AJPH, 92(2), 246-49.

Young, L. & Nestle, M, [2007]. Portion sizes and obesity: Responses of fast food companies. JPHP, 28(2), 238-48.

CDC, Advance Data, No.347, Oct. 27, 2004.

CDC, National Health Statistics Reports, No. 10, Oct. 22, 2008.

Without such a gauge readily at hand, consumers most often underestimate the calories in restaurant foods.[1]*

When portions seem excessively large or calorie-rich, use creative solutions to cut them down to size: order a half portion, ask that half of a regular portion be packaged for a later meal, order a child's portion, or split an entrée with a friend. Another proven strategy is to cook at home more often. People who do so control their own portions and often comply better with the Dietary Guidelines, while saving substantial money as a bonus.[2]

Moving Ahead

Portion control is a habit—and a way to defend against overeating. When cooking at home, have measuring tools at the ready. When dining out, your tools are your practiced abilities to judge portion sizes. Then, when the waiter asks, "Are you ready to order?" the savvy consumer, armed with portion size know-how, answers confidently, "Yes."

Review Questions[†]

1. American restaurant portions are stable and consistent; you can rely on them as a guide when choosing portion sizes. T F

2. Experimenting with portion sizes at home is a valuable exercise in self-education. T F

3. When consumers guess at the calorie values in restaurant food portions, they generally overestimate. T F

* Reference notes are in Appendix F.

[†] Answers to Consumer's Guide questions are in Appendix G.

Unlike the USDA Eating Patterns (presented earlier), which sort foods primarily by their vitamin and mineral contents, these lists group foods primarily by their energy-nutrient contents—carbohydrate, fat, and protein. Consequently, foods do not always appear where you might expect to find them on the lists in Appendix D. For example, cheeses are grouped with meats on the "Proteins" list because, like meats, cheeses contribute negligible carbohydrate, but abundant fat and protein. The USDA groups cheeses with milk because they are similar to other milk products in terms of the vitamins and minerals they provide. Another difference is that starchy vegetables such as corn, green peas, and potatoes are listed with grains on the "Starch" list in the food list system, rather than with the vegetables as in the USDA patterns. The carbohydrate content of starchy vegetables is more like that of cereal than celery.

KEY POINTS

- The Food Lists for Diabetes and Weight Management assign foods to groups based on their carbohydrate, fat, protein, and calorie contents.
- The lists facilitate control of energy nutrient and calorie consumption.

The Last Word on Diet Planning

All of the dietary changes required to improve nutrition may seem daunting or even insurmountable at first, and taken all at once, they may be. However, small steps taken each day can add up to substantial dietary changes over time. If everyone would begin, today, to take such steps, the rewards in terms of lower risks of diabetes, obesity, heart disease, and cancer along with a greater quality of life with better health would prove well worth the effort.

Checking Out Food Labels

LO 2.5   Describe the information that appears on food labels.

A potato is a potato and needs no label to tell you so. But what can a package of potato chips tell you about its contents? By law, its label must list the chips' ingredients—potatoes, oil, and salt—and its **Nutrition Facts** panel must also reveal details about their nutrient composition. If the oil is high in saturated fat, the label will reveal it (more about fats in Chapter 5). In addition to required information, labels may make optional statements about the food being delicious, or good for you in some way, or a great value. Some of these comments, especially some that are regulated by the Food and Drug Administration (FDA), are reliable. Many others are marketing tools, based more on salesmanship than science.

What Food Labels Must Include

The Nutrition Education and Labeling Act of 1990 set the requirements for certain label information to ensure that food labels truthfully inform consumers about the nutrients and ingredients in the package. Every packaged food must state the following:

- The common or usual name of the product.
- The name and address of the manufacturer, packer, or distributor.
- The net contents in terms of weight, measure, or count.
- The nutrient contents of the product (Nutrition Facts panel).
- The ingredients in descending order of predominance by weight and in ordinary language.
- Essential warnings, such as alerts about ingredients that often cause allergic reactions or other problems.

Not every package need display information about every vitamin and mineral. A large package, such as a box of cereal, must provide all of the information just listed. A smaller label, such as the label on a can of tuna, provides some of the information in abbreviated

Nutrition Facts on a food label, the panel of nutrition information required to appear on almost every packaged food. Grocers may also provide the information for fresh produce, meats, poultry, and seafood.

form. The tiniest of labels, such as on a roll of candy rings, provides only a phone number to call or a website to visit for nutrient information.

The Nutrition Facts Panel Most shoppers read food labels, and when they do, they often rely on a Nutrition Facts panel, as shown in Figure 2–13. The original food label, shown on the left, first appeared 20 years ago; the updated label on the right has been approved and may soon appear in the marketplace. In addition to food labels, grocers also voluntarily post placards or offer handouts in produce and other departments to provide consumers with similar nutrition information for the most popular fresh fruit, vegetables, and seafoods.

Notice in Figure 2–13 that only the top portion of a food's Nutrition Facts panel conveys information specific to the food inside the package. The bottom portion is identical on every label—it stands as a reminder of the Daily Values.

Figure 2–13

What's on a Food Label?

This cereal label illustrates the information needed to make wise food purchases. The text provides details about each label section. The updated food label (right panel) is easier to use and reflects current nutrition science, such as updated serving sizes.

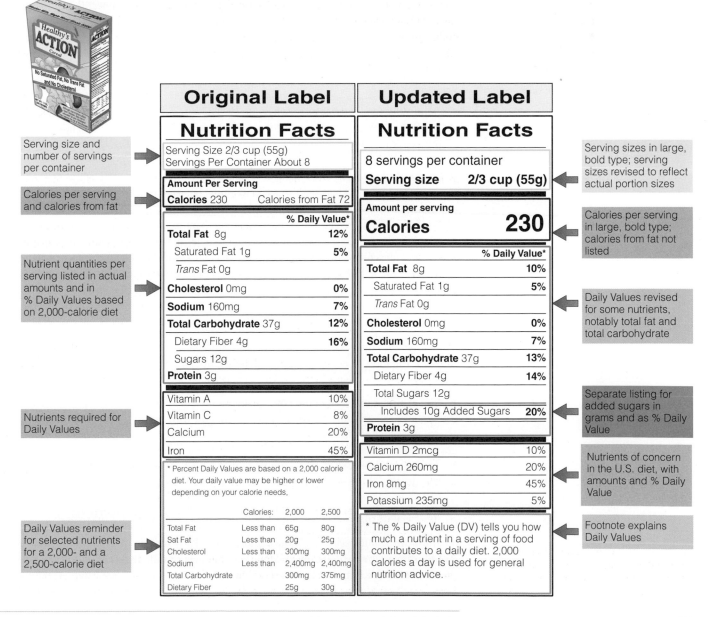

Serving size and number of servings per container

Calories per serving and calories from fat

Nutrient quantities per serving listed in actual amounts and in % Daily Values based on 2,000-calorie diet

Nutrients required for Daily Values

Daily Values reminder for selected nutrients for a 2,000- and a 2,500-calorie diet

Original Label

Nutrition Facts

Serving Size 2/3 cup (55g)
Servings Per Container About 8

Amount Per Serving

Calories 230   Calories from Fat 72

	% Daily Value*
Total Fat 8g	12%
Saturated Fat 1g	5%
Trans Fat 0g	
Cholesterol 0mg	0%
Sodium 160mg	7%
Total Carbohydrate 37g	12%
Dietary Fiber 4g	16%
Sugars 12g	
Protein 3g	

Vitamin A	10%
Vitamin C	8%
Calcium	20%
Iron	45%

* Percent Daily Values are based on a 2,000 calorie diet. Your daily value may be higher or lower depending on your calorie needs.

	Calories:	2,000	2,500
Total Fat	Less than	65g	80g
Sat Fat	Less than	20g	25g
Cholesterol	Less than	300mg	300mg
Sodium	Less than	2,400mg	2,400mg
Total Carbohydrate		300mg	375mg
Dietary Fiber		25g	30g

Updated Label

Nutrition Facts

8 servings per container

Serving size   **2/3 cup (55g)**

Amount per serving

Calories   **230**

	% Daily Value*
Total Fat 8g	10%
Saturated Fat 1g	5%
Trans Fat 0g	
Cholesterol 0mg	0%
Sodium 160mg	7%
Total Carbohydrate 37g	13%
Dietary Fiber 4g	14%
Total Sugars 12g	
Includes 10g Added Sugars	20%
Protein 3g	

Vitamin D 2mcg	10%
Calcium 260mg	20%
Iron 8mg	45%
Potassium 235mg	5%

* The % Daily Value (DV) tells you how much a nutrient in a serving of food contributes to a daily diet. 2,000 calories a day is used for general nutrition advice.

Serving sizes in large, bold type; serving sizes revised to reflect actual portion sizes

Calories per serving in large, bold type; calories from fat not listed

Daily Values revised for some nutrients, notably total fat and total carbohydrate

Separate listing for added sugars in grams and as % Daily Value

Nutrients of concern in the U.S. diet, with amounts and % Daily Value

Footnote explains Daily Values

The following information is located on the Nutrition Facts panel:

- *Serving size.* A common household and metric measure of a single serving that provides the calorie and nutrient amounts listed. A serving of chips may be 10 chips, so if you eat 50 chips, you will have consumed five times the calorie and nutrient amounts listed on the label. Keep in mind that label serving sizes are not recommendations. They simply reflect amounts that people typically consume in a serving.
- *Servings per container.* Number of servings per box, can, or package.
- *Calories/calories from fat.* Total food energy per serving and energy from fat per serving.
- *Nutrient amounts and percentages of Daily Values*, including:
  - *Total fat.* Grams of fat per serving with a breakdown showing grams of *saturated fat* and *trans fat* per serving.
  - *Cholesterol.* Milligrams of cholesterol per serving.
  - *Sodium.* Milligrams of sodium per serving.
  - *Total carbohydrate.* Grams of carbohydrate per serving, including starch, fiber, and sugars, with a breakdown showing grams of dietary *fiber* and *sugars*. The sugars listed on the original label include those that occur naturally in the food plus any added during processing; the updated label specifies how much of the sugar is added sugar.[10]
  - *Protein.* Grams of protein per serving.

Other nutrients present in significant amounts in the food may also be listed on the label. The percentages of the Daily Values are given for a 2,000-calorie diet (see the back of the book, p. E).

- *Daily Values and calories-per-gram reminder.* The original label spelled out the Daily Values for a person needing 2,000 or 2,500 calories a day; the updated label simply explains their meaning.

Ingredients List   An often neglected but highly valuable body of information is the list of ingredients. The product's ingredients must be listed in descending order of predominance by weight.

Knowing how to read an ingredients list puts you many steps ahead of naïve buyers. Anyone diagnosed with a food allergy quickly learns to use these lists for spotting "off-limits" ingredients in foods. In addition, you can glean clues about the nature of the food. For example, consider the ingredients list on an orange drink powder whose first three entries are "sugar, citric acid, orange flavor." You can tell that sugar is the chief ingredient. Now consider a canned juice whose ingredients list begins with "water, orange juice concentrate, pineapple juice concentrate." This product is clearly made of reconstituted juice. Water is first on the label because it is the main constituent of juice. Sugar is nowhere to be found among the ingredients because no sugar has been added. Sugar occurs naturally in juice, though, so the label does specify sugar grams; details are in Chapter 4.

Now consider a cereal whose entire list contains just one item: "100 percent shredded wheat." No question, this is a whole-grain food with nothing added. Finally, consider a cereal whose first six ingredients are "puffed milled corn, corn syrup, sucrose, honey, dextrose, salt." If you recognize that corn syrup, sucrose, honey, and dextrose are all different versions of sugar (and you will after Chapter 4), you might guess that this product contains close to half its weight as added sugar.

More about Percentages of Daily Values   The nutrient percentages of Daily Values ("% Daily Value") on labels are for a single serving of food, and they are based on the Daily Values set for a 2,000-calorie diet. For example, if a food contributes 4 milligrams of iron per serving and the Daily Value is 18 milligrams, then a serving of that food provides 22 percent of the Daily Value for iron.

Of course, though the Daily Values are based on a 2,000-calorie diet, people's actual calorie and nutrient needs vary widely. This makes the Daily Values most useful for comparing one food with another and less useful as nutrient intake targets for individuals. Still, by examining a food's general nutrient profile, you can determine whether the food contributes "a little" or "a lot" of a nutrient and whether it contributes "more" or "less" than another food.

What Food Labels *May* Include

So far, this section has presented the accurate and reliable food label facts. Another group of reliable statements are the **nutrient claims**.

Nutrient Claims: Reliable Information   A food that meets specified criteria may display certain approved nutrient claims on its label. These claims—for example, that a food is "low in cholesterol" or a "good source of vitamin A"—are based on the Daily Values. Table 2–6 provides a list of these regulated, valid label terms along with their definitions.

Health Claims: Reliable and Not So Reliable   In the past, the FDA held manufacturers to the highest standards of scientific evidence before allowing them to place **health claims** on food labels. A health claim describes a relationship between a food or its components and a disease or health condition. When a label stated "Diets low in sodium may reduce the risk of high blood pressure," for example, consumers could be sure that the FDA had substantial scientific support for the claim.

Today, however, the FDA also allows similar-sounding health claims that are backed by weaker evidence. These are "qualified" claims in the sense that labels bearing them must also state the strength of the scientific evidence backing them up. Unfortunately, consumers cannot distinguish between scientifically valid claims and those that are less so.

Structure-Function Claims: Best Ignored   Even less reliable are **structure-function claims**. A label-reading consumer is much more likely to encounter this kind of claim on a food or supplement label than the more regulated health claims just described. For food manufacturers, printing a *health claim* involves acquiring FDA permission, a time-consuming and expensive process. Instead, manufacturers can print a similar-looking structure-function claim that requires only FDA notification and no prior approval. Figure 2–14 compares claims on food labels.

nutrient claims FDA-approved food label statements that describe the nutrient levels in food. Examples: "fat free" or "less sodium."

health claims FDA-approved food label statements that link food constituents with disease or health-related conditions. Examples: "Soluble fiber from daily oatmeal in a diet low in saturated fat and *trans* fat may reduce the risk of heart disease" or "A diet low in total fat may reduce the risk of some cancers."

structure-function claims legal but largely unregulated statements permitted on labels of foods and dietary supplements, describing the effect of a substance on the structure or function of the body, but that omit references to diseases. Examples: "Supports immunity and digestive health" or "Builds strong bones."

Figure 2–14
Label Claims

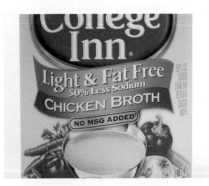

Nutrient claim

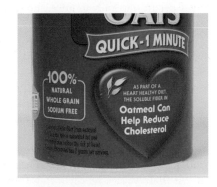

Health claim

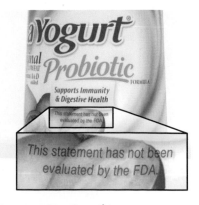

Structure-function claim

Table 2–6

Some Scientifically Valid Nutrient Claims on Food Labels

Energy Terms

- **low calorie** 40 calories or fewer per serving.
- **reduced calorie** at least 25% lower in calories than a "regular," or reference, food.
- **calorie free** fewer than 5 calories per serving.

Fat Terms (Meat and Poultry Products)

- **extra lean**[a]
  less than 5 g of total fat *and*
  less than 2 g of saturated fat and *trans* fat combined, *and*
  less than 95 mg of cholesterol per serving.
- **lean**[a]
  less than 10 g of total fat *and*
  less than 4.5 g of saturated fat and *trans* fat combined, *and*
  less than 95 mg of cholesterol per serving.

Fat Terms (All Products)

- **fat free** less than 0.5 g of fat per serving.
- **less saturated fat** 25% or less saturated fat and *trans* fat combined than the comparison food.
- **low fat** 3 g or less of total fat per serving.[a]
- **low saturated fat** 1 g or less of saturated fat and less than 0.5 g of *trans* fat per serving.
- **reduced saturated fat**
  at least 25% less saturated fat *and*
  reduced by more than 1 g of saturated fat per serving compared with a reference food.
- **saturated fat free or *trans* fat free**
  less than 0.5 g of saturated fat *and*
  less than 0.5 g of *trans* fat per serving.

Fiber Terms

- **high fiber** 5 g or more per serving. (Foods making high-fiber claims must fit the definition of low fat, or the level of total fat must appear next to the high-fiber claim.)
- **good source of fiber** 2.5 g to 4.9 g per serving.
- **more** or **added fiber** at least 2.5 g more per serving than a reference food.

Sodium Terms

- **low sodium** 140 mg or less of sodium per serving.
- **reduced sodium** at least 25% lower in sodium than the regular product.
- **sodium free** less than 5 mg per serving.
- **very low sodium** 35 mg or less of sodium per serving.

Other Terms

- **good source** 10 to 19% of the Daily Value per serving.
- **high in** 20% or more of the Daily Value for a given nutrient per serving; synonyms include "rich in" and "excellent source."
- **less, fewer, reduced** containing at least 25% less of a nutrient or calories than a reference food. This may occur naturally or as a result of altering the food. For example, pretzels, which are usually low in fat, can claim to provide less fat than potato chips, a comparable food.
- **light** this descriptor has three meanings on labels:
  1. A serving provides one-third fewer calories or half the fat of the regular product.
  2. A serving of a low-calorie, low-fat food provides half the sodium normally present.
  3. The product is light in color and texture, so long as the label makes this intent clear, as in "light brown sugar."

[a]*The word* lean *as part of the brand name (as in "Lean Supreme") indicates that the product contains fewer than 10 g of total fat per serving.*

A problem is that, to reasonable consumers, the two kinds of claims may appear identical:

- "Lowers cholesterol" (FDA-approved health claim)
- "Helps maintain normal cholesterol levels" (less-regulated structure-function claim)

Such valid-appearing but unreliable structure-function claims diminish the credibility of all health-related claims on labels. In the world of marketing, current label laws put the consumer on notice: "Let the buyer beware."

Front-of-Package Shortcuts Some consumers find the detailed Nutrition Facts panels on food labels to be daunting. For them, easy-to-read nutrient information icons posted on the fronts of packages can speed comparisons among packaged foods.[11] Without regulations or oversight, food companies developed all sorts of front-of-package symbols to convey whatever information suited them. To try to unify the symbols, a major grocery association and their advertising industry consulted with the FDA to develop Facts Up Front, as shown in Figure 2–15.[12] In general, consumers say they like using front-of-package labeling to help them select health-promoting foods.

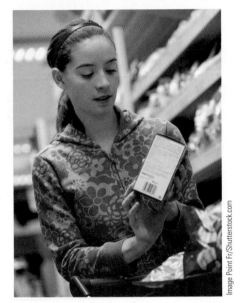

Image Point Fr/Shutterstock.com

Food labels provide clues for nutrition sleuths.

KEY POINTS

- Food labels may contain reliable nutrient claims and approved health claims but may also contain structure-function claims of varying reliability.
- Front-of-package icons speed consumers' comprehension of nutrient information.

Figure 2–15
Facts Up Front

Facts Up Front is a voluntary labeling initiative, developed by food manufacturing and marketing groups.

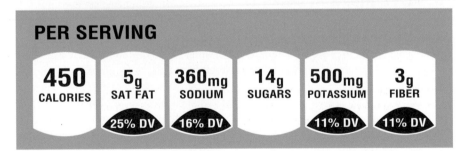

PER SERVING

| **450** CALORIES | **5g** SAT FAT 25% DV | **360mg** SODIUM 16% DV | **14g** SUGARS | **500mg** POTASSIUM 11% DV | **3g** FIBER 11% DV |

Source: FactsUpFront/GMA

FOOD FEATURE

Getting a Feel for the Nutrients in Foods

LO 2.6   Compare one day's nutrient-dense meals with meals not planned for nutrient density.

Figures 2–16 and 2–17 (pages 57–58) illustrate a playful contrast between two days' meals. Monday's meals were selected according to the recommendations of this chapter and follow the sample menu of Table 2–4, shown earlier, p. 45. Tuesday's meals were chosen more for convenience and familiarity than out of concern for nutrition.

Comparing the Nutrients

How can a person compare the nutrients that these sets of meals provide? One way is to look up each food in a table of food composition, write down the food's nutrient values, and compare each one to a standard such as the DRI, as we've done in Figures 2–16 and 2–17. By this measure, Monday's meals are the clear winners in terms of meeting nutrient needs within a calorie budget. Tuesday's meals oversupply calories and saturated fat while undersupplying fiber and critical vitamins and minerals.

Another useful exercise is to compare the total amounts of foods provided by a day's meals with the recommended amounts from each food group. A tally of the cups and ounces of foods consumed is provided in both Figures 2–16 and 2–17. The totals are then compared with USDA Eating Patterns in the tabular portion of the figures.

Monday's Meals in Detail

Monday's meals provide the necessary servings from each food group along with a small amount of oil needed for health. The energy provided falls well within the 2,000-calorie allowance. A closer look at Monday's foods reveals that the whole-grain cereal at breakfast, whole-grain sandwich roll at lunch, and whole-grain crackers at snack time meet the recommendation to obtain at least half of the day's grain servings from whole grains.

For the Vegetable subgroups, dark green vegetables, orange vegetables, and legumes are represented in the dinner salad, and "other vegetables" are prominent throughout. To repeat: it isn't necessary to choose vegetables from each subgroup every day, and people eating this day's meals will need to include vegetables from other subgroups throughout the week. In addition, Monday's eating plan has room to spare for additional servings of favorite foods or for some sweets or fats.

Tuesday's Meals in Detail

Tuesday's meals completely lack fruit and whole grains and are too low in vegetables and milk to provide adequate nutrients. In addition, they supply too much saturated fat and sugar, as well as excessive meats, oils, and refined grains, pushing the calorie total well above the day's allowance. A single day of such fare poses little threat to eaters, but a steady diet of Tuesday's meals presents a high probability of nutrient deficiencies and weight gain and greatly increases the risk of developing chronic diseases in later life.

Using Programs and Apps—or Not

If you have access to a computer or a "smart" cellular phone with a diet-planning application, it can be a time saver. Diet analysis programs and apps perform all of these calculations at lightning speed. Working them out for yourself, using paper and a sharp pencil with a big eraser, may seem a bit old-fashioned. But there are times when using electronic gadgets may not be practical—such as when hurrying to make decisions in the cafeteria or at a fast-food counter—where real-life food decisions must be made quickly.

People who work out diet analyses for themselves on paper and those who put extra time into studying, changing, and reviewing their computer diet analysis often learn to "see" the nutrients in foods. (This is a skill you can develop by the time you reach Chapter 10). They can quickly assess their food options and make informed choices at mealtimes, without electronic assistance. People who fail to develop such skills must wait until they can input their food data into their computer programs or apps to find out after the fact how well they did.

Figure 2-16

Monday's Meals—Nutrient-Dense Choices

Breakfast

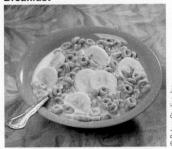

Lunch

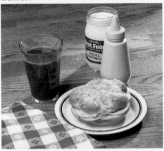

Afternoon snack

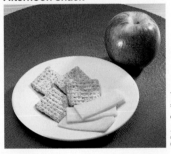

Dinner

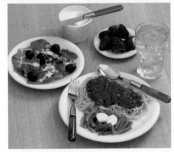

Bedtime snack

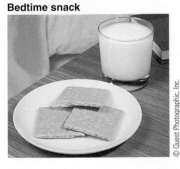

Foods	Food Group Amounts	Energy (cal)	Saturated Fat (g)	Fiber (g)	Vitamin C (mg)	Calcium (mg)
Before heading off to class, a student eats breakfast:						
1 c whole-grain cold cereal	1 oz grains	108	—	3	14	95
1 c fat-free milk	1 c milk	100	—	—	2	306
1 medium banana (sliced)	1/2 c fruit	105	—	3	10	6
Then goes home for a quick lunch:						
1 roasted turkey sandwich on 2-oz whole-grain roll with 1 1/2 tsp low-fat mayonnaise	2 oz meat 2 oz grains 1 1/2 tsp oils	343	4	2	—	89
1 c low-salt vegetable juice	1 c vegetables	50	—	1	60	27
While studying in the afternoon, the student eats a snack:						
4 whole-wheat reduced-fat crackers	1/2 oz grains	86	1	2	—	—
1 1/2 oz low-fat cheddar cheese	1 c milk	74	2	—	—	176
1 medium apple	1/2 c fruit	72	—	3	6	8
That night, the student makes dinner:						
A salad:						
1 3/4 c raw spinach leaves						
1/4 c shredded carrots	1 c vegetables	19	—	2	18	61
1/4 c garbanzo beans	1 oz legumes	71	—	3	2	19
5 lg olives and 2 tbs oil-based salad dressing	2 tsp oils	76	1	1	—	2
A main course:						
1 c spaghetti with meat and tomato sauce	2 oz grains 2 1/2 oz meat	425	3	5	15	56
1/2 c green beans	1 c vegetables	22	—	2	6	29
2 tsp soft margarine	2 tsp oils	67	1	—	—	—
And for dessert:						
1 c strawberries	1 c fruit	49	—	3	89	24
Later that evening, the student enjoys a bedtime snack:						
3 graham crackers	1/2 oz grains	90	—	—	—	—
1 c fat-free milk	1 c milk	100	—	—	2	306
Totals:		**1,857**	**12**	**30**	**224**	**1,204**
DRI:[a]		2,000	<20[b]	25	75	1,000
Percentage of DRI:		93%	60%	120%	299%	120%

Intakes Compared with Recommended Amounts

Food Group	Breakfast	Lunch	Snack	Dinner	Snack	Monday's Totals	Recommended Amounts
Fruit	1/2 c		1/2 c	1 c		2 c	2 c
Vegetables		1 c		2 c		3 c	2 1/2 c
Grains	1 oz	2 oz	1/2 oz	2 oz	1/2 oz	6 oz	6 oz
Protein foods		2 oz		3 1/2 oz		5 1/2 oz	5 1/2 oz
Milk	1 c		1 c		1 c	3 c	3 c
Oils		1 1/2 tsp		4 tsp		5 1/2 tsp	6 tsp
Calorie allowance						1,857 cal	2,000 cal

[a]DRI values for a sedentary woman, age 19–30.

[b]The 20-g value listed is the maximum allowable saturated fat for a 2,000-cal diet. The DRI recommends consuming less than 10% of calories from saturated fat.

Figure 2–17

Tuesday's Meals—Less-Nutrient-Dense Choices

Breakfast

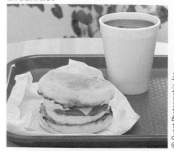

Lunch

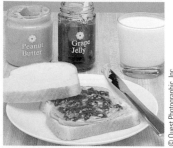

Afternoon snack

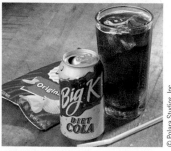

Dinner

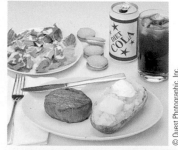

Bedtime snack

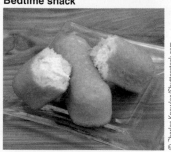

Foods	Food Group Amounts	Energy (cal)	Saturated Fat (g)	Fiber (g)	Vitamin C (mg)	Calcium (mg)
Today, the student starts the day with a fast-food breakfast:						
1 c coffee	2 oz grains	5	—	—	—	—
1 English muffin with egg, cheese, and bacon	2 oz protein foods 1 c milk	436	9	2	—	266
Between classes, the student returns home for a quick lunch:						
1 peanut butter and jelly sandwich on white bread	2 oz grains 1 oz protein foods	426	4	3	—	93
1 c whole milk	1 c milk	156	6	—	4	290
While studying, the student has:						
12 oz diet cola		—	—	—	—	—
Bag of chips (14 chips)[a]		105	2	—	4	—
That night for dinner, the student eats:						
A salad:						
1c lettuce						
1 tbs blue cheese dressing	½ c vegetables	84	2	1	2	23
A main course:						
6 oz steak	6 oz protein foods	349	6	—	—	27
½ baked potato	½ c vegetables	161	—	4	17	26
1 tbs butter		102	7	—	—	3
1 tbs sour cream[b]		31	2	—	—	17
12 oz diet cola		—	—	—	—	—
And for dessert:						
4 sandwich-type cookies	1 oz grains	158	2	1	—	—
Later on, a bedtime snack:						
2 cream-filled snack cakes	2 oz grains	250	2	2	—	20
1 c herbal tea		—	—	—	—	—
Totals:		**2,263**	**42**	**13**	**27**	**765**
DRI:[c]		2,000	<20[d]	25	75	1,000
Percentage of DRI:		113%	210%	52%	36%	77%

Intakes Compared with Recommended Amounts

Food Group	Breakfast	Lunch	Snack	Dinner	Snack	Tuesday's Totals	Recommended Amounts
Fruit						0 c	2 c
Vegetables			a	1 c		1 c	2½ c
Grains	2 oz	2 oz		1 oz	2 oz	7 oz	6 oz
Protein foods	2 oz	1 oz		6 oz		9 oz	5½ oz
Milk	1 c	1 c				2 c	3 c
Oils						7½ tsp[b]	6 tsp
Calorie allowance						2,263 cal	2,000 cal

[a]The potato in 14 potato chips provides less than ½ c vegetables.

[b]The saturated fats of steak, butter, and sour cream are among the solid fats and do not qualify as oils.

[c]DRI values for a sedentary woman, age 19–30.

[d]The 20-g value listed is the maximum allowable saturated fat for a 2,000-cal diet. The DRI recommends consuming less than 10% of calories from saturated fat.

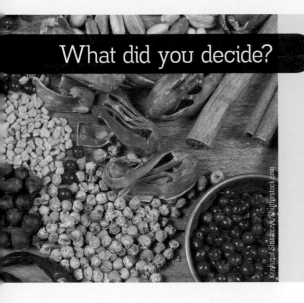
Krzysztof Slusarczyk/Shutterstock.com

What did you decide?

How can you tell **how much of each nutrient** you need to consume daily?

Can we trust the **government's dietary recommendations**?

Are the health claims on food labels **accurate and reliable**?

Can certain "**superfoods**" boost your health with more than just nutrients?

What's online?

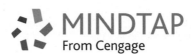 **MINDTAP**
From Cengage

Visit www.Cengage.com to access MindTap, a complete digital course that includes Diet & Wellness Plus, interactive quizzes, videos, and more.

Self Check

1. (LO 2.1) The nutrient standards in use today include all of the following *except* _____.
   a. Adequate Intakes (AI)
   b. Daily Minimum Requirements (DMR)
   c. Daily Values (DV)
   d. a and c

2. (LO 2.1) The Dietary Reference Intakes (DRI) were devised for which of the following purposes?
   a. to set nutrient goals for individuals
   b. to suggest upper limits of intakes, above which toxicity is likely
   c. to set average nutrient requirements for use in research
   d. all of the above

3. (LO 2.1) The energy intake recommendation is set at a level predicted to maintain body weight.
   T   F

4. (LO 2.1) The DRI are for all people, regardless of their medical history.
   T   F

5. (LO 2.2) Which of the following is *not* an action that could help meet the ideals of the Dietary Guidelines for Americans?
   a. increase intakes of vegetables
   b. increase intakes of nutrient-dense foods
   c. reduce intakes of artificial ingredients
   d. increase intakes of whole grains

6. (LO 2.2) The Dietary Guidelines for Americans recommend physical activity to help balance calorie intakes to achieve and sustain a healthy body weight.
   T   F

7. (LO 2.3) According to the USDA Eating Patterns, which of the following vegetables should be limited?
   a. carrots
   b. avocados
   c. baked beans
   d. potatoes

8. (LO 2.3) The USDA Eating Patterns recommend a small amount of daily oil from which of these sources?
   a. olives
   b. nuts
   c. vegetable oil
   d. all of the above

9. (LO 2.3) People who choose not to eat meat or animal products need to find an alternative to the USDA Eating Patterns when planning their diets.
   T   F

10. (LO 2.4) To plan a healthy diet that correctly assigns the needed amounts of food from each food group, diet planners should start by consulting
    a. USDA Eating Patterns.
    b. Dietary Reference Intakes.
    c. sample menus.
    d. none of the above.

11. (LO 2.4) A properly planned diet controls calories by excluding snacks.
    T   F

12. (LO 2.5) Which of the following values is found on food labels?
    a. Recommended Dietary Allowances
    b. Dietary Reference Intakes
    c. Daily Values
    d. Estimated Average Requirements

13. (LO 2.5) By law, food labels must name the ingredients in descending order of predominance by weight and in ordinary language.
    T   F

14. (LO 2.5) To be labeled "low fat," a food must contain 3 grams of fat or less per serving.
    T   F

15. (LO 2.6) One way to evaluate any diet is to compare the total food servings that it provides from each food group with those recommended by the USDA Eating Patterns.
    T   F

16. (LO 2.6) A carefully planned diet has which of these characteristics?
    a. It contains sufficient raw oil.
    b. It contains no solid fats or added sugars.
    c. It contains all of the Vegetable subgroups.
    d. a and c

17. (LO 2.7) Various whole foods contain so many different phytochemicals that consumers should focus on eating a wide variety of foods instead of seeking out a particular phytochemical.
    T   F

18. (LO 2.7) Because they arise as natural constituents of foods, phytochemicals are safe to consume in large amounts as supplements.
    T   F

Answers to these Self Check questions are in Appendix G.

CONTROVERSY 2 | Are Some Foods Superfoods for Health?

LO 2.7 Summarize the potential health effects of phytochemicals from both food sources and supplements.

Are some foods superfoods for health? Headlines certainly say so: "Forgetful? Blueberries sharpen brain function!" "Too many colds? Supercharge your immune system with soybeans!" "Worried about cancer? Eat tomatoes!" Can the produce aisle double as a medicine chest? Although headlines often overstate their talents, **functional foods** do supply **phytochemicals**—nonnutrient components of plants, some of which are under study for their potential to influence human health and disease. (Functional food terms are defined in Table C2–1.)

A Scientist's View of Phytochemicals

At one time, phytochemicals were known only for their sensory properties in foods, such as taste, aroma, texture, and color. Thank phytochemicals for the burning sensation of hot peppers, the pungent flavors of onions and garlic, the bitter tang of chocolate, the aromatic qualities of herbs, and the beautiful colors of tomatoes, spinach, pink grapefruit, and watermelon.

Today, many phytochemicals are believed to be **bioactive food components**—

food constituents other than the nutrients (defined in Chapter 1) that alter body processes. Many phytochemicals are known to have antioxidant activity, and **antioxidants** in the body protect DNA and other cellular compounds from oxidative damage. Some others may interact with genes, affecting protein synthesis; a few others mimic the body's own hormones; and many seem to have no effects or effects awaiting discovery.

Of the tens of thousands of phytochemicals known to exist, few have been studied for health effects, and only a sampling are mentioned in this Controversy—enough to illustrate the wide array of foods that supply them and their potential roles in human health. People eat foods, not individual phytochemicals, so this section focuses on a few well-known suppliers of these interesting compounds.

Blueberries and the Brain

When researchers fed chow rich in blueberry powder to a group of rats, they exhibited fewer age-related mental declines than rats on plain chow, a result that has been repeated in research.[1*] This finding set

govindji/Shutterstock.com

*Reference notes are in Appendix F.

off a flurry of excitement about blueberries as a potential superfood for the brain. To explain their results, the researchers suggest that the **flavonoids** of blueberries, along with grapes and walnuts, may act as antioxidants in the brain and thus limit damage to brain cells by oxidation (phytochemical definitions are in Table C2–2.). Some human studies support the idea that eating a diet high in fruit and vegetables, and therefore high in flavonoids, may help people stay mentally sharper as they age.[2] When researchers evaluated the mental status of groups of older women, they found that higher flavonoid intakes, especially from berries, accompanied less cognitive decline. Further, when healthy older adults were given a blueberry concentrate for 12 weeks, the blood flow through their brains increased and they scored better on a test of memory.[3]

Is it safe to say, then, that blueberries are a true superfood for brainpower? Blueberries currently bear well in flavonoid and brain research, but confirmation of their effects in people outside the laboratory are still needed. If future research supports their effectiveness, additional questions arise. How many blueberries might be enough? Can a steady diet of fast-food hamburgers,

---

Table C2–1

Functional Food Terms

- **antioxidants** (anti-OX-ih-dants) compounds that protect other compounds from damaging reactions involving oxygen by themselves reacting with oxygen (*anti* means "against"; *oxy* means "oxygen"). *Oxidation* is a potentially damaging effect of normal cell chemistry involving oxygen (see details in Chapters 5 and 7).
- **bioactive food components** compounds in foods, either nutrients or phytochemicals, that alter physiological processes.
- **drug** any substance that, when taken into a living organism, may modify one or more of its functions.
- **functional foods** whole or modified foods that contain bioactive food components believed to provide health benefits, such as reduced disease risks, beyond the benefits that their nutrients confer.

All whole foods are functional in some ways because they provide at least some needed substances, but certain foods stand out as rich sources of bioactive food components. Also defined in Chapter 1.

- **nutraceutical** a term that has no legal or scientific meaning but that is sometimes used to refer to foods, nutrients, or dietary supplements believed to have medicinal effects. Often used to sell unnecessary or unproven supplements.
- **phytochemicals** (FYE-toe-KEM-ih-cals) compounds in plants that confer color, taste, and other characteristics. Often, the bioactive food components of functional foods. Also defined in Chapter 1. *Phyto* means "plant."

Phytochemical Terms

- **broccoli sprouts** the sprouted seed of *Brassica italica*, or the common broccoli plant; believed to be a functional food by virtue of its high phytochemical content.
- **edamame** fresh green soybeans, a source of phytoestrogens.
- **flavonoids** (FLAY-von-oyds) a common and widespread group of phytochemicals, with over 6,000 identified members; physiologic effects may include antioxidant, antiviral, anticancer, and other activities. Some flavonoids are yellow pigments in foods; *flavus* means "yellow."
- **flaxseed** small brown seed of the flax plant; used in baking, cereals, or other foods. Valued in nutrition as a source of fatty acids, lignans, and fiber.
- **genistein** (GEN-ih-steen) a phytoestrogen found primarily in soybeans that both mimics and blocks the action of estrogen in the body; a type of flavonoid.
- **kefir** (KEE-fur) a liquid form of yogurt, based on milk, probiotic microorganisms, and flavorings.
- **lignans** phytochemicals present mostly in seeds, particularly flaxseed, that are converted to phytoestrogens by intestinal bacteria and are under study as possible anticancer agents.
- **lutein** (LOO-teen) a plant pigment of yellow hue; a phytochemical believed to play roles in eye functioning and health.
- **lycopene** (LYE-koh-peen) a pigment responsible for the red color of tomatoes and other red-hued vegetables; a phytochemical that may act as an antioxidant in the body.
- **miso** fermented soybean paste used in Japanese cooking. Soy products are considered to be functional foods.

- **organosulfur compounds** a large group of phytochemicals containing the mineral sulfur. Organosulfur phytochemicals are responsible for the pungent flavors and aromas of foods belonging to the onion, leek, chive, shallot, and garlic family and are thought to stimulate cancer defenses in the body.
- **phytoestrogens** (FYE-toe-ESS-troh-gens) phytochemicals structurally similar to the female sex hormone estrogen. Phytoestrogens weakly mimic estrogen or modulate hormone activity in the human body.
- **plant sterols** phytochemicals that resemble cholesterol in structure but that lower blood cholesterol, possibly by interfering with cholesterol absorption in the intestine. Plant sterols include sterol esters and stanol esters, formerly called *phytosterols*.
- **prebiotic** a substance that may not be digestible by the host, such as fiber, but that serves as food for probiotic bacteria and thus promotes their growth.
- **probiotic** a live microorganism that, when administered in adequate amounts, alters the bacterial colonies of the body in ways believed to confer a health benefit on the host.
- **resveratrol** (rez-VER-ah-trol) a phytochemical of grapes under study for potential health benefits.
- **soy milk** a milklike beverage made from soybeans, claimed to be a functional food. Soy drinks should be fortified with vitamin A, vitamin D, riboflavin, and calcium to approach the nutritional equivalency of milk.
- **tofu** a white curd made of soybeans, popular in Asian cuisines, and considered to be a functional food.

French fries, and colas be offset by a handful of blueberries? (Probably not.) Would a pill made of blueberries suffice? People seem to benefit most from a variety of flavonoid sources: artichokes, beans, coffee, pomegranates, seeds, spinach, strawberries and other berries, and in fact most fruit and vegetables, whole grains, food mixtures, and even nuts, maple syrup, and seaweed.[4] By focusing only on blueberries, a person could easily miss out on potential benefits of the nutrients and phytochemicals in a variety of foods.[5] Blueberries, of course, make a delicious contribution, and as complex whole foods, they probably confer other benefits as well.

Chocolate, Heart, and Mood

Imagine the delight of young research subjects who were paid to eat 3 ounces of dark chocolate for an experiment. Less appealingly, researchers then drew blood from the subjects to test whether an antioxidant flavonoid in chocolate could be absorbed into the bloodstream.

The tests were positive: the flavonoid had been absorbed, and at the same time, potentially harmful oxidizing compounds in the blood had dropped by 40 percent.

The story of chocolate and health is complex, but some evidence suggests that chocolate or its flavonoids may improve blood vessel functioning, but only when eaten in moderation. Associations with heart health vanish in those consuming more than one serving of chocolate per day.[6]

People often believe that eating chocolate lifts their spirits—it makes them happy. However, in a study of about 1,000 people, greater chocolate intakes were associated with *more* depressive symptoms, not fewer. It may be that depressed people in this study were seeking relief by self-medicating with chocolate. Too little is known about the effects of chocolate on mood to allow conclusions.

One proven medical use of chocolate is weight gain. Each 3-ounce piece of chocolate candy offers 400 calories of added sugar and solid fat, calories that most people can little afford to consume. Most people are better off obtaining phytochemicals from nutrient-dense, low-calorie fruit and vegetables—and savoring chocolate as an occasional treat.

Flaxseed

Long valued for relieving constipation and digestive distress, **flaxseed** is showing potential for other health benefits. Flaxseeds are rich in **lignans**, cholesterol-like phytochemicals that bacteria of the digestive tract convert into **phytoestrogens**, compounds that mimic the human hormone estrogen. In the U.S. diet, lignans are supplied mostly by other seeds, as well as whole wheat and vegetables.

Valentyn Volkov/Shutterstock.com

Max Lashcheuski/Shutterstock.com

When given to rats in huge amounts, flax lignans have been shown to lower blood pressure and inflammation, thus reducing potential heart disease risk.[7] However, population studies linking lignan intake with reduced incidence of heart disease are not convincing, reporting only mixed results.

Lignans are also under study for potential effects on certain cancers. Some recent research findings include these:

- Rat chow high in flaxseed reversed cancerous changes in rat mammary tissue.
- Breast cancer cells treated with flaxseed oil were slower to replicate and died off faster than untreated cells.[8]
- Women with the highest blood levels of a marker for intake of lignans have lower risks of both developing breast cancer and dying of the disease.[9]

Including a little flaxseed in the diet may not be a bad idea, even if research fails to bear out its status as a superfood. Flaxseed richly supplies linolenic acid, an essential fatty acid often lacking in the U.S. diet (see Chapter 5). To benefit from flaxseed, choose ground flaxseed or grind it yourself. When flaxseeds are consumed whole, they often pass intact right through the digestive tract.

Garlic

For thousands of years, people have consumed garlic for medicinal purposes. Early Egyptian medical writings report its use for headache, heart disease, and tumors.

Guitar Studio/Shutterstock.com

Today, garlic is studied because its antioxidant **organosulfur compounds** may inhibit cancer development. When oxidizing compounds damage DNA in cells, cancerous changes can occur. Antioxidants of garlic quench these oxidizing compounds, at least in test tubes. Whether garlic affects cancers in people is unknown. Although garlic is credited with opposing allergies, heart disease, infections, and ulcers, these effects are unsupported. For disease prevention, evidence is limited, and research does not support taking garlic supplements.[10] If you like garlicky foods, you can consume them with confidence: history and some research are on your side.

Soybeans and Soy Products

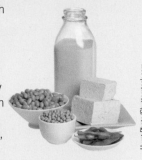

Hurst Photo/Shutterstock.com

Compared with people in the West, Asians consume far more soybeans and soy products, such as **edamame**, **miso**, **soy milk**, and **tofu**, and they suffer less frequently from obesity, heart disease, and certain cancers.[†] When Asian populations adopt Western diets and habits, however, their rates of obesity and chronic diseases increase.[11]

In research, evidence concerning soy and heart health seems promising.[12] Soy's cholesterol-like **plant sterols** may inhibit cholesterol absorption in the intestine and thus lower blood cholesterol.[13] Soy protein may also speed up excretion of cholesterol from the body.[14]

With regard to cancer, breast, colon, and prostate cancers can be estrogen-sensitive—that is, they grow when exposed to estrogen. In addition to plant sterols, soy contains phytoestrogens that may mimic or oppose estrogen's effects. Girls who eat soy foods during childhood and adolescence may have reduced breast cancer risk as young adults, a finding attributed to effects of soy phytoestrogens.[15] Soy intake may also lower the risk of breast cancer for adult women in Asian countries, but for women in Western nations, evidence does not suggest a benefit.[16] Scientists continue to search for cellular mechanisms that might explain these relationships.[17]

Soy's Potential Downsides

Low doses of the soy phytoestrogen **genistein** appear to speed up division of breast cancer cells in laboratory cultures and in mice, whereas high doses seemed to do the opposite. However, it seems unlikely that moderate intakes of soy foods cause harm in people. If they did, soy-eating peoples would have higher incidences of these cancers. In fact, the opposite is true.

The opposing actions of soy phytoestrogens should raise a red flag against taking supplements, especially by people who have had cancer or have

†Among the cancers occurring less often in Asia are breast, colon, and prostate cancers.

close relatives with cancer. The American Cancer Society recommends that breast cancer survivors and those under treatment for breast cancer consume moderate amounts of soy foods as part of a healthy plant-based diet but should not take supplemental soy phytoestrogens.[18]

Tea

People in Asia who drink two cups or more of green tea each day die less often from digestive tract cancers than nondrinkers, possibly due to the antioxidant activity of polyphenols found in green tea.[19] Black tea, the type most U.S. consumers drink, is a major contributor of flavonoids to the diet. In one study, drinking more than three cups of black tea each day was associated with fewer serious bone fractures.[20] Evidence also suggests that tea may influence cancers in women by altering the workings of genes associated with estrogen metabolism.[21]

Green tea, the kind widely consumed in Asia, is associated with reduced risk of death, and particularly deaths from heart disease, among the Chinese.[22] Indeed, compiled evidence from human studies suggests that green tea may improve blood pressure levels and reduce blood lipid concentrations, and therefore reduce chronic disease risks.[23] Long-term controlled human studies are needed to confirm these findings. As for cancer, when researchers search for links between green tea consumption and cancer reduction, the results are inconsistent.[24]

High-dose supplements of green tea extract have been linked with liver toxicity and high intakes of green tea with kidney problems.[25] When USDA analyzed popular green tea supplements, they reported a wide range of quality: some authentic, some lacking any trace of green tea components, and others containing undeclared additives. Supplement quality cannot be judged from label information, even in leading brand-name pills.

Grapes and Wine

Purple grape juice and red wine contain a number of flavonoids, and among them is a small amount of **resveratrol**. Resveratrol shows promise in research as

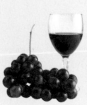

Rafael Angel Garcia Dobarganes/Shutterstock.com

a disease fighter.[26] In laboratory studies, resveratrol demonstrates the potential to reduce harmful tissue inflammation that often accompanies cancer, diabetes, obesity, and heart disease and to oppose heart disease development in other ways. Also to its credit are studies in which resveratrol seemed to extend the life of fish and worms.[27] In people, resveratrol is poorly absorbed, and evidence is lacking to conclude that any of these effects occur in human beings. Controversy 3 compares the potential risks and benefits of drinking alcohol.

Yogurt

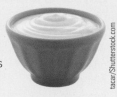

tacar/Shutterstock.com

Yogurt is a special case among superfoods. Being a milk product, yogurt lacks typical flavonoids or other phytochemicals from plants. Instead, it contains living *Lactobacillus* or other bacteria that ferment milk into products like yogurt or the liquid yogurt beverage **kefir**. Such microorganisms, called **probiotics**, can set up residence in the digestive tract and alter its functioning in ways that may reduce colon cancer, ulcers, and other digestive problems; reduce allergies; or improve immunity and resistance to infections. The types and ratios of organisms that make up the microbial colonies of the intestine are also under investigation for their roles in diseases such as diabetes and obesity.[28] *Lactobacillus* and other bacteria may help correct the diarrhea that often follows antibiotic drug use. However, there is cause for concern when it comes to the safety of probiotic supplementation among certain groups of people. Read Table C2–3 to learn more.

Table C2–3

Phytochemical and Functional Supplements: Point, Counterpoint

Arguments arise about whether large intakes of phytochemicals in superfoods or supplements might help or harm health. The arguments for loading up on certain phytochemicals are listed on the left; the opposing evidence, which calls for moderation, is offered on the right.

Points Made In Favor	Counterpoints and Opposing Evidence
1. *Protection from oxidation*. In levels obtainable from foods, certain phytochemicals may protect DNA and other cellular structures from oxidative damage.	1. *Damage from oxidation*. At high levels, obtainable only from supplements, these same phytochemicals may increase oxidative damage to DNA and other structures.
2. *Disease prevention*. Diets rich in phytochemicals are shown to benefit health through their anti-inflammatory and anticancer properties; they also may protect against cardiovascular and neurodegenerative diseases.	2. *Disease progression*. No benefits are associated with supplements of phytochemicals. In large doses, phytochemicals also inhibit absorption of certain vitamins or minerals and thus may promote disease progression.
3. *Safe for people*. Phytochemicals are safe because they are "natural"—they arise in food. Examples: ▪ *Lignans support health*. Dietary lignans may have protective effects against cancers, including breast and prostate cancers. ▪ *Probiotic benefits*. Probiotics, the microorganisms of the large intestine, may have beneficial effects, including improvements in antibiotic-induced diarrhea, digestive diseases, obesity, and immunity.	3. *Unproven safety*. "Natural" does not mean "safe." All substances, even water and vitamins, are hazardous in large amounts. Examples: ▪ *Lignans impede health*. High daily lignan intakes, particularly from supplements, can interfere with vitamin and mineral absorption, posing a risk of nutrient deficiencies. Digestive distress is also likely. ▪ *Probiotic harms*. Probiotic supplements may be safe for most healthy people, but patients with pancreatic diseases and those with weakened immunity have contracted serious infections after consuming them.
4. *Just a few foods*. Certain "superfoods" are the richest sources of phytochemicals. These few foods should be eaten every day.	4. *A variety of foods*. Focusing on a few select "superfoods" to the exclusion of other whole foods may limit the expected health benefits. Tens of thousands of phytochemicals exist in virtually all foods from plants, but only a few have been studied, making variety the best strategy. Also, foods from plants often contain natural toxins, another reason to choose a wide variety of foods.
5. *Evidence is good enough*. Existing evidence is good enough to recommend that people take supplements of purified phytochemicals.	5. *Not enough evidence*. Evidence for the safety of isolated phytochemical supplements is lacking, and evidence for potential harm is mounting.
6. *Healthy label claims*. Product labels on phytochemical supplements claim potent health benefits, so they must be true.	6. *Unreliable label claims*. Phytochemical labels can make structure-function claims that sound good but are generally based on weak or nonexistent scientific evidence.
7. *Sufficient regulation and oversight*. Phytochemical supplements must be safe because reliable businesses—even pharmacies—sell them.	7. *Lack of oversight*. No regulatory body oversees the safety of phytochemicals sold to consumers. No studies are required to prove their safety or effectiveness before they are sold.

Chapter 2 Nutrition Tools—Standards and Guidelines

Additional research is needed to clarify potential benefits or risks from probiotics.

Other foods provide **prebiotics**—that is, nondigestible carbohydrates or other constituents upon which bacteria in the digestive tract can feed. A fed colony multiplies rapidly, creating by-products that are associated with certain health benefits, such as a decrease in disease-related inflammation of the colon.

Phytochemical Supplements

No doubt exists that diets rich in legumes, vegetables, fruit, and other whole foods reduce the risks of heart disease and cancer, but isolating the responsible food, nutrient, or phytochemical has proved difficult. Foods deliver thousands of bioactive food components, all within a food matrix that maximizes their availability and effectiveness.[29] Broccoli, and particularly **broccoli sprouts**, may contain as many as 10,000 different phytochemicals—each with the potential to influence some action in the body. These foods are under study for their potential to defend against cancers

at the DNA level, and Chapter 11 comes back to them.

Even if it were known with certainty which foods protect against which diseases, most isolated supplements, even the most promising ones, fail to actually prevent diseases when they are administered in research.[30] Worse, some such supplements can interfere with and reduce the effectiveness of standard drugs given to people with serious illnesses. Such food and drug interactions are of critical importance, and the Controversy section of Chapter 14 is devoted to them.

Users and sellers of phytochemical supplements argue that people have been consuming foods containing phytochemicals for tens of thousands of years and because the body can handle phytochemicals in foods, it stands to reason that supplements of those phytochemicals are safe as well. Such thinking raises concerns among scientists, though. The latter point out that the body is equipped to handle the dilute phytochemicals of whole foods but not concentrated supplement doses. As often proves true in nutrition, it may be that too much is as bad as too little.

The Concept of Functional Foods

Virtually all whole foods have some special value in supporting health and are therefore functional foods. Modest evidence suggests that cranberries may help to prevent some urinary tract infections, for example.[31] Manufactured functional foods, however, often consist of ultra-processed foods that are fortified with bioactive food components (often from herbs) for which little or no supporting evidence of benefit exists (some examples are depicted in Figure C2–1).

Such novel foods raise questions:

- *Is it safe?* Functional foods can act like **drugs**. They contain ingredients that can alter body functions and cause allergies, drug interactions, drowsiness, and other side effects. Yet, unlike drugs, functional food packages do not provide instructions for the dosage, frequency, or duration of treatment.

- *Is it a healthful choice?* Adding phytochemicals to a food does not magically make it a healthy choice. A candy bar fortified with phytochemicals is still made mostly of sugar and fat.

The Final Word

In light of all of the evidence for and against phytochemicals and functional foods, a moderate approach is warranted. People who eat abundant and varied fruit and vegetables each day may cut their risk for many diseases by as much as half. Replacing some meat with soy foods may reduce those risks further. Table C2–4 offers some tips for consuming the whole foods known to provide phytochemicals.

A piece of advice: don't try to single out a few superfoods or phytochemicals for their magical health effects, and ignore the hype about packaged products—no evidence exists to support their use. Instead, take a no-nonsense approach and choose a wide variety of whole grains, legumes, nuts, fruit, and vegetables in the context of an adequate, balanced, and varied diet to receive all of the health benefits these foods can offer.

Figure C2–1

A Sampling of Functional Foods

Functional foods currently on the market promise to "enhance mood," "promote relaxation and good karma," "support alertness," and "benefit memory," among other claims.

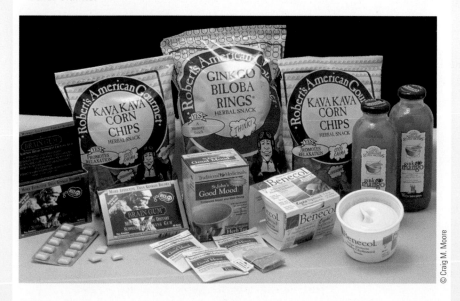

© Craig M. Moore

Tips for Consuming Phytochemicals

- Eat more fruit. The average U.S. diet provides little more than ½ cup of fruit a day. Remember to choose juices and raw, dried, or cooked fruit at mealtimes, as well as for snacks. Choose dried fruit in place of candy.
- Increase vegetable portions. Double the normal portion of cooked plain, nonstarchy vegetables. Dip cut raw vegetables into yogurt-based dips for snacks.
- Use herbs and spices. Cookbooks offer ways to include parsley, basil, garlic, hot peppers, oregano, turmeric, and other phytochemical-rich seasonings.
- Replace some meat. Replace some of the meat in the diet with grains, legumes, and vegetables. Oatmeal, soy meat replacer, or grated carrots mixed with ground meat and seasonings make a luscious, nutritious meat loaf, for example.
- Add grated vegetables. Carrots in chili or meatballs, celery and squash in spaghetti sauce, and similar combinations add phytochemicals without greatly changing the taste of the food.
- Try new foods. Try a new fruit, vegetable, or whole grain each week. Walk through vegetable aisles and visit farmers' markets. Read recipes. Try tofu, fortified soy milk, or soybeans in cooking.

Critical Thinking

1. Divide into two groups. One group will argue in support of using superfoods, and one group will argue against the use of superfoods. During the debate, be sure to answer the following questions:

   - What is a superfood, and is it appropriate to classify a given food as a superfood?
   - Are there foods that you can reliably say have the characteristics of a superfood? Describe the research you have consulted to support the classification of a food as a superfood.

2. Describe a situation when the intake of a phytochemical supplement or a functional food would be appropriate. Give reasons for using a phytochemical supplement or functional food, and also give reasons against its use.

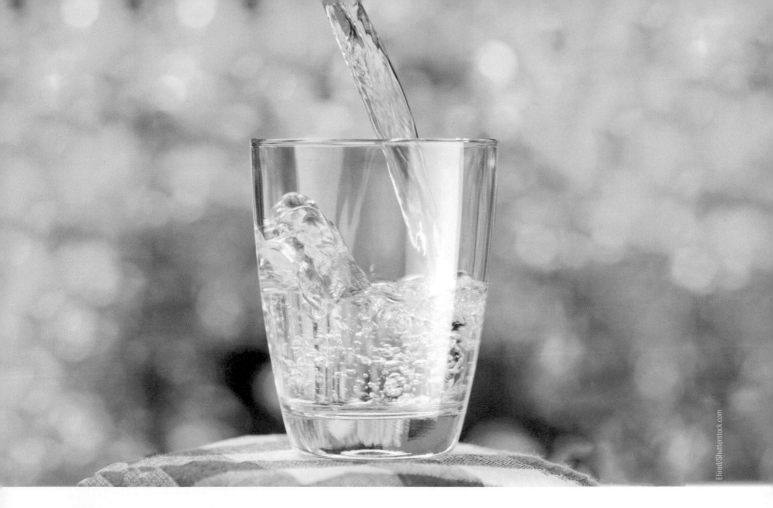

3 The Remarkable Body

Learning Objectives

After reading this chapter, you should be able to accomplish the following:

LO 3.1 Name six basic needs of the body's cells.

LO 3.2 Summarize the exchange of materials that takes place as body fluids circulate around the tissues.

LO 3.3 Summarize the interactions between the hormonal and nervous systems and nutrition.

LO 3.4 Summarize how the digestive system provides nutrients to the body tissues.

LO 3.5 Outline the symptoms of eight common digestive problems related to nutrition.

LO 3.6 Specify the excretory functions of the lungs, liver, kidneys, and bladder.

LO 3.7 Explain how body tissues store excess nutrients.

LO 3.8 Compare the effects of moderate and heavy alcohol consumption.

What do you think?

Is it true that "**you are what you eat**"?

How does food on the plate become **nourishment** for your body?

What does **bacteria in the intestine** have to do with nutrition?

Should you take antacids to relieve **heartburn**?

At the moment of conception, you received genes in the form of DNA from your mother and father, who, in turn, had inherited them from their parents, and so on into ancient history. Since that moment, your genes have been working invisibly, directing your body's development and functioning. Many of your genes are ancient in origin and are little changed from genes of thousands of centuries ago, but here you are—living with the food, luxuries, smog, contaminants, and all the other pleasures and problems of the 21st century. There is no guarantee that a diet haphazardly chosen from today's foods will meet the needs of your "prehistoric" body. Unlike your ancestors, who nourished themselves from the wild plants and animals surrounding them, you must learn how your body works, what it needs, and how to select foods to meet its needs.

The Body's Cells

LO 3.1   Name six basic needs of the body's cells.

The human body is composed of trillions of **cells**, and none of them knows anything about food. *You* may get hungry for fruit, milk, or bread, but each cell of your body needs nutrients—the vital components of foods. The ways in which the body's cells cooperate to obtain and use nutrients are the subjects of this chapter.

Each of the body's cells is a self-contained, living entity (see Figure 3–1), but at the same time, it depends on the rest of the body's cells to supply its needs. Among the cells' most basic needs are energy and the oxygen with which to burn it. Cells also need water to maintain the environment in which they live. They need building blocks and control systems. They especially need the nutrients they cannot make for themselves—the essential nutrients first described in Chapter 1—which

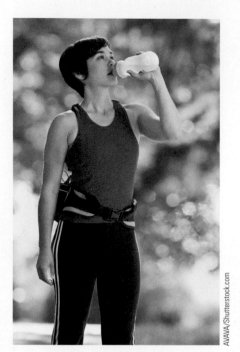
All the body's cells live in water.

AVAVA/Shutterstock.com

Figure 3–1

A Cell (Simplified Diagram)

This cell has been greatly enlarged; real cells are so tiny that 10,000 can fit on the head of a pin.

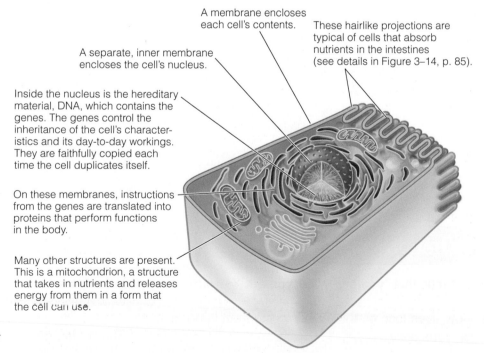

A membrane encloses each cell's contents.

These hairlike projections are typical of cells that absorb nutrients in the intestines (see details in Figure 3–14, p. 85).

A separate, inner membrane encloses the cell's nucleus.

Inside the nucleus is the hereditary material, DNA, which contains the genes. The genes control the inheritance of the cell's characteristics and its day-to-day workings. They are faithfully copied each time the cell duplicates itself.

On these membranes, instructions from the genes are translated into proteins that perform functions in the body.

Many other structures are present. This is a mitochondrion, a structure that takes in nutrients and releases energy from them in a form that the cell can use.

cells the smallest units in which independent life can exist. All living things are single cells or organisms made of cells.

Figure 3-2

From DNA to Living Cells

DNA is the large molecule that encodes all genetic information in its structure; genes are units of a cell's inheritance situated along the DNA strands.

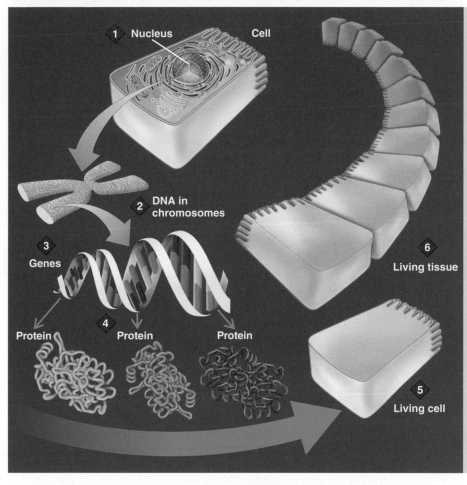

1 Nucleus Cell

2 DNA in chromosomes

3 Genes

4 Protein Protein Protein

6 Living tissue

5 Living cell

1 Each cell's nucleus contains DNA—the material of heredity in all living things.

2 Long strands of human DNA coil into 23 pairs of chromosomes. If the strands of DNA in all the body's cells were uncoiled and laid end to end, they would stretch to the sun and back four hundred times. Yet DNA strands are so tiny that about 5 million of them could be threaded at once through the eye of a needle.

3 Genes contain instructions for making proteins. Genes are sections along the strands of DNA that serve as templates for the building of proteins. Some genes are involved in building just one protein; others are involved in building more than one.

4 Many other steps are required to make a protein. See Figure 6–6 of Chapter 6.

5 Proteins do the work of living cells. Cells employ proteins to perform essential functions and provide structures.

6 Communities of functioning cells make up the living tissue.

must be supplied from food. The first principle of diet planning is that the foods we choose must provide energy and the essential nutrients, including water.

Being living things, cells also die off, although at varying rates. Some skin cells and red blood cells must replace themselves every 10 to 120 days, respectively. Cells lining the digestive tract replace themselves every 3 days. Under ordinary conditions, many muscle cells reproduce themselves only once every few years. Liver cells have the ability to reproduce quickly and do so whenever repairs to the organ are needed. Certain brain cells do not reproduce at all; if damaged by injury or disease, they are lost forever.

The cells work in cooperation with each other to support the whole body. Gene activity within each cell determines the nature of that work.

Genes Control Functions

Each gene is a blueprint that directs the production of one or more proteins, such as **enzymes** that performs cellular work, and **structural proteins** that provide the architecture of the cells. Genes also provide the instructions for all of the structural components cells need to survive (see Figure 3–2). Each cell contains a complete set of genes, located in the **chromosomes**, but different ones are active in different types of cells. For example, in some intestinal cells, the genes for making digestive

Connections between nutrition and gene activities are emerging in the field of nutritional genomics, described in **Controversy 11**.

enzymes working proteins that speed up specific chemical reactions, such as releasing energy from nutrient molecules, without themselves being altered in the process. Enzymes and their actions are described in Chapter 6.

structural proteins non-enzyme proteins of cells, such as the proteins of the cell membrane and of its interior structures.

chromosomes structures of mostly coiled DNA and proteins, housed in the nucleus of every cell. The DNA carries the genes for making cellular proteins; the protein and other constituents influence the configuration and functioning of the DNA.

enzymes are active, but the genes for making keratin in nails and hair are silent; in some of the body's **fat cells**, the genes for making enzymes that metabolize fat are active, but the digestive enzyme genes are silent. Certain nutrients are involved in activating and silencing genes in ways that are just starting to be revealed.

Genes affect the way the body handles its nutrients. Certain variations in some of the genes alter the way the body absorbs, metabolizes, or excretes nutrients from the body. Occasionally, a gene variation can cause a lifelong malady—that is, an **inborn error of metabolism**—in which the gene for a critical piece of cellular machinery, usually an enzyme, is defective or missing. As a result, the body's chemistry is disrupted. The disorder **phenylketonuria (PKU)** is one such inborn error. A defective gene produces a defective enzyme that cannot handle the substance phenylalanine (which comes from dietary protein) in the normal way. Toxic products accumulate in the body and cause a host of symptoms, including seizures, tremors, stunted growth, eczema, and mental retardation. A special diet that is free of phenylalanine must be provided beginning in infancy to prevent damage from this malady that, once present, cannot be reversed. To help facilitate treatment, food manufacturers are required to print warning labels on foods, such as certain artificial sweeteners, that contain phenylalanine.

Cells, Tissues, Organs, Systems

Cells are organized into **tissues** that perform specialized tasks. For example, individual muscle cells are joined together to form muscle tissue, which can contract. Tissues, in turn, are grouped together to form whole **organs**. In the organ we call the heart, for example, muscle tissues, nerve tissues, connective tissues, and others all work together to pump blood. Some body functions are performed by several related organs working together as part of a **body system**. For example, the heart, lungs, and blood vessels cooperate as parts of the cardiorespiratory system to deliver oxygen to all the body's cells. The next few sections present the body systems with special significance to nutrition.

KEY POINTS

- The body's cells need energy, oxygen, and nutrients, including water, to remain healthy and do their work.
- Genes direct the making of each cell's protein machinery, including enzymes.
- Specialized cells are grouped together to form tissues and organs; organs work together in body systems.

The Body Fluids and the Circulatory System

LO 3.2   Summarize the exchange of materials that takes place as body fluids circulate around the tissues.

Body fluids supply the tissues continuously with energy, oxygen, and nutrients, including water. The fluids constantly circulate to pick up fresh supplies and deliver wastes to points of disposal. Every cell continuously draws oxygen and nutrients from those fluids and releases carbon dioxide and other waste products into them.

The Body's Fluids   The body's circulating fluids are the **blood** and the **lymph**. Blood travels within the **arteries**, **veins**, and **capillaries**, as well as within the heart's chambers (see Figure 3–3). Lymph travels in separate vessels of its own.

Circulating around the cells are other fluids such as the **plasma** of the blood, which surrounds the white and red blood cells, and the fluid surrounding muscle cells (see Figure 3–4, p. 72). The fluid surrounding cells (**extracellular fluid**) is derived

fat cells cells that specialize in the storage of fat and form the fat tissue. Fat cells also produce fat-metabolizing enzymes; they also produce hormones involved in appetite and energy balance (see Chapter 9).

inborn error of metabolism a genetic variation present from birth that may result in disease.

phenylketonuria (PKU) an inborn error of metabolism that interferes with the body's handling of phenylalanine (from dietary protein) and, left untreated, results in serious harm to the brain and nervous system.

tissues groups of cells working together to perform specialized tasks. Examples are muscles, nerves, blood, and bone.

organs discrete structural units made of tissues that perform specific jobs. Examples are the heart, liver, and brain.

body system a group of related organs that work together to perform a function. Examples are the circulatory system, respiratory system, and nervous system.

blood the fluid of the cardiovascular system; composed of water, red and white blood cells, other formed particles, nutrients, oxygen, and other constituents.

lymph (LIMF) the fluid that moves from the bloodstream into tissue spaces and then travels in its own vessels, which eventually drain back into the bloodstream.

arteries blood vessels that carry blood containing fresh oxygen supplies from the heart to the tissues (see Figure 3–3).

veins blood vessels that carry blood, with the carbon dioxide it has collected, from the tissues back to the heart (see Figure 3–3).

capillaries minute, weblike blood vessels that connect arteries to veins and permit transfer of materials between blood and tissues (see Figures 3–3 and 3–4).

plasma the cell-free fluid part of blood and lymph.

extracellular fluid fluid residing outside the cells that transports materials to and from the cells.

Figure 3–3

Blood Flow in the Cardiovascular System

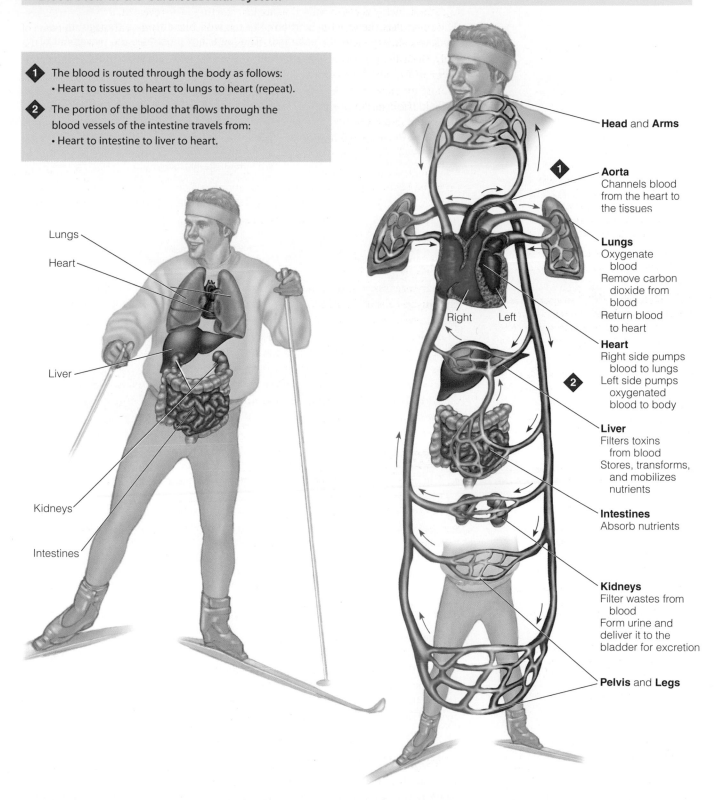

1 The blood is routed through the body as follows:
- Heart to tissues to heart to lungs to heart (repeat).

2 The portion of the blood that flows through the blood vessels of the intestine travels from:
- Heart to intestine to liver to heart.

Lungs
Heart
Liver
Kidneys
Intestines

Head and **Arms**

1

Aorta
Channels blood from the heart to the tissues

Lungs
Oxygenate blood
Remove carbon dioxide from blood
Return blood to heart

Right   Left

Heart
Right side pumps blood to lungs
Left side pumps oxygenated blood to body

2

Liver
Filters toxins from blood
Stores, transforms, and mobilizes nutrients

Intestines
Absorb nutrients

Kidneys
Filter wastes from blood
Form urine and deliver it to the bladder for excretion

Pelvis and **Legs**

Figure 3–4

How the Body Fluids Circulate around Cells

The upper box shows a tiny portion of tissue with blood flowing through its network of capillaries (greatly enlarged). The lower box illustrates the movement of the extracellular fluid. Exchange of materials also takes place between cell fluid and extracellular fluid.

1 Fluid filters out of blood through the capillary, whose walls are made of cells with small spaces between them.

2 Fluid may enter a capillary and rejoin the bloodstream.
3 Fluid may enter a lymph vessel to join the lymphatic fluids. Lymph flows through the vessels and ultimately into the bloodstream through a large lymph vessel that empties into a large vein.

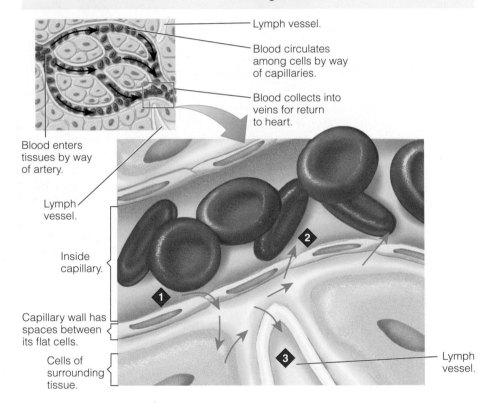

Lymph vessel.

Blood circulates among cells by way of capillaries.

Blood collects into veins for return to heart.

Blood enters tissues by way of artery.

Lymph vessel.

Inside capillary.

Capillary wall has spaces between its flat cells.

Cells of surrounding tissue.

Lymph vessel.

from the blood in the capillaries; it squeezes out through the capillary walls and flows around the outsides of cells, permitting exchange of materials.

Some of the extracellular fluid returns directly to the bloodstream by reentering the capillaries. The fluid remaining outside the capillaries forms lymph, which travels around the body by way of lymph vessels. The lymph eventually returns to the bloodstream near the heart where a large lymph vessel empties into a large vein. In this way, all cells are served by the cardiovascular system.

The fluid inside cells (**intracellular fluid**) provides a medium in which all cell reactions take place. Its pressure also helps the cells to hold their shape. The intracellular fluid is drawn from the extracellular fluid that bathes the outsides of the cells.

Blood and Lymph Circulation   All the blood circulates to the lungs, where it picks up oxygen and releases carbon dioxide wastes from the cells. Then the blood returns to the heart, where the pumping heartbeats push this freshly oxygenated blood through the **aorta**, the large artery leading from the heart, and then out to all body tissues.

intracellular fluid fluid residing inside the cells that provides the medium for cellular reactions.

aorta the large artery that conducts oxygenated blood away from the heart to the rest of the circulatory system.

As the blood travels through the rest of the cardiovascular system, it delivers materials cells need and picks up their wastes.

As it passes through the digestive system, the blood delivers oxygen to the cells there and picks up most nutrients, with the exceptions of fats and their relatives, from the **intestine** for distribution elsewhere.

Blood leaving the digestive system is routed directly to the **liver**, which has the special task of chemically altering the absorbed materials to make them better suited for use by other tissues. Later, in passing through the **kidneys**, the blood is cleansed of wastes (look again at Figure 3–3). Note that the blood carries nutrients from the intestine to the liver, which releases them to the heart, which pumps them to the waiting body tissues.

As for lymph, it takes a one-way ride through its own set of vessels that originate in the tissues and end at a duct in a large blood vein near the heart. Lymph vessels in the intestine pick up most of the fats present in a meal and conduct them along the lymph vessel route to the bloodstream. In addition, the lymphatic system plays critical roles in the body's extensive **immune system**. The lymphatic system transports and helps activate **lymphocytes**, white blood cells that defend against invading **microbes**. The digestive tract employs a large network of lymphatic cells and tissues to quash infections that could otherwise occur from among the millions of microbes that normally reside there (you will learn later that most of these microbes pose no threat).

Keeping the System Healthy To ensure efficient circulation of fluids to and from all your cells, you need an ample fluid intake. This means consuming sufficient water to replace the water lost each day. Cardiovascular fitness is essential, too, and it requires attention to both nutrition and physical activity. Healthy red blood cells also play a role, for they carry oxygen to all the other cells, enabling them to use fuels for energy. Because red blood cells arise, live, and die within about four months, your body replaces them constantly, a manufacturing process that requires many essential nutrients from food. Consequently, the blood is very sensitive to malnutrition and often serves as an indicator of disorders caused by dietary deficiencies or imbalances of vitamins or minerals.

KEY POINTS

- Blood and lymph deliver needed materials to all the body's cells and carry waste materials away from them.
- The cardiovascular system ensures that these fluids circulate properly among all tissues.

The Hormonal and Nervous Systems

LO 3.3   Summarize the interactions between the hormonal and nervous systems and nutrition.

In addition to fluid, blood cells, nutrients, oxygen, and wastes, the blood also carries chemical messengers, **hormones**, from one system of cells to another. Hormones communicate changing conditions that demand responses from the body's organs.

What Do Hormones Have to Do with Nutrition?

Hormones are secreted and released directly into the blood by organs known as **glands**. Glands and hormones abound in the body. Each gland monitors a condition and produces one or more hormones to regulate it. Each hormone acts as a messenger that stimulates various organs to take appropriate actions.

intestine the body's long, tubular organ of digestion and the site of nutrient absorption.

liver a large, lobed organ that lies just under the ribs. It filters the blood, removes and processes nutrients, manufactures materials for export to other parts of the body, and destroys toxins or stores them to keep them out of the circulatory system.

kidneys a pair of organs that filter wastes from the blood, make urine, and release it to the bladder for excretion from the body.

immune system a large system of tissues and organs that defend the body against microbes or foreign materials that have penetrated the skin or body linings.

lymphocytes (LIM-foh-sites) white blood cells that participate in the immune response.

microbes bacteria, viruses, fungi, or other organisms invisible to the naked eye, some of which cause diseases. Also called *microorganisms*.

hormones chemicals that are secreted by glands into the blood in response to conditions in the body that require regulation. These chemicals serve as messengers, acting on other organs to maintain appropriate conditions.

glands body organs that produce and release needed compounds, such as sweat, saliva, and hormones.

For example, hormones are produced to regulate the body's blood **glucose** concentration, a condition that is vitally important to the functioning of many other organs, including the brain. The **pancreas**, a gland, produces two hormones: **insulin**, which lowers the blood glucose level when it is too high, and **glucagon**, which raises blood glucose when it is too low. The pancreas, together with the liver and other major organs are diagrammed in a later figure (see Figure 3–7, p. 78).

Nutrition affects the hormonal system. In people who become very thin, for example, an altered hormonal balance causes their bones to lose minerals and weaken. Overly thin women may also cease to menstruate, a process regulated by hormones.

The hormonal system also affects nutrition. Hormones:

- Carry messages to regulate the digestive system in response to meals or fasting.
- Inform the brain about the degree of body fatness.
- Help to regulate hunger and appetite.
- Influence appetite changes during a woman's menstrual cycle and in pregnancy.
- Regulate the body's reaction to stress, suppressing hunger and digestion.

In addition, an altered hormonal state contributes to the loss of appetite that sick people often experience. When there are questions about a person's nutrition or health, the state of that person's hormones is often part of the answer.

KEY POINT

- Glands secrete hormones that act as messengers to help regulate body processes.

How Does the Nervous System Interact with Nutrition?

The body's other major communication system is, of course, the nervous system. With the brain and spinal cord as central controllers, the nervous system receives and integrates information from sensory receptors all over the body—sight, hearing, touch, smell, taste, and others—which communicate to the brain the state of both the outer and the inner worlds, including the availability of food and the appetite for it. The nervous system also sends instructions to the muscles and glands, telling them what to do.

The nervous system's role in hunger regulation is coordinated by the brain. The sensations of hunger and appetite are perceived by the brain's **cortex**, the thinking, outer layer. Deep inside the brain, the **hypothalamus** (see Figure 3–5) monitors many body conditions, including the availability of nutrients and water. To signal hunger, the physiological need for food, the digestive tract sends messages to the hypothalamus by way of hormones and nerves. The signals also stimulate the stomach to intensify its contractions and secretions, causing hunger pangs (and gurgling sounds). When your brain's cortex perceives these hunger sensations, you want to eat. The conscious mind of the cortex, however, can override such signals, and a person can choose to delay eating despite hunger or to eat when hunger is absent.

In a marvelous adaptation of the human body, the hormonal and nervous systems work together to enable a person to respond to physical danger. Known as the **fight-or-flight reaction**, or the *stress response*, this adaptation is present with only minor variations in all animals, showing how universally important it is to survival. When danger is detected, nerves release **neurotransmitters**, and glands supply the compounds **epinephrine** and **norepinephrine**. Every organ of the body responds, and **metabolism** speeds up. The pupils of the eyes widen so that you can see better; the muscles tense up so that you can jump, run, or struggle with maximum strength; breathing quickens and deepens to provide more oxygen. The heart races to rush the oxygen to the muscles, and the blood pressure rises

glucose a carbohydrate fuel present in the bloodstream. For optimal functioning and health, the blood glucose concentration must be maintained within a range neither too high nor too low. Also defined in Chapter 4.

pancreas a gland that produces the hormones insulin and glucagon, which regulate blood glucose concentrations. It also produces digestive enzymes, which it releases through a duct into the small intestine.

insulin a hormone from the pancreas that prompts cells to withdraw glucose from the blood (see details in Chapter 4).

glucagon a hormone from the pancreas that stimulates the liver to release glucose into the blood when necessary to raise its concentration.

cortex the outermost layer of something. The brain's cortex is the part of the brain where conscious thought takes place.

hypothalamus (high-poh-THAL-uh-mus) a part of the brain that senses a variety of conditions in the body, such as temperature, glucose content, salt content, and others. It signals other parts of the brain or body to adjust those conditions when necessary.

fight-or-flight reaction the body's instinctive hormone- and nerve-mediated reaction to danger. Also known as the *stress response*.

neurotransmitters chemicals that are released at the end of a nerve cell when a nerve impulse arrives there. They diffuse across the gap to the next cell and alter the membrane of that second cell to either inhibit or excite it.

epinephrine (EP-ih-NEFF-rin) the major hormone that elicits the stress response.

norepinephrine (NOR-EP-ih-NEFF-rin) a compound related to epinephrine that helps elicit the stress response.

metabolism the sum of all physical and chemical changes taking place in living cells; includes all reactions by which the body obtains and spends the energy from food.

Figure 3–5

Cutaway Side View of the Brain Showing the Hypothalamus and Cortex

The hypothalamus monitors the body's conditions and sends signals to the brain's thinking portion, the cortex, which decides on actions. The pituitary gland is called the body's master gland, referring to its roles in regulating the activities of other glands and organs of the body.

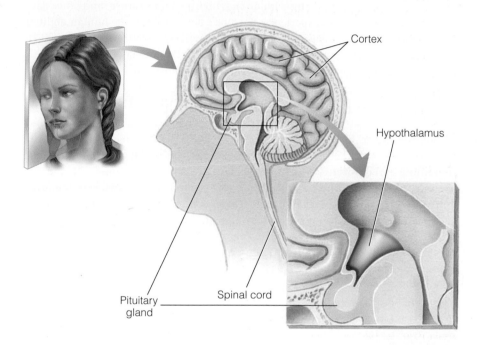

so that the fuel the muscles need for energy can be delivered efficiently. The liver pours forth glucose from its stores, and the fat cells release fat. The digestive system shuts down to permit all the body's systems to serve the muscles and nerves. With all action systems at peak efficiency, the body can respond with amazing speed and strength to whatever threatens it.

In ancient times, stress usually involved physical danger, and the response to it was violent physical exertion. In the modern world, stress is seldom physical, but the body reacts the same way. What stresses you today may be a checkbook out of control or a teacher who suddenly announces a pop quiz. Under these stresses, you are not supposed to fight or run, as your ancient ancestors did. You smile at the "enemy" and suppress your fear. But your heart races, you feel it pounding, and hormones still flood your bloodstream with glucose and fat.

Your number-one enemy today is not a saber-toothed tiger prowling outside your cave but a disease of modern civilization: heart disease. Years of fat and other constituents accumulating in the arteries and stresses that strain the heart often lead to heart attacks, especially when a body accustomed to chronic underexertion experiences sudden high blood pressure. Daily exercise as part of a healthy lifestyle releases pent-up stress and helps to protect the heart.

KEY POINT

- The nervous system and hormonal system regulate body processes, respond to the need for food, govern the act of eating, regulate digestion, and call for the stress response when needed.

The Digestive System

LO 3.4   Summarize how the digestive system provides nutrients to the body tissues.

When your body needs food, your brain and hormones alert your conscious mind by producing the sensation of hunger. Then, when you eat, your taste buds guide you in judging whether foods are acceptable.

Taste buds on the tongue contain surface structures that detect five basic chemical tastes: sweet, sour, bitter, salty, and umami (ooh-MOM-ee), the Asian name for *savory*. These basic tastes, along with aroma, texture, temperature, and other flavor elements, affect a person's experience of a food's flavor. In fact, the human ability to detect a food's aroma is thousands of times more sensitive than the sense of taste. The nose can detect just a few molecules responsible for the aroma of frying bacon, for example, even when they are diluted in several rooms full of air.

Why Do People Like Sugar, Salt, and Fat?

Sweet, salty, and fatty foods are almost universally desired, but most people have aversions to bitter and sour tastes (see Figure 3–6). The enjoyment of sugars is inborn and encourages people to consume ample energy, especially in the form of foods containing carbohydrates, which provide energy fuel for the brain.[1*] The pleasure of a salty taste prompts eaters to consume sufficient amounts of two very important minerals—sodium and chloride. Likewise, foods containing fats provide concentrated energy and essential nutrients needed by all body tissues. The aversion to bitterness, universally displayed in infants, discourages consumption of potentially dangerous substances containing bitter toxins. Unfortunately, an aversion to bitter tastes in infancy may persist in later life as an aversion to health-promoting vegetables with only slightly bitter flavors, such as turnips and broccoli.

Figure 3–6

The Innate Preference for Sweet Taste

This newborn baby is (a) resting; (b) tasting distilled water; (c) tasting sugar; (d) tasting something sour; and (e) tasting something bitter

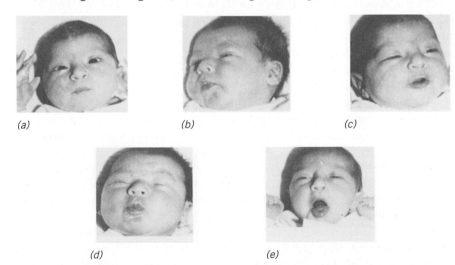

(a)   (b)   (c)

(d)   (e)

Source: Courtesy of Classic studies of J. E. Steiner, in Taste and Development: The Genesis of Sweet Preference, *ed. J. M. Weiffenbach, HHS publication no. NIH 77-1068 (Bethesda, MD: U.S. Department of Health and Human Services, 1977), pp. 173–189, with permission of the author.*

---

* Reference notes are in Appendix F.

The instinctive liking for sugar, salt, and fat can lead to drastic overeating of these substances. Sugar has become widely available in pure form only in the last hundred years, so it is relatively new to the human diet. Salt and fat have been around for much longer, but our tastes have not evolved to resist any of the three. Today, all three substances are added liberally to foods by manufacturers to tempt us to eat their products.

BW Folsom/Shutterstock.com

KEY POINT

- The preference for sweet, salty, and fatty tastes is inborn and can lead to overconsumption of foods that offer them.

The Digestive Tract Structures

Once you have eaten, your nervous system and hormones direct the many organs of the **digestive system** to **digest** and **absorb** the complex mixture of chewed and swallowed food. A diagram showing the digestive tract and associated organs appears in Figure 3–7, p. 78. The tract itself is a flexible, muscular tube extending from the mouth through the throat, esophagus, stomach, small intestine, large intestine, and rectum to the anus, for a total length of about 26 feet. The human body surrounds this digestive canal. When you swallow something, it still is not inside your body—it is only inside the inner bore of this tube. Only when a nutrient or other substance passes through the wall of the digestive tract does it actually enter the body's tissues. Many things pass into the digestive tract and out again, unabsorbed. A baby playing with beads may swallow one, but the bead will not really enter the body. It will emerge from the digestive tract within a day or two.

The digestive system's job is to digest food to its components and then to absorb the nutrients and some nonnutrients, leaving behind the substances, such as fiber, that are appropriate to excrete. To do this, the system works at two levels: one, mechanical; the other, chemical.

KEY POINTS

- The digestive tract is a flexible, muscular tube that digests food and absorbs its nutrients and some nonnutrients.
- Ancillary digestive organs, such as the pancreas and gallbladder, aid digestion.

The Mechanical Aspect of Digestion

The job of mechanical digestion begins in the mouth, where large, solid food pieces such as bites of meat are torn into shreds that can be swallowed without choking. Chewing also adds water in the form of saliva to soften rough or sharp foods, such as fried tortilla chips, to prevent them from injuring the esophagus. Saliva also moistens and coats each bite of food, making it slippery so that it can pass easily down the esophagus.

Nutrients trapped inside indigestible skins, such as the hulls of seeds, must be liberated by breaking these skins before they can be digested. Chewing bursts open kernels of corn, for example, which would otherwise traverse the tract and exit undigested. Once food has been mashed and moistened for comfortable swallowing, longer chewing times provide no additional advantages to digestion. In fact, for digestion's sake, a relaxed, peaceful attitude during a meal aids digestion much more than chewing for an extended time.

The stomach and intestines then take up the task of liquefying foods through various mashing and squeezing actions. The best known of these actions is **peristalsis**, a series of squeezing waves that start with the tongue's movement during a swallow and pass all the way down the esophagus (see Figure 3–8, p. 79). The stomach and intestines also push food through the tract by waves of peristalsis. Besides these actions, the **stomach** holds swallowed food for a while and mashes it into a fine paste; the stomach and intestines also add water so that the paste becomes more fluid as it moves along.

digestive system the body system composed of organs that break down complex food particles into smaller, absorbable products. The *digestive tract* and *alimentary canal* are names for the tubular organs that extend from the mouth to the anus. The whole system, including the pancreas, liver, and gallbladder, is sometimes called the *gastrointestinal*, or *GI*, system.

digest to break molecules into smaller molecules; a main function of the digestive tract with respect to food.

absorb to take in, as nutrients are taken into the intestinal cells after digestion; the main function of the digestive tract with respect to nutrients.

peristalsis (perri-STALL-sis) the wavelike muscular squeezing of the esophagus, stomach, and small intestine that pushes their contents along.

stomach a muscular, elastic, pouchlike organ of the digestive tract that grinds and churns swallowed food and mixes it with acid and enzymes, forming chyme.

Figure 3-7

The Digestive System

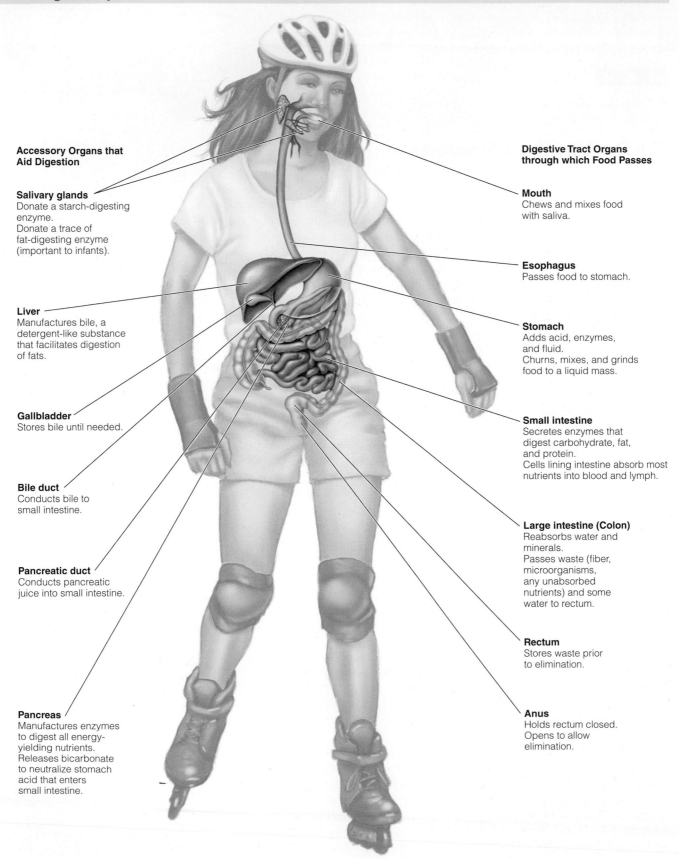

Accessory Organs that Aid Digestion

Salivary glands
Donate a starch-digesting enzyme.
Donate a trace of fat-digesting enzyme (important to infants).

Liver
Manufactures bile, a detergent-like substance that facilitates digestion of fats.

Gallbladder
Stores bile until needed.

Bile duct
Conducts bile to small intestine.

Pancreatic duct
Conducts pancreatic juice into small intestine.

Pancreas
Manufactures enzymes to digest all energy-yielding nutrients.
Releases bicarbonate to neutralize stomach acid that enters small intestine.

Digestive Tract Organs through which Food Passes

Mouth
Chews and mixes food with saliva.

Esophagus
Passes food to stomach.

Stomach
Adds acid, enzymes, and fluid.
Churns, mixes, and grinds food to a liquid mass.

Small intestine
Secretes enzymes that digest carbohydrate, fat, and protein.
Cells lining intestine absorb most nutrients into blood and lymph.

Large intestine (Colon)
Reabsorbs water and minerals.
Passes waste (fiber, microorganisms, any unabsorbed nutrients) and some water to rectum.

Rectum
Stores waste prior to elimination.

Anus
Holds rectum closed.
Opens to allow elimination.

Figure 3–8

Peristaltic Wave Passing Down the Esophagus and Beyond

Peristalsis moves the digestive tract contents.

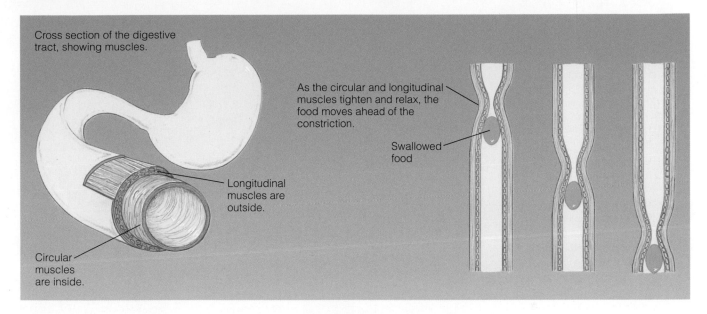

Cross section of the digestive tract, showing muscles.

As the circular and longitudinal muscles tighten and relax, the food moves ahead of the constriction.

Swallowed food

Longitudinal muscles are outside.

Circular muscles are inside.

Figure 3–9 shows the muscles of the stomach. Notice the circular **sphincter** muscle at the base of the esophagus. It squeezes the opening at the entrance to the stomach to narrow it and prevent the stomach's contents from creeping back up the esophagus as the stomach contracts. Swallowed food remains in a lump in the stomach's upper portion, squeezed little by little to its lower portion. There the food is ground and churned thoroughly, ensuring that digestive chemicals mix with the entire thick, liquid mass, now called **chyme**. Chyme bears no resemblance to the original food. The starches have been partly split, proteins have been uncoiled and clipped, and fat has separated from the mass.

The stomach also acts as a holding tank. The muscular **pyloric valve** at the stomach's lower end (look again at Figure 3–9) controls the exit of the chyme, allowing only a little at a time to be squirted forcefully into the **small intestine**. Within a few hours after a meal, the stomach empties itself by means of these powerful squirts. The small intestine contracts rhythmically to move the contents along its length.

By the time the intestinal contents have arrived in the **large intestine** (also called the **colon**), digestion and absorption are nearly complete. The colon's task is mostly to reabsorb the water donated earlier by digestive organs and to absorb minerals, leaving a paste of fiber and other undigested materials, the **feces**, suitable for excretion. The fiber provides bulk against which the muscles of the colon can work. The rectum stores this fecal material to be excreted at intervals. From mouth to rectum, the transit of a meal is accomplished in as short a time as a single day or as long as three days.

Some people wonder whether the digestive tract works best at certain hours in the day and whether the timing of meals can affect how a person feels. Timing of meals is important to feeling well, not because the digestive tract is unable to digest food at certain times but because the body requires nutrients to be replenished every few hours. Digestion is virtually continuous, slowing only during sleep and exercise. For some people, eating late may interfere with normal sleep. As for exercise, it is best pursued a few hours after eating because digestion can inhibit physical work (see Chapter 10 for details).

sphincter (SFINK-ter) a circular muscle surrounding, and able to constrict, a body opening.

chyme (KIME) the fluid resulting from the actions of the stomach upon a meal.

pyloric (pye-LORE-ick) **valve** the flap of muscle tissues of the lower stomach that regulates the flow of partly digested food into the small intestine and prevents backflow. Also called *pyloric sphincter*.

small intestine the 20-foot length of small-diameter intestine, below the stomach and above the large intestine, which is the major site of food digestion and nutrient absorption.

large intestine the portion of the intestine that completes the absorption process.

colon the large intestine.

feces waste material remaining after digestion and absorption are complete; eventually discharged from the body.

Table 3–1

Digestive Enzyme Terms

Over 30 digestive enzymes reduce food in the human digestive tract into nutrients that can be absorbed. Naming them all is beyond the scope of this book, but some general enzyme terms may prove useful.

- **-ase** (ACE) a suffix meaning *enzyme*. Categories of digestive and other enzymes and individual enzyme names often contain this suffix.
- **carbohydrase** (car-boh-HIGH-drace) any of a number of enzymes that break the chemical bonds of carbohydrates.
- **lipase** (LYE-pace) any of a number of enzymes that break the chemical bonds of fats (lipids).
- **protease** (PRO-tee-ace) any of a number of enzymes that break the chemical bonds of proteins.

Figure 3–9

The Muscular Stomach

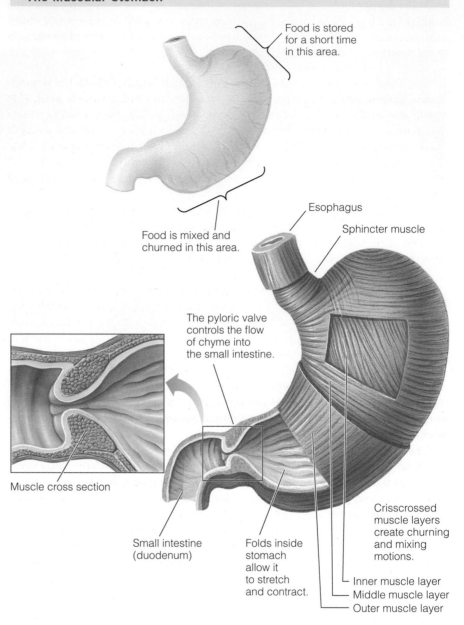

Food is stored for a short time in this area.

Food is mixed and churned in this area.

Esophagus

Sphincter muscle

The pyloric valve controls the flow of chyme into the small intestine.

Muscle cross section

Small intestine (duodenum)

Folds inside stomach allow it to stretch and contract.

Crisscrossed muscle layers create churning and mixing motions.

Inner muscle layer
Middle muscle layer
Outer muscle layer

gastric juice the digestive secretion of the stomach.

hydrochloric acid a strong, corrosive acid of hydrogen and chloride atoms, produced by the stomach to assist in digestion.

pH a measure of acidity on a point scale. A solution with a pH of 1 is a strong acid; a solution with a pH of 7 is neutral; a solution with a pH of 14 is a strong base.

mucus (MYOO-cus) a slippery coating of the digestive tract lining (and other body linings) that protects the cells from exposure to digestive juices (and other destructive agents). The adjective form is *mucous* (same pronunciation). The digestive tract lining is a *mucous membrane*.

KEY POINTS

- The mechanical digestive actions include chewing, mixing by the stomach, adding fluid, and moving the tract's contents by peristalsis.
- After digestion and absorption, wastes are excreted.

The Chemical Aspect of Digestion

Several organs of the digestive system secrete special digestive juices that perform the complex chemical processes of digestion. Digestive juices contain enzymes that break down nutrients into their component parts. (Table 3–1 presents some enzyme terms.) The digestive organs that release digestive juices are the salivary glands, the stomach, the pancreas, the liver, and the small intestine. Their secretions were listed in Figure 3–7 (p. 78).

In the Mouth Digestion begins in the mouth. An enzyme in saliva starts rapidly breaking down starch, and another enzyme initiates a little digestion of fat, especially the digestion of milk fat (important in infants). Saliva also helps maintain the health of the teeth in two ways: by washing away food particles that would otherwise create decay and by neutralizing decay-promoting acids produced by bacteria in the mouth.

In the Stomach In the stomach, protein digestion begins. Cells in the stomach release **gastric juice**, a mixture of water, enzymes, and **hydrochloric acid**. This strong acid mixture is needed to activate a protein-digesting enzyme and to initiate digestion of protein—protein digestion is the stomach's main function. The strength of an acid solution is expressed as its **pH**. The lower the pH number, the more acidic the solution; solutions with higher pH numbers are more basic. As Figure 3–10 demonstrates, saliva is only weakly acidic; the stomach's gastric juice is much more strongly acidic.

Upon learning of the powerful digestive juices and enzymes within the digestive tract, students often wonder how the tract's own cellular lining escapes being digested along with the food. The answer: specialized cells secrete a thick, viscous substance known as **mucus**, which coats and protects the digestive tract lining.

In the Intestine In the small intestine, the digestive process gets under way in earnest. The small intestine is *the* organ of digestion and absorption; it finishes what the mouth and stomach have started. The small intestine works with the precision of a laboratory chemist. As the thoroughly liquefied and partially digested nutrient mixture arrives there, hormonal messengers signal the gallbladder to contract and to squirt the right amount of **bile**, an **emulsifier**, into the intestine. Other hormones notify the pancreas to release **pancreatic juice**, containing the alkaline compound **bicarbonate**, in amounts precisely adjusted to neutralize the stomach acid that has reached the small intestine. All these actions adjust the intestinal environment to perfectly support the work of the digestive enzymes.

Meanwhile, as the pancreatic and intestinal enzymes act on the chemical bonds that hold the large nutrients together, smaller and smaller pieces are released into the intestinal fluids. The cells of the intestinal wall also hold some digestive enzymes on their surfaces; these enzymes perform last-minute breakdown reactions required before nutrients can be absorbed. Finally, the digestive process releases pieces small enough for the cells to absorb and use. Digestion by human enzymes and absorption of carbohydrate, fat, and protein are essentially complete by the time the intestinal contents enter the colon. Water, fiber, and some minerals, however, remain in the tract. And the bead swallowed by the baby mentioned earlier? It's in the colon, awaiting excretion with the feces.

KEY POINTS

- Chemical digestion begins in the mouth, where food is mixed with an enzyme in saliva that acts on carbohydrates.
- Digestion continues in the stomach, where stomach enzymes and acid break down protein.
- Digestion progresses in the small intestine, where the liver and gallbladder contribute bile that emulsifies fat, and the pancreas and small intestine donate enzymes that break down food to nutrients.

Microbes in the Digestive Tract

Certain remnants of food, largely fibers, not digested by human enzymes in the small intestine are often broken down by billions of living inhabitants in the colon, collectively called the **microbiota** (Table 3–2 defines microbe terms, p. 82). A healthy digestive tract is home to *trillions* of microbes of many species (Figure 3–11, p. 82, shows one of them). The bacteria alone outnumber the cells of the body tenfold.[2] Bacteria in the colon are so efficient at fermenting and breaking down substances from food that they have been

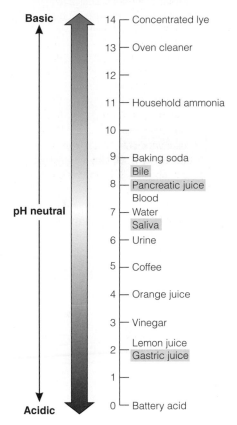

Figure 3–10

pH Values of Digestive Juices and Other Common Fluids

A substance's acidity or alkalinity is measured in pH units. Each step down the scale indicates a tenfold increase in concentration of hydrogen particles, which determine acidity. For example, a pH of 2 is 1,000 times stronger than a pH of 5.

Basic		14 — Concentrated lye
		13 — Oven cleaner
		12
		11 — Household ammonia
		10
		9 — Baking soda
		Bile
		8 — Pancreatic juice
		Blood
pH neutral		7 — Water
		Saliva
		6 — Urine
		5 — Coffee
		4 — Orange juice
		3 — Vinegar
		Lemon juice
		2 — Gastric juice
		1
Acidic		0 — Battery acid

bile a digestive fluid made by the liver, stored in the gallbladder, and released into the small intestine when needed. It emulsifies fats and oils to ready them for enzymatic digestion (described in Chapter 5).

emulsifier (ee-MULL-sih-fire) a compound with both water-soluble and fat-soluble portions that can attract fats and oils into water, dispersing them.

pancreatic juice fluid secreted by the pancreas that contains both enzymes to digest carbohydrates, fats, and proteins and sodium bicarbonate, an acid-neutralizing agent.

bicarbonate a common alkaline chemical; a secretion of the pancreas. (Sodium bicarbonate is baking soda.)

Table 3–2

Microbe Terms

intestinal flora intestinal bacteria.
microbiome the collective genes of a specific bacterial sample; for example, the particular array of bacterial species present in an individual's fecal sample.
microbiota any collection of microbes; for example, all of the bacteria, fungi, and viruses present in a person's digestive tract.

Figure 3–11

A Bacterium of the Digestive Tract

Enterococcus faecalis, one of the thousands of bacterial species living in the human digestive tract.

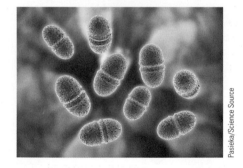

Pasieka/Science Source

adipose tissue the body's fat tissue, consisting of masses of fat-storing cells and blood vessels to nourish them.

likened to a body organ specializing in nutrient salvage. Table 3–3 (p. 83) presents a summary of digestion, including the actions of the bacteria.

Bacterial Activities   Digestive tract bacteria harvest energy from undigested food substances and use it to sustain themselves and to proliferate. In the process, they yield smaller molecules that the body can absorb and use.[3] For example, bacteria:

- Ferment many indigestible fibers, producing short fatty acids that many cells of the colon rely on for energy.
- Break down any undigested protein or unabsorbed amino acids that reach the colon, producing ammonia and other compounds.[†]
- Break down and help to recycle components of bile.
- Chemically alter certain drugs and phytochemicals, changing their effects on the body.

Bacteria produce several vitamins, too, but in amounts insufficient to meet the body's needs, so these vitamins must be obtained from the diet.

Good or Bad Bacteria?   The intestinal bacteria may affect the health and functioning of many body systems.[4] Microbes generate compounds that communicate with such diverse tissues as muscle, **adipose tissue** (see Chapter 9), and even the brain.[5] They also deliver messages to the immune system, that may facilitate immune defenses. Research suggests that, when the mix of bacterial species falls out of balance, potentially harmful bacteria proliferate, producing substances that increase inflammation and that are associated with obesity, diabetes, several intestinal conditions, fatty liver disease, certain cancers, and even asthma.[6]

Food intake largely controls the mix of species in intestinal bacteria. A steady diet of meats, fats, and ultra-processed foods (defined in Chapter 1) lacks the beneficial bacterial hitchhikers that ride into the digestive system in yogurt or other foods that contain live cultures. Such a diet is also stripped of the fibers upon which beneficial bacteria feed, and lacking proper food, beneficial colonies collapse. Then, unhindered by competition, less helpful and even harmful species rapidly multiply. Maintaining healthful microbiota is simple: include sources of beneficial bacteria in the diet and consume mostly whole foods to provide the fiber upon which beneficial bacteria can thrive.

Chapter 4 lists fiber-containing foods that support intestinal health.

KEY POINTS

- A substantial population of intestinal bacteria scavenges and breaks down fibers and other undigested compounds.
- The colon absorbs and uses products of bacterial metabolism; the bacteria and their products also interact with other organs and tissues.
- Diet strongly influences the composition and metabolism of the intestinal bacteria.

Are Some Food Combinations More Easily Digested than Others?

People sometimes wonder if the digestive tract has trouble digesting certain foods in combination—for example, fruit and meat. Proponents of fad "food-combining" diets claim that the digestive tract cannot perform more than one digestive task at a time, but this is a gross underestimation of the tract's capabilities. The digestive system adjusts to whatever mixture of foods is presented to it. The truth is that all foods, regardless of identity, are broken down by enzymes into the basic molecules that make them up. The next section reviews the major processes of digestion by showing how the nutrients in a mixture of foods are handled.

KEY POINT

- The healthy digestive system can adjust to almost any diet and handle any combination of foods with ease.

[†]Bacterial action on lipid is insignificant.

Table 3-3

Summary of Digestion

Food Constituent	Mouth	Stomach	Small Intestine, Pancreas, Liver, and Gallbladder	Large Intestine (Colon)
Sugar and Starch	The salivary glands secrete saliva to moisten and lubricate food; chewing crushes and mixes it with a salivary enzyme that initiates starch digestion.	Digestion of starch continues while food remains in the upper storage area of the stomach. In the lower digesting area of the stomach, hydrochloric acid and an enzyme in the stomach's juices halt starch digestion.	The pancreas produces a starch-digesting enzyme and releases it into the small intestine. Cells in the intestinal lining possess enzymes on their surfaces that break sugars and starch fragments into simple sugars, which then are absorbed.	Undigested carbohydrates reach the large intestine and are partly broken down by intestinal bacteria.
Fiber	The teeth crush fiber and mix it with saliva to moisten it for swallowing.	No action.	Fiber binds cholesterol and some minerals.	Most fiber is excreted with the feces; some fiber is digested by bacteria in the large intestine.
Fat	Fat-rich foods are mixed with saliva. The tongue produces traces of a fat-digesting enzyme that accomplishes some breakdown, especially of milk fats. The enzyme is stable at low pH and is important to digestion in nursing infants.	Fat tends to rise from the watery stomach fluid and foods and float on top of the mixture. Only a small amount of fat is digested. Fat is last to leave the stomach.	The liver secretes bile; the gallbladder stores it and releases it into the small intestine. Bile emulsifies the fat and readies it for enzyme action. The pancreas produces fat-digesting enzymes and releases them into the small intestine to split fats into their component parts (primarily fatty acids), which then are absorbed.	Some fatty materials escape absorption and are carried out of the body with other wastes.
Protein	Chewing crushes and softens protein-rich foods and mixes them with saliva.	Stomach acid (hydrochloric acid) works to uncoil protein strands and to activate the stomach's protein-digesting enzyme. Then the enzyme breaks the protein strands into smaller fragments.	Enzymes of the small intestine and pancreas split protein fragments into smaller fragments or free amino acids. Enzymes on the cells of the intestinal lining break some protein fragments into free amino acids, which then are absorbed. Some protein fragments are also absorbed.	Resident bacteria break down small amounts of undigested protein and amino acids; any remaining residue is carried out of the body with the feces. Normally, almost all food protein is digested and absorbed.
Water	The mouth donates watery, enzyme-containing saliva.	The stomach donates acidic, watery, enzyme-containing gastric juice.	The liver donates a watery juice containing bile. The pancreas and small intestine add watery, enzyme-containing juices.	The large intestine reabsorbs water and some minerals.

If "I Am What I Eat," Then How Does a Peanut Butter Sandwich Become "Me"?

The process of rendering foods into nutrients and absorbing them into the body fluids is remarkably efficient. Within about 24 to 48 hours of eating, a healthy body digests and absorbs about 90 percent of the carbohydrate, fat, and protein in a meal. Figure 3–12 illustrates a typical 24-hour transit time through the digestive system.[7] Next, we follow a peanut butter and banana sandwich on whole-wheat sesame-seed bread through the tract.

Figure 3–12

Typical Digestive System Transit Times

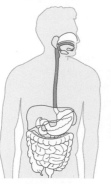

Time in mouth, less than a minute.

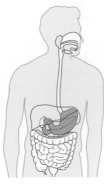

Time in stomach, about 1–2 hours.

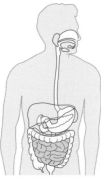

Time in small intestine, about 7–8 hours.*

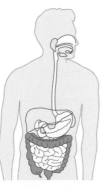

Time in colon, about 12–14 hours.*

Based on a 24-hour transit time. Actual times vary widely.

Figure 3–13

Microvilli on an Intestinal Villus Cell

This photomicrograph shows the microvilli on a single cell of an intestinal villus.

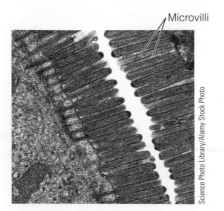

Microvilli

Science Photo Library/Alamy Stock Photo

In the Mouth In each bite, the teeth and tongue crush, mash, and mix food components with saliva. The sesame seeds are crushed and torn open by the teeth, which break through the indigestible fiber coating so that digestive enzymes can reach the nutrients inside the seeds. The peanut butter is the "extra crunchy" type, but the teeth grind the chunks to a paste before swallowing. The carbohydrate-digesting enzyme of saliva begins to break down the starch of the bread, banana, and peanut butter to sugars. Each swallow triggers a peristaltic wave that travels the length of the esophagus and carries one chewed bite of sandwich to the stomach.

In the Stomach The stomach collects bite after swallowed bite in its upper storage area, where starch continues to be digested until the gastric juice mixes with the salivary enzymes and halts their action. Small portions of the mashed sandwich are pushed into the digesting area of the stomach, where gastric juice mixes with the mass. Acid in the gastric juice unwinds proteins from the bread, seeds, and peanut butter; then an enzyme clips the protein strands into pieces. The sandwich has now become chyme. The watery, carbohydrate- and protein-rich part of the chyme enters the small intestine first; a layer of fat follows closely behind.

In the Small Intestine Some of the sweet sugars in the banana require so little digesting that they begin to cross the linings of the small intestine immediately on contact. Nearby, the liver donates bile through a duct into the small intestine. The bile blends the fat from the peanut butter and seeds with the watery, enzyme-containing digestive fluids. The nearby pancreas squirts enzymes into the small intestine to break down the fat, protein, and starch in the chemical soup that just an hour ago was a sandwich. The cells of the small intestine itself produce enzymes that complete these processes. As the enzymes do their work, smaller and smaller chemical fragments are liberated from the chemical soup and are absorbed into the blood and lymph through the cells of the small intestine's wall. Vitamins and minerals are absorbed here, too. They all eventually enter the bloodstream to nourish the tissues.

In the Large Intestine (Colon) Only fiber fragments, fluid, and some minerals are absorbed in the large intestine. The fibers from the seeds, whole-wheat bread, peanut butter, and banana are partly digested by the bacteria living in the colon, and some of the products are absorbed. Most fiber is not digested, however, and it passes out of the colon along with some other components, excreted as feces.

KEY POINT

- The mechanical and chemical actions of the digestive tract efficiently break down foods to nutrients and then large nutrients to their smaller building blocks.

Absorption and Transport of Nutrients

Once the digestive system has broken down food to its nutrient components, the rest of the body awaits their delivery. First, though, every molecule of nutrient must traverse one of the cells of the intestinal lining. These cells absorb nutrients from the mixture within the intestine and deposit the water-soluble compounds in the blood and the fat-soluble ones in the lymph. The cells are selective: they recognize that some nutrients may be in short supply in the diet. Take the mineral calcium, for example. The less calcium in the diet, the greater the percentage of calcium the intestinal cells absorb from the intestinal contents. The cells are also extraordinarily efficient: they absorb enough nutrients to nourish all the body's other cells.

The Intestine's Absorbing Surface The cells of the intestinal tract lining are arranged in sheets that poke out into millions of finger-shaped projections (**villi**). Every cell on every villus has a brushlike covering of tiny hairlike projections (**microvilli**) that entrap the nutrient particles. Each villus (projection) has its own capillary network and a lymph vessel, so that as nutrients move across the cells, they can immediately mingle with the body fluids. Figure 3–13 provides a

Chapter 3 The Remarkable Body

Figure 3–14

Details of the Small Intestinal Lining

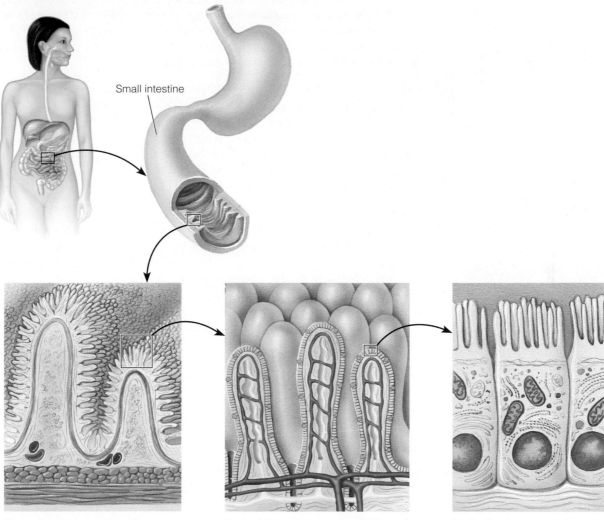

Small intestine

The walls of the small intestine are wrinkled into thousands of folds covered with villi.

Each villus contains a network of capillaries and lymphatic vessels for transporting nutrients out of the intestinal cells.

Each villus is made of absorptive cells that are covered with even smaller projections—the microvilli—that trap and absorb the nutrients.

Bill Crew/Superstock

close look at a single cell's microvilli, and Figure 3–14 gives an overview of the whole system.

The small intestine's lining, villi and all, is wrinkled into thousands of folds, so its absorbing surface is enormous. If the folds, and the villi that poke out from them, were spread out flat, they would cover a third of a football field. The billions of cells of that surface weigh only 4 to 5 pounds, yet they absorb enough nutrients to nourish the other 150 or so pounds of body tissues.

Nutrient Transport in the Blood and Lymph Vessels After the nutrients pass through the cells of the villi, the blood and lymph vessels transport the nutrients to their ultimate consumers, the body's cells. The lymph vessels initially transport most of the products of fat digestion and the fat-soluble vitamins, ultimately conveying them into a large blood vessel near the heart, as illustrated in Figure 3–15. The blood vessels directly transport the products of carbohydrate and protein digestion, most vitamins, and the minerals from the digestive tract to the liver. Thanks to these two transportation systems, every nutrient soon arrives at the place where it is needed.

villi (VILL-ee, VILL-eye) fingerlike projections of the sheets of cells lining the intestinal tract. The villi make the surface area much greater than it would otherwise be (*singular*: villus).

microvilli (MY-croh-VILL-ee, MY-croh-VILL-eye) tiny, hairlike projections on each cell of every villus that greatly expand the surface area available to trap nutrient particles and absorb them into the cells (*singular*: microvillus).

Figure 3–15

Lymph Vessels and the Bloodstream—Nutrient Flow through the Body

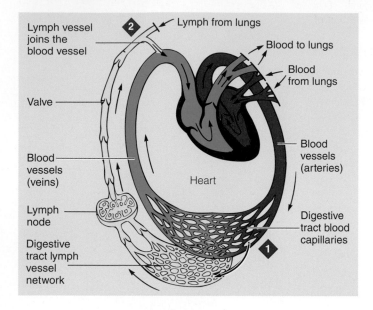

Lymph vessel joins the blood vessel

 Lymph from lungs

Blood to lungs

Blood from lungs

Valve

Blood vessels (arteries)

Heart

Blood vessels (veins)

Lymph node

Digestive tract blood capillaries

Digestive tract lymph vessel network

1. Nutrients are absorbed via two kinds of vessels in the intestines: blood capillaries and small lymph vessels. The capillaries lead to larger blood vessels that lead to the liver.

2. The lymph in the lymph vessels carries most of the absorbed dietary fat to the large vein near the heart. From there, the fat-laden lymph flows into the bloodstream.

Nourishment of the Digestive Tract The digestive system's millions of specialized cells are themselves highly sensitive to an undersupply of energy, nutrients, or dietary fiber. In cases of severe undernutrition with too little energy and nutrients, the absorptive surface of the small intestine shrinks. The surface may be reduced to a tenth of its normal area, preventing it from absorbing what few nutrients a limited food supply may provide. Without sufficient fiber to provide an undigested bulk for the tract's muscles to push against, the muscles become weak from lack of exercise. Malnutrition that impairs digestion is self-perpetuating because impaired digestion makes malnutrition worse.

The digestive system's needs are few, but important. The body has much to say to the attentive listener, stated in a language of symptoms and feelings that you would be wise to study. The next section takes a lighthearted look at what your digestive tract might be trying to tell you.

KEY POINTS

- The digestive system feeds the rest of the body and is itself sensitive to malnutrition.
- The folds and villi of the small intestine enlarge its surface area to facilitate nutrient absorption through countless cells to the blood and lymph, which deliver nutrients to all the body's cells.

A Letter from Your Digestive Tract

LO 3.5 Outline the symptoms of eight common digestive problems related to nutrition.

To My Owner,

You and I are so close; I hope that I can speak frankly without offending you. I know that sometimes I *do* offend with my gurgling noises and belching at quiet times and, oh yes, the gas. But, as you can read for yourself in Table 3–4, when you chew gum, drink carbonated beverages, or eat hastily, you gulp air with each swallow. I can't help making some noise as I move the air along my length or release it upward in a

Table 3–4

Foods and Intestinal Gas

Recent experiments have shed light on the causes and prevention of intestinal gas. Here are some recent findings.

Problem	Solution
Milk intake causes gas in those who cannot digest the milk sugar lactose. Most people, however, can consume up to a cup of milk without producing excessive gas.	Drink up to 4 ounces of fluid milk at a sitting, or substitute reduced-fat cheeses or yogurt without added milk solids. Use lactose-reduced milk, or treat regular milk with lactose-reducing enzyme products.
Beans cause gas because some of their carbohydrates are indigestible by human enzymes, but are broken down by intestinal bacteria. The amount of gas may not be as much as most people fear, however.	Use rinsed canned beans or dried beans that are well cooked, because cooked carbohydrates are more readily digestible. Try enzyme drops or pills that can help break down the carbohydrate before it reaches the intestine.
Air swallowed during eating or drinking can cause gas, as can the gas of carbonated beverages. Each swallow of a beverage can carry three times as much gas as fluid, which some people belch up.	Slow down during eating and drinking, and don't chew gum or suck on hard candies that may cause you to swallow air. Limit carbonated beverages.
Vegetables may or may not cause gas in some people, but research is lacking.	If you feel that certain vegetables cause gas, try eating small portions, cooked. Try the vegetable again: maybe the gas came from something else.

noisy belch. And if you eat or drink too fast, I can't help getting **hiccups** (definitions of common digestive problems appear in Table 3–5, p. 88). Please sit and relax while you dine. You will ease my task, and we'll both be happier.

Also, when someone offers you a new food, you gobble away, trusting me to do my job. I try. It would make my life easier, and yours less gassy, if you would start with small amounts of new foods, especially those high in fiber. The breakdown of fiber by bacteria produces gas, so introduce fiber-rich foods slowly. But, please, if you do notice more gas than normal from a specific food, avoid it. If the gas becomes excessive, check with a physician. The problem could be something simple—or serious.

When you eat or drink too much, it just burns me up. Overeating causes **heartburn** because the acidic juice from my stomach backs up into my esophagus. Acid poses no problem to my healthy stomach, whose walls are coated with thick mucus to protect them. But when my too-full stomach squeezes some of its contents back up into the esophagus, the acid burns its unprotected surface. Also, those tight jeans you wear constrict my stomach, squeezing the contents up into the esophagus. Just leaning over or lying down after a meal may do the same thing because the muscular sphincter separating the two spaces is much looser than other sphincters. And if we need to lose a few pounds, let's get at it—excess body fat can squeeze my stomach, too. When heartburn is a problem, do me a favor: try to eat smaller meals; drink liquids an hour before or after, but not during, meals; wear reasonably loose clothing; and relax after eating, but sit up (don't lie down). Don't smoke, and go easy on the alcohol and carbonated beverages, too—they all make heartburn likely.

Sometimes your food choices irritate me. Specifically, chemical irritants in foods, such as the "hot" component of chili peppers and the chemicals in coffee, as well as fat, chocolate, carbonated soft drinks, and alcohol, may worsen heartburn in some people. Avoid the ones that cause trouble. Above all, do not smoke. Smoking makes my heartburn worse—and you should hear your lungs bellyache about it.

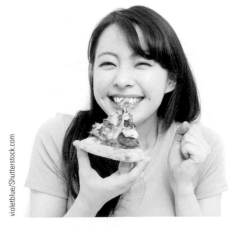

violetblue/Shutterstock.com

What is your digestive tract trying to tell you?

Table 3-5

Definitions of Selected Common Digestive Problems

These conditions occur frequently in the U.S. population.

constipation infrequent, difficult bowel movements, generally fewer than three per week, often caused by diet, inactivity, dehydration, or medication. Also defined in Chapter 4.

diarrhea frequent, watery bowel movements usually caused by diet, stress, or irritation of the colon. Severe, prolonged diarrhea robs the body of fluid and certain minerals, causing dehydration and imbalances that can be dangerous if left untreated.

gastroesophageal (GAS-tro-eh-SOFF-ahjeel) **reflux disease (GERD)** severe and chronic splashing of stomach acid and enzymes into the esophagus, throat, mouth, or airway that causes injury to those organs. Untreated GERD may increase the risk of esophageal cancer; treatment may require surgery or management with medication.

heartburn a burning sensation in the chest (in the area of the heart) caused by backflow of stomach acid into the esophagus.

hemorrhoids (HEM-or-oids) swollen, hardened (varicose) veins in the rectum, usually caused by pressure resulting from constipation.

hernia a protrusion of an organ or part of an organ through the wall of the body chamber that normally contains the organ. An example is a *hiatal* (high-AY-tal) *hernia*, in which part of the stomach protrudes up through the diaphragm into the chest cavity, which contains the esophagus, heart, and lungs.

hiccups spasms of both the vocal cords and the diaphragm, causing periodic, audible, short, inhaled coughs. These can result from irritation of the diaphragm, indigestion, or other causes. Hiccups usually resolve in a few minutes but can have serious effects if prolonged. Breathing into a paper bag (inhaling carbon dioxide) or dissolving a teaspoon of sugar in the mouth may stop them.

irritable bowel syndrome (IBS) intermittent disturbance of bowel function, especially diarrhea or alternating diarrhea and constipation, often with abdominal cramping or bloating; managed with diet, physical activity, or relief from psychological stress. The cause is uncertain, but inflammation is often involved, and a role for an altered intestinal microbiome is suspected. IBS does not permanently harm the intestines or lead to serious diseases.

ulcer an eroded spot in the topmost, and sometimes underlying, layers of cells that form a lining. Ulcers of the digestive tract commonly form in the esophagus, stomach, or upper small intestine.

Note: Other conditions, such as celiac disease and diverticulosis, are defined in later chapters—check the index at the back of the book.

By the way, I can tell you've been taking heartburn medicines again. You need to know that **antacids** are designed only to temporarily relieve pain caused by heartburn by neutralizing stomach acid for a while. But when the antacids reduce my normal stomach acidity, I respond by producing *more* acid to restore the normal acid condition. Also, the ingredients in antacids can interfere with my ability to absorb nutrients. Please check with our doctor if heartburn occurs more than just occasionally and certainly before you decide that we need to take the heavily advertised **acid reducers**; these restrict my normal ability to produce acid so much that my job of digesting food becomes harder.

Given a chance, my powerful stomach acid helps fight off many bacterial infections—most disease-causing bacteria won't survive a bath in my caustic juices. Acid-reducing drugs reduce acid (I'll bet you knew that), so they allow more bacteria to pass through.[8] And, even worse, self-prescribed heartburn medicine can mask the symptoms of **ulcer, hernia,** or the destructive form of chronic heartburn known as **gastroesophageal reflux disease (GERD).** This can be serious; the bacterium *H. pylori* that causes most ulcers responds to antibiotic drugs, but some ulcers have other causes, such as frequent use of certain painkillers—the *cause* of the ulcer must

antacids medications that react directly and immediately with the acid of the stomach, neutralizing it. Antacids are most suitable for treating occasional heartburn.

acid reducers prescription and over-the-counter drugs that reduce the acid output of the stomach; effective for treating severe, persistent forms of heartburn but not for neutralizing acid already present. Side effects are frequent and include diarrhea, other gastrointestinal complaints, and reduction of the stomach's capacity to destroy alcohol, thereby producing higher-than-expected blood alcohol levels from each drink (see this chapter's Controversy section). Also called *acid controllers*.

Chapter 3 The Remarkable Body

Figure 3–16

Normal Swallowing and Choking

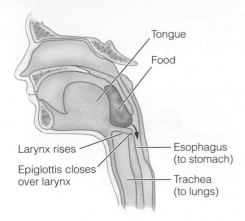

Tongue

Food

Larynx rises

Epiglottis closes over larynx

Esophagus (to stomach)

Trachea (to lungs)

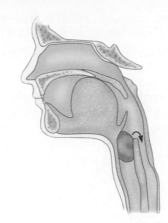

A normal swallow. The epiglottis acts as a flap to seal the entrance to the lungs (trachea) and direct food to the stomach via the esophagus.

Choking. A choking person cannot speak or gasp because food lodged in the airway (trachea) shuts off airflow. The red arrow points to where the food should have gone to prevent choking.

be treated, as well as its symptoms. A hernia can cause food to back up into the esophagus, so it can feel like heartburn, but many times hernias require corrective treatment by a physician, not antacids. GERD can feel like heartburn, too, but requires the correct drug therapy to prevent respiratory problems or damage to the esophagus that can lead to cancer.[9] So please don't wait too long to get medical help for chronic or severe heartburn—it may not be simple indigestion.

When you eat too quickly, I worry about choking (see Figure 3–16). Please take time to cut your food into small pieces and chew it until it is crushed and moistened with saliva. Also, refrain from talking or laughing before swallowing, and never attempt to eat when you are breathing hard. Also, for our sake and the sake of others, learn first aid for choking. An illustration is offered in Figure 3–17, p. 90.

When I'm suffering, you suffer, too, and when **constipation** or **diarrhea** strikes, neither of us is having fun. Slow, hard, dry bowel movements can be painful, and failing to have a movement for too long brings on headaches, backaches, stomachaches, and other ills. If chronic, constipation may cause **hemorrhoids**.[10] Most people suffer occasional harmless constipation, and laxatives may help, but too frequent use of laxatives and enemas can lead to dependency; can upset our fluid, salt, and mineral balances; and, in the case of mineral oil laxatives, can interfere with the absorption of fat-soluble vitamins. (Mineral oil, which is not absorbed, dissolves the vitamins and carries them out of the body with it.)

Instead of relying on laxatives, listen carefully for my signal that it is time to defecate, and make time for it even if you are busy. The longer you ignore my signal, the more time the colon has to extract water from the feces, hardening them. Also, please choose foods that provide enough fiber (some high-fiber foods are listed in Chapter 4, p. 133).‡ Fiber attracts water, creating softer, bulkier stools that stimulate my muscles to contract, pushing the contents along. Fiber helps my muscles to stay fit, too, making elimination easier. Be sure to drink enough water because dehydration causes the colon to absorb all the water it can get from the feces. And please make time to be physically active; exercise strengthens not just the muscles of arms, legs, and torso but those of the colon, too.

---

‡Rarely, a spastic, constricted bowel causes constipation; this condition requires medical attention, not fiber.

Figure 3–17

First Aid for Choking

First aid for choking relies on abdominal thrusts, sometimes called the Heimlich maneuver. If abdominal thrusts are not successful and the person loses consciousness, lower him to the floor, call 911, remove the object blocking the airway if possible, and begin CPR. Because there is no time for hesitation when called upon to perform this death-defying act, you would do well to take a life-saving course to learn these techniques.

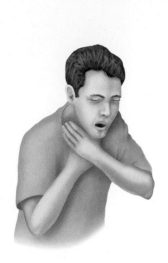

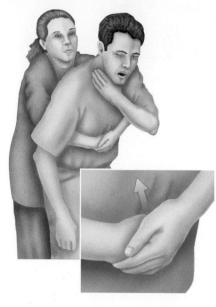

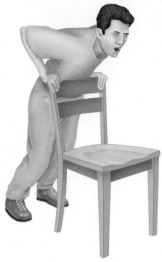

The universal signal for choking alerts others to the need for assistance.

Stand behind the person with your arms wrapped around him. Make a fist with one hand and place the thumb side snugly against the body, slightly above the navel and below the breastbone.

Grasp the fist with your other hand and make a quick upward and inward thrust. Repeat thrusts until the object is dislodged.

To perform abdominal thrusts on yourself, make a fist and place the thumb below your breast-bone and above your navel. Grasp your fist with your other hand and press inward with a quick upward thrust. Alternatively, quickly thrust your upper body against a table edge, chair, or railing.

When I have the opposite problem, diarrhea, my system will rob you of water and salts. In diarrhea, my intestinal contents have moved too quickly, drawing water and minerals from your tissues into the contents. When this happens, please rest a while and drink fluids (I prefer clear juices and broths). However, if diarrhea is bloody, or if it worsens or persists, call our doctor—severe diarrhea can be life-threatening.

To avoid diarrhea, try not to change my diet too drastically or quickly. I'm willing to work with you and learn to digest new foods, but if you suddenly change your diet, we're both in for it. I hate even to think of it, but one likely cause of diarrhea is food-borne illness. (*Please* read, and use, the tips in Chapter 12 to keep us safe.) Also, if diarrhea and abdominal pain occur more often than once a week, or if diarrhea alternates with constipation, it may signify **irritable bowel syndrome (IBS)**, and you should see a physician. In IBS, strong contractions speed up the intestinal contents, causing gas, bloating, diarrhea, and frequent or severe abdominal pain.[11] Weakened and slowed contractions may then follow, causing constipation. When you're stressed out, so am I, and stress may contribute to IBS. Try eating smaller meals, avoiding onions or other irritating foods, and using relaxation techniques or exercise to relieve mental stress.‡

---

‡Onions and certain other foods, along with sugar alcohols, contribute poorly digested carbohydrates known by the abbreviation FODMAP (fermentable oligosaccharides, disaccharides, monosaccharides, and polyols), which have been associated with IBS symptoms in some people.

If those don't work, by all means, call our doctor—IBS may respond to exercise, antibiotics, or antispasmodic drugs.[12]

By the way, I trust you not to believe false claims that health troubles can be solved by washing the colon with a powerful enema machine—in fact, this "colonic irrigation" is unnecessary and has caused illness and even some deaths from equipment contamination, electrolyte depletion, and intestinal perforation.

Thank you for listening. I know we'll both benefit from communicating like this because you and I are in this together for the long haul.

Affectionately,

Your Digestive Tract

KEY POINT

- Maintenance of a healthy digestive tract requires preventing or responding to symptoms with a carefully chosen diet and, when problems arise, sound medical care.

The Excretory System

LO 3.6   Specify the excretory functions of the lungs, liver, kidneys, and bladder.

Cells generate a number of wastes, and all of them must be eliminated. Many of the body's organs play roles in removing wastes. Carbon dioxide waste from the cells travels in the blood to the lungs, which exchange it for oxygen. Other wastes are pulled out of the bloodstream by the liver. The liver processes these wastes and either tosses them out into the digestive tract with bile, to leave the body with the feces, or prepares them to be sent to the kidneys for disposal in the urine. Organ systems work together to dispose of the body's wastes, but the kidneys are waste- and water-removal specialists.

The kidneys straddle the cardiovascular system and filter the passing blood. Waste materials, dissolved in water, are collected by the kidneys' working units, the **nephrons**. These wastes become concentrated as urine, which travels through tubes to the urinary **bladder**. The bladder collects the urine continuously and empties periodically, removing wastes from the body. Thus, the blood is purified continuously throughout the day, and dissolved materials are excreted as necessary. One dissolved mineral, sodium, helps regulate blood pressure, and its excretion or retention by the kidneys is a vital part of the body's blood pressure–controlling mechanism.

Though they account for just 0.5 percent of the body's total weight, the kidneys use up 10 percent of the body's oxygen supply, indicating intense metabolic activity. The kidney's waste-excreting function rivals breathing in its importance to life, but the kidneys act in other ways as well. By sorting among dissolved substances, retaining some while excreting others, the kidneys regulate the fluid volume and concentrations of substances in the blood and extracellular fluid with great precision. Through these mechanisms, the kidneys help regulate blood pressure (see Chapter 11 for details). As you might expect, the kidneys' work is regulated by hormones secreted by glands that respond to conditions in the blood (such as the sodium concentration). The kidneys also release certain hormones.

Because the kidneys remove toxins that could otherwise damage body tissues, whatever supports the health of the kidneys supports the health of the whole body. A strong cardiovascular system and an abundant supply of water are important to keep blood flushing swiftly through the kidneys. In addition, the kidneys need sufficient energy to do their complex sifting and sorting job, and many vitamins and minerals serve as the cogs of their machinery. Exercise and nutrition are vital to healthy kidney function.

KEY POINT

- The kidneys adjust the blood's composition in response to the body's needs, disposing of everyday wastes and helping remove toxins.

nephrons (NEFF-rons) the working units of the kidneys, consisting of intermeshed blood vessels and tubules.

bladder the sac that holds urine until time for elimination.

Storage Systems

The human body is designed to eat at intervals of about four to six hours, but cells need nutrients around the clock. Providing the cells with a constant flow of the needed nutrients requires the cooperation of many body systems. These systems store and release nutrients to meet the cells' needs between meals. Among the major storage sites are the liver and muscles, which store carbohydrate, and the fat cells, which store fat and other related substances.

When I Eat More than My Body Needs, What Happens to the Extra Nutrients?

Nutrients collected from the digestive system sooner or later all move through a vast network of capillaries that weave among the liver cells. This arrangement ensures that liver cells have access to newly arriving nutrients for processing.

The liver collects excess energy-yielding nutrients and converts them into two storage forms—**glycogen** (a form of carbohydrate) and several kinds of lipids, or fats (details follow in later chapters). The liver stores a supply of glycogen, which it can release to sustain the body's cellular activities when the intervals between meals become long. Should no food be available, the liver's glycogen supply dwindles; it can be effectively depleted within as few as three to six hours. Muscle cells take up glucose and make glycogen, too, but reserve it for their own use.

As for the fats, the liver packages these to be shipped out to other parts of the body (see details in Chapter 5.) All body cells may withdraw the fat they need from these packages, and the cells of adipose tissue pick up the remainder and store it to meet long-term energy needs. Unlike the liver, fat tissue can store virtually infinite quantities of fat. It can continue to supply the body's cells with fat for days, weeks, or possibly even months when no food is eaten.

These storage systems for carbohydrate and fat ensure that the body's cells will not go without energy even if the body is hungry for food. Body stores also exist for many other nutrients, each with a characteristic capacity. For example, liver and fat cells store many vitamins, and bones provide reserves of calcium and other minerals. Stores of nutrients are available to keep the blood levels constant and to meet cellular demands.

Variations in Nutrient Stores

Some nutrients are stored in the body in much larger quantities than others. For example, certain vitamins are stored without limit, even if they reach toxic levels. Other nutrients are stored in only small amounts, regardless of the amount taken in, and these can readily be depleted. As you learn how the body handles various nutrients, pay particular attention to their storage so that you can know your tolerance limits. For example, you needn't eat fat at every meal because fat is stored abundantly. On the other hand, you normally do need to have a source of carbohydrate at intervals throughout the day because the liver stores less than one day's supply of glycogen.

KEY POINTS

- The body stores limited amounts of carbohydrate as glycogen in muscle and liver cells.
- The body stores large quantities of fat in fat cells.
- Various nutrients are stored by the body in differing quantities.

Conclusion

In addition to the systems just described, the body has many more: bones, muscles, and reproductive organs, among others. All of these cooperate, enabling each cell to carry on its own life. For example, the skin and body linings defend other tissues

glycogen a storage form of carbohydrate energy (glucose); described in more detail in Chapter 4.

Chapter 3 The Remarkable Body

against microbial invaders while being nourished and cleansed by tissues specializing in these tasks. Each system needs a continuous supply of many specific nutrients to maintain itself and carry out its work. Calcium is particularly important for bones, for example; iron for muscles; and glucose for the brain. But all systems need all nutrients, and every system is impaired by an undersupply or oversupply of them.

While external events clamor and vie for attention, the body quietly continues its life-sustaining work. Most of the body's work is directed automatically by the unconscious portions of the brain and nervous system, and this work is finely regulated to achieve a state of well-being. But you need to involve your brain's cortex—your conscious, thinking brain—to cultivate an understanding and appreciation of your body's needs. In doing so, attend to nutrition first. The rewards are liberating—ample energy to tackle life's tasks, a robust attitude, and the glowing appearance that comes from the best of health. Read on, and learn to let nutrition principles guide your food choices.

KEY POINT

- To nourish a body's systems, nutrients from outside must be supplied through a human being's conscious food choices.

What did you decide?

Is it true that "**you are what you eat**"?

How does food on the plate become **nourishment** for your body?

What does **bacteria in the intestine** have to do with nutrition?

Should you take antacids to relieve **heartburn**?

What's online?

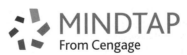

Visit www.Cengage.com to access MindTap, a complete digital course that includes Diet & Wellness Plus, interactive quizzes, videos, and more.

Self Check

1. (LO 3.1) Cells
   a. are self-contained, living units.
   b. serve the body's needs but have few needs of their own.
   c. remain alive throughout a person's lifetime.
   d. b and c.

2. (LO 3.1) Each gene is a blueprint that directs the production of one or more of the body's organs.
   T   F

3. (LO 3.2) After circulating around the cells of the tissues, all extracellular fluid then
   a. evaporates from the body.
   b. becomes urine.
   c. returns to the bloodstream.
   d. a and b.

4. (LO 3.2) Blood carries nutrients absorbed from food
   a. from the intestine to the liver.
   b. from the lungs to the extremities.
   c. from the kidneys to the liver.
   d. Nutrients do not travel in blood.

5. (LO 3.3) Hormones
   a. are rarely involved in disease processes.
   b. are chemical messengers that travel from one system of cells to affect another.
   c. are produced and remain inside single cells for intracellular communications.
   d. are unaffected by nutrition status of the body.

6. (LO 3.3) The nervous system sends messages to the glands, telling them what to do.
   T   F

7. (LO 3.4) Chemical digestion of all nutrients mainly occurs in which organ?
   a. mouth
   b. stomach
   c. small intestine
   d. large intestine

8. (LO 3.4) Which of the following passes through the large intestine mostly unabsorbed?
   a. starch
   b. vitamins
   c. minerals
   d. fiber

9. (LO 3.4) Absorption of the majority of nutrients takes place across the mucus-coated lining of the stomach.
   T   F

10. (LO 3.5) Which of the following increases the production of intestinal gas?
    a. chewing gum
    b. drinking carbonated beverages
    c. eating or drinking hastily
    d. all of the above

11. (LO 3.5) Concerning ulcers, which of the following statements is *not* correct:
    a. They usually occur in the large intestine.
    b. Some are caused by a bacterium.
    c. If not treated correctly, they can lead to stomach cancer.
    d. Their symptoms can be masked by using antacids regularly.

12. (LO 3.6) The kidneys' working units are _____.
    a. photons
    b. genes
    c. nephrons
    d. villi

13. (LO 3.6) The bladder straddles the cardiovascular system and filters the blood.
    T   F

14. (LO 3.7) The body's stores of _____ can sustain cellular activities when the intervals between meals become long.
    a. vitamins
    b. fat
    c. phytochemicals
    d. minerals

15. (LO 3.7) The body's adipose tissue has a virtually infinite capacity to store fats.
    T   F

16. (LO 3.8) A drinker may delay intoxication somewhat by
    a. eating plenty of snacks.
    b. quickly finishing drinks.
    c. drinking on an empty stomach.
    d. drinking undiluted drinks.

17. (LO 3.8) Alcohol is a natural substance and therefore does no real damage to body tissues.
    T   F

Answers to these Self Check questions are in Appendix G.

Alcohol Use: Risks and Benefits

LO 3.8 Compare the effects of moderate and heavy alcohol consumption.

Virtually everyone has heard media reports about positive associations between moderate alcohol consumption and a number of potential health benefits. Equally widely known, however, are alcohol's destructive effects. In the United States, alcohol-related deaths top 88,000 each year, making alcohol a top contributor to illness and mortality.[1]*

Should nondrinkers take up drinking for their health's sake? Or should drinkers stop now to avoid problems? This Controversy presents evidence on both sides of the issue.

U.S. Alcohol Consumption

On a given day, an average adult drinker consumes about 16 percent of total calories from alcoholic beverages, with men drinking more than women by far. Users of alcohol come in all stripes: some people drink no alcohol, many take a glass of wine with meals, many others drink mainly at social functions, and still others take in large quantities of **hard liquor** or other alcoholic beverages daily because of a life-shattering **addiction**.

Both **heavy drinking** and **heavy episodic drinking** (**binge drinking**) are common drinking patterns, particularly among college-age people. These patterns cause serious health and social consequences for drinkers and nondrinkers alike.[2] Among U.S. adults, one in six is a binge drinker, a pattern accounting for more than half of the annual deaths attributed to alcohol consumption.[3] In contrast, people who engage in **moderate drinking** limit their alcohol intakes to one drink each day for women and two for men—no more—and therefore minimize their risks. Table C3–1 defines "a drink" and drinking terms; Figure C3–1 depicts servings of alcoholic beverages that

*Reference notes are in Appendix F.

Table C3–1

Drinks and Drinking Terms

- **a drink** any alcoholic beverage that delivers 0.6 ounce of pure ethanol. See also *proof*.
- **addiction** a chronic, relapsing brain disease that is characterized by compulsive drug seeking and use, despite harmful consequences; addiction is classified as a brain disease because addictive drugs change the brain's structure and functioning.
- **alcohols** chemical compounds that consist of a carbon atom or chain of carbons to which a hydroxyl (oxygen-hydrogen) group is attached. The alcohol of alcoholic beverages is *ethanol*, which has two carbon atoms.
- **alcohol abuse** *see problem drinking*.
- **alcoholism** dependency on alcohol characterized by compulsive, uncontrollable drinking with negative effects on physical health, family relationships, and social health.
- **Antabuse** a drug that increases acetaldehyde, which produces such misery in combination with alcohol that a drinker will refrain from drinking after taking it. (Acetaldehyde is a product formed during alcohol metabolism.) The generic form is *disulfiram*.
- **antidiuretic** (AN-tee-dye-you-RET-ick) **hormone** a hormone of the brain that signals the kidneys to conserve water; alcohol suppresses this hormone, increasing urination.
- **binge drinking** *see heavy episodic drinking*.
- **drug** any substance that, when taken into a living organism, modifies one or more of its functions. Also defined in Controversy 2.
- **ethanol** the alcohol of alcoholic beverages, often called simply "alcohol"; a drug.
- **euphoria** (you-FOR-ee-uh): a state of intense happiness induced by an extremely pleasurable experience or by a drug such as ethanol.
- **hangover** a delayed, usually morning-after, reaction to drinking too much alcohol too fast the night before, characterized by a headache and sometimes nausea.
- **hard liquor** a beverage that is made by distilling a product such as wine or beer, which arose from fermentation; one that contains a higher percentage of alcohol. Examples are brandy, gin, rum, vodka, and whiskey.
- **heavy drinking** drinking five or more drinks on each of five or more days per month.
- **heavy episodic drinking** (**binge drinking**) engaging in heavy consumption of alcohol over a short time period, with the intention of becoming intoxicated; for a man: drinking five or more drinks; or for a woman: drinking four or more drinks on at least one occasion within a 30-day period.
- **intoxication** a condition of diminished mental and physical ability, hyperexcitability, or stupor induced by intake of alcohol or other drug.
- **moderate drinking** drinking no more than one drink per day (for a woman) or no more than two drinks per day (for a man) and behaving normally while drinking.
- **problem drinking** (**alcohol abuse**) drinking behavior that causes social, emotional, family, job-related, or other problems because of alcohol overuse; a step on the way to alcoholism.
- **proof** the percentage of alcohol in a beverage; a term used on labels. Water is the main ingredient in alcoholic beverages; proof equals twice the percentage of alcohol. Examples: Most beers and malt beverages are about 5 to 10 percent ethanol (10 to 20 proof). Most wines contain about 13 to 15 percent (26 to 30 proof), whereas "hard" liquors (whiskey, vodka, rum, and brandy) have about 50 percent (100 proof).

equal one drink. Be aware, however, that most wine glasses hold 6 to 8 rather than 5 ounces of wine; wine coolers may come packaged 12 rather than 10 ounces to a bottle; a large beer stein can hold 20 or more rather than 12 ounces; and a strong liquor drink may contain 2 or 3 ounces of various liquors rather than the standard $1\frac{1}{2}$ ounces total.

Servings of Alcoholic Beverages that Equal One Drink

Each of these beverage servings is one standard drink, containing 0.6 oz of pure ethanol.

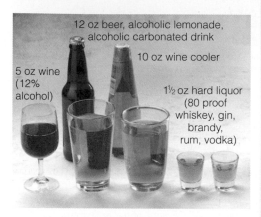

12 oz beer, alcoholic lemonade, alcoholic carbonated drink

10 oz wine cooler

5 oz wine (12% alcohol)

1½ oz hard liquor (80 proof whiskey, gin, brandy, rum, vodka)

© Polara Studios, Inc.

Alcohol's Chemistry and Handling by the Body

The **alcohols** are a set of compounds, all of which have the same reactive chemical group at one end.[†] The smallest alcohol is methanol, which has one carbon atom; the next-larger one is **ethanol** (two carbons), the alcohol of alcoholic beverages (you can see its structure on the first page of Appendix A). Glycerol (three carbons) is next, and shows up again in Chapter 5 in regard to fats. The suffix -ol identifies the alcohols.

Alcohols affect living things profoundly, partly because they dissolve lipids. Most kinds are toxins that can injure or kill cells. Alcohol can easily penetrate a cell's outer lipid membrane and, once inside, disrupt the cell's structures and kill the cell. Because some alcohols kill microbial cells, they make useful disinfectants and antiseptics.

The ethanol of alcoholic beverages is somewhat less toxic than other alcohols. Sufficiently diluted, taken slowly and in moderation, its action in the brain eases social interactions and produces **euphoria**, a pleasant sensation that people seek.

[†]The chemical group at the reactive end of an alcohol is a hydroxyl group (oxygen and hydrogen).

Because it can be used this way, alcohol can be considered a **drug**, and like many drugs, it presents both benefits and hazards to users.

From the moment one starts to drink an alcoholic beverage, the body gives it special attention. Unlike food, which requires digestion before it can be absorbed, ethanol starts diffusing right through the stomach walls into the bloodstream. When the stomach is full of food, molecules of alcohol are less readily absorbed into the bloodstream; also food delays the flow of alcohol into the small intestine. Drinkers who want to drink socially and not become intoxicated eat snacks both before and during drinking.

The stomach possesses an enzyme (*alcohol dehydrogenase*, abbreviated *ADH*) that alters some of the alcohol consumed, leaving its major breakdown product, acetaldehyde (ASS-set-AL-deh-hyde). Liver ADH also produces acetaldehyde from alcohol that is absorbed. Acetaldehyde is even more toxic than alcohol, but a second enzyme (*acetaldehyde dehydrogenase*, found in the liver) can break it down further to a nontoxic substance that ultimately becomes harmless water and carbon dioxide. Most of the body's ADH occurs in the liver, and the liver metabolizes the most alcohol by far.

Women make less stomach ADH than men do, and therefore absorb more alcohol from each drink than do men of equal weight. Experts often warn that women should not try to keep up drink for drink with males for this reason.

Alcohol's next stop beyond the stomach is the small intestine. There, absorption into the blood takes place promptly. The capillaries that surround the small intestine merge into veins that carry the alcohol-laden blood to the liver. The liver, with its large quantities of ADH, is the major site for alcohol breakdown. If a person drinks slowly enough, the liver will collect nearly all of the alcohol available from the passing

blood and process it without much affecting the other parts of the body.

The liver can process about $\frac{1}{2}$ ounce of blood ethanol (about one standard drink's worth) per hour, depending on the person's body size, previous drinking experience, gender, general health, and food intake. Going without food for as little as one day causes degradation of body proteins, including ADH enzymes, and this cuts the rate of alcohol metabolism by half, hence the maxim "Don't drink on an empty stomach."

Drinking Patterns

Drinking patterns influence alcohol's effects on the body. Occasional drinkers who take a glass of wine or two, perhaps once or twice a month, may not be affected at all. A moderate daily drinker, that is, a woman taking a single drink or a man two drinks a day, may be affected by this choice, for better or worse. People who drink more than this often suffer the consequences of dehydration (alcohol suppresses **antidiuretic hormone**), and the famous **hangover** of the morning after. Those who drink excessively suffer significant harm to all the body's organs. Alcohol is an addictive drug, and an alcohol addiction is **alcoholism**.

Abstinence from Drinking

People who abstain from alcohol may make this choice for cultural, religious, or health reasons. Some people should not drink because it poses special risks to them.[4] You shouldn't drink at all if:

- You are under the legal drinking age limit. Drowning, car accidents, and traumatic injuries are common causes of death in children and teens, and alcohol use intensifies these risks.

- You are pregnant or may be pregnant. No safe level of alcohol consumption during pregnancy has been established.

- You are breastfeeding (you may consume one drink if you then wait four hours before breastfeeding).

- You are taking medications that interact with alcohol. Such medications come with labels that warn you of the risks.

Table C3–2

Drinking Behaviors of Moderate and Problem Drinkers

Moderate Drinkers Typically	Problem Drinkers Typically
▪ Drink slowly, casually. ▪ Eat food while drinking or beforehand. ▪ Don't binge drink; know when to stop. ▪ Respect nondrinkers. ▪ Avoid drinking when solving problems or making decisions. ▪ Do not admire or encourage drunkenness. ▪ Remain peaceful, calm, and unchanged by drinking. ▪ Cause no problems to others or themselves by drinking.	▪ Gulp or "chug" drinks. ▪ Drink on an empty stomach. ▪ Binge-drink; drink to get drunk. ▪ Pressure others to drink. ▪ Turn to alcohol when facing problems or decisions. ▪ Consider drunks to be funny or admirable. ▪ Become loud, angry, violent, or silent when drinking. ▪ Physically or emotionally harm themselves, family members, or others when drinking.

- You have liver disease, high blood lipids, pancreatitis, or other conditions that amplify the harmful effects of alcohol.

- You plan to drive, operate machinery, or take part in other activities that require attention, skill, or coordination such as swimming, biking, or boating.

- You cannot limit your drinking to moderate levels.

Nonalcoholic drinks can also produce some of the pleasant sensations that drinkers seek (these contain, at most, 0.5% alcohol). Nonalcoholic beers and wines that elevate mood and ease social interactions are available—as are coffee and sodas. People who don't drink alcohol can drink these beverages instead.

Moderate Drinking

Many people drink moderately, sticking within defined limits. Moderate drinkers will not present the liver with more than it can handle, and a night of restful sleep after a pleasant social evening is all that is needed to restore the original healthy state. The key to achieving this result, of course, is to stop before drinking too much. It is worth repeating that alcohol intake shown to do no immediate damage is:

- One standard drink a day for women.

- Two standard drinks a day for men.

The left column of Table C3–2 shows how moderate drinkers manage alcohol. You will be invited to visit the right column in a later section.

Excessive Drinking

Excessive drinkers drink more than half an ounce of alcohol per hour. The euphoria that comes on at first is transient and is soon superseded by alcohol's large-dose effects of impeding social interactions and diminishing euphoria. Rapid drinkers will quickly manifest **intoxication**, especially when drinking on an empty stomach.

If a person drinks more than can be metabolized by the stomach and liver, the excess flows in to the bloodstream to the brain and the rest of the body. The lungs and kidneys then excrete some 10 percent of the blood alcohol in the breath and urine. The alcohol in the breath is directly proportional to that in the blood, so a breathalyzer test administered by law enforcement officers can accurately determine the degree of intoxication.

There is no way to hasten the liver's rate of alcohol clearance: only time restores sobriety. Walking around will not help because muscles cannot metabolize alcohol. Nor will drinking coffee: caffeine is a stimulant, but it won't speed up the metabolism of alcohol. The police say that a cup of coffee only makes a sleepy drunk into a wide-awake drunk. Table C3–3 presents other alcohol myths.

Binge Drinking

Heavy episodic drinking, often called *binge drinking*, is a problematic

Table C3–3

Myths and Truths Concerning Alcohol

Myth:	A shot of alcohol warms you up.
Truth:	Alcohol diverts blood flow to the skin, making you feel warmer, but it actually cools the body.
Myth:	Wine and beer are mild; they do not lead to addiction.
Truth:	Wine and beer drinkers worldwide have high rates of death from alcohol-related illnesses. It's not what you drink but how much that makes the difference.
Myth:	Mixing drinks is what gives you a hangover.
Truth:	Too much alcohol in any form produces a hangover.
Myth:	Alcohol is a stimulant.
Truth:	Alcohol depresses the brain's activity.
Myth:	Alcohol is legal; therefore, it is not a drug.
Truth:	Alcohol is legal, but it alters body functions and is medically defined as a depressant drug.

drinking style for a large and growing number of people.[5] Young adults enjoy parties, sports events, and other social occasions, but these settings often encourage binge drinking. Binge drinking skews national statistics, making alcohol use on college campuses appear to be more common than it is. The median number of drinks consumed by all college students is 1.5 per week, but for binge drinkers it is 14.5 per week. This destructive drinking pattern is observed in the greatest numbers among people 18 to 34 and is responsible for most of this group's alcohol-related accidents and illnesses.

The harms grow worse with age. In the United States, six binge drinkers die per day—mostly men aged 35 to 64. Compared with nondrinkers and moderate drinkers, binge drinkers are also more likely to damage property, assault other people, or cause fatal accidents. They are also more likely to engage in unprotected sex, resulting in sexually transmitted diseases and unplanned pregnancies.[6] Female binge drinkers are more likely to be victims of rape. Binge drinkers on and off campus may not recognize themselves as problem drinkers until their drinking behavior causes a crisis such as a car crash, or until enough years have passed to cause substantial, potentially irreversible, damage to their health.

Short-Term Effects of Too Much Alcohol

A person who drinks too much experiences negative effects on the body, some transient, others more damaging. The short-term effects of alcohol toxicity are often reversible, but the long-term effects may not be.

Dehydration

Excess alcohol exerts impacts on every other body organ. It penetrates all the tissues and dehydrates them—an effect familiar to anyone who drinks too much. Alcohol depresses the brain's production of a hormone (*antidiuretic hormone*) that curbs excretion of body water—so urine output increases. The resulting dehydration leads to thirst, and unwary drinkers who respond by drinking more alcohol only make matters worse. The only fluid that relieves thirst is water.

Water lost due to dehydration takes with it important minerals, such as magnesium, potassium, calcium, and zinc, depleting the body's reserves. These minerals are vital to nerve and muscle coordination and fluid balance. When drinking incurs mineral losses, minerals must be made up in subsequent meals to prevent deficiencies.

Hangover

The hangover—the next morning's miserable headache and nausea—is the result of drinking too much. Dehydration of the brain is a major cause of a hangover. Alcohol depletes the brain's cells of water; when they rehydrate, they swell and cause pain.

In addition, several chemicals in the body contribute to the hangover. Recall that the stomach and liver are busy converting alcohol to acetaldehyde, a toxic compound that accumulates in the body for a while, awaiting further breakdown. The later breakdown steps require the participation of still other liver compounds (*glutathione*, an important antioxidant, and *cysteine*, an amino acid), and these run out before the job is done. Time alone can clear the hangover-producing toxins from the body.

Paradoxically, because it is toxic, acetaldehyde offers a benefit to drinkers who want to quit. It is the active ingredient in a drug known as **Antabuse**, and it produces aldehyde toxicity symptoms so severe that people addicted to alcohol choose not to drink when they have it in their systems.

Heart and Brain

So long as excess alcohol is in the body, toxic effects are felt by every organ. The heart, stomach, and brain are examples. Emergency room nurses describe a condition in intoxicated people called "holiday heart syndrome," marked by life-threatening, irregular heartbeats.[7] This syndrome can occur in people of any age who take more than a few drinks in too short a time. But the stomach may come to the drinker's rescue, because a major overdose triggers the vomiting reflex, one of the body's primary defenses against ingested poisons.

In the brain, small quantities of alcohol selectively sedate inhibitory nerves, producing a false impression of stimulation. Some people use alcohol to achieve this "high," believing that it helps relieve anxiety and enables them to relax, but additional alcohol counteracts the high and then, in many people, produces tension and stress. When the blood alcohol concentration rises high enough, it sedates all of the nerve cells.

Figure C3–2 displays the impacts on the brain of progressively higher blood alcohol concentrations. At 0.08 percent, judgment, reasoning, and emotional control are impaired. At 0.1 percent, speech centers in the midbrain are sedated. At 0.15 percent, control of muscles and reflexes becomes impaired. At higher levels still, unconsciousness ensues and, if the person has drunk fast enough to ingest a lethal dose before vomiting or passing out, respiration and heartbeat cease. Most highway safety ordinances set the legal limit for intoxication at 0.08 percent, but driving ability may be impaired at lower concentrations.

Abstinence from alcohol, together with good nutrition, reverses some of the brain damage caused by heavy drinking if it has not continued for too many years. Prolonged drinking beyond a person's capacity to recover, however, can severely and irreversibly damage vision, memory, learning, reasoning, speech, and other brain functions.

Clearly, there is a marked contrast in risk between moderate drinking and excessive drinking. Studies show that although the former may in some ways benefit drinkers, the latter is extremely harmful.

Effects of Rising Blood Alcohol Levels on the Brain

The higher the blood alcohol, the more severe its effect on brain tissues. This is a typical progression, but individual responses vary to some degree.

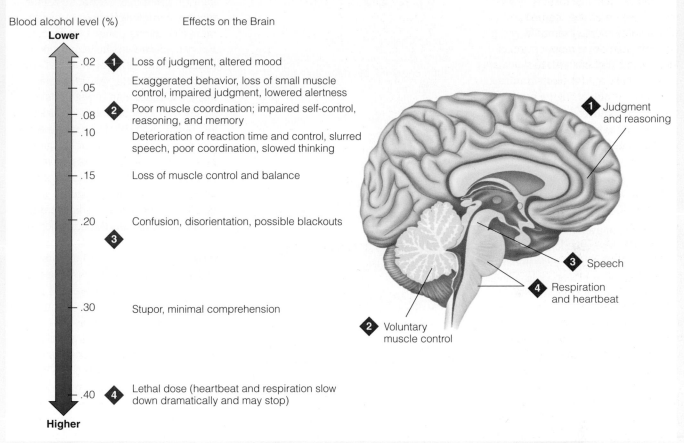

Blood alcohol level (%)

Lower

Effects on the Brain

1 .02 — Loss of judgment, altered mood

.05 — Exaggerated behavior, loss of small muscle control, impaired judgment, lowered alertness

2 .08 — Poor muscle coordination; impaired self-control, reasoning, and memory

.10 — Deterioration of reaction time and control, slurred speech, poor coordination, slowed thinking

.15 — Loss of muscle control and balance

.20 — Confusion, disorientation, possible blackouts

3

.30 — Stupor, minimal comprehension

4 .40 — Lethal dose (heartbeat and respiration slow down dramatically and may stop)

Higher

1 Judgment and reasoning

3 Speech

4 Respiration and heartbeat

2 Voluntary muscle control

Source: Centers for Disease Control and Prevention.

Potential Benefits of Moderate Alcohol Use

Some studies show that moderate drinking correlates with benefits to health, but these studies are tricky to interpret. Four types of studies are of particular interest: studies of adult populations, studies that compare drinking patterns of different countries, studies that focus on young people, and studies that compare effects of wine with other types of drinks.

Population studies are suggestive, but they cannot yield proof of cause. They reveal only correlations. Simply stated, if "A" often goes with "B," this doesn't prove that "A" causes "B" or vice versa. It may be that a third factor, "C," causes both "A" and "B."

Among the correlations found: populations of moderate drinkers often have reduced risks of heart attacks, strokes, and diabetes.[8] They also have improved blood lipids and blood-clotting factors.[9] These studies suggest, but cannot prove, that moderate drinking reduces heart disease risks; they show that the two occur together. It may be that moderate alcohol consumption simply reflects higher socioeconomic status, which is also characterized by better diet, less stress, more exercise, less smoking, and more accessible medical care.

Population studies made in France shed light on the relationship between drinking and health. In France, light and moderate daily drinking dispersed throughout the week is the norm, and this drinking pattern correlates with indicators

of above-average heart health and lower-than-average mortality. In other countries, people who consume the same amounts of alcohol have higher disease risks. They often drink in heavy episodes. For example, they may abstain on most weekdays but then consume four or five drinks or more each weekend day. Because the total alcohol consumed is within the "moderate" range when averaged over time, researchers may accidentally count these people among moderate drinkers in surveys, but they are in fact heavy episodic drinkers who are incurring high risks of heart disease and mortality.[10]

Studies of alcohol use by teens and young adults yield evidence that is crystal clear. Whether or not young people drink, their highest mortality rates are not from disease, but from car crashes, homicides, and other violence. Drinking, even just a little, raises the risks of young people's deaths from these causes. For them, the question whether moderate alcohol use benefits heart health becomes irrelevant.

As for the benefits of drinking wine, research is continuing. Anyone you ask will probably tell you that red wine is good for health. Labels on red wines sold in the United States often make statements such as "We encourage you to consult your family doctor about the health effects of wine consumption." Such statements seem to promise some good news about wine and health, but the science on wine and health is mixed. For example:

- Some good news: Some population studies show that a glass or two of wine each day often correlates with a lower-than-average risk of heart attacks.[11] The credit for this effect may be owed to the grape juice from which the wine is made: grape juice contains potassium and the phytochemical resveratrol (see Controversy 2, p. 61), which may help maintain normal blood pressure; and these ingredients persist when the juice is made into wine.

- Bad news: Alcohol in large amounts, even from red wine, raises blood pressure and increases inflammation, effects detrimental to the heart.

- More good news: Some of the phytochemicals in wine seem to oppose certain cancers.[12]

- More bad news: Such phytochemicals are poorly absorbed; only tiny amounts reach body tissues.

And the good news about cancers is counterbalanced by the finding that consuming alcohol, even in amounts of less than one drink per day, can cause or contribute to cancers of the the breast, colon, esophagus, liver, and throat; the greater the intake and the longer the exposure, the greater the risk.[13]

To conclude, then, although researchers would like to be able to report definitive findings on the possible benefits of moderate drinking, the scientific evidence is not persuasive. *The Dietary Guidelines for Americans* recommends that no one begin drinking or drink more frequently in hopes of benefitting their health.

Long-Term Consequences of Excessive Drinking

A term that describes self-destructive, excessive drinking is **problem drinking**, also known as **alcohol abuse**. Typical behaviors of problem drinkers can be recognized by looking at the *right* side of Table C3–2, on page 97, which provides

a kind of mirror for problem drinking behavior.

Alcoholism is the most severe form of self-destructive drinking. Many people who start out drinking moderately find that they cannot sustain a moderate drinking pattern but slide into harmful and dangerous excess. For people with alcoholism, drinking leads to many forms of irrational and dangerous behavior including driving while intoxicated, arguments and violence, and unplanned and risky sexual behavior. With continued drinking, such people face psychological depression, physical illness, severe malnutrition, and demoralizing erosion of self-esteem. Making matters worse, because alcohol is an addictive drug, denial accompanies the addiction. "I'm not an alcoholic," say many with an alcohol addiction, and the first step toward recovery is admitting the problem. If you are wondering about the possibility that you may have a drinking problem, refer to Table C3–4. If you conclude that you do, you should seek a professional evaluation right away.[‡]

‡*If you need to talk with someone right away, call (24 hours a day) the federal Substances Abuse and Mental Health Services Administration (SAMHSA): (800) 662-4357.*

Table C3–4

Symptoms of Problem Drinking and Alcoholism

A health professional can diagnose and evaluate problem drinking or alcohol addiction with the answers to these questions. In the past year, have you:

- Ever ended up drinking more or for longer than you intended?
- Wanted to cut down or stop drinking, or tried to, but couldn't on more than one occasion?
- Felt a strong urge or craving for a drink?
- Endangered yourself more than once while or after drinking (such as driving, swimming, using machinery, walking in a dangerous area, or having unsafe sex)?
- Noticed that you need more than your regular number of drinks to feel the effect?
- Continued to drink even though it made you feel depressed, anxious, or physically ill?
- Spent a lot of time drinking, or being sick, or getting over other aftereffects?

- Continued to drink even though it was causing trouble with your family or friends?
- Found that drinking—or being sick from drinking—often interfered with taking care of your home or family? Or caused job troubles? Or school problems?
- Given up or cut back on activities that were important or interesting to you or that gave pleasure in order to drink?
- Found that, when the effects of alcohol were wearing off, you had withdrawal symptoms, such as trouble sleeping, shakiness, restlessness, nausea, sweating, racing heartbeat, or seizure? Or sensed things that were not there?
- Found yourself drinking to hold off withdrawal symptoms?

If you have any of these symptoms, or if people close to you are concerned about your drinking, then alcohol may be a cause for concern. The more symptoms you have and the more often you have them, the more urgent the need for change. See a health professional.

Note: These questions are based on symptoms for alcohol use disorders in the American Psychiatric Association's Diagnostic and Statistical Manual of Mental Disorders, Fifth Edition, 2013. *The DSM is the most commonly used system in the United States for diagnosing mental health disorders.*

Alcohol Damage to the Liver

Left, normal liver; center, fatty liver; right, cirrhosis

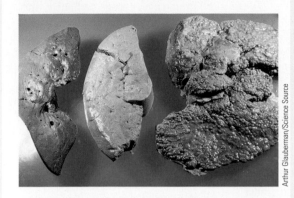

Arthur Glauberman/Science Source

Prolonged, excessive drinking produces cumulative, irreversible damage to the brain, the liver, kidneys, heart, and all other body systems. The progression of liver damage is shown in

Figure C3–3. The figure presents a classic photo of the stages of liver degeneration associated with prolonged excessive drinking, demonstrating the potential severity of the damage. Many more details about the harms from excessive alcohol intakes are known, and many people die of them each year.

Nutrition and Alcohol Use

Nutrition and alcohol interact in many ways, some beneficial, some harmful. Among the beneficial ones, a small dose of alcohol (such as a small glass of wine) may stimulate the appetite in a person who is too anxious to eat or an elderly person

who has lost interest in food. Research shows that moderate use of wine in later life also improves morale, stimulates social interactions, and promotes restful sleep among people who drink. In nursing homes, improved patient and staff relations have been attributed to offering one drink of wine or an afternoon cocktail to elderly patients who drink.

On the negative side, alcohol may burden the body with unwanted body fat. Alcohol itself is caloric, and alcoholic beverages can be very high in calories. Ethanol yields 7 calories of energy per gram (compared with 4 for carbohydrate, 4 for protein, and 9 for fat). Only a small percentage of the calories of ingested ethanol escape from the body in breath and urine. Also, drink mixers, such as piña colada mix, often present many additional calories. Table C3–5 offers some examples of the calories in alcoholic beverages and mixers.

Fat and alcohol interact in the body. Presented with both fat and alcohol, the body stores the comparatively harmless fat and rids itself of the toxic alcohol by using it preferentially for energy. As a result, alcohol promotes fat storage, often in the central abdominal area—the "beer belly" often seen in drinkers.

The use of alcohol increases the likelihood of developing vitamin and mineral imbalances. Like sugar, alcohol constitutes "empty calories"—that is, it delivers energy without bringing any nutrients along. A 2,000-calorie diet consisting of nutritious foods, is bound to deliver more nutrients than one in which 500 calories of food have been displaced by alcohol. In addition, alcohol alters the metabolism or promotes the excretion of several important vitamins.[14] When minerals become unbalanced, the blood's sensitive acid-base balance can falter, creating a medical emergency.[15]

Alcohol abuse also disrupts every tissue's metabolism of nutrients. In the presence of alcohol, stomach cells oversecrete both acid and histamine, the latter an agent of the immune system that produces inflammation. Intestinal cells fail to absorb thiamin, folate, vitamin B_{12}, and other vitamins. Liver cells lose efficiency in activating vitamin D. Cells

Table C3–5

Calories in Alcoholic Beverages and Mixers

Labels of alcoholic beverage containers need not list calorie amounts, but calories in alcoholic drinks, such as cocktails, may soon appear on many restaurant menus.

Beverage	Amount (oz)	Energy (cal)
Malt beverage (sweetened, such as hard lemonade)	16[a]	350
Malt beverage (unsweetened)	16	175
Wine cooler	12	170
Pina colada mix (no alcohol)	4	160
Beer	12	150
Dessert wine	3½	140
Fruit-flavored soda, Tom Collins mix	8	115
Gin, rum, vodka, whiskey (86 proof)	1½	105
Cola, root beer, tonic, ginger ale	8	100
Margarita mix (no alcohol)	4	100
Light beer	12	100
Table wine	3½	85
Tomato juice, Bloody Mary mix (no alcohol)	8	45
Club soda, plain seltzer, diet drinks	8	1

[a]Typical container size, but up to 32-oz containers are common.

of the eye's retina, which normally process the alcohol form of vitamin A (retinol) to the form needed in vision (retinal), must process ethanol instead. Liver cells, too, suffer a reduced capacity to process and use vitamin A. The kidneys excrete needed minerals: magnesium, calcium, potassium, and zinc.

The inadequate food intake and impaired nutrient absorption of alcohol abuse lead to a deficiency of the B vitamin thiamin in about 80 percent of people with alcohol addiction.[16] In fact, the cluster of thiamin-deficiency symptoms commonly seen in chronic alcoholism has its own name—the *Wernicke-Korsakoff syndrome*. This syndrome is characterized by paralysis of the eye muscles, poor muscle coordination, impaired memory, and damaged nerves. Thiamin supplements may help to repair some of the damage, especially if the person stops drinking.

Another dramatic example is alcohol's effect on folate. When an excess of alcohol is present, the body actively expels folate from its sites of action and storage. The liver, which normally contains enough folate to meet all needs, leaks its folate into the blood. As blood folate rises, the kidneys excrete it, as if it were in excess. The intestine normally releases and retrieves folate continuously, but it becomes so damaged by folate deficiency and alcohol toxicity that it fails to absorb folate. Alcohol also interferes with the action of what little folate is left. This interference inhibits the production of new cells, especially the rapidly dividing cells of the intestine and the blood.

Nutrient deficiencies and imbalances are thus an inevitable consequence of alcohol abuse not only because alcohol displaces food but also because alcohol interferes directly with the body's use of nutrients. People treated for alcohol addiction also need nutrition therapy to reverse deficiencies and to treat deficiency diseases rarely seen in others: night blindness, beriberi, pellagra, scurvy, and acute malnutrition.

The Final Word

This discussion has explored some of the ways alcohol affects health and nutrition. In the end, each person must decide individually whether or not to consume alcohol, a decision that can change at any time. Table C3–6 sums up both sides of selected issues.

As for drinking wine or other alcoholic beverages for health's sake, most researchers conclude that, although people who drink moderately may gain some small benefits, far greater benefits come from engaging in regular physical activity and maintaining a healthy body weight. Alcohol also poses some serious risks, so nondrinkers should not start drinking with the thought of improving their health. If you do choose to drink, do so with care and strictly in moderation.

Critical Thinking

1. Moderate alcohol use has been credited with providing possible health benefits. Construct an argument for why moderate alcohol use to provide protection from heart disease or other health problems may not be a good idea.

2. Your daughter is leaving for college in the fall. Recently, there has been disturbing news about the excessive drinking on college campuses and even a report about the death of one student who had been drinking excessively at the college your daughter is planning to attend. Form a group of four or five people. Each group has an imaginary daughter who is leaving for college. Each member of the group will choose one of the following topics and prepare a short (one-minute) speech that attempts to educate your daughter on the dangers of excessive drinking. To facilitate the speaker's delivery, a group member takes on the role of "daughter," rotating the role with each speaker. Be sure to emphasize facts as much as possible with your argument.

- Explain the physiology of the hangover.
- Discuss the role of alcohol in weight gain.
- Describe alcohol's effect on vitamins.
- Describe the effect of alcohol on the heart and brain.
- Describe alcohol's effect on the liver and other organs.

Table C3–6

Moderate Drinking: Point, Counterpoint

Many people debate the merits and demerits of drinking alcohol on many levels. This table outlines some of the arguments made for and against drinking.

Point: Arguments in Favor of Drinking Alcohol	Counterpoint: Arguments against Drinking Alcohol
1. *Ease social interactions.* Alcohol removes inhibitions, making it easier to interact socially.	1. *Removes social inhibitions.* Alcohol removes inhibitions, permitting socially unacceptable behaviors and interactions.
2. *Relieve stress.* Drinking alcohol relieves stress and produces euphoria.	2. *Increased depression and anxiety.* Regular drinking can deepen depression and cause anxiety. Removing the source of stress provides more lasting relief.
3. *Heart health.* Population studies suggest that moderate drinking can benefit the heart in older adults.	3. *Correlation, not cause.* Controlled clinical trials are lacking to support the heart health theory. Other factors may confound these results, and even moderate drinking has been associated with heart damage in some people.
4. *Brain protection.* A small amount of preliminary research associates moderate drinking with less dementia and improved memory in aging.	4. *Brain cell destruction.* Research is inconclusive about dementia or memory in aging, but firmly concludes that alcohol kills brain cells, and heavy drinking causes dementia.
5. *Reduced mortality.* In large populations, moderate drinking is sometimes associated with reduced mortality.	5. *Increased mortality.* For young people, alcohol increases risks of car crashes and violence, negating any potential health benefits. *Increased cancer.* For women, even one drink a day raises breast cancer risks significantly. Other cancers may also be affected.
6. *Natural equals harmless.* Alcoholic beverages have been used for centuries as natural tonics to "fix what ails you."	6. *Natural toxin.* Alcohol is a toxin that can be lethal when overconsumed. Safe, effective medications achieve the same things with less risk.
7. *Phytochemicals.* Red wine provides beneficial phytochemicals.	7. *Not the only source.* Ordinary foods, such as grapes and whole grains, are also good sources.
8. *Taste.* Many people perceive alcoholic beverages to taste good; they like the flavors.	8. *Taste.* Safer beverages are equally tasty. Alcohol is addictive and toxic in large doses.
9. *Thirst quencher.* Cold beer, coolers, or malt beverages are thirst quenchers.	9. *Diuretic.* Alcohol is a diuretic that causes water loss. Other beverages hydrate more efficiently.
10. *Ubiquitous.* Everyone drinks.	10. *Not everyone.* More than a third of U.S. adults do not drink alcohol.
11. *Nutrient source.* Alcoholic beverages are claimed to "provide B vitamins and minerals."	11. *Nutrient poor.* Alcoholic beverages are generally poor nutrient sources, and alcohol in large doses causes nutrient losses from the body.

Sources: Point: J. Ilomaki and coauthors, Alcohol consumption, dementia and cognitive decline: An overview of systematic reviews, Current Clinical Pharmacology 10 (2015): 204–212; J. H. O'Keefe and coauthors, Alcohol and cardiovascular health: The dose makes the poison . . . or the remedy, Mayo Clinic Proceedings 89 (2014): 382–393; E. Nova and coauthors, Potential health benefits of moderate alcohol consumption: Current perspectives in research, Proceedings of the Nutrition Society 71 (2012): 307–315; M. Krenz and R. J. Korthius, Moderate ethanol ingestion and cardiovascular protection: From epidemiologic associations to cellular mechanisms, Journal of Molecular and Cellular Cardiology 52 (2012): 93–104. Counterpoint: C. S. Knott and coauthors, All cause mortality for age specific alcohol consumption guidelines: Pooled analyses of up to 10 population based cohorts, British Medical Journal 350 (2015), epub, doi: 10.1136/bmj.h384; A. Gonçalves and coauthors, Relationship between alcohol consumption and cardiac structure and function in the elderly, Circulation Cardiovascular Imaging (2015), epub, doi:10.1161/circimaging.114.002846; M. Stahre and coauthors, Contribution of excessive alcohol consumption to deaths and years of potential life lost in the United States, Preventing Chronic Disease 11 (2014), epub, doi: http://dx.doi.org/10.5888/pcd11.130293; K. Gonzales and coauthors, Alcohol-attributable deaths and years of potential life lost—11 states, 2006–2010, Morbidity and Mortality Weekly Report 63 (2014): 213–216.

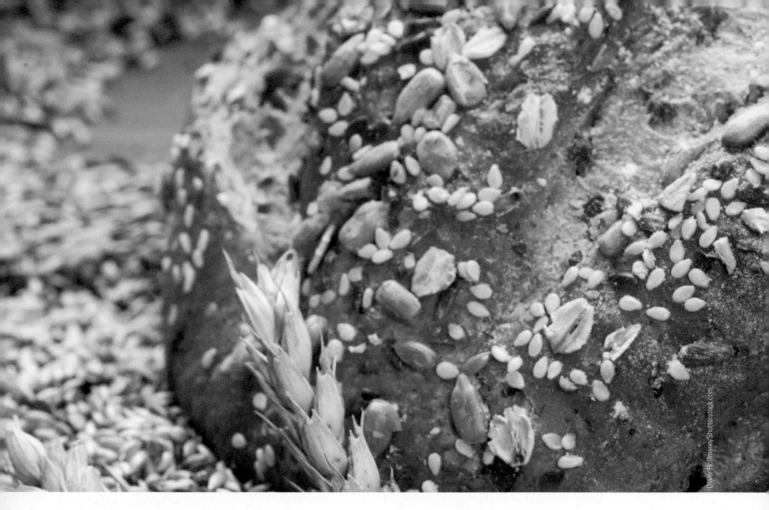

4 The Carbohydrates: Sugar, Starch, Glycogen, and Fiber

Learning Objectives

After completing this chapter, you should be able to accomplish the following:

LO 4.1 Explain how plants synthesize carbohydrates.

LO 4.2 Explain why carbohydrates are needed in the diet.

LO 4.3 Describe how carbohydrates are converted to glucose in the human body.

LO 4.4 Describe the body's handling of glucose.

LO 4.5 Briefly summarize the differences among type 1 diabetes, type 2 diabetes, and hypoglycemia.

LO 4.6 Identify foods that are rich in carbohydrates.

LO 4.7 Itemize the effects of added sugars on health.

What do you think?

Do carbohydrates provide only **unneeded calories** to the body?

Why do nutrition authorities unanimously recommend **whole grains**?

Are **low-carbohydrate diets** the best way to lose weight?

Should people with **diabetes** stop eating sugar?

Carbohydrates are ideal nutrients to meet your body's energy needs, to feed your brain and nervous system, to keep your digestive system fit, and, within calorie limits, to help fuel physical activity and keep your body lean. Digestible carbohydrates, together with fats and protein, add bulk to foods and provide energy and other benefits for the body. Indigestible carbohydrates, which include most of the fibers in foods, yield little or no energy but provide other important benefits.

All carbohydrates are not equal in terms of nutrition. This chapter invites you to learn the differences between foods containing **complex carbohydrates** (starch and fiber) and those made of **simple carbohydrates** (sugars) and to consider the effects of both on the body. Controversy 4 goes on to explore current theories about how consumption of certain carbohydrates may affect human health.

This chapter on the carbohydrates is the first of three on the energy-yielding nutrients. Chapter 5 deals with the fats and Chapter 6 with protein. Controversy 3 already addressed one other contributor of energy to the human diet, alcohol.

A Close Look at Carbohydrates

LO 4.1   Explain how plants synthesize carbohydrates.

Carbohydrates contain the sun's radiant energy, captured in a form that living things can use to drive the processes of life. Green plants make carbohydrate through **photosynthesis** in the presence of **chlorophyll** and sunlight. In this process, water (H_2O) absorbed by the plant's roots donates hydrogen and oxygen. Carbon dioxide gas (CO_2) absorbed into its leaves donates carbon and oxygen. Water and carbon dioxide combine to yield the most common of the **sugars**, the single sugar **glucose**. Scientists know the reaction in the minutest detail but have yet to fully reproduce it—living things are required to make it happen (see Figure 4–1, p. 106).

Light energy from the sun drives the photosynthesis reaction. The light energy becomes the chemical energy of the bonds that hold six atoms of carbon together in the sugar glucose. Glucose provides energy for the work of all the cells of the stem, roots, flowers, and fruit of the plant. For example, in the roots, far from the energy-giving rays of the sun, each cell draws upon some of the glucose made in the leaves, breaks it down (to carbon dioxide and water), and uses the energy thus released to fuel its own growth and water-gathering activities.

Plants do not use all of the energy stored in their sugars, so it remains available for use by the animals or human beings that consume the plants. Thus, carbohydrates form the first link in the food chain that supports all life on earth. Carbohydrate-rich foods come almost exclusively from plants; milk is the only animal-derived food that contains significant amounts of carbohydrate. The next few sections describe the forms assumed by carbohydrates: sugars, starch, glycogen, and fibers.

KEY POINTS

- Through photosynthesis, plants combine carbon dioxide, water, and the sun's energy to form glucose.
- Carbohydrates are made of carbon, hydrogen, and oxygen held together by energy-containing bonds: *carbo* means "carbon"; *hydrate* means "water."

Sugars

Six sugar molecules are important in nutrition. Three of these are single sugars, or **monosaccharides**. The other three are double sugars, or **disaccharides**. All of their chemical names end in *ose*, which means "sugar." Although they all sound alike

carbohydrates compounds composed of single or multiple sugars. The name means "carbon and water," and a chemical shorthand for carbohydrate is CHO, signifying carbon (C), hydrogen (H), and oxygen (O).

complex carbohydrates long chains of sugar units arranged to form starch or fiber; also called *polysaccharides*.

simple carbohydrates sugars, including both single sugar units and linked pairs of sugar units. The basic sugar unit is a molecule containing six carbon atoms, together with oxygen and hydrogen atoms.

photosynthesis the process by which green plants make carbohydrates from carbon dioxide and water using the green pigment chlorophyll to capture the sun's energy (*photo* means "light"; *synthesis* means "making").

chlorophyll the green pigment of plants that captures energy from sunlight for use in photosynthesis.

sugars simple carbohydrates; that is, molecules of either single sugar units or pairs of those sugar units bonded together. By common usage, *sugar* most often refers to sucrose.

glucose (GLOO-cose) a single sugar used in both plant and animal tissues for energy; sometimes known as blood sugar or *dextrose*. Also defined in Chapter 3.

monosaccharides (mon-oh-SACK-ah-rides) single sugar units (*mono* means "one"; *saccharide* means "sugar unit").

disaccharides pairs of single sugars linked together (*di* means "two").

Figure 4–1

Carbohydrate Is Made by Photosynthesis

The sun's energy becomes part of the glucose molecule—its calories, in a sense. In the molecule of glucose on the leaf here, black dots represent the carbon atoms; bars represent the chemical bonds that contain energy.

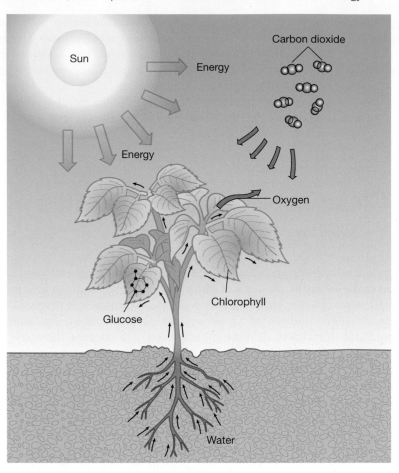

fructose (FROOK-tose) a monosaccharide; sometimes known as fruit sugar (*fruct* means "fruit"; *ose* means "sugar").

galactose (ga-LACK-tose) a monosaccharide; part of the disaccharide lactose (milk sugar).

added sugars sugars and syrups added to a food for any purpose, such as to add sweetness or bulk or to aid in browning (baked goods). Also called *carbohydrate sweeteners*, they include concentrated fruit juice, glucose, fructose, high-fructose corn syrup, sucrose, and other sweet carbohydrates. Also defined in Chapter 2.

lactose a disaccharide composed of glucose and galactose; sometimes known as milk sugar (*lact* means "milk"; *ose* means "sugar").

maltose a disaccharide composed of two glucose units; sometimes known as malt sugar.

sucrose (SOO-crose) a disaccharide composed of glucose and fructose; sometimes known as table, beet, or cane sugar and, often, as simply *sugar*.

at first, they exhibit distinct characteristics once you get to know them as individuals. Figure 4–2 shows the relationships among the sugars.

Monosaccharides   The three monosaccharides are glucose, **fructose**, and **galactose**. Fructose or fruit sugar, the intensely sweet sugar of fruit, is made by rearranging the atoms in glucose molecules. Fructose occurs naturally in fruit, in honey, and as part of table sugar. However, most fructose is consumed in sweet beverages, desserts, and other foods sweetened with **added sugars**. Glucose and fructose are the most common monosaccharides in nature.

The other monosaccharide, galactose, has the same number and kind of atoms as glucose and fructose but in another arrangement. Galactose is one of two single sugars that are bound together to make up the sugar of milk. Galactose rarely occurs free in nature but is tied up in milk sugar until it is freed during digestion.

Disaccharides   The three other sugars important in nutrition are disaccharides, which are linked pairs of single sugars. The disaccharides are **lactose**, **maltose**, and **sucrose**. All three contain glucose. In lactose, the milk sugar just mentioned, glucose is linked to galactose. Malt sugar, or maltose, has two glucose units. Maltose appears wherever starch is being broken down. It occurs in germinating seeds and arises during the digestion of starch in the human body.

Figure 4–2

How Monosaccharides Join to Form Disaccharides

Single sugars are monosaccharides, while pairs of sugars are disaccharides.

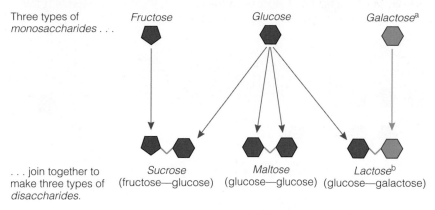

Three types of *monosaccharides . . .*

Fructose   Glucose   Galactose[a]

. . . join together to make three types of *disaccharides.*

Sucrose
(fructose—glucose)

Maltose
(glucose—glucose)

Lactose[b]
(glucose—galactose)

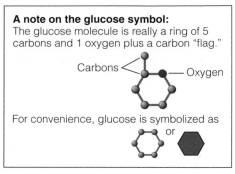

A note on the glucose symbol:
The glucose molecule is really a ring of 5 carbons and 1 oxygen plus a carbon "flag."

Carbons ← → Oxygen

For convenience, glucose is symbolized as ___ or ⬡

[a]*Galactose does not occur in foods singly but only as part of lactose.*
[b]*The chemical bond that joins the monosaccharides of lactose differs from those of other sugars and makes lactose hard for some people to digest—lactose intolerance (see later section, p. 124). Appendix A presents more detailed structures.*

The last of the six sugars, sucrose, is familiar table sugar, the product most people think of when they refer to *sugar*. In sucrose, fructose and glucose are bonded together. Table sugar is obtained by refining the juice from sugar beets or sugar cane, but sucrose also occurs naturally in many vegetables and fruit. It tastes sweet because it contains the sweetest of the monosaccharides, fructose.

When you eat a food containing monosaccharides, you can absorb them directly into your blood. When you eat disaccharides, though, you must digest them first. Enzymes in your intestinal cells must split the disaccharides into separate monosaccharides so that they can enter the bloodstream. The blood delivers all products of digestion first to the liver, which possesses enzymes to modify nutrients, making them useful to the body. Glucose is the monosaccharide used for energy by all the body's tissues, so the liver releases abundant glucose into the bloodstream for delivery to all of the body's cells. Galactose can be converted into glucose by the liver, adding to the body's supply. Fructose, however, is normally used for fuel by the liver or broken down to building blocks for fat or other needed molecules.

Although it is true that the energy of fruit and many vegetables comes from sugars, this doesn't mean that eating them is the same as eating concentrated sweets such as candy or drinking cola beverages. From the body's point of view, fruit are vastly different from purified sugars (as later sections make clear) except that both provide glucose in abundance.

KEY POINTS

- Glucose is the most important monosaccharide in the human body.
- Monosaccharides can be converted by the liver to other needed molecules.

Starch

In addition to occurring in sugars, the glucose in food occurs in long strands of thousands of glucose units. These are the **polysaccharides** (see Figure 4–3, p. 108). **Starch** is a polysaccharide, as are glycogen and most of the fibers.

Starch is a plant's storage form of glucose. As a plant matures, it not only provides energy for its own needs but also stores energy in its seeds for the next generation. For example, after a corn plant reaches its full growth and has many leaves manufacturing glucose, it links glucose together to form starch, stores packed clusters of starch molecules in **granules**, and packs the granules into its seeds. These giant starch clusters are packed side by side in the kernels of corn. For the plant, starch is useful because it is an insoluble substance that will stay with the seed in the ground and nourish it until it forms shoots

polysaccharides another term for complex carbohydrates; compounds composed of long strands of glucose units linked together (*poly* means "many").

starch a plant polysaccharide composed of glucose. After cooking, starch is highly digestible by human beings; raw starch often resists digestion.

granules small grains. Starch granules are packages of starch molecules. Various plant species make starch granules of varying shapes.

Figure 4–3

How Glucose Molecules Join to Form Polysaccharides

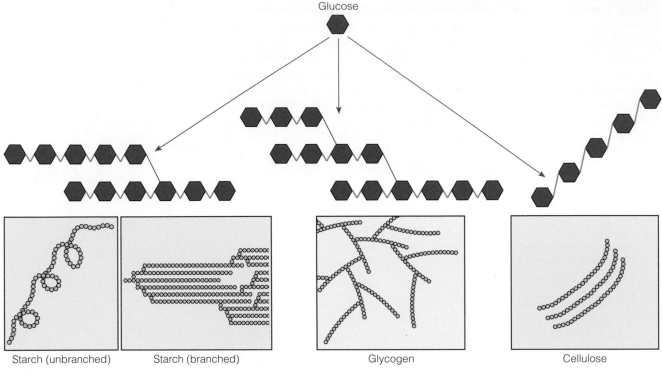

Glucose

| Starch (unbranched) | Starch (branched) | Glycogen | Cellulose |

Starch Glucose units are linked in long, occasionally branched chains to make starch. Human digestive enzymes can digest these bonds, retrieving glucose. Real glucose units are so tiny that you cannot see them, even with the highest-power light microscope.

Glycogen Glycogen resembles starch in that the bonds between its glucose units can be broken by human enzymes, but the chains of glycogen are more highly branched.

Cellulose (fiber) The bonds that link glucose units together in cellulose are different from the bonds in starch or glycogen. Human enzymes cannot digest them.

Figure 4–4

Model of A Glycogen Molecule

One glycogen molecule stores tens of thousands of glucose units nested in an easy-to-retrieve form. In this photo, individual glucose molecules are depicted as black dots linked together with white sticks.

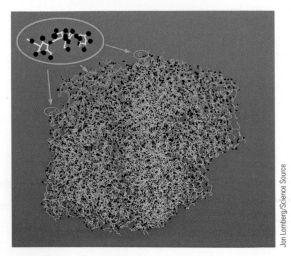

Jon Lomberg/Science Source

with leaves that can catch the sun's rays. Glucose, in contrast, is soluble in water and would be washed away by the rains while the seed lay in the soil. The starch of corn and other plant foods is nutritive for people, too, because people can digest the starch to glucose and extract the sun's energy stored in its chemical bonds. A later section describes starch digestion in detail.

KEY POINT

- Starch is the storage form of glucose in plants and also yields glucose for the body's use.

Glycogen

Just as plant tissues store glucose in long chains of starch, animal liver and muscle tissues store glucose in long chains that clump together to form **glycogen** (depicted in Figure 4–3).[1]* Glycogen resembles starch in that it consists of glucose molecules linked together to form chains, but its chains are longer and more highly branched (see Figure 4–4). Unlike starch, which is abundant in grains, potatoes, and other foods from plants, glycogen is nearly undetectable in meats because it breaks down rapidly when the animal is slaughtered. A later section describes how the human body handles its own packages of stored glucose.

KEY POINT

- Glycogen is the storage form of glucose in the body.

*Reference notes are in Appendix F.

Fibers

Some of the **fibers** of a plant form the supporting structures of its leaves, stems, and seeds. Other fibers play other roles; for example, they retain water and thus protect seeds from drying out. Like starch, most fibers are polysaccharides—chains of sugars—but they differ from starch in that the sugar units are held together by bonds that human digestive enzymes cannot break. Most fibers therefore pass through the human body intact, without providing energy for its use. A little energy arises, however, when certain fibers encounter the colon's bacterial colonies, which do possess fiber-digesting enzymes. This digestion involves **fermentation**, a form of breakdown that produces tiny products, mainly fat fragments, which the human colon absorbs. Many animals, such as cattle, depend heavily on their digestive-system bacteria to make the energy of glucose available from the abundant cellulose, a form of fiber, in their fodder. Thus, when we eat beef, we indirectly receive some of the sun's energy that was originally stored in the fiber of the plants. Beef itself, like other animal products, contains no fiber.

KEY POINTS

- Fibers lend structure to plants and perform other functions.
- Human digestive enzymes cannot break the chemical bonds of fibers.
- Some fiber is susceptible to fermentation by bacteria in the colon.

Summary

Plants combine carbon dioxide, water, and the sun's energy to form glucose, which they can store as the polysaccharide starch. Then animals or people eat the plants and retrieve the glucose. In the body, the liver and muscles may store the glucose as the polysaccharide glycogen, but ultimately it yields glucose again. Thus, glucose delivers the sun's energy to fuel the body's activities. In the process, glucose breaks down to the waste products carbon dioxide and water, which are excreted. Later, plants use these compounds again as raw materials to make carbohydrate. Fibers are plant constituents that are not digested directly by human enzymes, but intestinal bacteria ferment some fibers, and dietary fiber contributes to the health of the body.

The Need for Carbohydrates

LO 4.2   Explain why carbohydrates are needed in the diet.

Glucose from carbohydrate is an important fuel for most body functions. Only two other nutrients provide energy to the body: protein and fats.[†] Protein-rich foods are usually expensive and, when used to make fuel for the body, provide no advantage over carbohydrates. Moreover, excess dietary protein has disadvantages, as Chapter 6 explains. Fats normally are not used as fuel by the brain and central nervous system; these tissues prefer glucose, and red blood cells use glucose exclusively. Thus, glucose is a critical energy source, and whole foods that supply carbohydrates—particularly the fiber-rich ones—are the preferred source of glucose in the diet.[‡]

Carbohydrates also play vital roles in the functioning of body tissues. For example, sugars that dangle from protein molecules, once thought to be mere hitchhikers, are now known to dramatically alter the shape and function of certain proteins. Such a sugar-protein complex is responsible for the slipperiness of mucus, the watery lubricant that coats and protects the body's internal linings and membranes. Sugars also bind to the outsides of cell membranes, where they facilitate cell-to-cell communication and nerve and brain cell functioning. Clearly, the body needs carbohydrates for more than just energy.

glycogen (GLY-co-gen) a highly branched polysaccharide that is made and held in liver and muscle tissues as a storage form of glucose. Glycogen is not a significant food source of carbohydrate and is not counted as one of the complex carbohydrates in foods.

fibers the indigestible parts of plant foods, largely nonstarch polysaccharides that are not digested by human digestive enzymes, although some are digested by resident bacteria of the colon. Fibers include cellulose, hemicelluloses, pectins, gums, mucilages, and a few non-polysaccharides such as lignin.

fermentation the anaerobic (without oxygen) breakdown of carbohydrates by microorganisms that releases small organic compounds along with carbon dioxide and energy.

[†]Ethanol, the alcohol in alcoholic beverages, also supplies calories, but alcohol is toxic to body tissues.

If I Want to Lose Weight and Stay Healthy, Should I Avoid Carbohydrates?

Carbohydrates have been wrongly accused of being the "fattening" ingredient of foods, thereby misleading millions of weight-conscious people into eliminating nutritious carbohydrate-rich foods from their diets. In truth, people who wish to lose fat, maintain lean tissue, and stay healthy can do no better than to attend closely to portion sizes and calorie intakes, and to design an eating plan around carbohydrate-rich fruit, legumes, vegetables, and **whole grains**.

Lower in Calories Gram for gram, carbohydrates donate fewer calories than do dietary fats, and converting excess glucose into fat for storage is inefficient, costing many calories. Still, it is possible to consume enough calories of carbohydrate to exceed the need for energy, and this reliably leads to weight *gain*. To lose weight, dieters must plan to consume fewer total calories from all foods and beverages each day.

Empty Calories of Added Sugars Recommendations to choose carbohydrate-rich foods do not extend to refined added sugars. Purified, refined sugars (mostly sucrose or fructose) contain no other nutrients—no protein, vitamins, minerals, or fiber—and thus are low in nutrient density. A person choosing 400 calories of sugar in place of 400 calories of whole-grain bread loses the nutrients, phytochemicals, and fiber of the bread. You can afford to do this only if you have already met all of your nutrient needs for the day and still have calories to spend.

Overuse of added sugars may have other effects as well. The Controversy section of this chapter considers evidence concerning added sugars, blood lipids, and chronic disease risks.

Guidelines For health's sake, then, most people should increase their intakes of fiber-rich whole-food sources of carbohydrates and reduce their intakes of foods high in refined grains and added sugars. Table 4–1 presents carbohydrate recommendations and guidelines from several authorities.

Note that recommendations for total carbohydrate and added sugars may be given as "percentages of total calories," a concept introduced in the Do the Math feature of Chapter 2 (p. 33). Percentages make sense in this regard because they apply proportionally to all calorie intakes, and individuals' calorie needs vary widely. For example, the recommended range of total carbohydrate intakes is from 45 to 65 percent of daily calories. This amounts to 900 to 1,300 calories of carbohydrate in a 2,000-calorie diet, but for a person needing just 1,200 calories a day, carbohydrate should provide only 540 to 780 calories. Likewise, the limit on added sugars also depends upon a person's daily calorie needs.

The recommended range for total carbohydrate intake is one of the three AMDR (see pp. 32–33). These ranges for energy nutrients ensure adequate intakes and are associated with low risks for developing chronic diseases. Figure 4–5 illustrates that when the contribution of one energy nutrient (for example, carbohydrate, shown by the blue bar) changes in a calorie-controlled diet, the other energy nutrients must increase or decrease proportionally to hold total calories constant.

This chapter's Consumer's Guide describes various whole-grain foods, and the Food Feature helps you "see" the carbohydrates in foods. For weight loss, authorities do not recommend omitting carbohydrates. In fact, the opposite is true.

The brain uses glucose as its primary fuel.

Unlike the added sugars in concentrated sweets, the sugars in fruit are diluted with water and naturally packaged with vitamins, minerals, phytochemicals, and fiber.

KEY POINTS

- The body tissues use carbohydrate for energy and other critical functions.
- The brain and nerve tissues prefer carbohydrate as fuel, and red blood cells can use nothing else.
- Intakes of refined carbohydrates should be limited.

whole grains grains or foods made from them that contain all the parts and naturally occurring nutrients of the entire grain seed, except the inedible husk.

‡Such combination molecules are known as *glycoproteins*.

Chapter 4 The Carbohydrates: Sugar, Starch, Glycogen, and Fiber

Table 4–1

Recommendations for Carbohydrate Intakes

1. Total carbohydrate
Dietary Reference Intakes (DRI)
- At a minimum, adults and children need 130 g/day to provide glucose to the brain.
- For optimal health, most people should consume between 45 and 65% of total calories from carbohydrate.

Dietary Guidelines for Americans
- Choose nutrient-dense grains, fruit, starchy vegetables, legumes, and milk to meet the day's total carbohydrate intake.

2. Added sugars
Dietary Guidelines for Americans
- Limit intakes of added sugars to a maximum of 10% of total calories.

American Heart Association
- A prudent daily upper limit is not more than 100 cal (about 6 teaspoons) of added sugars for most women and children or 150 cal for most men.

World Health Organization (WHO)
- *Strong recommendation*[a] Both adults and children should reduce the intake of added sugars to less than 10% of total energy intake.
- *Conditional recommendation*[b] Both children and adults should further reduce the intake of added sugars to below 5% of total energy intake.

3. Whole grains
Dietary Guidelines for Americans
- A healthy eating pattern includes grains, at least half of which are whole grains.

4. Fiber
Dietary Reference Intakes (DRI)
- 38 g of total fiber per day for men through age 50; 30 g for men 51 and older.
- 25 g of total fiber per day for women through age 50; 21 g for women 51 and older.

[a]*Strong recommendations indicate that desirable effects of adherence to the recommendation outweigh undesirable consequences. The recommendation can be applied in most situations.*

[b]*Conditional recommendations are made with less certainty, but with some scientific support.*

Figure 4–5

Percentages of Energy Nutrients

The three energy nutrients—carbohydrate, fat, and protein—all contribute to the total energy (calorie) intake. Whenever the percentage of one energy nutrient increases or decreases, the percentages from the others must change as well to keep calories constant.

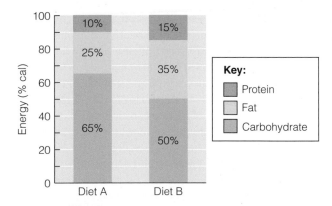

Key:
- Protein
- Fat
- Carbohydrate

Why Do Nutrition Experts Recommend Fiber-Rich Foods?

People who regularly eat fiber-rich fruit, legumes, vegetables, nuts, seeds, and whole grains are often reported to be healthier than those who do not, and the fibers in those foods deserve some of the credit.[2] Researchers often classify dietary fibers according to their solubility in water. This section introduces the fibers and explores their health effects.

Soluble Fibers   Fibers that readily dissolve in water are the **soluble fibers**. In foods, soluble fibers add a pleasing consistency. Examples are pectin that puts the gel

soluble fibers food components that readily dissolve in water, become viscous, and often impart gummy or gel-like characteristics to foods. An example is pectin from fruit, which is used to thicken jellies.

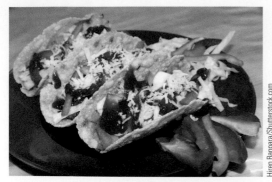

A delicious high-fiber meal.

in jelly and gums that make bottled salad dressings **viscous**. Soluble fibers are naturally abundant in oats, barley, legumes, okra, and citrus fruit. In addition to food sources, extracted single soluble fiber preparations are used as medications or as food additives.

In the body, soluble fibers are best known for their ability to modulate blood glucose levels, lower blood cholesterol, and promote the health of the colon.[3] Many kinds are readily fermented by colonic bacteria, and products of their fermentation:

- nourish cells of the colon and promote resistance to colon cancer,
- reduce inflammation, and
- support immunity.[4]

Clearly, an eating pattern that supplies ample soluble fibers helps maintain the body's health.

KEY POINTS

- Soluble fibers dissolve in water, form viscous gels, and many are readily fermented by colonic bacteria.
- Soluble fibers and products of their fermentation play roles in maintaining the body's health.

Insoluble Fibers   Other fibers are **insoluble fibers**. These do not dissolve in water, do not form gels, are not viscous, and resist fermentation. Insoluble fibers, such as cellulose, form structures of plants, such as the outer layers of whole grains (bran), the strings of celery, the hulls of seeds, and the skins of corn kernels. These fibers retain their shape and rough texture even after hours of cooking. In the digestive system, they ease elimination, as described later.

Figure 4–6 shows the diverse effects of different fibers, and generally where they are found in foods. Most unrefined plant foods contain a mix of fiber types.

KEY POINTS

- Insoluble fibers do not dissolve in water; they form structural parts of plants and resist fermentation by colonic bacteria.
- Insoluble fibers support digestive tract health.

Heart Disease and Stroke   Evidence suggests that diets rich in fruit, legumes, vegetables, nuts, seeds, and whole grains—and therefore rich in fibers and other complex carbohydrates—are protective against heart disease and stroke.[5] Such diets are also generally low in added sugars, saturated fat, and *trans* fat, and are high in nutrients and phytochemicals—all factors associated with a reduced risk of heart disease. Oatmeal was first to be identified among cholesterol-lowering foods.[6] Apples, barley, carrots, and legumes are also rich in gel-forming fibers that can lower blood cholesterol. In contrast, diets high in refined grains and added sugars may push blood lipids toward elevated heart disease risks.

Soluble, gel-forming fibers may lower blood cholesterol by binding bile, a digestive juice that contains cholesterol compounds. Bile is made by the liver and secreted into the intestine (see Chapter 3). Normally, much of bile's cholesterol would be reabsorbed from the intestine for reuse, but the fiber carries some of it out with the feces (Figure 4–7, p. 114). These bile compounds are needed in digestion, so the liver responds to a lack of them by drawing on the body's cholesterol stocks to synthesize more.

KEY POINT

- Foods rich in soluble fibers help control blood cholesterol.

Blood Glucose Control   The soluble fibers of foods such as oats and legumes help regulate blood glucose following a carbohydrate-rich meal. Soluble fibers delay digestion of nutrients, thus slowing glucose absorption from the digestive tract.[7] People with **diabetes** are urged to consume fiber-rich foods to help improve their blood glucose control.[8]

Diabetes is a topic of Chapter 11.

viscous (VISS-cuss) having a sticky, gummy, or gel-like consistency that flows relatively slowly.

insoluble fibers the tough, fibrous structures of fruit, vegetables, and grains; indigestible food components that do not dissolve in water.

diabetes (dye-uh-BEET-eez) metabolic diseases that impair a person's ability to regulate blood glucose.

Figure 4–6

Characteristics, Sources, and Health Effects of Fibers

Most plant-derived foods provide a mixture of soluble and insoluble fibers.

People who eat these foods...		obtain these types of fibers...	with these actions in the body...	and receive these probable health benefits.
		Soluble, viscous, often fermentable and gel-forming		
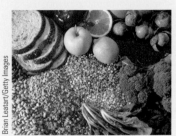	• Barley, oats, oat bran, rye, fruit (apples, citrus), legumes (especially young green peas and black-eyed peas), seaweeds, seeds, many vegetables, fibers used as food additives[b]	• Beta-glucans • Gums • Inulin[a] • Pectins • Psyllium[b] • Some hemicellulose	• Reduce blood cholesterol by binding bile • Slow glucose absorption • Slow transit of food through upper GI tract; delay nutrient absorption • Hold moisture in stools, softening them (less fermentable soluble fibers) • Nourish beneficial bacterial colonies in the colon • Yield small fat molecules after fermentation that the colon can use for energy • Increase satiety	• Alleviate constipation (less fermentable soluble fibers) • Lower risk of heart disease • Lower risk of diabetes • Lower risk of colon and rectal cancer • Increase satiety (improve weight management)
		Insoluble, nonviscous, mostly unfermentable		
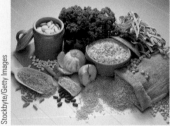	• Brown rice, fruit, legumes, seeds, vegetables (cabbage, carrots, brussels sprouts), wheat bran, whole grains, extracted fibers used as food additives	• Cellulose • Lignins • Resistant starch • Hemicellulose	• Stimulate colon lining, increase fecal weight, and speed fecal passage through colon • Provide bulk and feelings of fullness	• Alleviate constipation • Lower risk of hemorrhoids and appendicitis • Reduce complications from diverticulosis • Lower risk of colon and rectal cancer

Brian Leatart/Getty Images

Stockbyte/Getty Images

[a]*Inulin, a soluble and fermentable but nonviscous fiber, is found naturally in a few vegetables, but is also purified from chicory root for use as a food additive.*
[b]*Psyllium, a soluble fiber derived from seed husks, resists fermentation and is used as a laxative and food additive.*

Sources: Information from J. W. McRorie, Evidence-based approach to fiber supplements and clinically meaningful health benefits, Part I, Nutrition Today 50 (2015): 82–89; J. W. McRorie, Evidence-based approach to fiber supplements and clinically meaningful health benefits, Part II, Nutrition Today 50 (2015): 90–97.

KEY POINT

■ Foods rich in soluble fibers help to modulate the rate of glucose absorption.

> The microbiota of the digestive tract is described in Chapter 3.

Digestive Tract Health Soluble and insoluble fibers, along with an ample fluid intake, support the colon's health and proper function. Fermentable soluble fibers of whole foods are of special importance in these roles.[9] Although human enzymes cannot digest these fibers, colonic bacteria readily ferment them, deriving sustenance that allows beneficial colonies to multiply and flourish.

People who suffer occasional constipation often find relief by taking fiber supplements. Specially manufactured soluble fiber in supplements resists fermentation by the colon's bacteria and remains intact in the digestive tract.[§] This fiber cannot nourish beneficial bacteria but swells with water, softening and giving weight to fecal matter, easing its passage from the system. Coarse insoluble fibers also relieve constipation by stimulating the colon lining to secrete mucus and water that enlarge and soften the stools.

Large, soft stools ease the task of elimination. Pressure is then reduced in the lower bowel (colon), helping to prevent swelling of the rectal veins (**hemorrhoids**). Fiber prevents compaction of the intestinal contents, which could obstruct the appendix and

hemorrhoids (HEM-or-oids) swollen, hardened (varicose) veins in the rectum, usually caused by pressure resulting from constipation.

[§]The unfermentable manufactured fibers are methylcellulose (from wood pulp) and psyllium (from seed husk).

Figure 4–7

One Way Fiber in Food May Lower Cholesterol in the Blood

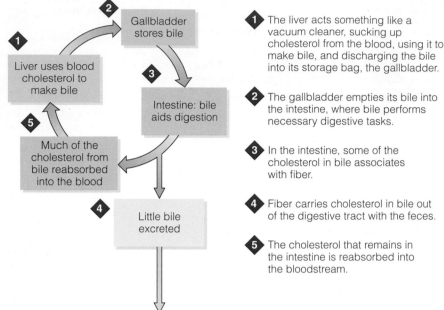

High-fiber diet: More cholesterol (in bile) is carried out of the body.

- Liver uses blood cholesterol to make bile ❶
- Gallbladder stores bile ❷
- Intestine: bile aids digestion; bound by fiber in colon ❸
- A little cholesterol from bile reabsorbed into the blood ❺
- Fiber and bile excreted in feces ❹

Low-fiber diet: More cholesterol (from bile) is reabsorbed and returned to the bloodstream.

- Liver uses blood cholesterol to make bile ❶
- Gallbladder stores bile ❷
- Intestine: bile aids digestion ❸
- Much of the cholesterol from bile reabsorbed into the blood ❺
- Little bile excreted ❹

❶ The liver acts something like a vacuum cleaner, sucking up cholesterol from the blood, using it to make bile, and discharging the bile into its storage bag, the gallbladder.

❷ The gallbladder empties its bile into the intestine, where bile performs necessary digestive tasks.

❸ In the intestine, some of the cholesterol in bile associates with fiber.

❹ Fiber carries cholesterol in bile out of the digestive tract with the feces.

❺ The cholesterol that remains in the intestine is reabsorbed into the bloodstream.

Figure 4–8

Diverticula

Diverticula are abnormally bulging pockets in the colon wall. These pockets can entrap feces and become painfully infected and inflamed, requiring hospitalization, antibiotic therapy, or surgery.

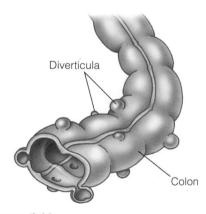

Diverticula

Colon

appendicitis inflammation and/or infection of the appendix. (The appendix is a sac about 4 inches long, protruding from the large intestine. It may become infected if fragments of the intestinal contents become trapped within it.)

diverticula (dye-ver-TIC-you-la) sacs or pouches that balloon out of the intestinal wall, caused by weakening of the muscle layers that encase the intestine. The painful inflammation of one or more of the diverticula is known as *diverticulitis*.

---

permit bacteria to invade and infect it (**appendicitis**). In addition, many people suffer from weaknesses in the wall of the large intestine that leads portions of the wall to bulge out into pouches known as **diverticula** (illustrated in Figure 4–8). Ample dietary fiber may help reduce complications of diverticula, but, contrary to long-held beliefs, it may not keep them from forming.[10]

KEY POINTS

- Soluble fibers help to sustain intestinal colonies of beneficial bacteria.
- Both soluble and insoluble fibers ease elimination by enlarging and softening stools, and maintain digestive tract health.

Digestive Tract Cancers   Cancers of the colon and rectum claim tens of thousands of lives each year.[11] The risks of these cancers are highest among people with low dietary fiber intakes. Evidence supports an inverse association between dietary fiber and cancers of the colon and rectum.[12] Subjects in one study who ate the most fiber (28 or more grams per day) had risks of colon and rectal cancer that were 17 percent lower than in subjects who ate the least. This study and others with similar results focus on fiber from grains, fruit, and vegetables and not from supplements. Fiber supplements lack the nutrients and phytochemicals of whole foods, which may also help protect against cancers.

All plant foods have attributes that may reduce the risks of colon and rectal cancers but researchers are still working out these relationships. Fibers dilute, bind, and rapidly remove potential cancer-causing agents from the colon. In addition, small fat molecules arising from the bacterial fermentation of fiber that takes place during digestion may activate cancer-destroying mechanisms and inhibit inflammation in the colon.[13] (Many other daily choices influence colon cancer risks, and you can read about them in Chapter 11.)

KEY POINTS

- Adequate dietary fiber may reduce the risks of colon and rectal cancers.
- Plant foods supply fiber, nutrients, and phytochemicals that oppose cancers in many ways.

Healthy Weight Management Foods rich in fibers tend to be low in fats, added sugars, and calories and can therefore help to prevent weight gain and promote weight loss by delivering less energy per bite. In addition, fibers absorb water from the digestive juices; as they swell, they create feelings of fullness and delay hunger. The small fat molecules formed during fermentation of soluble fibers may shift the body's hormones in ways that promote feelings of fullness, but no one yet knows if daily food intake is reduced by this mechanism.[14] The opposite is certainly true of low fiber intakes: as populations eat more refined low-fiber grains and concentrated sweets, body fat stores expand.

To achieve the fiber intakes that are best for you, follow the eating patterns of the Dietary Guidelines for Americans. Choose the recommended servings of whole, nutrient-dense fruit and vegetables, make at least half the grain choices whole grains, and choose legumes several times per week. That way, you'll obtain all of the benefits that plant foods have to offer. Eating a diet of highly refined foods and adding a fiber supplement is simply not the same.

KEY POINT

- A diet with adequate fiber-rich whole foods may help to manage body weight.

Fiber Intakes and Excesses

Few people in the United States or Canada consume sufficient fiber. The DRI value for fiber is 14 grams per 1,000 calories, or 25 grams per day for most women and 38 grams for most men—almost twice the average current intake of about 15 grams (women) and 18 grams (men).[15] Fiber recommendations (in the back pages, p. A) are made in terms of total fiber with no distinction among fiber types because most fiber-rich foods supply a mixture of fibers.

An effective way to add fiber while lowering saturated fat is to substitute plant sources of protein (legumes) for some of the animal sources of protein (meats and cheeses) in the diet. Another way is to focus on consuming the recommended amounts of fruit, vegetables, legumes, and whole grains each day. (Figure 4–16 of the Food Feature provides some tips for increasing fiber intake.) You can make a quick approximation of a day's fiber intake by following the instructions in Table 4–2. People choosing high-fiber foods are also wise to drink extra fluids to help the fiber do its job.

Can My Diet Have Too Much Fiber? No Tolerable Upper Intake Level has been established for fiber, but consuming purified fiber added to foods or supplements can be taken to extremes. One overly enthusiastic eater of oat bran muffins required emergency surgery for a blocked intestine; too much oat bran and too little fluid overwhelmed his digestive system. Use bran and other purified fibers with moderation, and remember to drink an extra beverage with them.

Fiber makes food bulky and takes up space in the stomach, so a person who eats only small amounts of food at a time may not meet energy or nutrient needs when the diet presents too much high-fiber food. The malnourished, the elderly, and young children adhering to all-plant (vegan) diets are especially vulnerable to this problem.

A by-product of fiber fermentation can be any of several odorous gases, an effect most noticeable with sudden increases in fiber intake. Don't give up on high-fiber foods if they cause gas. Instead, start with small servings and gradually increase the serving size over several weeks; chew foods thoroughly to break up hard-to-digest lumps that can ferment in the intestine; and try a variety of fiber-rich foods until you find some that do not cause the problem. Some people also find relief from excessive gas by using commercial enzyme preparations sold for use with beans. Such products contain enzymes that help break down some of the indigestible fibers in foods before they reach the colon.

Binders in Fiber Binders in some fibers act as **chelating agents**. This means that they link chemically with important nutrient minerals (iron, zinc, calcium, and others)

Table 4–2

A Quick Method for Estimating Fiber Intake

1. Multiply servings (½ c cut up or 1 medium piece) of any fruit or vegetable (excluding juice) by 1.5 g.[a] *Example:* 5 servings of fruit and vegetables × 1.5 = 7.5 g fiber

2. Multiply ½ c servings of refined grains by 1.0 g. *Example:* 4 servings of refined grains × 1.0 = 4.0 g fiber

3. Multiply ½ c servings of whole grains by 2.5 g. *Example:* 3 servings of whole grains × 2.5 = 7.5 g fiber

4. Add fiber values for servings of legumes, nuts, seeds, and high-fiber cereals and breads; look these up online.[b] *Example:* ½ c navy beans = 6.0 g fiber

5. Add up the grams of fiber from the previous lines. *Example:* 7.5 + 4.0 + 7.5 + 6.0 = 25 g fiber

Day's total fiber = 25 g fiber

[a]*Most cooked and canned fruit and vegetables contain about this amount, while whole raw fruit and some vegetables contain more.*

[b]*Find fiber values of foods in USDA's What's in the Foods You Eat Search Tool, available at https://ndb.nal.usda.gov/ndb/.*

chelating agents (KEY-late-ing) molecules that attract or bind with other molecules and are therefore useful in either preventing or promoting movement of substances from place to place.

Table 4-3

Usefulness of Carbohydrates

Carbohydrates in the Body	Carbohydrates in Foods
■ *Energy source.* Sugars and starch from the diet provide energy for many body functions; they provide glucose, the preferred fuel for the brain and nerves.	■ *Flavor.* Sugars provide sweetness.
■ *Glucose storage.* Muscle and liver glycogen store glucose.	■ *Browning.* When exposed to heat, sugars undergo browning reactions, lending appealing color, aroma, and taste.
■ *Raw material.* Sugars can be partly broken down to fragments that are used in making other compounds, such as certain amino acids (the building blocks of proteins), as needed.	■ *Texture.* Sugars help make foods tender. Cooked starch lends a smooth, pleasing texture.
■ *Structures and functions.* Sugars interact with protein molecules, affecting their structures and functions.	■ *Gel formation.* Starch molecules expand when heated and trap water molecules, forming gels. The fiber pectin forms the gel of jellies when cooked with sugar and acid from fruit.
■ *Digestive tract health.* Fibers help maintain healthy bowel function (reduce risk of bowel diseases).	■ *Bulk and viscosity (thickness).* Carbohydrates lend bulk and increased viscosity to foods. Soluble, viscous fibers lend thickness to foods such as salad dressings.
■ *Blood cholesterol.* Fibers promote normal blood cholesterol concentrations (reduce risk of heart disease).	■ *Moisture.* Sugars attract water and keep foods moist.
■ *Blood glucose.* Fibers modulate blood glucose concentrations (help control diabetes).	■ *Preservative.* Sugar in high concentrations dehydrates bacteria and preserves the food.
■ *Satiety.* Fibers and sugars contribute to feelings of fullness.	■ *Fermentation.* Carbohydrates are fermented by yeast, a process that causes bread dough to rise and beer to brew.
■ *Body weight.* A fiber-rich diet is conducive to a healthy body weight.	

and then carry them out of the body. The mineral iron is mostly absorbed at the top of the intestinal tract, and excess insoluble fibers may limit its absorption by speeding foods along the upper part of the tract. Chelating agents are often sold by supplement vendors to "remove toxins" from the body. Some valid medical uses exist, such as the treatment of lead poisoning, but most chelating agents sold over the counter are unnecessary.

A later section focuses on the handling of carbohydrates by the digestive system. Table 4–3 sums up the points made so far concerning the functions of carbohydrates in the body and in foods.

KEY POINTS

- Few people consume sufficient fiber.
- The best fiber sources are whole foods from plants.
- Fluid intake should increase along with fiber.
- Very-high-fiber all-plant diets can pose nutritional risks for people who are old or malnourished, and for young children.

Whole Grains

The Dietary Guidelines for Americans urge everyone to make at least half of their daily grain choices *whole* grains, an amount equal to at least three 1-ounce servings of whole grains a day. To do this, you must distinguish among grain foods that are **refined**, **enriched**, **fortified**, and whole grain (see Table 4–4). This chapter's Consumer's Guide (p. 120) explains how to find whole-grain foods.

Flour Types   The part of a typical grain plant, such as wheat, that is made into flour (and then into bread, cereals, and pasta) is the seed, or kernel. The kernel has four main parts: the **germ**, the **endosperm**, the **bran**, and the **husk**, as shown in Figure 4–9. The germ is the part that grows into a new plant, in this case wheat, and therefore contains concentrated food to support the new life—it is especially rich in oils, vitamins, and minerals. The endosperm is the soft, white inside portion of the kernel, containing starch and proteins that help nourish the seed as it sprouts. The kernel is encased in the bran, a protective coating that is similar in function to the shell of a nut;

Table 4–4

Terms that Describe Grain Foods

- **bran** the protective fibrous coating around a grain; the chief fiber constituent of a grain.
- **brown bread** bread containing ingredients such as molasses that lend a brown color; these breads may be made with any kind of flour, including white flour.
- **endosperm** the bulk of the edible part of a grain, the starchy part.
- **enriched, fortified** refers to the addition of nutrients to a refined food product. As defined by U.S. law, these terms mean that specified levels of thiamin, riboflavin, niacin, folate, and iron have been added to refined grains and grain products. The terms *enriched* and *fortified* can refer to the addition of more nutrients than just these five; read the label.[a]
- **germ** the nutrient-rich inner part of a grain.
- **husk** the outer, inedible part of a grain.
- **multi-grain** a term used on food labels to indicate a food made with more than one kind of grain. Not an indicator of a whole-grain food.
- **refined** refers to the process by which the coarse parts of food products are removed. For example, the refining of wheat into white enriched flour involves removing three of the four parts of the kernel—the chaff, the bran, and the germ—leaving only the endosperm, which is composed mainly of starch and a little protein.
- **refined grains** grains and grain products from which the bran, germ, or other edible parts of whole grains have been removed; not a whole grain. Many refined grains are low in fiber and are enriched with vitamins, as required by U.S. regulations.
- **stone-ground** refers to a milling process using limestone to grind any grain, including refined grains, into flour.
- **unbleached flour** a beige-colored refined endosperm flour with texture and nutritive qualities that approximate those of regular white flour.
- **wheat bread** bread made with any wheat flour, including refined enriched white flour.
- **wheat flour** any flour made from wheat, including refined white flour.
- **white flour** an endosperm flour that has been refined and bleached for maximum softness and whiteness.
- **white wheat** a wheat variety developed to be paler in color than common red wheat (most familiar flours are made from red wheat). White wheat is similar to red wheat in carbohydrate, protein, and other nutrients, but it lacks the dark and bitter, although potentially beneficial, phytochemicals of red wheat.
- **100% whole grain** a label term for food in which the grain is entirely whole grain, with no added refined grains.
- **whole-wheat flour** flour made from intact wheat kernels; a whole-grain flour. Also called *graham flour*.

[a]*Formerly,* enriched *and* fortified *carried distinct meanings with regard to the nutrient amounts added to foods, but a change in the law has made these terms virtually synonymous.*

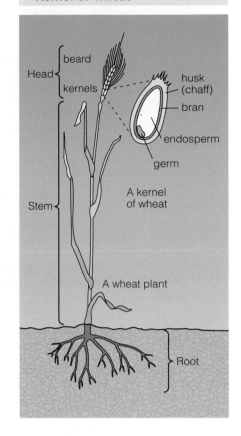

Figure 4–9

A Wheat Plant and a Single Kernel of Wheat

the bran is also rich in nutrients and fiber. The husk, commonly called chaff, is the dry outermost layer that is inedible by human beings but can be consumed and digested by many plant-eating animals, so it is used in animal feed.

In earlier times, people milled wheat by grinding it between two stones, blowing or sifting out the tough outer chaff, but retaining all the nutrient-rich bran and germ, as well as the endosperm. With advances in milling machinery, it became possible to remove the dark, heavy bran and germ, leaving a whiter, smoother-textured flour with a higher starch content and far less fiber. An advantage of this flour, besides producing soft, white baked goods, is its durability—white flour "keeps" much longer than whole-grain flour because the nutrient-rich, oily germ of whole grains turns rancid over time. As food production became more industrialized, suppliers realized that customers also favored this refined, soft, white flour over the crunchy, dark brown, "old-fashioned" flour.

KEY POINT

- Whole-grain flours retain all edible parts of grain kernels.

Enrichment of Refined Grains In turning to highly refined grains, many people suffered deficiencies of iron, thiamin, riboflavin, and niacin—nutrients formerly obtained from whole grains. To reverse this tragedy, Congress passed the U.S. Enrichment Act of 1942, requiring that iron, niacin, thiamin, and riboflavin be added to all refined grain products before they were sold. In 1996, the vitamin folate (often called *folic acid* on labels) was added to the list. Today, all refined grain products are enriched with at least the nutrients mandated by the act.

A single serving of enriched grain food is not "rich" in the enrichment nutrients, but people who eat several servings a day obtain significantly more of these nutrients than they would from unenriched refined products, as the bread example of Figure 4–10 shows.

Figure 4–10

Nutrients in Whole-Grain, Enriched White, and Unenriched White Breads

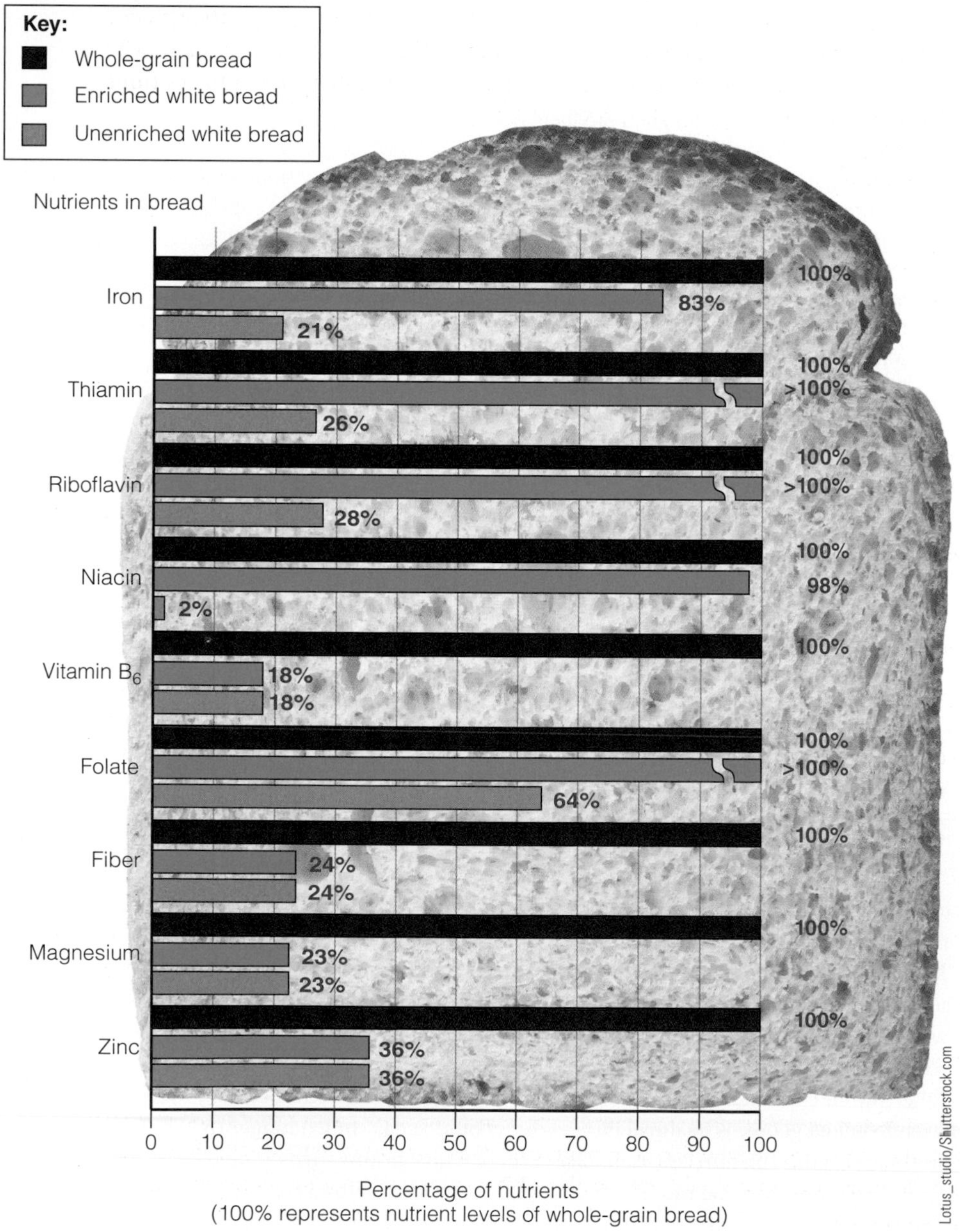
Key:
Whole-grain bread
Enriched white bread
Unenriched white bread
Nutrients in bread
Iron
100%
83%
21%
Thiamin
100%
>100%
26%
Riboflavin
100%
>100%
28%
Niacin
100%
98%
2%
Vitamin B_6
100%
18%
18%
Folate
100%
>100%
64%
Fiber
100%
24%
24%
Magnesium
100%
23%
23%
Zinc
100%
36%
36%
0 10 20 30 40 50 60 70 80 90 100
Percentage of nutrients
(100% represents nutrient levels of whole-grain bread)
Lotus_studio/Shutterstock.com

Enriched grain foods are nutritionally comparable to whole-grain foods only with respect to their added nutrients; whole grains provide greater amounts of vitamin B_6 and the minerals magnesium and zinc that refined grains lack. Whole grains also provide substantial fiber (see Table 4–5), along with a wide array of potentially beneficial phytochemicals in the bran and the essential oils of the germ.

KEY POINT

- Refined grain products are less nutritious than whole grains.

Health Effects of Whole Grains   Whole-grain intakes provide health benefits beyond just nutrients and fiber. People who take in just three daily servings of whole grains often have healthier body weights and less body fat than other people.[16] It could be that whole grains fill up the stomach, slow down digestion, or promote longer-lasting feelings of fullness than refined grains. A higher intake of whole grains also correlates with lower risks of heart disease, type 2 diabetes, and death from all causes.[17] Finally, people who make a habit of eating whole grains may have lower than average risks of certain cancers, particularly of the colon. It may be that the fiber, phytochemicals, or nutrients of whole grains improve body tissue health, but these issues need clarification.

Refined grains in amounts of up to one-half of the daily grain intake (without added sugars, fats, or sodium) seem to pose little risk to health. Clearly, however, those who choose to ignore the Dietary Guidelines for Americans recommendation to consume sufficient whole grains do so at their peril.

KEY POINT

- A diet rich in whole grains is associated with reduced risks of overweight and certain chronic diseases.

Table 4–5

Grams of Fiber in One Cup of Flour

Dark rye, 31 g
Barley, 15 g
Whole wheat, 13 g
Buckwheat, 12 g
Oat, 12 g
Whole-grain cornmeal, 9 g
Light rye, 8 g
Enriched white, 3 g

From Carbohydrates to Glucose

LO 4.3   Describe how carbohydrates are converted to glucose in the human body.

You may eat bread or a baked potato, but the body's cells cannot use foods or even whole molecules of lactose, sucrose, or starch for energy. They need the glucose in those molecules. The various body systems must make glucose available to the cells, not all at once when it is eaten but at a steady rate all day.

Digestion and Absorption of Carbohydrate

To obtain glucose from newly eaten food, the digestive system must first render the starch and disaccharides from the food into monosaccharides that can be absorbed through the cells lining the small intestine. The largest of the digestible carbohydrate molecules, starch, requires the most extensive breakdown. Disaccharides, in contrast, need be split only once before they can be absorbed.

Starch   Digestion of most starch begins in the mouth, where an enzyme in saliva mixes with food and begins to split starch into shorter units. While chewing a bite of bread, you may notice that a slightly sweet taste develops—the disaccharide maltose is being liberated from starch by the enzyme. The salivary enzyme continues to act on the starch in the bite of bread until it is pushed downward and mixed with the stomach's acid and other juices. The salivary enzyme (made of protein) is deactivated by the stomach's protein-digesting acid.

With the breakdown of the salivary enzyme in the stomach, starch digestion ceases, but it resumes at full speed in the small intestine, where another starch-splitting enzyme is delivered by the pancreas. This enzyme breaks starch down into disaccharides and small polysaccharides. Other enzymes liberate monosaccharides for absorption.

Finding Whole-Grain Foods

"OK, it's time to take action." A consumer, ready to switch to some whole-grain foods, may find these good intentions derailed in the tricky terrain of the grocery store. Even experienced shoppers may feel bewildered in store-length aisles bulging with breads that range from light-as-a-feather, refined enriched white loaves to the heaviest, roughest-textured whole-grain varieties. Baffling arrays of label claims vie for shoppers' attention, too—and although some are trustworthy, others are not.

Not Every Choice Must Be 100 Percent Whole Grain

If you are just now starting to include whole grains in your diet, keep in mind that various combinations of whole and refined grains can meet the Dietary Guidelines recommendation that half of the day's grains be whole grains.[1]* Until your taste buds adjust, you may prefer breads, cereals, pastas, and other grain foods made from a half-and-half blend of whole and refined grains for all of your day's choices. The addition of some refined enriched white flour smoothes the texture of whole grain foods and provides a measure of folate, an important enrichment vitamin in the U.S. diet. Alternatively, you might choose 100 percent whole grains half of the time and refined grains for the other half, or any other combination to meet the need.

In addition to whole-grain blends, a variety of white durum wheat has been developed to mimic the taste and appearance of ordinary enriched refined white flour while offering nutrients similar to those of whole grains. Such **white wheat** products lack the dark-colored and strong-flavored phytochemicals associated with ordinary whole-wheat products, however, and research has not established whether their effects on

the health of the body are equivalent.[†] (Look back at Table 4–4, p. 117, for definitions.)

High Fiber Does Not Equal Whole Grain

An important distinction exists between foods labeled "high-fiber" and those made of whole grains. High-fiber breads or cereals may derive their fiber from the addition of wheat bran or even purified cellulose, and not from whole grains. Label readers can distinguish one kind from the other by scanning the food's ingredients list for words like *bran, cellulose, methylcellulose, gums,* or *psyllium.* Such high-fiber foods may be nutritious and useful in their own way, but they cannot substitute for whole-grain foods in the diet.

Brown Color Does Not Equal Whole Grain

"**Brown bread**" may sound healthy, and white bread less so, but the term *brown* simply refers to color that may derive from brown ingredients, such as molasses. Similarly, whole-grain rice, commonly called brown rice, cannot be judged by color alone. Whole-grain rice comes in red and other colors, too. Also, many rice dishes appear brown because they contain brown-colored ingredients, such as soy sauce, beef broth, or seasonings. Pasta comes in a rainbow of colors, and whole-grain noodles and blends are increasingly available—just read the ingredients list on the label to check that any descriptors on the outside of the package accurately reflect the food inside.

Label Subtleties

A label proclaiming "Multi-Grain Goodness" or "Natural Wheat Bread" may

imply healthfulness but can mislead uninformed shoppers, who assume, falsely, that such terms mean "whole grain." Tricky descriptors such as **multi-grain**, **wheat bread**, and **stone-ground** do not indicate whole grains. To find the real whole grains, look for the words *whole* or *whole grain* preceding the name of a grain in the ingredients list. Learn to recognize individual whole grains by name, too. Many are listed in Table 4–6.

Table 4–6

A Sampling of Whole Grains

If a food has at least 8 grams of whole grains per ounce, it is at least half whole grains.

- Amaranth, a grain of the ancient Aztec people[a]
- Barley (hulled but not pearled)[b]
- Buckwheat[a]
- Bulgur wheat
- Corn, including whole cornmeal and popcorn
- Millet
- Oats, including oatmeal
- Quinoa (KEEN-wah), a grain of the ancient Inca people[a]
- Rice, including brown, red, and others
- Rye
- Sorghum (also called milo), a drought-resistant grain
- Teff, popular in Ethiopia, India, and Australia
- Triticale, a cross of durum wheat and rye
- Wheat, in many varieties such as spelt, emmer, farro, einkorn, durum; and forms such as bulgur, cracked wheat, and wheatberries
- Wild rice[a]

[a]Although not botanical grains, these foods are similar to grains in nutrient contents, preparation, and use.

[b]Hulling removes only inedible husk; pearling removes beneficial bran.

*Reference notes are in Appendix F.

[†]In 2005, ConAgra began marketing white wheat as UltraGrain.

Look at the bread labels in Figure 4–11 below, and recall from Chapter 2 that ingredients must be listed in descending order of predominance on an ingredients list. It's easy to see from the label of the "Natural Wheat Bread" in the figure that this bread contains no whole grains whatsoever. This loaf is made entirely of refined enriched wheat flour, another name for white flour. The word "Natural" in the name is a marketing gimmick and has no meaning in nutrition.

Now read the label of "Multi-Grain, Honey Fiber Bread." It does contain multiple whole grains, but the major ingredient is still unbleached enriched wheat flour. The key here is the refinement of the wheatberries to yield refined "white" flour that requires enrichment, that is, enriched wheat flour. The bleaching status is irrelevant. Most of the fiber of this bread's name comes from added cellulose and not from its tiny amounts of "multigrains." Now focus on the bread labeled "Whole Grain, Whole Wheat." This, at last, is a 100 percent whole-grain food.

After the Salt

Here's a trick: a loaf of bread generally contains about one teaspoon of salt. Therefore, if an ingredient is listed *after* the salt, you'll know that the entire loaf contains less than a teaspoonful of that ingredient, not enough to make a significant contribution to the eater's whole-grain intake. In the "Multi-Grain" bread of the figure, all of the whole grains are listed after the salt.

A Word about Cereals

Ready-to-eat breakfast cereals, from toasted oat rings to granola, are a pleasant way to include whole grains in almost anyone's diet. Like breads, cereals vary widely in their contents of whole grains, but, also like breads, they can be evaluated by reading their ingredients lists.

Oatmeal in all its forms—old-fashioned, quick cooking, and even microwavable instant—qualifies as whole grain, but be careful: some instant oatmeal packets contain more sugar than grain. Limit intake of any cereal, hot or cold, with a high sugar, sodium, or saturated fat content, even if it touts "whole grains" on the label.

Moving Ahead

"I've tried buckwheat pancakes, and they're pretty tasty. But what on earth is quinoa?" Admittedly, certain whole grains may be unavailable in

---

Figure 4–11

Bread Labels Compared

Natural Wheat Bread

Nutrition Facts
Serving size 1 slice (30g)
Servings Per Container 15

Amount per serving

Calories 90	Calories from Fat 14

	% Daily Value*
Total Fat 1.5g	2%
Trans Fat 0g	
Sodium 220mg	9%
Total Carbohydrate 15g	5%
Dietary fiber less than 1g	2%
Sugars 2g	
Protein 4g	

INGREDIENTS: UNBLEACHED ENRICHED WHEAT FLOUR [MALTED BARLEY FLOUR, NIACIN, REDUCED IRON, THIAMIN MONONITRATE (VITAMIN B1), RIBOFLAVIN (VITAMIN B2), FOLIC ACID], WATER, HIGH FRUCTOSE CORN SYRUP, MOLASSES, PARTIALLY HYDROGENATED SOYBEAN OIL, YEAST, CORN FLOUR, SALT, GROUND CARAWAY, WHEAT GLUTEN, CALCIUM PROPIONATE (PRESERVATIVE), MONOGLYCERIDES, SOY LECITHIN.

Multi-Grain Honey Fiber

Nutrition Facts
Serving size 1 slice (43g)
Servings Per Container 18

Amount per serving

Calories 120	Calories from Fat 15

	% Daily Value*
Total Fat 1.5g	2%
Trans Fat 0g	
Sodium 170mg	7%
Total Carbohydrate 9g	3%
Dietary fiber 4g	16%
Sugars 2g	
Protein 5g	

INGREDIENTS: UNBLEACHED ENRICHED WHEAT FLOUR, WATER, WHEAT GLUTEN, CELLULOSE, YEAST, SOYBEAN OIL, HONEY, SALT, BARLEY, NATURAL FLAVOR PRESERVATIVES, MONOCALCIUM PHOSPHATE, MILLET, CORN, OATS, SOYBEAN FLOUR, BROWN RICE, FLAXSEED.

Whole Grain Whole Wheat

Nutrition Facts
Serving size 1 slice (30g)
Servings Per Container 18

Amount per serving

Calories 90	Calories from Fat 14

	% Daily Value*
Total Fat 1.5g	2%
Trans Fat 0g	
Sodium 135mg	6%
Total Carbohydrate 15g	5%
Dietary fiber 2g	8%
Sugars 2g	
Protein 4g	

MADE FROM: UNBROMATED STONE GROUND 100% WHOLE WHEAT FLOUR, WATER, CRUSHED WHEAT, HIGH FRUCTOSE CORN SYRUP, PARTIALLY HYDROGENATED VEGETABLE SHORTENING (SOYBEAN AND COTTONSEED OILS), RAISIN JUICE CONCENTRATE, WHEAT GLUTEN, YEAST, WHOLE WHEAT FLAKES, UNSULPHURED MOLASSES, SALT, HONEY, VINEGAR, ENZYME MODIFIED SOY LECITHIN, CULTURED WHEY, UNBLEACHED WHEAT FLOUR AND SOY LECITHIN.

(continued)

mainstream grocery stores. It may take a trip to a "health-food" store to find quinoa, for example. In a welcome trend, larger chain stores are responding to increased consumer demand by stocking more brown rice, wild rice, bulgur, and other whole-grain goodies on their shelves.

Once people begin to enjoy the added taste dimensions of whole grains, they may be less drawn to the bland refined foods formerly eaten out of habit. More than 90 percent of Americans are stuck in this rut, failing to eat the whole grains they need. Be adventurous with health in mind, and give the hearty flavors of a variety of whole-grain foods a try.

Review Questions‡

1. When searching for whole-grain bread, a consumer should search the labels _____.

   a. for words like *multigrain*, *wheat bread*, *brown bread*, or *stone-ground*

   b. for the order in which whole grains appear on the ingredients list

   c. for the word *unbleached*, which indicates that the food is primarily made from whole grains

   d. b and c

‡*Answers to Consumer's Guide review questions are found in Appendix G.*

2. Whole-grain rice, often called brown rice, _____.

   a. can be recognized by its characteristic brown color

   b. cannot be recognized by color alone

   c. is often more refined than white rice

   d. b and c

3. A bread labeled "high-fiber" _____.

   a. may not be a whole-grain food

   b. is a good substitute for whole-grain bread

   c. is required by law to contain whole grains

   d. may contain the dangerous chemical cellulose

Pommer Irina/Shutterstock.com

Most forms of starch are easily digested. The starch of refined white flour, for example, breaks down rapidly to glucose that is absorbed high up in the small intestine. Other starch, such as that of cooked beans, digests more slowly and releases its glucose later in the digestion process. The least digestible starch, called **resistant starch**, is technically a kind of fiber because much of it passes undigested through the small intestine into the colon where bacteria eventually ferment it.[18] Barley, raw or chilled cooked potatoes, cooked dried beans and lentils, oatmeal, popcorn and raw corn, intact seeds and kernels, and underripe bananas all contain resistant starch.

Sugars Sucrose and lactose from food, along with maltose and small polysaccharides freed from starch, undergo one more split to yield free monosaccharides before they are absorbed. This split is accomplished by digestive enzymes attached to the cells of the lining of the small intestine. The conversion of a bite of bread to nutrients for the body is completed when monosaccharides cross these cells and are washed away in a rush of circulating blood that carries them to the waiting liver. Figure 4–12 presents a review of carbohydrate digestion.

The absorbed carbohydrates (glucose, galactose, and fructose) travel in the bloodstream to the liver, which can convert fructose and galactose to glucose. The circulatory system transports the glucose and other products to the cells. Liver and muscle cells store circulating glucose as glycogen; all cells split glucose for energy.

Fiber As explained earlier, although molecules of most fibers are not changed by human digestive enzymes, many of them can be fermented by the bacterial inhabitants of the human colon. The fermentation process breaks down carbohydrate components of fiber into other products, including the small fats important to the health of the colon.

KEY POINTS

- A main task of the human digestive system is to convert starch and sugars to glucose for absorption.
- Other body systems transport and store glucose; all cells can split glucose for energy.

resistant starch the fraction of starch in a food that is digested slowly, or not at all, by human enzymes.

Chapter 4 The Carbohydrates: Sugar, Starch, Glycogen, and Fiber

Figure 4–12

How Carbohydrate in Food Becomes Glucose in the Body

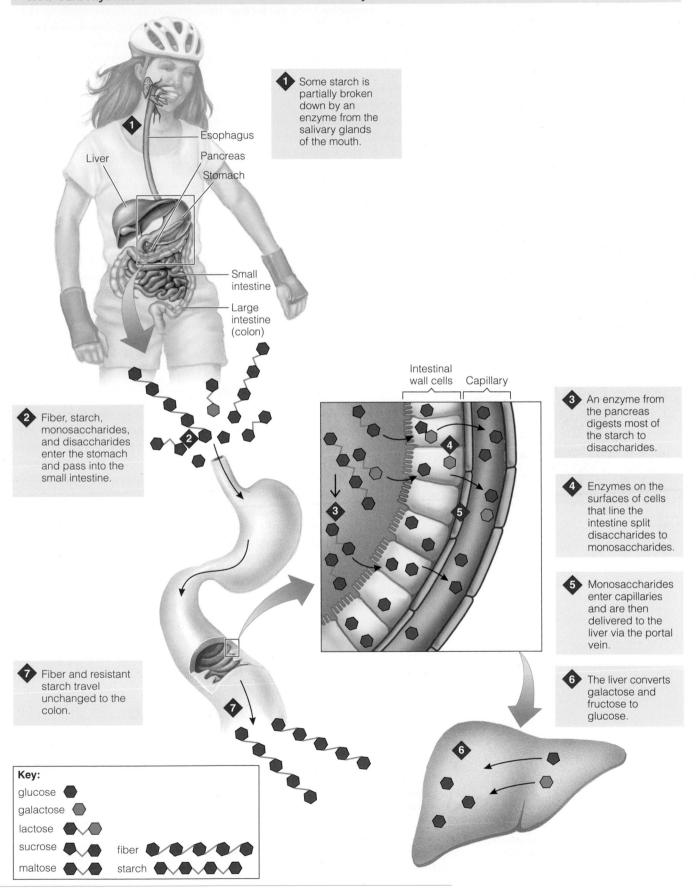

1 Some starch is partially broken down by an enzyme from the salivary glands of the mouth.

Esophagus

Liver

Pancreas

Stomach

Small intestine

Large intestine (colon)

2 Fiber, starch, monosaccharides, and disaccharides enter the stomach and pass into the small intestine.

Intestinal wall cells

Capillary

3 An enzyme from the pancreas digests most of the starch to disaccharides.

4 Enzymes on the surfaces of cells that line the intestine split disaccharides to monosaccharides.

5 Monosaccharides enter capillaries and are then delivered to the liver via the portal vein.

7 Fiber and resistant starch travel unchanged to the colon.

6 The liver converts galactose and fructose to glucose.

Key:

glucose

galactose

lactose

sucrose

maltose

fiber

starch

Why Do Some People Have Trouble Digesting Milk?

Persistent painful gas may herald a change in the digestive tract's ability to digest the sugar in milk, a condition known as **lactose intolerance**. Its cause is insufficient production of **lactase**, the enzyme of the small intestine that splits the disaccharide lactose into its component monosaccharides glucose and galactose, which are then absorbed.

Nearly all infants produce abundant lactase, which helps them absorb the sugar of breast milk and milk-based formulas; a very few suffer inborn lactose intolerance and must be fed solely on lactose-free formulas. Among adults, the ability to digest the carbohydrate of milk varies widely. As they age, an estimated 65 to 75 percent of the world's people lose much of their ability to produce lactase.

The number of people in the United States with lactose intolerance is unknown, but most people who report having the condition are of African, Asian, Hispanic, or Native American descent. People with a long history of consuming unfermented milk, such as northern Europeans, are least likely to have lactose intolerance—only about 5 percent of their descendants develop it.[19]

Symptoms of Lactose Intolerance People with lactose intolerance experience nausea, pain, diarrhea, and excessive gas upon drinking milk or eating lactose-containing products. The undigested lactose remaining in the intestine demands dilution with fluid from surrounding tissue and the bloodstream. Intestinal bacteria use the undigested lactose for their own energy, a process that produces gas and intestinal irritants.

Sometimes sensitivity to milk is due not to lactose intolerance but to an allergic reaction to either of the two proteins in milk.** The immune system overreacts when it encounters the offending milk protein. When people avoid milk for any reason, care must be taken to replace its protein, calcium, and vitamin D in the diet, particularly for growing children. Later chapters point out alternative sources of these nutrients.

Milk Tolerance and Strategies The failure to digest lactose affects people to differing degrees, and total elimination of milk products is rarely necessary. Yogurt may be tolerated because the bacterial strains that change milk into yogurt also help digest lactose.[20] Many affected people can consume up to 6 grams of lactose (½ cup of milk) without symptoms. The most successful strategies seem to be increasing intakes of milk products gradually, spreading them out through the day, and consuming them with meals. Table 4–7 offers more strategies for including milk products and substitutes. Often, people overestimate the severity of their lactose intolerance, blaming it for symptoms most probably caused by something else—a mistake that could cost them the health of their bones (see details in Chapter 8).

KEY POINTS

- In lactose intolerance, the body fails to produce sufficient amounts of the enzyme lactase, needed to digest the sugar of milk, leading to uncomfortable symptoms.
- People with lactose intolerance or milk allergy need alternatives that provide the nutrients of milk.

The Body's Use of Glucose

LO 4.4   Describe the body's handling of glucose.

Glucose is the basic carbohydrate unit used for energy by each of the body's cells. The body handles its glucose judiciously—maintaining an internal store to be used when needed and tightly controlling its blood glucose concentration to ensure a steady supply. Recall that carbohydrates serve functional roles, too, such as forming part of mucus, but they are best known for providing energy.

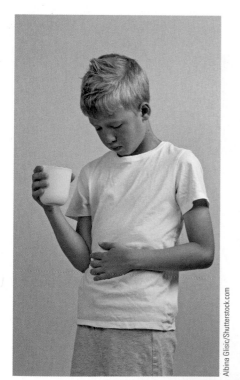

Children who cannot drink milk must receive its nutrients from other sources.

lactose intolerance impaired ability to digest lactose due to reduced amounts of the enzyme lactase.

lactase the intestinal enzyme that splits the disaccharide lactose to monosaccharides during digestion.

**The two proteins of milk are casein and whey protein.

Table 4-7

Lactose Intolerance Strategies

People with lactose intolerance can experiment with milk-based foods to find a strategy that works for them. The trick is to find ways of splitting lactose to glucose and galactose before a food is consumed, rather than providing a lactose feast for colonic bacteria.

Product	Effects/Strategies
Aged cheeses	Bacteria or molds used to create cheeses ferment lactose during the aging process. Use in moderation.
Lactase pills and drops	Lactase added to milk products by consumers or pills taken before milk product consumption split lactose molecules in the digestive tract. Harmless when used as directed by the manufacturer.
Lactase-treated milk products	Lactase added to milk products during manufacturing splits lactose before purchase. Use freely in place of ordinary milk products.
Milk substitutes (soy, pea, nut, or grain beverages), cheese and yogurt substitutes	Nonmilk replacements for milk products may or may not be fortified with the nutrients of milk. Compare Nutrition Facts panels for calcium, protein, and vitamin D in particular.
Yogurt (live culture type)	Yogurt-making bacteria can survive in the human digestive tract; the bacteria possess an enzyme to split lactose.
Yogurt (with added milk solids listed on the label)	These contain *extra* lactose and can overwhelm the system.

Splitting Glucose for Energy

Glucose fuels the work of every cell in the body to some extent, but the cells of the brain and nervous system depend almost exclusively on glucose, and the red blood cells use only glucose. When a cell splits glucose for energy, it performs an intricate sequence of maneuvers that are of great interest to biochemists—and of no interest at all to most people who eat bread and potatoes. What everybody needs to understand, though, is that there is no good substitute for carbohydrate. Carbohydrate is *essential*, as the following details illustrate.

The Point of No Return   At a certain point in the process of splitting glucose for energy, glucose itself is forever lost to the body. First, glucose is broken in half, releasing some energy. Then two pathways open to these glucose halves. They can be put back together to make glucose again, or they can be broken into smaller molecules. If they are broken further, they cannot be reassembled to form glucose.

The smaller molecules can also take different pathways. They can continue along the breakdown pathway to yield still more energy and eventually break down completely to just carbon dioxide and water. Or they can be used as a raw material needed to make certain amino acids. They may also be hitched together into units of body fat. Figure 4–13 (p. 126) shows how glucose is broken down to yield energy and carbon dioxide.

Below a Healthy Minimum   Although glucose can be converted into body fat, body fat cannot be converted into glucose to feed the brain adequately. When the body faces a severe carbohydrate deficit, it has two problems. Having no glucose, it must turn to protein to make some (the body has this ability), diverting protein from its own critical functions, such as maintaining immune defenses. When body protein is used, it is taken from blood, organ, or muscle proteins; no surplus of protein is stored specifically for such emergencies. Protein is indispensable to body functions, and carbohydrate should be kept available precisely to prevent the use of protein for energy. This is called the **protein-sparing action** of carbohydrate. As for fat, it regenerates a small amount of glucose—but not enough to feed the brain and nerve tissues.

protein-sparing action the action of carbohydrate and fat in providing energy that allows protein to be used for purposes it alone can serve.

Figure 4–13

The Breakdown of Glucose Yields Energy and Carbon Dioxide

Cell enzymes split the bonds between the carbon atoms in glucose, liberating the energy stored there for the cell's use. ❶ The first split yields two 3-carbon fragments. The two-way arrows mean that these fragments can also be rejoined to make glucose again. ❷ Once they are broken down further into 2-carbon fragments, however, they cannot rejoin to make glucose. ❸ The carbon atoms liberated when the bonds split are combined with oxygen and released into the air, via the lungs, as carbon dioxide. Although not shown here, water is also produced at each split.

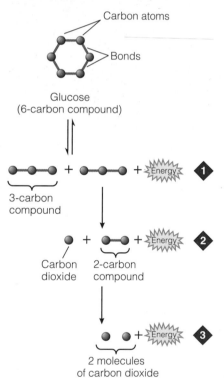

Carbon atoms

Bonds

Glucose
(6-carbon compound)

3-carbon compound + 3-carbon compound + Energy ❶

Carbon dioxide + 2-carbon compound + Energy ❷

+ Energy ❸

2 molecules of carbon dioxide

ketone (kee-tone) **bodies** acidic, water-soluble compounds that arise during the breakdown of fat when carbohydrate is not available. Also called by the broader term *ketones*, although some of these compounds vary chemically.

ketosis (kee-TOE-sis) an undesirably high concentration of ketone bodies, such as acetone, in the blood or urine.

Ketosis With too little carbohydrate flowing to the brain, the body shifts to a mode of metabolism in which it uses fat products, known as **ketone bodies**, for energy in place of some of its glucose. Instead of producing energy by following its main metabolic pathway, fat takes another route in which fat fragments combine with each other. This shift cause an accumulation of the normally scarce acidic ketone bodies.

Ketone bodies can accumulate in the blood, causing **ketosis**. When they reach high levels, they can disturb the normal acid-base balance, a rare but life-threatening situation. Over time, people eating diets that produce ketosis may develop deficiencies of vitamins and minerals, loss of bone minerals, elevated blood cholesterol, impaired mood, and other adverse outcomes. In addition, glycogen stores become too scanty to meet a metabolic emergency or to support vigorous muscular work.

Ketosis isn't all bad, however. Ketone bodies provide a fuel alternative to glucose for brain and nerve cells when glucose is lacking, such as in periods of fasting or in starvation. Not all brain tissues can use ketones—some rely exclusively on glucose, so the body must still sacrifice some protein to provide it—but at a slower rate. A therapeutic ketogenic diet has substantially reduced seizures in children and adults with epilepsy, although many find the diet difficult to follow for long periods and substantial side effects have been reported.[21]

The DRI Minimum Recommendation for Carbohydrate To feed the brain, the DRI committee recommends at least 130 grams of carbohydrate a day for an average-sized person.[22] Much more than this minimum is recommended to maintain health and glycogen stores (explained in the next section). By design, the USDA eating patterns of Chapter 2 deliver more than enough carbohydrates to meet recommendations.

KEY POINTS

- Lacking glucose, the body is forced to alter its uses of protein and fat.
- To help supply the brain with glucose, the body breaks down its protein to make glucose and converts its fats into ketone bodies, incurring ketosis.

How Is Glucose Regulated in the Body?

Should your blood glucose ever climb abnormally high, you might become confused or have difficulty breathing. Should your glucose supplies ever fall too low, you would feel dizzy and weak. A healthy body guards against both conditions with two safeguard activities:

- Siphoning off excess blood glucose into the liver and muscles for storage as glycogen and into the adipose tissue for storage as body fat.
- Replenishing diminished blood glucose from liver glycogen stores.

Two hormones prove critical to these processes. The hormone **insulin** stimulates glucose storage as glycogen, while the hormone **glucagon** helps release glucose from storage.

Insulin After a meal, as blood glucose rises, the pancreas is the first organ to respond. It releases insulin, the hormone that signals body tissues to remove glucose from the blood. Muscle tissue responds to insulin by taking up excess blood glucose and using it to build the polysaccharide glycogen. The liver takes up excess blood glucose, too, but it needs no help from insulin to do so. Instead, liver cells respond to insulin by speeding up their glycogen production. (Figure 4–14 shows glycogen stored in a liver cell.) Adipose tissue also responds to insulin by taking up excess blood glucose. Simply put, insulin regulates blood glucose by:

- Facilitating blood glucose uptake by the muscles and adipose tissue.
- Stimulating glycogen synthesis in the liver.

Figure 4–15 (p. 128) provides an overview of these relationships.

Glucagon   When blood glucose starts to fall too low, the hormone glucagon flows into the bloodstream and triggers the breakdown of liver glycogen to single glucose molecules. The glycogen molecule is highly branched, with hundreds of ends bristling from each molecule's surface (review this structure in Figure 4–3 on p. 108). Enzymes in liver cells respond to glucagon by attacking a multitude of glycogen ends simultaneously to release a surge of glucose into the blood for use by all the body's cells. Thus, the highly branched structure of glycogen uniquely suits the purpose of releasing glucose on demand.

Tissue Glycogen Stores   The muscles hoard two-thirds of the body's total glycogen to ensure that glucose, a critical fuel for physical activity, is available for muscular work. The brain stores a tiny fraction of the total as an emergency reserve to fuel the brain for an hour or two in severe glucose deprivation. The liver stores the remainder and is generous with its glycogen, releasing glucose into the bloodstream for the brain or other tissues when the supply runs low. Without carbohydrate from food to replenish it, the glycogen stores in the liver can be depleted in less than a day. Figure 4–14 shows a liver cell full of the glycogen it stored from a carbohydrate-containing meal.

Be Prepared: Eat Carbohydrate   Another hormone, epinephrine, also triggers the breakdown of liver glycogen as part of the body's defense mechanism to provide extra glucose for quick action in times of danger.[††] To store glucose for emergencies, we are well advised to eat carbohydrate at each meal.

You may be asking, "What kind of carbohydrate?" Candy, "energy bars," and sugary beverages are quick sources of abundant sugar energy, but they provide mostly empty calories and are not the best choices. Balanced meals and snacks, eaten on a regular schedule, help the body maintain its blood glucose. Meals with starch and soluble fiber combined with some protein and a little fat slow digestion so that glucose enters the blood gradually at an ongoing, steady rate.

KEY POINTS

- The muscles and liver store glucose as glycogen; the liver can release glucose from its glycogen into the bloodstream.
- The hormones insulin and glucagon regulate blood glucose concentrations.

Excess Glucose and Body Fatness

Suppose you have eaten dinner and are now sitting on the couch, munching pretzels and drinking cola as you watch a ball game on television. Your digestive tract is delivering molecules of glucose to your bloodstream, and your blood is carrying these molecules to your liver, adipose tissue, and other body cells. The body cells use as much glucose as they can for their energy needs of the moment. Excess glucose molecules are linked together and stored as glycogen until the muscle and liver stores are full to overflowing with glycogen. Still, the glucose keeps coming.

Two Ways to Handle Excess Glucose   To handle the excess, tissues shift to burning more glucose for energy in place of fat. As a result, more fat is left to circulate in the bloodstream until it is picked up by the fat tissues and stored there. If these measures still do not accommodate all of the incoming glucose, the liver, the body's major site of nutrient metabolism, has no choice but to handle the overflow because

---

Figure 4–14

Full Glycogen Stores after a Meal

This photo shows the inside of a single liver cell after a meal (magnified over 100,000 times). The clusters of dark-colored dots are glycogen granules. (The blue structures at the bottom are cellular organelles.)

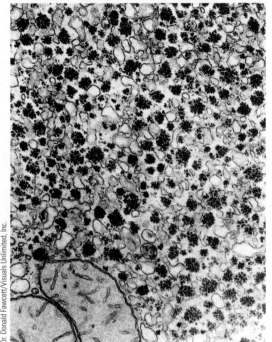

insulin   a hormone secreted by the pancreas in response to a high blood glucose concentration. It assists cells in drawing glucose from the blood.

glucagon   (GLOO-cah-gon)   a hormone secreted by the pancreas that stimulates the liver to release glucose into the blood when blood glucose concentration dips.

[††] Epinephrine is also called adrenaline.

Figure 4–15

Blood Glucose Regulation—An Overview

The pancreas monitors blood glucose (blue hexagons) and adjusts its concentration with two opposing hormones, insulin and glucagon. When glucose is high, the pancreas releases insulin which stimulates body tissues to take up glucose from the bloodstream. When glucose is low, it releases glucagon, which stimulates the liver to release glucose. When glucose concentration is restored to the normal range, the pancreas slows its hormone output in an elegant feedback system.

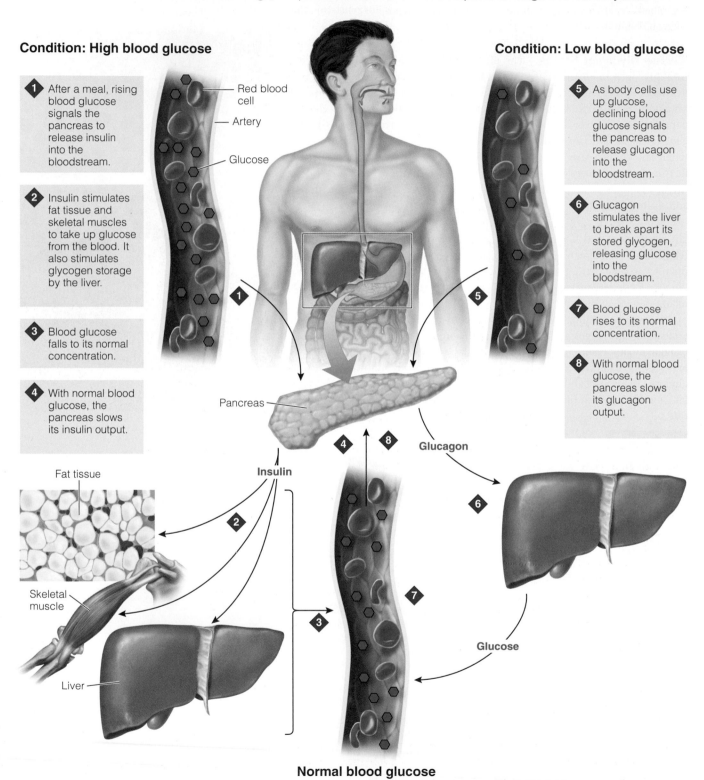

Condition: High blood glucose

1. After a meal, rising blood glucose signals the pancreas to release insulin into the bloodstream.

2. Insulin stimulates fat tissue and skeletal muscles to take up glucose from the blood. It also stimulates glycogen storage by the liver.

3. Blood glucose falls to its normal concentration.

4. With normal blood glucose, the pancreas slows its insulin output.

Red blood cell

Artery

Glucose

Fat tissue

Skeletal muscle

Insulin

Liver

Pancreas

Condition: Low blood glucose

5. As body cells use up glucose, declining blood glucose signals the pancreas to release glucagon into the bloodstream.

6. Glucagon stimulates the liver to break apart its stored glycogen, releasing glucose into the bloodstream.

7. Blood glucose rises to its normal concentration.

8. With normal blood glucose, the pancreas slows its glucagon output.

Glucagon

Glucose

Normal blood glucose

A working body needs carbohydrate fuel to replenish glycogen, and when it runs low, physical activity can seem more difficult. If your workouts seem to drag and never get easier, take a look at your eating pattern. Are your meals regularly timed? Do they provide abundant carbohydrate from nutritious whole foods to fill up glycogen stores so they last through a workout?

Here's a trick: at least an hour before your workout, eat a small snack of about 300 calories of foods rich in complex carbohydrates and drink some extra fluid (see Chapter 10 for ideas). Remember to cut back your intake at other meals by an equivalent amount to prevent unwanted weight gain. The snack provides glucose at a steady rate to spare glycogen, and the fluid helps maintain hydration.

start now! Choose a one-week period and have a healthy carbohydrate-rich snack of about 300 calories, along with a bottle of water, about an hour before you exercise. Be sure to track your diet in Diet & Wellness Plus in MindTap during this period so that you can accurately determine your total calorie intake. Did you have more energy for exercise after you changed your eating plan?

---

excess glucose left circulating in the blood can harm the tissues. The liver breaks the extra glucose into smaller molecules and puts them together into a more permanent energy-storage compound—fat.[23] Newly made fat travels in the blood to the adipose tissues and is stored there. (Fat that builds up in the liver instead can cause injury; see the Controversy.) Unlike the liver cells, which store only about 2,000 calories of glycogen, the fat cells of an average-size person store over 70,000 calories of fat, and their ability to expand their fat storage capacity over time is almost limitless. Moral: you had better play the game if you are going to eat the food. (The Think Fitness feature offers tips to help you play.)

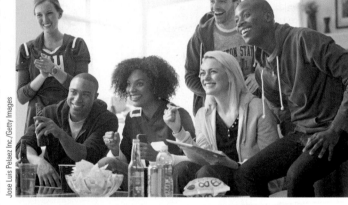

You had better play the game if you are going to eat the food.

Carbohydrate and Weight Maintenance A balanced eating pattern that provides the recommended complex carbohydrates from whole foods can help control body weight and maintain lean tissue. Bite for bite, complex carbohydrate-rich foods contribute less to the body's available energy than do fat-rich foods, and they best support physical activity to promote a lean body. Thus, if you want to stay healthy and remain lean, you should make every effort to follow a calorie-appropriate eating pattern providing 45 to 65 percent of its calories from mostly unrefined sources of carbohydrates.

This chapter's Food Feature provides the first set of tools required for the job of choosing such a diet. Once you have learned to identify the food sources of various carbohydrates, you must then set about learning which fats are which (Chapter 5) and how to obtain adequate protein without overdoing it (Chapter 6). By Chapter 9, you can put it all together to meet the goal of achieving and maintaining a healthy body weight.

KEY POINT

- The liver has the ability to convert glucose into fat, but most excess glucose is stored as glycogen or used to meet the body's immediate needs for fuel.

The Glycemic Index of Food

Carbohydrate-rich foods vary in the degree to which they elevate both blood glucose and insulin concentrations. A food's average effect in laboratory tests can be ranked on a scale known as the **glycemic index (GI)**. It can then be compared with the score of a reference dose of pure glucose, taken by the same person. A food's ranking may surprise you. For example, baked potatoes rank higher than ice cream, partly because ice cream contains

glycemic index (GI) a ranking of foods according to their potential for raising blood glucose relative to a reference dose of glucose.

Table 4–8

Glycemic Index of Selected Common Foods

Glycemic Index	Grains	Fruit	Vegetables	Milk Products	Protein Foods[a]	Other
Low	Barley, chapati, corn tortilla, rice noodles, rolled oats, pasta	Apple, apple juice, banana, dates, mango, orange, orange juice, peaches (canned), strawberry jam	Carrots, corn	Ice cream, milk, soy milk, yogurt	Legumes	Chocolate candy
Medium	Brown rice, couscous	Pineapple	Potatoes (French fries), sweet potatoes			Popcorn, potato chips, soft drinks
High	Breads, breakfast cereals, white rice	Watermelon	Potatoes (boiled)			Rice crackers

Note: Using the glucose reference scale, foods are classified as low (55 or less), medium (56 to 69), or high (70 or greater).

[a]Protein foods that contain little or no carbohydrate (such as meats, poultry, fish, and eggs) do not raise blood glucose, and therefore do not have a glycemic index.

Source: Adapted from F. S. Atkinson, K. Foster-Powell, and J. C. Brand-Miller, International tables of glycemic index and glycemic load values: 2008, Diabetes Care 31 (2008): 2281–2283.

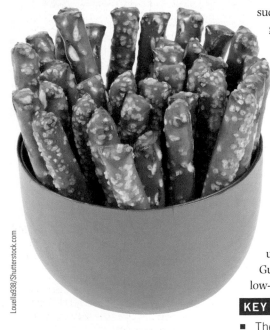

Louella938/Shutterstock.com

sucrose, made of equal parts fructose and glucose. Fructose only slightly raises blood glucose. In contrast, the starch of potatoes is all glucose. The milk fat of ice cream also slows digestion and glucose absorption, factors that lower its GI ranking. Protein in food lowers its GI, too.[24] Table 4–8 shows generally where some foods have been ranked, but test results often vary widely between laboratories, depending on food ripeness, processing, and seasonal and varietal differences.

In addition to food factors, an individual's own metabolism affects the body's insulin response to carbohydrate. The glycemic response to any one food often varies widely among individual people.[25]

Research supports a link between higher chronic disease risks and a steady diet of high-glycemic ultra-processed foods, such as refined grains, sugary drinks, and snack cakes.[26] However, categorizing foods as good or bad on the basis of their GI ranking alone is often not the best choice nutritionally—chocolate candy, for example, has a lower GI than does nutritious brown rice. For people with diabetes, the glycemic index is not of primary concern.[27] In fact, research suggests it may be unnecessary in the context of a diet that follows the eating patterns of the Dietary Guidelines for Americans, and is based on whole grains, legumes, vegetables, fruit, low-fat protein foods, and milk and milk products.[28]

KEY POINTS

- The glycemic index reflects the degree to which a food raises blood glucose.
- A steady diet of high-glycemic ultra-processed foods may be linked with chronic diseases.
- The concept of good and bad foods based solely on the glycemic response is an oversimplification.

What Happens If Blood Glucose Regulation Fails?

LO 4.5   Briefly summarize the differences among type 1 diabetes,
         type 2 diabetes, and hypoglycemia.

In some people, blood glucose regulation fails. When this happens, either of two conditions can result: diabetes or **hypoglycemia**.

Diabetes

This section serves as a brief introduction to this serious and widespread metabolic disease. Chapter 11 presents the details concerning diabetes prevention, diagnosis, consequences, and treatment.

In diabetes, blood glucose rises after a meal and remains above normal because insulin is either inadequate or ineffective. Abnormally high blood glucose is a characteristic of two main types of diabetes. In the less common **type 1 diabetes**, the pancreas fails to produce insulin. The immune system attacks and destroys insulin-producing cells in the pancreas as if they were foreign cells. In the more common **type 2 diabetes**, the body cells fail to respond to insulin by taking up blood glucose. This condition tends to occur as a consequence of obesity, and the best preventive measure is often to maintain a healthy body weight.

Diabetes was defined earlier on p. 112.

Achieving stable blood glucose is the goal of diabetes treatment. Three approaches work together: controlling carbohydrate and calorie intakes, exercising appropriately, and taking insulin injections or medications that modulate blood glucose. To control the amount of carbohydrate presented to the body at one time, it helps to eat regularly timed meals and snacks, to eat similar amounts of food at each meal and snack, and to choose nutritious foods that support a healthy body weight. Small amounts of added sugars are permissible, but nutrition suffers if the empty calories of sugar displace needed whole foods, such as fruit or vegetables, from the diet.[29] (Other reasons to limit added sugars are discussed in the Controversy.) Dietitians commonly rely on the Food Lists for Diabetes to help plan healthy meals for people with diabetes (see Appendix D).

KEY POINTS

- In type 1 diabetes, blood glucose stays too high because insulin is lacking.
- In type 2 diabetes, blood glucose stays too high because the cells do not respond to normal insulin levels.

Hypoglycemia

In healthy people, blood glucose rises after eating and then gradually falls back into the normal range without attracting notice. In hypoglycemia, blood glucose drops below normal, bringing on unpleasant symptoms such as weakness, irregular heartbeats, sweating, anxiety, hunger, trembling, and, rarely, seizures and loss of consciousness.

Hypoglycemia rarely occurs in healthy people, whose hormones maintain normal blood glucose concentrations. It most often happens as a consequence of poorly managed diabetes. Blood glucose can plummet with too much insulin, too much strenuous physical activity, inadequate food intake, or illness.[30] If the person is conscious, administering glucose in the form of fruit juice, hard candies, or glucose tablets can raise the blood glucose concentration. An unconscious person needs immediate medical intervention.

KEY POINT

- In hypoglycemia, blood glucose falls below normal, usually as a result of poorly controlled diabetes or other diseases.

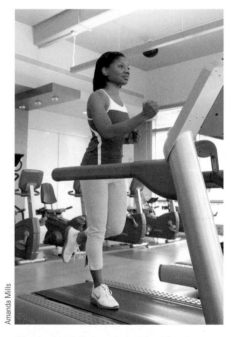

Physical activity, control of food intake, and medications play key roles in diabetes management.

hypoglycemia (HIGH-poh-gly-SEE-mee-ah) an abnormally low blood glucose concentration, often accompanied by symptoms such as anxiety, rapid heartbeat, and sweating.

type 1 diabetes the type of diabetes in which the pancreas produces no or very little insulin; often diagnosed in childhood, although some cases arise in adulthood.

type 2 diabetes the type of diabetes in which the pancreas makes plenty of insulin but the body's cells resist insulin's action; often diagnosed in adulthood.

Conclusion

Part of eating right is choosing wisely among the many foods available. Largely without your awareness, the body responds to the carbohydrates supplied by your diet. Now you take the controls by learning how to integrate carbohydrate-rich foods into an eating pattern that meets your body's needs.

FOOD FEATURE

Finding the Carbohydrates in Foods

LO 4.6 Identify foods that are rich in carbohydrates.

To support optimal health, an eating pattern must supply enough of the right kinds of carbohydrate-rich foods. A health-promoting 2,000-calorie diet should provide in the range of 45 to 65 percent of calories from carbohydrates (225 to 325 grams), mostly from whole foods, each day. This amount more than meets the minimum DRI amount of 130 grams needed to feed the brain and ward off ketosis. People needing more or less energy require proportionately more or less carbohydrate.

If you are curious about your own carbohydrate need, find your DRI estimated energy requirement (see the back of the book, p. A), and multiply by 45 percent to obtain the bottom of your carbohydrate intake range and then by 65 percent for the top. Then divide both answers by 4 calories per gram (see the example in the margin).

Breads and cereals, starchy vegetables, fruit, and milk are all good contributors of starch and dilute sugars. Many foods also provide fiber in varying amounts, as Figure 4–16 (p. 133) demonstrates. Concentrated sweets provide sugars but little else, as the last section demonstrates.

Fruit

A fruit portion of ½ cup of juice, a small banana or apple or orange, ½ cup of canned or fresh fruit, or ¼ cup of dried fruit supplies an average of about 15 grams of carbohydrate, mostly as sugars, including the fruit sugar fructose. Fruit vary greatly in their water and fiber contents and in their sugar concentrations. Juices should contribute no more than half of a day's intake of fruit. Except for avocados and olives, which are high in healthful fats, fruit contain insignificant amounts of fat and protein.

Vegetables

Starchy vegetables are major contributors of starch in the diet. Just one small white or sweet potato or ½ cup of cooked dry beans, corn, peas, plantain, or winter squash provides 15 grams of carbohydrate, as much as in a slice of bread, though as a mixture of sugars and starch. One-half cup of carrots, okra, onions, tomatoes, cooked greens, or most other nonstarchy vegetables or a cup of salad greens provides about 5 grams as a mixture of starch and sugars.

Grains

Breads and other starchy foods are famous for their carbohydrate contributions. Nutrition authorities encourage people to reduce intakes of refined grains and to make at least half of the grain choices whole grains. A slice of bread, half an English muffin, a 6-inch tortilla, ⅓ cup of rice or pasta, or ½ cup of cooked cereal provides about 15 grams of carbohydrate, mostly as starch. Ready-to-eat cereals, particularly those that children prefer, can derive over half their weight from added sugars, so consumers must read labels.

Most grain choices should also be low in solid fats and added sugar. When extra calories are required to meet energy needs, some selections higher in unsaturated fats (see Chapter 5) and added sugar can supply needed calories and provide pleasure in eating.

Do the Math

The carbohydrate intake recommended in a 2,700-calorie eating pattern ranges between about 300 and 440 grams per day. Example for 45% of calories in a 2,700-calorie diet:

- 2,700 cal × 0.45 = 1,215 cal
- 1,215 cal ÷ 4 cal/g = 304 g

Example for 65% of calories in a 2,700-calorie diet:

- 2,700 cal × 0.65 = 1,755 cal
- 1,775 cal ÷ 4 cal/g = 439 g

Using this information, find the carbohydrate range for a 1,600-calorie diet.

Chapter 4 The Carbohydrates: Sugar, Starch, Glycogen, and Fiber

Figure 4–16

Fiber in the Food Groups

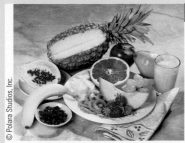

Fruit

Fiber Tips:
- Add dried or chopped fresh fruit to salads.
- Leave skins on peaches and pears (wash well).
- Eat a fresh peeled orange instead of drinking juice.

Food[a]	Fiber (g)	Food	Fiber (g)
Pear, raw, 1 medium	6	Other berries, raw, 1/2 c	2
Blackberries/raspberries, raw, 1/2 c	4	Peach, raw, 1 medium	2
Prunes, cooked, 1/4 c	4	Strawberries, sliced, 1/2 c	2
Figs, dried, 3	3	Cantaloupe, raw, 1/2 c	1
Apple, 1 medium	3	Cherries, raw, 1/2 c	1
Apricots, raw, 4	3	Fruit cocktail, canned, 1/2 c	1
Banana, raw, 1	3	Peach half, canned	1
Orange, 1 medium	3	Raisins, dry, 1/4 c	1
		Orange juice, 3/4 c	<1

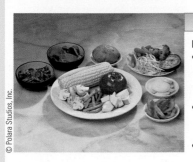

Vegetables

Fiber Tips:
- Leave the skins on most vegetables (wash well).
- Snack on raw vegetable sticks.
- Add extra chopped vegetables to chili or other stews.

Food	Fiber (g)	Food	Fiber (g)
Baked potato with skin, 1	4	Mashed potatoes, home recipe, 1/2 c	2
Broccoli, chopped, 1/2 c	3	Bell peppers, 1/2 c	1
Brussels sprouts, 1/2 c	3	Broccoli, raw, chopped, 1/2 c	1
Spinach, 1/2 c	3	Carrot juice, 1/2 c	1
Asparagus, 1/2 c	2	Celery, 1/2 c	1
Baked potato, no skin, 1	2	Dill pickle, 1 whole	1
Cabbage, red, 1/2 c	2	Eggplant, 1/2 c	1
Carrots, 1/2 c	2	Lettuce, romaine, 1 c	1
Cauliflower, 1/2 c	2	Onions, 1/2 c	1
Corn, 1/2 c	2	Tomato, raw, 1 medium	1
Green beans, 1/2 c	2	Tomato juice, canned, 3/4 c	1

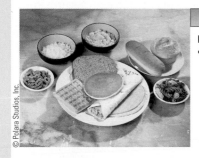

Grains

Fiber Tips:
- Choose whole-grain breads, buns, cereals, crackers, pasta, rice, and tortillas.

Food	Fiber[a] (g)	Food	Fiber (g)
100% bran cereal, 1 oz	10	Pumpernickel bread, 1 slice	2
Barley, pearled, 1/2 c	3	Shredded wheat, 1 large biscuit	2
Cheerios, 1 oz	3	Cornflakes, 1 oz	1
Whole-wheat bread, 1 slice	3	Muffin, blueberry, 1	1
Whole-wheat pasta,[b] 1/2 c	3	Puffed wheat, 1 1/2 c	1
Wheat flakes, 1 oz	3	White pasta,[b] 1/2 c	1
Brown rice, 1/2 c	2	Cream of wheat, 1/2 c	<1
Light rye bread, 1 slice	2	White bread, 1 slice	<1
Muffin, bran, 1 small	2	White rice, 1/2 c	<1
Oatmeal, 1/2 c	2		
Popcorn, 2 c	2		

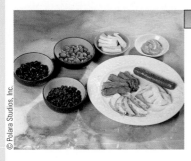

Protein Foods

Fiber Tips:
- Add cooked or canned beans or lentils to soups, stews, and salads.
- Snack on nuts or peanuts with skins.
- Try a soy burger or soy crumbles in recipes that call for meat.

Food	Fiber (g)	Food	Fiber (g)
Lentils, 1/2 c	8	Soybeans, 1/2 c	5
Kidney beans, 1/2 c	8	Soy burger or soy crumbles, 3 oz	4
Pinto beans, 1/2 c	8	Almonds or mixed nuts, 1/4 c	4
Black beans, 1/2 c	7	Peanuts, with skins, 1/4 c	3
Black-eyed peas, 1/2 c	6	Peanut butter, 2 tbs	2
Lima beans, 1/2 c	5	Cashew nuts, 1/4 c	1
		Meat, poultry, fish, and eggs	0

[a]All values are for ready-to-eat or cooked foods unless otherwise noted. Fruit values include edible skins. All values are rounded values.
[b]Pasta includes spaghetti noodles, lasagna, macaroni, and other noodles.

(continued)

These choices might include biscuits, cookies, croissants, muffins, ready-to-eat sweetened cereals, and snack crackers.

Protein Foods

With two exceptions, foods of this group provide almost no carbohydrate to the diet. The exceptions are nuts, which provide a little starch and fiber along with their abundant fat, and legumes (dried beans), revered by diet-watchers as high-protein, low-fat sources of both starch and fiber that can reduce feelings of hunger. Just ½ cup of cooked beans, peas, or lentils provides 15 grams of carbohydrate, an amount equaling the richest carbohydrate sources. Among sources of fiber, legumes are peerless, providing as much as 8 grams in ½ cup.

Milk and Milk Products

A cup of milk or plain yogurt is a generous contributor of carbohydrate, donating about 12 grams. Cottage cheese provides about 6 grams of carbohydrate per cup, but most other cheeses contain little, if any, carbohydrate. These foods also contribute high-quality protein (a point in their favor), as well as several important vitamins and minerals. Calcium-fortified soy beverages (soy milk) and soy yogurts approximate the nutrients of milk, providing some amount of added calcium and 14 grams of carbohydrate. Milk and soy milk products vary in fat content, an important consideration in choosing among them. Sweetened milk and soy products contain added sugars.

Butter and cream cheese, though dairy products, are not equivalent to milk because they contain little or no carbohydrate and insignificant amounts of the other nutrients important in milk. They are appropriately associated with the solid fats.

Oils, Solid Fats, and Added Sugars

Oils and solid fats are devoid of carbohydrate, but added sugars provide almost pure carbohydrate. Most people enjoy sweets, so it is important to learn something of their nature and to account for them in an eating pattern. First, the definitions of "sugar" come into play (Table 4–9 defines sugar terms).

Table 4–9

Terms that Describe Sugar

Note: The term *sugars* here refers to monosaccharides and disaccharides. On a label's ingredients list, the term *sugar* means sucrose. See Chapter 12 for terms related to noncaloric, nonnutritive sweeteners.

- **added sugars** sugars and syrups added to a food for any purpose, such as to add sweetness or bulk or to aid in browning (baked goods). Also called carbohydrate sweeteners, they include glucose, fructose, corn syrup, concentrated fruit juice, and other sweet carbohydrates.
- **agave syrup** a carbohydrate-rich sweetener made from a Mexican plant; a high fructose content gives some agave syrups a greater sweetening power per calorie than sucrose.
- **brown sugar** white sugar with molasses added, 95% pure sucrose.
- **coconut sugar** a granulated sugar composed of sucrose, glucose, and fructose; made by evaporating the sap of the flower buds of coconut palm trees.
- **concentrated fruit juice sweetener** a concentrated sugar syrup made from dehydrated, deflavored fruit juice, commonly grape juice; used to sweeten products that can then claim to be "all fruit."
- **confectioner's sugar** finely powdered sucrose, 99.9% pure.
- **corn sweeteners** corn syrup and sugar solutions derived from corn.
- **corn syrup** a syrup, mostly glucose, partly maltose, produced by the action of enzymes on cornstarch. Includes corn syrup solids.
- **dextrose, anhydrous dextrose** forms of glucose.
- **evaporated cane juice** raw sugar from which impurities have been removed.
- **fructose, galactose, glucose** the monosaccharides important in nutrition.
- **granulated sugar** common table sugar, crystalline sucrose, 99.9% pure.
- **high-fructose corn syrup** a commercial sweetener used in many foods, including soft drinks. Composed almost entirely of the monosaccharides fructose and glucose, its sweetness and caloric value are similar to those of sucrose.

- **honey** a concentrated solution composed primarily of glucose and fructose, produced by enzymatic digestion of the sucrose in nectar by bees.
- **invert sugar** a mixture of glucose and fructose formed by the splitting of sucrose in an industrial process. Sold only in liquid form and sweeter than sucrose, invert sugar forms during certain cooking procedures and works to prevent crystallization of sucrose in soft candies and sweets.
- **lactose, maltose, sucrose** the disaccharides important in nutrition.
- **levulose** an older name for fructose.
- **malt syrup** a sweetener made from sprouted barley.
- **maple syrup** a concentrated solution of sucrose derived from the sap of the sugar maple tree. This sugar was once common but is now usually replaced by sucrose and artificial maple flavoring.
- **molasses** a thick brown syrup left over from the refining of sucrose from sugar cane. The major micronutrient in molasses is iron, a contaminant from the machinery used in processing it.
- **naturally occurring sugars** sugars that are not added to a food but are present as its original constituents, such as the sugars of fruit or milk.
- **nectars** concentrated juice and pulp of peach, pear, or other fruit.
- **raw sugar** the first crop of crystals harvested during sugar processing. Raw sugar cannot be sold in the United States because it contains too much filth (dirt, insect fragments, and the like). Sugar sold as U.S. "raw sugar" is actually evaporated cane juice.
- **turbinado** (ter-bih-NOD-oh) **sugar** raw sugar from which the filth has been washed; legal to sell in the United States.
- **white sugar** granulated sucrose, produced by dissolving, concentrating, and recrystallizing raw sugar. Also called *table sugar*.

Chapter 4 The Carbohydrates: Sugar, Starch, Glycogen, and Fiber

All sugars originally develop by way of photosynthesis in plants. A sugar molecule inside a grape (one of the **naturally occurring sugars**) is chemically indistinguishable from one extracted from sugar beets, sugar cane, grapes, or corn and added to sweeten strawberry jam. Honey added to food is also an added sugar with similar chemical makeup. All arise naturally and, through processing, are purified to remove most or all of the original plant material—bees process honey and machines process the other types. The body handles all the sugars in the same way, whatever their source.

Added sugars, when consumed in large amounts, may be linked with health problems (see the Controversy section), and they bring only empty calories into the diet, with no other significant nutrients. Conversely, the naturally occurring sugars of, say, an orange provide calories but also the vitamins, minerals, fiber, and phytochemicals of oranges. Added sugars can contribute to nutrient deficiencies by displacing nutritious food from the diet. Most people can afford only a little added sugar in their diets if they are to meet nutrient needs within calorie limits. The Dietary Guidelines for Americans suggest a limit of about 8 teaspoons of sugar, or almost one soft drink's worth, in a nutrient-dense 2,200-calorie eating pattern. Table 4–10 provides some tips for limiting intakes of added sugar while still enjoying its sweet taste.

The Nature of Sugar

Each teaspoonful of any sweet can be assumed to supply about 16 calories and 4 grams of carbohydrate. An exception is honey, which packs more calories into each teaspoon

Table 4–10

Tips for Reducing Intakes of Added Sugars

These tricks can help reduce added sugar intake by changing old habits:

- A good use of sugar is to make nutrient-dense but bland or sharp-tasting foods (such as oatmeal or grapefruit) more palatable. Use the smallest amount that does the job.
- Add sweet spices such as cinnamon, nutmeg, allspice, or clove.
- Add a tiny pinch of salt; it will make food taste sweeter.
- Nonnutritive sweeteners add sweetness without calories. Read about them in Chapter 12.
- Choose fruit for dessert most often.
- Choose smaller portions of cake, cookies, ice cream, other desserts, and candy, or skip them.
- Compare sugar contents of similar foods on their Nutrition Facts panels, and choose those with less sugar.
- Reduce sugar added to recipes or foods at the table by a third—the difference in taste generally isn't noticeable.
- Replace empty-calorie-rich regular sodas, sports drinks, energy drinks, and fruit drinks with water, fat-free milk, 100% fruit juice, or unsweetened tea or coffee.
- Warm up sweet foods before serving (heat enhances sweet tastes).

because its crystals are dissolved in water; the dry crystals of sugar take up more space. If you use ketchup liberally, remember that each tablespoon of it contains a teaspoon of sugar. And for soft-drink users, a 12-ounce can of sugar-sweetened cola contains at least 8 teaspoons of added sugar.

What about the nutritional value of a product such as molasses or concentrated fruit juice sweetener as compared with white sugar? Molasses, a by-product of sugar manufacturing, contains 1 milligram of iron per tablespoon. (A man's DRI is 8 milligrams; a young woman's is 18 milligrams.) The iron of molasses comes from the machinery in which molasses is made, however, and is in the form of an iron salt not easily absorbed by the body. The nutrients of added sugars simply do not add up as fast as their calories.

As for concentrated juice sweeteners, such as the concentrated grape or pear "juice" used to sweeten foods and beverages, these are highly refined and have lost virtually all of the beneficial nutrients and phytochemicals of the original fruit. A child's fruit punch sweetened with grape juice concentrate, for example, may claim to be "100 percent fruit juice" and sounds nutritious but can contain as much sugar as punches sweetened with sucrose or high-fructose corn syrup. No form of sugar, even honey, is any "more healthy" than white sugar, as Table 4–11, page 136, shows.

Sugar Alcohols

Sugar alcohols are manufactured sweet-tasting carbohydrates that are poorly absorbed and metabolized by the body, and so present fewer

sugar alcohols sugarlike compounds derived from fruit or manufactured from carbohydrates; sugar alcohols are absorbed more slowly than sugars, are metabolized differently, and do not elevate the risk of dental caries. Also called polyols.

(continued)

Table 4–11

The Empty Calories of Sugar

These data demonstrate the absurdity of trying to rely on added sugars for nutrient contributions. The 64 calories of honey (1 tablespoon) listed bring 0.1 mg of iron into the diet, but it would take 11,500 calories of honey (180 tablespoons) to provide the needed 18 mg of iron for a young woman; even for molasses, a thousand calories of it could meet her iron need, but she would still lack most other needed nutrients.

Food	Energy (cal)	Protein (g)	Fiber (g)	Calcium (mg)	Iron (mg)	Magnesium (mg)	Potassium (mg)	Zinc (mg)	Vitamin A (μg)	Thiamin (mg)	Riboflavin (mg)	Niacin (mg)	Vitamin B$_6$ (mg)	Folate (μg)	Vitamin C (mg)
Sugar (1 tbs)	46	0	0	0	0	0	0	0	0	0	0	0	0	0	0
Honey (1 tbs)	64	0	0	1	0.1	0	11	0	0	0	0	0	0	<1	0
Molasses (1 tbs)	55	0	0	42	1.0	50	300	0.1	0	0	0	0.2	0.1	0	0
Concentrated grape or fruit juice sweetener (1 tbs)	30	0	0	0	0	0	0	0	0	0	0	0	0	0	0
Daily Values	2,000	50	25	1,000	18	400	3,500	15	1,000	1.5	1.7	20	2	400	60

calories (0 to about 3 calories per gram) than sugars do, and they produce a lower glycemic response.[31] Table 4–12 names some common ones, and points out that most sugar alcohols taste less sweet than sugar. Products sweetened with sugar alcohols, such as cookies, sugarless gum, hard candies, and jams and jellies, are safe in moderation, but in large amounts, they can cause gas, abdominal discomfort, and diarrhea. Sugar alcohols don't cause **dental caries** so they are advisedly used in chewing gums, breath mints, and other products that people keep in their mouths for a while. Other types of man-made sweeteners, the non-caloric sweeteners, sweeten foods without calories, and their nature and safety are topics of Chapter 12.

dental caries decay of the teeth (*caries* means "rottenness"). Also called *cavities.*

Table 4–12

Sugar Alcohol	Sweetness Relative to Sucrose
Erythritol	70%
Isomalt	55%
Lactitol	35%
Maltitol	75%
Mannitol	60%
Sorbitol	60%
Xylitol	100%

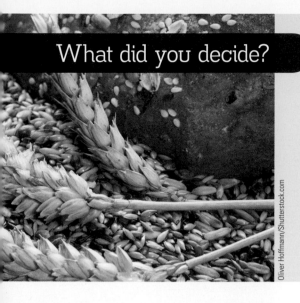

What did you decide?

Do carbohydrates provide only **unneeded calories** to the body?

Why do nutrition authorities unanimously recommend **whole grains**?

Are **low-carbohydrate diets** the best way to lose weight?

Should people with **diabetes** stop eating sugar?

What's online?

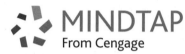

MINDTAP
From Cengage

Visit www.Cengage.com to access MindTap, a complete digital course that includes Diet & Wellness Plus, interactive quizzes, videos, and more.

Self Check

1. (LO 4.1) The dietary monosaccharides include _____.
   a. sucrose, glucose, and lactose
   b. fructose, glucose, and galactose
   c. galactose, maltose, and glucose
   d. glycogen, starch, and fiber

2. (LO 4.1) The polysaccharide that helps form the supporting structures of plants is _____.
   a. cellulose
   b. maltose
   c. glycogen
   d. sucrose

3. (LO 4.2) Foods rich in soluble fiber lower blood cholesterol.
   T   F

4. (LO 4.2) The fiber-rich portion of the wheat kernel is the bran layer.
   T   F

5. (LO 4.3) Digestible carbohydrates are absorbed as _____ through the small intestinal wall and are delivered to the liver, which releases _____ into the bloodstream.
   a. disaccharides; sucrose
   b. glucose; glycogen
   c. monosaccharides; glucose
   d. galactose; cellulose

6. (LO 4.3) Around the world, most people are lactose intolerant.
   T   F

7. (LO 4.4) When blood glucose concentration rises, the pancreas secretes _____, and when blood glucose levels fall, the pancreas secretes _____.
   a. glycogen; insulin
   b. insulin; glucagon
   c. glucagon; glycogen
   d. insulin; fructose

8. (LO 4.4) The body's use of fat for fuel without the help of carbohydrate results in the production of _____.
   a. ketone bodies
   b. glucose
   c. starch
   d. galactose

9. (LO 4.4) Ketosis is the result of too much carbohydrate in the body tissues.
   T   F

10. (LO 4.4) The liver's capacity to store glycogen is virtually unlimited.
    T   F

11. (LO 4.5) Type 1 diabetes is often prevented by successful weight-loss management.
    T   F

12. (LO 4.5) To manage diabetes, it helps to:
    a. eat a diet as low in carbohydrate as possible.
    b. eat a diet as low in fat as possible.
    c. eat regularly timed meals and snacks.
    d. a and b

13. (LO 4.5) Achieving stable blood glucose is the goal of diabetes treatment.
    T   F

14. (LO 4.5) Hypoglycemia among healthy people is relatively rare.
    T   F

15. (LO 4.6) Protein foods provide almost no carbohydrate to the U.S. diet, with these exceptions:
    a. chicken and turkey
    b. beef and pork
    c. fish and eggs
    d. milk, nuts, and legumes

16. (LO 4.7) Fruit punch sweetened with grape juice concentrate can contain as much sugar as fruit punch sweetened with high-fructose corn syrup.
    T   F

17. (LO 4.7) In the United States, diets high in refined carbohydrate intakes, particularly added sugars from soft drinks, are often associated with increased body fatness.
    T   F

18. (LO 4.7) When added sugar is consumed in excess of calorie need,
    a. it alters blood lipids in potentially harmful ways.
    b. it suppresses the insulin response and so is more fattening.
    c. it provides more calories per gram than fat and so is more fattening.
    d. its metabolism in the body diminishes chronic disease risks.

Answers to these Self Check questions are in Appendix G.

Are Added Sugars "Bad" for You?

LO 4.7   Itemize the effects of added sugars on health.

Authorities around the world urge people to strictly limit their intakes of added sugars.[1]* Does this mean that sugary soft drinks and snack cakes constitute a health hazard? This Controversy addresses some of the accusations made against added sugars and demonstrates a scientific response via peer-reviewed, published research.

Do Added Sugars Cause Obesity?

Over the past several decades, people in the United States have grown dramatically fatter (Figure C4–1). During the same period, total calorie intakes and intakes of sugary foods and drinks also

* Reference notes are in Appendix F

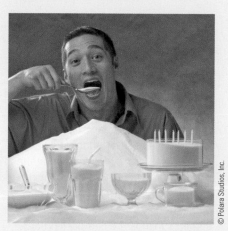

Most people are unaware of how much added sugar they consume in foods and beverages.

© Polara Studios, Inc.

climbed sharply. The sharp increase in energy consumption, estimated at more than 300 calories a day (see Figure C4–2), was more than enough

to cause an average weight gain of two pounds *every month*.[†] In addition, as calorie intakes went up, physical activity declined, and most people were not active enough to use up those extra calories.[2] This is important because excess body weight raises a person's risk of harm from chronic diseases.

Intakes of Added Sugars

Added sugars of many kinds are commonplace in the U.S. diet, and average sugar consumption weighs in at about double the recommended upper limit (refer back to Table 4–1 of the chapter, p.111).[3] Sugar intakes have declined somewhat in recent years, but they are

[†] *Based on a gain of 1 lb of body weight per 3,500 excess calories; actual amounts vary widely among individuals.*

Figure C4–1

Increases in Adult Body Weight over Time

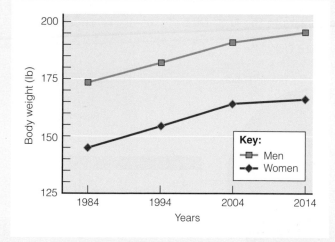

Source: C. D. Fryar and coauthors, National Center for Health Statistics, Anthropometric reference data for children and adults: United States, 2011–2014 Vital and Health Statistics 38 (2016), available at www.cdc.gov/nchs/data/series /sr_03/sr03_039.pdf.

Figure C4–2

Daily Energy Intake over Time

Carbohydrates, and mostly added sugars, account for almost all of the increase in energy intakes during this period. The recent dip in calorie intakes parallels a slight reduction in added sugar intakes and a slowing of the rate of increase in obesity prevalence.

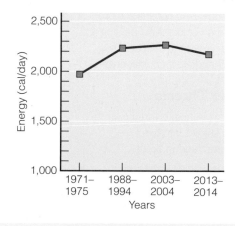

Source: U.S. Department of Agriculture, Agricultural Research Service Energy Intakes, Percentages of energy from protein, carbohydrate, fat, and alcohol, by gender and age, What We Eat in America, NHANES 2013–2014, (2016), available at https://www.ars .usda.gov/ARSUserFiles/80400530/pdf/1314/Table_5_EIN_GEN_13.pdf; E. S. Ford and W. H. Dietz, Trends in energy intake among adults in the United States: Findings from NHANES, American Journal of Clinical Nutrition 97 (2013): 848–853.

---

still high (see Table C4–1).[4] For example, adolescent boys, the top sugar consumers, take in about a half cup of added sugars in foods and beverages each day, or almost 90 pounds of sugar per year.

Sugary foods and beverages taste delicious, cost little money, and are constantly available, making their overconsumption extremely likely. More than 95 percent of the sugars in the U.S. diet are now added to foods and beverages by manufacturers (Figure C4–3 depicts sugar sources). In comparison, very little sugar is added from the sugar bowl at home. When added sugars are prepackaged into foods, consumers easily lose track of how much they are eating.

Sugar or Carbohydrates?

In the United States, observational studies often link intakes of added sugars, particularly from soft drinks, with increased body fatness. At the same time, studies of other cultures report an *inverse* relationship between total carbohydrate intake and body weight. For example, the world's leanest peoples are often those eating traditional low-sugar diets that are high in carbohydrate-rich rice or root vegetables, such as Japanese, Chinese, or African. When such people abandon their traditional diets in favor of "Western"-style foods and beverages, they take in far more sugars and calories, and their rates of obesity and chronic diseases soar. As a society gains wealth, however, its people also consume more meat, grains, and cooking fats, making it difficult to tease apart the effects of sugars from the other dietary constituents.

Sugar's Two Threats

Researchers divide health threats attributed to added sugars into two categories—direct and indirect:

1. Direct effects include metabolic disruptions from high sugar intakes that may lead to diseases, such as cardiovascular disease (CVD) and diabetes.

2. Indirect effects arise when added sugars in the diet cause the accumulation of body fat that, in turn, elevates the risks of many chronic diseases (see Chapter 9).[5]

Table C4–1				
U.S. Average Daily Added Sugars Intakes, 2004 and 2014				
	Age 2–5 yr	**Age 6–11 yr**	**Age 12–19 yr**	**Age 20+ yr**
2004	15 tsp	23 tsp	27 tsp	20 tsp
2014	11 tsp	17 tsp	20 tsp	18 tsp

Sources: National Council on Health Statistics, Data Briefs 122 and 87, reviewed 2015; U.S. Department of Health and Human Services and U.S. Department of Agriculture, 2015–2020 Dietary Guidelines for Americans, 8th edition, 2015.

Does Sugar Cause Diabetes?

Diabetes involves blood sugar, so people once believed that eating sugar *caused* diabetes by "overstraining the pancreas." Now we know that this is not the case. Excess body fatness is more strongly implicated in causing diabetes than is the composition of the diet.

Still, type 2 diabetes often gains ground in populations as they take in more added sugars. A striking example is the rapid increase in diabetes observed among some Native American tribes when added sugars and refined flour replaced traditional roots, gourds, whole corn, and seeds as staple foods in their diets.[6] No simple cause-and-effect conclusion about sugar is possible, however, because at the same time these people ate more processed meats and fats, increased total calorie intakes, and gained body fatness. Excess weight gain could explain their high rate of diabetes, but excess sugar could also contribute directly through its effects on metabolism.[7] It may cause the liver and other tissues to resist the effects of insulin, thereby raising blood glucose.[8] Today, more clinical research is needed to help resolve these issues.

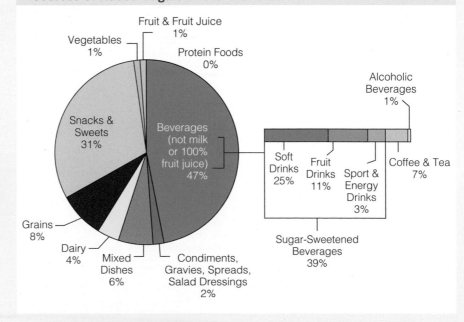

Figure C4–3
Sources of Added Sugars in the U.S. Diet

Sources: U.S. Department of Health and Human Services and U.S. Department of Agriculture, 2015–2020 Dietary Guidelines for Americans, 8th edition (2015), available at http://health.gov/dietaryguidelines/2015/guidelines/.

Chapter 4 The Carbohydrates: Sugar, Starch, Glycogen, and Fiber

The most valid conclusion may be that maintaining a healthy body weight and eating according to the *Dietary Guidelines for Americans* reduces diabetes risk, and that people who are physically active, limit alcohol, and refrain from smoking dramatically reduce their disease risks.[9] Limiting sugar intake is part of a healthy lifestyle.

Do Added Sugars Cause High Blood Pressure?

Added sugars may raise blood pressure, and blood pressure plays a critical role in the health of the heart.[10] Body weight reliably affects blood pressure—the higher the weight, the greater the risk. However, even when body weight was taken into account, a recent systematic review exposed a significant link between higher sugar intakes and higher blood pressure.[11] Another review revealed a trend toward increasing blood pressure with increasing intakes of sugar-sweetened beverages, such as soft drinks, punches, and fruit drinks.[12] More evidence, this time in children, adds to the story: sugar intake is positively associated with increased blood pressure, even in the very young.[13] Given this and other evidence, the American Heart Association recommends a limit of 25 grams (about 6 teaspoons) or less of added sugars for children older than two years, and no added sugars for younger children.[14]

Do Liquid Calories Pose Special Risks?

Research often links the consumption of sugar-sweetened beverages, particularly soft drinks, with overweight.[15] It may be that the liquid nature of sugar calories in beverages eludes normal appetite control mechanisms that apply to solid foods. To test this idea, subjects were given jelly beans (solid sugar) before a meal. At mealtime, they automatically compensated by eating fewer calories of food. But when liquid sugar was substituted for the jelly beans, subjects did not compensate—

they ate the full meal. These results seem to indicate that sugar-sweetened beverages may be particularly fattening, but subsequent studies have yielded only mixed results.[16]

It may be that people's expectations modify their intakes: if they do not expect a clear, caloric liquid to make them feel full, that expectation may influence their subsequent eating. In addition, the liquid sugars of fruit punches and soft drinks are easily gulped down—no chewing required. Few people realize that a sugary 16-ounce soft drink can easily deliver 200 calories, and many young people drink several each day. When overweight people substituted water or diet beverages for caloric beverages, they dropped significant amounts of weight with no other dietary changes.

Hints of Metabolic Mayhem

Some important metabolic links exist among added sugars, obesity, and chronic diseases.[17] Such links have held researchers' attention since the mid-20th century, when a professor called sugar, "pure, white, and deadly."[‡]

Is It the Insulin?

All digestible carbohydrates, including sugars, elevate blood glucose to varying degrees, and blood glucose triggers the release of insulin into the bloodstream. Then insulin interacts with many tissues to promote storage of energy nutrients, including storage of body fat in the adipose tissue.

So does sugar cause obesity through insulin's actions? In healthy, normal-weight people who eat a reasonable diet, insulin works in balance with other hormones and mechanisms to regulate the appetite and maintain a normal

‡ The professor was the late John Yudkin, as reported in G. A. Bray, Fructose: Pure, white, and deadly? Fructose, by any other name, is a health hazard, Journal of Diabetes Science and Technology 4 (2010): 1003–1007.

body weight. In people with insulin resistance, however, the body cells fail to respond to insulin's effects, upsetting the normal balance. (Insulin resistance is discussed in Chapter 11, p. 418.) In healthy people, insulin itself is unlikely to trigger obesity. Other metabolic mechanisms involving the monosaccharide fructose, however, may be in play.

Is It the Fructose?

Figure C4-4 (p. 142) illustrates that most added sugars are composed of about half fructose. The exception is regular corn syrup, made by splitting apart the glucose molecules of starch (cornstarch) to yield a glucose syrup. High-fructose corn syrup (HFCS) is also made from cornstarch but about half of its glucose is changed chemically into fructose to increase the sweetness of the syrup. As sugar intakes increase, so do fructose intakes.

Glucose and fructose, despite both being monosaccharides, are handled differently in the body. In digestion, the intestine avidly absorbs glucose, but restricts absorption of fructose to half or less. Inside the body, all the cells pick up glucose from the bloodstream and use it as such. In contrast, the liver soaks up almost all the absorbed fructose and quickly converts it to other compounds. When energy is abundant, the primary compound the liver makes from fructose is fat.

Fructose and Appetite

Glucose and fructose affect appetite differently, too. Glucose creates appetite-regulating signals directly in the brain, and it also triggers release of insulin, a hormone that curbs the appetite.[18] Fructose, in contrast, cannot enter the brain and does not raise blood insulin by much, and so does not affect the appetite in these ways.[19]

Fructose, Other Sugars, and Fatness

In rodents, a diet high in fructose or sucrose often leads to obesity, diabetes, and altered blood lipids. For example, when groups of rats are given free access to solutions of glucose, fructose, or sucrose in addition to their chow, all gain body fatness, but the fructose-fed rats gain the most. Fructose-fed rats also consistently develop insulin resistance a condition related to diabetes. In people, when calories are held constant and fructose is *substituted* for other carbohydrates, no effect on body weight is observed.[20] However, most people do not reduce calories from other foods when they have a sweet treat, particularly a sugary beverage. The calories of the sugar are extra.

Fructose intake bears a special connection with obesity.[21] As mentioned earlier, intake of fructose stimulates the liver to synthesize new fat molecules that can be stored in adipose tissue. Adipose tissue is the safest storage depot for excess fat; when stored in other tissues, it causes health problems.

Two properties of fructose could also *oppose* obesity. Recall that some portion of ingested fructose is not absorbed by the intestine, and fructose metabolism by the liver is energy costly. However, these factors clearly do not prevent weight gain from excess added sugars in the diet.

Fructose and Fatty Liver

When fat levels in the blood exceed the capacity of adipose tissue to absorb more, the liver stores much of the excess. Over time, this can cause damaging non-alcoholic fatty liver disease (NAFLD), an increasingly common malady associated with obesity and metabolic disorders. The liver readily converts fructose to fat, so fructose intakes may contribute to NAFLD causation.[22] For example, in men fed calorie-controlled diets, substituting fructose for complex carbohydrates caused a significant increase in newly made fat in the blood. In children,

reducing fructose intakes reduced new fats in their blood by half.[23]

Fructose and Blood Lipids

The balance between the body's fat-making and fat-clearing mechanisms plays critical roles in CVD development. In research, both children and adults with higher sugar intakes often have blood lipid values that indicate an elevated risk of CVD.[24] It may not take an unrealistic amount of added sugars to cause this effect. Consuming as little as the equivalent of one or two sugar-sweetened soft drinks a day for two weeks significantly shifts blood lipids in an unhealthy direction, and the greater the intake, the greater the response.[25]

Is High-Fructose Corn Syrup Hazardous to Health?

Is HFCS more harmful to consumers than sucrose? When the effects of HFCS and sucrose are compared, most studies observe virtually identical metabolic effects of HFCS and sucrose—an expected result, given their similar chemical makeups. The Dietary Guidelines committee concludes that U.S. intakes of all types of added sugars are too high and increase health risks for many people.[26] Until research

proves otherwise, it can be assumed that all common added sugars are similar from the body's point of view, and that none should be consumed in excess of recommendations.

Conclusion

Investigation into the potential health effects of carbohydrates is ongoing. The idea that complex problems, such as obesity or diabetes, might be easily resolved by removing a single class of ingredients, such as added sugars, from the diet is attractive but simplistic. Table C4–2 provides a sampling of the ongoing scientific debates about the health effects of added sugars.

What is clear is that the *source* of sugars matters to disease risks. By one estimate, ultra-processed foods contribute 90 percent of the added sugars to the U.S. diet but few of the nutrients that people need.[27] In contrast, fruit and vegetables package their naturally occurring sugars with fiber, vitamins, minerals, and protective phytochemicals. Therefore, limiting intakes of ultra-processed foods is a prudent step in reducing intake of sugar, while any advice to eliminate fruit and vegetables from the diet should be ignored by healthy people.

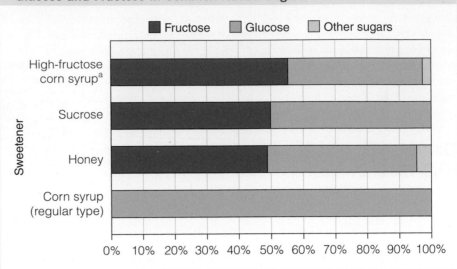

Figure C4–4

Glucose and Fructose in Common Added Sugars

Fructose · Glucose · Other sugars

Sweetener: High-fructose corn syrup[a], Sucrose, Honey, Corn syrup (regular type)

0% 10% 20% 30% 40% 50% 60% 70% 80% 90% 100%

[a]A typical mixture; others exist.

Chapter 4 The Carbohydrates: Sugar, Starch, Glycogen, and Fiber

Table C4–2

Harms from Added Sugars: Point, Counterpoint

Scientists, politicians, food and beverage manufacturers, sugar industry representatives, and others debate issues surrounding the safety of added sugars. This table presents some of the arguments.

Point: Added Sugars Cause Harm	Counterpoint: Added Sugars Are Safe
1. *Increased obesity risk.* Obesity rates are growing rapidly throughout the world. This trend parallels dramatic increases in world intakes of added sugars.	1. *Correlation, not cause.* Worldwide, meat, oil, and grain intakes have also increased. It could be calories or another factor causing obesity, not sugars.
2. *Sugars and gain of body weight.* When sugars are added to the diet, they cause weight gain, particularly in the abdomen.	2. *Excess calories and weight gain.* Excess calories from any source cause weight gain.
3. *Dental caries.* No doubt remains that added sugars cause dental caries, particularly when consumed in excess of 10% of calories.	3. *Dental caries.* True, added sugars can cause dental caries, but brushing the teeth after consuming sugar and drinking fluoridated water prevent caries development.
4. *Less satiety value.* Fructose fails to trigger the body's appetite control mechanisms, but glucose suppresses the appetite.	4. *No real-life application.* People rarely consume isolated fructose or glucose. Most sugars are half glucose.
5. *Increased disease risks.* In populations, greater intakes of added sugars correlate with higher rates of metabolic diseases, such as diabetes, heart disease, high blood pressure, and metabolic syndrome.	5. *Correlation, not cause.* Research is insufficient to prove causation, and factors other than added sugars may be at fault.
6. *Metabolic disturbances.* Fructose, in large quantities, disturbs lipid and glucose metabolism and causes fatty liver disease.	6. *Safe moderate intakes.* Agree, but fructose in small amounts is harmless to health.
7. *Nutrient lack.* Sugar provides only empty calories, displacing nutritious foods and beverages from the diet and increasing the risk of nutrient deficiencies.	7. *Deficiency diseases rare.* Nutrient deficiency diseases are rare in the United States; even many sugary foods and beverages are fortified with certain vitamins and minerals.

Sources: Point: World Health Organization, Guideline: Sugars Intake for Adults and Children (Geneva: World Health Organization, 2015), available at http://who.int/nutrition/publications/guidelines/sugars_intake/en/; USDA, Scientific Report of the 2015 Dietary Guidelines Advisory Committee (2015): D-6, 20–23, available at www.health.gov; G. A. Bray and B. M. Popkin, Dietary sugar and body weight: Have we reached a crisis in the epidemic of obesity and diabetes? Health be damned! Pour on the sugar, Diabetes Care 37 (2014): 950–956; G. A. Bray, Energy and fructose from beverages sweetened with sugar or high-fructose corn syrup pose a health risk for some people, Advances in Nutrition 4 (2013): 220–225; R. H. Lustig, Fructose: It's "alcohol without the buzz," Advances in Nutrition 4 (2013): 226–235; A. Rebollo and coauthors, Way back for fructose and liver metabolism: Bench side to molecular insights, World Journal of Gastroenterology 18 (2012): 6552–6559. Counterpoint: J. M. Rippe, The metabolic and endocrine response and health implications of consuming sugar-sweetened beverages: Findings from recent randomized controlled trials, Advances in Nutrition 4 (2013): 677–686; J. S. White, Challenging the fructose hypothesis: New perspectives on fructose consumption and metabolism, Advances in Nutrition 4 (2013): 246–256.

Tastes adapt over time, and soon, foods and beverages lower in sugar can be as pleasing to the palate as the highly sweetened ones once were.[28] Still, the pleasure of sweet foods and beverages is part of the enjoyment of life. Just remember to keep them in their place—as occasional treats in the context of a nutritious diet, not as staple foods or drinks at every meal.

Critical Thinking

1 This Controversy addresses accusations leveled against sugars in foods and beverages as causes of health problems. Break into groups of five. Have one person in each group take one accusation from the following list and present a one-minute argument in support of the accuracy of that accusation. When each person has completed his or her argument, vote as a group to determine which is most likely to cause health problems:

- Added sugars are making us fat.
- Added sugars cause diabetes.
- Added sugars cause obesity and illness.
- High-fructose corn syrup harms health.
- Blood insulin is to blame.

2 Recommendations about carbohydrate intake can seem to be contradictory. Nutrition experts recommend that the bulk of the diet be carbohydrates (fruit, vegetables, and whole grains), yet some research indicates that certain carbohydrates may be bad for you. Explain this discrepancy in three paragraphs. Use one paragraph to explain why the bulk of the diet should be carbohydrates, including a description of the types of foods that should be eaten. The second paragraph should explain in detail why carbohydrates can be bad for you (give at least three examples). Finally, use the third paragraph to summarize how carbohydrates should be consumed in a way that makes them part of a healthy diet.

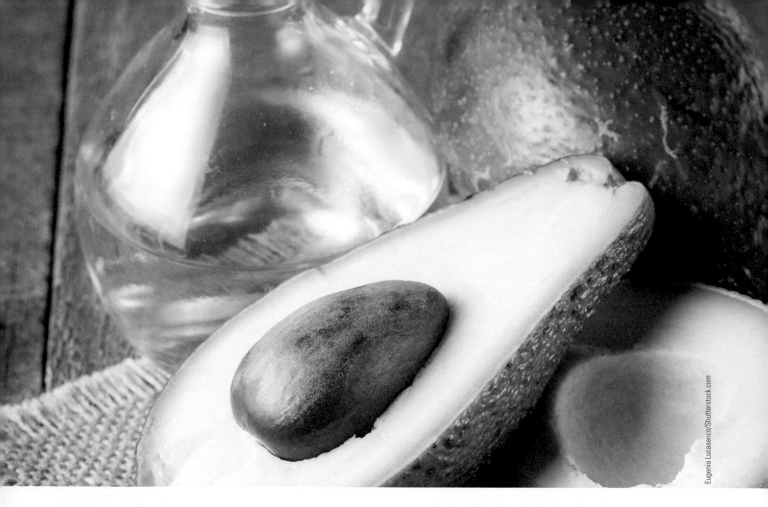

5 The Lipids: Fats, Oils, Phospholipids, and Sterols

Learning Objectives

After completing this chapter, you should be able to accomplish the following:

LO 5.1 Describe the usefulness of lipids in the body and in food.

LO 5.2 Compare the physical and chemical properties and the functions of the three categories of lipids.

LO 5.3 Describe the processes of digestion, absorption, and transportation of lipids in the body.

LO 5.4 Describe how fats are stored and used by the body.

LO 5.5 State the significance of blood lipoproteins and dietary fats to health.

LO 5.6 Summarize the functions of essential fatty acids.

LO 5.7 Outline the process of hydrogenation and its effects on health.

LO 5.8 Identify the sources of fats among the food groups.

LO 5.9 Describe ways to reduce solid fats in an average diet.

LO 5.10 Discuss both sides of the scientific debate about current lipid guidelines.

Are **fats** unhealthy food constituents that are best eliminated from the diet?

What are the differences between **"bad" and "good" cholesterol**?

Why is choosing **fish** recommended in a healthy diet?

If you trim all **visible fats** from foods, will your diet meet lipid recommendations?

Your bill from a medical laboratory reads "Blood **lipid** profile—$250." A health-care provider reports, "Your blood **cholesterol** is high." Your physician advises, "You must cut down on the saturated **fats** in your diet and replace them with **oils** to lower your risk of **cardiovascular disease (CVD)**." Blood lipids, cholesterol, saturated fats, and oils—what are they, and how do they relate to health?

No doubt you are expecting to hear that fats have the potential to harm your health, but lipids are also valuable. In fact, lipids are absolutely necessary, and the diet recommended for health is by no means a "no-fat" diet. Luckily, at least traces of fats and oils are present in almost all foods, so you needn't make an effort to eat any extra. The trick is to choose the right ones.

Introducing the Lipids

LO 5.1   Describe the usefulness of lipids in the body and in food.

The lipids in foods and in the human body, though many in number and diverse in function, generally fall into three classes. About 95 percent are **triglycerides**. The other major classes of the lipids are the **phospholipids** (of which **lecithin** is one) and the **sterols** (cholesterol is the best known of these). Some of these names may sound unfamiliar, but most people will recognize at least a few functions of lipids in the body and in the foods that are listed in Table 5–1 (p. 146). More details about each class of lipids follow later.

How Are Fats Useful to the Body?

When people speak of fat, they are usually talking about triglycerides. The term *fat* is more familiar, though, and we will use it in this discussion.

Fuel Stores   Fat provides most of the energy needed to perform the body's muscular work. Fat is also the body's chief storage form for the energy from food eaten in excess of need. The storage of fat is a valuable survival mechanism for people who live a feast-or-famine existence: stored during times of plenty, fat helps keep them alive during times of famine.

Most body cells can store only limited fat, but some cells are specialized for fat storage. These fat cells seem able to expand almost indefinitely—the more fat they store, the larger they grow. An obese person's fat cells may be many times the size of a thin person's. Far from being a collection of inert sacks of fat, adipose (fat) tissue secretes a huge variety of hormones and other compounds that help regulate appetite and influence other body functions in ways critical to health.[1]* A fat cell is shown in Figure 5–1 (p. 147).

---

*Reference notes are in Appendix F.

lipid (LIP-id) a family of organic (carbon-containing) compounds soluble in organic solvents but not in water. Lipids include triglycerides (fats and oils), phospholipids, and sterols.

cholesterol (koh-LESS-ter-all) a member of the group of lipids known as sterols; a soft, waxy substance made in the body and also found in animal-derived foods.

fats lipids that are solid at room temperature (70°F or 21°C).

oils lipids that are liquid at room temperature (70°F or 21°C).

cardiovascular disease (CVD) disease of the heart and blood vessels. Disease of the arteries of the heart is called *coronary heart disease* (*CHD*). Also defined in Chapter 11.

triglycerides (try-GLISS-er-ides) one of the three main classes of dietary lipids and the chief form of fat in foods and in the human body. A triglyceride is made up of three units of fatty acids and one unit of glycerol (*fatty acids* and *glycerol* are defined later).

phospholipids (FOSS-foh-LIP-ids) one of the three main classes of dietary lipids. These lipids are similar to triglycerides, but each has a phosphorus-containing structure in place of one of the fatty acids. Phospholipids are present in all cell membranes.

lecithin (LESS-ih-thin) a phospholipid manufactured by the liver and also found in many foods; a major constituent of cell membranes.

sterols (STEER-alls) one of the three main classes of dietary lipids. Sterols have a structure similar to that of cholesterol.

Table 5–1

The Usefulness of Fats

Fats in the Body	Fats in Food
■ *Energy fuel.* Fats provide 80 to 90 percent of the resting body's energy and much of the energy used to fuel muscular work.	■ *Nutrients.* Food fats provide essential fatty acids, fat-soluble vitamins, and other needed compounds.
■ *Energy stores.* Fats are the body's chief form of stored energy.	■ *Transport.* Fats carry fat-soluble vitamins A, D, E, and K along with some phytochemicals and assist in their absorption.
■ *Emergency reserve.* Fats serve as an emergency fuel supply in times of severe illness and starvation.	
■ *Padding.* Fats protect the internal organs from shock, cushioning them with fat pads inside the body cavity.	■ *Energy.* Food fats provide a concentrated energy source.
■ *Insulation.* The layer of fat under the skin insulates the internal tissues against cold temperatures.	■ *Sensory appeal.* Fats contribute to the taste and smell of foods.
■ *Cell membranes.* Fats form the major material of cell membranes.	■ *Appetite.* Fats stimulate the appetite.
	■ *Texture.* Fats make fried foods crisp and other foods tender.
■ *Raw materials.* Lipids are converted to other compounds, such as hormones, bile, and vitamin D, as needed.	■ *Satiety.* Fats in foods contribute to feelings of fullness.

Efficiency of Fat Stores You may be wondering why the carbohydrate glucose is not the body's major form of stored energy. As mentioned in Chapter 4, glucose is stored in the form of glycogen. Because glycogen holds a great deal of water, it is quite bulky and heavy, and the body cannot store enough to provide energy for very long. Fats, however, pack tightly together without water and can store much more energy in a small space. Gram for gram, fats provide more than twice the energy of carbohydrate or protein, making fat the most efficient storage form of energy. The body fat found on a normal-weight person contains more than enough energy to fuel an entire marathon run or to battle prolonged illness.

Cushions, Climate, and Cell Membranes Fat serves many other purposes in the body. Pads of fat surrounding the vital internal organs serve as shock absorbers. Thanks to these fat pads, you can play sports or ride a motorcycle for many hours with no serious internal injuries. A fat blanket under the skin also insulates the body and slows heat loss in cold temperatures, thus assisting with internal climate control. Lipids also play critical roles in all of the body's cells as part of their surrounding envelopes, the cell membranes.

Transport and Raw Material Lipids move around the body in association with other lipids, as described in later sections. Once a lipid arrives at its destination, it may serve as raw material for making a number of needed products, among them vitamin D, which helps build and maintain the bones; bile, which assists in digestion; and lipid hormones, which regulate tissue functions.

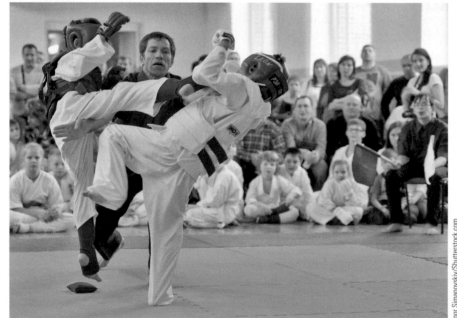

Internal fat pads help cushion vital organs from shock.

Igor Simanovskiy/Shutterstock.com

KEY POINT

■ Lipids provide and store energy, cushion vital organs, insulate against cold temperatures, form cell membranes, transport fat-soluble substances, and serve as raw materials.

Figure 5–1

A Fat Cell

Within the fat cell, lipid is stored in a droplet. This droplet can greatly enlarge, and the fat cell membrane will expand to accommodate its swollen contents. More about adipose tissue and body functions in Chapter 9.

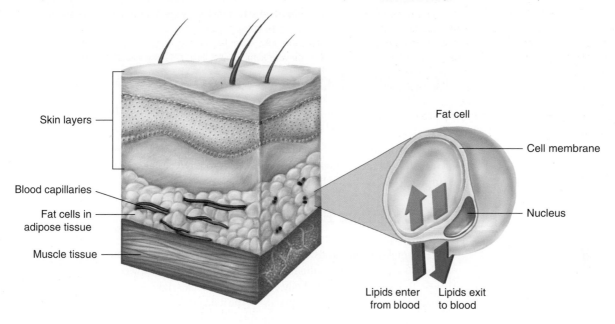

Skin layers

Blood capillaries

Fat cells in adipose tissue

Muscle tissue

Fat cell

Cell membrane

Nucleus

Lipids enter from blood   Lipids exit to blood

How Are Fats Useful in Food?

Fats in foods are valuable in many ways. They provide concentrated energy and needed substances to the body, and they are pleasingly tempting to the palate.

Concentrated Calorie Source   Energy-dense fats are uniquely valuable in many situations. A hunter or hiker must consume a large amount of food energy to travel long distances or to survive in intensely cold weather. An athlete must meet often enormous energy needs to avoid weight loss that could impair performance. As Figure 5–2 (p. 148) demonstrates, for such a person fat-rich foods most efficiently provide the needed energy in the smallest package. But for a person who is not expending much energy in physical work, those same high-fat foods may deliver many unneeded calories in only a few bites.

Fat-Soluble Nutrients and Their Absorption   Some essential nutrients are lipid in nature and therefore soluble in fat. They often occur in foods that contain fat, and some amount of fat in the diet is necessary for their absorption. These nutrients are the fat-soluble vitamins: A, D, E, and K. Other lipid nutrients are **fatty acids** themselves, including the **essential fatty acids**. Fat also aids in the absorption of some phyto-chemicals, plant constituents that may be of benefit to health.

Sensory Qualities   People naturally like high-fat foods. Fat carries with it many dissolved compounds that give foods enticing aromas and flavors, such as the aroma of frying bacon or French fries. In fact, when a sick person refuses food, dietitians offer foods flavored with some fat to spark the appetite and tempt that person to eat again. Fat also lends crispness to fried foods and tenderness to foods such as meats and baked goods. Around the world, as fats become less expensive and more available in a given food supply, people increasingly choose fatty foods.

A Role in Satiety   Fat also contributes to **satiety**, the satisfaction of feeling full after a meal.[2] The fat of swallowed food triggers a series of physiological events that helps to suppress the desire to eat.[3] Still, people can easily overeat on fat-rich foods before the

Do the Math

Fats are energy-dense nutrients:

- 1 g fat = 9 cal
- 1 g carbohydrate = 4 cal
- 1 g protein = 4 cal

Following the general formula given on page 33, find the percentage of calories from fat in a day's meals providing 1,950 calories and 80 g fat.

fatty acids organic acids composed of carbon chains of various lengths. Each fatty acid has an acid end and hydrogens attached to all of the carbon atoms of the chain.

essential fatty acids fatty acids that the body needs but cannot make and so must be obtained from the diet.

satiety (sat-EYE-uh-tee) the feeling of fullness or satisfaction that people experience after meals.

Figure 5–2

Two Lunches

Both lunches contain the same number of calories, but the fat-rich lunch takes up less space and weighs less.

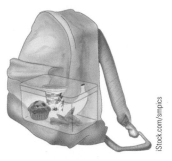

iStock.com/smpics

Carbohydrate-rich lunch
1 low-fat muffin
1 banana
2 oz carrot sticks
8 oz fruit yogurt

calories = 550
weight (g) = 500

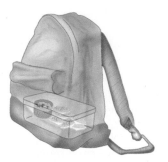

Fat-rich lunch
6 butter-style crackers
1 1/2 oz American cheese
2 oz trail mix with candy

calories = 550
weight (g) = 115

iStock.com/smpics

glycerol (GLISS-er-all) an organic compound, three carbons long, of interest here because it serves as the backbone for triglycerides.

sensation stops them because the delicious taste of fat stimulates eating, and each bite of a fat-rich food delivers many calories. Over time, a chronically high-fat diet may weaken the satiety responses to fat, at least in rats.[4] Chapter 9 revisits the body's complex system of appetite control.

KEY POINT

- Lipids provide abundant food energy in small packages, enhance aromas and flavors of foods, and contribute to satiety.

A Close Look at Lipids

LO 5.2 Compare the physical and chemical properties and the functions of the three categories of lipids.

Each class of lipids—triglycerides, phospholipids, and sterols—possesses unique characteristics. As mentioned, the term *fat* refers to triglycerides, the major form of lipid found in food and in the body.

Triglycerides: Fatty Acids and Glycerol

Very few fatty acids are found free in the body or in foods; most are incorporated into large, complex compounds: triglycerides. The name almost explains itself: three fatty acids (*tri*) are attached to a molecule of **glycerol** to form a triglyceride molecule (see Figure 5–3). Tissues all over the body can easily assemble triglycerides or disassemble them as needed. Triglycerides make up most of the lipid present both in the body and in food.

Fatty acids can differ from one another in two ways: in chain length and in degree of saturation (explained next). Triglycerides usually include mixtures of various fatty acids. Depending on which fatty acids are incorporated into a triglyceride, the resulting fat will be softer or harder at room temperature. Triglycerides containing mostly the shorter-chain fatty acids or the more unsaturated ones are softer and melt more readily at lower temperatures.

Each species of animal (including people) makes its own characteristic kinds of triglycerides, a function governed by genetics. Fats in the diet, though, can affect the types

Figure 5–3

Triglyceride Formation

Glycerol, a small, water-soluble carbohydrate derivative, plus three fatty acids equals a triglyceride.

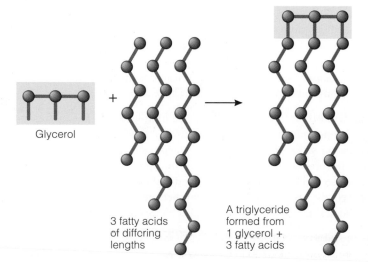

Glycerol

3 fatty acids of differing lengths

A triglyceride formed from 1 glycerol + 3 fatty acids

148   **Chapter 5** The Lipids: Fats, Oils, Phospholipids, and Sterols

More details about lipid chemical structures are found in **Appendix A**.

of triglycerides made because dietary fatty acids are often incorporated into triglycerides in the body. For example, many animals raised for food can be fed diets containing specific triglycerides to give the meat the types of fats that consumers demand.

- The body combines three fatty acids with one glycerol to make a triglyceride, its storage form of fat.
- Fatty acids in food influence the composition of fats in the body.

Saturated vs. Unsaturated Fatty Acids

Saturation refers to whether or not a fatty acid chain is holding all of the hydrogen atoms it can hold. If every available bond from the carbons is holding a hydrogen, the chain is a **saturated fatty acid**; it is filled to capacity with hydrogen. The zigzag structure on the left in Figure 5–4 represents a saturated fatty acid.

Saturation of Fatty Acids   Sometimes, especially in the fatty acids of plants and fish, the chain has a place where hydrogens are missing: an "empty spot," or **point of unsaturation**.[†] A fatty acid carbon chain that possesses one or more points of unsaturation is an **unsaturated fatty acid**. With one point of unsaturation, the fatty acid is a **monounsaturated fatty acid** (see the second structure in Figure 5–4). With two or more points of unsaturation, it is a **polyunsaturated fatty acid**, often abbreviated **PUFA** (see the third structure in Figure 5–4. Other examples are given later in this chapter). Often, a single triglyceride contains both saturated and unsaturated fatty acids of varying lengths, making it a mixed triglyceride.

Figure 5–4

Three Types of Fatty Acids

The more carbon atoms in a fatty acid, the longer it is. The more hydrogen atoms attached to those carbons, the more saturated the fatty acid is.

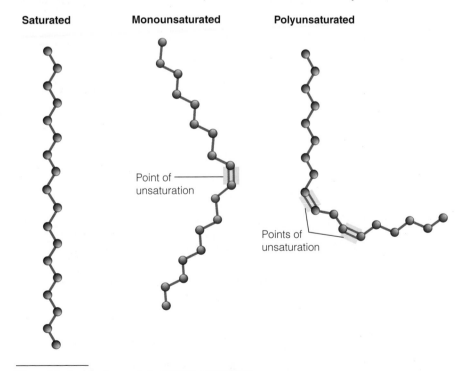

Saturated   **Monounsaturated**   **Polyunsaturated**

Point of unsaturation

Points of unsaturation

saturated fatty acid a fatty acid carrying the maximum possible number of hydrogen atoms (having no points of unsaturation). A saturated fat is a triglyceride with three saturated fatty acids.

point of unsaturation a site in a molecule where the bonding is such that additional hydrogen atoms can easily be attached.

unsaturated fatty acid a fatty acid that lacks some hydrogen atoms and has one or more points of unsaturation. An unsaturated fat is a triglyceride that contains one or more unsaturated fatty acids.

monounsaturated fatty acid a fatty acid containing one point of unsaturation.

polyunsaturated fatty acid (PUFA) a fatty acid with two or more points of unsaturation.

[†]These points of unsaturation can also be referred to as double bonds.

Figure 5–5

Saturation Affects a Fat's Melting Point

The high saturated fat content of a stick of butter keeps it solid at room temperature, but unsaturated oil stays in the liquid state.

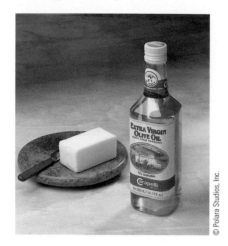

© Polara Studios, Inc.

Melting Point and Fat Hardness The degree of saturation of the fatty acids in a fat affects the temperature at which the fat melts. Generally, the more unsaturated the fatty acids, the more liquid the fat will be at room temperature. Conversely, the more saturated the fatty acids, the more solid the fat will be at room temperature. Figure 5–5 illustrates this concept. The butter and oil are both at room temperature, but the saturated fats of the butter keep it solid—it has a higher melting point. Thus, looking at three fats—beef tallow (a type of beef fat), chicken fat, and safflower oil—beef tallow is the most saturated and the hardest; chicken fat is less saturated and somewhat soft; and safflower oil, which is the most unsaturated, is a liquid at room temperature.

If a health-care provider recommends replacing **solid fats**, **saturated fats**, and *trans* **fats** (a topic of a later section) with **monounsaturated fats** and **polyunsaturated fats** to protect your health, you can generally judge by the hardness of the fats which ones to choose. Figure 5–6 compares the percentages of saturated, monounsaturated, and polyunsaturated fatty acids in various fats and oils. To determine the degree of saturation of the fats in the oil you use, place it in a clear container in the refrigerator and watch how solid it becomes. The least saturated oils, such as polyunsaturated vegetable

Figure 5–6

Fatty Acid Composition of Common Food Fats

Most fats are a mixture of saturated, monounsaturated, and polyunsaturated fatty acids.

Key:

- Saturated fatty acids
- Monounsaturated fatty acids
- Polyunsaturated, omega-6 fatty acids[a]
- Polyunsaturated, omega-3 fatty acids[a]

Tropical oils (coconut and palm) and animal fats contain mostly saturated fatty acids.

Coconut oil	
Butter	
Beef tallow (beef fat)	
Palm oil	
Lard (pork fat)	
Chicken fat	

Some vegetable oils, such as olive and canola, are rich in monounsaturated fatty acids.

Avocado oil	
Olive oil	
Canola oil	
Peanut oil	

Many vegetable oils are rich in omega-6 polyunsaturated fatty acids.[a]

Safflower oil[b]	
Sunflower oil	
Corn oil	
Soybean oil	
Walnut oil	
Cottonseed oil	

Only a few oils provide significant omega-3 polyunsaturated fatty acids.[a]

Flaxseed oil	
Fish oil[c]	

[a]These families of polyunsaturated fatty acids are explained in a later section.
[b]Salad or cooking type more than 70% linoleic acid.
[c]Fish oil average values derived from USDA data for salmon, sardine, and herring oils.
Note: The USDA Nutrient Database (http://ndb.nal.usda.gov) lists the fatty acid contents of many other foods.

solid fats fats that are high in saturated fatty acids and are usually solid at room temperature. Solid fats are found naturally in most animal foods and tropical oils and arise when vegetable oils are hydrogenated. Also defined in Chapter 2.

saturated fats triglycerides in which most of the fatty acids are saturated.

***trans* fats** fats that contain any number of unusual fatty acids—*trans*-fatty acids—formed during processing.

monounsaturated fats triglycerides in which most of the fatty acids have one point of unsaturation (are monounsaturated).

polyunsaturated fats triglycerides in which most of the fatty acids have two or more points of unsaturation (are polyunsaturated).

Chapter 5 The Lipids: Fats, Oils, Phospholipids, and Sterols

oils, remain clear. Olive oil, mostly monounsaturated fat, is an exception. It may turn cloudy when chilled, but olive oil is still an excellent choice from the standpoint of the health of the heart, as a later section reveals.

Another exception is the solid fat of homogenized milk. Highly saturated milk fat normally collects and floats as a layer of cream (butterfat) on top of the watery milk fluids. Once skimmed from the milk and churned into butter, the solid fat quickly hardens in the refrigerator. During **homogenization**, heated milk and cream are forced under high pressure through tiny nozzle openings to finely divide and disperse the fat droplets evenly throughout the milk. Thus, fluid milk can be a source of solid fat that remains liquid at cold temperatures.

Where the Fatty Acids Are Found Most vegetable and fish oils are rich in polyunsaturated fatty acids. Some vegetable oils are also rich in monounsaturated fatty acids. Animal fats are generally the most saturated. But you have to know your oils—it is not enough to choose foods with plant oils over those containing animal fats. Coconut oil, for example, comes from a plant, but its fatty acids—even those of the heavily advertised "virgin" types—are more saturated than those of cream.[5] (By the way, no solid evidence supports claims made by advertisers for special curative powers of coconut oil.) Palm oil, a vegetable oil used in food processing, is also highly saturated. Likewise, **shortening**, stick margarine, and commercially fried or baked products may claim to be or use "all vegetable fat," but much of their fat may be saturated (see details in a later section).

KEY POINTS

- Fatty acids are energy-rich carbon chains that can be saturated (filled with hydrogens) or monounsaturated (with one point of unsaturation) or polyunsaturated (with more than one point of unsaturation).
- The degree of saturation of the fatty acids in a fat determines the fat's softness or hardness.

Phospholipids and Sterols

Thus far, we have dealt with the largest of the three classes of lipids—the triglycerides and their component fatty acids. The other two classes—phospholipids and sterols—play important structural and regulatory roles in the body.

Phospholipids A phospholipid, like a triglyceride, consists of a molecule of glycerol with fatty acids attached, but it contains two, rather than three, fatty acids. In place of the third is a molecule containing phosphorus, which makes the phospholipid soluble in water, while its fatty acids make it soluble in fat. This versatility permits any phospholipid to play a role in keeping fats dispersed in water—it can serve as an **emulsifier**.

Food manufacturers blend fat with watery ingredients by way of **emulsification**. Some salad dressings separate to form two layers—vinegar on the bottom, oil on top, as shown in Figure 5–7. Other dressings, such as mayonnaise, are also made from vinegar and oil, but they never separate. The difference lies in a special ingredient of mayonnaise, the emulsifier lecithin (LESS-ih-thin) of egg yolks. Lecithin, a phospholipid, blends the vinegar with the oil to form a stable **emulsion**: spreadable mayonnaise.

Health-promoting properties, such as the ability to lower blood cholesterol, are sometimes attributed to lecithin, but the people making the claims profit from selling supplements. Lecithin supplements have no special ability to promote health—the body makes all of the lecithin it needs.

Phospholipids also play key structural and regulatory roles in the cells. Phospholipids bind together in a strong double layer that forms the membranes of cells. Because phospholipids have both water-loving and fat-loving characteristics, they help fats travel back and forth across the lipid membranes of cells into the watery fluids on both sides. In addition, some phospholipids generate signals inside the cells in response to hormones, such as insulin, to help modulate body conditions.

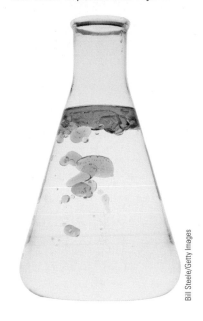

Bill Steele/Getty Images

Figure 5–7

Oil and Water

Without help from emulsifiers, fats and water separate into layers.

homogenization a process by which milk fat is evenly dispersed within fluid milk; under high pressure, milk is passed through tiny nozzles to reduce the size of fat droplets and reduce their tendency to cluster and float to the top as cream.

shortening a semi-solid fat made from vegetable oil commonly used for frying foods, or in baked goods to achieve a "short," or flaky, texture.

emulsifier a substance with both water-soluble and fat-soluble portions that mixes with both fat and water and permanently disperses the fat in the water, forming an emulsion.

emulsification the process of mixing lipid with water by adding an emulsifier.

emulsion a mixture of two liquids that do not usually mix, in which tiny particles of one liquid are held suspended in the other.

Sterols   Sterols such as cholesterol are large, complicated molecules consisting of interconnected *rings* of carbon atoms with side chains of carbon, hydrogen, and oxygen attached. Cholesterol serves as the raw material for making emulsifiers in **bile** (see the next section for details), important to fat digestion. Cholesterol is also important in the structure of the cell membranes of every cell, making it necessary to the body's proper functioning. Like lecithin, cholesterol can be made by the body, so it is not an essential nutrient. Other sterols include vitamin D, which is made from cholesterol, and the familiar steroid hormones, including the sex hormones.

Cholesterol forms the major part of the plaques that narrow the arteries in **atherosclerosis**, the underlying cause of heart attacks and strokes. Sterols other than cholesterol exist in the cells of plants. These plant sterols resemble cholesterol in structure and can inhibit cholesterol absorption in the human digestive tract, lowering the cholesterol concentration in the blood.[6] Plant sterols occur naturally in nuts, seeds, legumes, whole grains, vegetables, and fruit and are added to margarine that can then bear a "heart-healthy" claim on the label.

KEY POINTS

- Phospholipids play key roles in cell membranes.
- Sterols play roles as part of bile, vitamin D, the sex hormones, and other important compounds.
- Plant sterols in foods inhibit cholesterol absorption.

Lipids in the Body

LO 5.3   Describe the processes of digestion, absorption, and transportation of lipids in the body.

From the moment they enter the body, lipids affect the body's functioning and condition. They also demand special handling because fat separates from water and body fluids consist largely of water.

How Are Fats Digested and Absorbed?

A bite of food in the mouth first encounters the enzymes of saliva. An enzyme produced by a gland at the base of the tongue plays a major role in digesting milk fat in infants but is of little importance to lipid digestion in adults.

Fat in the Stomach   After being chewed and swallowed, the food travels to the stomach, where droplets of fat separate from the watery components and tend to float as a layer on top. Even the stomach's powerful churning cannot completely disperse the fat, so little fat digestion takes place in the stomach.

Fat in the Small Intestine   As the stomach contents empty into the small intestine, the digestive system faces a problem: how to thoroughly mix fats, which have separated into a layer, with its own watery fluids. The solution is an emulsifier: bile. Bile, made by the liver, is stored in the gallbladder and released into a duct that leads to the small intestine when it is needed for fat digestion. Bile contains compounds made from cholesterol that work as emulsifiers; one end of each molecule attracts and holds fat, while the other end is attracted to and held by water.

Bile emulsifies and suspends fat droplets within the watery fluids (see Figure 5–8) until the fat-digesting enzymes contributed by the pancreas can split them into smaller molecules for absorption. These fat-splitting enzymes act on triglycerides to split fatty acids from their glycerol backbones. Free fatty acids, phospholipids, and **monoglycerides** all cling together in balls surrounded by bile emulsifiers.

To review: first, the digestive system mixes fats with bile-containing digestive juices to emulsify the fats. Then fat-digesting enzymes break down the fats into absorbable pieces. The pieces then assemble themselves into balls that remain emulsified by bile.

---

bile an emulsifier made by the liver from cholesterol, stored in the gallbladder, and released into the small intestine when needed. Bile does not digest fat as enzymes do but emulsifies it so that enzymes in the watery fluids may contact it and split the fatty acids from their glycerol for absorption.

atherosclerosis (ATH-er-oh-scler-OH-sis) a disease of the arteries characterized by lipid deposits known as plaques along the inner walls of the arteries; a major cause of cardiovascular disease. Chapter 11 provides details.

monoglycerides (mon-oh-GLISS-er-ides) products of the digestion of lipids; a monoglyceride is a glycerol molecule with one fatty acid attached (*mono* means "one"; *glyceride* means "a compound of glycerol").

152

Best_photo_studio/Shutterstock.com

Figure 5–8

The Action of Bile in Fat Digestion

Bile and detergents are both emulsifiers and work the same way, which is why detergents are effective in removing grease spots from clothes. Molecule by molecule, the grease is dissolved out of the spot and suspended in the water, where it can be rinsed away.

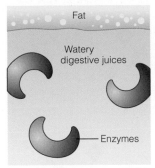

Fat and watery digestive juices tend to separate. Enzymes are in the water and can't get at the fat.

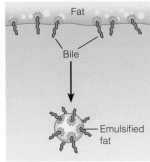

When fat enters the small intestine, the gallbladder secretes bile. Bile compounds have an affinity for both fat and water, so bile can mix the fat into the water.

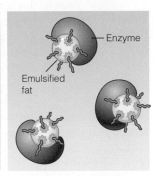

After emulsification, more fat is exposed to the enzymes, and fat digestion proceeds efficiently.

People sometimes wonder how a person without a gallbladder can digest food. The gallbladder is just a storage organ. Without it, the liver still produces bile but delivers it to the small intestine instead of into the gallbladder.

Fat Absorption   Once split and emulsified, the fats face another barrier: the watery layer of mucus that coats the absorptive lining of the digestive tract. Fats must traverse this layer to enter the cells of the digestive tract lining. The solution again depends on bile, this time in the balls of digested lipids. The bile shuttles the lipids across the watery mucus layer to the waiting absorptive surfaces on cells of the intestinal villi. The cells then extract the lipids. The bile may be absorbed and reused by the body, or it may flow back into the intestinal contents and exit with the feces, as shown in Figure 4–7 (p. 114).

The digestive tract absorbs triglycerides from a meal with remarkable efficiency: up to 98 percent of fats consumed are absorbed. Very little fat is excreted by a healthy system. The process of fat digestion takes time, though, so the more fat taken in at a meal, the slower the digestive system action becomes. The efficient series of events just described is depicted in Figure 5–9 (p. 154).

KEY POINTS
- In the stomach, fats separate from other food components.
- In the small intestine, bile emulsifies the fats, enzymes digest them, and the intestinal cells absorb them.

Transport of Fats

Glycerol and shorter-chain fatty acids pass directly through the cells of the intestinal lining into the bloodstream, where they travel unassisted to the liver. The larger lipids, however, present a problem for the body. As mentioned, fat floats in water. Without some mechanism to keep them dispersed, large lipid globules would separate out of the watery blood as it circulates around the body, disrupting the blood's normal functions. The solution to this problem lies in an ingenious use of proteins: many fats travel from place to place in the watery blood as passengers in **lipoproteins**, assembled packages of lipid and protein molecules.

The larger digested lipids, monoglycerides and long-chain fatty acids, must form lipoproteins before they can be released into the lymph in vessels that lead to the bloodstream. Inside the intestinal cells, these lipids re-form into triglycerides and cluster

lipoproteins (LYE-poh-PRO-teens, LIH-poh-PRO-teens) clusters of lipids associated with protein, which serve as transport vehicles for lipids in blood and lymph.

Figure 5–9

The Process of Lipid Digestion and Absorption

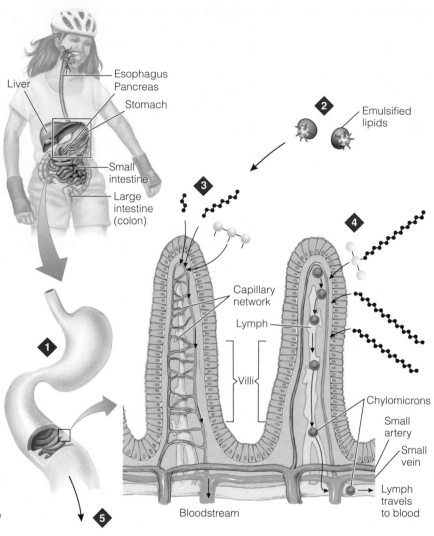

1 In the mouth and stomach:

Little fat digestion takes place.

2 In the small intestine:

Digestive enzymes accomplish most fat digestion in the small intestine. There, bile emulsifies fat, making it available for enzyme action. The enzymes cleave triglycerides into free fatty acids, glycerol, and monoglycerides.

3 At the intestinal lining:

The parts are absorbed by intestinal villi. Glycerol and short-chain fatty acids enter directly into the bloodstream.

4 The cells of the intestinal lining convert large lipid fragments, such as monoglycerides and long-chain fatty acids, back into triglycerides and combine them with protein, forming chylomicrons (a type of lipoprotein) that travel in the lymph vessels to the bloodstream.

5 In the large intestine:

A small amount of cholesterol trapped in fiber exits with the feces.

Note: In this diagram, molecules of fatty acids are shown as large objects, but, in reality, molecules of fatty acids are too small to see even with a powerful microscope, while villi are visible to the naked eye.

together with proteins and phospholipids to form **chylomicrons** that can safely carry lipids from place to place in the watery blood. Chylomicrons form one type of lipoprotein (as shown in Figure 5–9) and are part of the body's efficient lipid transport system. Other lipoproteins are discussed later with regard to their profound importance to health.

KEY POINTS

- Glycerol and short-chain fatty acids travel in the bloodstream unassisted.
- Other lipids need special transport vehicles—the lipoproteins—to carry them in watery body fluids.

Storing and Using the Body's Fat

LO 5.4   Describe how fats are stored and used by the body.

The conservative body wastes no energy. It methodically stores fat molecules not immediately required for energy. Stored fat serves as a sort of "rainy day" fund to fuel the body's activities at times when food is unavailable, when illness impairs the appetite, or when energy expenditures increase.

chylomicrons (KYE-low-MY-krons) lipoproteins formed when lipids from a meal cluster with carrier proteins in the cells of the intestinal lining. Chylomicrons transport food fats through the watery body fluids to the liver and other tissues.

Figure 5–10

Glucose to Fat

Glucose can be used for energy, or it can be changed into fat and stored.

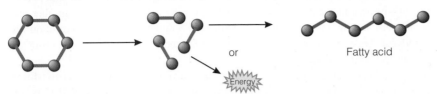

Glucose is broken down into fragments.

The fragments can provide immediate energy for the tissues.

Or, if the tissues have sufficient energy, the fragments can be reassembled, not back into glucose but into fatty acid chains.

or

Fatty acid

The Body's Fat Stores   Many triglycerides eaten in foods are transported by the chylomicrons to the fat depots—the **subcutaneous** fat layer under the skin, the internal fat pads of the abdomen, the breasts, and others—where they are stored by the body's fat cells for later use. When a person's body starts to run out of available fuel from food, it begins to retrieve this stored fat to use for energy. (It also draws on its stored glycogen, as the last chapter described.)

With sufficient food energy, the body can convert excess carbohydrate to fat, but this conversion is not energy-efficient. Figure 5–10 illustrates a simplified series of conversion steps from carbohydrate to fat. Before excess glucose can be stored as fat, it must first be broken into tiny fragments by enzymes and then reassembled into fatty acids, steps that require energy to perform. (The body also possesses enzymes to convert excess protein to fat or to glucose, but these processes are even less efficient.) Storing fat itself is most efficient; fat requires the fewest chemical steps before storage. This does not mean that excess calories from carbohydrate- and protein-rich foods do not contribute to energy stores in the body, however—far from it. Excess calorie intakes reliably lead to weight gain, and overfatness often correlates with diets high in sweets and meats.

What Happens When the Tissues Need Energy?   Fat cells respond to the call for energy by dismantling stored fat molecules (triglycerides) and releasing fatty acids into the blood. Upon receiving these fatty acids, the energy-hungry cells break them down further into small fragments. Finally, each fat fragment is combined with a fragment derived from glucose, and the energy-releasing process continues, liberating energy, carbon dioxide, and water. The way to use more of the energy stored as body fat, then, is to create a greater demand for it in the tissues by reducing the intake of food energy, by increasing the body's expenditure of energy, or both.

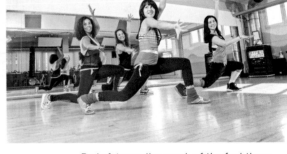

Body fat supplies much of the fuel these muscles need to do their work.

Val Thoermer/Shutterstock.com

Carbohydrate in Fat Breakdown   When fat is broken down to provide cellular energy, carbohydrate helps the process run most efficiently. Without carbohydrate, products of incomplete fat breakdown (ketones) build up in the tissues and blood, and they spill out into the urine.

Carbohydrate's role in fat metabolism is discussed on page 126.

For weight-loss dieters who want to use their body fat for energy, knowing these details of energy metabolism is less important than remembering what research and common sense tell us: successful weight loss simply depends on taking in less energy than the body needs. The distribution of calories among energy nutrients doesn't matter much in this regard (see Chapter 9). For the body's health, however, the proportions of certain lipids in the diet matter greatly, as the next section makes clear.

KEY POINTS

- The body draws on its stored fat for energy.
- Carbohydrate is necessary for the complete breakdown of fat.

subcutaneous (sub-cue-TAY-nee-us) located beneath the skin.

Dietary Fat, Cholesterol, and Health

LO 5.5   State the significance of blood lipoproteins and dietary fats to health.

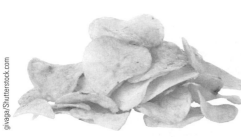

High intakes of saturated and *trans* fats are associated with serious diseases, and particularly with heart and artery disease (cardiovascular disease, or CVD), the number-one cause of death among adults in the United States.[7] So much research is focused on the links between diet and diseases that the whole of Chapter 11 is devoted to presenting the details of these connections.

People who center their diets on foods rich in saturated fatty acids and **trans-fatty acids** often have blood lipid profiles that indicate higher risks of developing CVD. When they replace these foods with those rich in polyunsaturated or monounsaturated fat, their blood lipids often shift toward a profile associated with good health.[8]

Reducing saturated fats is important, but what replaces them in the diet matters, too. When added sugars and refined carbohydrates take the place of saturated or *trans* fats, little benefit to health is observed. The greatest benefits can be expected from focusing the diet on protein-rich nuts, seafood, and soy foods; fiber–rich legumes, barley, and oatmeal; and a variety of fruit, vegetables, and other whole foods, with little solid fat, refined grain, or added sugars.

If you are a woman, take note: these observations apply to you. Heart disease kills more women in the United States than any other cause, and the old myth that heart disease is a "man's disease" should be forever put to rest.

Recommendations for Lipid Intakes

As mentioned, some fat is essential to good health. The Dietary Guidelines for Americans recommend that a portion of each day's total fat intake come from a few teaspoons of raw oil, such as found in nuts, avocados, olives, or vegetable oils. A little peanut butter on toast or mayonnaise in tuna salad, for example, can easily meet this need. In addition, the DRI committee sets specific recommended intakes for the essential fatty acids, **linoleic acid** and **linolenic acid**, and they are listed in Table 5–2.

A Healthy Range of Fat Intakes   Defining an upper limit—the exact gram amount of fat, saturated fat, or *trans* fat that begins to harm people's health—is difficult, so no Tolerable Upper Intake Level for the lipids is set. Instead, the DRI committee suggests an intake range of 20 to 35 percent of daily energy from total fat, less than 10 percent of daily energy intake from saturated fat, and as little *trans* fat as possible. Older recommendations also limited dietary cholesterol to less than 300 milligrams a day. In practical terms, for a 2,000-calorie diet, 20 to 35 percent represents 400 to 700 calories from total fat (roughly 45 to 75 grams, or about 9 to 15 teaspoons).

U.S. Fat Intakes   According to surveys, the average U.S. diet provides about 35 percent of total energy from fat, with saturated fat contributing more than 11 percent of the total.[9] As Figure 5–11 shows, "mixed dishes" (burgers, pizza, tacos, and others) are the top providers of saturated fat, but snacks and sweets (chips, cookies, snack cakes), protein foods (red meats, fried chicken, fried fish), and dairy (butter, cheeses, ice cream) all contribute substantially.

Traditional Mediterranean Fat Intakes   In the mid-20th century, people eating the traditional diets of the Mediterranean Sea regions were observed to achieve a rare feat: they consumed a relatively large amount of dietary fat (about 40 percent of calories) while having low rates of cardiovascular diseases.[10] Their diets also provided abundant nutrients from vegetables, legumes, nuts and seeds, fruit, whole grains, fish, other seafood, and some cheeses and yogurt, but little red meat, few added sugars, and no ultra-processed foods. Today, the Dietary Guidelines for Americans recommend this healthy Mediterranean-style eating pattern for meeting nutrient needs and lowering disease risks.

The fats of healthy Mediterranean-style diets derive mostly from avocados, **extra virgin olive oil**, olives, nuts, and seeds. These foods are rich in unsaturated fatty acids and phytochemicals, and when they replace the solid fats of butter, stick margarine, coconut and palm oil, or meats, improvements in markers of heart disease risks, such as blood clotting and **inflammation**, often follow.[11]

---

trans-fatty acids fatty acids with unusual shapes that can arise when hydrogens are added to the unsaturated fatty acids of polyunsaturated oils (a process known as *hydrogenation*).

linoleic (lin-oh-LAY-ic) **acid** an essential polyunsaturated fatty acid of the omega-6 family.

linolenic (lin-oh-LEN-ic) **acid** an essential polyunsaturated fatty acid of the omega-3 family. The full name of linolenic acid is *alpha-linolenic acid*.

extra virgin olive oil minimally processed olive oil produced by mechanical means, such as pressing (not chemical extraction), to preserve phytochemicals, green color, and flavor from the original olives. The highest grade of olive oil.

inflammation an immune response to cellular injury that produces an increase in white blood cells, redness, heat, pain, and swelling. Chronic inflammation accompanies many diseases.

Table 5–2

Lipid Intake Recommendations for Healthy People

1. **Total fat[a]**

   Dietary Reference Intakes
   - An acceptable range of fat intake is estimated at 20 to 35% of total calories.

2. **Saturated fat**

   American Heart Association
   - For adults who would benefit from lowering blood LDL cholesterol:
     - Reduce percentage of calories from saturated fat to between 5 and 6%.

   Dietary Reference Intakes
   - Keep saturated fat intake low, less than 10% of calories, within the context of an adequate diet.

   Dietary Guidelines for Americans[b]
   - Consume less than 10% of calories per day from saturated fats.

3. **Trans fat**

   American Heart Association
   - For adults who would benefit from lowering blood LDL cholesterol:
     - Reduce percentage of calories from *trans* fat.

   Dietary Guidelines for Americans[b]
   - A healthy eating pattern limits *trans* fats.

4. **Polyunsaturated fatty acids**

   Dietary Reference Intakes[c]
   - Linoleic acid (5 to 10% of total calories):
     17 g/day for young men.
     12 g/day for young women.
   - Linolenic acid (0.6 to 1.2% of total calories):
     1.6 g/day for men.
     1.1 g/day for women.

   Dietary Guidelines for Americans
   - A healthy eating pattern includes oils.

5. **Cholesterol**

   Dietary Reference Intakes
   - Minimize cholesterol intake within the context of a healthy diet.

[a]Includes monounsaturated fatty acids.

[b]The Dietary Guidelines for Americans 2015 use the term solid fats to describe sources of saturated and trans-fatty acids. Solid fats include milk fat, fats of high-fat meats and cheeses, hard margarines, butter, lard, and shortening.

[c]For DRI values set for various life stages, see the back of the book, p. A.

Figure 5–11

Sources of Saturated Fats in the U.S. Diet

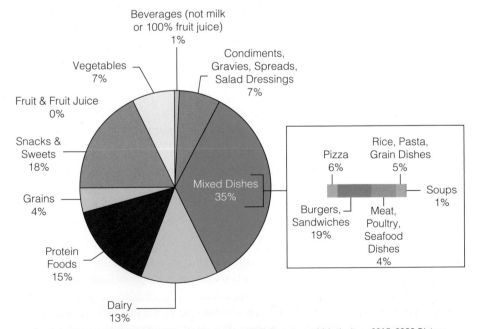

Source: U.S. Department of Health and Human Services and U.S. Department of Agriculture, 2015–2020 Dietary Guidelines for Americans, 8th edition (2015), available at http://health.gov/dietaryguidelines/2015/guidelines/.

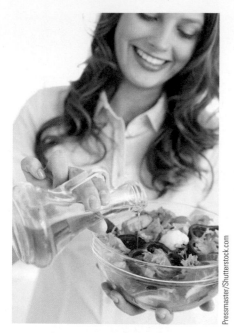

People who eat the Mediterranean way rely on avocado, fatty fish, olive oil, olives, nuts, and seeds for most of their fats.

Appendix E offers eating patterns for USDA's Healthy Mediterranean-Style diet.

Eating the Mediterranean way involves more than just adding olives to your taco salad or drizzling olive oil like a magic potion on a cheesy sausage pizza. The right way is to *replace* sources of solid fat with foods rich in unsaturated oils to keep calories constant and avoid unneeded weight gain that could worsen disease risks.

Too Little Lipid   A very few people manage to eat too little fat to support health. Among them are people with eating disorders who eat too little of all foods and misguided athletes hoping to improve performance. When fat intake falls short of the 20 percent minimum, energy, vitamins, and essential fatty acids may also be lacking, and the eater's health may suffer.

Some points about lipids and heart health are presented next because they form the foundation of lipid intake recommendations. The lipoproteins take center stage because they play important roles in the health of the heart.

KEY POINTS

- A small amount of raw oil is recommended each day.
- Energy from fat should provide 20 to 35 percent of the total energy in the diet.
- The high-fat foods of a Mediterranean eating pattern present mostly unsaturated fats.

Lipoproteins and Heart Disease Risk

Recall that monoglycerides and long-chain fatty acids from digested food fat depend on chylomicrons, a type of lipoprotein, to transport them around the body. Chylomicrons and other lipoproteins are clusters of protein and phospholipids that act as emulsifiers—they attract both water and fat to enable their large lipid passengers to travel dispersed in the watery body fluids.[12] The tissues of the body can extract whatever fat they need from chylomicrons passing by in the bloodstream. The remnants are then picked up by the liver, which dismantles them and reuses their parts.

Major Lipoproteins: Chylomicrons, VLDL, LDL, HDL   The body makes four main types of lipoproteins, distinguished by their size and density. Each type contains different kinds and amounts of lipids and proteins: the more lipids, the less dense; the more proteins, the more dense. In addition to chylomicrons, the lipoprotein with the least density, the body makes three other types of lipoproteins to carry its fats:

- **Very-low-density lipoproteins (VLDL)**, which transport triglycerides and other lipids made in the liver to the body cells for their use.
- **Low-density lipoproteins (LDL)**, which transport cholesterol and other lipids to the tissues for their use. LDL are what is left after VLDL have donated many of their triglycerides to body cells.
- **High-density lipoproteins (HDL)**, which pick up cholesterol from body cells and carry it to the liver for disposal.[13]

Figure 5–12 depicts typical lipoproteins and demonstrates how a lipoprotein's density changes with its lipid and protein contents.

The LDL and HDL Difference   The separate functions and effects of LDL and HDL are worth a moment's attention because they carry important implications for the health of the heart and blood vessels:

- Both LDL and HDL carry lipids in the blood, but LDL are larger, lighter, and richer in cholesterol; HDL are smaller, denser, and packaged with more protein.
- LDL deliver cholesterol to the tissues; HDL scavenge excess cholesterol and other lipids from the tissues, transport them via the bloodstream, and deposit them in the liver.
- When LDL cholesterol is too high, it contributes to lipid buildup in tissues, particularly in the linings of the arteries, that can trigger inflammation and lead to heart disease; HDL cholesterol opposes these effects, and when HDL in the blood drops below the recommended level, heart disease risks rise in response.

very-low-density lipoproteins (VLDL) lipoproteins that transport triglycerides and other lipids from the liver to various tissues in the body.

low-density lipoproteins (LDL) lipoproteins that transport lipids from the liver to other tissues such as muscle and fat; contain a large proportion of cholesterol.

high-density lipoproteins (HDL) lipoproteins that return cholesterol from the tissues to the liver for dismantling and disposal; contain a large proportion of protein.

Chapter 5 The Lipids: Fats, Oils, Phospholipids, and Sterols

Figure 5–12

Lipoproteins

As the graph shows, the density of a lipoprotein is determined by its lipid-to-protein ratio. All lipoproteins contain protein, cholesterol, phospholipids, and triglycerides in varying amounts. An LDL has a high ratio of lipid to protein (about 80 percent lipid to 20 percent protein) and is especially high in cholesterol. An HDL has more protein relative to its lipid content (about equal parts lipid and protein).

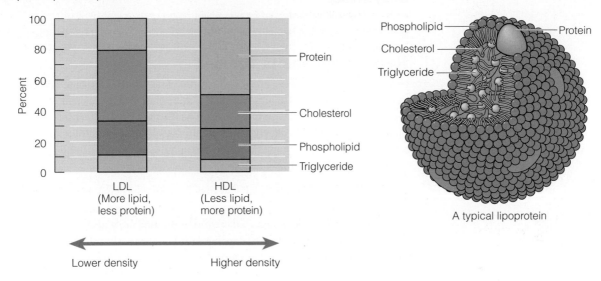

A typical lipoprotein

Both LDL and HDL carry cholesterol, but *high* blood *LDL* warns of an increased risk of heart attack, and so does *low* blood *HDL* (Chapter 11 has details). Thus, some people refer to LDL as "bad" cholesterol and HDL as "good" cholesterol—yet they carry the same kind of cholesterol. The key difference to health between LDL and HDL lies in the proportions of lipids they contain and the tasks they perform, not in the *type* of cholesterol they carry.

The Importance of Cholesterol Testing The importance of blood cholesterol concentrations to heart health cannot be overstated.[‡] The blood lipid profile, a medical test mentioned at the beginning of this chapter, tells much about a person's blood cholesterol and the lipoproteins that carry it.[14] High blood LDL cholesterol and low blood HDL cholesterol account for two major risk factors for CVD (see Table 5–3).

> Chapter 11 lists the standards for blood lipid profile testing.

KEY POINTS

- The chief lipoproteins are chylomicrons, VLDL, LDL, and HDL.
- High blood LDL and low blood HDL are major heart disease risk factors.

What Does *Food* Cholesterol Have to Do with *Blood* Cholesterol?

The answer may be "Not as much as most people think." Most saturated food fats and *trans* fats raise harmful blood cholesterol, but food *cholesterol* has little effect on blood cholesterol values in most people.[15] Even eating an egg each day, a notoriously rich source of cholesterol, does not appear to raise the risk of heart disease.[16] When told that dietary cholesterol doesn't matter much, people may then jump to the wrong conclusion—that blood cholesterol doesn't matter. It does matter. High *blood* LDL cholesterol is a major indicator of CVD risk. The two main food lipids associated with raising it are saturated fat and *trans* fat when intakes exceed recommendations.

Table 5–3

Modifiable Lifestyle Factors in Heart Disease Risk

The more of these factors present in a person's life, the more urgent the need for changes in diet and lifestyle to reduce heart disease risk:

- High blood LDL cholesterol
- Low blood HDL cholesterol
- High blood pressure (hypertension)
- Diabetes (insulin resistance)
- Obesity
- Physical inactivity
- Cigarette smoking
- A diet high in saturated fats, including *trans* fats, and low in fish, vegetables, legumes, fruit, and whole grains

Family history, older age, and male gender are risk factors that cannot be changed.

[‡]*Blood*, *plasma*, and *serum* all refer to about the same thing; this book uses the term *blood* cholesterol. Plasma is blood with the cells removed; in serum, the clotting factors are also removed. The concentration of cholesterol is not much altered by these treatments.

The 2015 Dietary Guidelines for Americans did not set a guideline for dietary cholesterol. The committee explains why: People who consume a healthy eating pattern that holds saturated fat to less than 10 percent of calories naturally take in less cholesterol because the same foods, such as fatty meats and cheeses, often provide both.[17] Genetic inheritance modifies everyone's ability to handle dietary cholesterol, however, so someone who tends to develop high blood cholesterol should follow the advice of a physician.

KEY POINTS

- Saturated fat and *trans* fat intakes raise blood cholesterol.
- Dietary cholesterol has little effect on blood cholesterol in most people.

Recommendations Applied

In a welcome trend, fewer people in the United States have high blood cholesterol than in past decades. Even so, a large number—more than a quarter of adults—still test too high for LDL cholesterol.[18] To repeat, dietary saturated fat and *trans* fat can trigger a rise in LDL in the blood. Conversely, trimming the saturated fat and *trans* fat from foods and replacing them with monounsaturated and polyunsaturated fats while keeping calories reasonable can lower LDL levels.

Lowering LDL Cholesterol A step toward improving blood lipids is to identify sources of saturated fat—that is, solid fats—in the diet and reduce their intakes. Figure 5–13 shows that, when food is trimmed of solid fat, it also loses saturated fat and calories. A pork chop trimmed of its border of fat drops almost 70 percent of its saturated fat and 220 calories. A plain baked potato has no saturated fat and contains about 40 percent of the calories of one with butter and sour cream. Choosing fat-free milk over whole milk provides large savings of saturated fat and calories. Then, with solid fats identified and eliminated, diners are free to replace them with unsaturated fats, or skip them altogether to reduce calories.

> Chapter 11 lists the standards for blood lipid profile testing.

Nutritionists know this: the best diet for health not only replaces saturated fats with polyunsaturated and monounsaturated oils but also is adequate, balanced, calorie-controlled, varied, and based mostly on nutrient-dense whole foods. The overall eating pattern is important, too.

Raising HDL As for blood HDL cholesterol, dietary measures are ineffective at raising its concentration. Regular physical activity raises it effectively and reduces heart disease risks, as the Think Fitness feature points out. Physically active people also reap many other benefits, as Chapter 10 makes clear.

THINK FITNESS

Why Exercise the Body for the Health of the Heart?

Every leading authority recommends physical activity to promote and maintain the health of the heart. The blood, arteries, heart, and other body tissues respond to exercise in these ways:

- Blood lipids shift toward higher HDL cholesterol.
- The muscles of the heart and arteries strengthen and circulation improves,

easing delivery of blood to the lungs and tissues.

- A larger volume of blood is pumped with each heartbeat, reducing the heart's workload.
- The body grows leaner, reducing the overall risk of cardiovascular disease.
- Blood glucose regulation is improved, reducing the risk of diabetes.

start now! Ready to make a change? Set a goal of exercising 30 minutes per day at least five days per week, then track your activity in Diet & Wellness Plus in MindTap.

Chapter 5 The Lipids: Fats, Oils, Phospholipids, and Sterols

Figure 5–13

Cutting Solid Fats Cuts Calories and Saturated Fat

The solid fats in these foods are easy to spot—you can see much of the solid fat on a pork chop and in a butter pat, and you can read about it on a milk label.

Savings:	**Savings:**	**Savings:**
110 cal, 10 g solid fat, 4 g saturated fat	150 cal, 14 g solid fat, 10 g saturated fat	60 cal, 8 g solid fat, 5 g saturated fat

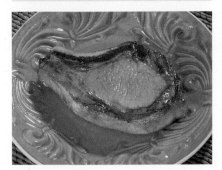

Pork chop with fat
- 340 cal
- 19 g solid fat
- 7 g saturated fat

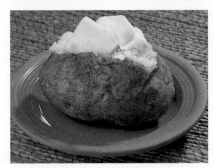

Potato with 1 tbs butter and 1 tbs sour cream
- 350 cal
- 14 g solid fat
- 10 g saturated fat

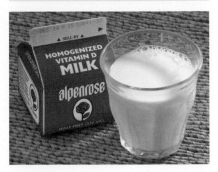

Whole milk, 1 c
- 150 cal
- 8 g solid fat
- 5 g saturated fat

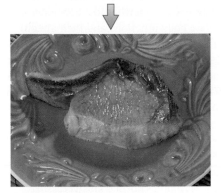

Pork chop trimmed of fat
- 230 cal
- 9 g solid fat
- 3 g saturated fat

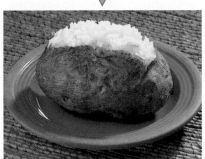

Plain potato
- 200 cal
- 0 g solid fat
- 0 g saturated fat

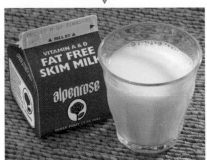

Fat-free milk, 1 c
- 90 cal
- 0 g solid fat
- 0 g saturated fat

© Polara Studios, Inc. (all photos)

KEY POINTS

- To lower LDL in the blood, follow a healthy eating pattern that replaces dietary saturated fat and *trans* fat with polyunsaturated and monounsaturated oils.
- To raise HDL in the blood and lower heart disease risks, be physically active.

Essential Polyunsaturated Fatty Acids

LO 5.6 Summarize the functions of essential fatty acids.

The human body needs fatty acids, and it can use carbohydrate, fat, or protein to synthesize nearly all of them. Two are well-known exceptions: linoleic acid and linolenic acid. Body cells cannot make these two polyunsaturated fatty acids from scratch, nor can the cells convert one to the other.

Table 5–4

Functions of the Essential Fatty Acids

Essential fatty acids:

- Provide raw material from which eicosanoids (biologically active lipids) are made.
- Serve as structural and functional parts of cell membranes.
- Contribute lipids to the brain and nerves.
- Promote normal growth and vision.
- Maintain health of the skin, thus protecting against water loss.
- Help regulate genetic activities affecting metabolism.
- Participate in immune cell functions.

omega-6 fatty acid a polyunsaturated fatty acid with its endmost double bond six carbons from the end of the carbon chain. Linoleic acid is an example.

arachidonic (ah-RACK-ih-DON-ik) **acid** an omega-6 fatty acid derived from linoleic acid.

eicosanoids (eye-COSS-ah-noyds) biologically active compounds that regulate body functions.

omega-3 fatty acid a polyunsaturated fatty acid with its endmost double bond three carbons from the end of the carbon chain. Linolenic acid is an example.

EPA, DHA eicosapentaenoic (EYE-cossa-PENTA-ee-NO-ick) acid, docosahexaenoic (DOE-cossa-HEXA-ee-NO-ick) acid; omega-3 fatty acids made from linolenic acid in the tissues of fish.

Why Do I Need Essential Fatty Acids?

Because the body cannot make linoleic or linolenic acids, they must be supplied by the diet and are therefore essential nutrients. For this reason, the DRI committee set recommended intake levels for them (see the back of the book, p. A). Table 5–4 summarizes their established roles in the body, but new functions continue to emerge.

A diet deficient in the essential polyunsaturated fatty acids produces symptoms such as skin abnormalities and poor wound healing. In infants, growth is retarded, and vision is impaired. The body stores some essential fatty acids, so deficiencies are seldom seen except when intentionally induced in research or on rare occasions when inadequate diets have been provided to infants or hospital patients by mistake. In the United States and Canada, such deficiencies are almost unknown among otherwise healthy adults. The story doesn't end there, however.

KEY POINT

- Deficiencies of the essential fatty acids are harmful but virtually unknown in the United States and Canada.

Omega-6 and Omega-3 Fatty Acid Families

Linoleic acid is the "parent" member of the **omega-6 fatty acid** family, so named for the chemical structure of these compounds. Given dietary linoleic acid, the body can produce other needed members of the omega-6 family. One of these is **arachidonic acid**, notable for its role as a starting material from which the body makes a number of biologically active lipids, known as **eicosanoids**.[19] Somewhat like hormones, eicosanoids arise in tissues where they help regulate body functions and then are quickly destroyed. Omega-6 fatty acids are supplied abundantly in the U.S. diet by vegetable oils.

Linolenic acid is the parent member of the **omega-3 fatty acid** family. Given dietary linolenic acid, the body can make other members of the omega-3 series. Two family members of great interest to researchers are **EPA** and **DHA**. The body makes only limited amounts of EPA and even less DHA, but they are found abundantly in the oils of certain fish. U.S. intakes of these oils are limited.

EPA (omega-3) forms its own eicosanoids that often oppose those from arachidonic acid (omega-6). For example, an omega-3 eicosanoid relaxes blood vessels and lowers the blood pressure, whereas an omega-6 eicosanoid constricts the vessels and increases pressure.[20] A balance between the two therefore promotes normal blood pressure.

KEY POINTS

- The essential fatty acids fall into two chemical families: omega-6 or omega-3 fatty acids.
- The omega-6 family of polyunsaturated fatty acids includes linoleic acid and arachidonic acid.
- The omega-3 family includes linolenic acid, EPA, and DHA.

Omega-3 Fatty Acids

An area of active research concerns links between intakes of omega-3 fatty acids and reduced risks of certain diseases. This section describes some of the findings.

Heart Health   Years ago, someone thought to ask why the native peoples of the extreme north, who eat a diet very high in animal fat, were reported to have low rates of heart disease. The trail led to their intakes of fish and marine foods, then to the oils in fish, and finally to EPA and DHA in fish oils. These early observations are now in question, but no one disputes the importance of omega-3 fatty acids in the body. EPA and DHA each play critical roles in regulating the heart rate, regulating blood pressure, reducing blood clot formation, reducing blood triglycerides, and reducing inflammation—all factors associated with heart health.[21]

Research often links higher EPA and DHA in the blood and greater intakes of fish in the diet with fewer deaths from heart attacks and strokes. Not every study reports lower cardiovascular risks with higher EPA and DHA intakes, however, partly because genetic inheritance influences the body's handling of these fatty acids.[22]

Cancer   Consuming seafood that provides omega-3 fatty acids has been associated with lower than average rates of some cancers, but evidence to indicate prevention or causation is lacking.[23] So little is known about the relationships between cancers and omega-3 fatty acids that people are wise to eat fish, and not to take supplements, to obtain them.

Cell Membranes   EPA and DHA tend to collect in cell membranes. Unlike straight-backed saturated fatty acids, which physically stack closely together, the kinked shape of unsaturated fatty acids demands more elbow room (look back at Figure 5–4, p. 149).[§] When the highly unsaturated EPA and DHA amass in cell membranes, they profoundly change cellular activities and structures in ways that may promote healthy tissue functioning.

Brain Function and Vision   The brain is a fatty organ. A quarter of its dry weight is lipid, and its cell membranes avidly collect DHA in their structures. Once there, DHA may assist in the brain's internal communication, and reduce inflammation associated with aging.[24] Likewise, the retina of the eye selectively gathers up and holds DHA for its use. In infants, breast milk and fortified formula provide abundant DHA, associated with normal growth, visual acuity, immune system functioning, and brain development. Many more details about these remarkable lipids are known.

Requirements and Sources

Authorities recommend choosing 8 to 12 ounces of a variety of seafood each week to provide an average of 250 mg of EPA and DHA per day, but few people in this country regularly consume this amount.[25] Common foods that provide essential fatty acids are listed in Table 5–5, and the Food Feature (pp. 171–175) suggests ways to include seafood

Table 5–5
Food Sources of Omega-6 and Omega-3 Fatty Acids

Omega-6	
Linoleic acid	Nuts and seeds (cashews, walnuts, sunflower seeds, others)
	Poultry fat
	Vegetable oils (corn, cottonseed, safflower, sesame, soybean, sunflower); margarines made from these oils
Omega-3	
Linolenic acid[a]	Nuts and seeds (chia seeds, flaxseeds, walnuts, soybeans)
	Vegetable oils (canola, flaxseed, soybean, walnut, wheat germ; liquid or soft margarine made from canola or soybean oil)
	Vegetables (soybeans)
EPA and DHA	Egg, enriched:
	75–100 mg DHA/egg (flaxseed-enriched)
	100–130 mg DHA/egg (fish oil-enriched)
	Human milk
	Fish and seafood:
	Top contributors: (500–1,800 mg/3.5 oz) Barramundi, Mediterranean seabass (bronzini), herring (Atlantic and Pacific), mackerel,[b] oyster (Pacific wild), salmon (wild and farmed), sardines, shark,[b] swordfish,[b] tilefish,[b] toothfish (includes Chilean seabass), lake trout (freshwater, wild, and farmed)
	Good contributors: (150–500 mg/3.5 oz) Black bass, catfish (wild and farmed), clam, crab (Alaskan king), croakers, flounder, haddock, hake, halibut, oyster (eastern and farmed), perch, scallop, shrimp (mixed varieties), sole
	Other contributors: (25–150 mg/3.5 oz) Cod (Atlantic and Pacific), grouper, lobster, mahi-mahi, monkfish, orange roughy,[b] red snapper, skate, tilapia, triggerfish, tuna, wahoo

[a]*Alpha-linolenic acid. Also found in the seed oil of the herb evening primrose.*

[b]*King mackerel, orange roughy, shark, swordfish, and tilefish are highest in mercury and should not be consumed by children or pregnant or lactating women (see the Consumer's Guide).*

[§]Triglyceride structures are depicted in Appendix A.

Weighing Seafood's Risks and Benefits

Do you ever stand at a seafood counter or sit in a restaurant imagining a healthy fish dinner but wondering what to choose? These days, seafood comes with some questions: Which fish provides the needed essential fatty acids? Which fish is lowest in toxins or microorganisms that may pose risks to health? Which is better—farmed or wild?

Finding the EPA and DHA

Fish in many forms—fresh, frozen, and canned—makes a nutritious choice because EPA and DHA, along with other key nutrients, survive most cooking and processing. However, the *type* of fish is critical. Among frozen selections, for example, pre-fried fish sticks and fillets are most often made of cod, a nutritious fish but one that provides little EPA and DHA (look again at the bottom of Table 5–5, p. 163).

In fast-food places, fried fish sandwiches are generally cod. These fried fillets derive more of their calories from their oily breading or batter than from the fish itself, and more still from fatty sauces that flavor the bun. Cod, like any fish, provides little solid fat when served grilled, baked, poached, or broiled. And if it displaces fatty meats from the diet, it provides a benefit to the heart—just don't count on cod for EPA and DHA. In sit-down restaurants, diners can almost always find EPA- and DHA-rich species, such as salmon, on menus—but only if they know which ones to look for.

Concerns about Toxins

Analyses of seafood samples have revealed widespread contamination by toxins, raising concerns about seafood safety, particularly regarding the heavy

methylmercury any toxic compound of mercury to which a characteristic chemical structure, a methyl group, has been added, usually by bacteria in aquatic sediments. Methylmercury is readily absorbed from the intestine and causes nerve damage in people.

metal mercury. Mercury escapes from many industries, power plants, and natural sources into the earth's waterways, where bacteria in the water convert it into a highly toxic form, **methylmercury**. Methylmercury then concentrates in the flesh of large predatory species of both saltwater and freshwater fish. Cooking and processing do not diminish mercury or other industrial toxins in seafood.

Mercury damages living tissues, and animal studies suggest that even a moderate exposure might harm the heart.[1]* Currently, for most people, the benefits of eating seafood far outweigh the risks, and parents and children alike are urged to eat fish.[2]

Special Populations

Children and pregnant and lactating women have a critical need for EPA and DHA, but they are also most susceptible to harm from the mercury that contaminates many food fish species. For children, the U.S. Food and Drug Administration (FDA) suggests one or two age-appropriate weekly servings of a variety of lower-mercury seafood.[3] For women who are pregnant or breastfeeding, eating 8 to 12 ounces weekly of a variety of lower-mercury seafood, including some EPA- and DHA-rich species, is compatible with good health. However, intakes of white albacore tuna, a high-mercury fish, should be limited to no more than 6 ounces per week, and tilefish, shark, swordfish, and king mackerel should be off the menu entirely because their mercury content is too high for children and pregnant and nursing women.

Cooked vs. Raw

Many people love sushi, but authorities never recommend eating raw fish and shellfish—doing so causes many cases of serious or fatal bacterial, viral, and other illnesses each year (Chapter 12 provides

Reference notes are in Appendix F.

many details). Cooking easily kills off all illness-causing microorganisms, making seafood safe to eat.

Fresh from the Farm

Are farm-raised fish safer? Compared with wild fish, farm-raised fish do tend to collect somewhat less methylmercury in their flesh, and the levels of other harmful pollutants generally test below the maximums set by the FDA.[4] However, fish "farms" are often giant ocean cages, exposed to whatever contaminants float by in the water. The contamination of fish serves as a reminder that our health is inextricably linked with the health of our planet (details in Chapter 15).

Moving Ahead

Keep these pointers in mind:

- Choose a variety of fish and shellfish (prepared without the addition of solid fats) instead of red meat several times a week—people who do generally stay healthier than those who don't.

- Apply the dietary principles of adequacy, moderation, and variety to obtain the benefits of seafood while minimizing risks.

- Don't eat raw seafood.

In conclusion, use a variety of seafood to meet your needs—just don't go overboard.

Review Questions**

1. Methylmercury is a toxic industrial pollutant that is easily destroyed by cooking. T F

2. Children and pregnant or lactating women should definitely not consume fish because of contamination. T F

3. Cod is one of the richest sources of the beneficial fatty acids, EPA and DHA. T F

**Answers to Consumer's Guide review questions are found in Appendix G.*

in the diet. Some eggs are enriched with EPA and DHA by feeding laying hens a diet rich in fish oil or algae oil; feeding flaxseed enriches eggs to a lesser degree.

As for fish oil supplements, evidence does not support taking them to prevent heart attacks or other maladies in most people, but physicians may still recommend them for those with certain forms of heart disease.[26] Large doses of fish oil from supplements carry risks, such as increased bleeding, delayed wound healing, and immune suppression, so supplements are not the preferred source of these oils for most people. This illustrates an important concept in nutrition: too much of a nutrient is often as harmful as too little.

KEY POINTS

- EPA and DHA may play roles in heart health, brain development, and vision.
- Most people should increase their seafood consumption.
- Supplements of omega-3 fatty acids or fish oil are not recommended for most people.

The Effects of Processing on Unsaturated Fats

LO 5.7   Outline the process of hydrogenation and its effects on health.

Vegetable oils make up most of the added fat in the U.S. diet because fast-food chains use them for frying, food manufacturers add them to processed foods, and consumers tend to choose margarine over butter. Consumers of vegetable oils may feel safe in choosing them because they are generally less saturated than animal fats. If consumers choose a liquid oil, they may be justified in feeling secure. If the choice is a processed food, however, their security may be questionable, especially if the words *hydrogenated* or *partially hydrogenated* appear on the label's ingredient list.

What Is "Hydrogenated Vegetable Oil," and What's It Doing in My Chocolate Chip Cookies?

When manufacturers process foods, they often alter the fatty acids in the fat (triglycerides) the foods contain through a process called **hydrogenation**. Hydrogenation of fats makes them resistant to **oxidation**, and helps them stay fresher longer. It changes their physical properties.

Hydrogenation of Oils   Points of unsaturation in fatty acids are weak spots that are vulnerable to attack by oxygen damage. When the unsaturated points in the oils of food are oxidized, the oils become rancid and the food tastes "off." This is why cooking oils should be stored in tightly covered containers that exclude air. If stored for long periods, they need refrigeration to retard oxidation.

One way to prevent spoilage of unsaturated fats and also to make them harder and more stable when heated to high temperatures is to change their fatty acids chemically by hydrogenation, as shown on the left side of Figure 5–14. When food producers want to use a polyunsaturated oil such as soybean oil to make a spreadable margarine, for example, they hydrogenate it by forcing hydrogen into the liquid oil. Some of the unsaturated fatty acids become more saturated as they accept the hydrogen, and the oil hardens. The resulting product is more saturated and more spreadable than the original oil. It is also more resistant to damage from oxidation or breakdown from high cooking temperatures. Hydrogenated oil has a high **smoking point**, so it is suitable for frying foods at high temperatures in restaurants.

Hydrogenated oils are thus easy to handle and easy to spread, and they store well. Makers of peanut butter often replace a small quantity of the liquid oil from the ground peanuts with hydrogenated vegetable oils to create a creamy paste that does not separate into layers of oil and peanuts as the "natural" types do. The saturated fat content of peanut butter increases a bit with the addition of hydrogenated oils, but the finished product still presents mostly unsaturated oils to the eater.

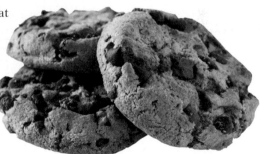

Baked goods with no trans fat may still contain a great deal of saturated fat from shortening.

hydrogenation (high-dro-gen-AY-shun) the process of adding hydrogen to unsaturated fatty acids to make fat more solid and resistant to the chemical change of oxidation.

oxidation interaction of a compound with oxygen; in this case, a damaging effect by a chemically reactive form of oxygen. Chapter 7 provides details.

smoking point the temperature at which fat gives off an acrid blue gas.

Figure 5–14

Hydrogenation Yields Both Saturated and *Trans*-Fatty Acids

Unsaturated fatty acid
Points of unsaturation are places on fatty acid chains where hydrogen is missing. The bonds that would normally be occupied by hydrogen in a saturated fatty acid are shared as a somewhat unstable double bond between two carbons.

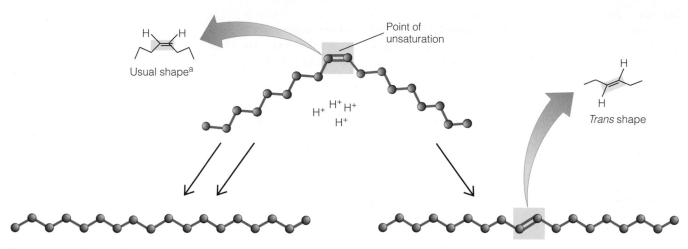

Usual shape^a

Point of unsaturation

Trans shape

Hydrogenated fatty acid (now fully saturated)
When a positively charged hydrogen is made available to an unsaturated bond, it readily accepts the hydrogen and, in the process, becomes saturated. The fatty acid no longer has a point of unsaturation.

Trans-fatty acid
The hydrogenation process also produces some *trans*-fatty acids. The *trans*-fatty acid retains its double bond but takes a twist instead of becoming fully saturated. It resembles a saturated fatty acid both in its shape and in its effects on health.

^a The usual shape of the double bond structure is known as a cis (pronounced sis) formation.

Nutrient Losses Once fully hydrogenated, oils lose their unsaturated character and the health benefits that go with it. Hydrogenation may affect not only the essential fatty acids in oils but also vitamins, such as vitamin K, decreasing their activity in the body. If you, the consumer, are looking for health benefits from polyunsaturated oils, hydrogenated oils such as those in shortening or stick margarine will not meet your needs.

An alternative to hydrogenation for extending a product's shelf life is to add a chemical preservative that will compete for oxygen and thus protect the oil. The additives are antioxidants, and they work by reacting with oxygen before it can do damage. Examples are the additives BHA and BHT** listed on snack food labels. Another alternative, already mentioned, is to keep the product refrigerated.

KEY POINTS

- Vegetable oils become more saturated when they are hydrogenated.
- Hydrogenated vegetable oils are useful, but they lose the health benefits of unsaturated oils.

What Are *Trans*-Fatty Acids, and Are They Harmful?

Trans-fatty acids form during hydrogenation. When polyunsaturated oils are hardened by hydrogenation, some of the unsaturated fatty acids end up changing their shapes instead of becoming saturated (look at the right side of Figure 5–14). This change in chemical structure creates *trans* unsaturated fatty acids that are similar in shape to saturated fatty acids. The change in shape changes their effects in the body.

Health Effects of *Trans*-Fatty Acids Consuming manufactured *trans* fat poses a risk to the heart and arteries by raising blood LDL cholesterol, worsening

---

**BHA and BHT are butylated hydroxyanisole and butylated hydroxytoluene.

atherosclerosis, exerting toxic effects on the heart, and increasing tissue inflammation; high intakes are associated with increased CVD and sudden death.[27] In addition, when hydrogenation changes essential fatty acids into their saturated or *trans* counterparts, consumers lose the health benefits of the original raw oil. The risk to health from *trans* fat is similar to or even greater than that from saturated fat, so guidelines suggest that people avoid *trans* fats as much as possible. A small amount of naturally occurring *trans* fat also comes from animal sources, such as milk and lean beef, but these *trans* fats have little effect on blood lipids.

In recent years, food manufacturers have employed new technologies to reduce the *trans* fat in their products but despite these efforts people's blood *trans*-fatty acid concentrations remain elevated.[28] *Trans* fats can still be found in processed foods, such as desserts, microwave popcorn, frozen pizza, some margarines, and coffee creamers, but the FDA aims to eliminate even this amount from the food supply by the year 2020. This move is expected to prevent thousands of fatal heart attacks each year.[29]

Swapping *Trans* Fats for Saturated Fats?   Newly formulated commercial oils and fats perform the same jobs as the old hydrogenated fats but with fewer *trans*-fatty acids.[30] If a fatty food is free of *trans* fats, is it safe for the heart? It may be, but some new fats merely substitute saturated fat for *trans* fat—and the risk to the heart and arteries from saturated fats is well established.

KEY POINTS

- The process of hydrogenation creates *trans*-fatty acids.
- *Trans* fats, like saturated fats, are harmful to the heart and arteries.

Fat in the Diet

LO 5.8   Identify the sources of fats among the food groups.

The remainder of this chapter will enlighten readers who are evaluating the fat contents of foods. A way to find lipid values of many foods is to access an online nutrient database, such as USDA's "What's in the Foods You Eat" search tool.[††]

Get to Know the Fats in Foods

Fats, naturally occurring or added, are widely distributed among foods. Learning their sources can help you choose wisely among them.

Essential Fats   Everyone needs the essential fatty acids and vitamin E provided by such foods as fish, nuts, and vegetable oils. Infants receive them indirectly via breast milk, but all others must choose the foods that provide them. Luckily, the amount of fat needed to provide these nutrients is small—just a few teaspoons of raw oil a day and two servings of seafood a week are sufficient. Most people consume more than this minimum amount. The goal is to choose unsaturated fats in liquid oils instead of saturated solid fats as often as possible.

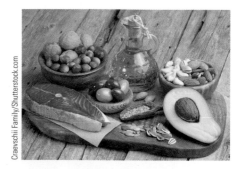

These foods provide mostly unsaturated oils, along with other important nutrients.

Visible vs. Invisible Solid Fats   The solid fat of some foods, such as the rim of fat on a steak, is visible (and therefore identifiable and removable). Other solid fats, such as those in candy, cheeses, coconut, hamburger, homogenized milk, and lunchmeats, are invisible (and therefore easily missed or ignored). Equally hidden are the solid fats blended into biscuits, cakes, cookies, chip dips, ice cream, mixed dishes, pastries, sauces, and creamy soups and in fried foods and spreads. Invisible fats supply most of the solid fats in the U.S. diet.

Replace, Don't Add   Keep in mind that, whether solid or liquid, essential or nonessential, all fats bring the same abundant calories to the diet and excesses contribute

---

††USDA's What's In The Foods You Eat Search Tool; search the USDA website (www.usda.gov) for "What's In The Foods You Eat."

to body fat stores. Each of the following provides about 5 grams of fat, 45 calories, and negligible protein and carbohydrate:

- 1 teaspoon oil or shortening
- 1½ teaspoons mayonnaise, butter, or margarine
- 1 tablespoon regular salad dressing, cream cheese, or heavy cream
- 1½ tablespoons sour cream

Remember to replace and not add. No benefits can be expected when oil is added to an already fat-rich diet.

Do the Math

A ground beef label may state "85% lean," but this number refers to *weight*. To calculate the percentage of *calories* from fat, use the general equation of Chapter 2 (p. 33 margin).

For a quarter pound of beef hamburger with 328 calories and 24 grams of fat:

24 × 9 cal/g = 216 cal from fat
(216 ÷ 328) × 100 = 66%

This hamburger patty derives almost two-thirds of its *calories* from fat. What percentage of calories from fat does a hamburger with 425 calories and 30 grams of fat provide?

Fats in Protein Foods

The marbling of meats and the fat ground into lunchmeat, chicken products, and hamburger conceal a hefty portion of the solid fat that people consume. All meats contain about equal amounts of protein, but their fat, saturated fat, and calorie amounts vary significantly. Figure 5–15 shows the fat and calorie data on packages of ground meats, and it depicts the amount of solid fat provided by a 3-ounce serving of each kind. Nutrition Facts panels list the fat contents of many packaged meats.

> Definitions of terms relating to the fat contents of meats were provided in **Chapter 2**.

The USDA Eating Patterns (see Chapter 2) suggest that most adults limit their intakes of protein foods to about 5 to 7 ounces a day. For comparison, the smallest fast-food hamburger weighs about 3 ounces. Steaks served in restaurants often run 8, 12, or 16 ounces, more than a whole day's meat allowance. You may have to weigh a serving or two of meat to see how much you are eating.

Meat: Mostly Protein or Fat?   People recognize meat as a protein-rich food, but a close look at some nutrient data reveals a surprising fact. A big (4-ounce) fast-food

---

Figure 5–15

Calories, Fat, and Saturated Fat in Cooked Ground Meat Patties[a]

Only the ground round, at 10 percent fat by raw weight, qualifies to bear the word *lean* on its label. To be called "lean," products must contain fewer than 10 grams of fat and 4 grams of saturated fat per 100 grams of food. (The red labels on these packages list rules for safe meat handling, explained in Chapter 12.)

Higher in fat →← Lower in fat

Regular ground beef 23% fat	Ground chuck 16% fat	Commercial ground turkey 15% fat	Ground round 10% fat

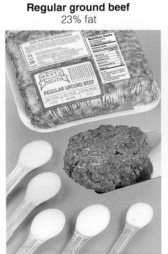 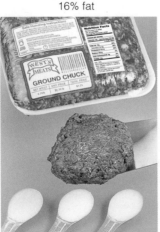 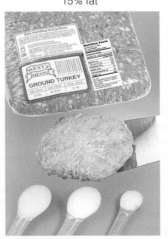 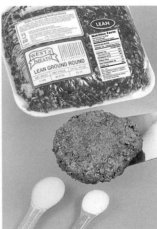

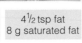 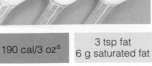 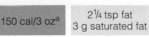

240 cal/3 oz[a]	4½ tsp fat 8 g saturated fat	190 cal/3 oz[a]	3 tsp fat 6 g saturated fat	150 cal/3 oz[a]	2¼ tsp fat 3 g saturated fat	150 cal/3 oz[a]	1½ tsp fat 4 g saturated fat

© Quest Photographic, Inc. (all photos)

[a]*All patties weigh three ounces, cooked. Larger servings will, of course, provide more fat, saturated fat, and calories than the values listed here.*

Chapter 5 The Lipids: Fats, Oils, Phospholipids, and Sterols

Figure 5–16

Lipids in Milk and Milk Products

Red boxes below indicate foods with lipid contents that warrant moderation in their use. Green indicates lower-fat choices.

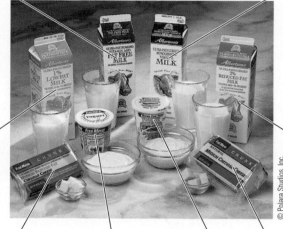

Nutrition Facts
Amount Per Serving

Fat-free, skim, zero-fat, no-fat, or nonfat milk, 8 oz (<0.5% fat by weight)

Calories 80	Calories from Fat 0
	% Daily Value*
Total Fat 0g	**0%**
Saturated Fat 0g	**0%**

Whole milk, 8 oz (3.3% fat by weight)

Calories 150	Calories from Fat 70
	% Daily Value*
Total Fat 8g	**12%**
Saturated Fat 5g	**25%**

Low-fat milk, 8 oz (1% fat by weight)

Calories 105	Calories from Fat 20
	% Daily Value*
Total Fat 2g	**3%**
Saturated Fat 1.5g	**8%**

Reduced-fat, less-fat milk, 8 oz (2% fat by weight)

Calories 120	Calories from Fat 45
	% Daily Value*
Total Fat 5g	**8%**
Saturated Fat 2g	**10%**

Low-fat cheddar cheese, 1.5 oz

Calories 70	Calories from Fat 30
	% Daily Value*
Total Fat 3g	**5%**
Saturated Fat 2g	**10%**

Strawberry yogurt, 8 oz

Calories 250	Calories from Fat 45
	% Daily Value*
Total Fat 5g	**8%**
Saturated Fat 3g	**15%**

Cheddar cheese, 1.5 oz

Calories 165	Calories from Fat 130
	% Daily Value*
Total Fat 14g	**22%**
Saturated Fat 9g	**45%**

Low-fat strawberry yogurt, 8 oz

Calories 240	Calories from Fat 20
	% Daily Value*
Total Fat 2.5g	**4%**
Saturated Fat 2g	**10%**

© Polara Studios, Inc.

hamburger sandwich contains 23 grams of protein and 23 grams of fat, more than 8 of them saturated fat.[31] Because protein offers 4 calories per gram and fat offers 9, the meat of the sandwich provides 92 calories from protein but 207 calories from fat. Hot dogs, fried chicken sandwiches, and fried fish sandwiches also provide hundreds of mostly invisible calories of solid fat. Because so much meat fat is hidden from view, meat eaters can easily and unknowingly consume a great many grams of solid fat from this source.

Tips for Limiting Fats from Meats   When choosing beef or pork, look for lean cuts named *loin* or *round* from which the fat can be trimmed, and eat small portions. Chicken and turkey flesh are naturally lean, but commercial processing and frying add solid fats, especially to "patties," "nuggets," "fingers," and wings. Watch out for ground turkey or chicken products. The skin is often ground in to add pleasing moistness, but the food ends up with more solid fat than the amount found in many cuts of lean beef. Also, some people (even famous chefs) misinterpret Figure 5–6 (p. 150), reasoning that, if poultry or pork fat is less saturated than beef fat, it must be harmless to the heart. Nutrition authorities emphatically state, however, that all sources of saturated fat pose a risk and that even the skin of poultry should be removed before eating the food.

KEY POINT

- Meats account for a large proportion of the hidden solid fat in many people's diets.

Milk and Milk Products

Milk products go by many names that reflect their varying fat contents, as shown in Figure 5–16. A cup of homogenized whole milk contains the protein and carbohydrate of fat-free milk, but in addition, it contains about 80 extra calories from butterfat, a

Figure 5–17

Saturated Fat in Popular Grain Foods

Plain cooked grains are naturally low in saturated fat, but manufacturers often add saturated-fat-rich ingredients to popular grain-based foods during processing. The values below are for one item; one doughnut, for example, delivers 40 percent of the Daily Value for saturated fat; two doughnuts deliver 80 percent, and so forth.

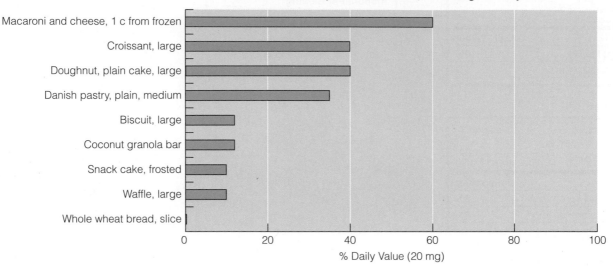

Saturated Fat in Popular Grain Foods, Percentage of Daily Value

% Daily Value (20 mg)

solid fat. A cup of reduced-fat (2 percent fat) milk falls between whole and fat-free, with 45 calories of fat. The fat of whole milk occupies only a teaspoon or two of the volume but nearly doubles the calories in the milk.

Milk and yogurt appear together in the Milk and Milk Products group, but cream and butter do not. Milk and yogurt are rich in calcium and protein, but cream and butter are not. Cream and butter are solid fats, as are whipped cream, sour cream, and cream cheese, and they are properly grouped together with other fats. Other cheeses, grouped with milk products, vary in their fat contents and are major contributors of saturated fat in the U.S. diet.

KEY POINT

- Milk products bear names that identify their fat contents.

Grains

Grain foods in their natural state are very low in fat, but fats of all kinds may be added during manufacturing, processing, or cooking (see Figure 5–17). In fact, today's leading single contributor of solid fats to the U.S. diet is grain-based desserts, such as cookies, cakes, and pastries, which are often prepared with butter, margarine, or hydrogenated shortening. Other grain foods made with solid fats include biscuits, cornbread, granola and other ready-to-eat cereals, croissants, doughnuts, fried rice, pasta with creamy or oily sauces, quick breads, snack and party crackers, muffins, pancakes, and homemade waffles. Packaged breakfast bars often resemble vitamin-fortified candy bars in their solid fat and added sugar contents.

Now that you know where the fats in foods are found, how can you reduce or eliminate the harmful ones? The Food Feature provides some pointers.

KEY POINT

- Solid fat in grain foods can be well hidden.

Defensive Dining

LO 5.9 Describe ways to reduce solid fats in an average diet.

Following today's lipid guidelines can be tricky. To reduce intakes of saturated and *trans*-fatty acids, for example, you need to identify food sources of these fatty acids in your diet—that is, foods rich in solid fats (see Table 5–6). Then, to replace them appropriately, you need to identify suitable replacements to include in your own eating pattern. Here are some tips to help simplify these feats:

1. Select the most nutrient-dense foods from all food groups. Warning: Solid fats and high-calorie choices lurk in every group.

2. Consume fewer and smaller portions of foods and beverages that contain solid fats.

3. Replace solid fats with liquid oils whenever possible.

4. Check Nutrition Facts labels and select foods with little saturated fat and no *trans* fat.

Such advice is easily dispensed but not easily followed, however. Here are some tips.

In the Grocery Store

The right choices in the grocery store can save you many grams of saturated and *trans* fats. Armed with label information,

Table 5–6

Solid Fat Ingredients on Labels

- Beef fat
- Butter
- Chicken fat
- Coconut oil
- Cream
- Hydrogenated oil
- Margarine
- Milk fat
- Palm kernel oil; palm oil
- Partially hydrogenated oil
- Pork fat (lard)
- Shortening

you can decide whether to use a food often as a staple item, limit it to an occasional treat, or reject it altogether. For example, plain frozen vegetables without butter or other high-fat sauces are a staple food—they are high in nutrient density and devoid of solid fats. Within calorie limits, vegetables with olive oil or other unsaturated oils are also low in solid fats.

Make the same distinctions among precooked meats. Avoid those that are coated and fried or prepared in fatty gravies. Try rotisserie chicken from the deli section—rotisserie cooking lets much of the solid fat drain away. Removing the skin leaves only the chicken—a nutrient-dense food.

Choosing Seafood

Grocery stores offer many kinds and forms of seafood, such as salmon (fresh, canned, or broiled in the deli), canned tuna, and many frozen fillets, scallops, or shrimp that can help meet your need for the omega-3 fatty acids. Look back at Table 5–5, p. 163, for a list of good sources. Limit fried fish sticks and breaded fillets, as well as seafood prepared in butter or creamy sauces. Stock pantry shelves with canned salmon, sardines, or tuna for a quick lunch; keep plain frozen fillets and seafood in the freezer for a week or two to sauté or bake from frozen (no defrosting necessary). (Use up fresh fish within a day or two after purchasing it.) Twice a week, try one of these quick meals:

- Tuna salad sandwich on whole-grain bread

- Tuna melt on a whole-wheat English muffin with low-fat cheddar cheese

- Grilled fish tacos with shredded coleslaw mix and salsa

- Crab cakes or salmon cakes with a sauce of Greek yogurt, capers, and dill

- Smoked or grilled salmon or other fish as a main dish or in pasta salad

- Manhattan-style clam chowder or other broth-based seafood soups for lunch or supper

- Sardines on whole-grain bread or crackers

- Sushi made with cooked seafood

- Shrimp marinated in Italian dressing or lime juice tossed with black beans, onion, and corn for a delicious salad

Choosing among Margarines

Soft or liquid margarines made from unhydrogenated vegetable oils are mostly unsaturated, so they make better choices than the saturated solid fats of butter or stick margarines. Some margarines are made with extra virgin olive oil or omega-3 fatty acids, which may provide extra benefits.

Diet margarines contain fewer calories than regular varieties because water, air, or fillers have been added. A few margarines advertised to "support heart health" contain added plant sterols, phytochemicals known to lower blood LDL cholesterol somewhat.[‡‡] Bottom line: read the Nutrition Facts panels. Choose margarines made with oils (but not hydrogenated oils) that have little saturated fat and no *trans* fats.

Choosing Unsaturated Oils

When choosing oils, try various types to obtain the benefits different oils offer. Peanut and safflower oils are especially rich in vitamin E. Olive oil presents naturally occurring antioxidant phytochemicals (see the next paragraph), and canola oil is rich with monounsaturated and essential fatty acids. High temperatures, such as those used in frying, destroy some omega-3 acids and other beneficial constituents, so treat your oils gently. Take care to *substitute* oils for saturated fats in the diet; do not add oils to an already fat-rich diet.

[‡‡]The brand name of the margarine is Benecol.

(continued)

Some oils are valued for their pleasing flavors or their phytochemicals believed to support health.[32] Virgin or extra virgin olive oils are mechanically pressed from olives, a process that retains the phytochemicals that confer a characteristic green color and full flavor. Less colorful "light" or regular olive oils may be extracted with chemicals or processed to remove some of the bitter-tasting phytochemicals to please consumer palates. These less costly, lower-quality oils lack many phytochemicals but are as rich in monounsaturated fatty acids as the more expensive kinds, so they still make good substitutes for saturated fats. Many people enjoy the interesting flavors of avocado oil, grape seed oil, sesame oil, and walnut oil, each with its own array of phytochemicals. Research about their health effects is ongoing.

Adding Nuts

Little doubt remains about the value of nuts for heart health—people who include nuts and peanuts in their diets often have lower rates of chronic diseases.[33] Try some traditional Mediterranean uses for nuts. Grind almonds or walnuts and add them to savory sauces. Chop, sliver, or shave them to sprinkle atop vegetables or salads. Mix them into grain dishes for crunch. Use them in desserts to add richness. Use restraint, however: a quarter cup of nuts can deliver up to 200 calories.

Fat-Free Products and Artificial Fats

Keep in mind that "fat-free" versions of normally high-fat foods, such as cakes

fat replacers ingredients that replace some or all of the functions of fat and may or may not provide energy.

artificial fats zero-energy fat replacers that are chemically synthesized to mimic the sensory and cooking qualities of naturally occurring fats but that are totally or partially resistant to digestion. Olestra (trade name *Olean*) is an example of a noncaloric artificial fat.

or cookies, do not necessarily provide fewer calories than the original and may not offer a health advantage if added sugars take the place of fats (explained in the Controversy). Some foods contain **fat replacers**—ingredients made from carbohydrate or protein that mimic the taste and texture of solid fats but with fewer calories and less saturated fat. Others contain **artificial fats**, synthetic compounds offering the sensory properties of fat but none of the calories or fat. Chapter 12 comes back to the topic of artificial fats and other food additives.

Revamp Recipes

At home, minimize solid fats used as seasonings. This means enjoying the natural flavor of steamed or roasted vegetables, seasoned with lemon pepper, garlic, and herbs or a squeeze of lemon, lime, or other citrus. You might also like vegetables with a teaspoon or two of tasty oils: olive oil or liquid margarine, sesame seed oil, nut oils, or some toasted nuts or seeds. Seek out recipes that replace solid shortening with liquid vegetable oil such as canola oil and that provide replacements for meat gravies and cheese or cream sauces. To prepare seafood, use tomatoes, onions, peppers, herbs, and other flavorful, nutrient-dense ingredients; frying in butter, shortening, or other solid fats negates some of the benefit that seafood offers.

Figure 5–18 illustrates how saturated fats are affected by some simple substitutions. Here are some other tips to help revise recipes:

- Grill, roast, broil, boil, bake, stir-fry, microwave, or poach foods. Don't fry in solid fats, such as shortening, lard, or butter. Try pan frying in a few teaspoons of olive or vegetable oil instead of deep-fat frying.
- Reduce or eliminate food "add-ons" such as buttery, cheesy, or creamy sauces; sour cream dressings; and

bacon bits that drive up the calories and saturated fat. Instead, add a small amount of olives, nuts, hummus (a tangy chickpea paste), or avocado for rich flavor.

- Prepared side dishes, such as noodles or potatoes, are convenient, but check the Nutrition Facts label and reject any that present high saturated fat contents.

For snacks, replace commercial "buttery" popcorn with the plain kind, and season it yourself with fat-free butter-flavored sprinkles, liquid or spray margarine, or a little grated parmesan cheese. The fats used in most popcorn brands are extraordinarily high in saturated fats.

Table 5–7 (p. 174) lists many practical ways to cut down on solid fats and replace them with liquid oils in foods. These replacements don't change the taste or appearance much, but they dramatically lower the saturated fat contents of the foods.

Feast on Fast Foods

All of these suggestions work well when a person plans and prepares each meal at home. But in the real world, people fall behind schedule and don't have time to shop or cook, so they eat fast food. Figure 5–19 (p. 175) compares some fast-food choices and offers tips to reduce the calories and saturated fat to make fast-food meals healthier.

Keep these facts about fast food in mind:

- Salads are a good choice, but beware of toppings such as fried noodles, bacon bits, grease-soaked croutons, sour cream, or shredded cheese that can drive up the calories and solid fat contents.
- If you are really hungry, order a small hamburger, broiled chicken sandwich, or "veggie burger" and a side salad. Hold the cheese (usually full-fat in fast-food restaurants); use mustard or ketchup as condiments.

Chapter 5 The Lipids: Fats, Oils, Phospholipids, and Sterols

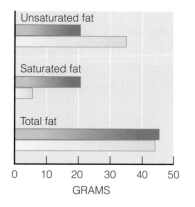

Figure 5–18

Fat Substitution in a Grilled Meal

These two meals are similar in total fat and calories and are equally delicious, but look at the graph to see what happens to saturated fat when olive oil, fish, and seeds replace butter, meat, and cheese. Importantly, the calories remain the same.

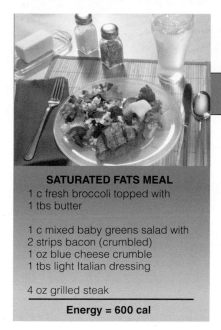

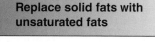
Replace solid fats with unsaturated fats

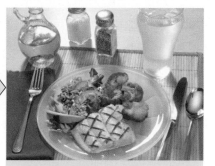

SATURATED FATS MEAL

1 c fresh broccoli topped with
1 tbs butter

1 c mixed baby greens salad with
2 strips bacon (crumbled)
1 oz blue cheese crumble
1 tbs light Italian dressing

4 oz grilled steak

Energy = 600 cal

UNSATURATED FATS MEAL

1 c fresh broccoli sautéed in
1 tbs olive oil

1 c mixed baby greens salad with
½ avocado
2 tbs sunflower seeds
1 tbs light Italian dressing

4 oz grilled salmon

Energy = 600 cal

(Graph: Unsaturated fat, Saturated fat, Total fat — GRAMS, scale 0 to 50)

- A small bowl of chili (hold the cheese and sour cream) poured over a plain baked potato can also satisfy a bigger appetite. Top it with chopped raw onions or hot sauce for spice, and pair it with a small salad and fat-free milk for a complete meal.

- Chicken or fish tacos, bean burritos, and other Mexican treats are delicious topped with salsa and onions instead of cheese and sour cream.

- Fast-food fried fish or fried chicken sandwiches can contain as much solid fat as hamburgers. Broiled chicken and fish sandwiches are far less fatty if you order them without cheese, bacon, or mayonnaise sauces.

- Chicken wings are mostly fatty skin, and the tastiest wing snacks are fried

in cooking fat (often a saturated type), smothered with a buttery, spicy sauce, and then dipped in blue cheese dressing, making wings an extraordinarily high-fat, high-calorie food.

Because fast foods are short on variety, let them be part of a lifestyle in which they complement the other parts. Eat differently, often, elsewhere.

Change Your Habits

The lipid guidelines offered in this chapter do not occur in isolation—they accompany recommendations to achieve and sustain a healthy body weight, to keep calories under control, and to eat a nutrient-dense diet with adequate fruit, vegetables, whole grains, and legumes, which provide cholesterol-lowering

soluble fiber as well. By this time, you may be wondering if you can realistically make all the changes recommended for your diet.

Be assured that even small changes can yield big dividends in terms of reducing solid fat intake, and most such changes can become habits after a few repetitions. You do not have to give up all high-fat treats, even chicken wings, nor should you strive to eliminate all fats. You decide what the treats should be and then choose them in moderation, just for pure pleasure. Meanwhile, make sure that your everyday, ordinary choices are the whole, nutrient-dense foods suggested throughout this book. That way you'll meet all your body's needs for nutrients and never feel deprived.

Table 5-7

Solid Fat Replacements

Select foods that replace solid fats with polyunsaturated or monounsaturated fats. Avoid foods that replace fats with refined white flour or added sugars, as these may present risks of their own. Remember that "light" on a label can refer to color or texture, so always compare the Nutrition Facts panel with the regular product.

Instead of these . . .	. . . try choosing these
Solid Fats and Oils	
Regular margarine and butter for spreading, cooking, or baking	Olive, nut, seed, and other vegetable oils; reduced-fat, diet, liquid, or spray margarine; granulated butter replacers; fruit butters, hummus, nut butters, or avocado for spreading
Shortening or lard in cooking	Nonstick cooking spray, olive oil, or vegetable oil for frying; applesauce or oil for baking
Solid fats as seasonings: bacon, bacon fat, butter; fried onion or greasy crouton salad toppers	Herbs, lemons, spices, liquid smoke flavoring, ham-flavored bouillon cubes, broth, wine; olive oil; olives; toasted nut or toasted whole-grain crouton toppers
Milk Products/Dairy Products	
Whole milk; half and half	Fat-free or reduced-fat milk; fat-free half and half
Regular ricotta cheese; mozzarella cheese; yogurt or sour cream	Part-skim ricotta or fat-free cottage cheese; part-skim mozzarella; fat-free sour cream, "zero" plain Greek-style yogurt[a]
Regular cheddar, American, or other cheeses; cream cheese	Low-fat or fat-free cheeses; fat-free or reduced-fat cream cheese, Neufchatel cheese
Large amounts of mild cheeses	Small amounts of strong-flavored aged cheeses (sharp cheddar; grated Asiago, Romano, or Parmesan)
Ice cream, mousse, cream custards	"Light" ice cream, frozen yogurt, or other frozen desserts; low-sugar sherbet or sorbet; skim milk low-sugar puddings
Protein Foods	
Bologna, salami, other sliced sandwich meats; hot dogs	Low-fat sandwich meats and hot dogs (95–97% lean, or "light")
Breakfast sausage or bacon	Canadian bacon, lean ham, or soy-based sausage or bacon-like products
High-fat beef, pork, or lamb; ground beef	Leaner cuts trimmed of fat, broiled salmon or other seafood; ground turkey breast (98% lean), soy-based "ground beef" crumbles; legume main dishes
Poultry with skin	Skinless poultry
Commercial fish sticks, breaded fried fish fillets	Plain fish fillets, broiled or rolled in seasoned whole-wheat breadcrumbs and pan sautéed in oil
Grains and Desserts	
Chips, such as tortilla or potato; appetizer crackers	Baked or "light" chips; reduced-fat crackers and cookies, saltine-type crackers; nut, seed, or whole-grain crackers low in saturated and *trans* fat
Cakes, cookies; doughnuts, pastries, other desserts	Fresh and dried fruit; whole-grain muffins, quick breads, or cakes made with oil (not shortening)
Granola, other cereals with saturated fat or hydrogenated fat	Cereals low in saturated fat, with no *trans* fat (compare the Nutrition Facts panel information)
Macaroni and cheese	Spaghetti and marinara sauce
Ramen-type noodles[b]	Soba noodles or other whole-grain noodles cooked in broth, with Asian seasonings
Other	
Frozen or canned main dishes with more than 2 or 3 g saturated fat per serving	Similar foods with less saturated fat per serving (compare the Nutrition Facts panel information)
Cream-based, cheese, or "loaded" soups	Broth-based, vegetable, or bean soups; poultry-based, meatless, or other low-fat chili

[a]If the food must be boiled, stabilize the cottage cheese or yogurt with a small amount of cornstarch or flour.
[b]Ramen noodles are often fried in saturated oils during processing.

Chapter 5 The Lipids: Fats, Oils, Phospholipids, and Sterols

Figure 5–19

Making Fast-Food Choices

Scan fast-food menus for lower-calorie options, and then make substitutions like these. Chapter 9 revisits calorie information on menus.

Key: ■ Calories ■ Grams saturated fat ■ % Daily Value (DV=20 g saturated fat)

Indulgent Choices

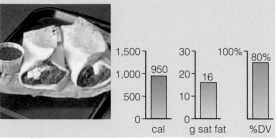

2 "grande" burritos with beef, beans, cheese, and sour cream; salsa

- cal: 950
- g sat fat: 16
- %DV: 80%

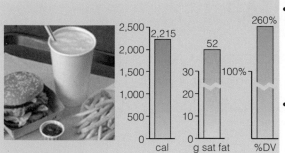

Big double cheeseburger, large fries, regular milkshake

- cal: 2,215
- g sat fat: 52
- %DV: 260%

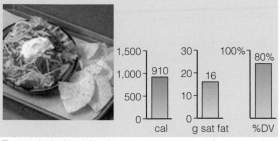

Taco salad with chili, cheese, sour cream, salsa, and taco chips

- cal: 910
- g sat fat: 16
- %DV: 80%

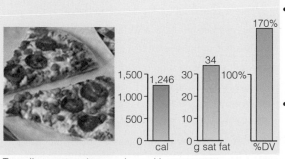

Two slices extra cheese pizza with sausage and pepperoni

- cal: 1,246
- g sat fat: 34
- %DV: 170%

Burrito choices
- Enjoy beans, cheese, and salsa.
- Omit beef and sour cream.

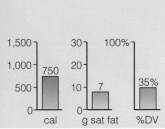

Sandwich choices
- Choose grilled (not fried) chicken with spicy mustard, lettuce, onion, and tomato; milk; and a crunchy side salad with reduced-calorie dressing.
- Omit beef, mayonnaise sauce, fries, and shake.

Salad choices
- Enjoy chili, onions, salsa, and a few chips on crispy salad vegetables. Use half the dressing.
- Omit cheese and sour cream.

Pizza choices
- Top with mushrooms, bell and hot peppers, onions, olives, artichokes, sun-dried tomatoes, and the regular amount of cheese.
- Omit fatty meats and extra cheese.

Enlightened Choices

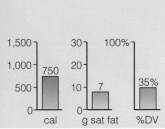

2 bean burritos; salsa

- cal: 750
- g sat fat: 7
- %DV: 35%

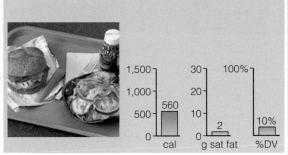

Big grilled chicken breast sandwich, pickle, side salad with reduced-calorie dressing, fat-free milk

- cal: 560
- g sat fat: 2
- %DV: 10%

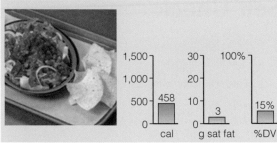

Taco salad with chili, salsa, and taco chips

- cal: 458
- g sat fat: 3
- %DV: 15%

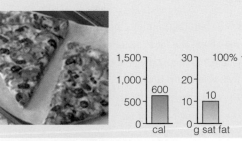

Two slices cheese pizza with mushrooms, olives, onions, and peppers

- cal: 600
- g sat fat: 10
- %DV: 48%

© Matthew Farruggio (all photos)

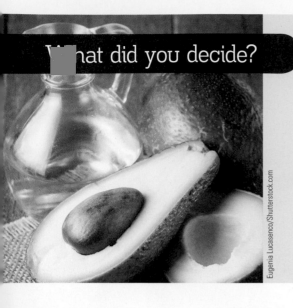

What did you decide?

Are **fats** unhealthy food constituents that are best eliminated from the diet?

What are the differences between **"bad" and "good" cholesterol**?

Why is choosing **fish** recommended in a healthy diet?

If you trim all **visible fats** from foods, will your diet meet lipid recommendations?

What's online?

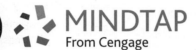
From Cengage

Visit www.Cengage.com to access MindTap, a complete digital course that includes Diet & Wellness Plus, interactive quizzes, videos, and more.

Self Check

1. (LO 5.1) Which of the following is *not* one of the ways fats are useful in foods?
   a. Fats contribute to the taste and smell of foods.
   b. Fats carry fat-soluble vitamins.
   c. Fats provide a low-calorie source of energy compared to carbohydrates.
   d. Fats provide essential fatty acids.

2. (LO 5.1) Fats play few roles in the body, apart from providing abundant fuel in the form of calories.
   T   F

3. (LO 5.2) Saturation refers to
   a. the ability of a fat to penetrate a barrier, such as paper.
   b. whether or not a fatty acid chain is holding all of the hydrogen atoms it can hold.
   c. the characteristic of pleasing flavor and aroma.
   d. the fattening power of fat.

4. (LO 5.2) Generally speaking, vegetable and fish oils are rich in saturated fat.
   T   F

5. (LO 5.2) A benefit to health is seen when _____ is used in place of _____ in the diet.
   a. saturated fat/monounsaturated fat
   b. saturated fat/polyunsaturated fat
   c. unsaturated fat/saturated fat
   d. triglycerides/cholesterol

6. (LO 5.3) Little fat digestion takes place in the stomach.
   T   F

7. (LO 5.3) Bile is essential for fat digestion because it
   a. splits triglycerides into fatty acids and glycerol.
   b. emulsifies fats in the small intestine.
   c. works as a hormone to suppress appetite.
   d. emulsifies fat in the stomach.

8. (LO 5.4) When energy from food is in short supply, the body
   a. dismantles its glycogen to release triglycerides for energy.
   b. dismantles its cholesterol and releases glucose for energy.
   c. converts its glucose to fat for more efficient energy.
   d. dismantles its stored triglycerides and releases fatty acids for energy.

9. (LO 5.4) Fat breakdown without carbohydrate causes ketones to build up in the tissues and blood and to be excreted in the urine.
   T   F

10. (LO 5.5) LDL, a class of lipoprotein, delivers triglycerides and cholesterol from the liver to the body's tissues.
    T   F

11. (LO 5.5) Chylomicrons, a class of lipoprotein, are produced in the liver.
    T   F

12. (LO 5.5) Consuming large amounts of saturated fatty acids lowers LDL cholesterol and thus lowers the risk of heart disease and heart attack.
    T   F

13. (LO 5.6) The roles of the essential fatty acids include
    a. forming parts of cell membranes.
    b. supporting infant growth and vision development.
    c. maintaining normal blood pressure.
    d. all of the above.

14. (LO 5.6) Taking supplements of fish oil is recommended for those who don't like fish.
    T   F

15. (LO 5.6) Fried fish from fast-food restaurants and frozen fried fish products are often low in omega-3 fatty acids and high in solid fats.
    T   F

16. (LO 5.7) A way to prevent spoilage of unsaturated fats and make them harder is to change their fatty acids chemically through _____.
    a. acetylation
    b. hydrogenation
    c. oxidation
    d. mastication

17. (LO 5.7) *Trans*-fatty acids arise when unsaturated fats are
    a. used for deep frying.
    b. hydrogenated.
    c. baked.
    d. used as preservatives.

18. (LO 5.8) An eating pattern with sufficient essential fatty acids includes
    a. nuts and vegetable oils.
    b. ¼ cup of raw oil each day.
    c. two servings of seafood a week.
    d. a and c.

19. (LO 5.8) Most solid fats in the U.S. diet are supplied by invisible fats.
    T   F

20. (LO 5.9) Solid fats and high-calorie choices lurk in every food group.
    T   F

21. (LO 5.10) The best way to apply the lipid advice from the Dietary Guidelines for Americans is to:
    a. Ignore it because the scientists keep changing their minds.
    b. Focus on individual fatty acids that are associated with diseases and eliminate those from the diet.
    c. Follow a low-fat diet except for butter, which presents healthy fats.
    d. Follow an eating pattern recommended by the Dietary Guidelines.

Answers to these Self Check questions are in Appendix G.

Is Butter Really Back? The Lipid Guidelines Debate

LO 5.10   Discuss both sides of the scientific debate about current lipid guidelines.

To consumers, advice about dietary fats appears to change almost daily. "Eat less fat—choose more margarine." "Give up butter and margarine—use soft margarine." "Forget soft margarine—replace it with olive oil." Then headlines seem to turn all the previous advice on its head. To researchers, however, the evolution of advice about fats reflects decades of research that have built a massive foundation of knowledge about the health effects of dietary fats. The details, however, have varied over time.

This Controversy explores changing lipid guidelines and the arguments surrounding them. It ends with the current opinion that, although specific lipids are associated with disease risks, a person's repeated daily food choices—that is, their entire eating pattern—seems to exert the greatest impact.[1]*

Shifting Guidelines

In years past, Dietary Guidelines urged all healthy people, not just those with heart disease, to cut their total fat intakes in everything from hot dogs to salad dressings to preserve their good health. This advice was straightforward: cut the fat and improve your health. Did this strategy work? Yes, but only for those few who consistently replaced all high-fat foods with whole grains, vegetables, fruit, fat-free milk products, and low-fat fish and poultry.

In response to total fat guidelines, food manufacturers flooded market shelves with an abundance of fat-free (but sugar-laden) cookies, candies, and ice cream and low-fat (but high-calorie) main courses. In the mistaken belief that "fat-free" means "no limits," consumers gobbled them up, often in addition to their regular diets.

*Reference notes are in Appendix F.

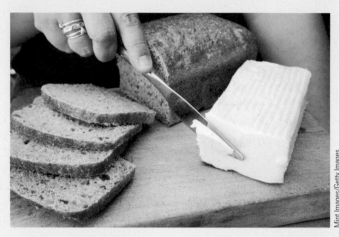

Mint Images/Getty Images

Calorie intakes from carbohydrates, mainly from added sugars and refined starches, climbed, and so did rates of obesity and heart disease. In the end, most consumers gave up in frustration and went back to their old ways of eating.

Research Revelations

A classic study, the Seven Countries Study, initially published in the 1960s, helped nudge national guidelines away from the total fat approach to heart health.[2] In the study, researchers compared death rates from cardiovascular diseases (CVD) with intakes of total fat and saturated fat in seven countries of the world. Study subjects reported their diet histories to dietitians who interviewed them at home, in the presence of the people who prepared their food, and then cross-checked the information with records of the food purchased by that family during the week to improve the accuracy. The researchers also collected personal, medical, and lifestyle information, and then repeated all of these processes 5 and 10 years afterward.

The results were, at the time, remarkable. Two of the seven countries, Finland and the Greek island of Crete,

emerged as having the highest intakes of total fat—40 percent of calories. Here's the unexpected finding: Finland also had the highest CVD death rate by far of all the countries, but Crete had the lowest. These findings suggested that total fat intake alone could not account for differences in rates of CVD—something else had to be responsible. On closer examination, the researchers discovered a difference in saturated fat intakes: the average Finnish diet was high in saturated fat (18 percent of calories), while the diet of Crete was much lower (less than 10 percent of calories). The people of Crete also preferred olive oil, rich in unsaturated fatty acids, over butter.

Soon, nutrition guidelines had singled out saturated fats for restriction to address soaring U.S. rates of heart disease. Again, food manufacturers acted quickly, replacing lard and butter in their formulations with partially hydrogenated vegetable shortenings and margarines. No one knew it at the time, but the replacements were rich in *trans*-fatty acids, now known to be as bad as or worse than saturated fatty acids with regard to CVD risk.[3] As you might expect, heart disease rates remained high during this period.

Dietary Guidelines for Americans 2015

Many studies in the decades that followed, including clinical, epidemiological, and animal studies, have largely supported the saturated fat theory.[4] After reviewing available evidence, the Dietary Guidelines 2015 committee concluded that saturated fat is a nutrient of concern for public health, because:

- Strong, consistent evidence shows that replacing saturated fats with unsaturated fats, especially polyunsaturated fats, significantly reduces total and LDL cholesterol in the blood, and

- Strong, consistent evidence shows that replacing saturated fats with polyunsaturated fats reduces the risk of developing CVD and of dying of heart disease (see Figure C5–1).[5]

The committee also stated that:

- Partially hydrogenated oils containing *trans* fat should be avoided.

The committee based these conclusions on multiple recent high-quality systematic reviews and meta-analyses (studies that combine priorly published data and reanalyze them) comparing saturated fat intakes with factors such as:

- Blood lipids,
- Blood pressure,
- CVD mortality,
- Heart attacks, and
- Strokes.

The results of a few studies do suggest no relationship between reducing saturated fat intake and heart disease or mortality.[6] The problem with these studies, however, is that when people reduce saturated fats, they typically increase carbohydrates, and a diet high in refined carbohydrates and added sugars is likely to raise heart disease risk (see Controversy 4).[7] The Dietary Guidelines committee concluded that replacing saturated fat with unspecified types of carbohydrate, which could be refined starches and added sugars, is not effective in reducing CVD risk. When carbohydrates from whole fruit, vegetables, legumes, or grains replace saturated fat in the diet, CVD risk is reliably reduced. The source matters.[8]

You can read more about the research that the committee used in setting the guidelines on the Internet—open a free copy of the *Scientific Report of the 2015 Dietary Guidelines Advisory Committee.*[†]

The American Heart Association and American College of Cardiologists Concur

Two venerable medical organizations, the American Heart Association and the American College of Cardiologists (AHA/ACC), on reviewing current research, reasserted with their strongest level of confidence that people who need to lower their blood LDL cholesterol should reduce their intakes of saturated fat. In addition to increasing blood LDL, a high intake of one saturated fatty acid in particular (**palmitic acid**; see Table C5–1) may worsen atrial fibrillation, a dangerous twitching of the heart muscle that impedes normal heartbeats.[9] The goal for people who must reduce LDL is therefore set at no more than 5 to 6 percent of total calories from saturated fat, lower than an earlier goal of 7 percent.[10]

[†] *Available at www.health.gov.*

Table C5–1
Saturated Fatty Acid Terms

palmitic acid a 16-carbon saturated fatty acid found in tropical palm oil, among other foods. Palmitic acid raises LDL cholesterol, increases CVD risk, and is associated with a dangerous form of irregular heartbeat.

stearic acid an 18-carbon saturated fatty acid found in most animal fats. Stearic acid intake increases heart risks, but does not raise blood LDL cholesterol.

So What's the Debate?

Most scientists generally agree with current lipid intake guidelines, but others argue that saturated fat is irrelevant to heart health.[11] They offer the following lines of research to defend their position.

Missing Mechanism

First, they argue that, other than raising LDL cholesterol, no biological mechanism has been firmly established to explain how, exactly, saturated fat leads to the formation of atherosclerosis, the hardening of the arteries that underlies CVD.[12] Before condemning saturated fat by association with CVD, they want to find the smoking gun, so to speak—the physiological mechanism by which these fats may cause the disease.

Actions of Genes

Second, they point out that a person's genetic inheritance strongly influences how his or her body handles fatty acids. Some people are more susceptible to forming particularly harmful types of LDL or less effective HDL, changing their CVD risks independently of diet.

Differing Actions of Saturated Fatty Acids

Third, the degree to which individual saturated fatty acids increase LDL varies somewhat. Almost all saturated fatty acids clearly elevate blood LDL, but one, **stearic acid**, does not; it does, however, increase the risk of CVD, and replacing it with polyunsaturated fat, whole grains, or plant proteins reduces the risk substantially.[13]

Figure C5–1
Saturated Fatty Acids and CVD Risk

Replacing saturated fat with unsaturated fat reduces in CVD risk. The reverse is also true: increasing saturated fat intakes increases the risk.

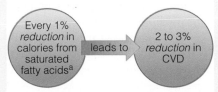

Every 1% *reduction* in calories from saturated fatty acids[a] → leads to → 2 to 3% *reduction* in CVD

[a] When replaced by polyunsaturated fat; the effect of carbohydrate is not clear and may depend on the type and source of carbohydrate.

Source: U.S. Department of Agriculture and U.S. Department of Health and Human Services, Scientific Report of the 2015 Dietary Guidelines Advisory Committee (2015): D-6-12-17, available at www.health.gov.

Headline Hype

Gleeful media headlines proclaiming "Butter Is Back," shocked (and often delighted) consumers with stories urging them to ignore the Dietary Guidelines for Americans and eat all the ice cream, marbled steaks, and butter that they desire. "Research," the journalists said, "has vindicated saturated fat—it plays no role in causing heart disease."[14]

These startling claims were spawned by the publication of a scientific meta-analysis that did, in fact, fail to find a correlation between dietary saturated fat intakes and elevated CVD risk.[15] This study included data from many previous observational studies—that is, studies that asked people what they ate and then tracked their health over time.

Authorities Weigh In

Challenges to this meta-analysis were immediate and vigorous.[16] One objection arose from the kinds of data that were included in the study. The data were drawn from observational research that relies on what people *say* they eat, which most often differs from what people *actually* eat. Apparently, something about human nature, perhaps memory lapses or fear of embarrassment, renders self-reports of food consumption inaccurate. The best studies rely not on self-reports but on verified intakes.

Another objection concerned the studies chosen for inclusion. The Dietary Guidelines committee pointed out that the analysis was based on a limited number of certain kinds of studies.[17] A subsequent study of over 125,000 people in the United States revealed a clear association between greater intakes of dietary saturated fat and increased mortality: the risk of death from all causes increased by 8 percent for every 5 percent increase in total calories from saturated fat.[18]

What about Butter?

People love butter and want to believe media stories claiming that its saturated fats are safe and that it is full of vitamins.

These are overstatements. It's a myth that butterfat is made up of mostly harmless fatty acids with limited ability to raise blood LDL cholesterol. In fact, butter's major saturated fatty acid is palmitic acid, which readily raises LDL cholesterol and causes damaging arterial inflammation.[19] And butter is a poor source of vitamins—calorie per calorie, fruit and vegetables are the best sources.

Solid evidence is lacking to say whether saturated fat from butter is safe or in what amounts, and interpreting study results can take some scientific sleuthing. For example, one study reporting no harm from saturated fat came from an area of the world with high fish intakes, and thus high intakes of EPA and DHA; its results are inapplicable to populations who eat little fish but abundant pizza, cookies, snack cakes, and fast foods, such as in the United States.[20] In a Dutch population, no harm was reported from saturated dairy fat, but subjects of this study received medical treatments that could have skewed the data.[21] Further, dairy foods, such as cheese and milk, deliver nutrients that can benefit the heart and this might affect the study results.[22]

Butter also contains naturally occurring *trans*-fatty acids, called CLA, which collect in the meat and milk of ruminant animals.[†] In rats, small dietary doses of CLA slightly trim body fatness but larger doses produce serious side effects.[23] Much is still unknown about CLA's effects on health.[24] Unless butter is exonerated by future research, it is best used in moderation.

Research Continues

Today, in the normal pace of science, studies are quietly probing into the roles of saturated and *trans* fats in CVD risk. For example, we now know that both saturated and *trans*-fatty acids worsen atherosclerosis and injure the arteries by increasing inflammation and oxidation, a plausible mechanism for CVD causation.[25] Also, diets high in *unsaturated*

[†] CLA stands for "conjugated linoleic acid," a mixture of *trans*-fatty acids.

fat reduce the most harmful type of LDL cholesterol.[26] A point of strong agreement today is that *trans*-fatty acids are associated with CVD and an increased rate of death.[27]

The Power of Eating Patterns

In the end, people choose foods, not individual nutrients such as saturated fat, and their choices form habitual eating patterns that affect their health.[28] For this reason, an eating pattern approach was used to set the 2015 Dietary Guidelines for Americans.[29] Following an eating pattern that meets the ideals of the Dietary Guidelines (see Chapter 2) reliably improves health in many ways, including controlling body fatness and reducing CVD risk factors, such as diabetes and hypertension. The individual components of such a pattern have synergistic and cumulative effects—that is, they work in harmony over decades to improve health beyond the effects of fats alone.

Figure C5–2 presents two meals that characterize two very different eating patterns—one associated with lower chronic disease risks and the other with increased risks. If most of your meals resemble the dinner on the left, you can be assured of obtaining the nutrients you need within a pattern that supports health superbly. Conversely, if most of your meals resemble the commercially prepared fried chicken fingers and french fries in the other meal, without a fruit or nonstarchy vegetable in sight, you may want to reconsider your choices for your health's sake.[30] This is not to say that an occasional treat of chicken fingers and fries or a corn dog and cola is forever off limits, but if your treats become a repeated pattern on most days, your disease risks will climb.

The Dietary Guidelines for Americans offer these three eating patterns that meet their ideals:

- A healthy vegetarian diet,
- A healthy U.S.-style diet, and
- A healthy Mediterranean diet.

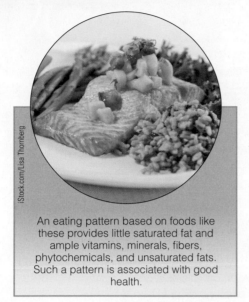

An eating pattern based on foods like these provides little saturated fat and ample vitamins, minerals, fibers, phytochemicals, and unsaturated fats. Such a pattern is associated with good health.

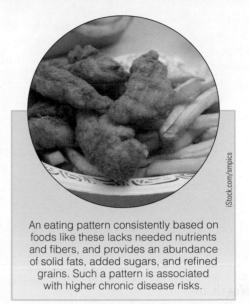

An eating pattern consistently based on foods like these lacks needed nutrients and fibers, and provides an abundance of solid fats, added sugars, and refined grains. Such a pattern is associated with higher chronic disease risks.

The details about all three are in Appendix E. Following any of these eating patterns can both meet nutrient needs and keep the risks of chronic diseases low.

Conclusion

It's easy for consumers to become confused when headlines howl for attention, particularly when they say what people want to hear. Keep in mind that no one study is sufficient to reverse decades of previous findings and that the best action may be no action while you wait and watch for other studies to examine the issue. Meanwhile, don't take chances with your health—follow the advice of the Dietary Guidelines for Americans.

Critical Thinking

1. Find an article in a newspaper or magazine or on the Internet that makes claims about saturated fat, particularly one that extols the safety of high intakes of butter, fatty meats, and cheeses. Based on what you know about the science behind national recommendations, analyze the article's talking points, and come to a conclusion about its veracity.

2. Discuss whether you believe that an eating pattern approach to dietary guidelines is best, or that specific nutrient limits, such as percentages of calories from fats, are most helpful. Defend your opinion.

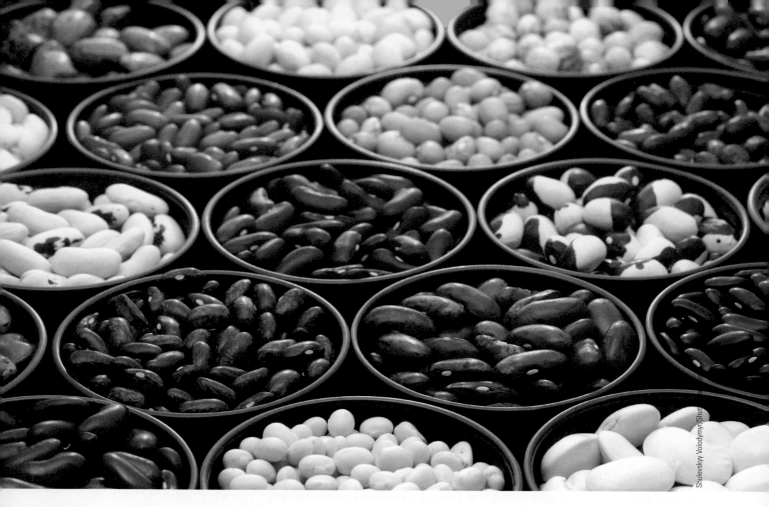

6 The Proteins and Amino Acids

Learning Objectives

After completing this chapter, you should be able to accomplish the following:

LO 6.1 Describe the nature of proteins and amino acids.

LO 6.2 Outline the processes of protein digestion and absorption of amino acids.

LO 6.3 Identify the roles of proteins and amino acids in the body.

LO 6.4 List the factors that determine the daily protein needs of an individual.

LO 6.5 List the potential health problems that are caused by eating patterns that are either too low or too high in protein.

LO 6.6 Identify the benefits and drawbacks of protein-rich foods in the diet.

LO 6.7 Compare the advantages and disadvantages of a vegetarian diet and a meat eater's diet.

What do you think?

Why does your body need **protein**?

How does heating an **egg** change it from a liquid to a solid?

Do protein or amino acid **supplements** bulk up muscles?

Will your diet lack protein if you don't eat **meat**?

The proteins are amazing, versatile, and vital molecules. Without them, life would not exist. First named 150 years ago after the Greek word *proteios* (meaning "of prime importance"), **proteins** have revealed countless secrets of the processes of life and have helped answer many questions in nutrition: How do we grow? How do our bodies replace the materials they lose? How does blood clot? How do wounds heal? What gives us immunity? What makes one person different from another? Understanding the nature of the proteins sheds light on these mysteries.

The Structure of Proteins

LO 6.1   Describe the nature of proteins and amino acids.

The structure of proteins enables them to perform many vital functions. One key difference from carbohydrates and fats is that proteins contain nitrogen atoms in addition to the carbon, hydrogen, and oxygen atoms that all three energy-yielding nutrients contain. These nitrogen atoms give the name *amino* (which means "nitrogen containing") to the **amino acids**, the building blocks of proteins. Another key difference is that in contrast to the carbohydrates—whose repeating units, glucose molecules, are identical—the amino acids in a strand of protein are different from one another. A strand of amino acids that makes up a protein may contain 20 *different* kinds of amino acids.

Amino Acids

All amino acids have the same simple chemical backbone consisting of a single carbon atom with both an **amine group** (the nitrogen-containing part) and an acid group attached to it. Each amino acid also has a distinctive chemical **side chain** attached to the center carbon of the backbone (see Figure 6–1). This side chain gives each amino acid its identity and chemical nature. About 20 amino acids, each with a different side chain, make up most of the proteins of living tissue.[1]* Other rare amino acids appear in a few proteins.

The side chains make the amino acids differ in size, shape, and electrical charge. Some are negative, some positive, some neutral. The first part of Figure 6–2 is a diagram of three amino acids, each with a different side chain attached to its backbone. The rest of the figure shows how amino acids link to form protein strands. Long strands of amino acids form large protein molecules, and the side chains of the amino acids ultimately help determine the protein's molecular shape and behavior.

Essential Amino Acids   The body can make more than half of the 20 amino acids for itself, given the needed parts: fragments derived from carbohydrate or fat to form the backbones, and nitrogen from other sources to form the amine groups. A body cannot make nine of the amino acids or makes them too slowly to meet its needs. These

*Reference notes are in Appendix F.

Figure 6–1

An Amino Acid

The "backbone" is the same for all amino acids. The side chain differs from one amino acid to the next. The nitrogen is in the amine group. (Amino acid structures are shown in Appendix A.)

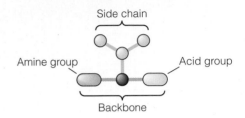

proteins compounds composed of carbon, hydrogen, oxygen, and nitrogen and arranged as strands of amino acids. (Some amino acids also contain the element sulfur.)

amino (a-MEEN-o) **acids** the building blocks of protein. Each has an amine group at one end, an acid group at the other, and a distinctive side chain.

amine (a-MEEN) **group** the nitrogen-containing portion of an amino acid.

side chain the unique chemical structure attached to the backbone of each amino acid that distiguishes one amino acid from another.

Figure 6–2

Different Amino Acids Join Together

This is the basic process by which proteins are assembled.

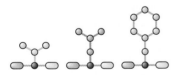

Valine   Leucine   Tyrosine

Single amino acids with different side chains ...

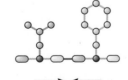

can bond to form ...

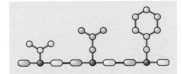

a strand of amino acids, part of a protein.

Table 6–1

Amino Acids Important in Nutrition

The left column lists amino acids that are essential for human beings—the body cannot make them, and they must be provided in the diet. The right column lists other, nonessential amino acids—the body can make these for itself.

Essential Amino Acids	Nonessential Amino Acids
Histidine (HISS-tuh-deen)	Alanine (AL-ah-neen)
Isoleucine (eye-so-LOO-seen)	Arginine (ARJ-ih-neen)
Leucine (LOO-seen)	Asparagine (ah-SPAR-ah-geen)
Lysine (LYE-seen)	Aspartic acid (ah-SPAR-tic acid)
Methionine (meh-THIGH-oh-neen)	Cysteine (SIS-tee-een)
Phenylalanine (fen-il-AL-ah-neen)	Glutamic acid (glu-TAM-ic acid)
Threonine (THREE-oh-neen)	Glutamine (GLU-tah-meen)
Tryptophan (TRIP-toe-fan, TRIP-toe-fane)	Glycine (GLY-seen)
Valine (VAY-leen)	Proline (PRO-leen)
	Serine (SEER-een)
	Tyrosine (TIE-roe-seen)

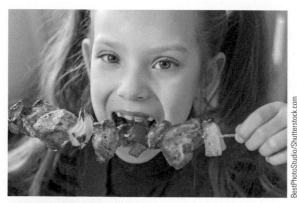

Hair, skin, eyesight, and the health of the whole body depend on proteins from food.

are the **essential amino acids** (listed in Table 6–1). Without these essential nutrients, the body cannot make the proteins it needs to do its work. Because the essential amino acids can be replenished only from foods, a person must frequently eat the foods that provide them.

Under special circumstances, a nonessential amino acid can become essential. For example, the body normally makes tyrosine (a nonessential amino acid) from the essential amino acid phenylalanine. If the diet fails to supply enough phenylalanine or if the body cannot make the conversion for some reason (as happens in the inherited disease phenylketonuria; see Chapter 3, p. 70), then tyrosine becomes a **conditionally essential amino acid**.

Recycling Amino Acids The body not only makes some amino acids but also breaks protein molecules apart and reuses their amino acids. Both food proteins after digestion and body proteins when they have finished their cellular work are dismantled to liberate their component amino acids. Amino acids from both sources provide the cells with raw materials from which they can build the protein molecules they need. Cells can also use the amino acids for energy and discard the nitrogen atoms as wastes. By reusing intact amino acids to build proteins, however, the body recycles and conserves nitrogen, a valuable commodity, while easing its nitrogen disposal burden.

This recycling system also provides access to an emergency fund of amino acids in times of fuel, glucose, or protein deprivation. At such times, tissues can break down their own proteins, sacrificing working molecules before the ends of their normal lifetimes, to supply amino acids and energy to the body's cells.

essential amino acids amino acids that either cannot be synthesized at all by the body or cannot be synthesized in amounts sufficient to meet physiological need.

conditionally essential amino acid an amino acid that is normally nonessential but must be supplied by the diet in special circumstances when the need for it exceeds the body's ability to produce it.

KEY POINTS

- Proteins are unique among the energy nutrients in that they are composed of amino acids, which contain nitrogen as well as carbon and oxygen.
- Of the 20 amino acids, nine are essential amino acids.
- Under special circumstances, a nonessential amino acid can become essential.

How Do Amino Acids Build Proteins?

In the first step of making a protein, each amino acid is hooked to the next (as shown in Figure 6–2, p. 183). A chemical bond, called a **peptide bond**, is formed between the amine group end of one amino acid and the acid group end of the next. The side chains bristle out from the backbone of the structure, giving the protein molecule its unique character. Figure 6–2 shows only the first step in making all proteins—the linking of amino acid units with peptide bonds until the strand contains from several dozen to hundreds or thousands of amino acids. A string of about 10 to 50 amino acids is known as a **polypeptide**.

The strand of protein does not remain a straight chain. Amino acids at different places along the strand are chemically attracted to each other, and this attraction can cause some segments of the strand to coil, somewhat like a metal spring. Also, each spot along the strand is attracted to, or repelled from, other spots along its length (demonstrated in Figure 6–3). These interactions often cause the entire protein coil to fold this way and that to form a globular structure, as shown in Figure 6–4 (p. 186). Other strands link together in other ways to form different structures that perform specific functions.

Figure 6–3

The Coiling and Folding of a Protein Molecule

1 The first shape of a strand of amino acids is a chain, which can be very long. This shows just a portion of the strand.

2 Coiling the strand. The strand of amino acids takes on a springlike shape as the side chains variously attract and repel each other.

3 Folding the coil. The coil then folds and flops over on itself to take a functional shape.

4 Once coiled and folded, the protein may be functional as is, or it may need to join with other proteins or to add a carbohydrate molecule or a vitamin or mineral.

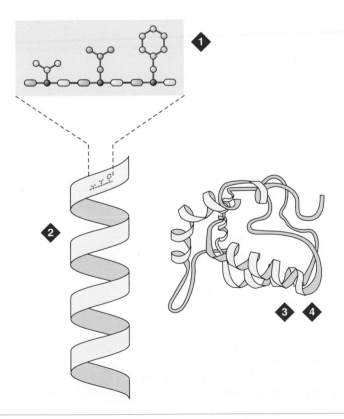

peptide bond a bond that connects one amino acid with another, forming a link in a protein chain. A peptide is a strand of amino acids.

polypeptide (POL-ee-PEP-tide) a protein fragment of about 10 to 50 amino acids bonded together (*poly* means "many").

The Structure of Proteins

The amino acids whose side chains are electrically charged are attracted to water. Therefore, in the body's watery fluids, they orient themselves on the outside of the protein structure. The amino acids whose side chains are neutral are repelled by water and are attracted to one another; these tuck themselves into the center away from the body fluids. All these interactions among the amino acids and the surrounding fluids fold each protein into a unique architecture, a form to suit its function.

Other final details may be needed for the protein to become functional. Several strands may cluster together into a functioning unit; a metal ion (mineral), a vitamin, or a carbohydrate molecule may also join to the unit.

KEY POINT

- Amino acids link into long strands that make a wide variety of different proteins.

The Variety of Proteins

The particular shapes of proteins enable them to perform different tasks in the body. Those of globular shape, such as some proteins of blood, are water-soluble. Some form hollow balls, which can carry and store materials in their interiors. Some proteins, such as those of tendons, are more than 10 times as long as they are wide, forming stiff, rod-like structures that are somewhat insoluble in water and very strong. A form of the protein **collagen** acts somewhat like glue between cells. The hormone insulin, a protein, helps regulate the blood glucose concentration. Among the most fascinating proteins are the **enzymes**, which act on other substances to change them chemically.

Some protein strands work alone, whereas others must associate in groups of strands to become functional. One molecule of **hemoglobin**—the large, globular protein molecule that is packed into the red blood cells by the billions and carries oxygen—is made of four associated protein strands, each holding the mineral iron (see Figure 6–4).

The great variety of proteins in the world is possible because an essentially infinite number of sequences of amino acids can be formed. To understand how so many different proteins can be designed from only 20 or so amino acids, think of how many words are in an unabridged dictionary—all of them constructed from just 26 letters. If you had only the letter "G," all you could write would be a string of Gs: G–G–G–G–G–G–G. But with 26 different letters available, you can create poems, songs, or novels. Similarly, the 20 amino

Figure 6–4

The Structure of Hemoglobin

Four highly folded protein strands form the globular hemoglobin protein.

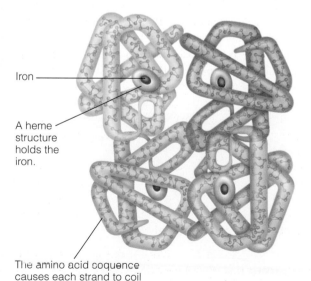

Iron

A heme structure holds the iron.

The amino acid sequence causes each strand to coil and loop, forming the globular protein structure.

collagen (KAHL-ah-jen) the chief protein of most connective tissues, including scars, ligaments, and tendons, and the underlying matrix on which bones and teeth are built.

enzymes (EN-zimes) proteins that facilitate chemical reactions without being changed in the process; protein catalysts. Also defined in Chapter 3.

hemoglobin the globular protein of red blood cells, whose iron atoms carry oxygen around the body via the bloodstream (more about hemoglobin in Chapter 8).

Chapter 6 The Proteins and Amino Acids

Figure 6–5

Normal Red Blood Cells and Sickle Cells

Normal red blood cells are disk-shaped. In sickle-cell disease, the amino acid valine displaces the amino acid glutamic acid at one site in the protein strand, causing the red blood cell to change shape and lose function.

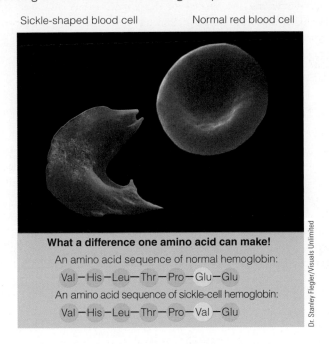

Sickle-shaped blood cell   Normal red blood cell

What a difference one amino acid can make!
An amino acid sequence of normal hemoglobin:
Val—His—Leu—Thr—Pro—Glu—Glu
An amino acid sequence of sickle-cell hemoglobin:
Val—His—Leu—Thr—Pro—Val—Glu

Dr. Stanley Flegler/Visuals Unlimited

acids can be linked together in a huge variety of sequences—many more than are possible for letters in a word, which must alternate consonant and vowel sounds. Thus, the variety of possible sequences for amino acid strands is tremendous.

Inherited Amino Acid Sequences   For each protein, there exists a standard amino acid sequence, and that sequence is specified by the genes. Often, if a wrong amino acid is inserted, the result can be disastrous to health.

Sickle-cell disease—in which hemoglobin, the oxygen-carrying protein of the red blood cells, is abnormal—is an example of an inherited variation in the amino acid sequence. Normal hemoglobin contains two kinds of protein strands. In sickle-cell disease, one of the strands is an exact copy of that in normal hemoglobin, but in the other strand, the sixth amino acid is valine rather than glutamic acid. This replacement of one amino acid so alters the protein that it is unable to carry and release oxygen. The red blood cells collapse from the normal disk shape into crescent shapes (see Figure 6–5). If too many crescent-shaped cells appear in the blood, the result is abnormal blood clotting, strokes, bouts of severe pain, susceptibility to infection, and early death.[2]

You are unique among human beings because of minute differences in your body proteins that establish everything from eye color and shoe size to susceptibility to certain diseases. These differences are determined by the amino acid sequences of your proteins, which are written into the genetic code you inherited from your parents and they from theirs. Ultimately, the genes determine the sequence of amino acids in each finished protein (how DNA directs protein synthesis and **RNA** molecules perform it is described in Figure 6–6, p. 188). When scientists completed the DNA sequence of the human genome, they realized that a still greater task lay ahead of them: the identification of every protein made by the human body.[†]

Nutrients and Gene Expression   When a cell makes a protein, as shown in Figure 6–6, scientists say that the gene for that protein has been "expressed." Every

RNA (ribonucleic acid) cellular nucleic acids that play key roles in the process and control of protein synthesis.

[†] The identification of the entire collection of human proteins, the *human proteome* (PRO-tee-ohme), is a work in progress.

Figure 6–6
Protein Synthesis

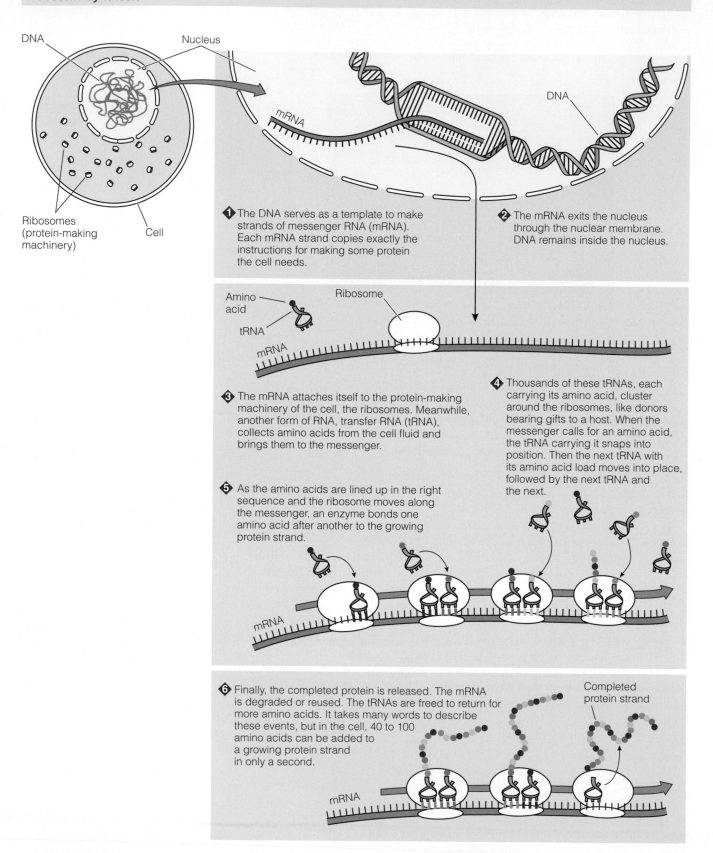

DNA
Nucleus

Ribosomes
(protein-making
machinery)
Cell

DNA

mRNA

❶ The DNA serves as a template to make strands of messenger RNA (mRNA). Each mRNA strand copies exactly the instructions for making some protein the cell needs.

❷ The mRNA exits the nucleus through the nuclear membrane. DNA remains inside the nucleus.

Amino acid
tRNA
Ribosome
mRNA

❸ The mRNA attaches itself to the protein-making machinery of the cell, the ribosomes. Meanwhile, another form of RNA, transfer RNA (tRNA), collects amino acids from the cell fluid and brings them to the messenger.

❹ Thousands of these tRNAs, each carrying its amino acid, cluster around the ribosomes, like donors bearing gifts to a host. When the messenger calls for an amino acid, the tRNA carrying it snaps into position. Then the next tRNA with its amino acid load moves into place, followed by the next tRNA and the next.

❺ As the amino acids are lined up in the right sequence and the ribosome moves along the messenger, an enzyme bonds one amino acid after another to the growing protein strand.

mRNA

❻ Finally, the completed protein is released. The mRNA is degraded or reused. The tRNAs are freed to return for more amino acids. It takes many words to describe these events, but in the cell, 40 to 100 amino acids can be added to a growing protein strand in only a second.

Completed protein strand

mRNA

The answer is mostly "no" but also a qualified "yes." Athletes and fitness seekers cannot stimulate their muscles to gain size and strength simply by consuming more protein or amino acids. Hard work is necessary to trigger the genes to build more of the muscle tissue needed for sport. The "yes" part of the answer reflects research suggesting that well-timed protein intakes can often further stimulate muscle growth. Protein intake cannot replace exercise in this regard, however, as many supplement sellers would have people believe. Exercise generates cellular messages that stimulate the DNA to begin synthesizing the muscle proteins needed to perform the work.

A protein-rich snack—say, a glass of skim milk or soy milk—consumed shortly after strength-building exercise (such as weight lifting) also stimulates muscle protein synthesis, but evidence is lacking for a benefit to athletic performance.

Athletes may need somewhat more dietary protein than other people do, and exercise authorities recommend higher protein intakes for athletes pursuing various activities (see Chapter 10 for details). Amino acid or protein supplements, however, offer no advantage over food, and amino acid supplements are more likely to cause problems (as the Consumer's Guide, p. 198, makes clear). Bottom line: the path to bigger muscles is well-planned, consistent physical training with adequate energy and nutrients from balanced, well-timed meals, snacks, and beverages. Research findings concerning dietary protein and muscles are interesting and important, but this truth remains: extra protein and amino acids without physical work add nothing but excess calories.

start now! Ready to make a change? Go to Diet & Wellness Plus in MindTap and generate an Intake Report for your three-day dietary tracking. What is your protein intake level? If it is low, create an alternate profile and substitute one 8-oz glass of skim or low-fat milk for other beverages at two meals (or one meal and one snack). What is the effect on your protein intake?

---

cell nucleus contains the DNA for making every human protein, but no one cell makes them all. Some cells specialize in making certain proteins; for example, cells of the pancreas express the gene for the protein hormone insulin. The gene for making insulin is present in all other cells of the body, but is silent.

Nutrients, including amino acids and proteins, do not change DNA structure, but they greatly influence gene expression.[3] As research in **nutritional genomics** advances, researchers hope to one day use nutrients to influence a person's genes in ways that reduce that individual's disease risks, but for now, that day is remote. The Think Fitness feature (p. 189) addresses a related concern of exercisers and athletes about whether extra dietary protein or amino acids can trigger the synthesis of muscle tissue and augment strength.

> Controversy 11 comes back to the facts and fiction of nutritional genomics.

KEY POINTS

- Each type of protein has a distinctive sequence of amino acids and so has great functional specificity.
- Certain proteins are common to all cells. In addition, specialized cells synthesize specific proteins that enable them to do distinct jobs.
- Nutrients do not alter genes, but they powerfully influence genetic expression.

Denaturation of Proteins

When a protein molecule loses its shape, it can no longer function as it was designed to do. This is how many agents damage living cells: they cause **denaturation** of their proteins. Among denaturing agents are heat, radiation, alcohol, acids, bases, the salts of heavy metals, and many more. In digestion, however, denaturation is useful: it unfolds and inactivates the proteins in food, and exposes their peptide bonds to the digestive enzymes that cleave them.

Denaturation also occurs during the cooking of foods. Cooking eggs denatures their proteins and makes them firm, as Figure 6–7 demonstrates. Among egg proteins that heat denatures, two are notable in nutrition. One binds the vitamin biotin and the mineral iron: when this protein is denatured, it releases biotin and iron, making them available to the body. The other slows protein digestion; denaturing this protein allows digestion to proceed normally.

Figure 6–7
Heat Denatures Protein

Heat unfolds and uncoils protein structures, causing eggs to become firm as they cook.

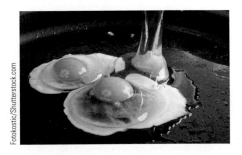

Fotokostic/Shutterstock.com

nutritional genomics the science of how food components, such as nutrients, interact with the body's genetic material.

denaturation the irreversible change in a protein's folded shape brought about by heat, acids, bases, alcohol, salts of heavy metals, or other agents.

Many well-known poisons are salts of heavy metals such as mercury and silver; these poisons denature protein strands wherever they touch them. The common first-aid antidote for swallowing a heavy-metal poison is to drink milk. The poison then acts on the protein of the milk rather than on the protein tissues of the mouth, esophagus, and stomach. Later, vomiting can be induced to expel the poison that has combined with the milk.

KEY POINTS

- Proteins can be denatured by heat, acids, bases, alcohol, the salts of heavy metals, or other agents.
- Denaturation begins the process of digesting food protein and can also destroy body proteins.

Digestion and Absorption of Dietary Protein

LO 6.2   Outline the processes of protein digestion and absorption of amino acids.

Each protein performs a special task in a particular tissue of a specific kind of animal or plant. When a person eats food proteins, whether from cereals, vegetables, beef, fish, or cheese, the body must first break them down into amino acids; only then can it rearrange them into specific human body proteins.

Protein Digestion

Other than being crushed and torn by chewing and moistened with saliva in the mouth, nothing happens to protein until it reaches the stomach. Then the action begins.

In the Stomach   Strong hydrochloric acid produced by the stomach denatures proteins in food. This acid helps uncoil the protein's tangled strands so that molecules of the stomach's protein-digesting enzyme can attack the peptide bonds. You might expect that the stomach enzyme, being a protein itself, would be denatured by the stomach's acid. Unlike most enzymes, though, the stomach enzyme functions best in an acid environment. Its job is to break *other* protein strands into smaller pieces. The stomach lining, which is also made partly of protein, is protected against attack by acid and enzymes by the coat of mucus secreted by its cells.

The whole process of digestion is an ingenious solution to a complex problem. Proteins (enzymes), activated by acid, digest proteins from food, denatured by acid. Digestion and absorption of other nutrients, such as iron, also rely on the stomach's ability to produce strong acid. The acid in the stomach is so strong (pH 1.5) that no food is acidic enough to make it stronger; for comparison, the pH of vinegar is about 3.

pH was defined in **Chapter 3** on page 80.

In the Small Intestine   By the time most proteins slip from the stomach into the small intestine, they are denatured and cleaved into smaller pieces. A few single amino acids have been released, but most of the original protein enters as long strands—polypeptides. In the small intestine, alkaline juice from the pancreas neutralizes the acid delivered by the stomach. The pH rises to about 7 (neutral), enabling the next enzyme team to accomplish the final breakdown of the strands. Protein-digesting enzymes from the pancreas and intestine continue working until almost all pieces of protein are broken into single amino acids or into strands of two or three amino acids, **dipeptides** or **tripeptides** (see Figure 6–8). Figure 6–9 summarizes the whole process of protein digestion.

Common Misconceptions   Consumers who fail to understand the basic mechanism of protein digestion are easily misled by advertisers of books and other products who urge, "Take enzyme A to help digest your food" or "Don't eat foods containing enzyme C, which will digest cells in your body." The writers of such statements fail to realize that enzymes (proteins) are digested before they are absorbed, just as all proteins are. Even the stomach's digestive enzymes are denatured and digested when

Figure 6–8

A Dipeptide and Tripeptide

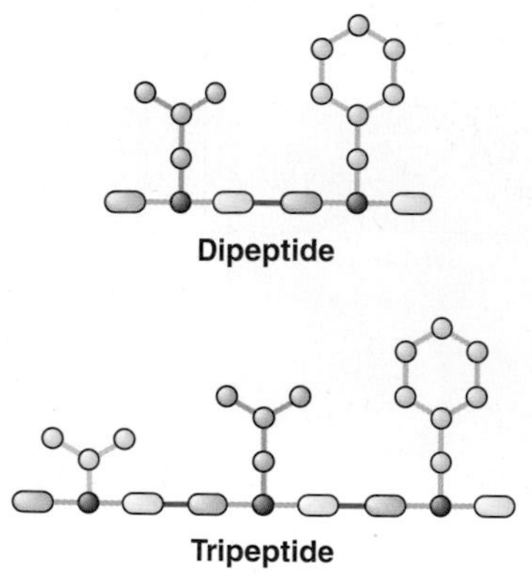

Dipeptide

Tripeptide

dipeptides (dye-PEP-tides) protein fragments that are two amino acids long (*di* means "two").

tripeptides (try-PEP-tides) protein fragments that are three amino acids long (*tri* means "three").

Chapter 6 The Proteins and Amino Acids

Figure 6–9

How Protein in Food Becomes Amino Acids in the Body

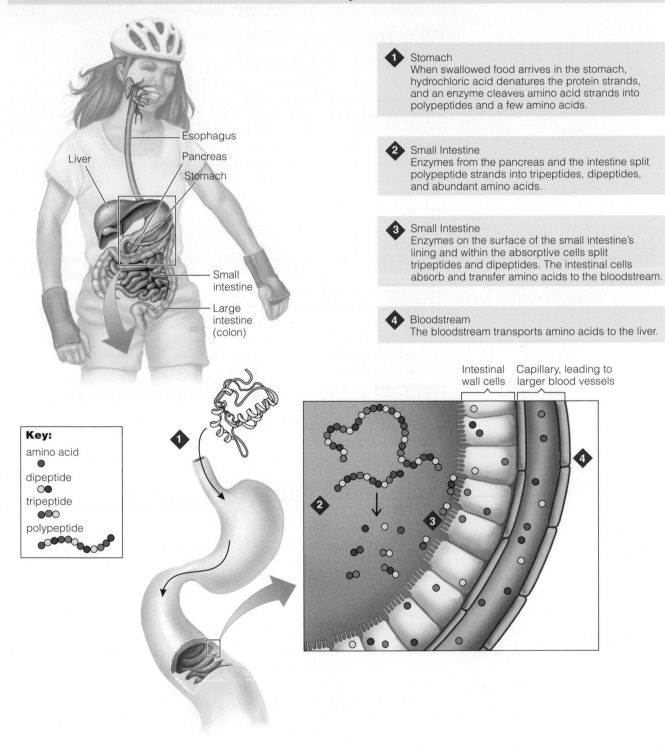

1. **Stomach**
When swallowed food arrives in the stomach, hydrochloric acid denatures the protein strands, and an enzyme cleaves amino acid strands into polypeptides and a few amino acids.

2. **Small Intestine**
Enzymes from the pancreas and the intestine split polypeptide strands into tripeptides, dipeptides, and abundant amino acids.

3. **Small Intestine**
Enzymes on the surface of the small intestine's lining and within the absorptive cells split tripeptides and dipeptides. The intestinal cells absorb and transfer amino acids to the bloodstream.

4. **Bloodstream**
The bloodstream transports amino acids to the liver.

Esophagus
Pancreas
Stomach
Liver
Small intestine
Large intestine (colon)

Intestinal wall cells   Capillary, leading to larger blood vessels

Key:
amino acid
dipeptide
tripeptide
polypeptide

their jobs are done. Similar false claims suggest that predigested proteins (amino acid supplements) are "easy to digest" and can therefore protect the digestive system from "overworking." Of course, a healthy digestive system is superbly designed to digest whole proteins with ease. In fact, it handles whole proteins better than predigested ones because it dismantles and absorbs the amino acids at rates that are optimal for the body's use.

Digestion and Absorption of Dietary Protein

- Digestion of protein involves denaturation by stomach acid and enzymatic digestion in the stomach and small intestine to amino acids, dipeptides, and tripeptides.

What Happens to Amino Acids after Protein Is Digested?

The cells all along the small intestine absorb single amino acids. As for dipeptides and tripeptides, enzymes on the cells' surfaces split most of them into single amino acids, and the cells absorb them, too. Dipeptides and tripeptides are also absorbed as-is into the cells, where they are split into amino acids and join with the others to be released into the bloodstream. A few larger peptide molecules can escape the digestive process altogether and enter the bloodstream intact. Scientists believe these larger particles may act as hormones to regulate body functions and provide the body with information about the external environment. The larger molecules may also stimulate an immune response and thus play a role in food allergy.

The cells of the small intestine possess separate sites for absorbing different types of amino acids. Chemically similar amino acids compete for the same absorption sites. Consequently, when a person ingests a large dose of any single amino acid, that amino acid may limit absorption of others of its general type. The Consumer's Guide (p. 198) cautions against taking single amino acids as supplements partly for this reason.

Once amino acids are circulating in the bloodstream, they are carried to the liver, where they may be used or released into the blood to be taken up by other cells of the body. The cells can then link the amino acids together to make proteins that they keep for their own use or liberate them into lymph or blood for other uses. When necessary, the body's cells can also use amino acids for energy.

- The cells of the small intestine complete digestion, absorb amino acids and some larger peptides, and release them into the bloodstream for use by the body's cells.

The Importance of Protein

LO 6.3   Identify the roles of proteins and amino acids in the body.

Amino acids must be continuously available to build the proteins of new tissue. The new protein may be in an embryo; in the muscles of an athlete in training; in a growing child; in new blood cells needed to replace blood lost in menstruation, hemorrhage, or surgery; in the scar tissue that heals wounds; or in new hair and nails.

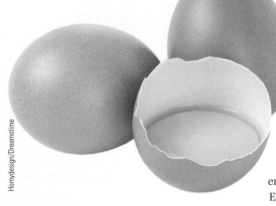

Hornydesign/Dreamstime

Less obvious is the protein that helps replace worn-out cells and internal cell structures. Each of your millions of red blood cells lives for only 3 or 4 months. Then it must be replaced by a new cell produced by the bone marrow. The millions of cells lining your intestinal tract live for only 3 days; they are constantly being shed and replaced. The cells of your skin die and rub off, and new ones grow from underneath. Nearly all cells arise, live, and die in this way, and while they are living, they constantly make and break down proteins. In addition, cells must continuously replace their own internal working proteins as old ones wear out. Amino acids conserved from these processes provide a great deal of the required raw material from which new structures are built. The entire process of breakdown, recovery, and synthesis is called **protein turnover**.

Each day, about a quarter of the body's available amino acids are irretrievably diverted to other uses, such as being used for fuel. For this reason, amino acids from food are needed each day to support the new growth and maintenance of cells and to make the working parts within them. The following sections spell out some of the critical roles that proteins play in the body.

protein turnover the continuous breakdown and synthesis of body proteins involving the recycling of amino acids.

- The body needs dietary amino acids to grow new cells and to replace old or damaged ones.

The Roles of Body Proteins

Only a sampling of the many roles proteins play can be described here, but these illustrate their versatility, uniqueness, and importance in the body. One important role was already mentioned: regulation of gene expression. Among their other roles, proteins serve as digestive enzymes, antibodies, tendons, ligaments, scars, filaments of hair, the materials of nails, and countless more. No wonder their discoverers called proteins the primary material of life.

Structure and Movement Much of the body's protein (about 40 percent) exists in muscle tissue. Specialized muscle protein structures allow the body to move. In addition, muscle proteins can release some of their amino acids, should the need for energy become dire, as in starvation. These amino acids are integral parts of the muscle structure, and their loss exacts a cost of functional protein. Other structural proteins confer shape and strength on bones, teeth, skin, tendons, cartilage, blood vessels, and other tissues. All are important to the workings of a healthy body.

Enzymes, Hormones, and Other Compounds Among proteins formed by living cells, enzymes are metabolic workhorses. An enzyme acts as a **catalyst**: it speeds up a reaction that would happen anyway, but much more slowly. Thousands of enzymes reside inside a single cell, and each one facilitates a specific chemical reaction. Figure 6–10 shows how a hypothetical enzyme works—this one synthesizes a compound from two chemical components. Other enzymes break compounds apart into two or more products or rearrange the atoms in one kind of compound to make another. A single enzyme can facilitate up to a hundred reactions in a second.

The body's **hormones** are messenger molecules, and many of them are made from amino acids. Various body glands release hormones when changes occur in the internal environment; the hormones then elicit tissue responses necessary to restore normal conditions. For example, the familiar pair of hormones, insulin and glucagon, oppose each other to maintain blood glucose levels. Both are built of amino acids. For interest, Figure 6–11 shows how many amino acids are linked in sequence to form human insulin. It also shows how certain side groups attract one another to complete the insulin molecule and make it functional.

In addition to serving as building blocks for proteins, amino acids perform other tasks in the body. For example, the amino acid tyrosine forms parts of the neurotransmitters epinephrine and norepinephrine, which relay messages throughout the nervous system.

Figure 6–10

Enzyme Action

Compounds A and B are attracted to the enzyme's active site and park there for a moment in the exact position that makes the reaction between them most likely to occur. They react by bonding together and leave the enzyme as a new compound, AB.

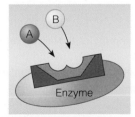

Enzyme plus two compounds A and B

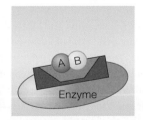

Enzyme complex with A and B

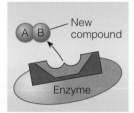

Enzyme plus new compound AB

catalyst a substance that speeds the rate of a chemical reaction without itself being permanently altered in the process. All enzymes are catalysts.

hormones chemical messengers secreted by a number of body organs in response to conditions that require regulation. Each hormone affects a specific organ or tissue and elicits a specific response. Also defined in Chapter 3.

Figure 6-11

Amino Acid Sequence of Human Insulin

This picture shows a refinement of protein structure not mentioned earlier. The amino acid cysteine (Cys) has a sulfur-containing side group. The sulfur groups on two cysteine molecules can bond together, creating a bridge between two protein strands or two parts of the same strand. Insulin contains three such bridges.

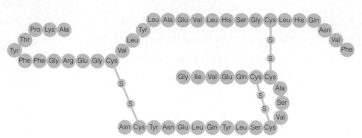

The body also uses tyrosine to make the brown pigment melanin, which gives a brown color to skin, hair, and eyes. In addition, tyrosine is converted into the thyroid hormone **thyroxine**, which regulates the body's metabolism. Another amino acid, tryptophan, serves as starting material for the neurotransmitter **serotonin** and the vitamin niacin.

Antibodies   Of all the proteins in living organisms, the **antibodies** best demonstrate that proteins are specific to one organism. Antibodies distinguish foreign particles (usually proteins) from all the proteins that belong in "their" body. When they recognize an intruder, they mark it as a target for attack. The foreign protein may be part of a bacterium, a virus, or a toxin, or it may be present in a food that causes an allergic reaction.

Each antibody is designed to help destroy one specific invader. An antibody active against one strain of influenza is of no help to a person ill with another strain. Once the body has learned how to make a particular antibody, it remembers. The next time the body encounters that same invader, it destroys the invader even more rapidly. In other words, the body develops **immunity** to the invader. This molecular memory underlies the principle of immunizations, injections of drugs made from destroyed and inactivated microbes or their products that activate the body's immune defenses. Some immunities are lifelong; others, such as that to tetanus, must be "boosted" at intervals.

Transport System   A large group of proteins specializes in transporting other substances, such as lipids, vitamins, minerals, and oxygen, around the body. To do their jobs, such substances must travel within the bloodstream and into and out of cells. Two familiar examples are the protein hemoglobin within the red blood cells, which carries oxygen from the lungs to the tissues, and the lipoproteins, which transport lipids in the watery blood.

Fluid and Electrolyte Balance   Proteins help maintain the **fluid and electrolyte balance** by regulating the quantities of fluids in body compartments. To remain alive, a cell must contain a constant volume of internal fluid. Too much fluid would rupture the cell; too little would shrink it, making it unable to function. Although water can diffuse freely into and out of cells, proteins cannot, and proteins attract water. In addition, proteins mounted on cell membranes act as pumps, constantly adjusting the cells' fluid and electrolyte balance.

By maintaining stores of internal proteins and electrolytes, cells retain the fluid they need. In a similar way, fluid is kept inside the blood vessels by proteins too large to move freely across the capillary walls. The proteins attract water, keeping it within the vessels, and preventing it from freely flowing into the spaces between the cells. Should any part of this system begin to fail, too much fluid will soon collect in the spaces between the cells of tissues, causing **edema**, the condition shown in Figure 6–12.

Not only is the quantity of the body fluids vital to life, but their composition is also. Cellular pumps control this composition by continuously transferring substances into

thyroxine (thigh-ROX-in) a principal peptide hormone of the thyroid gland that regulates the body's rate of energy use.

serotonin (SARE-oh-TONE-in) a compound related in structure to (and synthesized from) the amino acid tryptophan. It serves as one of the brain's principal neurotransmitters.

antibodies (AN-te-bod-ees) large proteins of the blood, produced by the immune system in response to an invasion of the body by foreign substances (antigens). Antibodies combine with and inactivate the antigens.

immunity protection from or resistance to a disease or infection by the development of antibodies and by the actions of cells and tissues in response to a threat.

fluid and electrolyte balance the proper distribution of fluid and dissolved particles (electrolytes) among body compartments (see also Chapter 8).

edema (eh-DEEM-uh) swelling of body tissue caused by leakage of fluid from the blood vessels; seen in protein deficiency (among other conditions).

Chapter 6 The Proteins and Amino Acids

Figure 6–12

Edema

Edema results when body tissues fail to control the movement of water.

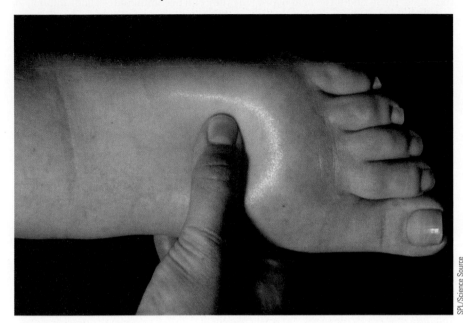

and out of cells (see Figure 6–13). For example, sodium is concentrated outside the cells, and potassium is concentrated inside. A disturbance of this balance can impair the action of the heart, lungs, and brain, triggering a major medical emergency. Cell proteins avert such a disaster by controlling the movement of fluids and electrolytes.

Acid-Base Balance   Normal processes of the body continually produce **acids** and their opposite, **bases**, that must be carried by the blood to the organs of excretion. The blood must do this without allowing its own **acid-base balance** to be affected. This feat is another trick of the blood proteins, which act as **buffers** to maintain the blood's normal pH. The protein buffers pick up hydrogens (acid) when there are too many in the bloodstream and release them again when there are too few. The secret is that negatively charged side chains of amino acids can accommodate additional hydrogens, which are positively charged.

acids   compounds that release hydrogens in a watery solution.

bases   compounds that accept hydrogens from solutions.

acid-base balance   equilibrium between acid and base concentrations in the body fluids.

buffers   compounds that help keep a solution's acidity or alkalinity constant.

Figure 6–13

Proteins Transport Substances into and out of Cells

A transport protein within the cell membrane acts as a sort of two-door passageway—substances enter on one side and are released on the other, but the protein never leaves the membrane. The protein differs from a simple passageway in that it actively escorts the substances in and out of cells. Therefore, this form of transport is often called active transport.

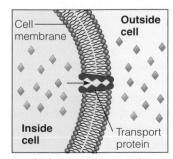
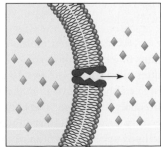
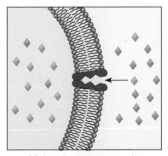
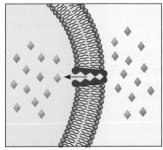

| Molecule enters protein from inside cell. | Protein changes shape; molecule exits protein outside the cell. | Molecule enters protein from outside cell. | Molecule exits protein; proper balance restored. |

Table 6–2

Summary of Protein Functions

- *Acid-base balance.* Proteins help maintain the acid-base balance of various body fluids by acting as buffers.
- *Antibodies.* Proteins form the immune system molecules that fight diseases.
- *Blood clotting.* Proteins provide the netting on which blood clots are built.
- *Energy and glucose.* Proteins provide some fuel for the body's energy needs.
- *Enzymes.* Proteins facilitate needed chemical reactions.
- *Fluid and electrolyte balance.* Proteins help to maintain the water and mineral composition of various body fluids.
- *Gene expression.* Proteins associate and interact with DNA, regulating gene expression.
- *Hormones.* Some hormones are proteins or are made from amino acids.
- *Structure and movement.* Proteins form integral parts of most body tissues and confer shape and strength on bones, skin, tendons, and other tissues. Structural proteins of muscles execute body movement.
- *Transport.* Proteins help transport needed substances, such as lipids, minerals, and oxygen, around the body.

acidosis (acid-DOH-sis) the condition of excess acid in the blood, indicated by a below-normal pH (*osis* means "too much").

alkalosis (al-kah-LOH-sis) the condition of excess base in the blood, indicated by an above-normal blood pH (*alka* means "base"; *osis* means "too much").

urea (yoo-REE-uh) the principal nitrogen-excretion product of protein metabolism; generated mostly by removal of amine groups from unneeded amino acids or from amino acids being sacrificed for energy.

Blood pH is one of the most rigidly controlled conditions in the body. If blood pH changes too much, **acidosis** or the opposite basic condition, **alkalosis**, can cause coma or death. These conditions constitute medical emergencies because of their effects on proteins. When the proteins' buffering capacity is filled—that is, when they have taken on all the acid hydrogens they can accommodate—additional acid pulls them out of shape, denaturing them and disrupting many body processes.

Blood Clotting   To prevent dangerous blood loss, special blood proteins respond to an injury by clotting the blood. In an amazing series of chemical events, these proteins form a stringy net that traps blood cells to form a clot. The clot acts as a plug to stem blood flow from the wound. Later, as the wound heals, the protein collagen finishes the job by replacing the clot with scar tissue.

The final function of protein, providing energy, depends on some metabolic adjustments, as described in the next section. Table 6–2 provides a summary of the functions of proteins in the body.

KEY POINT

- Proteins help regulate gene expression; provide structure and movement; serve as enzymes, hormones, and antibodies; provide molecular transport; help regulate fluid and electrolyte balance; buffer the blood; contribute to blood clotting; and provide energy.

Providing Energy and Glucose

Only protein can perform all the functions just described, but protein will be surrendered to provide energy if need be. Under conditions of inadequate carbohydrate or energy, protein breakdown speeds up.

Amino Acids to Glucose   The body must have energy to live from moment to moment, so obtaining that energy is a top priority. Not only can amino acids supply energy, but also many of them can be converted to glucose, as fatty acids can never be. Thus, if the need arises, protein can help to maintain a steady blood glucose level and help meet the glucose need of the brain.

When amino acids are degraded for energy or converted into glucose, their nitrogen-containing amine groups are stripped off and used elsewhere or are incorporated by the liver into **urea** and sent to the kidneys for excretion in the urine. The fragments that remain are composed of carbon, hydrogen, and oxygen, as are carbohydrate and fat, and can be used to build glucose or fatty acids or can be metabolized like them.

Drawing Amino Acids from Tissues   Glucose is stored as glycogen and fat as triglycerides, but no specialized storage compound exists for protein. Body protein is present only as the active working molecular and structural components of body tissues. When protein-sparing energy from carbohydrate and fat is lacking and the need becomes urgent, as in starvation, prolonged fasting, or severe calorie restriction, the body must dismantle some of its tissue proteins to obtain amino acids for building the most essential proteins and for energy. Each protein is taken in its own time: first, small proteins from the blood, then proteins from the muscles. The body guards the structural proteins of the heart and other organs until forced, by dire need, to relinquish them. Thus, energy deficiency (starvation) always incurs wasting of lean body tissue as well as loss of fat.

Using Excess Amino Acids   When amino acids are oversupplied, the body cannot store them. It has no choice but to remove and excrete their amine groups and then use the residues in one of three ways: to meet immediate energy needs, to make glucose for storage as glycogen, or to make fat for energy storage. The body readily converts amino acids to glucose. The body also possesses enzymes to convert amino acids into fatty acids. An indirect contribution of amino acids to fat stores also exists—the body speeds up its use of excess amino acids for fuel, burning them instead of fat, making fat more abundantly available for storage in the fat tissue.

Chapter 6 The Proteins and Amino Acids

Figure 6–14
Three Different Energy Sources

Carbohydrate offers energy; fat offers concentrated energy; and protein, if necessary, can offer energy plus nitrogen. The compounds at the left yield the 2-carbon fragments shown at the right. These fragments oxidize quickly in the presence of oxygen to yield carbon dioxide, water, and energy.

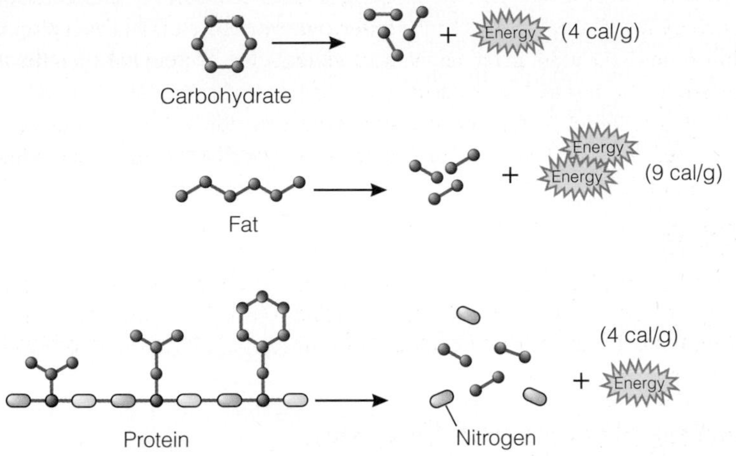

The similarities and differences of the three energy-yielding nutrients should now be clear. Carbohydrate offers energy; fat offers concentrated energy; and protein can offer energy plus nitrogen (see Figure 6–14).

KEY POINTS
- Amino acids can be used as fuel or converted to glucose or fat.
- No storage form of protein exists in the body.

The Fate of an Amino Acid

To review the body's handling of amino acids, let us follow the fate of an amino acid that was originally part of a protein-containing food. When the amino acid arrives in a cell, it can be used in one of several ways, depending on the cell's needs at the time:

- The amino acid can be used as-is to build part of a growing protein.
- The amino acid can be altered somewhat to make another needed compound, such as the vitamin niacin.
- The cell can dismantle the amino acid to use its amine group to build a different amino acid. The remainder can be used for fuel or, if fuel is abundant, converted to glucose or fat.

When a cell is starved for energy and has no glucose or fatty acids, it strips the amino acid of its amine group (the nitrogen part) and uses the remainder of its structure for energy. The amine group is excreted from the cell and then from the body in the urine. In a cell that has a surplus of energy and amino acids, the cell takes the amino acid apart, excretes the amine group, and uses the rest to meet immediate energy needs or converts it to glucose or fat for storage.

When not used to build protein or make other nitrogen-containing compounds, amino acids are "wasted" in a sense. This wasting occurs under any of four conditions:

1. When the body lacks energy from other sources.
2. When the diet supplies more protein than the body needs.

Evaluating Protein and Amino Acid Supplements

Nature provides protein abundantly in foods, but many people become convinced that they need extra protein and amino acids from supplements. Sorting truth from wishful thinking in advertisements can be tricky: "Take this protein supplement to build muscle," "This one will help you lose weight," "Take an amino acid to get to sleep, grow strong fingernails, cure herpes, build immunity . . . " Can these products really do these things?

Protein Powders

Dietary protein is needed to build muscle protein, so many athletes take protein powders in hopes of building bigger muscles. It's true that protein eaten soon after lifting weights or other exertion increases protein synthesis for a while (Chapter 10 describes this effect), but this detail of metabolism does not improve athletic ability. Protein supplements are not "muscles in a bottle," as they are often advertised—physical work is required to build muscle.

What a boon it would be to overweight people if they could add the right protein or amino acids to a milkshake and lose weight effortlessly, but both evidence and common sense oppose this idea. Protein in a meal contributes to satiety, but "protein drinks" and shakes often add many calories to a day's intake.[1]* In addition, any excess nitrogen, including nitrogen from a protein supplement, must be metabolized and excreted. This places a burden on the kidneys, particularly if they are weakened by disease.

gelatin a protein product of collagen breakdown. In foods, it confers structure, such as in gelatin desserts; in nutrition, it supplies low-quality protein that lacks certain essential amino acids.

Reference notes are in Appendix F.

Bone Broth and Collagen

Bone broth is a long-simmered **gelatin**-rich soup, also sold in powdered form, and marketed with comforting images of home. Gelatin arises when collagen, a protein present in bones, dissolves into the broth during long, moist cooking (despite claims, broth contains no actual collagen). Because collagen in human skin and joints diminishes with age, bone broth advocates claim that it restores youthful-looking skin and pain-free joints, but consuming collagen or gelatin cannot do these things. Nor can it make hair glossy or reduce "cellulite." As a protein source, gelatin is low in quality—it lacks many essential amino acids (a later section comes back to protein quality).

Many people try to treat soft, dry, weak, easily breakable fingernails with collagen or gelatin supplements but this doesn't work, either. Made largely of protein, nails depend on sulfur bonds between amino acids for flexible strength, fatty acids for water resistance, and sufficient water for proper hydration. In addition, the living tissues that form nails need many minerals and vitamins to put these materials into place. Nails, hair, and skin all depend upon a nutritious diet to look their best, not protein supplements.

Amino Acids

Athletes and others often take supplements of branched-chain amino acids (valine, leucine, and isoleucine) in hopes of building muscle or losing fat. Like protein, leucine stimulates muscle protein synthesis following exercise, but ordinary protein-rich foods do the same thing. Some evidence suggests that supplemental branched-chain amino acids, taken in the context of a high-fat diet, may cause a buildup of metabolic products that disturbs normal energy

systems, particularly concerning insulin action.[2] Theoretically, such disturbances could worsen chronic diseases, such as diabetes, in people who take the supplements and eat a typical high-fat U.S. diet.

In two other cases, claims for single amino acid supplements have led to widespread use—lysine to prevent or relieve the infections that cause herpes cold sores on the mouth or genital organs and tryptophan to relieve depression and insomnia. Research has not determined that lysine suppresses herpes infections, but it appears safe in doses up to 3 grams per day.[3] Tryptophan may be effective for inducing drowsiness, but daily large doses can have side effects, such as temporary nausea or skin problems. People taking antidepressant drugs should consult with their physicians before taking tryptophan supplements.

Food Is Often Best

The body handles whole proteins best. It breaks them into manageable pieces (dipeptides and tripeptides) and then splits these, a few at a time, simultaneously releasing them into the blood. This slow, bit-by-bit assimilation is ideal because groups of chemically similar amino acids compete for the carriers that absorb them into the blood. An excess of one amino acid can tie up a carrier and interfere with the absorption of another, creating a temporary imbalance.

Within the cells' nuclei, amino acids play key roles in gene regulation. Amino acid imbalances may alter these processes in unpredictable ways. In mice, feeding excess methionine causes the buildup of an amino acid associated with heart disease (homocysteine) and worsens heart and liver disease.[4] No one knows if the same is true in people.

In cases of disease or malnutrition, a registered clinical dietitian may employ a special protein or amino acid supplement.[5] Not every patient is a candidate for such therapy, though, because the supplements may stimulate inflammation, which can worsen the condition, or draw water into the digestive tract, which causes diarrhea. Protein supplements can also worsen kidney disease or interfere with the actions of certain medications, allowing diseases to advance unchecked.

A lack of research prevents the DRI committee from setting Tolerable Upper Intake Levels for amino acids.[6] Therefore, no level of amino acid supplementation can be assumed safe. The people most likely to be harmed are listed in Table 6–3. Take heed: much is still unknown, and those who take amino acid supplements cannot be certain of safety or effectiveness, despite convincing marketing materials.

Table 6–3

People Most Likely to Be Harmed by Amino Acid Supplements

Growth or altered metabolism makes these people especially likely to be harmed by self-prescribed amino acid supplements:

- All women of childbearing age, especially those who are pregnant or lactating
- Infants, children, and adolescents
- Elderly people
- People with inborn errors of metabolism that affect their bodies' handling of amino acids
- Smokers
- People on low-protein diets
- People with chronic or acute mental or physical illnesses

Moving Ahead

Even with all that we've learned from science, it is hard to improve on nature. In almost every case, the complex balance of amino acids and other nutrients found together in whole foods is best for nutrition. Keep it safe and simple: select a variety of protein-rich foods that are low in saturated fat each day, and reject unnecessary protein and amino acid supplements.

Review Questions*

1. Commercial shakes and energy bars have proven to be the best protein sources to support weight-loss efforts. **T F**

2. Gelatin supplements cannot strengthen fingernails or restore a youthful look to the skin. **T F**

3. In high doses, tryptophan can improve nausea and skin disorders. **T F**

*Answers to Consumer's Guide review questions are found in Appendix G.

3. When the body has too much of any single amino acid—for example, from a supplement.

4. When the diet supplies protein of low quality, with too few essential amino acids, as described in the next section.

To prevent the wasting of dietary protein and permit the synthesis of needed body protein, the dietary protein must be of adequate quality: it must supply all essential amino acids in the proper amounts. It must also be accompanied by enough energy-yielding carbohydrate and fat to permit the dietary protein to be used as such.

To review, amino acids in a cell can be:

- Used to build protein.
- Converted to other amino acids or small nitrogen-containing compounds.

Stripped of their nitrogen, amino acids can be:

- Burned as fuel.
- Converted to glucose or fat.

KEY POINTS

- Amino acids can be metabolized to protein, nitrogen plus energy, glucose, or fat.
- Amino acids will be metabolized to protein only if sufficient energy is present from other sources.
- When energy is lacking, the nitrogen part is removed from each amino acid, and the resulting fragment is oxidized for energy.

The DRI for protein (adult) = 0.8 g/kg. To find your protein recommendation:

1. Look up the healthy weight for a person of your height (back of the book, p. E). If your weight falls within the range, use it; if outside the range, use the midpoint of the range.
2. Convert pounds to kilograms (by dividing pounds by 2.2).
3. Multiply kilograms by 0.8 to find total grams of protein recommended.

For example:

Weight = 130 lb
130 lb ÷ 2.2 = 59 kg
59 kg × 0.8 = 47 g

Table 6–4

Protein Intake Recommendations for Healthy Adults

DRI[a]
■ 0.8 g protein/kg body weight/day.
■ Women: 46 g/day; men: 56 g/day.
■ Acceptable intake range: 10 to 35% of calories from protein.

Dietary Guidelines for Americans 2015–2020
■ A healthy eating pattern includes a variety of protein foods, including seafood, lean meats and poultry, eggs, legumes (peas and beans), and nuts, seeds, and soy products.

[a] Protein recommendations for infants, children, and pregnant and lactating women are higher; see the back of the book, page A.

Food Protein: Need and Quality

LO 6.4   List the factors that determine the daily protein needs of an individual.

A person's need for and use of dietary protein depend on many factors. To know whether, say, 60 grams of protein is enough to meet a person's daily needs, one must consider the effects of factors discussed in this section, some pertaining to the body and some to the nature of the protein.

How Much Protein Do People Need?

The DRI value for protein intake is designed to cover the need to replace protein-containing tissue that healthy adults break down every day. Therefore, it depends on body size: larger people have a higher protein need. For adults of healthy body weight, the DRI is set at 0.8 grams for each kilogram (or 2.2 pounds) of body weight (see back of the book, p. A). The minimum amount is set at 10 percent of total calories, although some evidence suggests that certain groups of people, such as the elderly, may need more than this minimum for optimal health.[4] Athletes, too, may need slightly more protein—1.2 to 1.7 grams per kilogram per day—but even this amount is provided by a well-chosen eating pattern with enough energy for athletes (see Chapter 10).

For infants and growing children, the protein recommendation, like all nutrient recommendations, is higher per unit of body weight. The DRI committee set an upper limit for protein intake of no more than 35 percent of total calories, an amount significantly higher than average intakes. The margin provides a method for determining your own protein need, and Table 6–4 reviews recommendations for protein intake. The following factors also modify protein needs.

The Body's Health   Malnutrition or infection may greatly increase the need for protein while making it hard to eat even normal amounts of food. In malnutrition, secretion of digestive enzymes slows as the tract's lining degenerates, impairing protein digestion and absorption. When infection is present, extra protein is needed for enhanced immune functions.

Other Nutrients and Energy   The need for ample energy, carbohydrate, and fat has already been emphasized. To be used efficiently by the cells, dietary protein must also be accompanied by the full array of vitamins and minerals.

Protein Quality   The remaining factor, protein quality, helps determine how well a diet supports the growth of children and the health of adults. Protein quality becomes crucial for people in areas where food is scarce, as described in a later section.

The DRI for protein assumes a normal mixed diet—that is, an eating pattern that provides sufficient nutrients and protein from a combination of animal and plant sources. Because not all proteins are used with 100 percent efficiency, the recommendation is generous. Many healthy people can consume less than the recommended amount and still meet their bodies' protein needs.

KEY POINTS

- The protein intake recommendation depends on size and stage of growth.
- The DRI for adults is 0.8 grams of protein per kilogram of body weight.
- Factors concerning both the body and food sources modify an individual's protein need.

Nitrogen Balance

Underlying the protein recommendation are **nitrogen balance** studies, which compare nitrogen lost by excretion with nitrogen eaten in food. In healthy adults,

nitrogen balance   the amount of nitrogen consumed compared with the amount excreted in a given time period.

Figure 6–15

Nitrogen Balance

● Nitrogen in   ● Nitrogen out

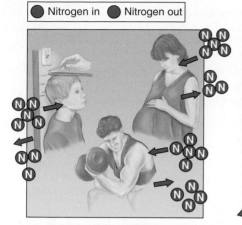

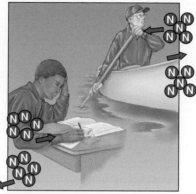

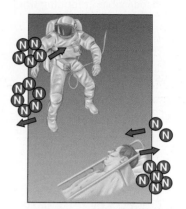

Positive Nitrogen Balance
These people—a growing child,
a person building muscle, and
a pregnant woman—all retain more
nitrogen than they excrete each day.

Nitrogen Equilibrium
These people—a healthy college
student and a young retiree—are in
nitrogen equilibrium.

Negative Nitrogen Balance
These people—an astronaut
and a surgery patient—lose
more nitrogen than they
take in.

nitrogen-in (consumed) must equal nitrogen-out (excreted). Scientists measure the body's daily nitrogen losses in urine, feces, sweat, and skin under controlled conditions and then estimate the amount of protein needed to replace these losses.[‡]

Under normal circumstances, healthy adults are in nitrogen equilibrium, or zero balance; that is, they have the same amount of total protein in their bodies at all times. When nitrogen-in exceeds nitrogen-out, people are said to be in positive nitrogen balance; somewhere in their bodies more proteins are being built than are being broken down and lost. When nitrogen-in is less than nitrogen-out, people are said to be in negative nitrogen balance; they are losing protein. Figure 6–15 illustrates these different states.

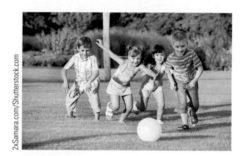

Growing children end each day with more bone, blood, muscle, and skin cells than they had at the beginning of the day.

Positive Nitrogen Balance   Growing children add new blood, bone, and muscle cells to their bodies every day, so children have more protein, and therefore more nitrogen, in their bodies at the end of each day than they had at the beginning. A growing child is therefore in positive nitrogen balance. Similarly, when a woman is pregnant, she must be in positive nitrogen balance until after the birth, when she once again reaches equilibrium.

Negative Nitrogen Balance   Negative nitrogen balance occurs when muscle or other protein tissue is broken down and lost: nitrogen excretion increases. Illness or injury triggers the release of powerful messengers that signal the body to break down some of the less vital proteins, such as those of the blood, skin, and muscle.[§] This action floods the blood with amino acids, which are then stripped of their nitrogen and used for energy to fuel the body's defenses and fight the illness. The result is greater nitrogen excretion and negative nitrogen balance. Astronauts, too, experience negative nitrogen balance. In the stress of space flight and with no need to support the body's weight against gravity, the astronauts' muscles waste and weaken. To minimize the inevitable loss of muscle tissue, the astronauts must do special exercises in space.

[‡] The average protein is 16 percent nitrogen by weight; that is, each 100 grams of protein contain 16 grams of nitrogen. Scientists can estimate the amount of protein in a sample of food, body tissue, or other material by multiplying the weight of the nitrogen in it by 6.25.

[§] The messengers are cytokines.

Figure 6-16

Limiting Amino Acids

Just as each letter of the alphabet is indispensable in forming whole words, each amino acid must be available to build finished proteins. If any essential amino acids are missing, their absence limits protein production.

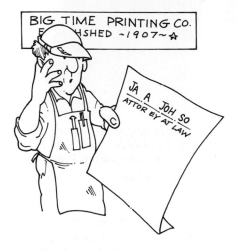

high-quality proteins dietary proteins containing all the essential amino acids in relatively the same amounts that human beings require. They may also contain nonessential amino acids.

limiting amino acid an essential amino acid that is present in dietary protein in an insufficient amount, thereby limiting the body's ability to build protein.

complementary proteins two or more proteins whose amino acid assortments complement each other in such a way that the essential amino acids missing from one are supplied by the other.

KEY POINT

- Protein recommendations are based on nitrogen balance studies, which compare nitrogen excreted from the body with nitrogen ingested in food.

Protein Quality

Put simply, **high-quality proteins** provide enough of all the essential amino acids needed by the body to create its own working proteins, whereas low-quality proteins don't. Two factors influence a protein's quality: its amino acid composition and its digestibility.

To make their required proteins, the cells need the full array of amino acids, including the essential amino acids. (Figure 6–16 takes a playful look at this concept.) If a nonessential amino acid (that is, one the cells can make) is unavailable from food, the cells synthesize it and continue attaching amino acids to the protein strands being manufactured. If the diet fails to provide enough of an essential amino acid (one the cells cannot make), the cells begin to adjust their activities. The cells:

- Break down more internal proteins to liberate the needed essential amino acid, and
- Limit their synthesis of proteins to conserve the essential amino acid.

As the deprivation continues, tissues make one adjustment after another in the effort to survive.

Limiting Amino Acids   The measures just described help the cells to channel the available **limiting amino acid** to its highest-priority use: making new proteins. Even so, the normally fast rate of protein synthesis slows to a crawl as cells make do with the proteins on hand. When the limiting amino acid once again becomes available in abundance, the cells resume their normal protein-related activities. If the shortage becomes chronic, however, the cells begin to break down their protein-making machinery. Consequently, when protein intakes become adequate again, protein synthesis lags behind until the needed machinery can be rebuilt. Meanwhile, the cells function less and less effectively as their proteins become depleted and are only partially replaced.

Thus, a diet that is short in any of the essential amino acids limits protein synthesis. An earlier analogy likened amino acids to letters of the alphabet. To be meaningful, words must contain all the right letters. For example, a print shop that has no letter "N" cannot make personalized stationery for Jana Johnson. No matter how many Js, As, Os, Hs, and Ss are in the printer's possession, the printer cannot use them to replace the missing Ns. Likewise, in building a protein molecule, no amino acid can fill another's spot. If a cell that is building a protein cannot find a needed amino acid, synthesis stops, and the partial protein is released.

Partially completed proteins are not held for completion at a later time when the diet may improve. Rather, they are dismantled, and the component amino acids are returned to the circulation to be made available to other cells. If they are not soon inserted into protein, their amine groups are removed and excreted, and the residues are used for other purposes. The need that prompted the call for that particular protein will simply not be met.

Complementary Proteins   It follows that, if a person does not consume all the essential amino acids in proportion to the body's needs, the body's pools of essential amino acids will dwindle until body organs are compromised. Consuming the essential amino acids presents no problem to people who regularly eat protein foods containing ample amounts of all of the essential amino acids, such as meat, fish, poultry, cheese, eggs, milk, and most soybean products.

An equally sound choice is to eat a variety of protein foods from plants so that amino acids that are low in some foods will be supplied by the others. The combination of such protein-rich foods yields **complementary proteins** (see Figure 6–17), or proteins containing all the essential amino acids in amounts sufficient to support health. This concept, often employed by vegetarians, is illustrated in Figure 6–18.

Figure 6–17

Complementary Protein Combinations

Healthful foods like these contribute substantial protein (42 grams total) to this day's meals without meat. Additional servings of nutritious foods, such as milk, bread, and eggs, can easily supply the remainder of the day's need for protein (14 additional grams for men and 4 for women).

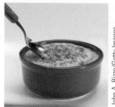
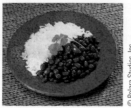
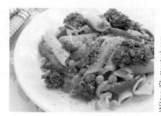

¾ c oatmeal =	5 g
Protein total	5 g

1 c rice	=	4 g
1 c beans	=	16 g
Protein total		20 g

1½ c pasta	= 11 g
1 c vegetables	= 2 g
2 tbs Parmesan cheese =	4 g
Protein total	17 g

The figure demonstrates that the amino acids of **legumes** and grains balance each other to provide all the needed amino acids. The complementary proteins need not be eaten together, so long as the day's meals supply all of them, along with sufficient energy and enough total protein from a variety of sources.

Protein Digestibility   In measuring a protein's quality, digestibility is also important. Simple measures of the total protein in foods are not useful by themselves—even animal hair and hooves would receive a top score by those measures alone. They are made of protein, but the protein is not in a form that people can use.

The digestibility of protein varies from food to food and bears profoundly on protein quality. The protein of oats, for example, is less digestible than that of eggs. In general, proteins from animal sources, such as chicken, beef, and pork, are most easily digested and absorbed (more than 90 percent). Those from legumes are next (about 80 to 90 percent). Those from grains and other plant foods vary (from 70 to 90 percent). Cooking with moist heat improves protein digestibility, as illustrated in Figure 6–19, whereas dry heat methods can impair it.

Figure 6–18

How Complementary Proteins Work Together

Legumes provide plenty of the amino acids isoleucine (Ile) and lysine (Lys) but fall short in methionine (Met) and tryptophan (Trp). Grains have the opposite strengths and weaknesses, making them a perfect match for legumes.

	Ile	Lys	Met	Trp
Legumes	✓	✓		
Grains			✓	✓
Together	✓	✓	✓	✓

Figure 6–19

Cooking Method Affects Protein Digestibility

Cooking with moist heat improves protein digestibility, whereas frying makes protein harder to digest.

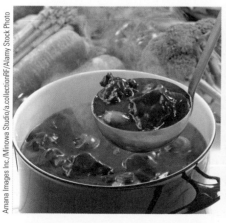
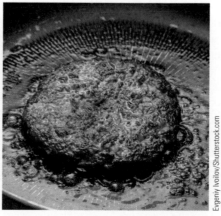

legumes (leg-GOOMS, LEG-yooms) plants of the bean, pea, and lentil family that have roots with nodules containing special bacteria. These bacteria can trap nitrogen from the air in the soil and convert it into a form that becomes part of the plant's seeds. The seeds are rich in protein compared with those of most other plant foods. Also defined in Chapter 1.

■ Digestibility of protein varies from food to food, and cooking can improve or impair it.

Perspective on Protein Quality Concern about the quality of individual food proteins is of only theoretical interest in settings where food is abundant. Healthy adults in these places would find it next to impossible *not* to meet their protein needs, even if they were to eat no meat, fish, poultry, eggs, or cheese products at all. Even healthy vegetarians need not pay attention to balancing amino acids so long as they follow an eating pattern that is varied, nutritious, and adequate in energy and other nutrients—not made up of, say, just cookies, crackers, potato chips, and juices.[5] Protein sufficiency follows effortlessly behind a balanced, nutritious eating pattern.

For people in areas where food sources are less reliable, protein quality can make the difference between health and disease. When food energy is restricted, where malnutrition is widespread, or when the variety of available foods is severely limited (where a single low-protein food, such as **fufu** made from cassava root,** provides 90 percent of the calories), the primary food source of protein must be checked because its quality is crucial.

KEY POINTS

■ A protein's amino acid assortment greatly influences its usefulness to the body.
■ Low-quality food proteins lack essential amino acids and so can be used to build body structures only if the missing amino acids are supplied by other sources.
■ The more severely food supplies are limited, the more important protein quality becomes.

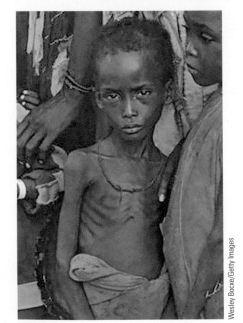

Wesley Bocxe/Getty Images

Malnutrition: too little food causes deficiencies of protein and many other nutrients. See Chapter 15.

fufu a low-protein staple food that provides abundant starch energy to many of the world's people; fufu is made by pounding or grinding root vegetables or refined grains and cooking them to a smooth, semisolid consistency.

Protein Deficiency and Excess

LO 6.5 List the potential health problems that are caused by eating patterns that are either too low or too high in protein.

When diets lack sufficient protein from food or sufficient amounts of any of the essential amino acids, symptoms of malnutrition appear. Health effects of protein excess are less well established, but high-protein diets, and particularly high-meat diets, have been implicated in several chronic diseases (see the Controversy section). Evidence is currently insufficient to establish a Tolerable Upper Intake Level for protein, but both deficiencies and excesses are of concern.

What Happens When People Consume Too Little Protein?

In protein deficiency, when the diet supplies too little protein or lacks a specific essential amino acid relative to the others (a limiting amino acid), the body slows its synthesis of proteins while increasing its breakdown of body tissue protein to liberate the amino acids it needs to build other proteins of more critical importance. Without its most critical proteins, many of the body's life-sustaining activities would come to a halt. The consequences of protein deficiency include slow growth in children, impaired brain and kidney functions, weakened immune defenses, and impaired nutrient absorption from the digestive tract. These conditions often occur in starvation wherein the diet lacks not only protein, but energy, vitamins, and minerals as

---

**Cassava is also called *manioc* or *yucca*.

well. The severe malnutrition of starvation and its clinical manifestations are a focus of Chapter 15's discussion of world hunger.

Is It Possible to Consume Too Much Protein?

Overconsumption of protein-rich foods offers no benefits and may pose a health risk for people with compromised kidney function. This section explores current protein intakes and considers the potential for harm from excesses.

How Much Protein Do People Take In?   Most people suspect that Americans eat far too much protein. In fact, the average protein intake for U.S. men is about 16 percent of total calories, with women consuming slightly less, or 15.5 percent.[6] These amounts are well within the DRI suggested range of between 10 and 35 percent of calories. Stated another way, the DRI range for protein intake in a 2,000-calorie diet is 50 to 175 grams; the average U.S. daily intake of protein amounts to about 78 grams.

Weight-Loss Dieting   Some popular weight-loss diet advice suggests 65 percent or more of calories from protein as a way to lose weight. True, meeting protein recommendations during weight loss is critical for preserving the body's working lean tissues, such as liver and muscles. Also, protein foods may help control the appetite, and may cost some extra energy for their metabolism.[7] However, as Chapter 9 explains, it is controlling calorie intake, not changing the proportions of energy nutrients in the diet, that brings about long-term weight loss.

Protein Sources in Heart Disease   Protein itself is not known to contribute to heart disease and mortality, but some of its food sources may do so. Selecting too many animal-derived protein-rich foods, such as fatty red meats, processed meats, and fat-containing milk products, adds a burden of saturated fat to the diet and crowds out fruit, vegetables, legumes, nuts, and whole grains. Consequently, it is not surprising that people who habitually take in a great deal of animal protein, and particularly processed meats such as lunchmeats and hot dogs, have higher body weights and greater risks of chronic diseases than those who take in less.[8] The Controversy section explores how substituting vegetable protein for at least some of the animal protein in the diet may improve risk factors for chronic diseases and mortality.

Kidney Disease   Animals fed experimentally on high-protein diets often develop enlarged kidneys or livers. In human beings, a high-protein diet increases the kidneys' workload, but research is insufficient to say whether this alone can damage healthy kidneys or cause kidney disease.[9] In people with kidney stones or other kidney diseases, however, a high-protein diet may speed the kidneys' decline.[10] For people with established kidney problems, a somewhat lower protein intake often improves the symptoms of their disease.[11] The challenge is to provide enough protein to support the body's health, but not more than the damaged kidneys can handle.

Cancer   The risk of cancer does not appear to increase with greater protein intakes. However, eating a diet high in red meats and **processed meats** correlates with certain cancers, particularly colon cancer.[12] Being overweight, being physically inactive, smoking, and drinking alcohol also raise cancer risks significantly. In contrast, people who eat just three servings of protein-rich legumes each week may lower their cancer risks. Chapter 11 discusses the known links between diet and cancer.

processed meats a general term for meat products preserved by smoking, curing, salting, or adding chemical preservatives—for example, ham, bacon, jerky, hot dogs (including chicken and turkey), luncheon meats, salami and other sausages, SPAM, and Vienna sausages.

Is a Gluten-Free Diet Best for Health?

Gluten, a protein that forms in grain foods, is best known for providing a pleasing stretchy texture to yeast breads. It also provides bulk and texture to many other foods made from wheat, triticale, barley, rye, and related grains.

Celiac Disease In people with **celiac disease**, gluten triggers an abnormal immune response that inflames the small intestine and erodes the intestinal villi, severely limiting nutrient absorption. The result is a lifelong battle against extreme weight loss accompanied by deficiencies of vitamins, minerals, essential fatty acids, and, in fact, all nutrients.[13] Symptoms often include chronic diarrhea or constipation, vomiting, bloating, and pain, or a long list of disparate symptoms that may delay an accurate diagnosis: anemia, fatigue, aches and pains, bone loss, depression, anxiety, infertility, mouth sores, or an itchy, blistering skin rash.

A blood test revealing high concentrations of certain antibodies can indicate celiac disease or the similar problem of gluten allergy. To heal their intestines, people with these conditions must eliminate all gluten-containing foods from their diets and then continue avoiding them for the rest of their lives. This is easier said than done because gluten can hide in foods that contain wheat-based additives, such as modified food starch and preservatives. Even corn and rice, naturally gluten-free foods, can be contaminated with gluten if they are milled in machines that also process wheat. The U.S. Food and Drug Administration (FDA) requires food labels to clearly identify ingredients containing wheat and related grains; foods labeled "gluten-free" are held to strict standards.[††]

Non-Celiac Gluten Sensitivity Physicians increasingly report a group of symptoms called **non-celiac gluten sensitivity** (NCGS).[14] Patients suffer from digestive symptoms resembling those of celiac disease or a gluten allergy, but test negative for these conditions. Some people with NCGS find relief when they eat a gluten-free diet, although the reasons why are not clear.[15]

> More on food allergies in **Chapters 13 and 14.**

Gluten-Free Hype Recently, popular media have blamed gluten for causing headaches, insomnia, obesity, and even cancer and Alzheimer's disease, but no evidence supports these accusations. Gluten-free diets have no special power to spur weight loss either, despite noisy claims made by diet sellers. In fact, the opposite is often true: many gluten-sensitive people become overweight when they begin eating more food on a a gluten-free diet that relieves their symptoms. Manufactured gluten-free foods are often higher in fats, added sugars, and calories than their regular counterparts, making overconsumption of calories likely (see Figure 6–20).

Most people with celiac disease are never diagnosed, and without treatment, they continue to suffer needlessly. Ironically, most people following a gluten-free diet may not have celiac disease, NCGS, or gluten allergy.[16] They eat expensive, high-calorie, processed specialty foods and unnecessarily omit nutritious whole grains because they believe the false claims of faddists.

Figure 6–20

Gluten-Free Foods

A gluten-free diet can bring relief to people with celiac disease, but a diet high in sugary ultra-processed foods like these does not support good health.

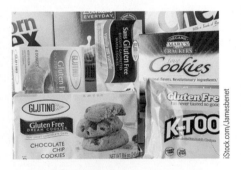

iStock.com/Jamesbenet

---

gluten (GLOO-ten) a type of protein in certain grain foods that is toxic to the person with celiac disease.

celiac (SEE-lee-ack) **disease** a disorder characterized by an abnormal immune response, weight loss, and intestinal inflammation on exposure to the dietary protein gluten; also called *gluten-sensitive enteropathy* or *celiac sprue*.

non-celiac gluten sensitivity a poorly defined collection of digestive symptoms that improves with elimination of gluten from the diet.

KEY POINTS

- Most U.S. protein intakes fall within the DRI range of 10 to 35 percent of calories.
- No Tolerable Upper Intake Level exists for protein, but health risks may accompany the overconsumption of protein-rich foods.
- Gluten-free diets often relieve symptoms of celiac disease, non-celiac gluten sensitivity, or gluten allergy, but no evidence supports claims that they cure other ills.

---

†† A food labeled "gluten-free" may not contain gluten-containing grains or ingredients derived from them (unless processed to remove gluten).

Chapter 6 The Proteins and Amino Acids

FOOD FEATURE

Getting Enough but Not Too Much Protein

LO 6.6 Identify the benefits and drawbacks of protein-rich foods in the diet.

Most foods contribute at least some protein to the diet. The most nutrient-dense selections among them are generally best for nutrition.

Protein-Rich Foods

Foods in the Protein Foods group (meat, poultry, fish, dry peas and beans, eggs, and nuts) and in the Milk and Milk Products group (milk, yogurt, and cheese) contribute an abundance of high-quality protein. Two others, the Vegetables group and the Grains group, contribute smaller amounts of protein, but they can add up to significant quantities. What about the Fruit group? Don't rely on fruit for protein; fruit contains only small amounts. Figure 6–21 (p. 208) demonstrates that a wide variety of foods contribute protein to the diet. Figure 6–22 (p. 209) lists the top protein contributors in the U.S. diet.

Protein is critical in nutrition, but too many protein-rich foods can displace other important foods from the diet. Foods richest in protein carry with them a characteristic array of vitamins and minerals, including vitamin B$_{12}$ and iron, but they lack others—vitamin C and folate, for example. In addition, many protein-rich foods such as meat are high in calories, and to overconsume them is to invite obesity.

Because American consumption of protein is ample, you can plan meatless or reduced-meat meals with pleasure. Meats are not always the best, or even the most desirable, sources of protein in a balanced, nutritious diet. Of the many interesting, protein-rich meat equivalents available, one has already been mentioned: the legumes.

The Nature of Legumes

The protein of some legumes, and soybeans in particular, is of a quality almost comparable to that of meat, an unusual trait in a fiber-rich vegetable. Figure 6–23 (p. 209) shows a legume plant's special root system that enables it to make abundant protein by obtaining nitrogen from the soil. Legumes are also excellent sources of many B vitamins, iron, and other minerals, making them exceptionally nutritious foods. On average, a cup of cooked legumes contains about 30 percent of the Daily Values for both protein and iron. Like meats, though, legumes do not offer every nutrient, and they do not make a complete meal by themselves. They contain no vitamin A, vitamin C, or vitamin B$_{12}$, and their balance of amino acids can be much improved by using grains and other vegetables along with them.

Soybeans are versatile legumes, and many nutritious products are made from them. Heavy use of soy products in place of meat, however, inhibits iron absorption. The effect can be alleviated by using small amounts of meat and/or foods rich in vitamin C in the same meal with soy products.

Vegetarians and others sometimes use convenience foods made from **textured vegetable protein** (soy protein) formulated to look and taste like hamburgers or breakfast sausages. Many of these are intended to match the known nutrient contents of animal protein foods, but they often fall short. Wise vegetarians use such foods in combination with whole foods to supply the entire array of needed nutrients. The nutrients of soybeans are

also available as bean curd, or **tofu**, a staple used in many Asian dishes. Thanks to the use of calcium salts when some tofu is made, it can be high in calcium. Check the Nutrition Facts panel on the label.

Food Label Trickery

Protein has become a marketing buzzword, and everything from cereal to supplements now sports the word *protein* on the label. Oftentimes, however, "protein" bars, cereals, and beverages would be more accurately labeled "sugar." A cereal bar named "Protein," for example, offers just 4 grams of protein per bar, not enough to qualify as a "good source," but provides added sugars in abundance: 14 grams per bar.* A serving of a "protein" beverage with 15 grams (60 calories) of protein also delivers more than 120 calories of added sugars. In contrast, plain, nonfat Greek yogurt (6-ounce container, see Figure 6-24, p. 210) provides 17 grams of protein but with just 100 calories and no added sugar. Another trick of marketing: a package banner may claim that a serving of cereal provides as much as 12 grams of protein, but the label

textured vegetable protein processed soybean protein used in products formulated to look and taste like meat, fish, or poultry.

tofu (TOE-foo) a curd made from soybeans that is rich in protein, often enriched with calcium, and variable in fat content; used in many Asian and vegetarian dishes in place of meat. Also defined in Controversy 2.

*A food is a "good source" if it provides ≥10% of a nutrient's Daily Value in a serving.

(continued)

Finding the Protein in Foods[a]

Fruit		
Food	**Protein g**	**%DV**[b]
Avocado	½ c	2	4
Cantaloupe	½ c	1	2
Orange sections	½ c	1	2
Strawberries	½ c	1	2

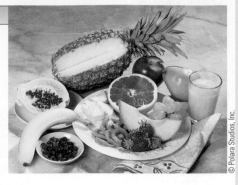

© Polara Studios, Inc.

Vegetables		
Food	**Protein g**	**%DV**[b]
Corn	½ c	3	6
Broccoli	½ c	2	4
Collard greens	½ c	2	4
Sweet potato	½ c	2	4
Baked potato	½ c	1	2
Bean sprouts	½ c	1	2
Winter squash	½ c	1	2

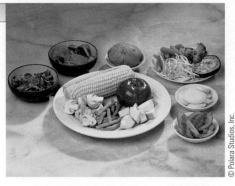

© Polara Studios, Inc.

Grains		
Food	**Protein g**	**%DV**[b]
Pancakes	2 sm	6	12
Bagel	½	4	8
Brown rice	½ c	3	6
Whole-grain bread	1 sl	3	6
Noodles, pasta	½ c	3	6
Oatmeal	½ c	3	6
Barley	½ c	2	4
Cereal flakes	1 oz	2	4

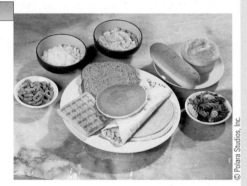

© Polara Studios, Inc.

Protein Foods		
Food	**Protein g**	**%DV**[b]
Roast beef	2 oz	19	33
Turkey leg	2 oz	16	32
Chicken breast	2 oz	15	30
Pork meat	2 oz	15	30
Tuna	2 oz	14	28
Lentils, beans, peas	½ c	9	18
Peanut butter	2 tbs	8	16
Almonds	¼ c	8	16
Hot dog	1 reg	7	14
Lunchmeat	2 oz	6	12
Egg	1 lg	6	12
Cashew nuts	¼ c	5	10

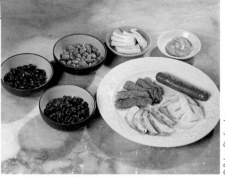

© Polara Studios, Inc.

Milk and Milk Products		
Food	**Protein g**	**%DV**[b]
Cheese, processed	2 oz	13	26
Milk, yogurt	1 c	10	20
Pudding	1 c	5	10

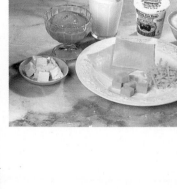

© Polara Studios, Inc.

Oils, Solid Fats, and Added Sugars

Not a significant source

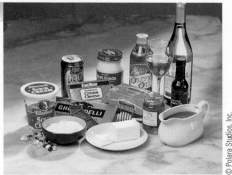

© Polara Studios, Inc.

[a]All foods are prepared and ready to eat.

[b]The Daily Value (DV) for protein is 50 g, based on an energy intake of 2,000 cal/day.

Figure 6–22

Top Contributors of Protein to the U.S. Diet[a]

In recent decades, poultry (largely chicken) intakes have been rising steadily, while beef intakes have been declining.

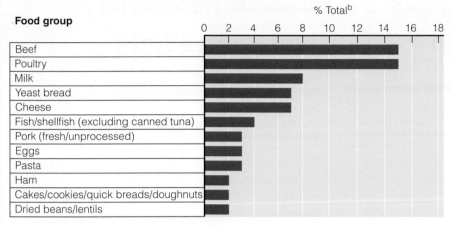

Food group	% Total[b]
Beef	15
Poultry	15
Milk	8
Yeast bread	7
Cheese	7
Fish/shellfish (excluding canned tuna)	4
Pork (fresh/unprocessed)	3
Eggs	3
Pasta	3
Ham	2
Cakes/cookies/quick breads/doughnuts	2
Dried beans/lentils	2

[a]These foods supply about 70 percent of the protein in the U.S. diet. The remainder comes from foods that each contribute less than 2 percent of the total.
[b]Rounded values.

makers counted the protein in a half-cup of milk, as well as the cereal. The cereal itself provides less than half this amount. Moral: ignore trendy labels and banners, and turn to the Nutrition Facts panel for the real story about protein, sugars, and calories in foods.

Conclusion

The Food Features presented so far show that the recommendations for the three energy-yielding nutrients occur in balance with each other. The diets of most people, however, supply too little fiber, too much fat, too many calories, and abundant protein. To bring their diets into line with recommendations, then, requires changing the bulk of intake from calorie-rich fried foods, fatty meats, and sweet treats to lower-calorie complex carbohydrates and fiber-rich choices, such as whole grains, legumes, and vegetables. With these changes, protein totals remain adequate, while other constituents automatically fall into place in a healthier eating pattern.

Figure 6–23

A Legume

Legumes include such plants as the kidney bean, soybean, green pea, lentil, black-eyed pea, and lima bean. Bacteria in the root nodules can "fix" nitrogen from the air, contributing it to the beans. Ultimately, thanks to these bacteria, the plant accumulates more nitrogen than it can get from the soil and also contributes more nitrogen to the soil than it takes out. Legumes are so efficient at trapping nitrogen that farmers often grow them in rotation with other crops to fertilize fields. Legumes are included with meat in the protein foods group in Figure 6–21.

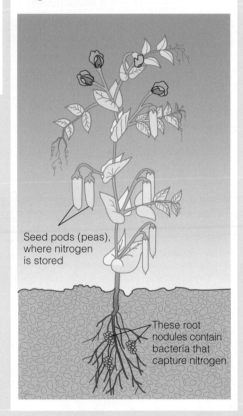

Seed pods (peas), where nitrogen is stored

These root nodules contain bacteria that capture nitrogen

(continued)

Figure 6-24

Two Protein Sources Compared

Plain, nonfat Greek yogurt provides more protein with fewer calories and less sodium and sugar than most products that shout "protein" on the label.

Greek Yogurt

Nutrition Facts

Serving Size 6 ounces (168 g)
Serving Per Container 1

Amount Per Serving

Calories 100	Calories from Fat 6

	% Daily Value
Total Fat 0.7g	1%
Cholesterol 9 mg	3%
Sodium 61 mg	2%
Potassium 240 mg	6%
Total Carbohydrate 6 g	2%
Dietary fiber 0 g	0%
Sugar 6 g	
Protein 17 g	34%

Commercial Protein Shake

Nutrition Facts

Serving Size 1 Bottle (296 ml)
Serving Per Container 1

Amount Per Serving

Calories 190	Calories from Fat 50

	% Daily Value
Total Fat 5 g	8%
Cholesterol <5 mg	1%
Sodium 240 mg	10%
Potassium 370 mg	11%
Total Carbohydrate 23 g	8%
Dietary fiber 5 g	20%
Sugar 18 g	
Protein 15 g	30%

LOVE_LIFE/Getty Images

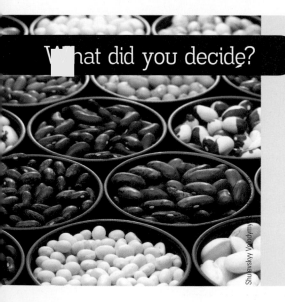

Shulevskyy Volodymyr/

What did you decide?

Why does your body need **protein**?

How does heating an **egg** change it from a liquid to a solid?

Do protein or amino acid **supplements** bulk up muscles?

Will your diet lack protein if you don't eat **meat**?

What's online?

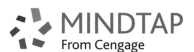
MINDTAP
From Cengage

Visit www.Cengage.com to access MindTap, a complete digital course that includes Diet & Wellness Plus, interactive quizzes, videos, and more.

Self Check

1. (LO 6.1) The basic building blocks for protein are
   _____.
   a. glucose units
   b. amino acids
   c. side chains
   d. saturated bonds

2. (LO 6.1) The roles of protein in the body include all but
   _____.
   a. blood clot formation
   b. tissue repair
   c. gas exchange
   d. immunity

3. (LO 6.1) Amino acids are linked together to form a protein strand by _____.
   a. peptide bonds
   b. essential amino acid bonds
   c. side chain attraction
   d. super glue

4. (LO 6.1) Some segments of a protein strand coil, are some-what like a metal spring, because
   a. amino acids at different places along the strand are chemically attracted to each other.
   b. the protein strand has been denatured by acid.
   c. the protein strand is missing one or more essential amino acids.
   d. a coil structure allows access by enzymes for digestion.

5. (LO 6.2) Protein digestion begins in the _____.
   a. mouth
   b. stomach
   c. small intestine
   d. large intestine

6. (LO 6.2) In the intestine, amino acids of the same general type compete for the same absorption sites, so a large dose of any one amino acid can limit absorption of another.
   T F

7. (LO 6.3) Under certain circumstances, amino acids can be con-verted to glucose and so serve the energy needs of the brain.
   T F

8. (LO 6.3) To prevent wasting of dietary protein, which of the following conditions must be met?
   a. Dietary protein must not exceed the body's need in quantity.
   b. Dietary protein must supply all essential amino acids in the proper amounts.
   c. The diet must supply enough carbohydrate and calories.
   d. All of the above.

9. (LO 6.4) For healthy adults, the DRI for protein has been set at
   a. 0.8 grams per kilogram of body weight.
   b. 2.2 pounds per kilogram of body weight.
   c. 12 to 15 percent of total calories.
   d. 100 grams per day.

10. (LO 6.4) An example of a person in positive nitrogen balance is a pregnant woman.
    T F

11. (LO 6.4) Partially completed proteins are not held for completion at a later time when the diet may improve.
    T F

12. (LO 6.4) Which of the following pairs of foods offers complementary protein?
    a. pot roast and chicken
    b. pot roast and carrots
    c. rice and French fries
    d. peanut butter on whole-wheat bread

13. (LO 6.5) Insufficient dietary protein can have severe consequences, but excess dietary protein cannot cause harm.
    T F

14. (LO 6.5) Insufficient dietary protein can cause
    a. slowed protein synthesis.
    b. hepatitis.
    c. accelerated growth in children.
    d. all of the above.

15. (LO 6.5) A diagnostic criterion for celiac disease is
    a. high levels of blood antibodies.
    b. high levels of blood gluten.
    c. weight gain.
    d. none of the above.

16. (LO 6.6) Two tablespoons of peanut butter offer about the same amount of protein as a hot dog.
    T F

17. (LO 6.6) Legumes are a particularly nutritious choice among protein-rich foods because they also provide
    a. vitamin C and vitamin E.
    b. fiber.
    c. B vitamins, iron, and other minerals.
    d. b and c.

18. (LO 6.7) Blood LDL values of people eating typical, meat-rich Western diets are generally higher than LDL values of vegetarians.
    T F

19. (LO 6.7) A vegetarian diet planner must make an effort to obtain adequate _____.
    a. carbohydrate
    b. vitamin C
    c. vitamin B_{12}
    d. vitamin E

20. (LO 6.7) Fried banana or vegetable snack chips make a healthy everyday snack choice for vegetarians.
    T F

Answers to these Self Check questions are in Appendix G.

Are Vegetarian or Meat-Containing Diets Better for Health?

LO 6.7   Compare the advantages and disadvantages of a vegetarian diet and a meat eater's diet.

In affluent countries, where heart disease and cancer claim many lives, people who eat well-planned **vegetarian** diets often have lower rates of chronic diseases, and a lower risk of dying from all causes, than people whose diets center on meat.[1]* Should everyone consider using a vegetarian eating pattern, then? If so, is it enough to simply omit meat, or is more demanded of vegetarian diet planners? What positive contributions do animal products make to the diet? This Controversy looks at these issues and ends with some practical advice for vegetarian diet planners. Table C6–1 defines vegetarian terms.

A vegetarian lifestyle may be immediately associated with a particular cultural, religious, political, or other belief system, but there are many reasons why people might choose it, such as concerns about health, the environment, or the human treatment of animals. Vegetarians are categorized not by motivation but by the foods they choose to eat. Distinctions among vegetarian diets are useful academically, but they do not represent uncrossable lines. Some people use meat or broth as a condiment or seasoning for vegetable or grain dishes. Some people eat meat only once or twice a week and use plant protein foods the rest of the time, a choice shown to be healthy by research.[2] Others eat mostly milk products and eggs for protein but will eat fish, too, and so forth. To force people into the categories of "vegetarians" and "meat eaters" leaves out all those in-between eating styles (aptly named *flexitarian* by the press) that have much to recommend them.

Positive Health Aspects of Vegetarian Diets

Today, nutrition authorities state with confidence that a well-chosen vegetarian diet can meet nutrient needs while supporting health superbly.[3] Although much evidence supports this choice,

*Reference notes are in Appendix F.

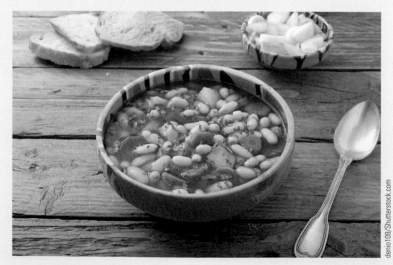

Can an eating pattern without animal products supply the needed nutrients?

denio109/Shutterstock.com

Table C6–1

Terms Used to Describe Vegetarian Diets

Some of the following terms are in common usage, but others are useful only to researchers.

- **fruitarian** includes only raw or dried fruit, seeds, and nuts in the diet.
- **lacto-ovo vegetarian** includes dairy products, eggs, vegetables, grains, legumes, fruit, and nuts; excludes flesh and seafood.
- **lacto-vegetarian** includes dairy products, vegetables, grains, legumes, fruit, and nuts; excludes flesh, seafood, and eggs; (*lacto* means "milk").
- **macrobiotic diet** a vegan diet composed chiefly of whole grains, beans, and certain vegetables; taken to extremes, macrobiotic diets can compromise nutrient status.
- **ovo-vegetarian** includes eggs, vegetables, grains, legumes, fruit, and nuts, and excludes flesh, seafood, and milk products; *ovo* means "egg").
- **partial vegetarian** a term sometimes used to mean an eating style that includes seafood, poultry, eggs, dairy products, vegetables, grains, legumes, fruit, and nuts; excludes or strictly limits certain meats, such as red meats. Also called *flexitarian*.
- **vegan** includes only food from plant sources: vegetables, grains, legumes, fruit, seeds, and nuts. Also called *strict vegetarian*.
- **vegetarian** includes plant-based foods and eliminates some or all animal-derived foods.

such evidence is not easily obtained. It would be easy if vegetarians differed from others only in the absence of meat, but they often have *increased* intakes of fruit, legumes, nuts, seeds, whole grains, and vegetables as well. Such eating patterns are rich contributors of carbohydrates, fiber, vitamins, minerals, and phytochemicals that also correlate with low disease risks.[4] For example, in one study, as servings of fruit and vegetables increased from fewer than one to more than five per day, overall risk of death decreased by 36 percent, risk from cancers decreased by 25 percent, and risk from heart disease decreased by 20 percent, regardless of meat consumption.[5]

Also, many vegetarians live healthy lifestyles: they avoid tobacco, use alcohol in moderation, if at all, and are more physically active than other adults. But when researchers take these and other lifestyle variables into account, they still find that vegetarian eating patterns favor disease resistance.

Defense against Obesity

Among both men and women and across many ethnic groups, vegetarians more often maintain a healthier body weight than nonvegetarians.[6] The converse is also true: meat consumption correlates with higher calorie intakes and increased obesity. It may be that many meat eaters overconsume daily calories by eating too much meat, a point illustrated in Figure 6-1 (p. 214).

Defense against Heart and Artery Disease

Vegetarians often have lower blood LDL cholesterol concentrations and die less often from heart disease than do meat eaters, but avoiding meat does not guarantee heart health—other dietary factors also affect it.[7] When vegetarians choose the unsaturated fats of soybeans, seeds, avocados, nuts, olives, and vegetable oils and shun the saturated fats of cheese, sour cream, butter, shortening, and other sources, their risks of heart disease are reduced. If their diets also contains

nuts and legumes, as most vegetarian diets do, then LDL cholesterol typically falls, and heart benefits accumulate. In contrast, even a plant-based diet that emphasizes sugar-sweetened beverages, refined baked goods, French fries, and sweets is associated with an increased risk of heart disease.[8]

Defense against High Blood Pressure

Vegetarians tend to have lower blood pressure and lower rates of hypertension than average. As mentioned, vegetarians often maintain healthy body weights, and appropriate body weight helps maintain healthy blood pressure. So does eating enough fiber, fruit, vegetables, low-fat milk products, and soy protein, which are usually amply supplied by a vegetarian diet. Other lifestyle factors such as not smoking, moderating alcohol intake, and being physically active all work together to keep blood pressure normal.

Defense against Cancer

Questions about diet and cancers are not easily answered, but the World Health Organization (WHO) has concluded that high intakes of red meats, such as beef, goat, lamb, pork, veal, venison, boar, and so forth raise the risk of colon and rectal cancers.[9] The group also lists processed meats, such as lunchmeats and hot dogs, among human carcinogens and concludes that eating about two ounces daily increases colon and rectal cancer risks by 18 percent.

In a study of over 60,000 people in the United Kingdom, those who ate fish or vegetables but not red meats had the lowest overall cancer rates—a finding that agrees with many other studies.[10] Accounting for smoking, exercise, and other lifestyle factors, the overall cancer risk (compared to meat eaters) was 19 percent lower in **vegans**, 12 percent lower in fish eaters, and 11 percent lower in **lacto-ovo vegetarians**.

All meats are not the same in this regard. When unprocessed "white meats" (fish or poultry) replace red

meats in the diet, deaths from cancer decline substantially, as do deaths from other chronic diseases.[11] Researchers suspect that the heme iron in red meats (previously shown in Figure 6–4, p. 186) or additives in processed meats may contribute to cancer causation.[12]

More details about diet and cancer appear in **Chapter 11**.

Other Health Benefits

In addition to opposing obesity, heart disease, high blood pressure, and cancer, vegetarian eating patterns may help prevent cataracts, diabetes, diverticular disease, gallstones, and osteoporosis. However, these effects may arise more from what vegetarians include in their diet—abundant fruit, legumes, vegetables, milk products, and whole grains—than from omission of meat. Table C6–2 (p. 215) spells out some arguments for and against eliminating meat from the diet.

Positive Health Aspects of the Meat Eater's Diet

With prudent choices, both meat eaters and lacto-ovo vegetarians can rely on their diets to support health during critical times of life. In contrast, a vegan eating pattern poses challenges. Protein is critical for building new tissues during growth, for fighting illnesses, for building bone during youth, and for maintaining bone and muscle in old age. Although protein from plant sources can meet most people's needs, very young children and very elderly vegans with small appetites may not consume enough legumes, whole grains, and nuts to supply the protein they need.

Chapter 6 made clear that protein from meat, fish, milk, and eggs is the clear winner in tests of digestibility and availability to the body, with soy protein a close second. Also, animal-derived foods provide abundant iron, zinc,

Perspective on a Meat Serving

This 5-ounce steak provides almost all of the meat recommended for an entire day's intake in a 2,000-calorie diet.

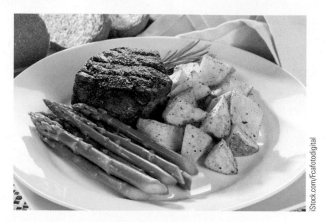

iStock.com/Fcafotodigital

vitamin D, calcium, and vitamin B_{12}, needed by everyone but particularly by pregnant women, infants, children, adolescents, and the elderly (details about these needs appear in later chapters). This is not to say that people need large amounts of meat to provide these nutrients. The USDA's Healthy U.S.-Style Eating Pattern recommends less meat for a whole day than most people eat at one sitting (look again at Figure C6-1.).

Iron and zinc are less readily absorbed from vegan sources, such as grains and legumes, than from meat, but iron and zinc from supplements or fortified foods can help prevent deficiencies. Vegans must also find and regularly consume alternate sources of vitamin D, calcium, vitamin B_{12}, and the omega-3 fatty acids EPA and DHA.

Concerns through Life

Nutrient needs change with different life stages. A vegetarian diet can support health throughout life, but only if it meets these nutrient needs.

In Pregnancy and Infancy

Women who eat seafood, eggs, or milk products can be sure of receiving enough energy, vitamin B_{12}, vitamin D, calcium, iron, and zinc, as well as protein, to support pregnancy and breastfeeding. A vegan woman can also meet her needs, provided she takes the appropriate supplements.[13] In contrast, a vegan woman who doesn't meet her nutrient needs may enter pregnancy too thin and with scant nutrient stores to draw on as the nutrient demands of the fetus increase.

Among nutrients of concern is vitamin B_{12}, a vitamin abundant in foods of animal origin but absent from plants. Obtaining enough vitamin B_{12} poses a substantial challenge to vegans of all ages, who often test low in the vitamin.[14] For pregnant or lactating women, obtaining vitamin B_{12} is critical to prevent serious disorders in mother and child.[15]

In Childhood

Children who eat eggs, milk, and fish receive abundant protein, iron, zinc, vitamin D, calcium, and vitamin B_{12}; such foods are reliable, convenient sources of nutrients needed for growth.[16] Likewise, children eating well-planned lacto-ovo vegetarian diets receive adequate nutrients and grow as well as their meat-eating peers. Child-sized servings of vegan foods, however, can fail to provide sufficient energy or several key nutrients needed for normal growth. A child's small stomach can hold only so

much food, and a vegan child may feel full before eating enough to meet his or her nutrient needs.

Small, frequent meals of fortified breads, cereals, or pastas with legumes, nuts, nut butters, and sources of unsaturated fats can help meet protein and energy needs in a smaller volume at each sitting. Because vegan children derive protein only from plant foods, their daily protein sources should be carefully chosen to provide sufficient essential amino acids and energy. Also, vegan children who rely on whole grains and vegetables for the minerals iron and zinc receive them, but in less absorbable forms, so fortified foods or a supplement may be needed.[17]

In Adolescence

The healthiest vegetarian adolescents choose balanced diets that are heavy in fruit and vegetables but light on the sweets, fast foods, and salty snacks that tempt the teenage palate. These healthy vegetarian teens often meet the goals of the Dietary Guidelines for Americans—a rare accomplishment in the United States.

Other teens, however, adopt poorly planned vegetarian eating patterns that provide too little energy and too few nutrients for health. Scant intakes of protein, calcium, and vitamin D, for example, lead to weak bone development at precisely the time when they must develop strength to protect their health through later life. If a vegetarian child or teen refuses sound parental advice, a registered dietitian nutritionist can help identify problems, dispense appropriate guidance, and put unwarranted parental worries to rest.

In Aging and in Illness

For elderly people with diminished appetites or impaired digestion, too little dietary protein compromises both bone and muscle strength, leading to bone fractures and infirmity. Providing frequent meals with high-quality protein, such as low-fat cheese, fish, or soft-cooked ground poultry or meat, may reduce these risks.[10] Vegetarians, and particularly vegans, may be at greater

Table C6-2

Should Meat Be Eliminated from the Diet? Point, Counterpoint

Arguments can be made for and against eliminating meats on all points, save one: inhumane treatment of animals. Many people choose a vegetarian diet on this point alone.

Point: Eliminating meat	Counterpoint: Including meat
1. *Reduced heart disease risk.* Vegetarians have reduced risks of developing heart disease and dying from heart disease.	1. *Reduced heart disease risk.* People who follow the Dietary Guidelines, and eat small portions of lean meat, fish, and poultry, have low rates of heart disease.
2. *Reduced cancer risks.* Vegetarians have reduced risks of developing certain cancers and dying from cancer.	2. *Reduced cancer risks.* Small daily intakes of meats, poultry, fish, and seafood are not associated with increased cancer risks, particularly when a diet follows the Dietary Guidelines for Americans.
3. *Reduced mortality risk.* Vegetarians have reduced risks of early death from all causes.	3. *Reduced mortality risk.* Ample fruit and vegetable intakes, regular physical activity, not smoking, and other healthy lifestyle choices reduce mortality risk without eliminating meat.
4. *Reduced obesity and diabetes risks.* Vegetarians are less likely to develop obesity or diabetes.	4. *Reduced obesity and diabetes risks.* A calorie-controlled diet of whole foods reduces the likelihood of developing obesity or diabetes without eliminating meat.
5. *Normal blood pressure.* Vegetarians have reduced risks of hypertension.	5. *Normal blood pressure.* Normal blood pressure can be maintained with a healthy eating pattern such as DASH (Chapter 8), which includes moderate amounts of meat.
6. *Ample nutrients.* Vegetarian diets reliably provide fiber, vitamin A, vitamin C, vitamin K, folate, and magnesium. Protein is generally sufficient.	6. *Ample nutrients.* Diets with meats, fish, poultry, eggs, and milk products reliably provide protein, EPA and DHA (fish), vitamin B_{12}, vitamin D (milk fortification), calcium, iron, and zinc.
7. *Honored traditions.* Vegetarianism is often part of religious, family, and cultural traditions.	7. *Honored traditions.* Hunting and fishing are often family and cultural traditions. Holidays often center on meat-containing meals, such as turkey at Thanksgiving.
8. *Ecological sustainability.* Nutrient-dense vegetarian diets require much less land, water, fuel, and other resources to produce than diets high in meats, cheeses, and highly processed foods. They also generate far less waste and pollution.	8. *Ecological sustainability.* Three eating patterns—Healthy U.S.-style, Healthy Mediterranean-style, and Healthy Vegetarian—are named by the Dietary Guidelines committee as having less environmental impact than the current U.S. diet. The first two contain significant amounts of meat.
9. *Treatment of animals.* Vegetarian diets are obtained without cruelty to or death of animals.	9. *Treatment of Animals.* Cruelty-free animal products are becoming more available as consumer demand for them increases.

risk for weakened bones and fractures than nonvegetarians.[19]

People battling life-threatening diseases may encounter testimonial stories of cures attributed to restrictive eating plans, such as **macrobiotic diets**. However, these diets often severely limit food selections and can fail to deliver the energy and nutrients needed for recovery.

Planning a Vegetarian Diet

Eating a nutritious vegetarian diet requires being aware of nutrient needs and sources of those nutrients, and then planning a diet that provides them every day. Grains, fruit, and vegetables are naturally abundant in a vegetarian diet and provide adequate amounts of the nutrients of plant foods: carbohydrate, fiber, thiamin, folate, and vitamins B_6, C, A, and E. Table C6–3 (p. 216) summarizes vegetarian sources for nutrients of concern in a vegetarian diet.

Choosing within the Food Groups

When selecting from the Vegetables and Fruit groups, vegetarians should emphasize sources of calcium and iron. Green leafy vegetables provide both calcium and iron. Similarly, dried fruit deserve special notice in the Fruit group because they can deliver more iron than other fruit. The Protein Foods group emphasizes legumes, soy products, nuts, and seeds. The Dietary Guidelines encourage the use of vegetable oils, nuts, and seeds rich in unsaturated fats and omega-3 fatty acids. To ensure adequate nutrient intakes, vegans need to select fortified foods or use supplements daily.

Milk Products and Protein Foods

It takes some planning to ensure adequate intakes from a variety of vegetarian foods in the Milk and

Vegetarian Sources of Key Nutrients

Nutrients	Grains	Vegetables	Fruit	Protein Foods	Milk	Oils
Protein	Whole grains			Legumes, seeds, nuts, soy products (tempeh, tofu, veggie burgers) Eggs (for ovo-vegetarians)	Milk, cheese, yogurt (for lacto-vegetarians)	
Iron	Fortified cereals, enriched and whole grains	Dark green leafy vegetables (spinach, turnip greens)	Dried fruit (apricots, prunes, raisins)	Legumes (black-eyed peas, kidney beans, lentils)		
Zinc	Fortified cereals, whole grains			Legumes (garbanzo beans, kidney beans, navy beans), nuts, seeds (pumpkin seeds)	Milk, cheese, yogurt (for lacto-vegetarians)	
Calcium	Fortified cereals	Dark-green leafy vegetables (bok choy, broccoli, collard greens, kale, mustard greens, turnip greens, watercress)	Fortified juices, figs	Fortified soy products, nuts (almonds), seeds (sesame seeds)	Milk, cheese, yogurt (for lacto-vegetarians) Fortified soy or pea milk	
Vitamin B$_{12}$	Fortified cereals			Eggs (for ovo-vegetarians) Fortified soy products	Milk, cheese, yogurt (for lacto-vegetarians) Fortified soy or pea milk	
Vitamin D		High-vitamin D mushrooms (wild types grown in sunlight or commercial types treated with ultraviolet light; see Chapter 7 for details)			Milk, cheese, yogurt (for lacto-vegetarians) Fortified soy or pea milk	
Omega-3 fatty acids				Flaxseed, walnuts, soybeans		Flaxseed oil, walnut oil, soybean oil

Milk Products group and the Protein Foods group. Figure C6–2 (p. 217) highlights these food groups. Note that the Milk and Milk Products group features fortified soy or pea milk and soy yogurt for vegans. Protein-rich soy and pea beverages are often fortified and match many of the nutrients of milk products. Other "milk" beverages and yogurts, based on almonds, coconuts, hemp, oats, or rice, generally lack protein and other nutrients. Smart planners compare the nutrients of substitutes with those of milk and dairy foods before choosing.

As for protein, the USDA Healthy Vegetarian Eating Pattern (Appendix E) specifies daily and weekly intakes at many calorie levels. For vegans, good protein sources include all legumes, seeds, nuts, and many products made from soy; other foods also make small protein contributions that increase the day's total.

Convenience Foods

Prepared frozen or packaged vegetarian foods make food preparation quick and easy—just be sure to scrutinize each label's Nutrition Facts panel when choosing among them. Some products offer a nutrition bargain, such as vegetarian "hot dogs" or "veggie burgers." Made of soy, these foods look and taste like the original meat product but contain much less fat and saturated fat. Some brands may be high in sodium or added sugars, however (read the labels). Soybeans in other forms, such as plain tofu (bean curd), edamame (cooked green soybeans, pronounced *ed-eh-MAH-may*), or soy flour, offer protein with fewer additives.

Among snack foods, banana or vegetable chips, often sold as "healthy" foods, are anything but: a quarter cup of banana chips fried in saturated coconut oil contains 150 calories with 7 grams of saturated fat (a big hamburger has 8 grams). In contrast, a plain banana has 100 calories and practically no fat. Look for freeze-dried fruit and vegetable "chips"—they have no added fats, and the freeze-drying process creates a pleasing crunch while preserving most nutrients.

Conclusion

This comparison has shown that both a meat-eater's diet and a vegetarian's

Filling the Vegetarian MyPlate

Each day, in a 2,000-calorie diet, both vegans and lacto-ovo vegetarians require 3 cups of Milk and Milk Product equivalents and 5½ ounces of Protein Foods. (For details and for other calorie levels, see Appendix E.)

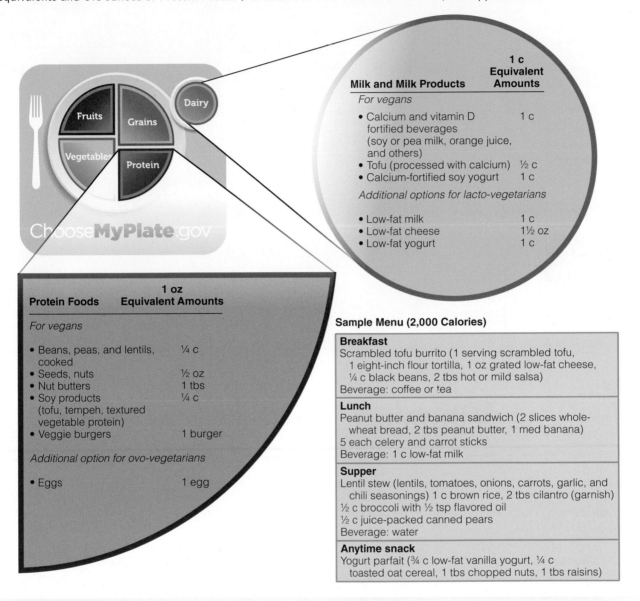

Milk and Milk Products	1 c Equivalent Amounts
For vegans	
• Calcium and vitamin D fortified beverages (soy or pea milk, orange juice, and others)	1 c
• Tofu (processed with calcium)	½ c
• Calcium-fortified soy yogurt	1 c
Additional options for lacto-vegetarians	
• Low-fat milk	1 c
• Low-fat cheese	1½ oz
• Low-fat yogurt	1 c

Protein Foods	1 oz Equivalent Amounts
For vegans	
• Beans, peas, and lentils, cooked	¼ c
• Seeds, nuts	½ oz
• Nut butters	1 tbs
• Soy products (tofu, tempeh, textured vegetable protein)	¼ c
• Veggie burgers	1 burger
Additional option for ovo-vegetarians	
• Eggs	1 egg

Sample Menu (2,000 Calories)

Breakfast
Scrambled tofu burrito (1 serving scrambled tofu, 1 eight-inch flour tortilla, 1 oz grated low-fat cheese, ¼ c black beans, 2 tbs hot or mild salsa)
Beverage: coffee or tea

Lunch
Peanut butter and banana sandwich (2 slices whole-wheat bread, 2 tbs peanut butter, 1 med banana)
5 each celery and carrot sticks
Beverage: 1 c low-fat milk

Supper
Lentil stew (lentils, tomatoes, onions, carrots, garlic, and chili seasonings) 1 c brown rice, 2 tbs cilantro (garnish)
½ c broccoli with ½ tsp flavored oil
½ c juice-packed canned pears
Beverage: water

Anytime snack
Yogurt parfait (¾ c low-fat vanilla yogurt, ¼ c toasted oat cereal, 1 tbs chopped nuts, 1 tbs raisins)

diet are best approached scientifically. If you are just beginning to study nutrition, consider adopting the attitude that the choice to make is not whether to be a meat eater or a vegetarian but where along the spectrum to locate yourself. Your preferences should be honored with these caveats: that you plan your own diet and the diets of those in your care to be adequate, balanced, controlled in calories, and varied and that you limit intakes of foods high in sodium, solid fats,

and added sugars. Whatever your eating style or reasons for choosing it, choose carefully: the foods that you eat regularly will exert major impacts on your health throughout your life.

Critical Thinking

1 Becoming a vegan takes a strong commitment and significant education to know how to combine foods and in what quantities to meet nutrient

requirements. Most of us will not choose to become vegetarians, but many of us would benefit from a diet of less meat. Identify ways you could alter your diet so that you eat less meat.

2 Identify two critical periods of life that demand high nutrient intakes, and defend the use of a vegetarian diet during those times. Discuss specific nutrient challenges and solutions for both of these life stages.

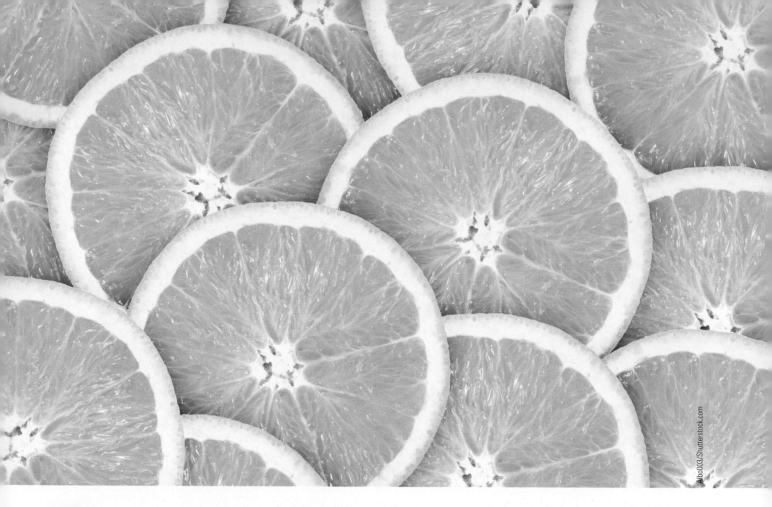

Albo003/Shutterstock.com

7 The Vitamins

How do **vitamins** work in the body?

Why is **sunshine** associated with good health?

Can **vitamin C tablets** ward off a cold?

Should you choose **vitamin-fortified foods** and take **supplements** for "insurance"?

At the beginning of the 20th century, the thrill of the discovery of the first **vitamins** captured the world's imagination as seemingly miraculous cures took place. In the usual scenario, a whole group of people was becoming unable to walk (or going blind or bleeding profusely) until an alert scientist stumbled onto the substance missing from their diets. The scientist confirmed the discovery by feeding vitamin-deficient chow to laboratory animals, which responded by becoming unable to walk (or going blind or bleeding profusely). When the missing ingredient was restored to their diets, they soon recovered. People, too, were quickly cured of such conditions when they received the vitamins they lacked.

In the decades that followed, advances in chemistry, biology, and genetics allowed scientists to isolate the vitamins, define their chemical structures, and reveal their functions in maintaining health and preventing deficiency diseases. Today, research hints that certain vitamins may influence the development of two major scourges of humankind: cardiovascular disease (CVD) and cancer. Many other conditions, from infections to cracked skin, bear relation to vitamin nutrition, details that unscrupulous sellers of vitamin supplements often use to market their wares (see the Controversy 7 section).

Can foods rich in vitamins protect us from life-threatening diseases? What about vitamin pills? For now, we can say this with certainty: the only disease a vitamin can *cure* is the one caused by a deficiency of that vitamin. As for chronic disease *prevention*, research is ongoing, but evidence so far supports the conclusion that vitamin-rich *foods* are protective. Vitamin supplements cannot make the same claim. The DRI values for vitamins are listed inside the front cover pages of this text.

According to the Dietary Guidelines 2015 committee, today's U.S. intakes of these vitamins may fall below recommended intakes:

- Vitamin A
- Vitamin D
- Vitamin E
- Vitamin C

Like all vitamins, these play critical roles in the body.

Definition and Classification of Vitamins

LO 7.1 Compare fat-soluble vitamins with water-soluble vitamins.

A child once defined a vitamin as "what, if you don't eat, you get sick." Although the grammar left something to be desired, the definition was accurate. Less imaginatively, a vitamin is defined as an essential, noncaloric, organic nutrient needed in tiny amounts in the diet. The role of many vitamins is to help make possible the processes by which

vitamins organic compounds that are vital to life and indispensable to body functions but that are needed only in minute amounts; essential, noncaloric nutrients.

Table 7–1

Vitamin Names[a]

Fat-Soluble Vitamins

Vitamin A
Vitamin D
Vitamin E
Vitamin K

Water-Soluble Vitamins

B vitamins
  Thiamin (B$_1$)
  Riboflavin (B$_2$)
  Niacin (B$_3$)
  Folate
  Vitamin B$_{12}$
  Vitamin B$_6$
  Biotin
  Pantothenic acid
Vitamin C

[a]Vitamin names established by the International Union of Nutritional Sciences Committee on Nomenclature. Other names are listed in Tables 7–8 and 7–9 (pp. 254–258).

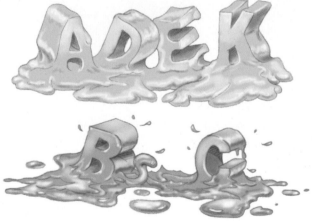

Vitamins fall into two classes—fat-soluble and water-soluble.

other nutrients are digested, absorbed, and metabolized or built into body structures. Although small in size and quantity, the vitamins accomplish mighty tasks.

As each vitamin was discovered, it was given a name, and some were given letters and numbers—vitamin A came before the B vitamins, then came vitamin C, and so forth. This led to the confusing variety of vitamin names that still exists today. This chapter uses the names in Table 7–1; alternative names are given in Tables 7–8 and 7–9 at the end of the chapter (pp. 254–258).

Vitamin Precursors

Some of the vitamins occur in foods in forms known as **precursors**. Once inside the body, these are transformed chemically to one or more active vitamin forms. Thus, to measure the amount of a vitamin found in food, we often must count not only the amount of the true vitamin but also the vitamin activity potentially available from its precursors.

Two Classes of Vitamins: Fat-Soluble and Water-Soluble

The vitamins fall naturally into two classes: fat-soluble and water-soluble (listed in Table 7–1). Solubility confers on vitamins many of their characteristics. It determines how the body absorbs, transports, stores, and excretes them.

Fat-soluble vitamins, like other lipids, are mostly absorbed into the lymph, and they travel in the blood and within the cells in association with protein carriers.[1]* Fat-soluble vitamins can be stored in the liver or with other lipids in fatty tissues, and some can build up to toxic concentrations. The water-soluble vitamins are absorbed directly into the bloodstream, where they travel freely. Most are not stored in tissues to any great extent; rather, excesses are excreted in the urine. Thus, the risks of toxicities are not as great as for fat-soluble vitamins.

Table 7–2 outlines the general features of the fat-soluble and water-soluble vitamins. The chapter then goes on to provide important details first about the fat-soluble vitamins and then about the water-soluble ones. At the end of the chapter, two summary tables (Tables 7–8 and 7–9) provide the basic facts about all of them.

KEY POINTS

- Vitamins are essential, noncaloric nutrients that are needed in tiny amounts in the diet and are indispensable for normal cellular processes.
- Vitamin precursors in foods are transformed into active vitamins by the body.
- The fat-soluble vitamins are vitamins A, D, E, and K.
- The water-soluble vitamins are vitamin C and the B vitamins.

The Fat-Soluble Vitamins

LO 7.2   Summarize the characteristics and functions of the fat-soluble vitamins.

The fat-soluble vitamins—A, D, E, and K—are found in the fats and oils of foods and require bile for absorption. Once absorbed, these vitamins are stored in the liver and fatty tissues until the body needs them.

Storage   Because they are stored, you need not eat foods containing each fat-soluble vitamin every day. If an eating pattern provides sufficient amounts of the fat-soluble vitamins on average over time, the body can survive for weeks at a time without consuming them.

precursors compounds that serve as starting material for other compounds. In nutrition, vitamin precursors are compounds that can be converted into active vitamins. Also called *provitamins*.

*Reference notes are in Appendix F.

Chapter 7 The Vitamins

Table 7–2

Characteristics of the Fat-Soluble and Water-Soluble Vitamins

Although each vitamin has unique functions and features, a few generalizations about the fat-soluble and water-soluble vitamins can aid understanding.

	Fat-Soluble Vitamins: Vitamins A, D, E, and K	Water-Soluble Vitamins: B Vitamins and Vitamin C
Absorption	Absorbed like fats, first into the lymph and then into the blood.	Absorbed directly into the blood.
Transport and Storage	Travel with protein carriers in watery body fluids; stored in the liver or fatty tissues.	Travel freely in watery fluids; most are not stored in the body.
Excretion	Not readily excreted; tend to build up in the tissues.	Readily excreted in the urine.
Toxicity	Toxicities are likely from supplements but occur rarely from food.	Toxicities are unlikely but possible with high doses from supplements.
Requirements	Needed in periodic doses (weekly or even monthly) depending on the extent of body stores.	Needed frequently (even daily) because the body does not store most of them to any extent.

Deficiencies   Deficiencies of the fat-soluble vitamins occur when the diet is consistently low in them. They also occur in people who undergo intestinal surgery for obesity treatment, which reduces energy nutrient absorption by design and vitamin absorption unintentionally. We also know that any disease that produces fat malabsorption (such as liver disease, which prevents bile production) can cause the loss of vitamins dissolved in undigested fat and so bring on deficiencies. In the same way, a person who uses mineral oil (which the body cannot absorb) as a laxative risks losing fat-soluble vitamins because they readily dissolve into the oil and are excreted with it. Deficiencies are also likely when people follow eating patterns that are extraordinarily low in fat because a little fat is necessary for absorption of these vitamins.

Toxicities   The capacity to be stored also sets the stage for toxic buildup if you take in too much. Excess vitamin A from high-dose supplements and highly fortified foods is especially likely to reach toxic levels.

Roles   Fat-soluble vitamins play diverse roles in the body. Vitamins A and D act somewhat like hormones, directing cells to convert one substance to another, to store this, or to release that. They also directly influence the genes, helping to regulate the production of enzymes and other proteins. Vitamin E protects tissues all over the body from destructive oxidative reactions. Vitamin K is necessary for blood to clot and for bone health. Each is worth a book in itself.

Vitamin A

LO 7.3   Describe the roles, food sources, and precursor of vitamin A, and the effects of vitamin A deficiency and toxicity.

Vitamin A has the distinction of being the first fat-soluble vitamin to be recognized. Today, after a century of scientific investigation, vitamin A and its plant-derived precursor, **beta-carotene**, are still very much a focus of research.

Three forms of vitamin A are active in the body. One of the active forms, **retinol**, is stored in specialized cells of the liver. The liver makes retinol available to the

beta-carotene an orange pigment with antioxidant activity; a vitamin A precursor made by plants and stored in human fat tissue.

retinol one of the active forms of vitamin A made from beta-carotene in animal and human bodies; an antioxidant nutrient. Other active forms are *retinal* and *retinoic acid*.

Figure 7–1

The Eye (Sectioned)

This eye is sectioned to reveal its inner structures.

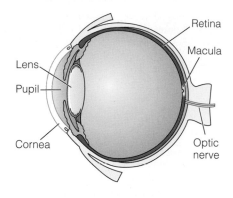

cornea (KOR-nee-uh) the transparent, hard outer covering of the front of the eye.

retina (RET-in-uh) the layer of light-sensitive nerve cells lining the back of the inside of the eye.

rhodopsin (roh-DOP-sin) the light-sensitive pigment of the cells in the retina; it contains vitamin A (*opsin* means "visual protein").

night blindness slow recovery of vision after exposure to flashes of bright light at night; an early symptom of vitamin A deficiency.

keratin (KERR-uh-tin) the normal protein of hair and nails.

keratinization accumulation of keratin in a tissue; a sign of vitamin A deficiency.

xerosis (zeer-OH-sis) drying of the cornea; a symptom of vitamin A deficiency.

xerophthalmia (ZEER-ahf-THALL-me-uh) progressive hardening of the cornea of the eye in advanced vitamin A deficiency that can lead to blindness (*xero* means "dry"; *ophthalm* means "eye").

epithelial (ep-ith-THEE-lee-ull) **tissue** the layers of the body that serve as selective barriers to environmental factors. Examples are the cornea, the skin, the respiratory tract lining, and the lining of the digestive tract.

cell differentiation (dih-fer-en-she-AY-shun) the process by which immature cells are stimulated to mature and gain the ability to perform functions characteristic of their cell type.

bloodstream and thereby to the body's cells. The cells convert retinol to its other two active forms, retinal and retinoic acid, as needed.

Foods derived from animals provide forms of vitamin A that are readily absorbed and put to use by the body. Foods derived from plants provide beta-carotene, which must be converted to active vitamin A before it can be used.[2]

Roles of Vitamin A and Consequences of Deficiency

Vitamin A is a versatile vitamin, with roles in gene expression, vision, maintenance of body linings and skin, immune defenses, growth of the body, and normal development of cells.[3] It is of critical importance for both male and female reproductive functions and for normal development of an embryo and fetus.[4] In short, vitamin A is needed everywhere. Its chief functions in the body are listed in Snapshot 7–1 on page 226). The following sections provide some details.

Eyesight   The most familiar function of vitamin A is to sustain normal eyesight. Vitamin A plays two indispensable roles: in the maintenance of a healthy, crystal-clear outer window, the **cornea**, and in the process of light perception at the **retina** (see Figure 7–1).

When light falls on the eye, it passes through the clear cornea and strikes the cells of the retina, bleaching many molecules of the pigment **rhodopsin** that lie within those cells. Vitamin A is a part of the rhodopsin molecule. When bleaching occurs, the vitamin is broken off, initiating the signal that conveys the sensation of sight to the optic center in the brain. The vitamin then reunites with the pigment, but a little vitamin A is destroyed each time this reaction takes place, and fresh vitamin A must replenish the supply.

Night Blindness   If the vitamin A supply begins to run low, a lag occurs before the eye can see again after a flash of bright light at night (see Figure 7–2). This lag in the recovery of night vision, termed **night blindness**, often indicates a vitamin A deficiency.[5] A bright flash of light can temporarily blind even normal, well-nourished eyes, but if you experience a long recovery period before vision returns, your health-care provider may want to check your vitamin A intake.

Xerophthalmia and Blindness   A more profound deficiency of vitamin A is exhibited when the protein **keratin** accumulates and clouds the eye's outer vitamin A–dependent part, the cornea. The condition is known as **keratinization**, and if the deficiency of vitamin A is not corrected, it can worsen to **xerosis** (drying) and then progress to thickening and permanent blindness, **xerophthalmia**.[6] Tragically, a half million of the world's vitamin A–deprived children become blind each year from this often preventable condition and about half die within a year after losing their sight. Vitamin A supplements given early to children developing vitamin A deficiency can reverse the process and save both eyesight and lives.[7] Better still, a child fed a variety of fruit and vegetables regularly is virtually assured protection.

Gene Regulation   Hundreds of genes are regulated by the retinoic acid form of vitamin A.[8] Genes direct the synthesis of proteins, including enzymes that perform the metabolic work of the tissues. Hence, through its influence on gene expression, vitamin A affects the metabolic activities of a vast array of tissues and, in turn, the health of the whole body. In the same way, retinoic acid may also affect the development and treatment of certain cancers, such as leukemia, breast cancer, prostate cancer, and others; research is ongoing.[9]

Cell Differentiation   Vitamin A is needed by all **epithelial tissue** (external skin and internal linings). The cornea of the eye, already mentioned, is such a tissue; so are skin and all of the protective linings of the lungs, intestines, vagina, urinary tract, and bladder. These tissues serve as barriers to infection and other threats.

An example of vitamin A's health-supporting work is the process of **cell differentiation**, in which each type of cell develops to perform a specific function. For example, when goblet cells (cells that populate the linings of internal organs) mature, they specialize in synthesizing and releasing mucus to protect delicate tissues from toxins or bacteria and other harmful elements.

If vitamin A is deficient, cell differentiation is impaired, and goblet cells fail to mature, fail to make protective mucus, and eventually die off. Goblet cells are then displaced by cells that secrete keratin, mentioned earlier with regard to the eye. Keratin is the same protein that provides toughness in hair and fingernails, but in the wrong place, such as skin and body linings, keratin makes the tissue surfaces dry, hard, and cracked. As dead cells accumulate on the surface, the tissue becomes vulnerable to infection (see Figure 7–3, p. 224). In the cornea, keratinization leads to xerophthalmia; in the lungs, the displacement of mucus-producing cells makes respiratory infections likely; in the urinary tract, the same process leads to urinary tract infections.

Immune Function   Vitamin A has gained a reputation as an "anti-infective" vitamin because so many of the body's defenses against infection depend on an adequate supply.[10] Much research supports the need for vitamin A in the regulation of the genes involved in immunity. Without sufficient vitamin A, these genetic interactions produce an altered response to infection that weakens the body's defenses. Vitamin A nutrition during fetal development may help set the stage for immune function throughout life.[11]

When the defenses are weak, especially in vitamin A–deficient children, an illness such as measles can become severe. A downward spiral of malnutrition and infection can set in. The child's body must devote its scanty store of vitamin A to the immune system's fight against the measles virus, but this destroys the vitamin. As vitamin A dwindles further, the infection worsens. Measles takes the lives of more than 330 of the world's children *every day*.[12] Even if a child survives the infection, permanent blindness is likely to occur. The corneas, already damaged by the chronic vitamin A shortage, degenerate rapidly as their meager supply of vitamin A is diverted to the immune system.

Reproduction and Growth   Vitamin A is essential for normal reproductive processes. In men, vitamin A participates in sperm development, and in women, it supports normal fetal development during pregnancy. In a developing embryo, vitamin A is crucial for the formation of the spinal cord, heart, and other organs.[13]

Vitamin A is also indispensable for growth in children. Normal children's bones grow longer, and the children grow taller, by remodeling each old bone into a new, bigger version. To do so, the body dismantles the old bone structures and replaces them with new, larger bone parts. Growth cannot take place just by adding on to the original small bone; vitamin A must be present for critical bone dismantling steps.[14] Failure to grow is one of the first signs of poor vitamin A status in a child. Restoring vitamin A to such children is imperative, but correcting dietary deficiencies may be more effective than giving vitamin A supplements alone because many other nutrients from nutritious foods are also needed for children to grow normally.

KEY POINTS

- Three active forms of vitamin A and one precursor are important in nutrition.
- Vitamin A plays major roles in gene regulation, eyesight, reproduction, cell differentiation, immunity, and growth.

Vitamin A Deficiency around the World   Vitamin A deficiency presents a vast problem worldwide, placing a heavy burden on society. An estimated 5 million of the world's preschool children suffer from obvious signs of vitamin A deficiency—not only night blindness but diarrhea, appetite loss, and reduced food intake that can rapidly worsen their condition. In addition, a staggering 190 million preschool children suffer from a milder deficiency that impairs immunity, leaving them open to infections.[15]

Figure 7–2

Night Blindness

This is one of the earliest signs of vitamin A deficiency.

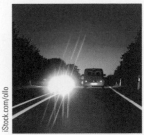

In dim light, you can see what's ahead on the road.

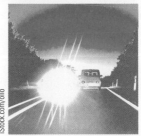

A flash of bright light, such as headlights, momentarily blinds you as the pigment in the retina is bleached.

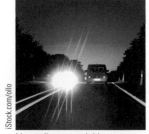

Normally, you quickly recover and can see the details again in a few seconds.

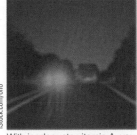

With inadequate vitamin A, you do not recover but remain blind for many seconds or minutes. This is night blindness.

Figure 7–3

The Skin in Vitamin A Deficiency

The hard lumps on the skin of this person's arm reflect accumulations of keratin in the epithelial cells.

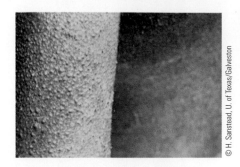

© H. Sanstead, U. of Texas/Galveston

In countries where such children receive vitamin A supplements, childhood rates of blindness, disease, and death have declined dramatically. Even in the United States, vitamin A supplements are recommended for children with measles to ward off deficiency.[16] The World Health Organization (WHO) and United Nations International Children's Emergency Fund (UNICEF) are working to eliminate vitamin A deficiency around the world; achieving this goal would greatly improve child survival.

KEY POINT

- Vitamin A deficiency causes blindness, sickness, and death, and is a major problem worldwide.

Vitamin A Toxicity

For people who take excess active vitamin A in supplements or fortified foods, toxicity is a real possibility. Figure 7–4 shows that toxicity compromises the tissues just as deficiency does and is equally damaging. Symptoms of vitamin A toxicity are many, and they vary depending partly on whether a sudden overdose occurs or too much of the vitamin is taken over time. The figure lists the best-known toxicity symptoms of both kinds. Hair loss, rashes, and a host of uncomfortable general symptoms are possible.

Ordinary vitamin supplements taken in the context of today's fortified food supply can add up to small daily excesses of vitamin A. Substantial amounts can be found in fortified cereals, water beverages, energy bars, and even chewing gum (see Table 7–3).

Pregnant women, especially, should be wary. Excessive vitamin A during pregnancy can injure the spinal cord and other tissues of a developing fetus, causing birth defects.[17] Even a single, massive vitamin A dose (100 times the need) can do so. Children, too, can be easily hurt by vitamin A excesses when they mistake chewable vitamin pills and vitamin-laced gum for treats. Even misinformed adolescents put themselves

Figure 7–4

Vitamin A Deficiency and Toxicity

Danger lies both above and below a normal range of intake of vitamin A.

Vitamin A intake, μg/day	Deficient 0–500		Normal 500–3,000		Toxic 3,000 and over	
	Effects on cells	**Health consequences**	**Effects on cells**	**Health consequences**	**Effects on cells**	**Health consequences**
	Slowed cell division and deficient cell development	Night blindness	Normal cell division and development	Normal body functioning	Overstimulated cell division	Skin rashes
		Keratinization				Hair loss
		Xerophthalmia				Hemorrhages
		Impaired immunity				Bone abnormalities
		Reproductive and growth abnormalities				Birth defects
		Exhaustion				Fractures
		Death				Liver failure
						Death

at risk when they take high doses of vitamin A in misguided attempts to cure acne. Some effective acne remedies are *derived* from vitamin A but they are chemically altered—vitamin A itself has no effect on acne (Chapter 14 comes back to acne).[18]

KEY POINT

- Vitamin A overdose and toxicity cause many serious symptoms.

Vitamin A Recommendations and Sources

You can meet your need for vitamin A in two ways: by consuming the active form in animal food sources, or by consuming beta-carotene in plants. Overdoses of the active form are toxic, so avoiding too much is as important as getting enough. Beta-carotene consumed in fruit and vegetables is harmless. The DRI for vitamin A is based on body weight. A typical man needs a daily average of about 900 micrograms of active vitamin A; a typical woman needs about 700 micrograms. During lactation, her need is higher. Children need less.

The ability of vitamin A to be stored in the tissues means that, although the DRI is stated as a daily amount, you need not consume vitamin A every day. An intake that meets the daily need when averaged over several months is sufficient.

As for vitamin A supplements, the DRI committee warns against exceeding the Tolerable Upper Intake Level (UL) of 3,000 micrograms/day (for adults older than age 18). The best way to ensure a safe intake of vitamin A is to steer clear of supplements that contain it and to rely on food sources instead.

Table 7–3	
Sources of Active Vitamin A	
Vitamin A from highly fortified foods and other rich sources can add up. The UL for vitamin A is 3,000 micrograms (μg) per day.	
High-potency vitamin pill	3,000 μg
Calf's liver, 1 oz cooked	2,300 μg
Regular multivitamin pill	1,500 μg
Vitamin gumball, 1	1,500 μg
Chicken liver, 1 oz cooked	1,400 μg
"Complete" liquid supplement drink, 1 serving	350–1,500 μg
Instant breakfast drink, 1 serving	600–700 μg
Cereal breakfast bar, 1	350–400 μg
"Energy" candy bar, 1	350 μg
Milk, 1 c	150 μg
Vitamin-fortified cereal, 1 serving	150 μg
Margarine, 1 tsp	55 μg

Food Sources of Vitamin A   As mentioned, active vitamin A is present in foods of animal origin. The richest sources are liver and fish oil, but milk and milk products and other vitamin A–fortified foods such as enriched cereals can also be good sources. Even butter and eggs provide some vitamin A. Beta-carotene is naturally present in many vegetable and fruit varieties. In food processing, beta-carotene is prized as a natural source of yellow coloring, and a tiny amount may be added to cheeses to change their color from white to the familiar yellow of cheddar and American-style cheese. The stereotypical fast-food meal—a hamburger, fries, and cola—lacks vitamin A, but most fast-food places also offer fortified milk, or salads with carrots that provide it.

Liver: A Lesson in Moderation   Foods naturally rich in vitamin A pose little risk of toxicity, with the possible exception of liver. When young laboratory pigs eat daily chow made from salmon parts, including the livers, their growth halts, and they fall ill from vitamin A toxicity. Inuit people and Arctic explorers know that polar bear livers are a dangerous food source because the bears eat whole fish (with the livers) and, in turn, concentrate large amounts of vitamin A in their own livers.

An *ounce* of ordinary beef or pork liver delivers three times the DRI for vitamin A intake, and a common portion is 4 to 6 ounces. An occasional serving of liver can provide abundant nutrients and boost nutrient status, but daily use may invite vitamin A toxicity, especially in young children and pregnant women who also routinely take supplements. Snapshot 7–1 shows a sampling of foods that provide more than 10 percent of the Daily Value for a vitamin in a standard-size portion and that therefore qualify as "good sources."

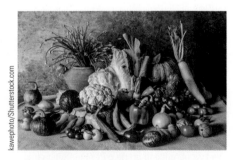
Colorful foods are often rich in vitamins.

kawephoto/Shutterstock.com

KEY POINT

- Vitamin A's active forms are supplied by foods of animal origin.

DRI
Men: 900 μg/day[a]
Women: 700 μg/day[a]

Tolerable Upper Intake Level
Adults: 3,000 μg vitamin A/day

Chief Functions
Vision; maintenance of cornea, epithelial cells, mucous membranes, skin; growth; regulation of gene expression; reproduction; immunity

Deficiency
Night blindness, corneal drying (xerosis), and blindness (xerophthalmia); impaired growth; keratin lumps on the skin; impaired immunity

Toxicity
Vitamin A:
Acute (single dose or short-term): nausea, vomiting, headache, vertigo, blurred vision, uncoordinated muscles, increased pressure inside the skull, birth defects
Chronic: birth defects, liver abnormalities, bone abnormalities, brain and nerve disorders
Beta-carotene: Harmless yellowing of skin

*These foods provide 10% or more of the vitamin A Daily Value in a serving. For a 2,000-cal diet, the DV is 900 μg/day.
[a]Vitamin A recommendations are expressed in retinol activity equivalents (RAE).
[b]This food contains preformed vitamin A.
[c]This food contains the vitamin A precursor, beta-carotene.

Good Sources*

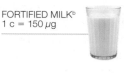
FORTIFIED MILK[b]
1 c = 150 μg

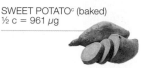
CARROTS[c] (cooked)
½ c = 671 μg

SWEET POTATO[c] (baked)
½ c = 961 μg

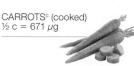
SPINACH[c] (cooked)
½ c = 472 μg

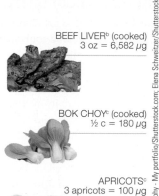
BEEF LIVER[b] (cooked)
3 oz = 6,582 μg

BOK CHOY[c] (cooked)
½ c = 180 μg

APRICOTS[c]
3 apricots = 100 μg

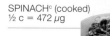

Daniel Gilbey Photography - My portfolio/Shutterstock.com; Elena Schweitzer/Shutterstock.com; Maks Narodenko/Shutterstock.com; Roxana Bashyrova/Shutterstock.com; hlphoto/Shutterstock.com; Jiang Hongyan/Shutterstock.com; Serghei Starus/Shutterstock.com

---

Beta-Carotene

dietary antioxidants compounds typically found in plant foods that counteract the adverse effects of oxidation on living tissues. The major antioxidant vitamins are vitamin E, vitamin C, and beta-carotene. Many phytochemicals are also antioxidants.

carotenoids (CARE-oh-ten-oyds) members of a group of pigments in foods that range in color from light yellow to reddish orange and are chemical relatives of beta-carotene. Many have a degree of vitamin A activity in the body. Also defined in Controversy 2.

macular degeneration a common, progressive loss of function of the part of the retina that is most crucial to focused vision (the macula was shown in Figure 7–1). This degeneration often leads to blindness.

retinol activity equivalents (RAE) a new measure of the vitamin A activity of beta-carotene and other vitamin A precursors that reflects the amount of retinol that the body will derive from a food containing vitamin A precursor compounds.

Beta-carotene is one of many **dietary antioxidants** present in foods. Others include vitamin E, vitamin C, the mineral selenium, and many phytochemicals (see Table 7–4). Bright orange fruit and vegetables derive their color from beta-carotene and are so colorful that they decorate the plate. Carrots, sweet potatoes, pumpkins, mango, cantaloupe, and apricots are all rich sources of beta-carotene—and therefore contribute vitamin A to the eyes and to the rest of the body—so, as an old saying goes, eating carrots is good for the eyes. Another colorful group, *dark* green vegetables, such as spinach, other greens, and broccoli, owes its deep dark green color to the blending of orange beta-carotene with the green leaf pigment chlorophyll.

Chemical relatives of beta-carotene, **carotenoids**, often occur with beta-carotene in plant foods and may also play roles in health. For example, diets lacking in dark green, leafy vegetables and orange vegetables are associated with the most common form of age-related blindness, **macular degeneration**.[†19] The macula, a yellow spot of pigment at the focal center of the retina (identified in Figure 7–1, p. 222), loses integrity, impairing the most important field of vision, the central focus. Evidence does not support taking supplements of carotenoids and other nutrients to prevent or slow the progression of this type of blindness, but many physicians prescribe them.[20]

Measuring Beta-Carotene The conversion of beta-carotene to retinol in the body entails losses, so vitamin A activity for precursors is measured in **retinol activity equivalents (RAE)**. It takes about 12 micrograms of beta-carotene from food

---

[†]The carotenoids associated with protection from macular degeneration are lutein (LOO-tee-in) and its close chemical relative zeaxanthin (zee-ZAN-thin).

to supply the equivalent of 1 microgram of retinol to the body. Some food tables and supplement labels express beta-carotene and vitamin A contents using **IU (international units)**. When comparing vitamin A in foods, be careful to notice whether a food table or supplement label uses micrograms or IU. To convert one to the other, use the factor provided in Appendix C.

Toxicity   Beta-carotene from food is not converted to retinol efficiently enough to cause vitamin A toxicity. A steady diet of abundant pumpkin, carrots, or carrot juice, however, has been known to turn light-skinned people bright yellow because beta-carotene builds up in the fat just beneath the skin and imparts a harmless yellow cast (see Figure 7–5). Likewise, red-colored carotenoids confer a rosy glow on those who consume the fruit and vegetables that contain them.[21] Food sources of the carotenoids are safe, but concentrated supplements may have adverse effects of their own.

Food Sources of Beta-Carotene   Plants contain no active vitamin A, but many vegetables and fruit provide beta-carotene in abundance. Snapshot 7–1 shows good sources of beta-carotene. Other colorful vegetables, such as red beets, red cabbage, and yellow corn, can fool you into thinking they contain beta-carotene, but these foods derive their colors from other pigments and are poor sources of beta-carotene. As for "white" plant foods such as grains and potatoes, they have none. Some confusion exists concerning the term *yam*. A white-fleshed Mexican root vegetable called "yam" is devoid of beta-carotene, but the orange-fleshed sweet potato called "yam" in the United States is one of the richest beta-carotene sources known.

KEY POINTS

- The vitamin A precursor in plants, beta-carotene, is an effective antioxidant in the body.
- Many brightly colored plant foods are rich in beta-carotene.

Vitamin D

LO 7.4   Describe the roles of vitamin D, its sources, and the consequences of its deficiency and toxicity.

Vitamin D is unique among nutrients in that, with the help of sunlight, the body can synthesize all it needs. In this sense, vitamin D is not an *essential* nutrient—given sufficient sun each day, most people can make enough to meet their need from this source.

As simple as it sounds to obtain vitamin D, many people may border on insufficiency. By one measure, an estimated 16 percent of the U.S. population has low blood concentrations of vitamin D.[22‡] The Dietary Guidelines 2015 report lists vitamin D among its nutrients of concern because most people's dietary intakes fall short of the DRI recommendation. Even so, most of the U.S. population has normal blood concentrations, presumably put there by sunshine.

Roles of Vitamin D

Once in the body, whether made from sunlight or obtained from the diet, vitamin D must undergo a series of chemical transformations in the liver and kidneys to be activated. Once activated, vitamin D exerts profound effects on the tissues.

Calcium Regulation   Vitamin D is the best-known member of a large cast of nutrients and hormones that interact to regulate blood calcium and phosphorus concentrations—and thereby maintain bone integrity.[23] Table 7–5 lists nutrients, including vitamin D, that are important for bone health. Calcium is indispensable to the proper functioning of cells in all body tissues, including muscles, nerves, and glands, which draw calcium from the blood as they need it.

---

‡Values <40 nmol/L; consensus about optimal thresholds for 25(OH)D is currently lacking.

Table 7-4

Functional Group of Antioxidants

Key antioxidant vitamins:
- Beta-carotene
- Vitamin E
- Vitamin C

A key antioxidant mineral:
- Selenium

Many antioxidant phytochemicals

Figure 7-5

Excess Beta-Carotene Symptom: Discoloration of the Skin

The hand on the right shows skin discoloration from excess beta-carotene. Another person's normal hand (left) is shown for comparison.

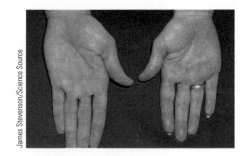

James Stevenson/Science Source

Table 7-5

Functional Group for Bone Health

Key vitamins:
- Vitamin D
- Vitamin K
- Vitamin C

Key minerals:
- Calcium
- Phosphorus
- Magnesium
- Fluoride

Key energy nutrient:
- Protein

IU (international units) a measure of fat-soluble vitamin activity sometimes used in food composition tables and on supplement labels.

When the blood calcium concentration is low, vitamin D acts on three body locations to raise it. First, the skeleton serves as a vast warehouse of stored calcium that can be tapped when blood calcium begins to fall. Second, the digestive tract increases absorption of calcium from food. Third, the kidneys recycle calcium that would otherwise be lost in urine.

Vitamin D and calcium are inextricably linked in nutrition—no matter how much vitamin D you take in, it cannot make up for a chronic shortfall of calcium. The reverse is also true: excess calcium cannot take the place of sufficient vitamin D for bone health.[24]

Other Vitamin D Roles   Activated vitamin D functions as a hormone—that is, a compound manufactured by one organ of the body that acts on other organs, tissues, or cells. Inside cells, for example, vitamin D acts at the genetic level to affect how cells grow, multiply, and differentiate. Vitamin D exerts its effects all over the body, from hair follicles, to reproductive system cells, to cells of the immune system.

Scientists are investigating whether vitamin D may offer protection against a wide variety of ailments, including cardiovascular disease and its risk factors, some cancers, infections, diabetes, autoimmune disorders, impaired brain development, cognitive decline, and more.[25] Vitamin D's impressive array of normal activities in the body may be linked with its numerous potential roles in preventing these diseases. Even so, research does not support taking vitamin D supplements to improve health or prevent diseases except those caused by vitamin D deficiency.[26] The well-established vitamin D roles concern calcium balance and the bones during growth and throughout life, and these form the basis for the DRI values.

KEY POINTS

- Low and borderline blood vitamin D concentrations are not uncommon in the United States.
- When exposed to sunlight, the skin makes vitamin D.
- Vitamin D helps regulate blood calcium and modifies genetic activities with far-reaching effects.

Too Little Vitamin D—A Danger to Bones

Although vitamin D insufficiency is relatively common in the population, overt signs of vitamin D deficiency are rarely reported. The most obvious sign occurs in early life—the abnormality of the bones in the disease **rickets** (as shown in Figure 7–6). Children with rickets develop bowed legs because they are unable to mineralize newly forming bone material, a rubbery protein matrix. As gravity pulls their body weights down against these weak bones, their legs bow.

Preventing Rickets   As early as the 1700s, rickets was known to be curable with cod-liver oil, now recognized as a rich source of vitamin D. More than a hundred years later, a physician linked ultraviolet light and sunlight exposure to prevention and cure of rickets.*

Today, in some areas of the world, such as Mongolia, Tibet, and the Netherlands, more than half of the children suffer the bowed legs, knock-knees, beaded ribs, and protruding pigeon chests of rickets. In the United States, rickets is uncommon but not unknown.[27] Many adolescents abandon vitamin D–fortified milk in favor of soft drinks and punches; they may also spend little time outdoors during daylight hours. Soon, their vitamin D values decline, and they may fail to develop the bone mineral density needed to offset bone loss in later life. To prevent rickets and support optimal bone health, the DRI committee recommends that all infants, children, and adolescents consume the recommended amounts of vitamin D each day.

Deficiency in Adults   In adults, poor mineralization of bone results in the painful bone disease **osteomalacia**.[28] The bones become increasingly soft, flexible, weak, and deformed. Older people can suffer painful joints if their vitamin D

rickets the vitamin D–deficiency disease in children; characterized by abnormal growth of bone and manifested in bowed legs or knock-knees, outward-bowed chest deformity (pigeon chest), and knobs on the ribs.

osteomalacia (OS-tee-o-mal-AY-shuh) the adult expression of vitamin D–deficiency disease, characterized by an overabundance of unmineralized bone protein (*osteo* means "bone"; *mal* means "bad"). Symptoms include bending of the spine and bowing of the legs.

---

*The physician was Kurt Huldschinsky, a German-born pediatrician of Polish heritage.

Chapter 7 The Vitamins

concentrations are low, a condition easily misdiagnosed as arthritis during examinations. Inadequate vitamin D also sets the stage for a loss of calcium from the bones, which can result in fractures from **osteoporosis**. For people with a low vitamin D blood concentration, a vitamin D supplement may help to normalize the blood value and maintain bone mineral density.

Researchers have spent decades asking whether supplemental vitamin D alone or with calcium might reduce the high numbers of bone fractures suffered by middle-aged and elderly people. Their evidence suggests that the simple act of taking a vitamin D and calcium pill could potentially save the life of an institutionalized elderly person who might otherwise fall and suffer a fracture. These benefits do not apply to people living in the community who get outdoors more often. A recent, well-controlled meta-analysis concludes that vitamin D supplements are ineffective for lowering the rate of fractures among community-dwelling adults.[29]

Who Should Be Concerned? People who restrict intakes of fish and dairy foods may not obtain enough vitamin D from food to meet recommendations. Strict vegetarians and people with milk allergies or lactose intolerance in particular must seek out other enriched foods or take supplements to be certain of obtaining enough vitamin D. People living in northern areas of North America; anyone lacking exposure to sunlight, such as office workers or institutionalized older people; and dark-skinned people, their breastfed infants, and their adolescent children often lack vitamin D. Some medications can also compromise vitamin D status.

Concentrations of circulating blood vitamin D have been falling among overweight U.S. adults.[30] Similarly, vitamin D is often reported to be low in the blood of overweight children.[31] Although vitamin sellers use this information to tout vitamin D pills as "obesity cures," scientists suggest that the opposite may be true: *obesity* may impair vitamin D status, and weight loss may help correct the situation.[32]

How can excess fat in the body cause low vitamin D in the blood? Two primary mechanisms have been suggested. First, extra fat tissue requires a great deal of extra blood flow, so vitamin D, even if amply provided, may become diluted in the larger blood volume of overweight people, yielding below-normal test results. Second, fat-soluble vitamin D may be taken up and sequestered in the fat tissue of overweight people, making it less available to the bloodstream.[33] Research concerning obesity and vitamin D deficiency is ongoing.

KEY POINTS

- A vitamin D deficiency causes rickets in childhood, low bone density in adolescence, and osteomalacia in later life.
- Vitamin D deficiency is likely in overweight people, those in northern climates, those who lack sun exposure, and among adults, breastfed infants, and adolescents with darker skin.

Too Much Vitamin D—A Danger to Soft Tissues

Vitamin D is the most potentially toxic among the vitamins. Vitamin D intoxication raises the concentration of blood calcium by withdrawing bone calcium, which can then collect in the soft tissues and damage them. With chronic high vitamin D intakes, kidney and heart function decline, blood calcium spins further out of control, and, when the kidneys and heart ultimately fail, death ensues.

High doses of vitamin D may bring on high blood calcium, nausea, fatigue, back pain, irregular heartbeat, and increased urination and thirst. Several reports of patients with high blood calcium have emerged as more and more people self-prescribe high-dose vitamin D supplements in response to preliminary reports of potential health benefits.[34]

KEY POINTS

- Vitamin D is the most potentially toxic vitamin.
- Overdoses raise blood calcium and damage soft tissues.

Figure 7–6
Rickets

This child has the bowed legs of the vitamin D–deficiency disease, rickets.

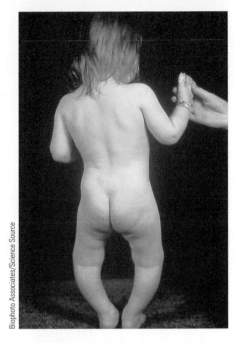

Biophoto Associates/Science Source

This child displays beaded ribs, a symptom of rickets.

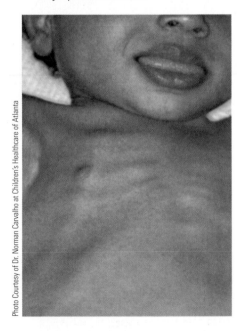

Photo Courtesy of Dr. Norman Carvalho at Children's Healthcare of Atlanta

osteoporosis a weakening of bone mineral structures caused by calcium loss that occurs commonly with advancing age. Also defined in Chapter 8.

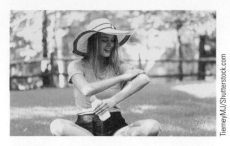
The sunshine vitamin: vitamin D.

Vitamin D from Sunlight

Sunlight supplies the needed vitamin D for most of the world's people. Sunlight presents no risk of vitamin D toxicity because after a certain amount of vitamin D collects in the skin, the sunlight itself begins breaking it down.

Vitamin D Synthesis and Activation   When ultraviolet (UV) light rays from the sun reach a cholesterol compound in human skin, the compound is transformed into a vitamin D precursor and is absorbed directly into the blood. Slowly, over the next day and a half, the liver and kidneys finish converting the inactive precursor to the active form of vitamin D. Diseases that affect either the liver or the kidneys can impair this conversion and therefore produce symptoms of vitamin D deficiency.

Like natural sunscreen, the pigments of dark skin protect against UV radiation. To synthesize several days' worth of vitamin D, dark-skinned people require up to 3 hours of direct sun (depending on the climate). Light-skinned people need much less time (an estimated 5 minutes without sunscreen or 10 to 30 minutes with sunscreen). Vitamin D deficiency is especially prevalent if sunlight is weak, such as in the winter months and in the extreme northern regions of the world. In fact, some scientists now suggest that seasonally different criteria should be considered when assessing vitamin D blood concentrations in a clinical setting.[35] The factors listed in Table 7–6 can all interfere with vitamin D synthesis.

KEY POINT

- Ultraviolet light from sunshine acts on a cholesterol compound in the skin to make vitamin D.

Table 7–6

Factors Affecting Vitamin D Synthesis

The more of these factors that are present in a person's life, the more critical it becomes to obtain vitamin D from food or supplements.

Factor	Effect on Vitamin D Synthesis
Advanced age	With age, the skin loses some of its capacity to synthesize vitamin D.
Air pollution	Particles in the air screen out the sun's rays.
City living	Tall buildings block sunlight.
Clothing	Most clothing blocks sunlight.
Cloudy skies	Heavy cloud cover reduces sunlight penetration.
Geography	Sunlight exposure is limited: • October through March at latitudes above 43 degrees (most of Canada) • November through February at latitudes between 35 and 43 degrees (many U.S. locations) In locations south of 35 degrees (much of the southern United States), direct sun exposure is sufficient for vitamin D synthesis year-round.
Homebound	Living indoors prevents sun exposure.
Season	Warmer seasons of the year bring more direct sun rays.
Skin pigment	Darker-skinned people synthesize less vitamin D per minute than lighter-skinned people.
Sunscreen	Proper use reduces or prevents skin exposure to sun's rays.
Time of day	Midday hours bring maximum direct sun exposure.

DRI

Adults: 15 µg (600 IU)/day (19–70 yr)
20 µg (700 IU)/day (> 70 yr)

Tolerable Upper Intake Level

Adults: 100 µg (4,000 IU)/day

Chief Functions

Mineralization of bones and teeth (raises blood calcium and phosphorus by increasing absorption from digestive tract, withdrawing calcium from bones, stimulating retention by kidneys)

Deficiency

Abnormal bone growth resulting in rickets in children, osteomalacia in adults; malformed teeth; muscle spasms

Toxicity

Elevated blood calcium; calcification of soft tissues (blood vessels, kidneys, heart, lungs, tissues of joints), excessive thirst, headache, nausea, weakness

*These foods provide 10% or more of the vitamin D Daily Value in a serving. For a 2,000-cal diet, the DV is 20 µg/day.
[a]Average value.
[b]Avoid prolonged exposure to sun.

Good Sources*

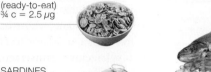
ENRICHED CEREAL
(ready-to-eat)
¾ c = 2.5 µg

SARDINES
3 oz = 4.1 µg

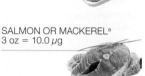
SALMON OR MACKEREL[a]
3 oz = 10.0 µg

SUNLIGHT
Promotes vitamin D
synthesis in
the skin.[b]

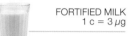
COD-LIVER OIL
1 tsp = 11 µg

FORTIFIED MILK
1 c = 3 µg

TUNA (light, canned)
3 oz = 5.7 µg

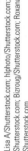
Lisa A/Shutterstock.com; hlphoto/Shutterstock.com; Picsfive/Shutterstock.com; starklem/Shutterstock.com; Bizroug/Shutterstock.com; Roxana Bashyrova/Shutterstock.com; tab62/Shutterstock.com

Vitamin D Intake Recommendations

The need for vitamin D remains remarkably steady throughout most of life. People ages 1 to 70 years old need 15 micrograms of vitamin D daily. For those 71 and older, the need jumps to 20 micrograms per day because this group faces an increased threat of bone fractures. The UL for vitamin D for adults of all ages is 100 micrograms (4,000 IU), above which the risk of harm from overdoses increases.

Vitamin D from the sun, while substantial, varies widely among people of different ages and living in different locations. Measuring the contribution of vitamin D from sunlight is difficult, and sun exposure increases skin cancer risks, so the DRI committee set its recommendations in terms of dietary vitamin D alone, with no contribution from the sun.[36] The recommendations do assume an adequate intake of calcium because vitamin D and calcium each alter the body's handling of the other.

The recommendations are set high enough to maintain blood vitamin D concentrations known to support healthy bones throughout life, but some research suggests that recommendations for some people should be set even higher. Some scientists suggest using mathematical equations that take into account factors such as ethnicity, body mass index (BMI), age, sex, seasonal variability, latitude location, and UV light exposure when determining vitamin D intake recommendations.[37]

KEY POINT

- The DRI for dietary vitamin D varies little through most of life.

Vitamin D Food Sources

Snapshot 7–2 shows the few significant naturally occurring food sources of vitamin D. In addition, egg yolks provide small amounts, along with butter and cream. Milk, whether fluid, dried, or evaporated, is fortified with vitamin D, so it constitutes a major food source for the United States. Yogurt and cheese products may lack vitamin D,

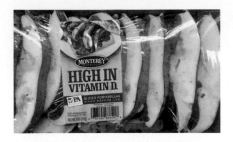

Mushrooms grown in sunlight or treated with UV light are rich sources of vitamin D. Mushrooms grown in the dark are poor sources.

however, whereas orange juice, cereals, margarines, and other foods may be fortified with it, so read the labels.

Many mushroom species, when grown in sunlight, produce substantial vitamin D; when grown without sunlight, the same species produce almost none, a variability that makes mushrooms an unreliable vitamin D source. Commercial producers may enrich common mushroom varieties by briefly exposing them to ultraviolet light. The vitamin D-rich mushrooms look and taste like the ordinary kind, but their labels often advertise their vitamin D content. Without UV light treatment, mushrooms are a poor source of vitamin D.[38]

Young adults who drink 3 cups of milk a day receive half of their daily requirement from this source; much of the rest comes from exposure to sunlight and other foods and supplements. Vegans can rely on vitamin D–fortified foods, such as cereals and beverages, along with supplements, to supply vitamin D. Importantly, feeding infants and young children unfortified "health beverages" instead of milk or infant formula can cause severe nutrient deficiencies, including rickets.

KEY POINT

- Food sources of vitamin D include a few naturally rich sources and many fortified foods.

Vitamin E

LO 7.5 Describe the roles, food sources, and effects of deficiency and toxicity of vitamin E.

Almost a century ago, researchers discovered a compound in vegetable oils essential for reproduction in rats. This compound was named **tocopherol** from *tokos*, a Greek word meaning "offspring." A few years later, the compound was named vitamin E.

Four tocopherol compounds have long been known to be of importance in nutrition, and each is designated by one of the first four letters of the Greek alphabet: alpha, beta, gamma, and delta. Of these, alpha-tocopherol is the gold standard for vitamin E activity, and the DRI values are expressed as alpha-tocopherol. Additional forms of vitamin E have also been identified and are of interest to researchers for potential roles in health.[§39]

Roles of Vitamin E

Vitamin E is an antioxidant and thus acts as a bodyguard against oxidative damage. Such damage occurs when highly unstable molecules known as **free radicals**, formed during normal cell metabolism, run amok. Left unchecked, free radicals create a destructive chain reaction that can damage the polyunsaturated lipids in cell membranes and lipoproteins, the DNA in genetic material, and the working proteins of cells. According to the theory of **oxidative stress**, this situation creates inflammation and cell damage associated with aging processes, cancer development, heart disease, diabetes, and a variety of other diseases.[40] Vitamin E, by being oxidized itself, quenches free radicals and reduces inflammation. Figure 7–7 (p. 233) provides an overview of the antioxidant activity of vitamin E and its potential role in disease prevention.[41]

The antioxidant protection of vitamin E is crucial, particularly in the lungs, where high oxygen concentrations would otherwise disrupt vulnerable membranes. Red blood cell membranes also need vitamin E's protection as they transport oxygen from the lungs to other tissues. White blood cells that fight diseases equally depend on vitamin E's antioxidant nature, as do blood vessel linings, sensitive brain tissues, and even bones.[42] Tocopherols also perform some nonantioxidant tasks that support the body's health.

Vitamin E Deficiency

A deficiency of vitamin E produces a wide variety of symptoms in laboratory animals, but these are almost never seen in otherwise healthy human beings. Deficiency of vitamin E, which dissolves in fat, may occur in people with diseases that cause fat malabsorption or in infants born prematurely. Disease or injury of the liver (which makes bile,

tocopherol (tuh-KOFF-er-all) a kind of alcohol. The active form of vitamin E is alpha-tocopherol.

free radicals atoms or molecules with one or more unpaired electrons that make the atom or molecule unstable and highly reactive.

oxidative stress a theory of disease causation involving cell and tissue damage that arises when free radical reactions exceed the capacity of antioxidants to quench them.

§The other forms of Vitamin E are tocotrienols: alpha, beta, gamma, and delta.

Figure 7-7

Free-Radical Damage and Antioxidant Protection

Free-radical formation occurs during metabolic processes, and it accelerates when diseases or other stresses strike.

Free radicals cause chain reactions that damage cellular structures.

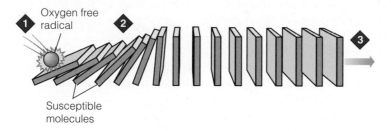

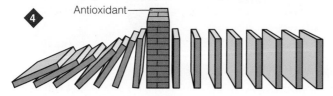

1 A chemically reactive oxygen free radical attacks fatty acid, DNA, protein, or cholesterol molecules, which form other free radicals in turn.

2 This initiates a rapid, destructive chain reaction.

3 The result is:
- Cell membrane lipid damage.
- Cellular protein damage.
- DNA damage.
- Oxidation of LDL cholesterol.
- Inflammation.

These changes may initiate steps leading to diseases such as heart disease, cancer, macular degeneration, and others.

4 Antioxidants, such as vitamin E, stop the chain reaction by changing the nature of the free radical.

necessary for digestion of fat), the gallbladder (which delivers bile into the intestine), or the pancreas (which makes fat-digesting enzymes) makes vitamin E deficiency likely. In people without diseases, low blood concentrations of vitamin E are most likely the result of years of consuming diets extremely low in fat.

A classic vitamin E deficiency occurs in babies born prematurely, before the transfer of the vitamin from the mother to the fetus, which occurs late in pregnancy. Without sufficient vitamin E, the infant's red blood cells rupture (**erythrocyte hemolysis**), and the infant becomes anemic. The few symptoms of vitamin E deficiency observed in adults include loss of muscle coordination, loss of normal reflexes, and impaired vision and speech. Vitamin E corrects all of these symptoms.

Toxicity of Vitamin E

Vitamin E in foods is safe to consume, and reports of vitamin E toxicity symptoms are rare across a broad range of intakes. However, vitamin E in supplements augments the effects of anticoagulant medication used to oppose unwanted blood clotting, so people taking such drugs risk uncontrollable bleeding if they also take vitamin E. Supplemental doses of vitamin E prolong blood clotting times and increase the risk of brain hemorrhages, a form of stroke that has been noted among people taking supplements of vitamin E.[43]

Pooled results from 78 experiments involving over a quarter-million people suggest that taking vitamin E supplements may increase mortality in both healthy and sick people.[44] Other studies find no effect or a slight decrease in mortality among groups taking low or moderate doses of vitamin E.[45] To err on the safe side, people who use vitamin E supplements should probably keep their dosages low, not exceeding the UL of 1,000 milligrams of alpha-tocopherol per day.

Vitamin E Recommendations and U.S. Intakes

The DRI (back of the book, p. B) for vitamin E is 15 milligrams a day for adults. This amount is sufficient to maintain healthy, normal blood values for vitamin E for most people. On average, U.S. intakes of vitamin E fall substantially below the recommendation (see Figure 7–8).[46] The need for vitamin E rises as people consume more polyunsaturated oil because the oil requires antioxidant protection by the vitamin. Luckily, most raw oils also contain vitamin E, so people who eat raw oils also receive the vitamin. Smokers may have higher needs.

Figure 7-8

Vitamin E Recommendations and Intakes Compared

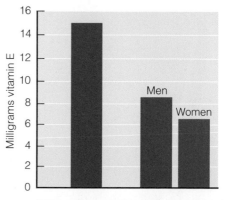

erythrocyte (eh-REETH-ro-sight)
hemolysis (hee-MOLL-ih-sis) rupture of the red blood cells that can be caused by vitamin E deficiency (*erythro* means "red"; *cyte* means "cell"; *hemo* means "blood"; *lysis* means "breaking"). The anemia produced by the condition is *hemolytic* (HEE-moh-LIT-ick) *anemia*.

Snapshot 7-3 Vitamin E

DRI
Adults: 15 mg/day

Tolerable Upper Intake Level
Adults: 1,000 mg/day

Chief Functions
Antioxidant (protects cell membranes, regulates oxidation reactions, protects polyunsaturated fatty acids)

Deficiency
Red blood cell breakage, nerve damage

Toxicity
Augments the effects of anticlotting medication

*These foods provide 10% or more of the vitamin E Daily Value in a serving. For a 2,000-cal diet, the DV is 22 IU or 15 mg/day.
[a]Cooking destroys vitamin E.*

Good Sources*

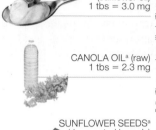

SAFFLOWER OIL[a] (raw)
1 tbs = 4.6 mg

WHEAT GERM
1 oz = 4.5 mg

MAYONNAISE (safflower oil)
1 tbs = 3.0 mg

CANOLA OIL[a] (raw)
1 tbs = 2.3 mg

SUNFLOWER SEEDS[a] (dry roasted kernels)
2 tbs = 4.18 mg

iStock.com/Aleaimage; Reika/Shutterstock.com; librakv/Shutterstock.com; Heike Brauer/Shutterstock.com; Robyn Mackenzie/Shutterstock.com

---

Vitamin E Food Sources

Vitamin E is widespread in foods (see Snapshot 7–3). Much of the vitamin E that people consume comes from vegetable oils and products made from them, such as margarine and salad dressings. Wheat germ oil is especially rich in vitamin E. Animal fats have almost none.

Vitamin E is readily destroyed by heat, as Figure 7–9 illustrates, and by oxidation—thus, fresh, raw oils and lightly processed vitamin E–rich foods are the best sources. As people choose more ultra-processed foods, fried fast foods, or "convenience" foods, they lose vitamin E because little vitamin E survives the heating and other processes used to make these foods. Authorities recommend increasing vitamin E–rich foods in the diet to close the gap between DRI amounts and average intakes.

KEY POINTS

- Vitamin E acts as an antioxidant in cell membranes.
- Average U.S. intakes fall short of DRI recommendations.
- Vitamin E–deficiency disease occurs rarely. Newborn premature infants may be deficient, however.
- Vitamin E supplements may carry risks but toxicity is rare.

Vitamin K

LO 7.6 Describe the roles of vitamin K, its food sources, and the effects of its deficiency and toxicity.

Have you ever thought about how remarkable it is that blood can clot? The liquid turns solid in a life-saving series of reactions. If blood did not clot, wounds would just keep bleeding, draining the blood from the body.

Roles of Vitamin K

The main function of vitamin K** is to help activate proteins that help clot the blood. Hospitals measure the clotting time of a person's blood before surgery and, if needed, administer vitamin K supplementation to reduce bleeding during the operation.

**K stands for the Danish word koagulation ("clotting").

Figure 7-9

High Temperatures Destroy Vitamin E

Restaurants typically reuse frying oil several times before replacing it, a practice that destroys most or all of its vitamin E.

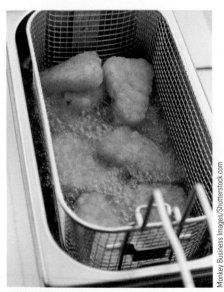

Source: Data from A. Chiou and N. Kalogeropoulos, Virgin olive oil as frying oil, Comprehensive Reviews in Food Science and Food Safety (2017), epub, doi: 10.1111/1541-4337.12268.

Monkey Business Images/Shutterstock.com

Supplemental vitamin K is of value only if a deficiency exists. Vitamin K does not improve clotting in those with other bleeding disorders, such as the inherited disease hemophilia.

Some people with heart problems need to *prevent* the formation of clots within their circulatory systems—this is popularly referred to as "thinning" the blood. One of the best-known medicines for this purpose is warfarin (pronounced WAR-fuh-rin), which interferes with vitamin K's clot-promoting action. Vitamin K therapy may be needed for people on warfarin if uncontrolled bleeding should occur.[47] People taking warfarin who self-prescribe vitamin K supplements risk causing dangerous clotting of their blood; those who suddenly stop taking vitamin K risk causing excess bleeding.

Vitamin K is also necessary for the synthesis of key bone proteins. With low blood vitamin K, the bones produce an abnormal protein that cannot effectively bind the minerals that normally form bones.[48] People who consume abundant vitamin K in the form of green leafy vegetables suffer fewer hip fractures than those with lower intakes.[49] Whether vitamin K supplementation is effective against bone loss, however, is unclear, and more research is needed to clarify the links between vitamin K and bone health.[50]

Vitamin K Deficiency

Few U.S. adults are likely to experience vitamin K deficiency, even if they seldom eat vitamin K–rich foods. This is because, like vitamin D, vitamin K can be obtained from a nonfood source—in this case, the intestinal bacteria. Billions of bacteria normally reside in the intestines, and some of them synthesize vitamin K.

Newborn infants present a unique case with regard to vitamin K because they are born with sterile intestinal tracts and the vitamin K–producing bacteria take weeks to establish themselves. To prevent hemorrhage, newborns are given a single dose of vitamin K at birth (as illustrated in Figure 7–10).[51] In an alarming trend, the number of parents who refuse vitamin K treatment for newborns has recently increased. This has led to increases in vitamin K deficiency–related vomiting, lethargy, and even bleeding, including bleeding of the brain in such babies.[52] Prospective parents should be informed that vitamin K injections at birth pose almost no risk but can avert major problems in newborns.

People who have taken antibiotics that have killed the bacteria in their intestinal tracts also may develop vitamin K deficiency. In other medical conditions, bile production falters, making lipids, including all of the fat-soluble vitamins, unabsorbable. Supplements of the vitamin are needed in these cases because a vitamin K deficiency can be fatal.

Vitamin K Toxicity

Reports of vitamin K toxicity among healthy adults are rare, and the DRI committee has not set a UL for vitamin K. For infants and pregnant women, however, vitamin K toxicity can result when supplements of a synthetic version of vitamin K are given too enthusiastically.[††] Toxicity induces breakage of the red blood cells and release of their pigment, which colors the skin yellow. A toxic dose of synthetic vitamin K causes the liver to release the blood cell pigment (bilirubin) into the blood (instead of excreting it into the bile) and leads to **jaundice**.

Vitamin K Requirements and Sources

The vitamin K requirement for men is 120 micrograms a day; women require 90 micrograms. As Snapshot 7–4 shows, vitamin K's richest plant food sources include dark green, leafy vegetables such as cooked spinach and other greens, which provide an average of 300 micrograms per half-cup serving. Lettuces, broccoli, brussels sprouts, and other members of the cabbage family are also good sources.

Among protein foods, soybeans, green and black-eyed peas, and split pea soup are rich sources. Canola and soybean oils (unhydrogenated liquid oils) provide smaller but still significant amounts; fortified cereals can also be rich sources of added vitamin K. Databases of food composition now include the vitamin K contents of many foods, thanks to improved methods of analysis.

[††]The version of vitamin K responsible for this effect is menadione.

Figure 7–10
Vitamin K in Newborns

Soon after birth, newborn infants receive a dose of vitamin K to prevent hemorrhage.

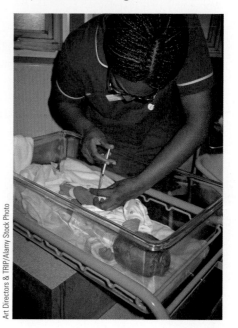

jaundice (JAWN-dis) yellowing of the skin due to spillover of the bile pigment bilirubin (bill-ee-ROO-bin) from the liver into the general circulation.

DRI
Men: 120 μg/day
Women: 90 μg/day

Chief Functions
Synthesis of blood-clotting proteins and bone proteins

Deficiency
Hemorrhage; abnormal bone formation

Toxicity
Opposes the effects of anticlotting medication

*These foods provide 10% or more of the vitamin K Daily Value in a serving. For a 2,000-cal diet, the DV is 120 μg/day.
ªAverage value.

Good Sources*

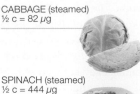
CABBAGE (steamed)
½ c = 82 μg

KALE (cooked)
1 c = 1062 μg

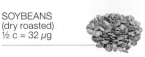
SPINACH (steamed)
½ c = 444 μg

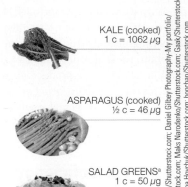
ASPARAGUS (cooked)
½ c = 46 μg

SOYBEANS
(dry roasted)
½ c = 32 μg

SALAD GREENSª
1 c = 50 μg

Jiri Hera/Shutterstock.com; Daniel Gilbey Photography-My portfolio/Shutterstock.com; Maks Narodenko/Shutterstock.com; Gaak/Shutterstock.com; Anna Hoychuk/Shutterstock.com; bonchan/Shutterstock.com

KEY POINTS

- Vitamin K is necessary for blood to clot.
- Vitamin K deficiency causes uncontrolled bleeding.
- Excess vitamin K can cause harm.
- The bacterial inhabitants of the digestive tract produce vitamin K.

The Water-Soluble Vitamins

LO 7.7   Summarize the characteristics and functions of the water-soluble vitamins.

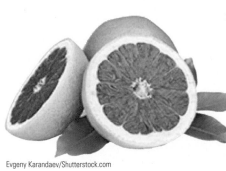
Evgeny Karandaev/Shutterstock.com

Vitamin C and the B vitamins dissolve in water, which has implications for their handling in food and by the body. In food, water-soluble vitamins easily dissolve and drain away with cooking water, and some are destroyed on exposure to light, heat, or oxygen during processing. Later sections examine vitamin vulnerability and provide tips for retaining vitamins in foods. Recall characteristics of water-soluble vitamins from Table 7–2.

In the body, water-soluble vitamins are easily absorbed and just as easily excreted in the urine. A few of the water-soluble vitamins can remain in the lean tissues for a month or more, but these tissues actively exchange materials with the body fluids all the time—no real storage tissues exist for any water-soluble vitamins. At any time, the vitamins may be picked up by the extracellular fluids, washed away by the blood, and excreted in the urine.

Advice for meeting the need for these nutrients is straightforward: choose foods rich in water-soluble vitamins frequently to achieve an average intake that meets the recommendation over a few days' time. The Snapshots in this section can help guide your choices. Foods never deliver toxic doses of the water-soluble vitamins, and their easy excretion in the urine protects against toxicity from all but the largest supplemental doses.

KEY POINTS

- Water-soluble vitamins are easily absorbed and excreted from the body, and foods that supply them must be consumed frequently.
- Water-soluble vitamins are easily lost or destroyed during food preparation and processing.

Do athletes who strive for top performance need more vitamins than foods can supply? Competitive athletes who choose their diets with reasonable care almost never need nutrient supplements. The reason is elegantly simple. The need for energy to fuel exercise requires that people eat extra calories of food, and if that extra food is of the kind shown in this chapter's Snapshots—fruit, vegetables, milk, eggs, whole or enriched grains, lean meats, and some oils—then the extra vitamins needed to support the activity flow naturally into the body. Chapter 10 comes back to the roles of vitamins in physical activity.

start now! If you haven't already done so, access Diet & Wellness Plus in MindTap and track your diet for three days, including one weekend day. After you have recorded your foods for three days, create an Intake Report to see how close you come to meeting the nutrient recommendations for a person of your age, weight, and level of physical activity.

Vitamin C

LO 7.8 Identify the roles of vitamin C, effects of its deficiency and toxicity, and its food sources.

More than 200 years ago, any man who joined the crew of a seagoing ship knew he had only half a chance of returning alive—not because he might be slain by pirates or die in a storm but because he might contract **scurvy**, a disease that often killed many members of a ship's crew on a long voyage. Ships that sailed on short voyages, especially around the Mediterranean Sea, were safe from this disease. The special hazard of long ocean voyages was that the ship's cook used up the perishable fresh fruit and vegetables early and relied on cereals and live animals for the duration of the voyage.

The first nutrition experiment to be conducted on human beings was devised more than 250 years ago to find a cure for scurvy. A physician divided some British sailors with scurvy into groups.[‡‡] Each group received a different test substance: vinegar, sulfuric acid, seawater, oranges, or lemons. Those receiving the citrus fruit were cured within a short time. Sadly, it took 50 years for the British navy to make use of the information and require all its vessels to provide lime juice to every sailor daily. British sailors were mocked with the term *limey* because of this requirement. The name later given to the vitamin that the fruit provided, **ascorbic acid**, literally means "no-scurvy acid." It is more commonly known today as vitamin C.

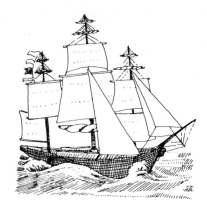

Long voyages without fresh fruit and vegetables spelled death by scurvy for the crew.

The Roles of Vitamin C

Vitamin C performs a variety of functions in the body. It is best known for two of them: its work in maintaining the connective tissues and as an antioxidant.

Connective Tissue   The enzymes involved in the formation and maintenance of the protein **collagen** depend on vitamin C for their activity, as do many other enzymes of the body. Collagen forms the base for all of the connective tissues: bones, teeth, skin, and tendons. Collagen forms the scar tissue that heals wounds, the reinforcing structure that mends fractures, and the supporting material of capillaries that prevents bruises. Vitamin C also participates in other synthetic reactions, such as in the production of carnitine, an important compound for transporting fatty acids within the cells, and in the creation of certain hormones.

Antioxidant Activity   Vitamin C also acts in a more general way as an antioxidant.[53] Vitamin C protects substances found in foods and in the body from oxidation by being oxidized itself. For example, cells of the immune system maintain high concentrations of vitamin C to protect themselves from free radicals that they generate to use

scurvy the vitamin C–deficiency disease.

ascorbic acid one of the active forms of vitamin C (the other is *dehydroascorbic* acid); an antioxidant nutrient.

collagen (COLL-a-jen) the chief protein of most connective tissues, including scars, ligaments, and tendons, and the underlying matrix on which bones and teeth are built.

[‡‡]The physician was James Lind.

Vitamin C

DRI
Men: 90 mg/day
Women: 75 mg/day
Smokers: add 35 mg/day

Tolerable Upper Intake Level
Adults: 2,000 mg/day

Chief Functions
Collagen synthesis (strengthens blood vessel walls, forms scar tissue, provides matrix for bone growth), antioxidant, restores vitamin E to active form, supports immune system, boosts iron absorption

Deficiency
Scurvy, with pinpoint hemorrhages, fatigue, bleeding gums, bruises; bone fragility, joint pain; poor wound healing, frequent infections

Toxicity
Nausea, abdominal cramps, diarrhea; rashes; interference with medical tests and drug therapies; in susceptible people, aggravation of gout or kidney stones

*These foods provide 10% or more of the vitamin C Daily Value in a serving. For a 2,000-cal diet, the DV is 90 mg/day.

Good Sources*

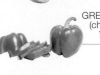

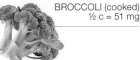
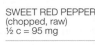

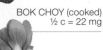

SWEET RED PEPPER (chopped, raw) ½ c = 95 mg

ORANGE JUICE ½ c = 62 mg

GREEN PEPPER (chopped, raw) ½ c = 60 mg

BRUSSELS SPROUTS (cooked) ½ c = 48 mg

BROCCOLI (cooked) ½ c = 51 mg

GRAPEFRUIT ⅓ c = 43 mg

STRAWBERRIES ½ c = 42 mg

SWEET POTATO ½ c = 20 mg

BOK CHOY (cooked) ½ c = 22 mg

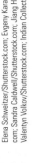
Elena Schweitzer/Shutterstock.com; Evgeny Karandaev/Shutterstock.com; Mayer Kleinostheim/Shutterstock.com; Sandra Caldwell/Shutterstock.com; Jiang Hongyan/Shutterstock.com; Denis Nata/Shutterstock.com; Valentyn Volkov/Shutterstock.com; Indian Collections/Shutterstock.com; Anna Kucherova/Shutterstock.com

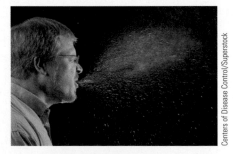
Centers of Disease Control/Superstock

Can vitamin C ease the suffering of a person with a cold?

prooxidant a compound that triggers reactions involving oxygen.

during assaults on bacteria and other invaders. After use, some oxidized vitamin C is degraded irretrievably and must be replaced by the diet. Most of the vitamin, however, is not lost but efficiently recycled back to its active form for reuse.

In the intestines, vitamin C protects iron from oxidation and so promotes its absorption. Once in the blood, vitamin C protects sensitive blood constituents from oxidation, reduces tissue inflammation, and helps to maintain the body's supply of vitamin E by protecting it and recycling it to its active form. The antioxidant roles of vitamin C are the focus of extensive study, especially in relation to prevention of chronic diseases.

In test tubes, a high concentration of vitamin C has the opposite effect from an antioxidant; that is, it acts as a **prooxidant** by activating oxidizing elements, such as iron and copper.[54] In the body, iron and copper are tightly bound to special proteins that normally control such interactions.[55]

Can Vitamin C Supplements Cure a Cold?   Many people hold that vitamin C supplements can prevent or cure a common cold, but research most often fails to support this long-lived belief.[56] In 29 trials of over 11,300 people, no relationship emerged between routine vitamin C supplementation and cold prevention. A few studies do report other modest potential benefits—fewer colds, fewer ill days, and shorter duration of severe symptoms, especially for those exposed to physical and environmental stresses, as well as those with low vitamin C status. *Sufficient* vitamin C intake is critically important to certain white blood cells of the immune system that act as primary defenders against infection.[57]

Experimentally, supplements of at least 1 gram of vitamin C per day and often closer to 2 grams (the UL and not recommended) seem to reduce blood histamine. Anyone who has ever had a cold knows the effects of histamine: sneezing, a runny or stuffy nose, and swollen sinuses. In drug-like doses, vitamin C may mimic a weak antihistamine drug, but studies vary in dosing and conditions; drawing conclusions is therefore difficult.

One other effect of taking pills might also provide relief. In one vitamin C study, some experimental subjects received a sugar pill but were told they were receiving vitamin C. These subjects reported having fewer colds than the group who had in fact received the vitamin but who thought they were receiving the placebo. At work was the healing effect of faith in a medical treatment—the placebo effect.

Deficiency Symptoms and Intakes

Most of the symptoms of scurvy can be attributed to the breakdown of collagen in the absence of vitamin C: loss of appetite, growth cessation, tenderness to touch, weakness, bleeding gums (as shown in Figure 7–11), loose teeth, swollen ankles and wrists, and tiny red spots in the skin where blood has leaked out of capillaries (also shown in the figure). One symptom, anemia, reflects an important role worth repeating—vitamin C helps the body to absorb and use iron. Table 7–9 (p. 256) summarizes deficiency symptoms and other information about vitamin C.

Vitamin C is listed among the nutrients of national concern because U.S. intakes may fall short of the DRI recommendations. People who smoke or have low incomes are particularly at risk for deficiency. The disease scurvy is seldom seen today except in a few elderly people, people addicted to alcohol or other drugs, sick people in hospitals, people with eating disorders who severely restrict food intake, and a few infants who are fed only cow's milk.[58] Breast milk and infant formula supply enough vitamin C, but infants who are fed cow's milk and receive no vitamin C in formula, fruit juice, or other outside sources are at risk. As for the elderly, poor appetites and low intakes of fruit and vegetables often lead to low vitamin C intakes.

Vitamin C Toxicity

The easy availability of vitamin C in pill form and the publication of books recommending vitamin C to prevent and cure colds and cancer have led thousands of people to take huge doses of vitamin C. These "volunteer" subjects enabled researchers to study potential adverse effects of large vitamin C doses. One effect observed with a 2-gram dose is alteration of the insulin response to carbohydrate in people with otherwise normal glucose tolerances. People taking anticlotting medications may unwittingly counteract the drug's effect if they also take massive doses of vitamin C. Those with kidney disease, a tendency toward gout, or abnormal vitamin C metabolism are prone to forming kidney stones if they take large doses of vitamin C.[59] Vitamin C supplements in any dosage may be unwise for people with an overload of iron in the body because vitamin C increases iron absorption from the intestine and releases iron from storage. Other adverse effects are mild, including digestive upsets, such as nausea, abdominal cramps, excessive gas, and diarrhea.

The safe range of vitamin C intakes seems to be broad, from the absolute minimum of 10 milligrams a day to the UL of 2,000 milligrams (2 grams), as Figure 7–12 demonstrates. Doses approaching 10 grams can be expected to be unsafe. Vitamin C from food is always safe.

Vitamin C Recommendations

The adult DRI for vitamin C is 90 milligrams for men and 75 milligrams for women. These amounts are far higher than the 10 or so milligrams per day needed to prevent the symptoms of scurvy. In fact, they are close to the amount at which the body's pool of vitamin C is full to overflowing: about 100 milligrams per day.

Tobacco use introduces oxidants that deplete the body's vitamin C. Thus, smokers generally have lower blood vitamin C concentrations than nonsmokers. Even "passive smokers" who live and work with smokers and those who regularly chew tobacco need more vitamin C than others. Intake recommendations for smokers are set high, at

Figure 7–11

Scurvy Symptoms—Gums and Skin

Vitamin C deficiency causes the breakdown of collagen, which supports the teeth.

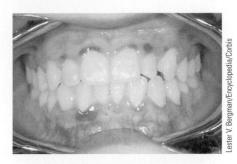

Small pinpoint hemorrhages (red spots) appear in the skin, indicating that invisible internal bleeding may also be occurring.

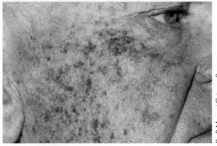

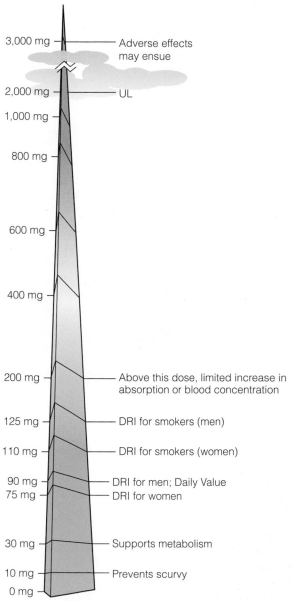

Figure 7–12

Vitamin C Tower of Recommendations

The DRI Tolerable Upper Intake Level (UL) for vitamin C is set at 2,000 mg (2 g)/day. Only 10 mg/day prevents scurvy.

3,000 mg — Adverse effects may ensue

2,000 mg — UL

1,000 mg

800 mg

600 mg

400 mg

200 mg — Above this dose, limited increase in absorption or blood concentration

125 mg — DRI for smokers (men)

110 mg — DRI for smokers (women)

90 mg — DRI for men; Daily Value
75 mg — DRI for women

30 mg — Supports metabolism

10 mg — Prevents scurvy
0 mg

coenzyme (co-EN-zime) a small molecule that works with an enzyme to promote the enzyme's activity. Many coenzymes have B vitamins as part of their structure (*co* means "with").

125 milligrams for men and 110 milligrams for women, in order to maintain blood concentrations comparable to those of nonsmokers. Importantly, vitamin C cannot reverse other damage caused by tobacco use. Physical stressors, including infections, burns, fever, toxic heavy metals such as lead, and certain medications, also increase the body's use of vitamin C.

Vitamin C Food Sources

Fruit and vegetables are the foods to remember for vitamin C, as Snapshot 7–5 shows. A cup of orange juice at breakfast, a salad for lunch, and a stalk of broccoli and a potato at dinner easily provide 300 milligrams, making pills unnecessary. People commonly identify orange juice as a source of vitamin C, but they often overlook other rich sources that may be lower in calories.

Vitamin C is vulnerable to heat and destroyed by oxygen, so for maximum vitamin C consumers should treat their fruit and vegetables gently. Losses occurring when a food is cut, processed, and stored may be large enough to reduce vitamin C's activity in the body. Fresh, raw, and quickly cooked fruit, vegetables, and juices retain the most vitamin C, and they should be stored properly and consumed within a week after purchase. The Consumer's Guide (p. 244) discusses the vitamin costs of food processing techniques and offers advice on how to minimize vitamin losses at home.

Because of their enormous popularity, white potatoes contribute significantly to vitamin C intakes, despite providing less than 10 milligrams per half-cup serving. The sweet potato, often ignored in favor of its paler cousin, is a gold mine of nutrients: a single half-cup serving provides about a third of many people's recommended intake for vitamin C, in addition to its lavish contribution of vitamin A.

KEY POINTS

- Vitamin C maintains collagen, protects against infection, acts as an antioxidant, and aids iron absorption.
- Ample vitamin C can be easily obtained from foods.

The B Vitamins in Unison

LO 7.9   Describe the collective roles of B vitamins in metabolism and the effects of their deficiencies.

The B vitamins function as parts of coenzymes. A **coenzyme** is a small molecule that combines with an enzyme (described in Chapter 6) and activates it. Figure 7–13 shows how a coenzyme enables an enzyme to do its job. The substance to be worked on is attracted to the active site (often the vitamin part) and snaps into place, enabling the reaction to proceed instantaneously. The shape of each enzyme predestines it to accomplish just one kind of job. Without its coenzyme, however, the enzyme is as useless as a car without its steering wheel.

Each of the B vitamins has its own special nature, and the amount of detail known about each one is overwhelming. To simplify things, this introduction describes the teamwork of the B vitamins and emphasizes the consequences of deficiencies. Many of these nutrients are so interdependent that it is sometimes difficult to tell which vitamin deficiency is the cause of which symptom; the presence or absence of one affects the absorption, metabolism, and excretion of others. Later sections present a few details about these vitamins as individuals.

Figure 7–13

Coenzyme Action

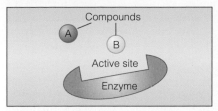

1. Without the coenzyme, compounds A and B don't respond to the enzyme.

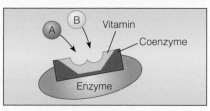

2. With the coenzyme in place, compounds A and B are attracted to the active site on the enzyme, and they react.

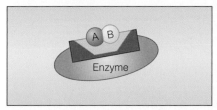

3. The reaction is completed with the formation of a new product. In this case, the product is AB.

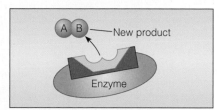

4. The product AB is released.

B Vitamin Roles in Metabolism

Figure 7–14 (p. 242) shows some body organs and tissues in which the B vitamins help the body metabolize carbohydrates, lipids, and amino acids. The purpose of the figure is not to present a detailed account of metabolism but to give you an impression of where the B vitamins work together with enzymes in the metabolism of energy nutrients and in the creation of new cells.

Many people mistakenly believe that B vitamins supply the body with energy. They do not, at least not directly. The B vitamins are "helpers." The energy-yielding nutrients—carbohydrate, fat, and protein—give the body fuel for energy; the B vitamins *help* the body to use that fuel. More specifically, active forms of five of the B vitamins— thiamin, riboflavin, niacin, pantothenic acid, and biotin—participate in the release of energy from carbohydrate, fat, and protein. Vitamin B_6 helps the body use amino acids to synthesize proteins; the body then puts the proteins to work in many ways—to build new tissues, to make hormones, to fight infections, or to serve as fuel for energy, to name only a few.

Folate and vitamin B_{12} help cells to multiply, which is especially important to cells with short life spans that must replace themselves frequently. Such cells include both the red blood cells (which live for about 120 days) and the cells that line the digestive tract (which replace themselves every 3 days). These cells absorb and deliver energy to all the others. In short, each and every B vitamin is involved, directly or indirectly, in energy metabolism.

B Vitamin Deficiencies

As long as B vitamins are present, their presence is not felt. Only when they are missing does their absence manifest itself in a lack of energy and a multitude of other symptoms, as you can imagine after looking at Figure 7–14. The reactions by which B vitamins facilitate energy release take place in every cell, and no cell can do its work without energy. Thus, in a B vitamin deficiency, every cell is affected. Among the symptoms of B vitamin deficiencies are nausea, severe exhaustion, irritability, depression, forgetful- ness, loss of appetite and weight, pain in muscles, impairment of the immune response, loss of control of the limbs, abnormal heart action, severe skin problems, swollen red

Figure 7–14

Some Roles of the B Vitamins in Metabolism: Examples

The purpose of this figure is to show a few of the many tissue functions that require a host of B vitamin–dependent enzymes working together in harmony. The B vitamins work in every cell, and this figure displays less than a thousandth of what they actually do.

Every B vitamin is part of one or more coenzymes that make possible the body's chemical work. For example, the niacin, thiamin, and riboflavin coenzymes are important in the energy pathways. The folate and vitamin B$_{12}$ coenzymes are necessary for making RNA and DNA and thus new cells. The vitamin B$_6$ coenzyme is necessary for processing amino acids and therefore protein. Although many other relationships are also critical to metabolism, this figure does not attempt to teach intricate biochemical pathways or names of B vitamin–containing enzymes.

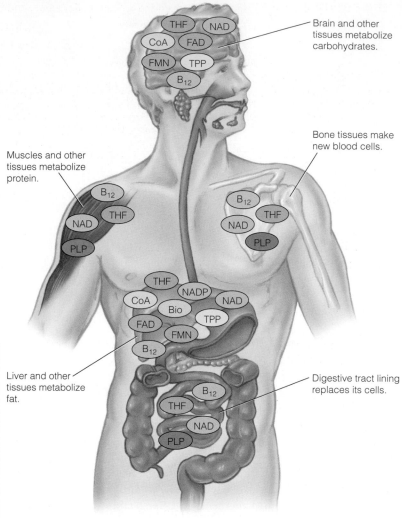

Brain and other tissues metabolize carbohydrates.

Bone tissues make new blood cells.

Muscles and other tissues metabolize protein.

Liver and other tissues metabolize fat.

Digestive tract lining replaces its cells.

Key:

Coenzyme		Vitamin
TPP	=	thiamin
FAD FMN	=	riboflavin
NAD NADP	=	niacin
PLP	=	vitamin B$_6$
THF	=	folate
CoA	=	pantothenic acid
Bio	=	biotin
B$_{12}$	=	vitamin B$_{12}$

tongue, cracked skin at the corners of the mouth, and teary or bloodshot eyes. Figure 7–15 shows two of these signs. Because cell renewal depends on energy and protein, which, in turn, depend on the B vitamins, the digestive tract and the blood are invariably damaged. In children, full recovery may be impossible. In the case of a thiamin deficiency during growth, permanent brain damage can result.

In academic discussions of the B vitamins, different sets of deficiency symptoms are given for each one. Such clear-cut sets of symptoms are found only in laboratory animals that have been fed fabricated diets that lack just one vitamin. In real life, a deficiency of any one B vitamin seldom shows up by itself because people don't eat nutrients singly; they eat foods that contain mixtures of nutrients. A diet low in one B vitamin is likely low in other nutrients, too. If treatment involves giving wholesome food rather than a single supplement, subtler deficiencies and impairments will be corrected along with the major one. The symptoms of B vitamin deficiencies and toxicities are listed in Table 7–9 (p. 256).

KEY POINTS

- As parts of coenzymes, the B vitamins help enzymes in every cell do numerous jobs.
- B vitamins help metabolize carbohydrate, fat, and protein.

Figure 7–15

B Vitamin–Deficiency Symptoms: Tongue and Mouth

The normally rough and bumpy tongue becomes smooth and swollen, and the corners of the mouth become inflamed and cracked.

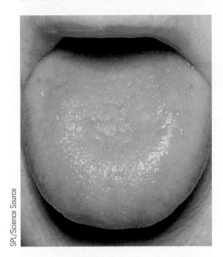
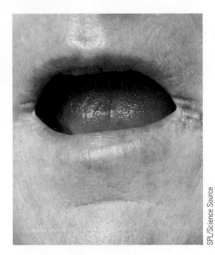

SPL/Science Source

SPL/Science Source

The B Vitamins as Individuals

LO 7.10 Describe the roles, the effects of deficiencies and toxicities, and food sources of each of the eight B vitamins.

Although the B vitamins all work as parts of coenzymes and share other characteristics, each B vitamin has special qualities. The next sections provide a few details.

Thiamin

Thiamin plays a critical role in the energy metabolism of all cells. Thiamin also occupies a special site on nerve cell membranes. Consequently, nerve processes and their responding tissues, the muscles, depend heavily on thiamin.

Thiamin Deficiency The classic thiamin-deficiency disease, **beriberi**, was first observed in East Asia, where rice provided 80 to 90 percent of the total calories most people consumed and was therefore their principal source of thiamin. When the custom of polishing rice (removing its brown coat, which contained the thiamin) became widespread, beriberi swept through the population like an epidemic. Scientists wasted years of effort hunting for a microbial cause of beriberi before they realized that the cause was not something present in the environment but something absent from it. Figure 7–16 depicts beriberi and describes its two forms.

Just before the year 1900, an observant physician working in a prison in East Asia discovered that beriberi could be cured with proper diet. The physician noticed that the chickens at the prison had developed a stiffness and weakness similar to that of the prisoners who had beriberi. The chickens were being fed the rice left on prisoners' plates. When the rice bran, which had been discarded in the kitchen, was given to the chickens, their paralysis was cured. The physician met resistance when he tried to feed the rice bran, the "garbage," to the prisoners, but it worked—it produced a miracle cure like those described at the beginning of this chapter. Later, extracts of rice bran were used to prevent infantile beriberi; still later, thiamin was identified.

In developed countries today, alcohol abuse often leads to a severe form of thiamin deficiency, **Wernicke-Korsakoff syndrome**. Alcohol contributes energy but carries almost no nutrients with it and often displaces food from the diet. In addition, alcohol impairs absorption of thiamin from the digestive tract and hastens its excretion in the urine,

Figure 7–16

Beriberi

Beriberi takes two forms: wet beriberi, characterized by edema (fluid accumulation), and dry beriberi, without edema. This person's ankle retains the imprint of the physician's thumb, showing the edema of wet beriberi.

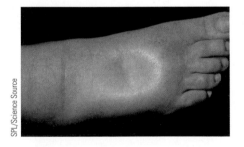

SPL/Science Source

thiamin (THIGH-uh-min) a B vitamin involved in the body's use of fuels.

beriberi (berry-berry) the thiamin-deficiency disease; characterized by loss of sensation in the hands and feet, muscular weakness, advancing paralysis, and abnormal heart action.

Wernicke-Korsakoff (VER-nik-ee KOR-sah-koff) **syndrome** a cluster of symptoms involving nerve damage arising from a deficiency of the vitamin thiamin in alcoholism. Characterized by mental confusion, disorientation, memory loss, jerky eye movements, and staggering gait.

The Effects of Food Processing on Vitamins

Consumers often wonder, "Do canned foods have any nutrient value left in them?" or "Is fresh or frozen food better than canned?" It is true, in general, that the more heavily processed a food, the less nutritious it may be. Ultra-processed foods (defined in Chapter 1) contribute much of the sodium, sugar, saturated fats, and calories found in the U.S. diet. Many forms of processing destroy vitamins, but the effect of processing on a food's nutrient value depends upon the nutrient and the process. Vitamin C in variously processed orange juice makes a convenient example:

- *Fresh squeezed, not from concentrate.* Juice extracted from the fibrous structures of whole oranges is quickly packaged, pasteurized, and refrigerated. (Almost all of the vitamin C is retained: 8 ounces provides 120 milligrams of vitamin C.)

- *Reconstituted, made from concentrate.* Fresh-squeezed juice is condensed by heat and pressure, and then frozen. After being reconstituted by adding water, it is packaged in cartons and refrigerated. The concentrate may also be sold frozen for reconstituting at home. (Condensing destroys a small amount of vitamin C: 8 ounces of reconstituted juice provides 97 milligrams of vitamin C.)

- *Canned 100% orange juice.* Fluid juice, most often reconstituted, is heated to sterilize it during canning. (Heating destroys more vitamin C: 8 ounces provides 75 milligrams of vitamin C.)

The numbers indicate that fresh juice is superior for vitamin C, but consider this: one eight-ounce serving of any of these choices meets or comes close to meeting an adult's entire daily need for this vitamin.

Canned or Frozen?

After harvest, cellular enzymes in fruit and vegetables continuously break down vitamins, causing significant losses over time. Freezing dramatically slows this enzymatic breakdown, and preserves almost all of the vitamins present at harvest. As for canning, it requires heating foods to a high enough temperature for long enough to destroy any illness-causing microbes that may be present. This heating process also denatures enzymes and so stops enzymatic vitamin destruction. However, heating itself destroys a small amount of vitamins, and about half of the water-soluble vitamins dissolve into the canning liquid, which is typically discarded. This doesn't make canned foods poor choices for vitamin nutrition—they can be good sources, particularly if their liquid is consumed—and they are inexpensive, convenient to store, and easily prepared.

Commercial Processing Mischief

Some processes are even harder on vitamins. As mentioned earlier, commercial frying can destroy virtually all of the vitamin E in oil. Another severe process involves **extrusion**, used to make many ultra-processed foods. Such foods may look pretty and taste delicious, but exposure to heat and oxidation during extrusion destroys an estimated 30 percent of the vitamin A, 50 percent of the vitamin K, and 90 percent of the vitamin C in the food, with similar losses for almost every other vitamin. Manufacturers may try to compensate by spraying on a few vitamins or minerals, but they cannot replace all of the nutrients,

fibers, and phytochemicals lost from the original whole foods. The nutrient density of processed foods exists on a continuum, from farm fresh to ultra-processed. The following are examples of the continuum from lesser to greater degrees of processing:

- Whole-grain bread > enriched white bread > packaged snack cakes.
- Milk > fruit-flavored yogurt > "yogurt" covered raisin candy.
- Fresh spinach > canned spinach > extruded green "vegetable" chips.
- Baked pork loin > ham lunch meat > fried bacon.

An occasional serving of an ultra-processed food is tolerable in nutrition. Just don't use it as a staple food.

Moving Ahead

Consumers often wrongly equate the terms *processed foods* and *junk foods*, but they are not synonymous. Thanks to commercial food processing, few people in this country must spend their days grinding grains for bread, making cheese, or curing ham before making a sandwich. Commercial processing also improves certain products, such as prewashed and cut fresh vegetables (they retain their vitamins, are convenient, and reduce waste) or canned fish (it costs much less than fresh, stores much longer, and retains most of the important vitamins). Making wise food choices is only half of the story, though; skillful food handling, storage, and preparation is the other half

extrusion processing techniques that transform grains, legumes, and other foods into fine particles that are cooked, shaped, colored, flavored, and often puffed, producing snacks, breakfast cereals, and other products.

(Table 7–7 offers some tips). With this information, you can make choices that deliver the bounty of the vitamins that foods contain.

Review Questions*

1. Freezing is better than canning for preserving vitamins in foods.   T   F
2. One eight-ounce serving of fresh, frozen, or canned orange juice provides most adults' daily need for vitamin C.   T   F
3. All processed foods can be classified as junk foods.   T   F

*Answers to Consumer's Guide review questions are in Appendix G.

tripling the risk of deficiency. The syndrome is characterized by symptoms almost indistinguishable from alcohol abuse itself: apathy, irritability, mental confusion, disorientation, memory loss, jerky eye movements, and a staggering gait (listed in Snapshot 7–6).[60] Unlike alcohol toxicity, the syndrome responds quickly to an injection of thiamin.

Snapshot 7–6   Thiamin

DRI
Men: 1.2 mg/day
Women: 1.1 mg/day

Chief Functions
Part of coenzyme active in energy metabolism

Deficiency[a]
Beriberi with possible edema or muscle wasting; enlarged heart, heart failure, muscular weakness, pain, apathy, poor short-term memory, confusion, irritability, difficulty walking, paralysis, jerky eye movements, anorexia, weight loss

Toxicity
None reported

*These foods provide 10% or more of the thiamin Daily Value in a serving. For a 2,000-cal diet, the DV is 1.2 mg/day.
[a]Severe thiamin deficiency is often related to heavy alcohol consumption.

Good Sources*

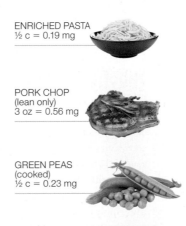

ENRICHED WHEAT BAGEL
½ bagel = 0.22 mg

ENRICHED PASTA
½ c = 0.19 mg

ENRICHED CEREAL
(ready-to-eat)
¾ c = 1.5 mg

PORK CHOP
(lean only)
3 oz = 0.56 mg

SUNFLOWER SEEDS
(raw kernels)
2 tbs = 0.26 mg

GREEN PEAS
(cooked)
½ c = 0.23 mg

BAKED POTATO
1 whole potato
= 0.22 mg

WAFFLE
1 waffle = 0.25 mg

BLACK BEANS
(cooked)
½ c = 0.21 mg

Riboflavin

Good Sources*

Daniel Gilbey Photography - My portfolio/Shutterstock.com; stavklem/Shutterstock.com; Africa Studio/Shutterstock.com; Serghei Starus/Shutterstock.com; Yasonya/Shutterstock.com; Joe Gough/Shutterstock.com; Gyorgy Barna/Shutterstock.com; Roxana Bashyrova/Shutterstock.com

DRI
Men: 1.3 mg/day
Women: 1.1 mg/day

Chief Functions
Part of coenzyme active in energy metabolism

Deficiency
Cracks and redness at corners of mouth; painful, smooth, purplish red tongue; sore throat; inflamed eyes and eyelids, sensitivity to light; skin rashes

Toxicity
None reported

*These foods provide 10% or more of the riboflavin Daily Value in a serving. For a 2,000-cal diet, the DV is 1.3 mg/day.

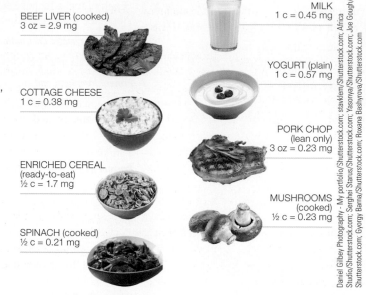

BEEF LIVER (cooked)
3 oz = 2.9 mg

COTTAGE CHEESE
1 c = 0.38 mg

ENRICHED CEREAL
(ready-to-eat)
½ c = 1.7 mg

SPINACH (cooked)
½ c = 0.21 mg

MILK
1 c = 0.45 mg

YOGURT (plain)
1 c = 0.57 mg

PORK CHOP
(lean only)
3 oz = 0.23 mg

MUSHROOMS
(cooked)
½ c = 0.23 mg

Recommended Intakes and Food Sources The DRI committee set the thiamin intake recommendation at 1.2 milligrams per day for men and at 1.1 milligrams per day for women. Pregnancy and lactation demand somewhat more thiamin (see the DRI, back of the book, p. B). Thiamin occurs in small amounts in many nutritious foods. Ham and other pork products, sunflower seeds, enriched and whole-grain cereals, and legumes are especially rich in thiamin. If you keep empty-calorie foods to a minimum and focus your meals on nutritious foods each day, you will easily meet your thiamin needs.

KEY POINTS

- Thiamin is a coenzyme important in energy metabolism and in nerve cell processes.
- The thiamin deficiency disease is beriberi.
- Many foods supply small amounts of thiamin.

Riboflavin Roles

Like thiamin, **riboflavin** plays a role as a coenzyme in the energy metabolism pathways of all cells.[61] When thiamin is deficient, riboflavin may be lacking, too, but its deficiency symptoms, such as cracks at the corners of the mouth, sore throat, or hypersensitivity to light, may go undetected because those of thiamin deficiency are more severe. Worldwide, riboflavin deficiency has been documented among children whose eating patterns lack milk products and meats, and researchers suspect that it occurs among some U.S. elders as well. An eating pattern that remedies riboflavin deficiency invariably contains some thiamin and so clears up both deficiencies.

Riboflavin recommendations are listed in Snapshot 7-7. People in this country obtain over a quarter of their riboflavin from enriched breads, cereals, pasta, and other grain products, while milk and milk products supply another 20 percent. Certain vegetables, eggs, and meats contribute most of the rest (see Snapshot 7-7). Ultraviolet light and irradiation destroy riboflavin. For these reasons, milk is sold in cardboard or opaque plastic containers, and precautions are taken if milk is processed by irradiation. Riboflavin is heat stable, so cooking does not destroy it.

riboflavin (RIBE-o-flay-vin) a B vitamin active in the body's energy-releasing mechanisms.

- Riboflavin's coenzymes are important in energy metabolism.
- Riboflavin is destroyed by ordinary light.

Niacin

The vitamin **niacin**, like thiamin and riboflavin, participates in the energy metabolism of every cell. A deficiency causes serious illness.

Niacin Deficiency The niacin-deficiency disease **pellagra** appeared in Europe in the 1700s when corn from the New World became a staple food. During the early 1900s in the United States, pellagra was devastating lives throughout the South and Midwest. Hundreds of thousands of pellagra victims were thought to be suffering from a contagious disease until this dietary deficiency was identified. The disease still occurs among poorly nourished people living in urban slums and particularly among those with alcohol addiction.[62] Pellagra is also still common in parts of Africa and Asia.[63] Its symptoms are known as the four "Ds": diarrhea, dermatitis, dementia, and, ultimately, death.

Figure 7–17 shows the skin disorder (dermatitis) associated with pellagra. For comparison, Figure 7–3 (p. 224) and Figure 7–21 (p. 252) show skin disorders associated with vitamin A and vitamin B₆ deficiencies, respectively. These figures serve as reminders that any nutrient deficiency affects the skin as well as all other cells; the skin just happens to be the organ you can see. Table 7–9 at the end of the chapter lists the symptoms of niacin deficiency.

Niacin Toxicity and Pharmacology For more than 50 years, large doses of a form of niacin have been prescribed to help improve blood lipids associated with cardiovascular disease.[64]§§ Its use is limited, however, by the most common side effect of large doses of niacin, the "niacin flush," a dilation of the capillaries of the skin with perceptible tingling that can be painful.[65] Today, effective, well-tolerated drugs are often used instead, and scientists question the effectiveness of niacin and debate its utility.[66] Reported risks from large doses of niacin include liver injury, digestive upset, impaired glucose tolerance, serious infection, muscle weakness, and, rarely, vision disturbances.[67] Anyone considering taking large doses of niacin on their own should instead consult a physician who can prescribe safe, effective alternatives.[68]

Niacin Recommendations and Food Sources Niacin recommendations are listed in Snapshot 7–8 (p. 248). The key nutrient that prevents pellagra is niacin, but any protein containing sufficient amounts of the amino acid tryptophan will serve in its place. Tryptophan, which is abundant in almost all proteins (but is limited in the protein of corn), is converted to niacin in the body, and it is possible to cure pellagra by administering tryptophan alone. Thus, a person eating adequate protein (as most people in developed nations do) will not be deficient in niacin. The amount of niacin in a diet is stated in terms of **niacin equivalents (NE)**, a measure that takes available tryptophan into account.

Early workers seeking the cause of pellagra observed that well-fed people never got it. From there, the researchers defined an eating pattern that reliably produced the disease—one of cornmeal, salted pork fat, and molasses. Corn not only is low in protein but also lacks tryptophan. Salt pork is almost pure fat and contains too little protein to compensate, and molasses is virtually protein-free. Snapshot 7–8 shows some good food sources of niacin.

- Niacin forms coenzymes important in energy metabolism.
- Niacin deficiency causes the disease pellagra, which can be prevented by adequate niacin intake or adequate dietary protein.
- The amino acid tryptophan can be converted to niacin in the body.

§§The form of niacin is nicotinic acid.

Figure 7–17

Pellagra

The typical "flaky paint" dermatitis of pellagra develops on skin that is exposed to light. The skin darkens and flakes away.

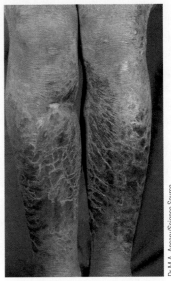

Dr M.A. Ansary/Science Source

niacin a B vitamin needed in energy metabolism. Niacin can be eaten preformed or made in the body from tryptophan, one of the amino acids. Other forms of niacin are *nicotinic acid*, *niacinamide*, and *nicotinamide*.

pellagra (pell-AY-gra) the niacin-deficiency disease (*pellis* means "skin"; *agra* means "rough"). Symptoms include the "4 Ds": diarrhea, dermatitis, dementia, and, ultimately, death.

niacin equivalents (NE) the amount of niacin present in food, including the niacin that can theoretically be made from its precursor tryptophan that is present in the food.

Snapshot 7–8 Niacin

DRI
Men: 16 mg/day[a]
Women: 14 mg/day

Tolerable Upper Intake Level
Adults: 35 mg/day

Chief Functions
Part of coenzymes needed in energy metabolism

Deficiency
Pellagra, characterized by flaky skin rash (dermatitis) where exposed to sunlight; mental depression, apathy, fatigue, loss of memory, headache; diarrhea, abdominal pain, vomiting; swollen, smooth, bright red or black tongue

Toxicity
Painful flush, hives, and rash ("niacin flush"); excessive sweating; blurred vision; liver damage, impaired glucose tolerance

These foods provide 10% or more of the niacin Daily Value in a serving. For a 2,000-cal diet, the DV is 16 mg/day. The DV values are for preformed niacin, not niacin equivalents.
[a]*Niacin DRI values are expressed in niacin equivalents (NE); the Tolerable Upper Intake Level refers to preformed niacin.*

Good Sources*

CHICKEN BREAST
3 oz = 8.9 mg
PORK CHOP
3 oz = 3.9 mg
BAKED POTATO
1 whole medium
potato = 2.4 mg
TUNA (in water)
3 oz = 11.3 mg
ENRICHED CEREAL
(ready-to-eat)
¾ c = 20 mg
MUSHROOMS
(cooked)
½ c = 3.5 mg

Joe Gough/Shutterstock.com; Joe Gough/Shutterstock.com; Mirka Markova/Shutterstock.com; Yasonya/Shutterstock.com; stavklem/Shutterstock.com; Bizroug/Shutterstock.com

Folate

To make new cells, tissues must have the vitamin **folate**. Each new cell must be equipped with new genetic material—copies of the parent cell's DNA—and folate helps synthesize DNA. Folate also participates in the metabolism of vitamin B_{12} and several amino acids.[69]

Folate Deficiency Folate deficiencies may result from following an eating pattern that is too low in folate or from illnesses that impair folate absorption, increase folate excretion, require medication that interacts with folate, or otherwise increase the body's folate need. However it occurs, folate deficiency has wide-reaching effects.

Immature red and white blood cells and the cells of the digestive tract divide most rapidly and therefore are most vulnerable to folate deficiency. Deficiencies of folate cause anemia, impaired immunity, and abnormal digestive function. The anemia of folate deficiency is related to the anemia of vitamin B_{12} malabsorption because the two vitamins work as teammates in producing red blood cells. Research links a chronic deficiency of folate with greater risks for developing breast cancer (particularly among women who drink alcohol), prostate cancer, and other cancers. The relationship between cancer and folate is not simple: research also suggests that high doses from supplements may speed up cancer progression.[70]

Of all the vitamins, folate is most likely to interact with medications. Many drugs, including antacids and aspirin and its relatives, have been shown to interfere with the body's use of folate. Occasional use of these drugs to relieve headaches or stomach upsets poses no concern, but frequent users may need to pay attention to their folate intakes. These include people with chronic pain or ulcers who rely heavily on aspirin or antacids, as well as those who smoke or take oral contraceptives or anticonvulsant medications.

Birth Defects and Folate Enrichment By consuming enough folate both before and during pregnancy, a woman can reduce her child's risk of having one of the devastating birth defects known as **neural tube defects (NTD)**. NTD range from slight

folate (FOH-late) a B vitamin that acts as part of a coenzyme important in the manufacture of new cells. The form added to foods and supplements is *folic acid.*

problems in the spine to mental retardation, severely diminished brain size, and death shortly after birth (an example of an NTD, spina bifida, is shown in Figure 7–18). NTD arise in the first days or weeks of pregnancy, long before most women suspect that they are pregnant. Adequate maternal folate may protect against other related birth defects, cleft lip, and miscarriages, as well.[71]

Most young women eat too few fruit and vegetables from day to day to supply even half the folate needed to prevent NTD.[72] In the late 1990s, the Food and Drug Administration (FDA) ordered that all enriched grain products such as bread, cereal, rice, and pasta sold in the United States be fortified with an absorbable synthetic form of folate, *folic acid*. Since this fortification began, typical folate intakes from fortified foods have increased dramatically, along with average blood folate values.[73] Among women of childbearing age, for example, prevalence of folate deficiency dropped from 21 percent before folate fortification to less than 1 percent afterward. During the same period, the U.S. incidence of NTD dropped by more than a third, a success story that sparked a worldwide trend toward folate fortification and many fewer infants born with NTD (see Figure 7–19).

Folate Toxicity A UL for synthetic folic acid from enriched foods and supplements is set at 1,000 micrograms a day for adults. The current level of folate fortification of the food supply appears to be safe for most people, but a question remains about the ability of folate to mask a **subclinical deficiency** of vitamin B_{12} (more about this effect later).[74] Less than 3 percent of the U.S. population exceeds the UL for folate, primarily young women who consume supplements.[75] Although a theoretical potential for harm from excess folic acid exists, this must be weighed against its resounding success in preventing NTD.[76]

Folate Recommendations The DRI for folate for healthy adults is set at 400 micrograms per day. With one voice, nutrition authorities advise all women of childbearing age to consume 400 micrograms of *folic acid*, a highly available form of folate, from supplements or enriched foods each day in addition to the folate that occurs naturally in their foods.[77]

Folate Food Sources The name *folate* is derived from the word *foliage*, and sure enough, leafy green vegetables such as spinach and turnip greens provide abundant folate. As Snapshot 7–9 shows, legumes and asparagus are also excellent sources.

Figure 7–18

Spina Bifida, a Neural Tube Defect

Spina bifida is characterized by incomplete closure of the bony encasement of the spinal cord. The cord may protrude abnormally from the spine, as shown.

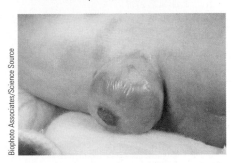

Biophoto Associates/Science Source

Figure 7–19

Effect of Folic Acid Fortification on the Prevalence of Neural Tube Defects

Far fewer neural tube defects have occurred since countries began fortifying their food supplies with folate.

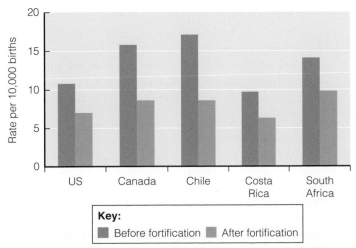

Key:
Before fortification ■ After fortification

Source: Centers for Disease Control and Prevention, Folic acid: Birth defects COUNT, (2017), available at www.cdc.gov/ncbddd/birthdefectscount/data.html.

neural tube defects (NTD) abnormalities of the brain and spinal cord apparent at birth and associated with low folate intake in women before and during pregnancy. The neural tube is the earliest brain and spinal cord structure formed during gestation. Also defined in Chapter 13.

subclinical deficiency a nutrient deficiency that has no outward clinical symptoms. Also called *marginal deficiency*.

DRI
Adults: 400 µg DFE/day[a]

Tolerable Upper Intake Level
Adults: 1,000 µg DFE/day

Chief Functions
Part of a coenzyme needed for new cell synthesis

Deficiency
Anemia, smooth, red tongue; depression, mental confusion, weakness, fatigue, irritability, headache; a low intake increases the risk of neural tube birth defects

Toxicity
Masks vitamin B_{12}–deficiency symptoms

*These foods provide 10% or more of the folate Daily Value in a serving. For a 2,000-cal diet, the DV is 400 µg/day.
[a]Folate recommendations are expressed in dietary folate equivalents (DFE). Note that for natural folate sources, 1 µg = 1 DFE; for enrichment sources, 1 µg = 1.7 DFE.
[b]Some highly enriched cereals may provide 400 µg or more in a serving.

Good Sources*

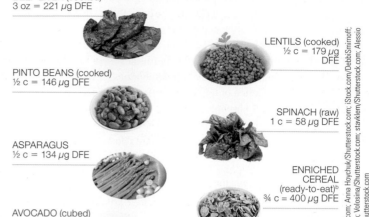

BEEF LIVER (cooked)
3 oz = 221 µg DFE

PINTO BEANS (cooked)
½ c = 146 µg DFE

ASPARAGUS
½ c = 134 µg DFE

AVOCADO (cubed)
½ c = 61 µg DFE

LENTILS (cooked)
½ c = 179 µg DFE

SPINACH (raw)
1 c = 58 µg DFE

ENRICHED CEREAL (ready-to-eat)[b]
¾ c = 400 µg DFE

BEETS
½ c = 68 µg DFE

Because the heat of cooking and the oxidation that occurs during long storage destroy much of the folate in foods, lightly cooked fresh vegetables are best.

A difference in absorption between naturally occurring food folate and synthetic folic acid necessitates compensation when measuring folate. The unit of measure, **dietary folate equivalent**, or **DFE**, converts all forms of folate into micrograms that are equivalent to the folate in foods. Appendix C demonstrates how to use the DFE conversion factor.

KEY POINTS

- Folate is part of a coenzyme necessary for making new cells.
- Low intakes of folate cause anemia, digestive problems, and birth defects in infants of folate-deficient mothers.
- High intakes can mask the blood symptom of a vitamin B_{12} deficiency.

Vitamin B_{12}

Vitamin B_{12} and folate are closely related: each depends on the other for activation. Vitamin B_{12} also functions as part of coenzymes needed in cell replication, and it helps maintain the protective sheaths that surround and protect nerve fibers, allowing them to function properly.

Vitamin B_{12} Deficiency Symptoms   Without sufficient vitamin B_{12}, folate fails to do its blood-building work, so vitamin B_{12} deficiency causes an anemia identical to that caused by folate deficiency. The blood symptoms of a deficiency of either folate or vitamin B_{12} include the presence of large, immature red blood cells. Administering extra folate often clears up this blood condition but allows the deficiency of vitamin B_{12} to continue undetected.[78] Vitamin B_{12}'s other functions then become compromised, and the results can be devastating: damaged nerve sheaths, creeping paralysis, and general malfunctioning of nerves and muscles. Even a marginal vitamin B_{12} deficiency may impair mental functioning in the elderly, worsening dementia.[79] Vitamin B_{12} deficiency

dietary folate equivalent (DFE) a unit of measure expressing the amount of folate available to the body from naturally occurring sources. The measure mathematically equalizes the difference in absorption between less absorbable food folate and highly absorbable synthetic folate (folic acid) added to enriched foods and found in supplements.

vitamin B_{12} a B vitamin that helps to convert folate to its active form and also helps to maintain the sheath around nerve cells. The vitamin's scientific name, not often used, is *cyanocobalamin*.

has also been associated with mental depression, but supplementation with vitamin B_{12} does not appear to improve symptoms of depression.[80] Research is ongoing.

A Special Case: Vitamin B_{12} Malabsorption   For vitamin B_{12}, deficiencies most often reflect poor absorption that occurs for one of two reasons:

- The stomach produces too little acid to liberate vitamin B_{12} from food.
- **Intrinsic factor**, a compound made by the stomach and needed for absorption, is lacking.

Once the stomach's acid frees vitamin B_{12} from the food proteins that bind it, intrinsic factor attaches to the vitamin, and the complex is absorbed into the bloodstream. The anemia of the vitamin B_{12} deficiency caused by lack of intrinsic factor is known as **pernicious anemia** (see Figure 7–20).

In a few people, an inborn defect in the gene for intrinsic factor begins to impair vitamin B_{12} absorption by mid-adulthood. With age, many others lose their ability to produce enough stomach acid and intrinsic factor to allow efficient absorption of vitamin B_{12}.*** Intestinal diseases, surgeries, or stomach infections with an ulcer-causing bacterium can also impair absorption.[81] Taking a common diabetes drug also makes vitamin B_{12} deficiency likely, although its symptoms have not been reported.†††[82] In cases of malabsorption, vitamin B_{12} must be supplied by injection or via nasal spray to bypass the defective absorptive system.

Vitamin B_{12} Food Sources   As Snapshot 7–10 (p. 252) shows, vitamin B_{12} is naturally supplied only by foods of animal origin, so strict vegetarians face a threat of vitamin B_{12} deficiency. Controversy 6 discussed vitamin B_{12} sources for vegetarians.

Perspective   The way folate masks the anemia of vitamin B_{12} deficiency underscores a point about supplements. It takes a skilled professional to correctly diagnose and treat a nutrient deficiency, and self-diagnosing or acting on advice from self-proclaimed experts poses serious risks. A second point: because vitamin B_{12} deficiency in the body may be caused by either a lack of the vitamin in the diet or a lack of the intrinsic factor necessary to absorb the vitamin, a dietary change alone may not correct the deficiency. A professional diagnosis can identify such problems.

KEY POINTS

- Vitamin B_{12} is critical for cell replication and proper nerve functioning.
- Vitamin B_{12} occurs only in foods of animal origin.
- Vitamin B_{12}–deficiency anemia mimics folate deficiency and arises with low intakes or, more often, poor absorption.
- Folate supplements can mask a vitamin B_{12} deficiency.

Vitamin B_6

Vitamin B_6 participates in more than 100 reactions in body tissues and is needed to help convert one kind of amino acid, which cells have in abundance, to other nonessential amino acids that the cells lack. In addition, vitamin B_6 functions in these ways:

- Aids in the conversion of tryptophan to niacin.
- Plays important roles in the synthesis of hemoglobin and neurotransmitters, the communication molecules of the brain. (For example, vitamin B_6 assists the conversion of the amino acid tryptophan to the mood-regulating neurotransmitter **serotonin**.)
- Assists in releasing stored glucose from glycogen and thus contributes to the maintenance of a normal blood glucose concentration.
- Plays roles in immune function and steroid hormone activity.
- Is critical to normal development of the fetal brain and nervous system; deficiency during this stage causes behavioral problems later.

***This condition is atrophic gastritis (a-TROH-fik gas-TRY-tis), chronic inflammation of the stomach accompanied by wasting and impaired function of the stomach's mucous membrane and glands.
†††The diabetes medication is metformin.

Figure 7–20

Anemic and Normal Blood Cells

The anemia of folate deficiency is indistinguishable from that of vitamin B_{12} deficiency.

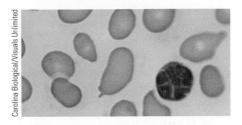

Carolina Biological/Visuals Unlimited

Blood cells of pernicious anemia. *The cells are larger than normal and irregular in shape.*

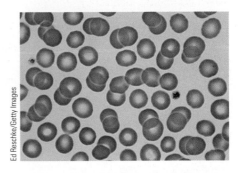

Ed Reschke/Getty Images

Normal blood cells. *The size, shape, and color of these red blood cells show that they are normal.*

intrinsic factor a factor made by the stomach that is necessary for absorption of vitamin B_{12} and prevention of pernicious anemia.

pernicious (per-NISH-us) **anemia** a vitamin B_{12}–deficiency disease, caused by lack of intrinsic factor and characterized by large, immature red blood cells and damage to the nervous system (*pernicious* means "highly injurious or destructive").

vitamin B_6 a B vitamin needed in protein metabolism. Its three active forms are *pyridoxine, pyridoxal,* and *pyridoxamine.*

serotonin (sare-oh-TONE-in) a neurotransmitter important in sleep regulation, appetite control, and mood regulation, among other roles. Serotonin is synthesized in the body from the amino acid tryptophan with the help of vitamin B_6.

Snapshot 7–10 Vitamin B₁₂

DRI
Adults: 2.4 µg/day

Chief Functions
Part of coenzymes needed in new cell synthesis; helps to maintain nerve cells

Deficiency
Pernicious anemia;[a] anemia (large-cell type);[b] smooth tongue; tingling or numbness; fatigue, memory loss, disorientation, degeneration of nerves progressing to paralysis

Toxicity
None reported

These foods provide 10% or more of the vitamin B₁₂ Daily Value in a serving. For a 2,000-cal diet, the DV is 2.4 µg/day.
[a]*The name **pernicious anemia** refers to the vitamin B₁₂ deficiency caused by a lack of stomach intrinsic factor but not to anemia from inadequate dietary intake.*
[b]*Large cell-type anemia is known as either macrocytic or megaloblastic anemia.*

Good Sources*

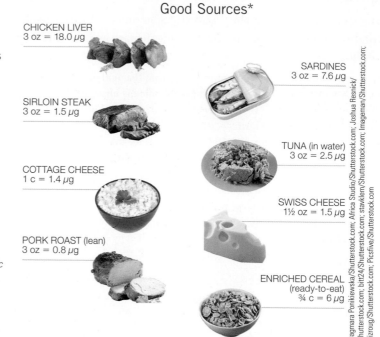

CHICKEN LIVER
3 oz = 18.0 µg

SIRLOIN STEAK
3 oz = 1.5 µg

COTTAGE CHEESE
1 c = 1.4 µg

PORK ROAST (lean)
3 oz = 0.8 µg

SARDINES
3 oz = 7.6 µg

TUNA (in water)
3 oz = 2.5 µg

SWISS CHEESE
1½ oz = 1.5 µg

ENRICHED CEREAL
(ready-to-eat)
¾ c = 6 µg

Dagmara Ponikiewska/Shutterstock.com; Africa Studio/Shutterstock.com; Joshua Resnick/Shutterstock.com; bitt24/Shutterstock.com; stawklem/Shutterstock.com; Imageman/Shutterstock.com; Bizroug/Shutterstock.com; Picsfive/Shutterstock.com

---

Figure 7–21

Vitamin B₆ Deficiency

In this dermatitis, the skin is greasy and flaky, unlike the skin affected by the dermatitis of pellagra.

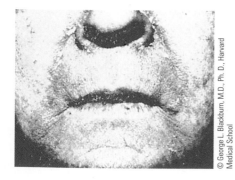

© George L. Blackburn, M.D., Ph. D., Harvard Medical School

Vitamin B₆ Deficiency Because of these diverse functions, vitamin B₆ deficiency is expressed in general symptoms, such as weakness, psychological depression, confusion, irritability, and insomnia. Other symptoms include anemia, the greasy dermatitis depicted in Figure 7–21, and, in advanced cases of deficiency, convulsions. A shortage of vitamin B₆ may also weaken the immune response. Some evidence links low vitamin B₆ intakes with increased risks of certain cancers and cardiovascular disease; more research is needed to clarify these relationships.[83]

Vitamin B₆ Toxicity Years ago, it was generally believed that, like most of the other water-soluble vitamins, vitamin B₆ could not reach toxic concentrations in the body. Then a report told of women who took more than 2 grams of vitamin B₆ daily for months (20 times the current UL of 100 *milligrams* per day), attempting to cure premenstrual syndrome (science doesn't support this use). The women developed numb feet, then lost sensation in their hands, and eventually became unable to walk or work. Withdrawing the supplement reversed the symptoms.

Food sources of vitamin B₆ are safe. Consider that one small capsule can easily deliver 2 grams of vitamin B₆ but it would take almost 3,000 bananas, more than 1,600 servings of liver, or more than 3,800 chicken breasts to supply an equivalent amount. Moral: stick with food. Table 7–9 (pp. 256–258) lists common deficiency and toxicity symptoms and food sources of vitamin B₆.

Vitamin B₆ Recommendations and Sources Vitamin B₆ plays so many roles in protein metabolism that the body's requirement for vitamin B₆ is roughly proportional to protein intakes. The DRI committee set the vitamin B₆ intake recommendation high enough to cover most people's needs, regardless of differences in protein intakes (see the back of the book, p. B). Meats, fish, and poultry (protein-rich foods); potatoes; leafy green vegetables; and some fruit are good sources of vitamin B₆ (see Snapshot 7–11). Other foods such as legumes and peanut butter provide smaller amounts.

Vitamin B$_6$

DRI
Adults (19–50 yr): 1.3 mg/day

Tolerable Upper Intake Level
Adults: 100 mg/day

Chief Functions
Part of a coenzyme needed in amino acid and fatty acid metabolism; helps to convert tryptophan to niacin and to serotonin; helps to make hemoglobin for red blood cells

Deficiency
Anemia, depression, confusion, convulsions; greasy, scaly dermatitis

Toxicity
Depression, fatigue, irritability, headaches, nerve damage causing numbness and muscle weakness progressing to an inability to walk and convulsions; skin lesions

These foods provide 10% or more of the vitamin B$_6$ Daily Value in a serving. For a 2,000-cal diet, the DV is 1.7 mg/day.

Good Sources*

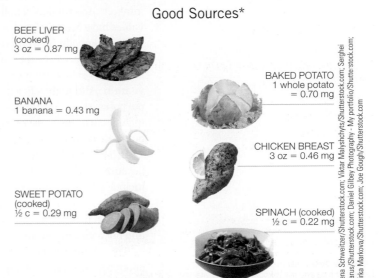

BEEF LIVER (cooked)
3 oz = 0.87 mg

BANANA
1 banana = 0.43 mg

SWEET POTATO (cooked)
½ c = 0.29 mg

BAKED POTATO
1 whole potato
= 0.70 mg

CHICKEN BREAST
3 oz = 0.46 mg

SPINACH (cooked)
½ c = 0.22 mg

Elena Schweitzer/Shutterstock.com; Viktar Malyshchyts/Shutterstock.com, Serghei Starus/Shutterstock.com; Daniel Gilbey Photography - My portfolio/Shutterstock.com; Mirka Markova/Shutterstock.com; Joe Gough/Shutterstock.com

KEY POINT

- Vitamin B$_6$ works in amino acid metabolism.

Biotin and Pantothenic Acid

Two other B vitamins, **biotin** and **pantothenic acid**, are, like thiamin, riboflavin, and niacin, important in energy metabolism. Biotin is a coenzyme for several enzymes in the metabolism of carbohydrate, fat, and protein. In addition, researchers are actively investigating new roles for biotin, particularly in gene expression.[84] Biotin is widespread in foods, so eating a variety of foods prevents deficiency. Also, intestinal bacteria release biotin that can be absorbed. No adverse effects from high biotin intakes have been reported, but some research indicates that high-dose biotin supplementation may damage DNA. No UL has yet been set for biotin.

Pantothenic acid is a component of a key coenzyme that makes possible the release of energy from the energy nutrients. It also participates in more than 100 steps in the synthesis of lipids, neurotransmitters, steroid hormones, and hemoglobin.

Although rare diseases may precipitate deficiencies of biotin and pantothenic acid, healthy people eating ordinary diets are not at risk for deficiencies. A steady diet of raw egg whites, which contain a protein that binds biotin, can produce biotin deficiency, but you would have to consume more than two dozen raw egg whites daily to produce the effect. Cooking eggs denatures the protein.

KEY POINTS

- Biotin and pantothenic acid are parts of coenzymes important in energy metabolism and in the synthesis of lipids, hormones, and other vital cell components.
- Biotin and pantothenic acid are adequately supplied in a well-balanced diet.

Non–B Vitamins

Choline, although not defined as a vitamin, might be called a conditionally essential nutrient. When the diet is devoid of choline, the body cannot make enough of the

biotin (BY-o-tin) a B vitamin; a coenzyme necessary for fat synthesis and other metabolic reactions.

pantothenic (PAN-to-THEN-ic) **acid** a B vitamin and part of a critical coenzyme needed in energy metabolism, among other roles.

choline (KOH-leen) a nutrient used to make the phospholipid lecithin and other molecules.

compound to meet its needs, and choline plays important roles in fetal development, particularly in the brain.[85] Choline is widely supplied by protein-rich foods (eggs are a particularly good source), yet recent data shows that less than 10 percent of U.S. adults and pregnant women consume enough choline to meet the recommended adequate intake.[86] Additionally, choline needs may rise in pregnancy (see Chapter 13).[87] DRI values have been set for choline (see the back of the book, p. B).

The compounds **carnitine**, **inositol**, and **lipoic acid** might appropriately be called *nonvitamins* because they are not essential nutrients for human beings. Carnitine, sometimes called "vitamin BT," is an important piece of cell machinery, but it is not a vitamin. Although deficiencies can be induced in laboratory animals for experimental purposes, these substances are abundant in ordinary foods. Vitamin companies often include carnitine, inositol, or lipoic acid to make their formulas appear more "complete," but there is no physiological reason to do so.

Other substances have been mistakenly thought to be essential in human nutrition because they are needed for growth by bacteria or other life-forms. These substances include PABA (para-aminobenzoic acid), bioflavonoids ("vitamin P" or hesperidin), and ubiquinone (coenzyme Q). Other names you may hear are "vitamin B_{15}" and pangamic acid (both hoaxes) or "vitamin B_{17}" (laetrile or amygdalin, not a cancer cure as claimed and not a vitamin by any stretch of the imagination).[‡‡‡]

This chapter has addressed all 13 of the vitamins. Table 7-8 sums up basic facts about the fat-soluble vitamins, and Table 7-9 deals with the water-soluble vitamins.

KEY POINTS

- Choline is needed in the diet, but it is not a vitamin.
- Many U.S. adults do not consume the DRI amount of choline, but effects on health are uncertain.
- Many other substances that people claim are vitamins are not.

carnitine a nonessential nutrient that functions in cellular activities. Also defined in Controversy 10.

inositol (in-OSS-ih-tall) a nonessential nutrient found in cell membranes.

lipoic (lip-OH-ic) **acid** a nonessential nutrient.

‡‡‡ Read about these and many other claims at the website of the National Council Against Health Fraud, www.ncahf.org.

Table 7–8

The Fat-Soluble Vitamins—Functions, Deficiencies, and Toxicities

VITAMIN A

Other Names
Retinol, retinal, retinoic acid; main precursor is beta-carotene

Chief Functions in the Body
Vision; health of cornea, epithelial cells, mucous membranes, skin; growth; regulation of gene expression; reproduction; embryonic development of spinal cord and heart; immunity
Beta-carotene: antioxidant

Deficiency Disease Name
Hypovitaminosis A

Significant Sources
Retinol: fortified milk, cheese, cream, butter, fortified margarine, eggs, liver
Beta-carotene: spinach and other dark, leafy greens; broccoli; deep orange fruit (apricots, cantaloupe) and vegetables (winter squash, carrots, sweet potatoes, pumpkin)

	Deficiency Symptoms	Toxicity Symptoms
Blood/Circulatory System	Anemia (small-cell type)[a]	Red blood cell breakage, cessation of menstruation, nosebleeds
Bones/Teeth	Cessation of growth, painful joints; impaired enamel formation, cracks in teeth, tendency toward tooth decay	Bone pain; growth retardation; difficulty gaining weight; increased pressure inside skull
Digestive System	Diarrhea, changes in intestinal and other body linings	Abdominal pain, nausea, vomiting, diarrhea, weight loss
Immune System	Frequent infections	Overreactivity
Nervous/Muscular System	Night blindness (retinal) Mental depression	Blurred vision, poor muscle coordination, fatigue, irritability, loss of appetite
Skin and Cornea	Keratinization, corneal degeneration leading to blindness[b], rashes	Dry skin, rashes; cracking and bleeding lips; brittle nails; hair loss; benign skin yellowing (beta-carotene)
Other	Kidney stones, impaired growth	Liver enlargement and liver damage; birth defects

(continued)

[a]Small-cell type anemia is termed microcytic anemia; large-cell type anemia is macrocytic or megaloblastic anemia.
[b]Corneal degeneration progresses from keratinization (hardening) to xerosis (drying) to xerophthalmia (thickening, opacity, and irreversible blindness).

Chapter 7 The Vitamins

VITAMIN D

Other Names
Calciferol, cholecalciferol, dihydroxy vitamin D; precursor is cholesterol

Chief Functions in the Body
Mineralization of bones (raises blood calcium and phosphorus via absorption from digestive tract and by withdrawing calcium from bones and stimulating retention by kidneys)

Deficiency Disease Name
Rickets, osteomalacia

Significant Sources
Self-synthesis with sunlight; fortified milk and other fortified foods, cod liver oil, sardines, salmon

	Deficiency Symptoms	Toxicity Symptoms
Blood/Circulatory System		Elevated blood calcium; calcification of blood vessels and heart tissues
Bones/Teeth	Abnormal growth, misshapen bones (bowing of legs), soft bones, joint pain, malformed teeth	Calcification of tooth soft tissues; thinning of tooth enamel
Nervous/Muscular System	Muscle spasms	Excessive thirst, headaches, irritability, loss of appetite, weakness, nausea
Other		Calcification and harm to soft tissues (kidneys, lungs, joints); heart damage

VITAMIN E

Other Names
Alpha-tocopherol, tocopherol

Chief Functions in the Body
Antioxidant (quenching of free radicals), stabilization of cell membranes, support of immune function, protection of polyunsaturated fatty acids; normal nerve development

Deficiency Disease Name
(No name)

Significant Sources
Polyunsaturated plant oils (margarine, salad dressings, shortenings), green and leafy vegetables, wheat germ, whole-grain products, nuts, seeds

	Deficiency Symptoms	Toxicity Symptoms
Blood/Circulatory System	Red blood cell breakage, anemia	Augments the effects of anticlotting medication
Digestive System		General discomfort, nausea
Eyes		Blurred vision
Nervous/Muscular System	Nerve degeneration, weakness, difficulty walking, leg cramps	Fatigue

VITAMIN K

Other Names
Phylloquinone, naphthoquinone

Chief Functions in the Body
Synthesis of blood-clotting proteins and proteins important in bone mineralization

Deficiency Disease Name
(No name)

Significant Sources
Bacterial synthesis in the digestive tract; green leafy vegetables, cabbage-type vegetables, soybeans

	Deficiency Symptoms	Toxicity Symptoms
Blood/Circulatory System	Hemorrhage	Interference with anticlotting medication
Bones	Poor skeletal mineralization	

Table 7–9

The Water-Soluble Vitamins—Functions, Deficiencies, and Toxicities

VITAMIN C

Other Names
Ascorbic acid

Chief Functions in the Body
Collagen synthesis (strengthens blood vessel walls, forms scar tissue, and matrix for bone growth), antioxidant, restores vitamin E to active form, hormone synthesis, supports immune cell functions, helps in absorption of iron

Deficiency Disease Name
Scurvy

Significant Sources
Citrus fruit, cabbage-type vegetables, dark green vegetables, cantaloupe, strawberries, peppers, lettuce, tomatoes, potatoes, papayas, mangoes

	Deficiency Symptoms	Toxicity Symptoms
Digestive System		Nausea, abdominal cramps, diarrhea, excessive urination
Immune System	Immune suppression, frequent infections	
Mouth, Gums, Tongue	Bleeding gums, loosened teeth	
Nervous/ Muscular System	Muscle degeneration and pain, depression, disorientation	Headache, fatigue, insomnia
Bones	Bone fragility, joint pain	Aggravation of gout
Skin	Pinpoint hemorrhages, rough skin, blotchy bruises	Rashes
Other	Anemia, failure of wounds to heal	Interference with medical tests; kidney stones in susceptible people

THIAMIN

Other Names
Vitamin B_1

Chief Functions in the Body
Part of a coenzyme needed in energy metabolism, supports normal appetite and nervous system function

Deficiency Disease Name
Beriberi (wet and dry)

Significant Sources
Occurs in all nutritious foods in moderate amounts; pork, ham, bacon, liver, whole and enriched grains, legumes, seeds

	Deficiency Symptoms	Toxicity Symptoms
Blood/Circulatory System	Edema, enlarged heart, abnormal heart rhythms, heart failure	(No symptoms reported)
Nervous/ Muscular System	Degeneration, wasting, weakness, pain, apathy, irritability, difficulty walking, loss of reflexes, jerky eye movements, mental confusion, paralysis	
Other	Anorexia; weight loss	

RIBOFLAVIN

Other Names
Vitamin B_2

Chief Functions in the Body
Part of a coenzyme needed in energy metabolism, supports normal vision and skin health

Deficiency Disease Name
Ariboflavinosis

Significant Sources
Milk, yogurt, cottage cheese, meat, liver, leafy green vegetables, whole-grain or enriched breads and cereals

	Deficiency Symptoms	Toxicity Symptoms
Mouth, Gums, Tongue	Cracks at corners of mouth[a], smooth magenta tongue[b], sore throat	(No symptoms reported)
Nervous System and Eyes	Hypersensitivity to light, reddening of cornea	
Skin	Skin rash	

(continued)

[a]Cracks at the corners of the mouth are termed cheilosis (kee-LOH-sis)
[b]Smoothness of the tongue is caused by loss of its surface structures and is termed glossitis (gloss-EYE-tis).

NIACIN

Other Names
Nicotinic acid, nicotinamide, niacinamide, vitamin B_3; precursor is dietary tryptophan

Chief Functions in the Body
Part of coenzymes needed in energy metabolism

Deficiency Disease Name
Pellagra

Significant Sources
Synthesized from the amino acid tryptophan; milk, eggs, meat, poultry, fish, whole-grain and enriched breads and cereals, nuts, and all protein-containing foods

	Deficiency Symptoms	Toxicity Symptoms
Digestive System	Diarrhea; vomiting; abdominal pain	Nausea, vomiting
Mouth, Gums, Tongue	Black or bright red swollen smooth tongue[b]	
Nervous System	Irritability, loss of appetite, weakness, headache, dizziness, mental confusion progressing to psychosis or delirium	
Skin	Flaky skin rash on areas exposed to sun	Painful flush and rash, sweating
Other		Liver damage; impaired glucose tolerance; vision disturbances

FOLATE

Other Names
Folic acid, folacin, pteroylglutamic acid

Chief Functions in the Body
Part of coenzymes needed for new cell synthesis

Deficiency Disease Name
(No name)

Significant Sources
Asparagus, avocado, leafy green vegetables, beets, legumes, seeds, liver; enriched bread, cereal, pasta, and grains

	Deficiency Symptoms	Toxicity Symptoms
Blood/Circulatory System	Anemia (large-cell type)[a], elevated homocysteine	Masks vitamin B_{12} deficiency
Digestive System	Heartburn, diarrhea, constipation	
Immune System	Suppression, frequent infections	
Mouth, Gums, Tongue	Smooth red tongue[b]	
Nervous/Muscular System	Increased risk of neural tube birth defects; depression, mental confusion, fatigue, irritability, headache	Depression, mental confusion, fatigue, irritability, headache

VITAMIN B_{12}

Other Names
Cyanocobalamin

Chief Functions in the Body
Part of coenzymes needed in new cell synthesis, helps maintain nerve cells

Deficiency Disease Name
(No name)c

Significant Sources
Animal products (meat, fish, poultry, milk, cheese, eggs), enriched foods

	Deficiency Symptoms	Toxicity Symptoms
Blood/Circulatory System	Anemia (large-cell type)[a,c]	(No toxicity symptoms known)
Mouth, Gums, Tongue	Smooth tongue[b]	
Nervous/Muscular System	Fatigue, nerve degeneration progressing to paralysis	
Skin	Tingling or numbness	

(continued)

[a]*Small cell–type anemia is termed* microcytic anemia; *large cell–type is* macrocytic *or* megaloblastic anemia.

[b]*Smoothness of the tongue is caused by loss of its surface structures and is termed* glossitis *(gloss-EYE-tis).*

[c]*The name* pernicious anemia *refers to the vitamin B_{12} deficiency caused by lack of intrinsic factor but not to that caused by inadequate dietary intake.*

VITAMIN B$_6$

Other Names
Pyridoxine, pyridoxal, pyridoxamine

Chief Functions in the Body
Part of a coenzyme needed in amino acid and fatty acid metabolism, helps convert tryptophan to niacin and to serotonin, helps make red blood cells

Deficiency Disease Name
(No name)

Significant Sources
Meats, fish, poultry, liver, legumes, fruit, potatoes, whole grains, soy products

	Deficiency Symptoms	Toxicity Symptoms
Blood/Circulatory System	Anemia (small-cell type)[a]	Bloating
Nervous/ Muscular System	Depression, confusion, convulsions	Depression, fatigue, irritability, headaches, numbness, damage to nerves, difficulty walking, loss of reflexes, restlessness, convulsions
Skin	Rashes; greasy, scaly dermatitis	Skin lesions

PANTOTHENIC ACID

Other Names
(None)

Chief Functions in the Body
Part of a coenzyme critical for energy metabolism

Deficiency Disease Name
(No name)

Significant Sources
Widespread in foods

	Deficiency Symptoms	Toxicity Symptoms
Digestive System	Vomiting, intestinal distress	Water retention (infrequent)
Nervous/ Muscular System	Insomnia, fatigue	
Other	Hypoglycemia, increased sensitivity to insulin	

BIOTIN

Other Names
(None)

Chief Functions in the Body
An enzyme needed in energy metabolism, fat synthesis, amino acid metabolism, and glycogen synthesis

Deficiency Disease Name
(No name)

Significant Sources
Widespread in foods; instestinal bacteria

	Deficiency Symptoms	Toxicity Symptoms
Blood/Circulatory System	Abnormal heart action	(No toxicity symptoms reported)
Digestive System	Loss of appetite, nausea	
Nervous/ Muscular System	Depression, muscle pain, weakness, fatigue, numbness of extremities	
Skin	Dry around eyes, nose, and mouth	

[a]*Small-cell type anemia is termed* microcytic anemia; *large-cell type is* macrocytic *or* megaloblastic anemia.

Choosing Foods Rich in Vitamins

LO 7.11 Describe how to choose foods to meet vitamin needs.

On learning how important the vitamins are to their health, most people want to choose foods that are vitamin-rich. How can they tell which are which? Not by food labels—these provide only limited vitamin information. A way to find out more about the vitamin contents of your foods is to search for them in an online nutrient database, such as USDA's What's in the Foods You Eat search tool or the USDA Food Composition Databases.* These websites provide lists of nutrients in specified amounts of the foods you select. Then, when you compare those nutrient amounts with the DRI, you'll find out, say, that cornflakes is a particularly good source of folate (manufacturers add folic acid), but a poor source of vitamin E.

Another way of looking at such data appears in Figure 7–22 (pp. 260–261)—the long bars show some foods that are rich sources of a particular vitamin and the short or nonexistent bars indicate poor sources. The colors of the bars represent the various food groups.

*Nutrient values of foods are listed in USDA's What's in the Foods You Eat Search Tool, available at https://reedir.arsnet.usda.gov/codesearchwebapp/(S(k3vwvz4wbmtp0seqwj3br3fj))/CodeSearch.aspx. Another excellent resource is the USDA Food Composition Databases, available at https://ndb.nal.usda.gov/ndb/.

Which Foods Should I Choose?

After looking at Figure 7–22, don't think that you must memorize the richest sources of each vitamin and eat those foods daily. That false notion would lead you to limit your variety of foods, while overemphasizing the components of a few foods. Although it is reassuring to know that your carrot-raisin salad at lunch provided more than your entire day's need for vitamin A, it is a mistake to think that you must then select equally rich sources of all the other vitamins. Such rich sources do not exist for many vitamins—rather, foods work in harmony to provide most nutrients. For example, a baked potato, not a star performer among vitamin C providers, contributes substantially to a day's need for this nutrient and contributes some thiamin and vitamin B_6, too. By the end of the day, assuming that your food choices were made with reasonable care, the bits of vitamin C, thiamin, and vitamin B_6 from each serving of food have accumulated to more than cover the day's need for them.

A Variety of Foods Works Best

The last two graphs of Figure 7–22 show sources of folate and vitamin C. These nutrients are both richly supplied by fruit and vegetables. The richest source of either one may be only a moderate source of the other, but the recommended amounts of fruit and vegetables in the USDA Food Intake Patterns of Chapter 2 cover both needs amply. As for vitamin E, vegetable oils and some seeds and nuts are the richest sources, but vegetables and fruit contribute a little, too.

By now, you should recognize a basic truth in nutrition. The eating pattern that best provides nutrients includes a wide variety of nutrient-dense foods that provide more than just isolated nutrients.[88] Moreover, phytochemicals, widespread among whole grains, nuts, fruit, and vegetables, play roles in human health, as do fiber and other constituents of whole foods. Therefore, when aiming for adequate intakes of vitamins, aim for a diet that meets the recommendations of Chapter 2. Even supplements cannot duplicate the benefits of such a diet, a point made in this chapter's Controversy section.

Phytochemicals are the topic of **Controversy 2**.

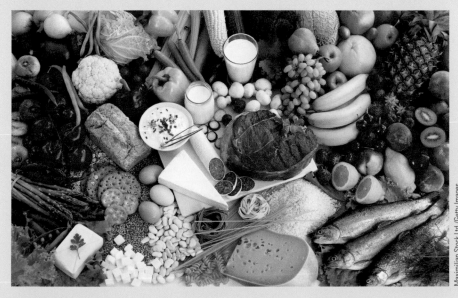

A variety of food like these provides more than just isolated nutrients to the body.

Figure 7–22

Food Sources of Vitamins Selected to Show a Range of Values

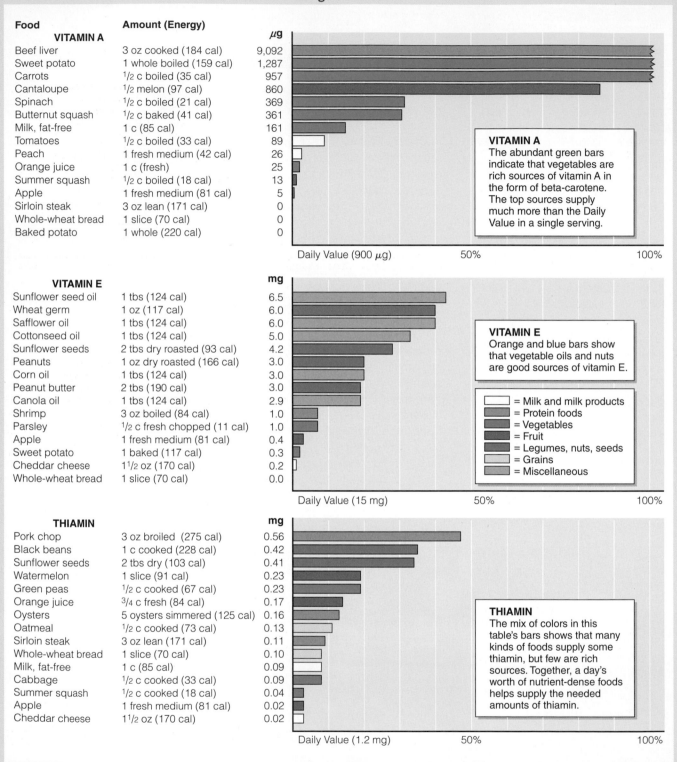

Food	Amount (Energy)	
VITAMIN A		μg
Beef liver	3 oz cooked (184 cal)	9,092
Sweet potato	1 whole boiled (159 cal)	1,287
Carrots	1/2 c boiled (35 cal)	957
Cantaloupe	1/2 melon (97 cal)	860
Spinach	1/2 c boiled (21 cal)	369
Butternut squash	1/2 c baked (41 cal)	361
Milk, fat-free	1 c (85 cal)	161
Tomatoes	1/2 c boiled (33 cal)	89
Peach	1 fresh medium (42 cal)	26
Orange juice	1 c (fresh)	25
Summer squash	1/2 c boiled (18 cal)	13
Apple	1 fresh medium (81 cal)	5
Sirloin steak	3 oz lean (171 cal)	0
Whole-wheat bread	1 slice (70 cal)	0
Baked potato	1 whole (220 cal)	0

VITAMIN A
The abundant green bars indicate that vegetables are rich sources of vitamin A in the form of beta-carotene. The top sources supply much more than the Daily Value in a single serving.

Daily Value (900 μg)   50%   100%

VITAMIN E		mg
Sunflower seed oil	1 tbs (124 cal)	6.5
Wheat germ	1 oz (117 cal)	6.0
Safflower oil	1 tbs (124 cal)	6.0
Cottonseed oil	1 tbs (124 cal)	5.0
Sunflower seeds	2 tbs dry roasted (93 cal)	4.2
Peanuts	1 oz dry roasted (166 cal)	3.0
Corn oil	1 tbs (124 cal)	3.0
Peanut butter	2 tbs (190 cal)	3.0
Canola oil	1 tbs (124 cal)	2.9
Shrimp	3 oz boiled (84 cal)	1.0
Parsley	1/2 c fresh chopped (11 cal)	1.0
Apple	1 fresh medium (81 cal)	0.4
Sweet potato	1 baked (117 cal)	0.3
Cheddar cheese	1 1/2 oz (170 cal)	0.2
Whole-wheat bread	1 slice (70 cal)	0.0

VITAMIN E
Orange and blue bars show that vegetable oils and nuts are good sources of vitamin E.

☐ = Milk and milk products
▨ = Protein foods
▨ = Vegetables
▨ = Fruit
▨ = Legumes, nuts, seeds
▨ = Grains
▨ = Miscellaneous

Daily Value (15 mg)   50%   100%

THIAMIN		mg
Pork chop	3 oz broiled (275 cal)	0.56
Black beans	1 c cooked (228 cal)	0.42
Sunflower seeds	2 tbs dry (103 cal)	0.41
Watermelon	1 slice (91 cal)	0.23
Green peas	1/2 c cooked (67 cal)	0.23
Orange juice	3/4 c fresh (84 cal)	0.17
Oysters	5 oysters simmered (125 cal)	0.16
Oatmeal	1/2 c cooked (73 cal)	0.13
Sirloin steak	3 oz lean (171 cal)	0.11
Whole-wheat bread	1 slice (70 cal)	0.10
Milk, fat-free	1 c (85 cal)	0.09
Cabbage	1/2 c cooked (33 cal)	0.09
Summer squash	1/2 c cooked (18 cal)	0.04
Apple	1 fresh medium (81 cal)	0.02
Cheddar cheese	1 1/2 oz (170 cal)	0.02

THIAMIN
The mix of colors in this table's bars shows that many kinds of foods supply some thiamin, but few are rich sources. Together, a day's worth of nutrient-dense foods helps supply the needed amounts of thiamin.

Daily Value (1.2 mg)   50%   100%

Figure 7–22

Food Sources of Vitamins Selected to Show a Range of Values *(continued)*

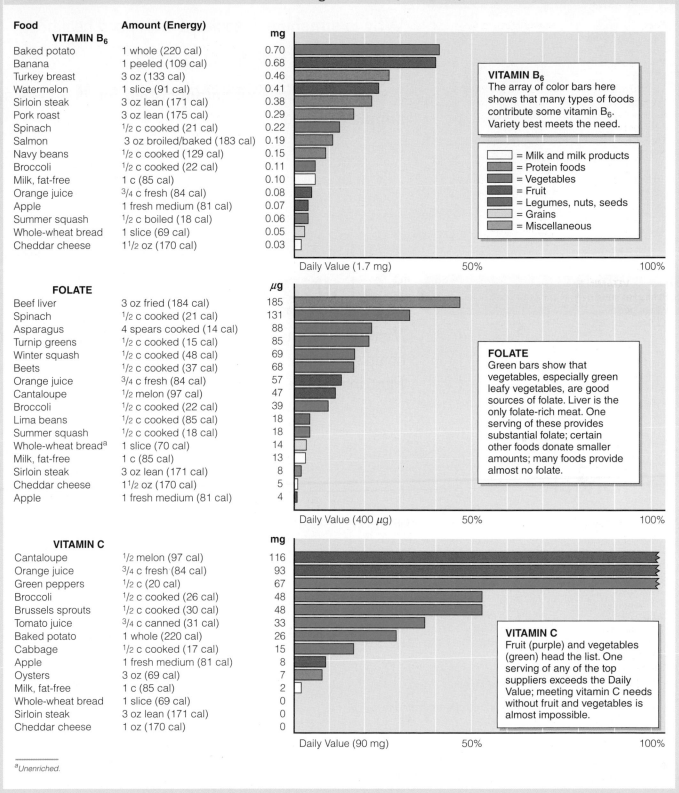

Food	Amount (Energy)	mg
VITAMIN B₆		
Baked potato	1 whole (220 cal)	0.70
Banana	1 peeled (109 cal)	0.68
Turkey breast	3 oz (133 cal)	0.46
Watermelon	1 slice (91 cal)	0.41
Sirloin steak	3 oz lean (171 cal)	0.38
Pork roast	3 oz lean (175 cal)	0.29
Spinach	1/2 c cooked (21 cal)	0.22
Salmon	3 oz broiled/baked (183 cal)	0.19
Navy beans	1/2 c cooked (129 cal)	0.15
Broccoli	1/2 c cooked (22 cal)	0.11
Milk, fat-free	1 c (85 cal)	0.10
Orange juice	3/4 c fresh (84 cal)	0.08
Apple	1 fresh medium (81 cal)	0.07
Summer squash	1/2 c boiled (18 cal)	0.06
Whole-wheat bread	1 slice (69 cal)	0.05
Cheddar cheese	1 1/2 oz (170 cal)	0.03

VITAMIN B₆
The array of color bars here shows that many types of foods contribute some vitamin B₆. Variety best meets the need.

☐ = Milk and milk products
■ = Protein foods
■ = Vegetables
■ = Fruit
■ = Legumes, nuts, seeds
☐ = Grains
■ = Miscellaneous

Daily Value (1.7 mg)   50%   100%

Food	Amount (Energy)	μg
FOLATE		
Beef liver	3 oz fried (184 cal)	185
Spinach	1/2 c cooked (21 cal)	131
Asparagus	4 spears cooked (14 cal)	88
Turnip greens	1/2 c cooked (15 cal)	85
Winter squash	1/2 c cooked (48 cal)	69
Beets	1/2 c cooked (37 cal)	68
Orange juice	3/4 c fresh (84 cal)	57
Cantaloupe	1/2 melon (97 cal)	47
Broccoli	1/2 c cooked (22 cal)	39
Lima beans	1/2 c cooked (85 cal)	18
Summer squash	1/2 c cooked (18 cal)	18
Whole-wheat bread[a]	1 slice (70 cal)	14
Milk, fat-free	1 c (85 cal)	13
Sirloin steak	3 oz lean (171 cal)	8
Cheddar cheese	1 1/2 oz (170 cal)	5
Apple	1 fresh medium (81 cal)	4

FOLATE
Green bars show that vegetables, especially green leafy vegetables, are good sources of folate. Liver is the only folate-rich meat. One serving of these provides substantial folate; certain other foods donate smaller amounts; many foods provide almost no folate.

Daily Value (400 μg)   50%   100%

Food	Amount (Energy)	mg
VITAMIN C		
Cantaloupe	1/2 melon (97 cal)	116
Orange juice	3/4 c fresh (84 cal)	93
Green peppers	1/2 c (20 cal)	67
Broccoli	1/2 c cooked (26 cal)	48
Brussels sprouts	1/2 c cooked (30 cal)	48
Tomato juice	3/4 c canned (31 cal)	33
Baked potato	1 whole (220 cal)	26
Cabbage	1/2 c cooked (17 cal)	15
Apple	1 fresh medium (81 cal)	8
Oysters	3 oz (69 cal)	7
Milk, fat-free	1 c (85 cal)	2
Whole-wheat bread	1 slice (69 cal)	0
Sirloin steak	3 oz lean (171 cal)	0
Cheddar cheese	1 oz (170 cal)	0

VITAMIN C
Fruit (purple) and vegetables (green) head the list. One serving of any of the top suppliers exceeds the Daily Value; meeting vitamin C needs without fruit and vegetables is almost impossible.

Daily Value (90 mg)   50%   100%

[a]Unenriched.

What did you decide?

How do **vitamins** work in the body?

Why is **sunshine** associated with good health?

Can **vitamin C tablets** ward off a cold?

Should you choose **vitamin-fortified foods** and take **supplements** for "insurance"?

What's online?

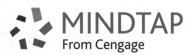

MINDTAP
From Cengage

Visit www.Cengage.com to access MindTap, a complete digital course that includes Diet & Wellness Plus, interactive quizzes, videos, and more.

Self Check

1. (LO 7.1) Which of the following vitamins are classified as fat-soluble?

   a. vitamins B and D
   b. vitamins A, D, E, and K
   c. vitamins B, E, D, and C
   d. vitamins B and C

2. (LO 7.1) Which of the following describes the fat-soluble vitamins?

   a. few functions in the body
   b. easily absorbed and excreted
   c. stored abundantly in tissues
   d. a and c

3. (LO 7.1) Most water-soluble vitamins are not stored in tissues to any great extent.
   T   F

4. (LO 7.2) Fat-soluble vitamins are mostly absorbed into

   a. the lymph.
   b. the blood.
   c. the extracellular fluid.
   d. b and c.

5. (LO 7.3) Which of the following foods is (are) rich in beta-carotene?

   a. sweet potatoes
   b. pumpkin
   c. spinach
   d. all of the above

6. (LO 7.3) Vitamin A supplements can help treat acne.
   T   F

7. (LO 7.4) Vitamin D functions as a hormone to help maintain bone integrity.
   T   F

8. (LO 7.4) In adults with vitamin D deficiency, poor bone mineralization can lead to _____.

   a. pellagra
   b. pernicious anemia
   c. scurvy
   d. osteomalacia

9. (LO 7.5) Which of the following is (are) rich source(s) of vitamin E?

   a. raw vegetable oil
   b. colorful foods, such as carrots

c. milk and milk products

d. raw cabbage

10. (LO 7.5) Vitamin E is famous for its role

    a. in maintaining bone tissue integrity.

    b. in maintaining connective tissue integrity.

    c. in protecting tissues from oxidation.

    d. as a precursor for vitamin C.

11. (LO 7.6) Vitamin K is necessary for the synthesis of key bone proteins.

    T F

12. (LO 7.6) Vitamin K

    a. can be made from exposure to sunlight.

    b. can be obtained from most milk products.

    c. can be made by digestive tract bacteria.

    d. b and c

13. (LO 7.7) Water-soluble vitamins are mostly absorbed into _____.

    a. the lymph   c. the extracellular fluid

    b. the blood   d. b and c

14. (LO 7.7) The water-soluble vitamins are characterized by all of the following except

    a. excesses are stored and easily build up to toxic concentrations.

    b. they travel freely in the blood.

    c. excesses are easily excreted and seldom build up to toxic concentrations.

    d. b and c.

15. (LO 7.8) The theory that vitamin C prevents or cures colds is well supported by research.

    T F

16. (LO 7.8) Vitamin C deficiency symptoms include _____.

    a. red spots   c. anemia

    b. loose teeth   d. all of the above

17. (LO 7.9) B vitamins often act as _____.

    a. antioxidants   c. coenzymes

    b. blood clotting factors   d. none of the above

18. (LO 7.9) A B vitamin often forms part of an enzyme's active site, where a chemical reaction takes place.

    T F

19. (LO 7.10) A deficiency of niacin may result in which disease?

    a. pellagra   c. scurvy

    b. beriberi   d. rickets

20. (LO 7.10) Which of these B vitamins is (are) present only in foods of animal origin?

    a. niacin   c. riboflavin

    b. vitamin B_{12} d. a and c

21. (LO 7.11) The eating pattern that best provides nutrients

    a. singles out a rich source for each nutrient and focuses on these foods.

    b. includes a wide variety of nutrient-dense foods.

    c. is a Western eating style that includes abundant meats and fats.

    d. singles out rich sources of certain phytochemicals and focuses on these foods.

22. (LO 7.12) The FDA has extensive regulatory control over supplement sales.

    T F

Answers to these Self Check questions are in Appendix G.

Vitamin Supplements: What are the Benefits and Risks?

LO 7.12 Debate for and against taking vitamin supplements.

More than half of the U.S. population takes dietary supplements, spending almost $38 *billion* each year to do so.[1]* Most take a daily multivitamin and mineral pill, hoping to make up for dietary shortfalls; others take single nutrient supplements hoping to ward off diseases; and many do both. Do people need all these supplements? If people do need supplements, which ones are best? Are there any health risks from supplements? This Controversy examines evidence surrounding these questions and concludes with some advice on choosing a supplement with the most benefit and least risk.

Dietary supplements were defined in **Chapter 1**.

Reference notes are in Appendix F.

Arguments in Favor of Taking Supplements

By far, most people can meet their nutrient needs from their diets alone. Indisputably, however, the people listed in Table C7–1 need supplements. For them, nutrient supplements can prevent or reverse illnesses. Because supplements are not risk-free, these people should consult health-care providers who are alert to potential adverse effects and nutrient-drug interactions.

People with Deficiencies

In the United States, few adults suffer nutrient-deficiency diseases such as scurvy, pellagra, and beriberi. When deficiency diseases do appear, prescribed supplements of the missing nutrients quickly stop or reverse most of the damage (exceptions include vitamin A–deficiency blindness, some vitamin B_{12}–deficiency nerve damage, and birth defects caused by folate deficiency in pregnant women).

Subtle subclinical deficiencies that do not cause classic symptoms are easily overlooked or misdiagnosed—and they often occur. People who diet habitually or elderly people with diminished appetite may eat so little nutritious food that they teeter on the edge of deficiency, with no reserves to handle any increase in demand. Similarly, people who omit entire food groups without proper diet planning or who are too busy or lack knowledge or lack money are likely to lack nutrients. For them, until they correct their diets, a low-dose, complete vitamin-mineral supplement may help them avoid deficiency diseases. This Controversy ends with advice on how to choose suitable supplements.

Life Stages with Increased Nutrient Needs

During certain stages of life, many people find it difficult or impossible to meet nutrient needs without supplements. For example, women who lose a lot of blood and therefore a lot of iron during menstruation each month generally need iron supplements. Similarly, pregnant and breastfeeding women have exceptionally high nutrient needs and routinely take special supplements to help meet them. A newborn needs a dose of vitamin K at birth, as this chapter pointed out.

Appetite and Physical Stress

Any interference with a person's appetite, ability to eat, or ability to absorb or use nutrients will impair nutrient status. Prolonged illnesses, extensive injuries or

Table C7–1

Some Valid Reasons for Taking Supplements

These people may need supplements:

- People with nutrient deficiencies.
- Women who are capable of becoming pregnant (supplemental or enrichment sources of folic acid are recommended to reduce risk of neural tube defects in infants).
- Pregnant women and lactating women (they may need iron and folate).
- Newborns (they are routinely given a vitamin K dose).
- Infants (they may need various supplements; see Chapter 13).
- People who undergo weight-loss surgery (incurs nutrient malabsorption).
- Those who are lactose intolerant (they need calcium to forestall osteoporosis).
- Habitual dieters (they may eat insufficient food).
- Elderly people often benefit from some of the vitamins and minerals in a balanced supplement (they may choose poor diets, have trouble chewing, or absorb or metabolize nutrients inefficiently; see Chapter 14).
- People living with HIV or other wasting illnesses (they lose nutrients faster than foods can supply them).
- Those addicted to drugs or alcohol (they absorb fewer and excrete more nutrients; nutrients cannot undo damage from drugs or alcohol).
- Those recovering from surgery, burns, injury, or illness (they need extra nutrients to help regenerate tissues).
- Strict vegetarians (vegans may need vitamin B_{12}, vitamin D, iron, and zinc).
- People taking medications that interfere with the body's use of nutrients.

burns, weight-loss or other surgery, and addictions to alcohol or other drugs all exert these effects, and such stressors increase nutrient requirements of the tissues. In addition, medications used to treat such conditions often increase nutrient needs. In all these cases, appropriate nutrient supplements can avert further decline.

Arguments against Taking Supplements

In study after study, well-nourished people are the ones found to be taking supplements, adding excess nutrients to already sufficient intakes.[2] Ironically, people with low nutrient intakes from food generally do not take supplements. As for risks, the most likely hazard to supplement takers is to the wallet—as an old saying goes, "If you take supplements of the water-soluble vitamins, you'll have the most expensive urine in town." Occasionally, though, supplement intake is both costly and harmful to health.

Toxicity

Foods rarely cause nutrient imbalances or toxicities, but supplements easily can—and the higher the dose, the greater the risk. Figure C7–1 illustrates this point. Supplement users are more likely to have excessive intakes of certain nutrients—notably iron, zinc, vitamin A, and niacin.

People's tolerances for high doses of nutrients vary, just as their risks of deficiencies do, and amounts tolerable for some may be harmful for others. The DRI Tolerable Upper Intake Levels (UL) define the highest intakes that appear safe for *most* healthy people. A few sensitive people may experience toxicities at lower doses, however.

In 2017, almost 275,000 calls to poison control centers across the nation resulted from adverse effects of taking vitamins, minerals, essential oils, herbs, and other supplements.[3] No upper intake guidelines exist for supplement add-ons, such as herbs or phytochemicals, so pills vary widely in their contents of these substances.[4] Many chronic, subclinical toxicities go unrecognized and unreported.

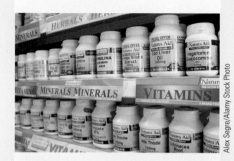

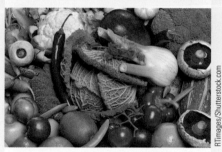

Supplement Contamination and Safety

More than 1,500 times since 2005, the FDA has warned consumers about contamination of dietary supplements, most often supplements sold over the Internet for weight loss, or enhanced athletic or sexual performance.[5] Today, illicit pharmaceutical drugs, such as steroid hormones or stimulants, still contaminate supplements, many of them ironically sold as "natural alternatives" to FDA-approved drugs. Manufacturers, once notified, must remove these dangerous products from the market but others quickly take their place. Athletes need to know that even accidental ingestion of banned drugs from a contaminated supplement can cause a potentially career-ending "positive" result on a drug test. Anyone who takes them risks liver injury, kidney failure, or stroke.

Plain multivitamin and mineral supplements from reputable sources, without herbs or add-ons, generally test free from contamination, although their contents may vary from those stated on the label. More than twice the label amount of vitamin A was found in a popular multivitamin, and several other brands contained more than the ULs of niacin and magnesium.[6] A prenatal multivitamin contained more than 140 percent of the chromium listed on the label.[7]

Many consumers wrongly believe that government scientists—in particular, those of the FDA—test each new dietary supplement to ensure its safety and effectiveness before allowing it to be sold. They do not. In fact, under the current Dietary Supplement Health and Education Act, the FDA has little control over supplement sales.[†] (It can act to remove *tainted* products from store shelves, however, and does so often.) Consumers can report adverse reactions to supplements directly to the FDA via its hotline or website.[‡]

Life-Threatening Misinformation

A person who is ill may come to believe that self-prescribed high doses of vitamins or minerals can be therapeutic. Such a person might postpone seeking a diagnosis, thinking, "I probably just need a supplement to make this go away." Meanwhile, without medical care, the disease worsens. Improper dosing can also cause problems. One man who suffered from mental illness arrived at an emergency room with dangerously low blood pressure. He had ingested 11 *grams* of niacin, on the advice of an Internet website. The UL for niacin is 35 *milligrams*.

Supplements are almost never effective for purposes other than those already listed in Table C7–1. This doesn't stop marketers from making enticing structure-function claims in materials of all kinds—in print, on labels, and on television or the Internet. Such sales pitches often fall far short of the FDA standard that claims should be "truthful and not misleading."

[†] *The Dietary Supplement Health and Education Act of 1994 regulates supplements, holding them to the same general labeling requirements that apply to foods (labeling terms were defined in Chapter 2).*

[‡] *Consumers should report suspected harm from dietary supplements to their health providers or to the FDA's MedWatch program at (800) FDA-1088 or on the Internet at www.fda.gov/medwatch/.*

Controversy 7 Vitamin Supplements: What are the Benefits and Risks?

265

False Sense of Security

Lulled into a false sense of security, a person might eat irresponsibly, thinking, "My supplement will cover my needs." However, no one knows exactly how to formulate the "ideal" supplement, and no standards exist for formulations. What nutrients should be included? How much of each? On whose needs should the choices be based? Which, if any, of the phytochemicals should be added?

Whole Foods Are Best for Nutrients

In general, the body assimilates nutrients best from foods that dilute and disperse them among other substances that facilitate their absorption and use by the body. Taken in pure, concentrated form, nutrients are likely to interfere with one another's absorption or with the absorption of other nutrients from foods eaten at the same time. Such effects are particularly well known among the minerals. For example, zinc hinders copper and calcium absorption, iron hinders zinc absorption, and calcium hinders magnesium and iron absorption. Among vitamins, vitamin C supplements *enhance* iron absorption, making iron overload likely in susceptible people. High doses of vitamin E interfere with vitamin K functions, delaying blood clotting and possibly raising the risk of brain hemorrhage (a form of stroke). These and other interactions represent drawbacks to supplement use.

Can Supplements Prevent Chronic Diseases?

Many people take supplements in the belief that they can prevent heart disease and cancer. Can taking supplements protect the takers from these killers?

Vitamin D and Cancer

Reports that vitamin D supplements might prevent cancers, particularly of the breast, colon, and prostate, have boosted sales. Low blood vitamin D intakes are generally associated with increased cancer risk in studies, and patients with higher serum vitamin D concentrations at the time of colorectal cancer diagnosis have better survival rates. Still, evidence does not support taking vitamin D supplements to prevent cancer from occurring.[8] The U.S. Preventive Services Task Force, a group that offers unbiased advice concerning medical treatments, has recommended against taking vitamin D for cancer prevention.[9]

Antioxidant Supplements

This chapter explained that normal activities of body cells produce free radicals (highly unstable molecules of oxygen) that can damage cell structures. Oxidative stress results when free-radical activity in the body exceeds its antioxidant defenses. When such damage accumulates, it triggers inflammation, which may lead to heart disease and cancer, among other conditions. **Antioxidant nutrients** help to quench these free radicals, rendering them harmless to cellular structures and stopping the chain of events. Antioxidant terms are defined in Table C7–2.

Taking antioxidant pills instead of making needed lifestyle changes may sound appealing, but evidence does not support a role for supplements against chronic diseases.[10] In some cases, supplements may even be harmful.[11]

Vitamin E and Chronic Disease

Hopeful early studies reported that taking vitamin E supplements reduced the rate of death from heart disease. It made sense because in the laboratory vitamin E opposes blood clotting, tissue inflammation, arterial injury, and lipid oxidation—all factors in heart disease development. After years of human studies, results are disappointing: neither help nor harm is consistently observed with vitamin E supplementation.

The Story of Beta-Carotene— A Case in Point

Again and again, population studies confirm that people who eat plenty of fruit and vegetables, particularly those rich in beta-carotene, have low rates of certain cancers. Years ago, researchers focused on beta-carotene, while supplement makers touted it as a powerful anticancer substance. Consumers eagerly bought and took beta-carotene supplements in response.

Then, in a sudden reversal, support for beta-carotene supplements crumbled overnight. Trials around the world were abruptly stopped when scientists noted no benefits but observed a 28 percent *increase* in lung cancer among smokers taking beta-carotene compared with a placebo. Today, other evidence supports these findings and beta-carotene supplements are not recommended.[12]

Such reversals might shock and frustrate the unscientific mind, but scientists expect them as research unfolds. In this case, a long-known and basic nutrition principle was reaffirmed: low disease risk accompanies a *diet* of nutritious whole foods, foods that present a balance of nutrients and other beneficial constituents. A pill provides only beta-carotene, a lone chemical.

For most people, taking an ordinary daily multivitamin and mineral supplement is generally safe, but probably offers no protection against chronic diseases.[13] Table C7–3 reviews the arguments for and against taking supplements.

Table C7–2

Antioxidant Terms

- **antioxidant nutrients** vitamins and minerals that oppose the effects of oxidants on human physical functions. The antioxidant vitamins are vitamin E, vitamin C, and beta-carotene. The mineral selenium also participates in antioxidant activities.
- **oxidants** compounds (such as oxygen itself) that oxidize other compounds. Compounds that prevent oxidation are called antioxidants, whereas those that promote it are called prooxidants (*anti* means "against"; *pro* means "for").

Table C7–3

Taking Dietary Supplements: Point, Counterpoint

Many people take dietary supplements either to counterbalance inadequate diets or to improve on their already abundant intakes of nutrients. This table considers some arguments for and against doing so.

Arguments in Support of Dietary Supplements	Arguments in Opposition to Dietary Supplements
1. *Prevent or correct deficiencies.* Supplements are important for people suffering from nutrient deficiencies, and in most cases, they can correct the problems and restore health.	1. *Cause toxicities.* Dietary supplements provide no benefits to well-nourished people. High-nutrient doses from single-nutrient supplements pose a threat of toxicity.
2. *Fill increased nutrient needs.* Adolescents of both genders, women of childbearing age, women who are pregnant or breast-feeding, newborn infants, people who are ill, smokers, and others all have increased needs for certain nutrients such as iron, folate, vitamin K, or vitamin C.	2. *Provide unneeded nutrients.* Most healthy children and adults who eat a nutritious diet consume adequate amounts of vitamins and minerals from food, making nutrients from supplements unnecessary.
3. *Improve nutrient status.* Certain groups of people, such as the elderly who may not eat enough food and vegetarians who omit entire food groups, can develop subclinical nutrient deficiencies that may produce no obvious symptoms but may impair health in subtle ways, such as reducing resistance to infection.	3. *Provide limited benefits.* A supplement can treat a single nutrient deficiency but cannot replace a nutritious diet to support health. A diet that lacks one nutrient surely lacks others, along with fiber, phytochemicals, and other constituents of whole, nutrient-dense foods.
4. *Provide nutritional insurance.* Vitamin pills are cheap to purchase, and taking them is easier than shopping, cooking, and planning an adequate diet.	4. *Create a false sense of security.* Research consistently shows that supplements cannot substitute for a nutritious diet in supporting the health of the body.
5. *Efficacy and safety of dietary supplements.* The FDA routinely recalls supplements containing harmful ingredients and removes them from the market. The FDA also prosecutes manufacturers violating the Dietary Supplement Health and Education Act, which requires supplements to be free of contaminants and ingredients that are not safe for human consumption.	5. *Efficacy and safety of dietary supplements.* Scientists and consumer groups agree that oversight policies are outdated and ineffective. The FDA does not regulate supplements as tightly as it does pharmaceutical drugs prior to marketing, but rather waits to remove products from the market until after they have proven unsafe by causing harm to consumers.

Sources: H. Ketha and coauthors, Iatrogenic vitamin D toxicity in an infant: A case report and review of literature, Journal of Steroid Biochemistry and Molecular Biology 148 (2015): 14–18; J. R. Genzen, Hypercalcemic crisis due to vitamin D toxicity, Lab Medicine 45 (2014): 147–150; S. M. Alsanad, E. M. Williamson, and R. L. Howard, Cancer patients at risk of herb/food supplement-drug interactions: A systematic review, Phytotherapy Research 28 (2014): 1749–1755; E. Fabian and coauthors, Vitamin status in elderly people in relation to the use of nutritional supplements, Journal of Nutrition 16 (2012): 206–212; P. A. Cohen, Assessing supplemental safety—The FDA's controversial proposal, New England Journal of Medicine 366 (2012): 389–391; M. E. Martinez and coauthors, Dietary supplements and cancer prevention: Balancing potential benefits against proven harms, Journal of the National Cancer Institute 104 (2012): 732–739.

SOS: Selection of Supplements

If you fall into one of the categories listed earlier in Table C7–1 and if you absolutely cannot meet your nutrient needs from foods, a supplement containing *nutrients only* can prevent serious problems. In these cases, the benefits outweigh the risks. (Table C7–4 on p. 268 provides some *invalid* reasons for taking supplements in which the risks clearly outweigh the benefits.) Remember, no standard formula for multivitamin and mineral preparations exists—the term *supplement* applies to any combination of nutrients in widely varying doses.

Choosing a Type

Which supplement to choose? The first step is to remain aware that sales of vitamin supplements often approach the realm of quackery because the profits are high and the industry is largely free of oversight. To escape the clutches of the health hustlers, use your imagination, and delete the label pictures of sexy, active people and the meaningless, glittering generalities like "Advanced Formula" or "Maximum Power." Also, ignore vague "structure-function claims" that refer to the functioning of body systems or common complaints, such as cramps or insomnia; most of these are distortions of the truth. Avoid "extras" such as herbs (see Chapter 11).

Don't be misled into buying and taking unneeded supplements, because none are risk-free.

Reading the Label

Now all you have left is the Supplement Facts panel, shown in Figure C7–2 (p. 268), that lists the nutrients, the ingredients, the form of the supplement, and the price—the plain facts. You have two basic questions to answer. The first question: What form do you want—chewable, liquid, or pills? If you'd rather drink your vitamins and minerals than chew them, fine. If you choose a fortified liquid meal replacer, a sugary vitamin drink, or an "energy bar" (a candy bar to which vitamins and

Some Invalid Reasons for Taking Supplements

Watch out for plausible-sounding, but false, reasons given by marketers trying to convince you, consumers, that you need supplements. The following invalid reasons have gained strength by repetition among friends, on the Internet, and by the media:

- You fear that foods grown on today's soils lack nutrients (a common false statement made by sellers of supplements).
- You feel tired and falsely believe that supplements can provide energy.
- You hope that supplements can help you cope with stress.
- You wish to build up your muscles faster or without physical activity.
- You want to prevent or cure self-diagnosed illnesses.
- You hope excess nutrients will produce unnamed mysterious beneficial reactions in your body.

People who should never take supplements without a physician's approval include those with kidney or liver ailments (they are susceptible to toxicities), those taking medications (nutrients can interfere with their actions), and smokers (who should avoid products with beta-carotene).

How to Read a Supplement Label

Check the Supplement Facts panel for a list of included nutrients, quantity per serving, and "% Daily Value." Less-reliable structure-function claims, shown on the bottom label, do not need FDA approval, but must be accompanied by a disclaimer.

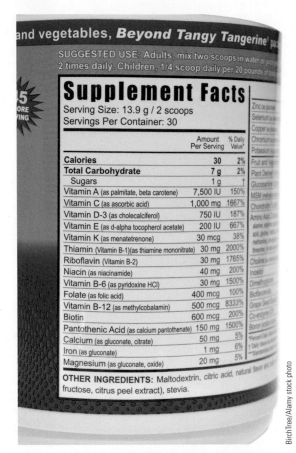

...and vegetables, *Beyond Tangy Tangerine*...		
SUGGESTED USE: Adults, mix two scoops in water or... 2 times daily. Children, 1/4 scoop daily per 20 pounds of...		

Supplement Facts
Serving Size: 13.9 g / 2 scoops
Servings Per Container: 30

	Amount Per Serving	% Daily Value*
Calories	30	2%
Total Carbohydrate	7 g	2%
Sugars	1 g	†
Vitamin A (as palmitate, beta carotene)	7,500 IU	150%
Vitamin C (as ascorbic acid)	1,000 mg	1667%
Vitamin D-3 (as cholecalciferol)	750 IU	187%
Vitamin E (as d-alpha tocopherol acetate)	200 IU	667%
Vitamin K (as menatetrenone)	30 mcg	38%
Thiamin (Vitamin B-1)(as thiamine mononitrate)	30 mg	2000%
Riboflavin (Vitamin B-2)	30 mg	1765%
Niacin (as niacinamide)	40 mg	200%
Vitamin B-6 (as pyridoxine HCl)	30 mg	1500%
Folate (as folic acid)	400 mcg	100%
Vitamin B-12 (as methylcobalamin)	500 mcg	8333%
Biotin	600 mcg	200%
Pantothenic Acid (as calcium pantothenate)	150 mg	1500%
Calcium (as gluconate, citrate)	50 mg	5%
Iron (as gluconate)	1 mg	6%
Magnesium (as gluconate, oxide)	20 mg	5%

OTHER INGREDIENTS: Maltodextrin, citric acid, natural flavor and other fructose, citrus peel extract), stevia.

BirchTree/Alamy stock photo

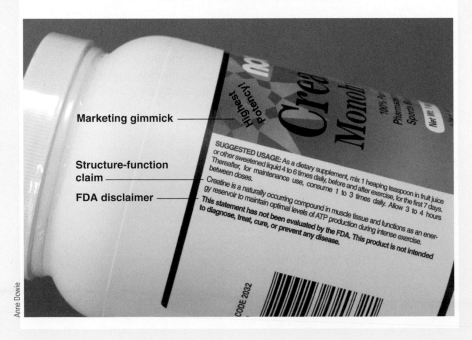

Marketing gimmick

Structure-function claim

FDA disclaimer

SUGGESTED USAGE: As a dietary supplement, mix 1 heaping teaspoon in fruit juice or other sweetened liquid 4 to 6 times daily, before and after exercise, for the first 7 days. Thereafter, for maintenance use, consume 1 to 3 times daily. Allow 3 to 4 hours between doses.

Creatine is a naturally occurring compound in muscle tissue and functions as an energy reservoir to maintain optimal levels of ATP production during intense exercise. This statement has not been evaluated by the FDA. This product is not intended to diagnose, treat, cure, or prevent any disease.

Anne Dowie

other nutrients are added), you must then proportionately reduce the calories you consume in food to avoid gaining unwanted weight. If you choose chewable pills, be aware that vitamin C can erode tooth enamel. Swallow promptly and swish the teeth with water.

Targeting Your Needs

The second question: Who are you? What vitamins and minerals do you actually need and in what amounts? Match your DRI values (at the back of the book, p. B) with the doses in supplement options. The DRI meet the needs of all reasonably healthy people.

Choosing Doses

As for doses of nutrients, for most people, an appropriate supplement provides all the vitamins and minerals in amounts smaller than, equal to, or very close to the DRI recommendations. Avoid any preparation that in a daily dose provides more than the DRI values of vitamin A, vitamin D, or any mineral or more than the UL of any nutrient. In addition, avoid high doses of iron (more than 10 milligrams per day) except for menstruating women. People who menstruate need more iron, but people who don't, don't. Warning: expect to reject about 80 percent of available preparations when you choose according to these criteria. Be choosy where your health is concerned.

Going for Quality

If you see a USP symbol on the label, it means that a manufacturer has voluntarily paid an independent laboratory to test the product, which confirms that it contains the ingredients listed and that it will dissolve in the digestive tract to make the ingredients available for absorption. The symbol does not imply that the supplement has been tested for safety or effectiveness with regard to health.

A high price also does not ensure the highest quality; generic brands are often as good as or better than expensive name-brand supplements. If they are less expensive, it may mean that their price doesn't have to cover the cost of national advertising. In any case, buy from a well-known retailer who stores them properly.

Avoiding Marketing Traps

In addition, avoid these:

- "For better metabolism." Preparations containing extra biotin may claim to improve metabolism, but no evidence supports this.

- "Organic" or "natural" preparations with added substances. They are no better than standard types, but they cost much more, and the added substances may add risks.

- "High-potency" or "therapeutic dose" supplements. More is not better.

- Items not needed in human nutrition, such as carnitine and inositol. These particular items won't harm you, but they reveal a marketing strategy that makes the whole mix suspect. The manufacturer wants you to believe that its pills contain the latest "new" nutrient that other brands omit, but in fact for every valid discovery of this kind, there are 999,999 frauds.

- "Time release." Medications such as some antibiotics or pain relievers often must be sustained at a steady concentration in the blood to be effective; nutrients, in contrast, are incorporated into the tissues where they are needed whenever they arrive.

- "Stress formulas." Although the stress response depends on certain B vitamins and vitamin C, the DRI provides all that is needed of these nutrients. If you are under stress (and who isn't?), generous servings of fruit and vegetables will more than cover your need.

- Claims that today's foods lack sufficient nutrients to support health. Plants make vitamins for their own needs, not ours. A plant lacking a needed mineral or failing to make a needed vitamin dies without yielding food for our consumption.

To get the most from a supplement of vitamins and minerals, take it with food. A full stomach retains the pill and dissolves it with its churning action.

Conclusion

People in developed nations are far more likely to suffer from *overnutrition* and poor lifestyle choices than from nutrient deficiencies. Yet, many of them wish that swallowing vitamin pills would boost their health or energy levels. The truth—that they need to improve their eating and exercise habits—is harder to swallow.

Critical Thinking

1. List three reasons why someone might take a multivitamin supplement that does not exceed 100 percent of the DRIs. Would you ever take an antioxidant supplement? Why or why not? Suppose you decided that you should take a vitamin supplement because you do not drink milk. How would you determine the best supplement to purchase?

2. Imagine that you are standing in a pharmacy comparing the Supplement Facts panels on the labels of two supplement bottles, one a "complete multivitamin" product and the other marked "high potency vitamins."

   What major differences in terms of nutrient inclusion and doses might you find between these two products? What differences in risk would you anticipate? If you were asked to pick one of these products for an elderly person with a poor appetite, which would you choose? Justify your answer.

Controversy 7 Vitamin Supplements: What are the Benefits and Risks?

269

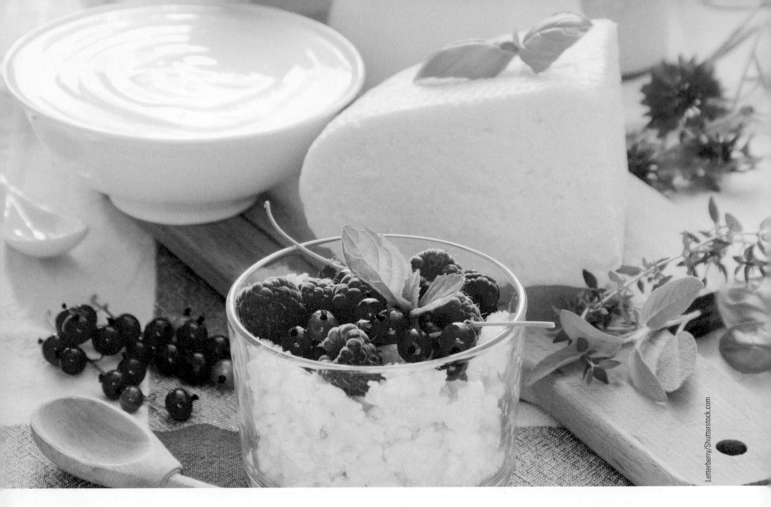

8 Water and Minerals

Learning Objectives

After completing this chapter, you should be able to accomplish the following:

LO 8.1 Explain the functions of water and the importance of maintaining the body's water balance.

LO 8.2 Compare the types and safety of drinking water from different sources.

LO 8.3 Describe the concepts of fluid and electrolyte balance and acid-base balance and their importance to health.

LO 8.4 Describe the functions of the seven major minerals, their food sources, and the effects of their deficiencies and toxicities.

LO 8.5 Discuss the functions of the nine known trace minerals, their food sources, and the effects of their deficiencies and toxicities.

LO 8.6 Itemize food choices that help to meet the need for calcium.

LO 8.7 Describe how osteoporosis develops and the actions that may help to prevent it.

Is **bottled water** better for you than tap water?

Can you blame **"water weight"** for extra pounds of body weight?

Do adults outgrow the need for **calcium**?

If you're feeling tired, do you need an **iron supplement**?

If you were to extract all of the **minerals** from a human body, they would form a small pile that weighs only about 5 pounds. The pile may not be impressive in size, but the work of those minerals is critical to living tissue.

Consider calcium and phosphorus. If you could separate these two minerals from the rest of the pile, you would take away about three-fourths of the total. Crystals made of these two minerals, plus a few others, form the structure of bones and so provide the architecture of the skeleton.

Run a magnet through the pile that remains and you pick up the iron. It doesn't fill a teaspoon, but it consists of billions and billions of iron atoms. As part of hemoglobin, these iron atoms are able to attach to oxygen and make it available at the sites inside the cells where metabolic work is taking place.

If you then extract all the other minerals from the pile, leaving only copper and iodine, you'll want to close the windows first. A slight breeze would blow these remaining bits of dust away. Yet the copper in the dust enables iron to hold and to release oxygen, and iodine is the critical mineral in the thyroid hormones. Figure 8–1 (p. 272) shows the amounts of the seven **major minerals** and a few of the **trace minerals** in the human body. Other minerals such as gold and aluminum are present in the body but are not known to have nutrient functions.

The distinction between major and trace minerals doesn't mean that one group is more important in the body than the other. A daily deficiency of a few micrograms of iodine is just as serious as a deficiency of several hundred milligrams of calcium. The major minerals are simply present in larger quantities in the body and are needed in greater amounts in the diet. All perform critical functions—some as parts of salts, which help to distribute the body's water; others form the bones and teeth, which lend structure to the body; and still others are cofactors which act, much as the vitamin coenzymes do, to enable enzymes to do their jobs.

The Dietary Guidelines for Americans committee names four minerals as shortfall nutrients—most people's intakes are too low:

- Potassium.
- Calcium.
- Magnesium.
- Iron (for some people).

Of the shortfall minerals, calcium and potassium are also named as nutrients of public health concern because their underconsumption has been convincingly linked with chronic diseases. In addition, one mineral stands out as being overconsumed by most people:

- Sodium.[1]*

Later sections present the key facts about these and other minerals important to nutrition.

---

* Reference notes are in Appendix F.

minerals naturally occurring, inorganic, homogeneous substances; chemical elements.

major minerals essential mineral nutrients required in the adult diet in amounts greater than 100 milligrams per day. Also called *macrominerals*.

trace minerals essential mineral nutrients required in the adult diet in amounts less than 100 milligrams per day. Also called *microminerals*.

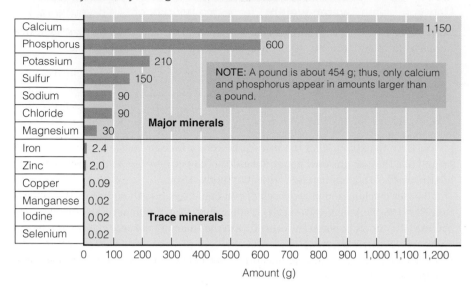

Figure 8–1

Minerals in a 60-Kilogram (132-Pound) Person, in Grams

The major minerals are present in the body in larger amounts and also are needed by the body in larger amounts than the trace minerals.

	Amount (g)
Calcium	1,150
Phosphorus	600
Potassium	210
Sulfur	150
Sodium	90
Chloride	90
Magnesium	30
Iron	2.4
Zinc	2.0
Copper	0.09
Manganese	0.02
Iodine	0.02
Selenium	0.02

Major minerals

Trace minerals

NOTE: A pound is about 454 g; thus, only calcium and phosphorus appear in amounts larger than a pound.

Amount (g): 0 100 200 300 400 500 600 700 800 900 1,000 1,100 1,200

Water, the first topic of this chapter, is unique among the nutrients and the most indispensable of all. The body needs more water each day than any other nutrient—50 times more water than protein and 5,000 times more water than vitamin C. You can survive a deficiency of any of the other nutrients for a long time, in some cases for months or years, but you can survive only a few days without water. In less than a day, a lack of water compromises the body's chemistry and metabolism.

Our discussion begins with water's many functions. Next we examine how water and the major minerals mingle to form the body's fluids and how cells regulate the distribution of those fluids. Then we take up the specialized roles of every one of the minerals. (Reminder: The DRI for water and minerals appear at the back of the book, pp. A and B.)

KEY POINTS

- Compared with trace minerals, major minerals are present in larger amounts in the body and in the diet.
- Major and trace minerals perform essential roles in the body.
- Potassium, calcium, magnesium, and iron may be lacking from U.S. diets, while sodium is overconsumed.

Water

LO 8.1   Explain the functions of water and the importance of maintaining the body's water balance.

You began as a single cell bathed in a nourishing fluid. As you became a beautifully organized, air-breathing body of trillions of cells, each of your cells had to remain next to water to stay alive.

Water makes up about 60 percent of an adult person's weight—that's almost 80 pounds of water in a 130-pound person. All this water in the body is not simply a river coursing through the arteries, capillaries, and veins. Soft tissues contain a great deal of water: the brain and muscles are 75 to 80 percent water by weight; and even bones contain 25 percent water. Some of the body's water is incorporated into the chemical structures of compounds that form cells, tissues, and organs of the body.

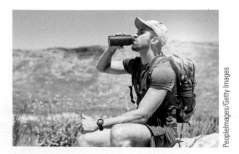

Water is the most indispensable nutrient.

For example, proteins hold water molecules within them, water that is locked in and not readily available for any other use. Water also participates actively in many chemical reactions.

Why Is Water the Most Indispensable Nutrient?

Water brings to each cell the exact ingredients the cell requires and carries away the end products of its life-sustaining reactions. The water of the body fluids is thus the transport vehicle for all the nutrients and wastes. Without water, cells quickly die.

Solvent   Water is a nearly universal **solvent**: it dissolves amino acids, glucose, minerals, and many other substances needed by the cells. Fatty substances, too, can travel freely in the watery blood and lymph because they are specially packaged in water-soluble proteins. In addition to transporting chemicals, water also reacts with them, thus participating in many of the reactions required to sustain life.

Cleansing Agent   Water is also the body's cleansing agent. Small molecules, such as the nitrogen wastes generated during protein metabolism, dissolve in the watery blood and then are removed before they build up to toxic concentrations. The kidneys filter these wastes from the blood and excrete them, mixed with water, as urine. When the kidneys become diseased, as can happen in diabetes and other disorders, toxins can build to life-threatening levels. Kidney **dialysis** must then be employed: the person's blood is routed, a little at a time, through a machine that removes the wastes and returns the cleansed blood to the body.

Lubricant and Cushion   Water molecules resist being crowded together. Thanks to this incompressibility, water can act as a lubricant and a cushion for the joints, and it can protect sensitive tissue such as the spinal cord from shock. The fluid within the eye serves in a similar way to keep optimal pressure on the retina and lens. From the start of human life, a fetus is cushioned against shock by the bag of amniotic fluid in the mother's uterus. Water also lubricates the digestive tract, the respiratory tract, and all tissues that are moistened with mucus.

Coolant   Yet another of water's special features is its ability to help maintain body temperature. The water of sweat is the body's coolant. Heat is produced as a by-product of energy metabolism and can build up dangerously in the body. To rid itself of this excess heat, the body routes its blood supply through the capillaries just under the skin. At the same time, the skin secretes sweat, and its water evaporates. Converting water to vapor takes energy; therefore, as sweat evaporates, heat energy dissipates, cooling the skin and the underlying blood. The cooled blood then flows back to cool the body's core. Sweat evaporates continuously from the skin, usually in slight amounts that go unnoticed. Thus, the skin is a major organ through which water is lost from the body. Lesser amounts are lost by way of exhaled breath and the feces.

To sum up, water:

- Carries nutrients throughout the body.
- Serves as the solvent for minerals, vitamins, amino acids, glucose, and other small molecules.
- Actively participates in many chemical reactions.
- Cleanses the tissues and blood of wastes.
- Acts as a lubricant and shock absorber around joints and organs.
- Aids in regulating the body's temperature.

KEY POINTS

- Water makes up about 60 percent of the body's weight.
- In the body, water transports, dissolves, and reacts with chemicals; provides lubrication and shock protection; and aids in temperature regulation.

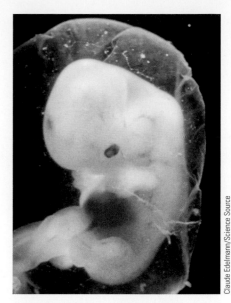

Human life begins in water.

Claude Edelmann/Science Source

solvent a substance that dissolves another and holds it in solution.

dialysis (dye-AL-ih-sis) a medical treatment for failing kidneys in which a person's blood is circulated through a machine that filters out toxins and wastes and returns cleansed blood to the body. More properly called *hemodialysis*, meaning "dialysis of the blood."

Figure 8–2

Water Balance—A Typical Example

Each day, water enters the body in liquids and foods, and some water arises as a by-product of the body's metabolic processes. Water leaves the body through the evaporation of sweat, in the moisture of exhaled breath, in the urine, and in the feces.

Water input (Total = 1,450–2,800 ml)

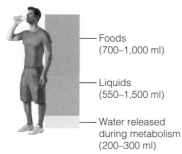

— Foods
(700–1,000 ml)

— Liquids
(550–1,500 ml)

— Water released
during metabolism
(200–300 ml)

Water output (Total = 1,450–2,800 ml)

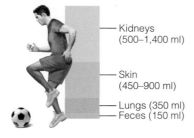

— Kidneys
(500–1,400 ml)

— Skin
(450–900 ml)

— Lungs (350 ml)
— Feces (150 ml)

water balance the balance between water intake and water excretion, which keeps the body's water content constant.

dehydration loss of water. The symptoms progress rapidly, from thirst to weakness to exhaustion and delirium, and end in death.

water intoxication a dangerous dilution of the body's fluids resulting from excessive ingestion of plain water. Symptoms are headache, muscular weakness, mental confusion, seizures, and coma; fatalities can occur.

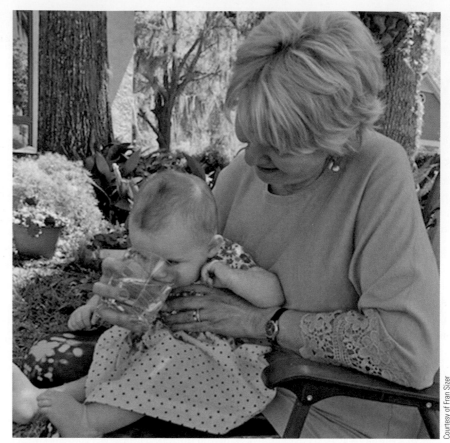

An extra drink of water benefits both young and old.

Courtesy of Fran Sizer

The Body's Water Balance

Water is such an integral part of us that people seldom are conscious of its importance unless they are deprived of it. Because the body loses some water every day, a person must consume at least the same amount to avoid life-threatening losses—that is, to maintain **water balance**. The total amount of fluid in the body is kept balanced by delicate mechanisms. Imbalances such as **dehydration** and **water intoxication** can occur, but the balance is restored as promptly as the body can manage it. The body controls both intake and excretion to maintain water equilibrium (see Figure 8–2).

The amount of the body's water varies by pounds at a time, especially in women who retain water during menstruation. Eating a meal high in salt can temporarily increase the body's water content; the body sheds the excess over the next day or so as the sodium is excreted. These temporary fluctuations in body water show up on the scale, but gaining or losing water weight does not reflect a change in body fat. Fat weight takes days or weeks to change noticeably, whereas water weight can change overnight.

KEY POINTS

- The body employs numerous tactics to balance water intake and output to maintain its water balance.
- A change in the body's water content can bring about a temporary change in body weight.

Quenching Thirst and Balancing Losses

Thirst and satiety govern water intake. When the blood is too concentrated (having lost water but not salt and other dissolved substances), the molecules and particles in the blood attract water out of the salivary glands, and the mouth becomes dry. Water is also drawn from the body's cells, causing them to collapse a little. Blood becomes more concentrated and blood pressure falls.

Table 8–1

Effects of Mild Dehydration, Severe Dehydration, and Chronic Lack of Fluid

Mild Dehydration (Loss of <5% Body Weight)	Severe Dehydration (Loss of >5% Body Weight)	Chronic Low Fluid Intake May Increase the Likelihood of:
Thirst	Pale or shriveled skin	Cardiac arrest (heart attack) and other heart problems
Sudden weight loss	Bluish lips and fingertips	Constipation
Dry, cool skin	Confusion; disorientation	Dental disease
Dry mouth, throat, body linings	Rapid, shallow breathing	Gallstones
Rapid pulse; low blood pressure	Weak, rapid, irregular pulse	Glaucoma (elevated pressure in the eye)
Lack of energy; weakness	Thickening of blood	Hypertension
Impaired kidney function	Scant urine; brown-colored urine	Kidney stones
Reduced quantity of urine; concentrated, dark yellow or amber-colored urine	Shock; seizures	Pregnancy/childbirth problems
Headache; reduced mental clarity	Coma; death	Stroke
Diminished muscular work and athletic performance		Urinary tract infections
Fever or increased internal temperature		
Fainting and delirium		

The brain center known as the hypothalamus (described in Chapter 3) responds to low cellular fluid, concentrated blood particles, and low blood pressure by initiating nerve impulses to the brain that register as "thirst." The hypothalamus also signals the pituitary gland to release a hormone that directs the kidneys to shift water back into the bloodstream from the fluid destined to become urine. (This is why, if you haven't drunk enough water, your urine has a darker hue; with proper hydration, urine ranges in color from very pale yellow to deep amber.) The kidneys themselves respond to the sodium concentration in the blood passing through them by secreting regulatory substances of their own. The net result is that the more water the body needs, the less it excretes.

Dehydration Thirst lags behind a lack of water. When too much water is lost from the body and is not replaced, dehydration can threaten survival. A first sign of dehydration is thirst, the signal that the body has already lost a cup or two of its total fluid and the need to drink is immediate. But suppose a thirsty person is unable to obtain fluid or, as in many elderly people, fails to recognize the thirst message. Instead of "wasting" precious water in sweat, the dehydrated body diverts most of its water into the blood vessels to maintain the life-supporting blood pressure. Meanwhile, body heat builds up because sweating has ceased, creating the possibility of serious consequences in hot weather (see Table 8–1).

To ignore the thirst signal is to invite dehydration. With a loss of just 1 percent of body weight as fluid, perceptible symptoms appear: headache, fatigue, confusion or forgetfulness, and an elevated heart rate. A loss of 2 percent impairs physical functioning and impedes a wide range of physical activities.[2] People should stay attuned to thirst and drink whenever they feel thirsty to replace fluids lost throughout the day. Older adults in whom thirst is blunted should drink regularly throughout the day, regardless of thirst.

A word about caffeine: people who drink caffeinated beverages lose a little more fluid than when they drink water because caffeine acts as a **diuretic**. The DRI committee concludes, however, that the mild diuretic effect of moderate caffeine intake does not lead to dehydration or keep people from meeting their fluid needs. Caffeinated beverages can therefore contribute to daily water intakes. The Controversy section of Chapter 14 discusses other effects of caffeine.

Water Intoxication At the other extreme from dehydration, water intoxication occurs when too much plain water floods the body's fluids and disturbs their normal composition. Typically, an adult with water intoxication has consumed several gallons of plain water in a few hours' time. Water intoxication is rare, but when it occurs, immediate action is needed to reverse dangerously diluted blood before death ensues.

Do the Math

Water loss can be expressed as a percentage of body weight. In a 150-lb person,

- A 3-lb loss of body fluid equals 2% of body weight.

  3 lbs ÷ 150 lbs × 100
  = 2% of body weight

- A 4½-lb loss equals 3% of body weight in the same 150-lb person.

  4.5 ÷ 150 × 100 = 3%

Now solve this: in a 180-lb person, find the percentage of body weight represented by 5 pounds of water.

diuretic (dye-you-RET-ic) a compound, usually a medication, causing increased urinary water excretion; a "water pill."

Table 8–2

Factors that Increase Fluid Needs

These conditions increase a person's need for fluids:

- Alcohol consumption
- Cold weather
- Dietary fiber
- Diseases that disturb water balance, such as diabetes and kidney diseases
- Forced-air environments, such as airplanes and sealed buildings
- Heated environments
- High altitude
- Hot weather, high humidity
- Increased protein, salt, or sugar intakes
- Ketosis
- Medications (diuretics)
- Physical activity
- Pregnancy and breastfeeding (see Chapter 13)
- Prolonged diarrhea, vomiting, or fever
- Surgery, blood loss, or burns
- Very young or old age

KEY POINTS

- Water losses from the body must be balanced by water intakes to maintain hydration.
- The brain regulates water intake; the brain and kidneys regulate water excretion.
- Dehydration and water intoxication can can arise with deficient or excessive water intake.

How Much Water Do I Need to Drink in a Day?

Water needs vary greatly, depending on the foods a person eats, the air temperature and humidity, the altitude, the person's activity level, and other factors (see Table 8–2). Fluid needs vary widely among individuals and also within the same person in various environmental conditions, so a specific water recommendation is hard to pin down.

Water from Fluids and Foods   A wide range of fluid intakes can maintain adequate hydration. As a general guideline, however, the DRI committee recommends that, given a normal diet and moderate environment, the reference man needs about 13 cups of fluid from beverages, including drinking water, and the reference woman needs about 9 cups.[3] This amount of fluid provides about 80 percent of the body's daily water need. On average, most people in the United States, with the exception of older adults, consume close to these amounts.[4] The fluids people choose to drink can affect daily calorie intakes, as the Consumer's Guide section makes clear.

Most of the rest of the body's needed daily fluid comes from the water in foods. Nearly all foods contain some water: water constitutes up to 95 percent of the volume of most fruit and vegetables and at least 50 percent of many meats and cheeses (see Table 8–3). A small percentage of the day's fluid is generated in the tissues themselves as energy-yielding nutrients release **metabolic water** as a product of chemical reactions.

Table 8–3

Water in Foods and Beverages

Many solid foods, such as broccoli and steak, are surprisingly high in water.

100%	water, diet soft drinks, seltzer (unflavored), plain tea
95–99%	sugar-free gelatin dessert, clear broth, Chinese cabbage, celery, cucumber, lettuce, summer squash, black coffee
90–94%	sports drinks, grapefruit, fresh strawberries, broccoli, tomatoes
80–89%	sugar-sweetened soft drinks, milk, yogurt, egg white, fruit juices, low-fat cottage cheese, cooked oatmeal, fresh apple, carrot
60–79%	low-calorie mayonnaise, instant pudding, banana, shrimp, lean steak, pork chop, baked potato, cooked rice
40–59%	diet margarine, sausage, chicken, macaroni and cheese
20–39%	bread, cake, cheddar cheese, bagel
10–19%	butter, margarine, regular mayonnaise
5–9%	peanut butter, popcorn
1–4%	ready-to-eat cereals, pretzels
0%	cooking oils, meat fats, shortening, white sugar

metabolic water water generated in the tissues during the chemical breakdown of the energy-yielding nutrients in foods.

Liquid Calories

Most ordinary beverages help meet the body's need for fluid. In developed nations such as ours, however, people encounter a constant stream of beverages that contain more than just water.

Mystery Pounds

Derek, an active college student, hasn't thought much about his fluid intake but is lamenting, "I'm exercising more and I've cut out the junk food, but I've still gained five pounds!" What has escaped Derek's attention is the calories that he's been drinking: a big glass of vitamin C–enriched orange punch at breakfast, a soda or two before lunchtime, sometimes a large mocha latte for an afternoon wake-up, and, of course, sports drinks when he works out.

Drinking without Thirst

Like Derek, most people choose beverages for reasons having little to do with thirst. They seek the stimulating effect

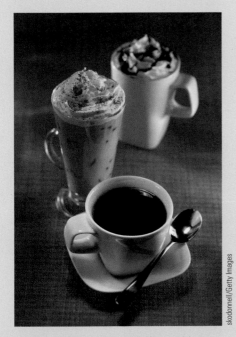

A fancy coffee drink can easily provide 400–700 calories; plain coffee contains zero calories.

of caffeine in coffee, tea, or sodas. They choose fluids such as milk, juice, or other beverages at mealtimes. They believe they need the added nutrients in sugar-sweetened "vitamin waters." They think they need the carbohydrate in sports drinks for all physical activities (few exercisers do; read Chapter 10). They drink hot beverages to warm up and cold ones to cool off. Or they drink for pleasure—for the aroma of coffee, the sweet taste of sugar, or the euphoria of alcohol. On each of these drinking occasions, with or without their awareness, people make choices among high-calorie and lower-calorie beverages.

Weighing In on Extra Fluids

Drinking extra fluid, and water in particular, may offer some health advantages, such as preventing minor dehydration and reducing the risk of developing kidney stones.[1]* Fluids such as fat-free milk and 100 percent fruit or vegetable juices provide needed nutrients and are thus included in the USDA eating patterns. Other beverages, such as sugary sodas and punches, provide many empty calories, and should be limited. Doing so could help many people to lose weight.[2]

Figure 8–3 shows that young men like Derek top the chart for energy intakes from beverages, with an average of almost 600 calories per day. Young women drink about 350 calories per day on average. High-calorie beverages, consistently chosen over water, can almost double a person's calorie intake in a day.[3]

Even among nutritious beverages, daily choices matter. For example, an 8-ounce glass of orange juice provides

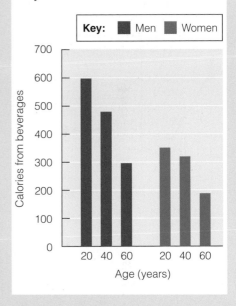

skodonnell/Getty Images

Figure 8–3

How Many Calories Do We Drink?

The daily intake of calories from beverages varies widely with age, with 20- to 30-year-old men consuming the greatest amounts by far.

about 110 calories; tomato juice, a similar choice with regard to vitamins and minerals, provides just 40. Calories in choices like these add up.

Seeking an Expert's Advice

"My advice is to track your intake of fluids and add up their calories," says the registered dietitian nutritionist at Derek's campus health clinic. "And watch serving sizes: your quart bottle of sports drink packs 200 calories of sugar and more than 400 milligrams of sodium, but its label lists much lower values for one 8-ounce serving, based on four servings per bottle" (see Figure 8–4).

*Reference notes are in Appendix F.

(continued)

Figure 8–4

What's in a Sports Drink?

When comparing labels, carefully note serving sizes. This Nutrition Facts panel lists calories and sodium for 8 ounces—one-fourth of the bottle.

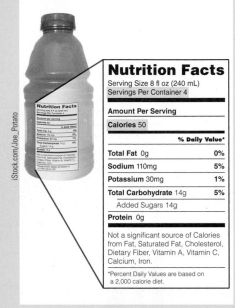

Nutrition Facts
Serving Size 8 fl oz (240 mL)
Servings Per Container 4

Amount Per Serving

Calories 50

	% Daily Value*
Total Fat 0g	0%
Sodium 110mg	5%
Potassium 30mg	1%
Total Carbohydrate 14g	5%
Added Sugars 14g	
Protein 0g	

Not a significant source of Calories from Fat, Saturated Fat, Cholesterol, Dietary Fiber, Vitamin A, Vitamin C, Calcium, Iron.

*Percent Daily Values are based on a 2,000 calorie diet.

iStock.com/Joe_Potato

Table 8–4

Ways to Add Flavor to Water

Here are some ideas for adding interest to the taste of plain water without artificial sweeteners, colors, or flavors or too much added sugar.

- Steep a cinnamon stick in a cup of water. Mix 1–2 tablespoons of this concentrate with a glass of ice and water to add flavor. For variety, add a slice or two of fresh apple to the mix.
- Add a splash of 100% fruit juice to flavor and color plain or sparkling water naturally.
- Infuse water with the flavor of fresh fruit, such as berries or melons. Simply add the fruit to your water and drink, or consider purchasing an infuser, a gadget that submerges flavoring agents in water, but holds them back during pouring.
- Crush fresh herbs and steep them in a glass or pitcher of water in the refrigerator overnight. Add fresh citrus slices, such as lemon or lime, before drinking.
- Try a mixture of herbs and fruit, such as strawberries and basil or watermelon and mint to add a more complex flavor to water.
- Add flavored ice cubes to your water. Freeze coffee, water with berries, pureed pineapple, or even whole grapes, and use them in place of regular ice cubes to cool and flavor your water.
- Add cucumber slices to your water to give it a subtle, refreshing taste.
- Brew extra coffee, tea, or herb tea, refrigerate, and enjoy it chilled or over ice.

And Derek's reply: "I counted at least 400 random calories that I *drank* every day . . . I'll switch out the sodas and sports drinks for water, and as for coffee, I'll just put some milk in it—it's cheaper than the fancy stuff, anyway."

Finding Calorie Information

Packaged drinks must carry a Nutrition Facts panel. But what about calories in unlabeled beverages? How many calories are in coffee drinks, iced teas, or fountain drinks served in restaurants? By law, most restaurants must provide calorie information on menus, tray liners, handouts, nearby posters, or even on computers. If you don't see it, ask for it.

Moving Ahead

All beverages (except alcohol) can readily meet the body's fluid needs, so the question becomes, "What else does this beverage supply?" A 500-calorie

smoothie or latte may be the right fluid choice for a person who needs to gain weight, but for most people, nutrition authorities often recommend plain water. Table 8–4 suggests flavorful additions for plain water. Other recommendations are plain tea, coffee, nonfat and low-fat milk and soy milk, artificially sweetened beverages, clear soups, 100 percent vegetable juices, and 100 percent fruit juices in moderation (see Chapter 2). If you enjoy regular soft drinks, sweet tea, creamy coffee drinks, punches, and other highly caloric beverages, limit yourself to the smallest sizes, and choose other beverages most of the time.

Review Questions**

1. The population group consuming the greatest number of daily calories from beverages is: _____.
   a. young men
   b. young women
   c. elderly people of both genders

**Answers to Consumer's Guide review questions are in Appendix G.*

2. When choosing a beverage, one should _____.
   a. read the label carefully, especially noting the number of servings in the container and the calories per serving
   b. consider how a beverage's calories fit into the day's calorie needs
   c. consider ingredients in addition to water supplied by the beverage
   d. all of the above

3. Nutrition authorities often recommend _____.
   a. drinking water, plain or lightly flavored, to quench thirst
   b. staying hydrated with plenty of regular soft drinks, sweet tea, creamy coffee drinks, punches
   c. drinking plain tea, coffee, nonfat and low-fat milk and soy milk, artificially sweetened beverages, and 100 percent fruit and vegetable juices, in addition to water
   d. a and c

The Effect of Sweating on Fluid Needs Sweating increases water needs. Especially when performing physical work outdoors in hot weather, people can lose 2 to 4 gallons of fluid in a day. An athlete training in the heat can sweat out more than a half gallon of fluid each hour. For athletes exercising in the heat, maintaining hydration is critical, and Chapter 10 provides detailed instructions for hydrating the exercising body.

KEY POINTS

- Many factors influence a person's need for water.
- Water is provided by beverages and foods and by cellular metabolism.
- Sweating increases fluid needs.
- High-calorie beverages affect daily calorie intakes.

Drinking Water: Types, Safety, and Sources

LO 8.2   Compare the types and safety of drinking water from different sources.

Clean, safe drinking water, could arguably be the earth's most precious natural resource. Just ask any of the almost 900 million of the world's people who struggle to stay alive in areas without access to safe drinking water.[5] This section offers perspective on our nation's supply. Chapter 15 comes back to the importance of clean water worldwide.

Hard Water or Soft Water—Which Is Best?

Water occurs as **hard water** or **soft water**, a distinction that affects your health with regard to three minerals. Hard water has high concentrations of calcium and magnesium. Soft water's principal mineral is sodium. In practical terms, soft water makes more bubbles with less soap; hard water leaves a ring on the tub, a jumble of rocklike crystals in the teakettle, and a gray residue in the wash.

Soft water may seem more desirable, and some homeowners purchase water softeners that remove magnesium and calcium and replace them with sodium. Several trade-offs attend this measure, though. The sodium of soft water, even when it bubbles naturally from the ground, may aggravate **hypertension**. Soft water also more easily dissolves certain contaminant metals, such as cadmium and lead, from pipes. Cadmium can harm the body, affecting enzymes by displacing zinc from its normal sites of action. Lead, another toxic metal, is absorbed more readily from soft water than from hard water, possibly because the calcium in hard water protects against its absorption. (Lead is particularly harmful to children; see Chapter 14 for details.) Old plumbing may contain cadmium or lead, so people living in old buildings should run the cold water tap for a minute to flush out harmful minerals before drawing water for the first use in the morning and whenever no water has been drawn for more than 6 hours.[6]

KEY POINTS

- Hard water is high in calcium and magnesium.
- Soft water is high in sodium and dissolves cadmium and lead from pipes.

Water Safety and Sources

What are consumers to drink? Tap water is treated for safety from microbial contamination and tested regularly for toxins, so most tap water is safe and wholesome. However, as municipal water systems age and water demand grows, the risk of contamination increases.[7] An extreme example was a widely reported incident in a Michigan city; government officials there failed to comply with regulations and many people were needlessly exposed to toxic levels of lead and other hazards.[8]

Home purifying equipment, costing from $50 to $10,000, can remove most of the lead, chlorine, and other contaminants from tap water, but be aware that some types improve only the water's taste. Also, not all sellers are legitimate—some perform dramatic-appearing but meaningless water tests to sell unneeded systems.

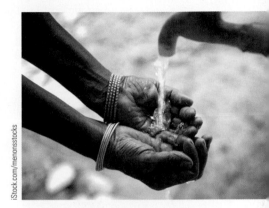

Clean water is precious and lifesaving in many areas of the world.

hard water water with high calcium and magnesium concentrations.

soft water water with a high sodium concentration.

hypertension high blood pressure; also defined in Chapter 11.

Table 8–5

Bottled Water Terms

- **baby water** ordinary bottled water treated with ozone to make it safe but not sterile.
- **bottled water** drinking water sold in single-use or reusable bottles commonly ranging in size from 5 ounces to 5 gallons.
- **caffeine water** bottled water with caffeine added.
- **carbonated water** water that contains carbon dioxide gas, either naturally occurring or added, that causes bubbles to form in it; also called bubbling or sparkling water. Seltzer, soda, and tonic waters are legally soft drinks and are not regulated as water.
- **coconut water** the fluid inside a young green coconut; heavily marketed for its substantial potassium content, it also provides about 45 calories per cup and little or no fat.
- **distilled water** water that has been vaporized and recondensed, leaving it free of dissolved minerals.
- **fitness water** lightly flavored bottled water enhanced with vitamins, supposedly to enhance athletic performance.

- **mineral water** water from a spring or well that typically contains at least 250 parts per million (ppm) of naturally occurring minerals. Minerals give water a distinctive flavor. Many mineral waters are high in sodium.
- **purified water** water that has been treated by distillation or other physical or chemical processes that remove dissolved solids. Because purified water contains no minerals or contaminants, it is useful for medical and research purposes.
- **spring water** water originating from an underground spring or well. It may be bubbly (carbonated) or "flat" or "still," meaning not carbonated. Spring water may be collected at the spring or through a man-made well some distance away that taps the underground formation feeding the spring. Brand names that include words such as "Spring" and "Pure" do not ensure that the water comes from a spring.
- **vitamin water** bottled water with a few vitamins added; does not replace vitamins from a balanced diet and may worsen overload in people receiving vitamins from enriched food, supplements, and other enriched products such as "energy" bars.

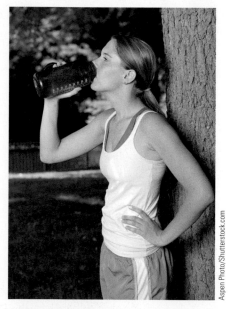

Aspen Photo/Shutterstock.com

Using refillable bottles saves money and cuts waste.

As an alternative to tap water, many U.S. households turn to **bottled water** and pay 250 to 10,000 times more for their water. (Table 8-5 defines bottled water terms.) Some bottled waters may taste fresher than tap because they are disinfected with ozone, which, unlike the chlorine used in most municipal water systems, leaves no flavor or odor. Other bottled waters are simply treated, packaged tap water.[9] All drinking water, tap or bottled, originates from **surface water** or **groundwater**, and both are vulnerable to contamination from industry and human activities. The USDA tightened bottled water standards after about a third of brand-name waters tested positive for bacteria, arsenic, or synthetic chemicals, and about half tested positive for the heavy metal lead.[10]

Disposable plastic water bottles require considerable fossil fuels (and many gallons of water) to produce and transport, and they pose serious disposal problems. Single-serving bottles can be recycled, but 80 percent of the 35 *billion* plastic water bottles purchased in the United States each year end up in landfills, in incinerators, or as litter on land and in rivers, lakes, and oceans. Disposal and cleanup of this waste costs, taxpayers hundreds of millions of dollars each year. By using stainless steel cups or reusable water bottles, consumers can save money for themselves and reduce waste in their communities. This choice also helps to protect ocean fish and other wildlife from harm caused by a buildup of discarded plastics.

Water is an important nutrient, and its sources must be kept clean and safe to protect human health. The following section describes water's activities inside the body.

KEY POINTS

- Public drinking water is tested and treated for safety, and with rare exceptions, systems are properly maintained.
- Bottled water is also tested, but single-use bottles create a disposal problem.

Body Fluids and Minerals

LO 8.3 Describe the concepts of fluid and electrolyte balance and acid-base balance and their importance to health.

surface water water that comes from lakes, rivers, and reservoirs.

groundwater water that comes from underground aquifers.

Most of the body's water weight is contained inside the cells, and some water bathes the outsides of the cells. The remainder fills the blood vessels. How do cells keep themselves from collapsing when water leaves them and from swelling up when too much water enters them?

Figure 8–5

How Electrolytes Govern Water Flow

Water flows in the direction of the more highly concentrated solution.

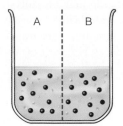 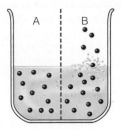 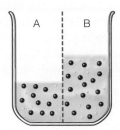

❶ With equal numbers of dissolved particles on both sides of a water-permeable divider, water levels remain equal.

❷ Now additional particles are added to increase the concentration on side B. Particles cannot flow across the divider. In the case of a cell, the divider (cell membrane) partitions fluids inside and outside the cell.

❸ Water can flow both ways across the divider but tends to move from side A to side B, where the concentration of dissolved particles is greater. The *volume* of water increases on side B, and the particle *concentrations* on sides A and B become equal.

Water Follows Salt

The cells cannot regulate the amount of water directly by pumping it in and out because water slips across membranes freely. The cells can, however, pump minerals across their membranes. The major minerals form **salts** that dissolve in the body fluids; the cells direct where the salts go, and this determines where the fluids flow because water follows salt.

When minerals (or other) salts dissolve in water, they separate into single, electrically charged particles known as **ions**. (Common table salt, for example, is sodium chloride, or NaCl, and in water it separates to form a sodium ion, Na^+, and a chloride ion, Cl^-.) Unlike pure water, which conducts electricity poorly, ions dissolved in water carry electrical current; for this reason, these electrically charged ions are called **electrolytes**.

As Figure 8–5 shows, when dissolved particles, such as electrolytes, are present in unequal concentrations on either side of a water-permeable membrane, water flows toward the more concentrated side to equalize the concentrations. Cells and their surrounding fluids work in the same way. Think of a cell as a sack made of a water-permeable membrane. The sack is filled with watery fluid and suspended in a dilute solution of salts and other dissolved particles. Water flows freely between the fluids inside and outside the cell but generally moves from the more dilute solution toward the more concentrated one (the photo of salted eggplant slices in Figure 8–6 shows this effect).

KEY POINT

- Cells regulate water movement by pumping minerals across their membranes; water follows the minerals.

Fluid and Electrolyte Balance

To control the flow of water, the body must spend energy moving its electrolytes from one compartment to another (see Figure 8–7). Transport proteins form the pumps that move mineral ions across cell membranes, as Chapter 6 described. The result is **fluid and electrolyte balance**, the proper amount and kind of fluid in every body compartment.

Figure 8–6

Salt Draws Water from Cells

The slices of eggplant on the right were sprinkled with salt. Notice their beads of "sweat," formed as cellular water moves across each cell's membrane (a water-permeable divider) toward the higher concentration of salt (dissolved particles) on the surface.

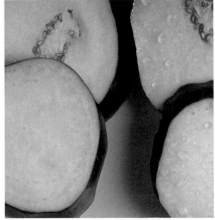

© Craig M. Moore

salts compounds composed of charged particles (ions). An example is potassium chloride (K^+Cl^-).

ions (EYE-ons) electrically charged particles, such as sodium (positively charged) or chloride (negatively charged).

electrolytes compounds that partly dissociate in water to form ions, such as the potassium ion (K^+) and the chloride ion (Cl^-).

fluid and electrolyte balance maintenance of the proper amounts and kinds of fluids and minerals in each compartment of the body.

Figure 8–7

Electrolyte Balance

Transport proteins in cell membranes maintain the proper balance of sodium (mostly outside the cells) and potassium (mostly inside the cells).

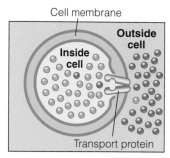

Cell membrane

Outside cell

Inside cell

Transport protein

Key
- Potassium
- Sodium

Table 8–6

Major Minerals[a]

The need for each of these is greater than 100 milligrams per day, in some cases far greater.

- Calcium
- Chloride
- Magnesium
- Phosphorus
- Potassium
- Sodium
- Sulfate

[a]*The major minerals are also called* macrominerals.

fluid and electrolyte imbalance failure to maintain the proper amounts and kinds of fluids and minerals in every body compartment; a medical emergency.

acid-base balance equilibrium between acid and base concentrations to maintain a proper pH in the body fluids. Also defined in Chapter 6.

buffers molecules that can help to keep the pH of a solution from changing by gathering or releasing H ions.

If the fluid balance is disturbed, severe illness can develop quickly because fluid can shift rapidly from one compartment to another. For example, in vomiting or diarrhea, the loss of water from the digestive tract pulls fluid from between the cells in every part of the body. Fluid then leaves the cell interiors to restore balance. Meanwhile, the kidneys detect the water loss and attempt to retrieve water from the pool destined for excretion. To do this, they raise the sodium concentration outside the cells, and this pulls still more water out of them. The result is **fluid and electrolyte imbalance**, a medical emergency. Water and minerals lost in vomiting or diarrhea ultimately come from all the body's cells. This loss disrupts the heartbeat and threatens life. It is a cause of death among those with eating disorders.

KEY POINT
- Mineral salts form electrolytes that help keep fluids in their proper compartments.

Acid-Base Balance

The minerals help manage still another balancing act, the **acid-base balance**, or the pH, of the body's fluids. In pure water, a small percentage of water molecules (H_2O) exists as positive (H^+) and negative (OH^-) ions, but they exist in equilibrium—the positive charges exactly equal the negatives. When dissolved in watery body fluids, some of the major minerals give rise to acids (H, or hydrogen, ions) and others to bases (OH ions). Excess H ions in a solution make it an acid; they lower the pH. Excess OH ions in a solution make it a base; they raise the pH.

Maintenance of body fluids at a nearly constant pH is critical to life. Even slight changes in pH drastically change the structure and chemical functions of most biologically important molecules. The body's proteins and some of its mineral salts help prevent changes in the acid-base balance of its fluids by serving as **buffers**—molecules that gather up or release H ions as needed to maintain the correct pH. The kidneys help control the pH balance by excreting more or less acid (H ions). The lungs also help by excreting more or less carbon dioxide. (Dissolved in the blood, carbon dioxide forms an acid, carbonic acid.) This tight control of the acid-base balance permits all other life processes to continue.

KEY POINT
- Minerals act as buffers to help maintain body fluids at the correct pH to support life's processes.

The Major Minerals

LO 8.4   Describe the functions of the seven major minerals, their food sources, and the effects of their deficiencies and toxicities.

All the major minerals help to maintain the fluid balance, but each one also has some special duties of its own. Table 8–6 lists the major minerals, and Table 8–14 (pp. 305–306) summarizes their roles.

Calcium

As Figure 8–1 showed, calcium is by far the most abundant mineral in the body. The roles of calcium are critical to body functioning, but many adults, adolescents, and even some children do not consume enough calcium-rich foods to meet the DRI for this mineral.[11] Most who do meet their needs are people who are taking calcium supplements.

Nearly all (99 percent) of the body's calcium is stored in the bones and teeth, where it plays two important roles. First, it is an integral part of bone structure. Second, bone calcium serves as a bank that can release calcium to the body fluids if even the slightest drop in blood calcium concentration occurs. Many people think

Figure 8–8

A Bone

Bone is active, living tissue. Blood travels in capillaries throughout the bone, bringing nutrients to the cells that maintain the bone's structure and carrying away waste materials from those cells. It picks up and deposits minerals as instructed by hormones.

Bone derives its structural strength from the lacy network of crystals that lie along its lines of stress. If minerals are withdrawn to cover deficits elsewhere in the body, the bone will grow weak and ultimately will bend or crumble.

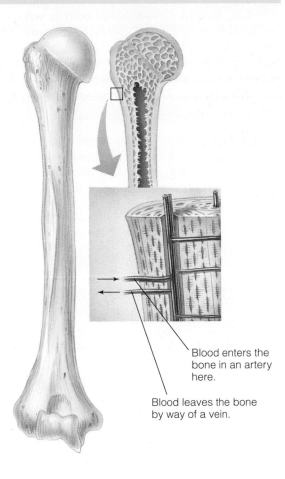

Blood enters the bone in an artery here.

Blood leaves the bone by way of a vein.

Figure 8–9

A Tooth

The inner layer of dentin is bonelike material that forms on a protein (collagen) matrix. The outer layer of enamel is harder than bone. Both dentin and enamel contain hydroxyapatite crystals (made of calcium and phosphorus). The crystals of enamel may become even harder when exposed to the trace mineral fluoride.

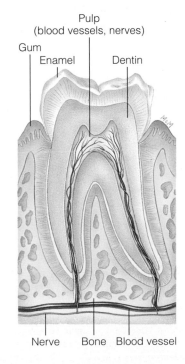

Pulp
(blood vessels, nerves)

Gum

Enamel

Dentin

Nerve   Bone   Blood vessel

hydroxyapatite (hi-DROX-ee-APP-uh-tight) the chief crystal of bone and teeth, formed from calcium and phosphorus.

that once deposited in bone, calcium (together with the other minerals of bone) stays there forever—that once a bone is built, it is inert, like a rock. Not so. The minerals of bones are in constant flux, with formation and dissolution taking place every minute of the day and night (see Figure 8–8). Almost the entire adult human skeleton is remodeled every 10 years. In addition, bone cells release hormones that work with other organs to help regulate several body functions.[12] The skeleton truly is a living body organ.

Calcium in Bone and Tooth Formation   Calcium and phosphorus are both essential to bone formation: calcium phosphate salts crystallize on a rubbery foundation material composed of the protein collagen. The resulting **hydroxyapatite** crystals invade the collagen and gradually lend more and more rigidity to a youngster's maturing bones until they are able to support the weight they will have to carry. If you could remove all of the minerals from bones, thereby eliminating the hydroxyapatite crystals, the remaining protein structures (mostly the protein collagen) would be so flexible that you could tie them in a knot.

Teeth are formed in a similar way: hydroxyapatite crystals form on a collagen matrix to create the dentin that gives strength to the teeth (see Figure 8–9). The turnover of minerals in teeth is not as rapid as in bone, but some withdrawals and deposits do take place throughout life.

Calcium in Body Fluids   The fluids that bathe and fill the cells contain the remaining 1 percent of the body's calcium, a tiny amount that is vital to life. It plays these major roles:

- Regulates the transport of ions across cell membranes and is particularly important in nerve transmission.
- Helps maintain normal blood pressure.
- Plays an essential role in the clotting of blood.
- Is essential for muscle contraction and therefore for the heartbeat.
- Activates cellular enzymes that regulate many processes.

Because of its importance, blood calcium concentration is tightly controlled.

Other roles for calcium are emerging as well. Adequate intakes of calcium may help protect against hypertension.[13] Some research also suggests protective relationships between calcium and blood cholesterol, diabetes, and colon and rectal cancers.[14] Large, well-designed clinical studies are needed to clarify these potential roles of calcium.[15]

Calcium Balance   The key to bone health lies in the body's calcium balance, directed by a system of hormones and vitamin D. Cells need continuous access to calcium, so the body maintains a constant calcium concentration in the blood. The body is sensitive to an increased need for calcium but sends no signals to the conscious brain to indicate a calcium need. Instead, three organ systems quietly respond:

1. The intestines increase their absorption of calcium.
2. The kidneys prevent calcium loss in the urine.
3. The bones release more calcium into the blood.

The skeleton serves as a bank from which the blood can borrow and return calcium as needed. Thus, a person can go for years with an inadequate calcium intake and still maintain normal blood calcium—but at the expense of **bone density**. It follows that a normal result on a laboratory test for *blood* calcium does not signify an adequate body calcium status. Bone density must be tested directly.

Calcium Absorption   Most adults absorb about 20 to 30 percent of the calcium they ingest.[16] When the body needs more calcium, the intestinal lining can substantially increase its absorption. The result is obvious in the case of a pregnant woman, who doubles her absorption.[17] Similarly, breastfed infants absorb about 60 percent of the calcium in breast milk. Children in puberty absorb almost 35 percent of the calcium they consume.

The body also absorbs and retains more calcium when habitual intakes are low.[18] Deprived of the mineral for years, an adult may double the calcium absorbed; conversely, when supplied for years with abundant calcium, the same person may absorb only about one-third the normal amount. Despite these adjustments, increases in calcium absorption cannot fully compensate for reduced intakes. A person who suddenly cuts back on calcium is likely to lose calcium from the bones.

Bone Loss   Some bone loss seems an inevitable consequence of aging.[19] Sometime around age 30, the skeleton no longer adds significantly to bone density. After about age 40, regardless of calcium intake, bones begin to lose density. Those who regularly meet calcium, protein, and other nutrient needs and who perform bone-strengthening physical activity may slow down the loss.[20] Table 8–7 lists nutrients that are critical to bone health and that work as a team to support it.

A person who reaches adulthood with an insufficient calcium savings account is likely to develop the fragile bones of **osteoporosis**. Osteoporosis along with its forerunner, **osteopenia**, constitute a major health problem for many older people—their possible causes and prevention are the topics of this chapter's Controversy. To protect

---

Table 8–7

Functional Group for Bones

The following are vitamins, minerals, and energy nutrients most important to bone health.

Key bone vitamins:
- Vitamin A
- Vitamin D
- Vitamin K
- Vitamin C

Key bone minerals:
- Calcium
- Phosphorus
- Magnesium

Key energy nutrient:
- Protein

---

bone density a measure of bone strength, the degree of mineralization of the bone matrix.

osteoporosis (OSS-tee-oh-pore-OH-sis) a reduction of the bone mass of older people in which the bones become porous and fragile (*osteo* means "bones"; *poros* means "porous"); also known as *adult bone loss*. (Also defined in Chapter 7.)

osteopenia (OS-tee-oh-PEE-nee-ah) a condition of low bone mass that often progresses to osteoporosis.

Chapter 8 Water and Minerals

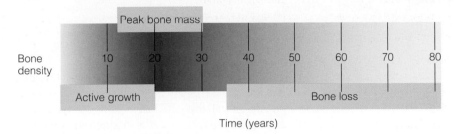

Figure 8–10

Bone throughout Life

From birth to about age 20, the bones are actively growing. Between the ages of 12 and 30 years, the bones achieve their maximum mineral density for life—the peak bone mass. Beyond those years, bone resorption exceeds bone formation, and bones lose density.

against bone loss, attention to calcium intakes during early life is crucial. Too few calcium-rich foods during the growing years may prevent a person from achieving **peak bone mass** (Figure 8–10 illustrates the timing).[21]

How Much Calcium Do I Need and Which Foods Are Good Sources?   Setting recommended intakes for calcium is difficult because absorption varies. The DRI committee took absorption into account and set recommendations for calcium at levels that produce maximum calcium retention (see the back of the book, p. B). At lower intakes, the body does not store calcium to capacity; at greater intakes, the excess calcium is excreted and thus is wasted. Because adverse effects, such as constipation and calcium buildup in soft tissues, are possible with supplemental doses, a Tolerable Upper Intake Level (UL) has been established (see the back of the book, p. C). The Controversy has more about calcium supplements.

Fiber and the binders phytate (in whole grains) and oxalate (in vegetables) interfere with calcium absorption, but their effects are only minor in typical U.S. eating patterns. Such patterns fall far short of the recommended intakes, so calcium is a nutrient of public health concern.[22] Snapshot 8–1 (p. 286) provides a look at some foods that are good or excellent sources of calcium, and the Food Feature at the end of this chapter focuses on foods that can help meet calcium needs.

KEY POINTS

- Calcium is the chief mineral of bones and teeth.
- Calcium plays roles in nerve transmission, muscle contraction, and blood clotting.
- Calcium absorption adjusts somewhat to dietary intakes and altered needs.

Phosphorus

Phosphorus is the second most abundant mineral in the body. More than 80 percent of the body's phosphorus is found combined with calcium in the crystals of the bones and teeth. The rest is everywhere else.

Roles in the Body   All body cells must have phosphorus for these functions:

- Phosphorous salts are critical buffers, helping to maintain the acid-base balance of cellular fluids. (Note that the mineral is phosphorus. The adjective form is spelled with an *-ous*, as in phosphorous salts.)
- Phosphorus is part of the DNA and RNA of every cell and thus is essential for growth and renewal of tissues.

peak bone mass the highest bone density attained by an individual; developed during the first three decades of life.

DRI

Adults: 1,000 mg/day (men and women, 19–50 yr; men, 51–70 yr)

1,200 mg/day (women, 51–70 yr; men and women, >70 yr)

Tolerable Upper Intake Level

Adults: 2,500 mg/day (19–50 yr)
2,000 mg/day (>50 yr)

Chief Functions

Mineralization of bones and teeth; muscle contraction and relaxation, nerve functioning, blood clotting

Deficiency

Stunted growth and weak bones in children; bone loss (osteoporosis) in adults

Toxicity

Elevated blood calcium; constipation; interference with absorption of other minerals; increased risk of kidney stone formation

These foods provide 10% or more of the calcium Daily Value in a serving. For a 2,000-cal diet, the DV is 1,300 mg/day.
[a]Broccoli, kale, and some other cooked green leafy vegetables are also important sources of bioavailable calcium. Almonds also supply calcium. Spinach and chard contain calcium in an unabsorbable form. Some calcium-rich mineral waters may also be good sources.

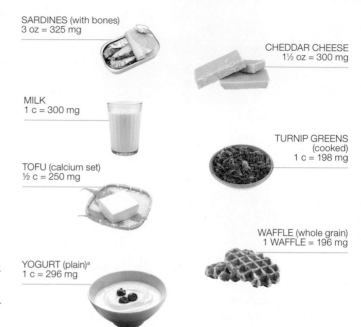

Good Sources*

SARDINES (with bones)
3 oz = 325 mg

CHEDDAR CHEESE
1½ oz = 300 mg

MILK
1 c = 300 mg

TURNIP GREENS
(cooked)
1 c = 198 mg

TOFU (calcium set)
½ c = 250 mg

WAFFLE (whole grain)
1 WAFFLE = 196 mg

YOGURT (plain)[a]
1 c = 296 mg

- Phosphorous compounds carry, store, and release energy during metabolism of energy nutrients.
- Phosphorous compounds act as cofactors, assisting many enzymes in extracting the energy from nutrients.
- Phosphorus forms part of the molecules of the phospholipids that are the principal components of cell membranes (discussed in Chapter 5).
- Phosphorus is present in some proteins.

Recommendations and Food Sources   Luckily, the body's need for phosphorus is easily met by almost any diet, deficiencies are unlikely, and most people in the United States meet their needs.[23] As Snapshot 8–2 shows, animal protein is the best source of phosphorus (because phosphorus is abundant in the cells of animals). Milk and cheese are also rich sources.

Phosphorus-based food additives, such as modified starches used in gravies, prepared meals, creamy desserts, and other processed foods, and phosphates added to colas also contribute phosphorus to the diet. Excess phosphorus in the *blood* is associated with indicators of heart and kidney diseases, but whether this bears a relationship to phosphorus in the diet is unknown.[24]

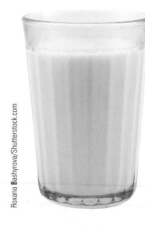

Roxana Bashyrova/Shutterstock.com

KEY POINTS

- Phosphorus is abundant in bones and teeth.
- Phosphorus helps maintain acid-base balance, is part of the genetic material in cells, assists in energy metabolism, and forms part of cell membranes.
- Phosphorus deficiencies are unlikely.

Phosphorus

DRI
Adults: 700 mg/day

Tolerable Upper Intake Level
Adults (19–70 yr): 4,000 mg/day

Chief Functions
Mineralization of bones and teeth; part of phospholipids, important in genetic material, energy metabolism, and buffering systems

Deficiency
Muscular weakness, bone pain[a]

Toxicity
Calcification of soft tissues, particularly the kidneys

*These foods provide 10% or more of the phosphorus Daily Value in a serving. For a 2,000-cal diet, the DV is 1,250 mg/day.
[a]Dietary deficiency rarely occurs, but some drugs can bind with phosphorus, making it unavailable.

Good Sources*

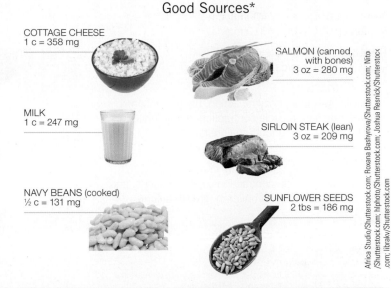

COTTAGE CHEESE
1 c = 358 mg

MILK
1 c = 247 mg

NAVY BEANS (cooked)
½ c = 131 mg

SALMON (canned, with bones)
3 oz = 280 mg

SIRLOIN STEAK (lean)
3 oz = 209 mg

SUNFLOWER SEEDS
2 tbs = 186 mg

Africa Studio/Shutterstock.com; Roxana Bashyrova/Shutterstock.com; Nito /Shutterstock.com; hlphoto/Shutterstock.com; Joshua Resnick/Shutterstock .com; iibravv/Shutterstock.com

Magnesium

Magnesium qualifies as a major mineral by virtue of its dietary requirement, but only about 1 ounce is present in the body of a 130-pound person, over half of it in the bones. Most of the rest is in the muscles, heart, liver, and other soft tissues, with only 1 percent in the body fluids. The body can tap the supply of magnesium in the bones to maintain a constant blood level whenever dietary intake falls too low. The kidneys can also act to conserve magnesium.

Roles in the Body Like phosphorus, magnesium is critical to many cell functions. Magnesium:

- Serves as a cofactor for hundreds of enzymes.
- Is needed for the release and use of energy from the energy-yielding nutrients.
- Is a necessary part of the cellular protein-making machinery.
- Is critical to normal nerve transmission, muscle contraction, and heart function.[25]

Magnesium and calcium work together for proper functioning of the muscles: calcium promotes contraction and magnesium helps relax the muscles afterward. In the teeth, magnesium promotes resistance to tooth decay by holding calcium in tooth enamel. Like most other nutrients, magnesium supports the normal functioning of the immune system.

Magnesium Deficiency U.S. magnesium intakes generally fall below recommendations, and chronically low intakes are associated with diabetes, heart failure, hypertension, inflammation, and stroke.[26] The Dietary Guidelines list magnesium among the shortfall nutrients for the U.S. population.

An acute magnesium deficiency may occur with alcoholism, prolonged diarrhea or vomiting, or severe malnutrition. It may also occur among people who take diuretics

DRI
Men (19–30 yr):   400 mg/day
Women (19–30 yr):   310 mg/day

Tolerable Upper Intake Level
Adults: 350 mg/day[a]

Chief Functions
Bone mineralization, enzyme action, heart function, immune function, muscle contraction, nerve function, protein synthesis, and tooth maintenance

Deficiency
Weakness, confusion; if extreme, convulsions, uncontrollable muscle contractions, hallucinations, and difficulty in swallowing; in children, growth failure

Toxicity
From nonfood sources only; diarrhea, pH imbalance, dehydration

These foods provide 10% or more of the magnesium Daily Value in a serving. For a 2,000-cal diet, the DV is 420 mg/day.
[a]*From nonfood sources, in addition to the magnesium provided by food.*
[b]*Whole wheat and wheat bran provides magnesium, but refined grain products are low in magnesium.*

Good Sources*

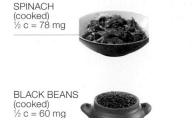

SPINACH (cooked) ½ c = 78 mg

BRAN CEREAL[b] (ready-to-eat) 1 c = 80 mg

BLACK BEANS (cooked) ½ c = 60 mg

SUNFLOWER SEEDS (dry roasted kernels) 2 tbs = 57 mg

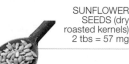

SOY MILK 1 c = 46 mg

YOGURT (plain) 1 c = 43 mg

---

or other medications that cause excessive magnesium loss in the urine. Its symptoms include a low blood calcium level, muscle cramps, and seizures. Magnesium deficiency also impairs brain functioning and may cause hallucinations that can be mistaken for mental illness or drunkenness.

Magnesium Toxicity   Magnesium toxicity is rare, but it can be fatal. Toxicity occurs only with high intakes from nonfood sources such as supplements. Accidental poisonings may occur in children with access to medicine chests and in older people who take too many magnesium-containing laxatives, antacids, and other medications. The symptoms can include diarrhea, acid-base imbalance, and dehydration.

Recommendations and Food Sources   Magnesium DRI values vary only slightly among adult age groups; see page B at the back of the book. Snapshot 8–3 shows magnesium-rich foods. Magnesium is easily washed and peeled away from foods during processing, so lightly processed or unprocessed foods are the best sources. The Dietary Guidelines 2015 committee recommends increasing fluid milk and yogurt consumption while reducing cheese intake to help increase magnesium in the diet. Fruit, vegetables, and whole grains are also important sources of magnesium. In some parts of the country, water augments magnesium intakes significantly, so people living in those regions need less from food.

KEY POINTS
- Magnesium stored in the bones can be drawn out for use by the cells.
- Magnesium is a shortfall nutrient for the U.S. population.

Sodium

Salt has been known and valued throughout recorded history. "You are the salt of the earth" means that you are valuable. If "you are not worth your salt," you are worthless. Even our word *salary* comes from the Latin word for *salt*. Chemically, sodium is the positive ion in the compound sodium chloride (table salt) and makes up 40 percent

Table 8–8

How Table Salt Is Formed

To chemists, a salt results from the reaction between a base and an acid.

- Sodium chloride (table salt) arises when the base sodium hydroxide reacts with hydrochloric acid.

Base + acid = salt + water
Sodium hydroxide + hydrochloric acid = sodium chloride + water

of its weight: a gram of salt contains 400 milligrams of sodium. Table 8–8 displays the chemical reaction that forms salt.

Roles of Sodium   Sodium is a major regulator of the body's fluid and electrolyte balance system because it is the chief ion used to maintain the volume of fluid outside cells. Sodium also helps maintain acid-base balance and is essential to muscle contraction and nerve transmission. About 30 to 40 percent of the body's sodium is stored in association with the bones, where the body can draw on it to replenish the blood concentration.[27]

Sodium Deficiency   A deficiency of sodium would be harmful, but no known human diet lacks sodium. Most foods include more salt than is needed, and the body absorbs it freely. The kidneys filter the surplus out of the blood into the urine. They can also sensitively conserve sodium. In the rare event of a deficiency, they can return to the bloodstream the exact amount needed. Small sodium losses occur in sweat, but the amount of sodium excreted in a day equals the amount ingested that day.

Overly strict use of low-sodium diets can deplete the body of needed sodium, as can vomiting, diarrhea, or extremely heavy sweating. If blood sodium drops, body water is lost, and both water and sodium must be replenished to avert an emergency.

Intense activities, such as endurance events performed over several days or in hot, humid conditions, can cause sodium losses that reach dangerous levels. Athletes in such events can lose so much sodium in sweat and drink so much plain water that they overwhelm the body's corrective actions and develop **hyponatremia**—the dangerous condition of having too little sodium in the blood. (Symptoms of hyponatremia are offered in Chapter 10, p. 388.)

How Are Salt and "Water Weight" Related?   Blood sodium levels are well controlled. If blood sodium begins to rise, as it will after a person eats salted foods, a series of events trigger thirst and ensure that the person will drink water until the sodium-to-water ratio is restored. Then the kidneys excrete the extra water along with the extra sodium.

Dieters sometimes think that eating too much salt or drinking too much water will make them gain weight, but they do not gain fat, of course. They gain water, but a healthy body excretes this excess water immediately. Excess salt is excreted as soon as enough water is drunk to carry the salt out of the body. From this perspective, then, the way to keep body salt (and "water weight") under control is to control salt intake and drink more, not less, water.

Sodium Recommendations and Intakes   A DRI for sodium adequacy has been set at 1,500 milligrams for healthy, active young adults; at 1,300 for people ages 51 through 70; and at 1,200 for the elderly. The UL is set at 2,300 milligrams per day (equivalent to about 1 tsp of salt), an amount met or exceeded daily by 90 percent of the U.S. adult population.[28] The average U.S. sodium intake nears 3,500 milligrams per day (Table 8–9 lists recommendations for limiting sodium intakes, and Figure 8–11 shows that most people's sodium intakes exceed these limits). An amount not much greater than this has been associated with damage to the pumping muscles of the heart.[29]

Do the Math

Salt is about 40% sodium and 60% chloride. (Reminder: 1g = 1,000 mg)

- 1 g of salt contains 400 mg of sodium.
- 1 tsp salt weighs 5.75 g.

Therefore, to find the milligrams of sodium in a teaspoon of salt:

400 × 5.75 = 2,300 mg

Now, find the milligrams of sodium in 1¾ tsp salt.

Table 8–9
Sodium Recommendations and Blood Pressure

These upper limits are recommended to help control blood pressure.

Dietary Guidelines for Americans, 2015–2020
- Consume less than 2,300 milligrams per day of sodium (ages 14 years and older).
- Further reductions to 1,500 milligrams of sodium may produce greater benefits in people with hypertension or prehypertension.

UL
- 2,300 mg/day, adults.
- For children age 14 years and younger, see the back of the book, p. C.

Figure 8–11
Average Daily Sodium Intakes, U.S. Adults

The solid red line indicates 2,300 mg of sodium, the current UL for healthy people. The broken red line beneath marks 1,500 mg, an adequate intake for young adults and the upper limit for people with hypertension and other conditions.

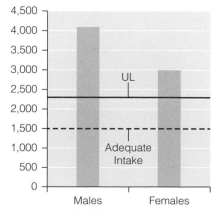

Source: Data from What We Eat In America, NHANES 2013–2014, available at www.ars.usda.gov/nea/bhnrc/fsrg.

hyponatremia (high-poh-nah-TREE-mee-ah) an abnormally low concentration of sodium in the blood. See also *water intoxication.*

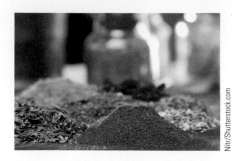

Herbs and spices add delicious flavors to foods without adding salt.

People who need to reduce their blood pressure for the sake of their health are urged to cut their sodium intakes.[30] For example, people with hypertension, diabetes, or chronic kidney disease should take in no more than 1,500 milligrams per day because this level of restriction often lowers blood pressure.[31] Even without meeting this recommendation, reducing sodium by at least 1,000 milligrams per day reduces blood pressure. This is a worthy goal—hypertension is a leading cause of death and disability in this country.

How Are Salt Intake and Hypertension Related? Over time, a high-salt diet can damage and stiffen the linings of arteries, making hypertension likely. As chronic sodium intakes increase, blood pressure rises in a stepwise fashion—the higher the intake, the higher the pressure. By one account, high intakes of salt account for almost a third of all cases of hypertension.[32] Excess salt may also damage and enlarge the heart muscle, increasing its workload along with the risk of heart problems.[33]

Too much salt can also aggravate kidney problems, and healthy kidneys play critical roles in regulating blood pressure.[34] Once hypertension sets in, a sharp increase in the risk of fatal heart attacks and strokes occurs; meanwhile, kidney disease and hypertension snowball, each worsening the other. When blood pressure is brought down, heart and kidney problems often improve.[35]

Genetic differences influence how readily people's blood pressure responds to sodium intakes.[36] These relationships are complex, but researchers suspect that genes controlling the kidneys' handling of sodium may be involved.[37]

Reducing Sodium Intakes Cutting down on sodium intake proves difficult within the current food supply. As Table 8–10 demonstrates, making meaningful salt reductions requires eliminating all salt, sauces, dressings, salty chips, pickles, and even piecrust from the diet. Choosing reduced-sodium, low-sodium, or salt-free products instead of their full-salt counterparts can help trim some sodium.[38] Another obvious step is controlling the saltshaker, but this source may contribute as little as 15 percent of the total salt consumed.

By far, the biggest contributor of sodium to the U.S. diet is processed and restaurant foods, so the Food and Drug Administration (FDA) has asked U.S. food manufacturers to voluntarily cut the sodium in their products.[39] Some progress is evident, but without oversight and enforcement, these efforts may not be sufficient to meet the national

Table 8–10

How to Trim Sodium from a Barbecue Lunch

Lunch #1 exceeds the whole day's Tolerable Upper Intake Level of 2,300 milligrams of sodium. With careful substitutions, the sodium drops dramatically in the second lunch, but it is still a high-sodium meal. In lunch #3, three additional changes—omitting the sauce, coleslaw dressing, and salt—cut the sodium by half again.

Lunch #1: Highest	Sodium (mg)	Lunch #2: Lower	Sodium (mg)	Lunch #3: Lowest	Sodium (mg)
■ Chopped pork sandwich, sauce and meat mixture	950	■ Sliced pork sandwich, with 1 tbs sauce	400	■ Sliced pork sandwich (no sauce)	210
■ Creamed corn, ½ c	460	■ Corn, 1 cob, soft margarine, salt	190	■ Corn, 1 cob, soft margarine	50
■ Potato chips, 2.5 oz	340	■ Coleslaw, ½ c	180	■ Green salad, oil and vinegar	10
■ Dill pickle, ½ medium	420	■ Watermelon, slice	10	■ Watermelon, slice	10
■ Milk, low-fat, 1 c	120	■ Milk, low-fat, 1 c	120	■ Milk, low-fat, 1 c	120
■ Pecan pie, slice	480	■ Ice cream, low-fat, ½ c	80	■ Ice cream, low-fat, ½ cup	80
Total 2,770		**Total 980**		**Total 480**	

Chapter 8 Water and Minerals

Figure 8–12

Major Sodium Sources in the U.S. Diet

Processed foods and foods from stores and restaurants contribute 75 percent of the sodium in the U.S. diet.

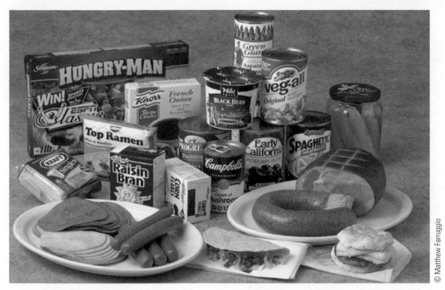

© Matthew Farruggio

Salts, about 2,000 mg/tsp
Salt, sea salt, seasoned salt, onion salt, garlic salt[a]
Dry soup mixes (prepared), about 1,000 to 2,000 mg/c
Bouillon, noodle, onion, ramen
Fast foods and frozen dinners, about 700 to 1,500 mg/serving
Breakfast biscuit (cheese, egg, ham), burger or cheeseburger, canned beans in sauce, chicken wings (10 spicy wings), deli sandwiches, frozen dinners, frozen or canned pasta, pizza, 2 tacos, chili dog, vegetarian soy burger (on bun)
Canned soups (prepared, most types), about 700 to 1,500 mg/c
Cold cuts/cured meats, about 500 to 700 mg/2 oz
Ham, lunchmeats, hot dogs, smoked sausages

Cheeses, processed, about 550 mg/oz
Pudding, instant, about 420 mg per $^1/_2$ c
Foods prepared in salt or brine, about 300 to 800 mg/serving
Anchovies (2 fillets), dill pickles (1), olives (5), sauerkraut ($^1/_2$ c), chipped beef (1 oz)
Canned vegetables, about 200 to 900 mg per $^1/_2$ c
Regular types[b]
Soy sauce, about 300 mg/tsp
Snack chips, puffs, crackers, about 200 to 300 mg/oz
Breads and rolls, about 125 mg/1 slice or $^1/_2$ roll
Condiments and sauces, about 100 to 200 mg/tbs
Barbecue sauce, ketchup, mustard, salad dressings, sweet pickle relish, taco sauce, Worcestershire sauce

[a]*Note that herb seasoning blends may or may not contain substantial sodium; read the labels.*
[b]*Some canned vegetables are reduced in salt; read the labels.*

objective of reducing the average sodium intake to below the UL by the year 2020.[40] Figure 8–12 lists foods high in sodium.

Finding Hidden Sodium   Foods high in sodium do not always taste salty. Who could guess by taste alone that a single half-cup serving of instant chocolate pudding provides almost one-fifth of the UL for sodium? Deceptively named "lemon pepper" seasoning often contains more salt than lemon or pepper. Additives other than salt also increase a food's sodium content: sodium benzoate, monosodium glutamate, sodium nitrite, and sodium ascorbate, to name a few. Moral: Read the Nutrition Facts labels (Figure 8–13).

The DASH Diet   An eating pattern proven to help people to reduce their sodium intake and control blood pressure is DASH (Dietary Approaches to Stop Hypertension).[41]

DASH diet details are in **Chapter 11** and **Appendix E**.

This pattern calls for greatly increased intakes of potassium-rich fruit and vegetables, adequate amounts of nuts, fish, whole grains, and low-fat dairy products, while

Figure 8–13

Sodium on a Food Label

Here's where to find the sodium content of a food—on the Nutrition Facts label. Table 2–6 (p. 54) defines sodium terms used on food labels.

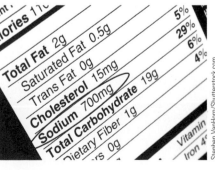

Stephen VanHorn/Shutterstock.com

restricting intakes of processed foods, red meat, solid fats, and sweets. You can read more about this remarkable diet in the Food Feature of Chapter 11 (p. 431) and Appendix E.

Remember that the recommendation is to limit sodium, not to eliminate it. Foods eaten without salt may seem less tasty at first, but with repetition, taste buds adjust, and the delicious natural flavors of unsalted foods and spices become the preferred tastes.[42]

KEY POINTS

- Sodium is the main positively charged ion outside the body's cells.
- Sodium attracts water.
- Too much dietary sodium raises blood pressure; few diets lack sodium.

Potassium

Outside the body's cells, sodium is the principle positively charged ion.[43] *Inside* the cells, potassium takes the role of the principal positively charged ion. All intact living cells contain potassium.

Roles in the Body   Potassium plays a major role in maintaining fluid and electrolyte balance and cell integrity. During nerve impulse transmission and muscle contraction, potassium and sodium briefly trade places across the cell membrane. The cell then quickly pumps them back into place. Controlling potassium distribution is a high priority for the body because it affects many critical functions, including maintaining a steady heartbeat.

Potassium Deficiency   Few people in the United States consume the DRI amount of potassium. Low potassium intakes, especially when combined with high sodium intakes, raise blood pressure and increase the risk of death from stroke. Higher intakes of dietary potassium may or may not lower blood pressure, but diets with ample potassium are associated with a reduced risk of cardiovascular disease and stroke. These effects, along with low U.S. consumption, earn potassium its status as a Dietary Guidelines nutrient of public health concern.[44]

Severe deficiencies are rare. In healthy people, almost any reasonable diet provides enough potassium to prevent dangerously low blood potassium under ordinary conditions. Dehydration leads to a loss of potassium from inside cells, dangerous partly because of potassium's role in maintaining regular heartbeats. The sudden deaths that occur with fasting, eating disorders, severe diarrhea, or severe malnutrition in children may be due to heart failure caused by potassium loss. Adults are warned not to take diuretics (water pills) that cause potassium loss or to give them to children except under a physician's supervision. Physicians prescribing diuretics will tell clients to eat potassium-rich foods to compensate for the losses.

Potassium Toxicity   Potassium from foods is safe, but potassium injected into a vein can stop the heart. Potassium overdoses from supplements normally are not life-threatening because the kidneys excrete small excesses and large doses trigger vomiting to expel the substance. A person with a weak heart, however, should not go through this trauma, and a baby may not be able to withstand it. Several infants have died when well-meaning parents overdosed them with potassium supplements.

Potassium Intakes and Food Sources   A typical U.S. eating pattern, with its low intakes of fruit and vegetables and high intakes of processed foods, provides far less potassium than the amount recommended by the DRI committee. Most vegetables and fruit are outstanding potassium sources (a few are shown in Snapshot 8–4). Bananas, despite their fame as the richest potassium source, are only one of many rich sources, which also include spinach, cantaloupe, and almonds. Nevertheless, bananas are readily available, conveniently portable, easy to chew, and have a likable sweet taste, so health-care professionals often recommend them. Potassium chloride, a salt substitute for people with hypertension, and potassium supplements provide potassium but do not reverse the hypertension associated with a lack of potassium-rich foods. Current guidelines do not recommend supplementing with potassium, but they do emphasize the importance of consuming a diet rich in fruit and vegetables.

DRI
Adults: 4,700 mg/day

Chief Functions
Maintains normal fluid and electrolyte balance; faciIitates chemical reactions; supports cell integrity; assists in nerve functioning and muscle contractions

Deficiency[a]
Muscle weakness, paralysis, confusion

Toxicity
Muscle weakness; vomiting; when given in a supplement to an infant or when injected into a vein in an adult, potassium can stop the heart

* These foods provide 10% or more of the potassium Daily Value in a serving. For a 2,000-cal diet, the DV is 4,700 mg/day.
[a]Deficiency accompanies dehydration.

Good Sources*

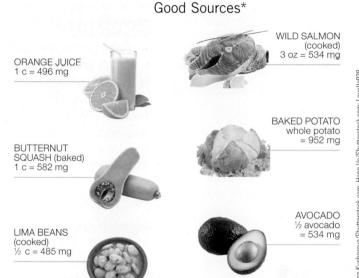

ORANGE JUICE
1 c = 496 mg

WILD SALMON (cooked)
3 oz = 534 mg

BAKED POTATO
whole potato = 952 mg

BUTTERNUT SQUASH (baked)
1 c = 582 mg

AVOCADO
½ avocado = 534 mg

LIMA BEANS (cooked)
½ c = 485 mg

Anna Kucherova/Shutterstock.com; Hong Vo/Shutterstock.com; Louella838 /Shutterstock.com; hiphoto/Shutterstock.com; Joe Gough/Shutterstock.com; Workmans Photos/Shutterstock.com

KEY POINTS

- Potassium, the major positive ion inside cells, plays vital roles in maintaining fluid and electrolyte balance and cell integrity.
- Americans take in too few potassium-rich fruit and vegetables.
- Potassium excess can be toxic.

Chloride

In its elemental form, chlorine forms a deadly green gas. In the body, the chloride ion plays important roles as the major negative ion. In the fluids outside the cells, it accompanies sodium and helps maintain the crucial fluid balances (acid-base and electrolyte balances). The chloride ion also plays a special role as part of hydrochloric acid, which maintains the strong acidity of the stomach necessary to digest protein. The principal food source of chloride is salt, both added and naturally occurring in foods, and no known diet lacks chloride.

KEY POINTS

- Chloride is the body's major negative ion, is responsible for stomach acidity, and assists in maintaining proper body chemistry.
- No known diet lacks chloride.

Sulfate

Sulfate is the oxidized form of sulfur as it exists in food and water. The body requires sulfate for synthesis of many important sulfur-containing compounds. Sulfur-containing amino acids play an important role in helping strands of protein assume their functional shapes. Skin, hair, and nails contain some of the body's more rigid proteins, which have high sulfur contents.

There is no recommended intake for sulfate, and deficiencies are unknown. Too much sulfate in drinking water, either naturally occurring or from contamination, causes diarrhea and may damage the colon. The summary table at the end of this chapter presents the main facts about sulfate and the other major minerals.

Table 8–11

Trace Minerals[a]

These minerals are needed by the body in tiny amounts.

- Iodine
- Iron
- Zinc
- Selenium
- Fluoride
- Chromium
- Copper
- Manganese
- Molybdenum

[a]*The trace minerals are also called* microminerals.

Figure 8–14

Goiter

In iodine deficiency, the thyroid gland enlarges—a condition known as goiter.

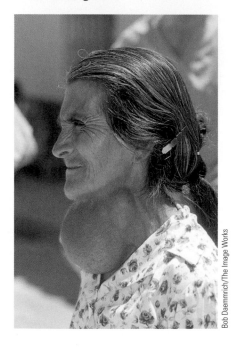

Bob Daemmrich/The Image Works

goiter (GOY-ter) enlargement of the thyroid gland due to an iodine deficiency is *goiter*; enlargement due to an iodine excess is *toxic goiter*.

cretinism (CREE-tin-ism) severe mental and physical retardation of an infant caused by the mother's iodine deficiency during pregnancy.

KEY POINT

- Sulfate is a necessary nutrient used to synthesize sulfur-containing body compounds.

The Trace Minerals

LO 8.5 Discuss the functions of the nine known trace minerals, their food sources, and the effects of their deficiencies and toxicities.

People require only miniscule amounts of the trace minerals, but these quantities are vital for health and life. Intake recommendations have been established for nine trace minerals—see Table 8–11. Others are recognized as essential nutrients for some animals but have not been proved to be required for human beings.

Iodine

The body needs only traces of iodine, but this amount is indispensable to life. Once absorbed, the form of iodine that does the body's work is the ionic form, iodide.

Iodine Roles Iodide is a cofactor that works with the hormone thyroxine, made by the thyroid gland. Thyroxine regulates the body's metabolic rate, temperature, reproduction, growth, heart functioning, and more. Iodine must be available for thyroxine to be synthesized.

Iodine Deficiency The ocean is the world's major source of iodine. In coastal areas, kelp, seafood, water, and even iodine-containing sea mist are dependable iodine sources. In many inland areas of the world, however, misery caused by iodine deficiency is all too common. In iodine deficiency, the cells of the thyroid gland enlarge in an attempt to trap as many particles of iodine as possible. Sometimes the gland enlarges to the point of making a visible lump in the neck, a **goiter**, as shown in Figure 8–14. People with iodine deficiency this severe may feel cold, may become sluggish and forgetful, and may gain weight. Iodine deficiency affects more than 2 billion people globally, including hundreds of millions of school-aged children.[45] This is a huge number but one that reflects some improvement over past decades.

Iodine deficiency during pregnancy causes fetal death, reduced infant survival, and extreme and irreversible mental and physical retardation in infants, known as **cretinism**. It constitutes one of the world's most common and preventable causes of mental retardation.[†] Much of this misery can be averted if the woman's deficiency is detected and treated within the first 6 months of pregnancy, but if treatment comes too late or not at all, the child's IQ and other developmental indicators are likely to be substantially below normal.[46] Children with even a mild iodine deficiency typically have goiters and may perform poorly in school; treatment with iodine relieves the deficiency.[47] Programs to provide iodized salt to the world's iodine-deficient areas now prevent much misery and suffering worldwide.[48]

Iodine Toxicity Excessive intakes of iodine can enlarge the thyroid gland just as a deficiency can.[49] Although average U.S. intakes are generally above the recommended intake of 150 micrograms, they are still below the UL of 1,100 micrograms per day for an adult. Like chlorine and fluorine, iodine is a deadly poison in large amounts.

Iodine Food Sources and Intakes The iodine in food varies with the amount in the soil in which plants are grown or on which animals graze.[50] Because iodine is plentiful in the ocean, seafood is a dependable source. In the central parts of the United States that were never beneath an ocean, the soil is poor in iodine. In those areas, once-widespread deficiencies have been wiped out by the use of iodized salt and the consumption of foods shipped in from iodine-rich areas. Surprisingly, sea salt delivers little iodine because iodine becomes a gas and flies off into the air during the salt-drying process. In the United States, salt labels like the ones shown in Figure 8–15 state whether the salt is iodized. Less than a half-teaspoon of iodized salt meets the daily recommendation.

[†]Collectively, the problems caused by iodine deficiency are sometimes referred to as *iodine deficiency disorder.*

Chapter 8 Water and Minerals

Figure 8–15

Iodized Salt Label

Iodized salt is a source of iodine; plain salt is not. The labels tell you which is which.

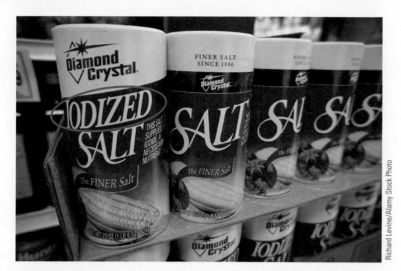

Most U.S. adults easily meet their iodine needs by consuming seafood, vegetables grown in iodine-rich soil, and iodized salt. Other sources are bakery products and milk. The baking industry uses iodine salts (iodates) as dough conditioners. Dairies often sanitize milking equipment and cow udders with iodine, which then migrates into the milk. Consumers in the United States rarely need extra iodine.

KEY POINTS

- Iodine is part of the hormone thyroxine, which helps regulate energy metabolism.
- Iodine deficiency diseases are goiter and cretinism.
- Large amounts of iodine are toxic.
- Most people in the United States meet their need for iodine.

Iron

Every living cell, whether plant or animal, contains iron. Most of the iron in the body is a component of two proteins: **hemoglobin** in red blood cells and **myoglobin** in muscle cells.

Roles of Iron Iron-containing hemoglobin in the red blood cells carries oxygen from the lungs to tissues throughout the body. Iron in myoglobin holds and stores oxygen in the muscles for their use.

All the body's cells need oxygen to combine with the carbon and hydrogen atoms released from energy nutrients during their metabolism. This generates carbon dioxide and water, which exit the cells; thus, body tissues constantly need fresh oxygen to keep the cells cleansed and functioning. As cells use up their oxygen, iron (in hemoglobin) shuttles fresh oxygen into the tissues from the lungs. In addition to this major task, iron is part of dozens of enzymes, particularly those involved in energy metabolism. Iron is also needed to make new cells, amino acids, hormones, and neurotransmitters.

Iron Stores Iron is clearly the body's gold, a precious mineral to be hoarded. The bone marrow uses large quantities of iron to make new red blood cells, which live only for about 4 months. When they die, the spleen and liver break them down, salvage their iron for recycling, and send it back to the bone marrow to be reused.

Once in the body, iron is difficult to excrete. The body does lose iron from the digestive tract, in nail and hair trimmings, and in shed skin cells—but only in tiny amounts. Bleeding, however, can cause significant iron loss from the body.

hemoglobin (HEEM-oh-globe-in) the oxygen-carrying protein of the blood; found in the red blood cells (*hemo* means "blood"; *globin* means "spherical protein").

myoglobin (MYE-oh-globe-in) the oxygen-holding protein of the muscles (*myo* means "muscle").

Figure 8–16

Nonheme Iron Absorption

Two constituents of this chili increase the absorption of nonheme iron from its legumes and ground beef: the vitamin C from its tomatoes and a peptide factor in meat.

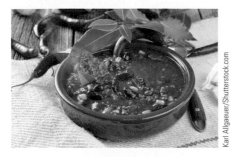

Karl Allgaeuer/Shutterstock.com

hepcidin (HEP-sid-in) a hormone secreted by the liver in response to elevated blood iron. Hepcidin reduces iron's absorption from the intestine and its release from storage.

heme (HEEM) the iron-containing portion of the hemoglobin and myoglobin molecules.

nonheme iron dietary iron not associated with hemoglobin; the iron of plants and other sources.

tannins compounds in tea (especially black tea) and coffee that bind iron. Tannins also denature proteins.

phytates (FYE-tates) compounds present in plant foods (particularly whole grains) that bind iron and may prevent its absorption.

iron overload the state of having more iron in the body than it needs or can handle, usually arising from a hereditary defect. Also called *hemochromatosis*.

iron deficiency the condition of having depleted iron stores, which, at the extreme, causes iron-deficiency anemia.

iron-deficiency anemia a form of anemia caused by a lack of iron and characterized by red blood cell shrinkage and color loss. Accompanying symptoms are weakness, apathy, headaches, pallor, intolerance to cold, and inability to pay attention. (For other anemias, see the index.)

anemia the condition of inadequate or impaired red blood cells; a reduced number or volume of red blood cells along with too little hemoglobin in the blood. The red blood cells may be immature and therefore too large or too small to function properly.

Special measures are needed to manage iron in the body. Left free, iron is a powerful oxidant that generates free-radical reactions. Free radicals increase oxidative stress and inflammation associated with diseases such as diabetes, heart disease, and cancer.[51] To guard against iron's renegade nature, special proteins transport and store the body's iron supply, and its absorption is tightly regulated.

An Iron-Regulating Hormone—Hepcidin In most well-fed people, only about 10 to 15 percent of iron in the diet is absorbed. However, if the body's iron supply is diminished or if the need for iron increases (say, during pregnancy), absorption can increase several-fold.[52] The reverse is also true: absorption declines when dietary iron is abundant. The hormone **hepcidin**, secreted by the liver, is an important regulator of blood iron.[53] Hepcidin reduces iron absorption from the small intestine and also reduces iron release from body stores, thereby keeping the blood iron concentration from rising too high. When the body needs more iron, the liver curbs its hepcidin output, allowing greater absorption of iron from food in the intestine and greater release of stored iron into the blood.

Iron Absorption Enhancers in Food Iron occurs in two forms in foods. Some is bound into **heme**, the iron-containing part of hemoglobin and myoglobin in meat, poultry, and fish. Some is **nonheme iron**, in plants and also in meats. The form affects absorption. Healthy people with adequate iron stores absorb heme iron at a rate of about 23 percent over a wide range of meat intakes. People absorb nonheme iron at rates of 2 to 20 percent, depending on dietary factors and iron stores. (A heme molecule was depicted in Figure 6–4 of Chapter 6.)

Meat, fish, and poultry also contain a peptide factor, sometimes called *MFP factor*, that promotes the absorption of nonheme iron from other foods, as depicted in Figure 8–16. Vitamin C also greatly improves absorption of nonheme iron, tripling iron absorption from foods eaten in the same meal. The bit of vitamin C in dried fruit, strawberries, or watermelon helps absorb the nonheme iron in these foods.

Iron Absorption Inhibitors Some food substances inhibit iron absorption. They include the **tannins** of tea and coffee, the calcium and phosphorus in milk, and the **phytates** that accompany fiber in lightly processed legumes and whole-grain cereals. Ordinary black tea excels at reducing iron absorption—clinical dietitians advise people with **iron overload** to drink it with their meals. For those who need more iron, the opposite advice applies—drink tea between meals, not with food. Thus, the amount of iron absorbed from a regular meal depends partly on the interaction between promoters and inhibitors, as listed in Table 8–12.

What Happens in Iron Deficiency? If absorption cannot compensate for losses or low dietary intakes, then iron stores are used up, and **iron deficiency** sets in. Iron deficiency and **iron-deficiency anemia** are not one and the same, though they often occur together. Anemia results from other nutrient deficiencies and causes unrelated to nutrition, such as blood loss. Anemia is not a disease but a symptom of another problem; its name literally means "too little blood."

Iron deficiency develops in stages, and the distinction between iron deficiency and its **anemia** is a matter of degree. People may be iron deficient, meaning that they have depleted iron stores, without being anemic. With worsening iron deficiency, they may become anemic.

A body severely deprived of iron becomes unable to make enough hemoglobin to fill new blood cells, and anemia results. A sample of iron-deficient blood examined under a microscope shows cells that are smaller and lighter red than normal (see Figure 8–17). These cells contain too little hemoglobin to deliver sufficient oxygen to the tissues. As iron deficiency limits the cells' oxygen and energy metabolism, the person develops fatigue, apathy, and a tendency to feel cold. The blood's lower concentration of its red pigment hemoglobin also explains the pale appearance of fair-skinned

Normal and Anemic Blood Cells

Well-nourished red blood cells, shown on the left, are normal in size and color. The cells on the right are typical of iron-deficiency anemia. These cells are small and pale because they contain less hemoglobin.

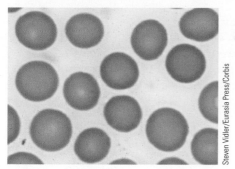 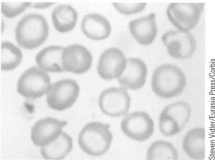

Steven Vidler/Eurasia Press/Corbis *Steven Vidler/Eurasia Press/Corbis*

iron-deficient people and the paleness of the normally pink tongue and eyelid linings of those with darker skin.

Symptoms of Iron Deficiency Long before the red blood cells are affected and anemia is diagnosed, a developing iron deficiency affects behavior. Even slightly lowered iron levels cause fatigue, mental impairments, and impaired physical work capacity and productivity.[54] Symptoms associated with iron deficiency are easily mistaken for behavioral or motivational problems (see Table 8–13). With reduced energy, people work less, play less, and think or learn less eagerly—symptoms that clear up reliably when iron is restored. Lack of energy does not always indicate a need for iron, however—see the Think Fitness feature. Taking iron supplements for fatigue without a deficiency will not increase energy levels, but can cause an iron overload in some people.

Children deprived of iron become restless, irritable, unwilling to work or play, and unable to pay attention, and they may fall behind their peers academically. Some symptoms in children, such as irritability, disappear when iron intake improves. More studies are needed to clarify whether replenished iron levels can improve cognitive function and reverse academic failure or whether these effects linger beyond treatment.

Promoters and Inhibitors of Iron Absorption

These dietary factors increase iron absorption:

- Heme form of iron
- Vitamin C
- Meat, fish, poultry (MFP) factor

These dietary factors hinder iron absorption:

- Nonheme form of iron
- Tea and coffee
- Calcium and phosphorus
- Phytates, tannins, and fiber

Mental Symptoms of Anemia

- Apathy, listlessness
- Behavior disturbances
- Clumsiness
- Hyperactivity
- Irritability
- Lack of appetite
- Learning disorders (vocabulary, perception)
- Lowered IQ
- Reduced physical work capacity
- Repetitive hand and foot movements
- Shortened attention span

Note: These symptoms are caused not by anemia itself but by iron deficiency in the brain. Children with much more severe anemias from other causes, such as sickle-cell anemia and thalassemia, show no reduction in IQ when compared with children without anemia.

THINK FITNESS Exercise-Deficiency Fatigue

On hearing about symptoms of iron deficiency, tired people may jump to the conclusion that they need to take iron supplements to restore their pep. More likely, they can obtain help by simply putting their diets in order, going to bed on time, and getting enough exercise. Few realize that too little exercise over weeks and months is as exhausting as too much—the less you do, the less

you're able to do, and the more fatigued you feel. The condition even has a name: "sedentary inertia."

Feeling fatigued, weak, and apathetic does not necessarily mean that you need iron or other supplements. Three actions are called for:

- Put your diet in order.
- Get some exercise.

- If fatigue persists for more than a week or two after making simple changes, consult a physician for a diagnosis.

start now! Using the Track Activity feature in Diet & Wellness Plus in MindTap, track your physical activity for one week, trying to increase your level of activity a little bit each day. See if you can walk briskly, bike, or jog for 30 minutes each day for a week.

Iron

DRI
Men: 8 mg/day
Women (19–50 yr):   18 mg/day
Women (51+):   8 mg/day

Tolerable Upper Intake Level
Adults: 45 mg/day

Chief Functions
Carries oxygen as part of hemoglobin in blood or myoglobin in muscles; required for cellular energy metabolism

Deficiency
Anemia: weakness, fatigue, headaches; impaired mental and physical work performance; impaired immunity; pale skin, nailbeds, and mucous membranes; concave nails; chills; pica

Toxicity
GI distress; with chronic iron overload, infections, fatigue, joint pain, skin pigmentation, organ damage

* These foods provide 10% or more of the iron Daily Value in a serving. For a 2,000-cal diet, the DV is 18 mg/day.
Note: Dried figs contain 0.6 mg per ¼ c; raisins contain 0.8 mg per ¼ c.
ᵃ Some clams may contain less, but most types are iron-rich foods.
ᵇ Legumes contain phytates that reduce iron absorption.
ᶜ Enriched cereals vary widely in iron content.

Good Sources*

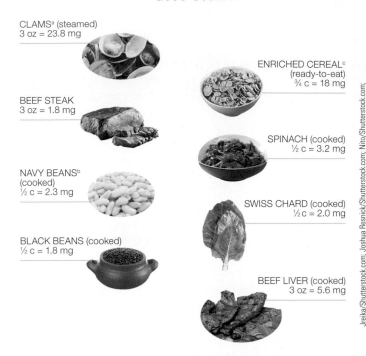

CLAMSᵃ (steamed)
3 oz = 23.8 mg

BEEF STEAK
3 oz = 1.8 mg

NAVY BEANSᵇ (cooked)
½ c = 2.3 mg

BLACK BEANS (cooked)
½ c = 1.8 mg

ENRICHED CEREALᶜ (ready-to-eat)
¾ c = 18 mg

SPINACH (cooked)
½ c = 3.2 mg

SWISS CHARD (cooked)
½ c = 2.0 mg

BEEF LIVER (cooked)
3 oz = 5.6 mg

A poorly understood behavior seen among some iron-deficient people, particularly low-income women and children, is **pica**—the craving for and intentional consumption of ice, chalk, starch, clay, soil, and other nonfood substances. These items contribute no iron to the body, and clay, soil, or starch can form a glaze over the intestinal surface that reduces nutrient absorption, including iron absorption.[55] Soil can also introduce parasites and heavy metals into the body.

Causes of Iron Deficiency and Anemia   Iron deficiency is usually caused by inadequate iron intake, either from sheer lack of food or from a steady diet of iron-poor foods or foods high in inhibitors of iron absorption. In developed nations, high-calorie foods that are rich in refined carbohydrates and fats and poor in nutrients often displace nutritious iron-rich foods from the diet and may impede iron absorption. In contrast, Snapshot 8–5 shows some foods that are good sources of iron.

The number-one nonnutritional factor that can cause anemia is blood loss. Because most of the body's iron is in the blood, losing blood entails losing iron. Menstrual losses increase women's iron needs to more than double those of men. Digestive tract problems such as ulcers and inflammation can also cause blood loss severe enough to cause anemia.

Who Is Most Susceptible to Iron Deficiency?   Women of childbearing age can easily develop iron deficiency because they not only lose more iron but also eat less food than men, on average. Pregnancy also demands additional iron to support the added blood volume, growth of the fetus, and blood loss during childbirth. Infants and toddlers receive little iron from their high-milk diets, yet they need extra iron to support

pica (PIE-ka) a craving and intentional consumption of nonfood substances. Also known as *geophagia* (gee oh FAY-gee-uh) when referring to clay eating and *pagophagia* (pag-oh-FAY-gee-uh) when referring to ice craving (*geo* means "earth"; *pago* means "frost"; *phagia* means "to eat").

their rapid growth. The rapid growth of adolescence, especially for males, and the menstrual losses of females also demand extra iron that a typical teen eating pattern may not provide.[56] Iron is of particular concern for the following groups of people:

- Women in their reproductive years.[57]
- Pregnant women.
- Infants and toddlers.
- Adolescents.

In addition, obesity at many life stages makes low blood iron more likely to occur.

In the United States, 2.4 million young children suffer from iron deficiency, while almost a half-million are diagnosed with iron-deficiency anemia. Most often, the children are from urban, low-income, or Hispanic families, but children from all groups can develop these conditions. As for women in childbearing years, the percentage of iron deficiency remains three times higher than the goal of Healthy People 2020: Objectives for the Nation. To combat iron deficiency, the Special Supplemental Feeding Program for Women, Infants, and Children (WIC) provides low-income families with credits redeemable for high-iron foods.

Worldwide, iron deficiency is the most common nutrient deficiency and the most common cause of anemia. Two billion people and almost half of preschool children and pregnant women have anemia, mostly due to iron deficiency.[58] In developing countries, parasitic infections of the digestive tract cause people to lose blood daily. For their entire lives, they may feel fatigued and listless but never know why. Iron supplements can reverse iron-deficiency anemia from dietary causes in short order, but they may also cause digestive upsets and other problems.

Can a Person Take in Too Much Iron? Iron is toxic in large amounts. Once absorbed inside the body, iron is difficult to excrete. A healthy body defends against iron overload by controlling its entry: the intestinal cells trap some of the iron and hold it within their boundaries. When they are shed, these cells carry out of the intestinal tract the excess iron that they collected during their brief lives. While present in the intestinal contents, excess iron may promote cancers of the colon and rectum.[59]

In healthy people, when iron stores fill up, hepcidin, the absorption-suppressing hormone, protects against iron overload. In people with a genetic failure of this protective system, mostly Caucasian men, excess iron builds up in the tissues.[60] Early symptoms include fatigue, mental depression, or abdominal pain; untreated, the condition can damage the liver, joints, or heart. Infections are also likely because excess iron can harm the immune system and bacteria thrive on iron-rich blood.[61] People with the condition must monitor and limit their iron intakes and forgo supplemental iron.

Iron-containing supplements can easily cause accidental poisonings in young children. As few as five ordinary iron tablets have proved fatal in young children. Keep iron-containing supplements out of children's reach.

Iron Recommendations and Sources The typical eating pattern in the United States provides about 6 to 7 milligrams of iron in every 1,000 calories. Men need 8 milligrams of iron each day, and so do women past age 51, so these people have little trouble meeting their iron needs. For women of childbearing age, the recommendation is higher—18 milligrams—to replace menstrual losses. During pregnancy, a woman needs even more—27 milligrams a day; to obtain this amount, pregnant women need a supplement. If a man has a low hemoglobin concentration, his health-care provider should examine him for a blood-loss site. Vegetarians, because iron from plant sources is poorly absorbed, should multiply the DRI value for their age and gender group by 1.8 (see the margin example).

Cooking foods in an old-fashioned iron pan adds iron salts, somewhat like the iron found in supplements. The iron content of 100 grams of spaghetti sauce simmered in a glass pan is 3 milligrams, but it increases to 87 milligrams when the

Do the Math

To calculate the iron RDA for vegetarians, multiply the regular RDA by 1.8:

8 mg × 1.8 = 14 mg/day
(vegetarian men)

18 mg × 1.8 = 32 mg/day
(vegetarian women, 19 to 50 years)

Older women need less iron. Turn to the back of this book, p. B, and find the iron RDA for a 60-year-old woman. Now, use it to calculate the iron RDA for a 60-year-old vegetarian woman.

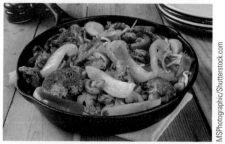

The old-fashioned iron skillet adds supplemental iron to foods.

sauce is cooked in a black iron pan. This iron salt is not as well absorbed as iron from meat, but some does get into the body, especially if the meal also contains meat or vitamin C.

Iron fortification of foods helps some people to fend off iron deficiency, but it can cause problems for others who tend toward iron overload. A single ounce of fortified cereal for breakfast, an ordinary ham sandwich at lunch, and a cup of chili with meat for dinner present almost twice the iron a man needs in a day but only about 800 calories. Most men need about 3,000 calories, and more food means still more iron. The U.S. love affair with vitamin C supplements makes matters worse because vitamin C enhances iron absorption. For healthy people, however, fortified foods pose virtually no risk for iron toxicity.

KEY POINTS

- Most iron in the body is in hemoglobin and myoglobin or occurs as part of enzymes in the energy-yielding pathways.
- Iron absorption is regulated in part by the hormone hepcidin, and affected by promoters and inhibitors in foods.
- Iron-deficiency anemia is a problem among many groups worldwide.
- Too much iron is toxic.

Zinc

Zinc occurs in a very small quantity in the human body, but it occurs in every organ and tissue. It acts as a cofactor for more than 300 enzymes to:

- Protect cell structures against damage from oxidation.[62]
- Make parts of the cells' genetic material.
- Make the heme of hemoglobin.

Zinc also assists the pancreas with its digestive and insulin functions and helps metabolize carbohydrate, protein, and fat.

Besides helping enzymes to function, special zinc-containing proteins associate with DNA and help regulate protein synthesis and cell division, functions critical to normal growth before and after birth.[63] Zinc is also needed to produce the active form of vitamin A in visual pigments. Even a mild zinc deficiency can impair night vision. Zinc also:

- Affects behavior, learning, and mood.
- Assists in proper immune functioning.[64]
- Is essential to wound healing, sperm production, taste perception, normal metabolic rate, nerve and brain functioning, bone growth, normal development in children, and many other functions.

When zinc deficiency occurs—even a slight deficiency—it packs a wallop to the body, impairing all of these functions.

Problem: Too Little Zinc   Zinc deficiency in human beings was first observed a half-century ago in children and adolescent boys in the Middle East who failed to grow and develop normally (see Figure 8–18). Their native diets were typically low in animal protein and high in whole grains and beans; consequently, the diets were low in zinc and high in fiber and phytates, which bind zinc as well as iron. Furthermore, their bread was not **leavened**. (In leavened bread, yeast breaks down phytates as the bread rises.) Since that time, zinc deficiency has been identified as a substantial contributor to illness throughout the developing world and is known to be responsible for almost a half-million deaths each year.[65]

Marginal declines in zinc status also cause widespread problems in pregnancy, infancy, and early childhood. Zinc deficiency alters digestive function profoundly and causes diarrhea, which accelerates the body's losses, not only of zinc but of all nutrients. It drastically impairs the immune response, making infections likely.[66] Infections of the intestinal tract then worsen the malnutrition and further increase

Figure 8–18

Zinc Deficiency

How old does the Egyptian boy in the picture appear to be? He is 17 years old but is only 4 feet tall, the height of a 7-year-old in the United States. His reproductive organs are like those of a 6-year-old. The retardation is rightly ascribed to zinc deficiency because it is partially reversible when zinc is restored to the diet.

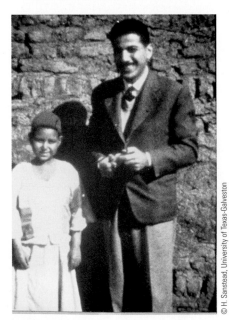

© H. Sanstead, University of Texas-Galveston

leavened (LEV-end) literally, "lightened" by yeast cells, which digest some carbohydrate components of the dough and leave behind bubbles of gas that make the bread rise.

susceptibility to infections—a classic cycle of malnutrition and disease. Zinc therapy often quickly reduces diarrhea and prevents death in malnourished children, but it can fail to restore normal weight and height if the child returns to the nutrient-poor diet after treatment.

Although zinc deficiencies are not common in developed countries, they do occur among some groups, including pregnant women, young children, the elderly, and the poor. When pediatricians or other health workers note poor growth accompanied by poor appetite in children, they should think zinc.

Problem: Too Much Zinc   Zinc is toxic in large quantities. High doses (more than 50 milligrams) of zinc may cause vomiting, diarrhea, headaches, exhaustion, and other symptoms. A UL for adults is set at 40 milligrams.

High doses of zinc inhibit iron absorption from the digestive tract. A blood protein that carries iron from the digestive tract to tissues also carries some zinc. If this protein is burdened with excess zinc, little or no room is left for iron to be picked up from the intestine. The opposite is also true: too much iron inhibits zinc absorption. Zinc from cold-relief lozenges, nasal gels, and throat spray products may shorten the duration of a cold, but they can upset the stomach and they contribute supplemental zinc to the body.[67]

Food Sources of Zinc   Meats, shellfish, poultry, and milk products are among the top providers of zinc in the U.S. diet (see Snapshot 8–6). Among plant sources, some legumes and whole grains are rich in zinc, but the zinc is not as well absorbed from plants as it is from meat. Most people in this country meet the recommended 11 milligrams per day for men and

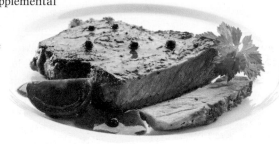

Dusan Zidar/Shutterstock.com

Snapshot 8–6   Zinc

DRI
Men: 11 mg/day
Women: 8 mg/day

Tolerable Upper Intake Level
Adults: 40 mg/day

Chief Functions
Activates many enzymes; associated with hormones; synthesis of genetic material and proteins, transport of vitamin A, taste perception, wound healing, reproduction

Deficiency[a]
Growth retardation, delayed sexual maturation, impaired immune function, hair loss, eye and skin lesions, loss of appetite

Toxicity
Loss of appetite, impaired immunity, reduced iron absorption, low HDL cholesterol (a risk factor for heart disease)

These foods provide 10% or more of the zinc Daily Value in a serving. For a 2,000-cal diet, the DV is 11 mg/day.
[a]*A rare inherited form of zinc malabsorption causes additional and more severe symptoms.*
[b]*Some oysters contain more or less than this amount, but all types are zinc-rich foods.*
[c]*Enriched cereals vary widely in zinc content.*

Good Sources*

OYSTERS[b] (steamed)
3 oz = 67 mg
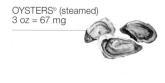

BEEF STEAK (lean)
3 oz = 4.9 mg
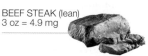

YOGURT (plain)
1 c = 2.2 mg
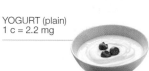

SHRIMP (cooked)
3 oz = 1.5 mg
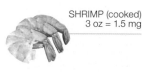

ENRICHED CEREAL[c]
(ready-to-eat)
¾ c = 15 mg
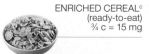

PORK CHOP
3 oz = 2.8 mg
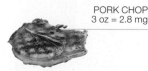

Olga Popova/Shutterstock.com; Joshua Resnick/Shutterstock.com; Gyorgy Barna /Shutterstock.com; Volosina/Shutterstock.com; stavklem/Shutterstock.com; Joe Gough /Shutterstock.com

8 milligrams per day for women. Vegetarians are advised to plan eating patterns that include zinc-enriched cereals or whole-grain breads well leavened with yeast, which helps make zinc available for absorption.[68] Unlike supplements, food sources of zinc never cause imbalances in the body.

KEY POINTS

- Zinc acts as a cofactor for hundreds of enzymes in protein, fat, and carbohydrate metabolism.
- Zinc plays roles in digestion, protein synthesis, cell division, and vision.
- Zinc deficiency impairs many vital body functions.
- Zinc supplements can interfere with iron absorption and can reach toxic doses; zinc in foods is nontoxic.

Selenium

Selenium has attracted the attention of the world's scientists. Hints of its relationships with chronic diseases make selenium a popular, but largely unnecessary, additive in supplements.

Roles in the Body Selenium works as a cofactor for many enzymes that, in concert with vitamin E, limits the formation of free radicals and prevents oxidative harm to cells and tissues.[69] In addition, selenium-containing enzymes are needed to assist the iodine-containing thyroid hormones that regulate metabolism.[70]

Relationship with Chronic Diseases Evidence is mixed on whether low dietary selenium plays a role in common forms of heart disease, but taking selenium supplements does not reduce the risk.[71] In cancer studies, adequate *blood* selenium seems protective against cancers of the prostate, colon, breast, and other sites.[72] Should everyone take selenium supplements to ward off cancer, then? No. Selenium *deficiency* may increase cancer risk, but U.S. intakes are generally sufficient, and excesses may harm healthy, well-fed people.[73]

Deficiency Severe selenium deficiencies cause muscle disorders with weakness and pain. A specific type of heart disease, prevalent in regions of China where the soil and foods lack selenium, is partly brought on by selenium deficiency. This condition prompted researchers to give selenium its status as an essential nutrient—adequate selenium prevents many cases from occurring.

Toxicity Toxicity is possible when people take selenium supplements and exceed the UL of 400 micrograms per day. Selenium toxicity brings on symptoms such as hair loss and brittle nails; diarrhea and fatigue; and bone, joint, and nerve abnormalities.[74]

Sources Selenium is widely distributed in meats and shellfish but varies greatly in vegetables, nuts, and grains, depending on whether they are grown on selenium-rich soil.[75] Soils in the United States vary in selenium, but foods from many regions mingle on supermarket shelves, ensuring that consumers are well supplied with selenium.

KEY POINTS

- Selenium works with an enzyme system to protect body compounds from oxidation.
- Deficiencies are rare in developed countries, but toxicities can occur from overuse of supplements.

Fluoride

Fluoride is present in virtually all soils, water supplies, plants, and animals. It is valued in the diet because of its ability to inhibit the development of dental caries in children and adults.

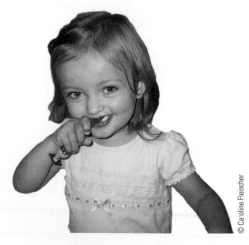

To prevent fluorosis, young children should not swallow toothpaste.

Chapter 8 Water and Minerals

Roles in the Body   In developing teeth and bones, fluoride replaces the hydroxy portion of hydroxyapatite, forming **fluorapatite**. During development, fluorapatite enlarges calcium crystals in bones and teeth, improving their resistance to demineralization.

Fluoride's primary role in health is prevention of dental caries throughout life. Once teeth have erupted through the gums, fluoride, particularly when applied to tooth surfaces, promotes the remineralization of early lesions of the enamel that might otherwise progress to form caries.[76] Fluoride also acts directly on the bacteria of plaque, suppressing their metabolism and reducing the amount of tooth-destroying acid they produce.

Deficiency   Where fluoride is lacking, dental decay is common, and fluoridation of public water is recommended for dental health (see Figure 8–19). Based on evidence of its benefits, fluoridation has been endorsed by the National Institute of Dental Health, the Academy of Nutrition and Dietetics, the American Medical Association, the National Cancer Institute, and the Centers for Disease Control and Prevention as beneficial and presenting no proven risks.

Toxicity   Too much fluoride can damage the teeth and bones, causing **fluorosis**. In mild cases, the teeth develop small white flecks; in severe cases, the enamel becomes pitted and permanently stained (as shown in Figure 8–20). Fluorosis in teeth occurs only during tooth development and it is permanent, making its prevention during the first 3 years of life a high priority. Fluorosis in bones makes them thick but weak and prone to fracture in later life. To limit fluoride ingestion, children should use just a pea-sized squeeze of toothpaste, and should be taught not to swallow it. The UL for fluoride is listed in the back of the book, p. B.

Sources of Fluoride   Drinking water is the usual source of fluoride. More than 70 percent of the U.S. population has access to public water supplies with an optimal fluoride concentration. Fluoride is rarely present in bottled waters unless it was added at the source, as in bottled municipal tap water. Fluoride supplements should be used only on the advice of a physician.

> **KEY POINTS**
> - Fluoride stabilizes bones and makes teeth resistant to decay.
> - Excess fluoride discolors teeth and weakens bones; large doses are toxic.

Chromium

Chromium is an essential mineral that acts as a cofactor for enzymes that mediate carbohydrate and lipid metabolism. Chromium in foods is safe and essential to health. Industrial chromium is a toxic contaminant, a known carcinogen that damages the DNA.[77]

Roles in the Body   Chromium helps regulate blood glucose by enhancing the activity of the hormone insulin, improving cellular uptake of glucose, and other actions.[78] When chromium is lacking, a diabetes-like condition can develop with elevated blood glucose and impaired glucose tolerance, insulin response, and glucagon response. Research results are mixed as to whether chromium supplements might improve glucose or insulin responses in diabetes.

Chromium Sources   Chromium is present in a variety of foods. The best sources are unrefined foods, particularly liver, brewer's yeast, and whole grains. The more refined foods people eat, the less chromium they receive.

Supplement advertisements may convince consumers that they can lose fat and build muscle by taking chromium picolinate. On the contrary, chromium supplements cannot reduce body fat or improve muscle strength more than diet and exercise alone.

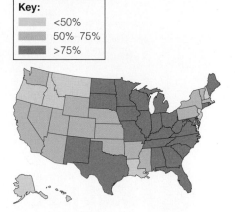

Key:
- <50%
- 50% 75%
- >75%

Source: Data from Centers for Disease Control and Prevention, National Water fluoridation statistics, 2014, available from www.cdc.gov/fluoridation/statistics/2014stats.htm.

Figure 8–20

Fluorosis

The mottled brown stains on these teeth indicate exposure to high concentrations of fluoride during development.

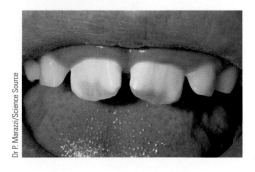

Dr. P. Marazzi/Science Source

fluorapatite (floor-APP-uh-tight) a crystal of bones and teeth, formed when fluoride displaces the "hydroxy" portion of hydroxyapatite. Fluorapatite resists being dissolved back into body fluid.

fluorosis (floor-OH-sis) discoloration of the teeth due to ingestion of too much fluoride during tooth development. *Skeletal fluorosis* is characterized by unusually dense but weak, fracture-prone, often malformed bones, caused by excess fluoride in bone crystals.

KEY POINTS

- Chromium is needed for normal blood glucose regulation.
- Whole, minimally processed foods are the best chromium sources.

Copper

Like most other trace minerals, copper plays vital roles as a cofactor for many enzymes. Among their tasks, these enzymes assist in the absorption and use of iron, and in synthesis of proteins such as hemoglobin and collagen. Another of these enzymes helps to control damage from free-radical activity in the tissues.§

Copper deficiency is rare but not unknown: it has been seen in severely malnourished infants fed a copper-poor milk formula. Deficiency can severely disturb growth and metabolism, and in adults, it can impair immunity and blood flow through the arteries. Excess zinc interferes with copper absorption and can cause deficiency. Two rare genetic disorders affect copper status in opposite directions—one causing a functional deficiency and the other toxicity.[79]

Copper toxicity from foods is unlikely, but supplements can cause it. The UL for adults is set at 10,000 micrograms (10 milligrams) per day. The best food sources of copper include organ meats, seafood, nuts, and seeds. Water may also supply copper, especially where copper plumbing pipes are used. In the United States, copper intakes are thought to be adequate.

KEY POINTS

- Copper is needed to form hemoglobin and collagen, and assists in many other body processes.
- Copper deficiency is rare.

Other Trace Minerals and Some Candidates

DRI values have been established for two other trace minerals: molybdenum and manganese. Molybdenum functions as part of several metal-containing enzymes, some of which are giant proteins. Manganese works with dozens of different enzymes that facilitate body processes and is widespread among whole grains, vegetables, fruit, legumes, and nuts.

Several other trace minerals are known to be important to health, but researching their roles in the body is difficult because their quantities are so small and because human deficiencies are unknown. For example, boron influences the activity of many enzymes and may play a key role in bone health, brain activities, and immune response. The richest food sources of boron are noncitrus fruit, leafy vegetables, nuts, and legumes. Cobalt is the mineral in the vitamin B_{12} molecule; the alternative name for vitamin B_{12}, *cobalamin*, reflects cobalt's presence. Nickel may serve as an enzyme cofactor; deficiencies harm the liver and other organs. Future research may reveal key roles played by other trace minerals, including barium, cadmium, lead, lithium, mercury, silver, tin, and vanadium. Even arsenic, a known poison and carcinogen, may turn out to be essential in tiny quantities.

All trace minerals are toxic in excess, and a UL exists for boron, nickel, and vanadium (see the back of the book, p. C). Overdoses are most likely to occur in people who take multiple nutrient supplements. Obtaining trace minerals from food is not hard to do—just eat a variety of whole foods in the amounts recommended in Chapter 2. Table 8–14 sums up what this chapter has said about the minerals and fills in some additional information.

KEY POINTS

- Many different trace elements play important roles in the body.
- All of the trace minerals are toxic in excess.

---

§ The enzyme is superoxide dismutase.

Chapter 8 Water and Minerals

Table 8–14

The Minerals—A Summary

MAJOR MINERALS

Chief Functions	Deficiency Symptoms	Toxicity Symptoms	Significant Sources
Calcium			
The principal mineral of bones and teeth. Also acts in normal muscle contraction and relaxation, nerve functioning, regulation of cell activities, blood clotting, blood pressure, and immune defenses.	Stunted growth and weak bones in children; adult bone loss (osteoporosis).	High blood calcium; abnormal heart rhythms; soft tissue calcification; kidney stones; kidney dysfunction; interference with absorption of other minerals; constipation.	Milk and milk products, oysters, small fish (with bones), calcium-set tofu (bean curd), certain leafy greens (bok choy, turnip greens, kale), broccoli.
Phosphorus			
Mineralization of bones and teeth; important in cells' genetic material, in cell membranes as phospholipids, in energy transfer, and in buffering systems.	Bone pain, muscle weakness, impaired growth.[a]	Calcification of nonskeletal tissues, particularly the kidney.	Foods from animal sources, some legumes.
Magnesium			
A factor involved in bone mineralization, the building of protein, enzyme action, normal heart and muscle function, transmission of nerve impulses, proper immune function, and maintenance of teeth.	Low blood calcium; muscle cramps; confusion; impaired vitamin D metabolism; if extreme, seizures, bizarre movements; hallucinations, and difficulty in swallowing. In children, growth failure.	Excess magnesium from abuse of laxatives (Epsom salts) causes diarrhea, nausea, and abdominal cramps with fluid and electrolyte and pH imbalances.	Nuts, legumes, whole grains, dark green vegetables, seafoods, chocolate, cocoa.
Sodium			
Sodium, chloride, and potassium (electrolytes) maintain normal fluid balance and acid-base balance in the body. Sodium is critical to nerve impulse transmission.	Muscle cramps, mental apathy, loss of appetite.	Hypertension, edema.	Salt, soy sauce, seasoning mixes, processed foods, condiments, fast foods.
Potassium			
Facilitates reactions, including protein formation; fluid and electrolyte balance; support of cell integrity; transmission of nerve impulses; and contraction of muscles, including the heart.	Deficiency accompanies dehydration; causes muscular weakness, paralysis, and confusion; can cause death.	Causes muscular weakness; triggers vomiting; if given into a vein, can stop the heart.	All whole foods: meats, milk, fruit, vegetables, grains, legumes.
Chloride			
Part of the hydrochloric acid found in the stomach, necessary for proper digestion. Helps maintain normal fluid and electrolyte balance.	Does not occur in normal circumstances, but can cause cramps, apathy, and death.	Normally harmless (the gas chlorine is a poison but evaporates from water); can cause vomiting.	Salt, soy sauce; moderate quantities in whole, unprocessed foods, large amounts in processed foods.
Sulfate			
A contributor of sulfur to many important compounds, such as certain amino acids, antioxidants, and the vitamins biotin and thiamin; stabilizes protein shape by forming sulfur-sulfur bridges (see Figure 6–11 in Chapter 6, p. 194).	None known; protein deficiency would occur first.	Would occur only if sulfur amino acids were eaten in excess; this (in animals) depresses growth.	All protein-containing foods.

(continued)

[a] Seen only rarely in infants fed phosphorus-free formula or in adults taking medications that interact with phosphorus.

Table 8–14, The Minerals—A Summary (continued)

TRACE MINERALS			
Chief Functions	**Deficiency Symptoms**	**Toxicity Symptoms**	**Significant Sources**
Iodine			
A component of the thyroid hormone thyroxine, which helps to regulate growth, development, and metabolic rate.	Goiter, cretinism.	Depressed thyroid activity; goiter-like thyroid enlargement.	Iodized salt, seafood, bread, plants grown in most parts of the country and animals fed those plants.
Iron			
Part of the protein hemoglobin, which carries oxygen in the blood; part of the protein myoglobin in muscles, which makes oxygen available for muscle contraction; necessary for the use of energy.	Anemia: weakness, fatigue, pale skin and mucous membranes, pale concave nails, headaches, inability to concentrate, impaired cognitive function (children), lowered cold tolerance.	Iron overload: fatigue, abdominal pain, infections, liver injury, joint pain, skin pigmentation, growth retardation in children, bloody stools, shock.	Red meats, fish, poultry, shellfish, eggs, legumes, green leafy vegetables, dried fruit.
Zinc			
Associated with hormones; needed for many enzymes; involved in making genetic material and proteins, immune cell activation, transport of vitamin A, taste perception, wound healing, the making of sperm, and normal fetal development.	Growth failure in children, dermatitis, sexual retardation, loss of taste, poor wound healing.	Nausea, vomiting, diarrhea, loss of appetite, headache, immune suppression, decreased HDL, reduced iron absorption.	Protein-containing foods: meats, fish, shellfish, poultry, grains, yogurt.
Selenium			
Assists a group of enzymes that defend against oxidation.	Predisposition to a form of heart disease characterized by fibrous cardiac tissue (uncommon).	Nausea; diarrhea; nail and hair changes; joint pain; nerve, liver, and bone damage; garlic breath odor.	Seafoods, organ meats, other meats, whole grains, and vegetables depending on soil content.
Fluoride			
Strengthens tooth enamel; confers decay resistance on teeth.	Susceptibility to tooth decay.	Fluorosis (discoloration) of teeth, skeletal fluorosis (weak, thickened bones), nausea, vomiting, diarrhea, chest pain, itching.	Drinking water if fluoride-containing or fluoridated, tea, seafood.
Chromium			
Associated with insulin; needed for energy release from glucose.	Abnormal glucose metabolism.	Possibly skin eruptions.	Meat, unrefined grains, vegetable oils.
Copper			
A cofactor for enzymes; assists in iron absorption and use; helps form hemoglobin and collagen.	Anemia; bone abnormalities.	Vomiting, diarrhea; liver damage.	Organ meats, seafood, nuts, seeds, whole grains, drinking water.

Meeting the Need for Calcium

LO 8.6 Itemize food choices that help to meet the need for calcium.

Some people behave as though calcium nutrition is of little consequence to their health—they neglect to meet their need. Yet a low calcium intake is associated with all sorts of major illnesses, including adult bone loss (see the following Controversy), high blood pressure, colon cancer (see Chapter 11), and even lead poisoning (Chapter 14).

Intakes of one of the best sources of calcium—milk—have declined in recent years, while consumption of other beverages, such as sweet soft drinks and fruit drinks, has increased dramatically. This Food Feature focuses on food and beverage sources of calcium and provides guidance about how to include them in an eating pattern that meets nutrient needs.

Milk and Milk Products

Milk and milk products are traditional sources of calcium for people who can tolerate them (see Figure 8–21). On average, people in the United States fall far short of the recommended intakes of milk, yogurt, or cheese (or replacements) each day. People who shun these foods because of lactose intolerance, allergy, a vegan diet, or other reasons can obtain calcium from other sources, but care is needed—*wise* substitutions must be made. This is especially true for children. Children who don't drink milk often have lower calcium intakes and poorer bone health than those who drink milk regularly. Most of milk's many relatives are good choices: yogurt, **kefir**, buttermilk, cheese (especially the low-fat or fat-free varieties), and, for people who can afford the calories, ice milk. Cottage cheese and frozen yogurt desserts contain about half the calcium of milk—2 cups are needed to provide the amount of calcium in 1 cup of milk. Butter, cream, and cream cheese are almost pure fat and contain negligible calcium.

Figure 8–21

Food Sources of Calcium in the U.S. Diet

Milk, cheese, and yogurt contribute much of the calcium in a typical U.S. diet.

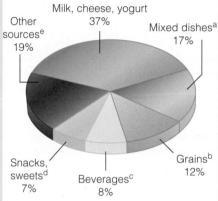

- Milk, cheese, yogurt 37%
- Mixed dishes[a] 17%
- Grains[b] 12%
- Beverages[c] 8%
- Snacks, sweets[d] 7%
- Other sources[e] 19%

[a]Includes pasta, macaroni and cheese, pizza, Mexican-style foods, fried rice.
[b]Includes breads, rolls, tortillas.
[c]Includes fortified juices and bottled drinks; excludes alcohol, milk.
[d]Includes ice cream, frozen dairy desserts, chocolate, cakes, pies, tortilla or corn chips.
[e]Meats, vegetables, fruit, condiments, other sources.

Source: M. K. Hoy and J. D. Goldman, Calcium intake of the U.S. population, USDA Dietary Data Brief No. 13, September 2014, available at www.ars.usda.gov/ARSUserFiles/80400530/pdf/DBrief/13_calcium_intake_0910.pdf.

Tinker with milk products to make them more appealing. Add cocoa to milk and fruit to yogurt, make your own fruit smoothies from fat-free milk or yogurt, or add fat-free milk powder to any dish. The cocoa powder added to make chocolate milk does contain a small amount of oxalic acid, which binds with some of milk's calcium and inhibits its absorption, but the effect on calcium balance is insignificant. Sugar lends both sweetness and calories to chocolate milk, so mix your chocolate milk at home where you control the amount of sugary chocolate added to the milk or choose a sugar-free product.

Figure 8–22

Calcium Absorption from Food Sources

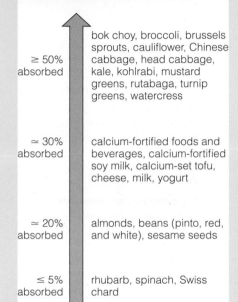

≥ 50% absorbed	bok choy, broccoli, brussels sprouts, cauliflower, Chinese cabbage, head cabbage, kale, kohlrabi, mustard greens, rutabaga, turnip greens, watercress
≈ 30% absorbed	calcium-fortified foods and beverages, calcium-fortified soy milk, calcium-set tofu, cheese, milk, yogurt
≈ 20% absorbed	almonds, beans (pinto, red, and white), sesame seeds
≤ 5% absorbed	rhubarb, spinach, Swiss chard

Vegetables

Among vegetables, beet greens, bok choy (a Chinese cabbage), broccoli, kale, mustard greens, rutabaga, and turnip greens provide some available calcium. So do collard greens, green cabbage, kohlrabi, parsley, watercress, and possibly some seaweeds, such as the **nori** popular in Japanese cookery. Certain other foods, including rhubarb, spinach, and Swiss chard, appear equal to milk in calcium content but provide very little or no calcium to the body because they contain binders that prevent calcium's absorption (see Figure 8–22).

A note in defense of spinach: The lack of absorbable calcium does

kefir a liquid form of yogurt, based on milk, probiotic microorganisms, and flavorings.

nori a type of seaweed popular in Asian, particularly Japanese, cooking.

not make spinach an inferior food. Spinach is rich in iron, beta-carotene, riboflavin, and dozens of other essential nutrients and potentially helpful phytochemicals. Just don't rely on it for calcium.

Calcium in Other Foods

For the many people who cannot use milk and milk products, a 3-ounce serving of small fish, such as canned sardines and other canned fishes eaten with their bones, provides as much calcium as a cup of milk. One-third cup of almonds supplies about 100 milligrams of calcium. Calcium-rich mineral water may also be a useful calcium source. The calcium from mineral water, including hard tap water, may be as absorbable as the calcium from milk but with zero calories. Many other foods contribute small but significant amounts of calcium to the diet.

stone-ground flour flour made by grinding kernels of grain between heavy wheels made of limestone, a kind of rock derived from the shells and bones of marine animals. As the stones scrape together, bits of the limestone mix with the flour, enriching it with calcium.

Calcium-Fortified Foods

Some foods contain large amounts of calcium salts by an accident of processing or by intentional fortification. Soybean curd (tofu) is in the processed category, and if calcium salts are used to coagulate it, then it's a rich source of calcium. Check the label. Canned tomatoes are a good calcium source because firming agents donate 63 milligrams of calcium per cup. Other unexpected sources include **stone-ground flour** and self-rising flour; stone-ground cornmeal and self-rising cornmeal; and blackstrap molasses.

Milk with extra calcium added can be an excellent source; it provides more calcium per cup than any natural milk, 450 milligrams per 8 ounces (Figure 8–23 provides a comparison). Next comes calcium-fortified orange juice, with 300 milligrams per 8 ounces, a good choice because the bioavailability of its calcium is comparable to that of milk. Calcium-fortified almond, pea, or soy milk can also be prepared so that it contains more calcium than whole cow's milk.

Finally, calcium supplements are available, sold mostly to people hoping to ward off osteoporosis. The Controversy following this chapter points out

that supplements are not magic bullets against bone loss, however.

Making Meals Rich in Calcium

For those who tolerate milk, many cooks slip extra calcium into meals by sprinkling a tablespoon or two of fat-free dry milk into almost everything. The added calorie value is small, and changes to the taste and texture of the dish are practically nil, but each 2 tablespoons adds about 100 extra milligrams of calcium. Dried buttermilk powder can also add flavor and calcium to baked goods and other dishes and keeps for a year or more when stored in the refrigerator. Table 8–15 provides some more tips for including calcium-rich foods in your meals.

Figure 8–23

Milk and Milk Replacers: Calcium and Protein Contents

	Pea milk, 8 oz	Soy milk, 8 oz	Almond milk, 8 oz	Dairy milk, 8 oz	Dairy milk with added calcium, 8 oz
Calcium (source)	450 mg (added fortification)	300 mg (added fortification)	460 mg (added fortification)	300 mg (naturally occurring)	450 mg (naturally occurring and added fortification)
Protein (source)	10 g (yellow peas)	7 g (soybeans)	1 g (almonds)	8 g (dairy milk)	8 g (dairy milk)

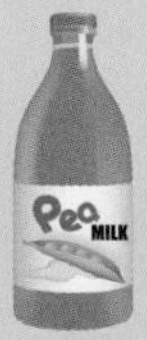

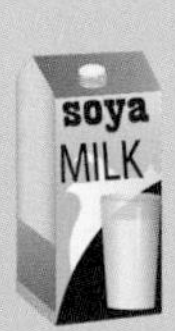

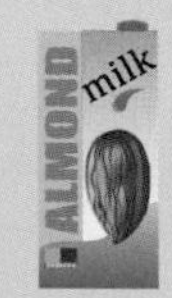

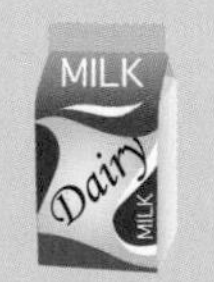

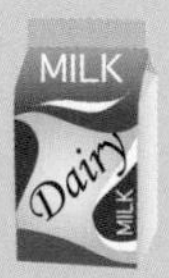

Chapter 8 Water and Minerals

Table 8–15

Calcium in Meals—Breakfast, Lunch, and Supper

Try the following techniques for meeting calcium needs.

At Breakfast	At Lunch	At Supper
▪ Choose calcium-fortified orange or vegetable juice. ▪ Lighten tea or coffee, hot or iced, with milk or calcium-fortified replacement, such as soy or pea milk. ▪ Eat cereals, hot or cold, with milk or calcium-rich replacement. ▪ Spread almond butter on toast (2 tbs provides 111 mg calcium, eight times the amount in peanut butter). ▪ Cook hot cereals with milk instead of water, then mix in 2 tbs of fat-free dry milk. ▪ Make muffins or quick breads with milk and extra fat-free powdered milk or dried buttermilk powder. ▪ Add milk to scrambled eggs. ▪ Moisten cereals with flavored yogurt.	▪ Add low-fat cheeses to sandwiches, burgers, or salads. ▪ Use a variety of green vegetables, such as watercress or kale, in salads and on sandwiches. ▪ Drink fat-free milk or calcium-fortified soy or pea milk as a beverage or in a smoothie. For tartness and extra calcium, add 2 tbs dried buttermilk powder. ▪ Drink calcium-rich mineral water as a beverage. ▪ Marinate cabbage shreds or broccoli spears in low-fat Italian dressing for an interesting salad that provides calcium. ▪ Choose coleslaw over potato and macaroni salads. ▪ Mix the mashed bones of canned salmon into salmon salad or patties. ▪ Eat sardines with their bones. ▪ Stuff potatoes with broccoli and low-fat cheese. ▪ Try pasta such as ravioli stuffed with low-fat ricotta cheese instead of meat. ▪ Sprinkle parmesan cheese on pasta salads.	▪ Toss a handful of thinly sliced green vegetables, such as kale or young turnip greens, with hot pasta; the greens wilt pleasingly in the steam of the freshly cooked pasta. ▪ Serve a green vegetable every night and try new ones—how about kohlrabi? It tastes delicious when cooked like broccoli. ▪ Remember your dark green, leafy vegetables—they can be good, low-calorie calcium sources. ▪ Learn to stir-fry Chinese cabbage and other Asian foods. ▪ Try tofu (the calcium-set kind); this versatile food has inspired whole cookbooks devoted to creative uses. ▪ Add fat-free powdered milk to almost anything—meat loaf, sauces, gravies, soups, stuffings, casseroles, blended beverages, puddings, quick breads, cookies, brownies. Be creative. ▪ Choose frozen yogurt, ice milk, or custards for dessert.

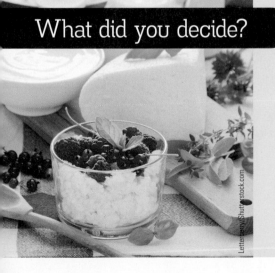

What did you decide?

Is **bottled water** better for you than tap water?

Can **"water weight"** explain extra pounds of body weight?

Do adults outgrow the need for **calcium**?

If you're feeling tired, do you need an **iron supplement**?

What's online?

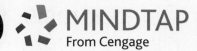

MINDTAP
From Cengage

Visit www.Cengage.com to access MindTap, a complete digital course that includes Diet & Wellness Plus, interactive quizzes, videos, and more.

Self Check

1. (LO 8.1) Water balance is governed by the _____.
   a. liver   b. kidneys   c. brain   d. b and c

2. (LO 8.1) Water intoxication cannot occur because water is so easily excreted by the body.
   T   F

3. (LO 8.2) Water from public water systems (tap water)
   a. requires frequent home testing for microorganisms.
   b. is less healthful than bottled water.
   c. is disinfected to kill most microorganisms.
   d. is less healthful than private well water.

4. (LO 8.2) On average, young men in the United States obtain _____ calories per day from beverages.
   a. 200   c. 1,200
   b. 600   d. 2,000

5. (LO 8.2) Whether from the tap or from a bottle, all water comes from the same sources.
   T   F

6. (LO 8.3) To temporarily increase the body's water content, a person need only
   a. consume extra salt.   b. consume extra sugar.
   c. take a diuretic.   d. consume extra potassium.

7. (LO 8.3) Vomiting or diarrhea
   a. causes fluid to be pulled from between the cells in every part of the body.
   b. causes fluid to leave the cell interiors.
   c. causes kidneys to raise the sodium concentration outside the cells.
   d. all of the above.

8. (LO 8.4) Which two minerals are the major constituents of bone?
   a. calcium and zinc   b. sodium and magnesium
   c. phosphorus and calcium   d. magnesium and calcium

9. (LO 8.4) Magnesium
   a. assists in the operation of enzymes.
   b. is needed for the release and use of energy.
   c. is critical to normal heart function.
   d. all of the above.

10. (LO 8.4) After about 60 years of age, bones begin to lose density.
    T   F

11. (LO 8.4) The best way to control salt intake is to cut down on processed and fast foods.
    T   F

12. (LO 8.5) The top food sources of zinc include _____.
    a. grapes   c. shellfish
    b. unleavened bread   d. potato

13. (LO 8.5) A deficiency of which mineral is a leading cause of mental retardation worldwide?
    a. iron   b. iodine   c. zinc   d. chromium

14. (LO 8.5) Which of these mineral supplements can easily cause accidental poisoning in children?
    a. iron   b. sodium   c. magnesium   d. potassium

15. (LO 8.5) The most abundant mineral in the body is iron.
    T   F

16. (LO 8.5) The Academy of Nutrition and Dietetics recommends fluoride-free water for the U.S. population.
    T   F

17. (LO 8.6) Dairy foods such as butter, cream, and cream cheese are good sources of calcium, whereas vegetables such as broccoli are poor sources.
    T   F

18. (LO 8.6) Children who don't drink milk often have lower bone density than those who do.
    T   F

19. (LO 8.7) Trabecular bone readily gives up its minerals whenever blood calcium needs replenishing.
    T   F

20. (LO 8.7) Too little _____ in the diet is associated with osteoporosis.
    a. vitamin B$_{12}$ c. sodium
    b. protein   d. niacin

Answers to these Self Check questions are in Appendix G.

Osteoporosis: Can Lifestyle Choices Reduce the Risk?

LO 8.7 Describe how osteoporosis develops and the actions that may help to prevent it.

Well over half of U.S. adults age 50 years and older have osteoporosis or low bone mass (osteopenia).[1]* Each year, millions of people break a hip, leg, arm, hand, ankle, or other bone as a result of osteoporosis. Of these, hip fractures prove most serious. The break is rarely clean—the bone explodes into fragments that cannot be reassembled. Just removing the pieces is a struggle, and replacing them with an artificial joint requires major surgery. Many people die of complications of such a fracture within a year; many more will never walk or live independently again. Both men and women are urged to do whatever they can to prevent fractures related to osteoporosis.

Development of Osteoporosis

Fractures from osteoporosis occur during the later years, but osteoporosis itself develops silently much earlier. Twenty-year-old adults are rarely aware of the strength ebbing from their bones until suddenly, 40 years later, a hip gives way. People say, "She fell and broke her hip," but in fact the hip may have been so fragile that it broke *before* she fell.

The causes of osteoporosis are tangled, and many are beyond a person's control. Insufficient dietary calcium, vitamin D, and physical activity certainly play roles, but age, gender, and genetics are also major players. No controversy exists as to the nature of osteoporosis; more controversial, however, are its causes and what people should do about it.

Bone Basics

To understand how the skeleton loses minerals in later years, you must first

* *Reference notes are in Appendix F.*

Table C8–1

Osteoporosis Terms

- **cortical bone** the ivorylike outer bone layer that forms a shell surrounding trabecular bone and that comprises the shaft of a long bone.
- **trabecular** (tra-BECK-you-lar) **bone** the weblike structure composed of calcium-containing crystals inside a bone's solid outer shell. It provides strength and acts like a calcium storage bank.

know a few things about bones. Table C8–1 offers definitions of relevant terms. Figure C8–1 shows a photograph of a healthy human leg bone sliced lengthwise, exposing the lattice of calcium-containing crystals (the **trabecular bone**) inside that are part of the body's calcium bank. Invested as savings during the milk-drinking years of youth, these deposits provide a nearly inexhaustible fund of calcium. **Cortical bone** is

Figure C8–1

A Healthy Bone

This healthy bone has been sectioned lengthwise to reveal its strong, dense crystal matrix.

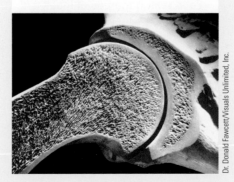

Dr. Donald Fawcett/Visuals Unlimited, Inc.

the dense, ivorylike bone that forms the exterior shell of a bone and the shaft of a long bone (look closely at the photograph). Both types of bone are crucial to overall bone strength. Cortical bone forms a sturdy outer wall, and trabecular bone provides strength along the lines of stress inside the bone.

The two types of bone handle calcium in different ways. The lacy crystals of the trabecular bone are tapped to raise blood calcium when the supply from the day's diet runs short, and are redeposited when dietary calcium is plentiful. The calcium of cortical bone fluctuates less.

Bone Loss

Trabecular bone, generously supplied with blood vessels, readily gives up its minerals at the necessary rate whenever blood calcium needs replenishing. Loss of trabecular bone begins to be significant for men and women around age 30. Calcium in cortical bone can also be withdrawn but more slowly.

As bone loss continues (see Figure C8–2), bone density declines. Soon, osteoporosis sets in, and bones become so fragile that the body's weight can overburden the spine. Vertebrae may suddenly disintegrate and crush down, painfully pinching major nerves. Or they may compress into wedges, forming what is insensitively called "dowager's hump," the bent posture of many older men and women as they "grow shorter" (see Figure C8–3). Wrists may break as trabecula-rich bone ends weaken, and teeth may loosen or fall out as the trabecular bone of the jaw recedes. As the cortical bone shell weakens as well, one or both hips may break.

Figure C8–2
Loss of Trabecular Bone

These bone sections are magnified to reveal details. The healthy trabecular bone shown on the left appears thick and strong. The bone on the right is thin and weak, reflecting osteoporosis.

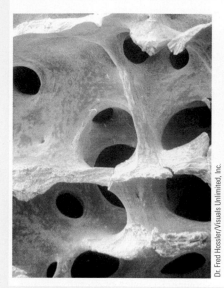

Dr. Fred Hossler/Visuals Unlimited, Inc.

Dr. Alan Boyde/Visuals Unlimited, Inc.

Figure C8–3
Loss of Height in a Woman with Osteoporosis

The woman on the left is about 50 years old. On the right, she is 80 years old. Her legs have not grown shorter; only her back has lost length, due to collapse of her spinal bones (vertebrae). When collapsed vertebrae cannot protect the spinal nerves, the pressure of bones pinching the nerves causes excruciating pain.

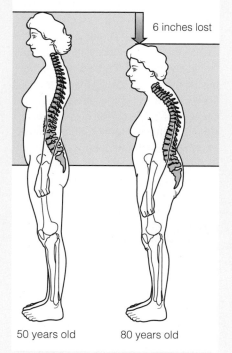

6 inches lost

50 years old   80 years old

Nondiet Factors that Affect Bone Health

Bones are affected by many factors. Lifestyle choices influence 20 to 40 percent of adult peak bone mass.[2] The remainder is determined by unalterable factors.

Bone Density and the Genes

A strong genetic component contributes to osteoporosis, bone density, and increased risk of fractures. Genes exert influence over:

- The activities of bone-forming cells and bone-dismantling cells;
- The cellular mechanisms that make collagen, a structural bone protein;
- The body's mechanisms for absorbing and employing vitamin D; and
- Many other contributors to bone metabolism.

Genes set a tendency for strong or weak bones, but diet and other lifestyle choices influence the final outcome, and anyone with risk factors for osteoporosis should take actions to prevent it.

Gender

Gender is a powerful predictor of osteoporosis: men have greater bone density than women at maturity, and women often lose more bone, particularly in the 6 to 8 years following menopause when the hormone estrogen diminishes. Thereafter, loss of bone minerals continues throughout the remainder of a woman's lifetime but not at the free-fall pace of the menopause years (refer again to Figure C8–3). If young women fail to produce enough estrogen, they lose bone rapidly, too, and going through menopause early almost doubles a woman's chance of developing osteoporosis.[3]

Each year, hundreds of thousands of men suffer fractures from osteoporosis.[4] Sex hormones, such as testosterone and the small amount of estrogen made by the male body, help to oppose men's osteoporosis.[5] Testosterone replacement therapy can help minimize bone loss in men with insufficient hormone production.[6]

Body Weight

After age and gender, the next risk factor for osteoporosis is being underweight or losing weight. Women who are thin throughout life or who lose 10 percent or more of their body weight after menopause face a doubled hip fracture rate. You might expect that, conversely, women who gain weight might have stronger bones than average, but in fact, it seems possible that at some point, excess body fatness may exert negative effects on bone health.[7]

Physical Activity

Physical activity supports bone strength and density during adolescence,

Table C8–2

Risk Factors for Osteoporosis

Nonmodifiable	Modifiable
■ Female gender	■ Sedentary lifestyle
■ Older age	■ Diet inadequate in calcium and vitamin D
■ Small frame	■ Diet excessive in protein, sodium, caffeine
■ Caucasian, Asian, or Hispanic/Latino heritage	■ Cigarette smoking
■ Family history of osteoporosis or fractures	■ Alcohol abuse
■ Personal history of fractures	■ Low body weight
■ Estrogen deficiency in women[a] testosterone deficiency in men	■ Certain medications, such as glucocorticoids and anticonvulsants
	■ Diet low in fruit and vegetables

particularly when calcium intake is adequate, and it may protect the bones later on.[8] Stronger muscles create denser, stronger bones by stressing, reshaping, and strengthening them.[9] When people lie idle—for example, when they are confined to bed—the bones lose strength just as the muscles do. The harm to the bones from a sedentary lifestyle equals the harm from nutrient deficiencies or cigarette smoking (see Table C8–2). The harms from a sedentary lifestyle can hardly be overstated.

Preventing falls is a critical focus for fracture prevention in the elderly. The best kind of exercise to keep bones and muscles healthy and thereby prevent falls is weight-bearing exercise such as jogging, doing jumping jacks, jumping rope, walking vigorously, or doing resistance (weight) training on most days throughout life.[10]

Tobacco Smoke and Alcohol

Smoking is hard on the bones. The bones of smokers are less dense than those of nonsmokers. Smoking also increases the risk of fractures and slows fracture healing.[11] Fortunately, quitting can reverse much of the damage. With time, the bone density of former smokers approaches that of nonsmokers.

Alcoholism is a major cause of osteoporosis in men. Heavy drinkers and people who regularly binge drink often have lower bone mineral density and experience more fractures than nondrinkers and light drinkers.[12]

Nutrients that Affect Bone Density

Obtaining the nutrients that build strong bones in youth helps prevent or delay osteoporosis later on. When people reach the bone-losing years of middle age, those who formed dense bones during youth can lose more bone tissue before suffering ill effects (see Figure C8–4). To a lesser degree, some nutrients can also help slow bone loss later in life.

Calcium and Vitamin D

Bone strength later in life is greatly affected by how well the bones were built during childhood and adolescence. Preteen children who consume enough calcium and vitamin D lay more calcium into the structure of their bones than children with less adequate intakes.[13] Unfortunately, most girls in their bone-building years fail to meet their calcium needs. Children who do not drink milk are unlikely to meet their calcium needs unless they use calcium-fortified foods or supplements. In adolescence, a critical time for gaining bone mass, soft drinks can displace milk from the diet, greatly reducing calcium and vitamin D intakes. Further, soft drink intake itself is associated with fractures in later life, but research has yet to say why.[14] It may be the carbonation or acids that they contain, or perhaps soft drinks are part of an eating pattern that lacks nutrients needed for bone strength.

Like calcium, sufficient vitamin D during the bone-forming years helps ensure that bones maximize their potential for density. Most milk products are fortified with vitamin D, so children who do not drink milk must

Figure C8–4

Two Women's Bone Mass History Compared

Bone density achieved during youth affects bone health in the later years.

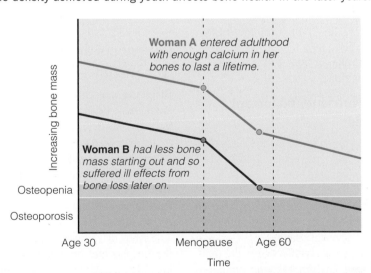

Woman A *entered adulthood with enough calcium in her bones to last a lifetime.*

Woman B *had less bone mass starting out and so suffered ill effects from bone loss later on.*

(Y axis) Increasing bone mass

Osteopenia

Osteoporosis

Age 30   Menopause   Age 60

Time

be provided with other sources to help them develop their bones.

In later life, calcium and vitamin D intakes cannot make up for earlier deficiencies, but they may help to slow the rate of bone loss. Additionally, calcium absorption declines with age, and older bodies become less efficient at making and activating vitamin D. For the elderly in nursing homes, low vitamin D status is associated with muscle weakness, and evidence suggests that taking supplemental vitamin D in the DRI amount may help to prevent injurious falls.[15]

Protein

When elderly people take in too little protein, their bones suffer.[16] Recall that the mineral crystals of bone form on a protein matrix—collagen. Restoring protein sources to the diet can often improve bone status and reduce the incidence of hip fractures even in the elderly. However, a diet lacking protein no doubt also lacks energy and other critical bone nutrients, so restoring a nutritious diet may be of highest importance. An opposite possibility, that a *high*-protein diet causes bone loss, has also been explored, but study results are inconsistent.[17]

Milk provides protein along with vitamin A, vitamin D, and calcium, all important nutrients for bone tissue. As might be expected, vegans, who do not consume milk products, generally have lower bone mineral density than people who do consume them.[18] Controversy 6 made the point that, for vegans, finding alternative sources of calcium is a must.

Other Nutrients Important to Bones

Vitamin K plays roles in the production of at least one bone protein important in bone maintenance. People with hip fractures often have low intakes of vitamin K.[19] Increasing vitamin K-rich vegetable intakes may improve both vitamin K status and skeletal health.

Sufficient vitamin A is needed in the bone-remodeling process, and vitamin C maintains bone collagen. Magnesium

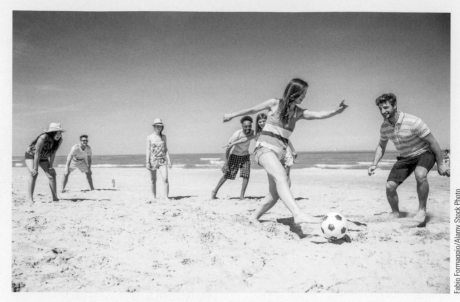

These young people are putting bone in the bank.

may help to maintain bone mineral density.[20] Omega-3 fatty acids may also help preserve bone integrity, and their effects are under study.[21] Clearly, a well-balanced diet that supplies a variety of abundant fruit, vegetables, protein foods, and whole grains along with a full array of nutrients is central to bone health.

The more risk factors of Table C8–2 (p. 313) that apply to you, the greater your chances of developing osteoporosis in the future, and the more seriously you should take the advice offered in this Controversy. Treatment, although continuously advancing, remains far from perfect.

Diagnosis and Medical Treatment

Diagnosis of osteoporosis includes measuring bone density using an advanced form of X-ray (DEXA; Figure C8–5) or ultrasound. Men with osteoporosis risk factors and all women should have bone density tests after age 50. A thorough examination also includes factors such as race, family history, and physical activity level.

Several drug therapies, including bisphosphonates (pronounced biz-FAHS foh-nates) that cause remineralization of bone, have worked minor

miracles in reversing even severe bone loss, but their side effects can be severe. Hormone replacement therapy can halt bone loss in nonmenstruating women, but safety questions must be weighed against its effectiveness for individual women with bone loss.[22] The mineral fluoride is less effective and poses the threat of skeletal fluorosis that damages bones. Clearly, prevention is far preferable to treatment; Figure C8–6 displays a lifetime plan to support bone health.

Figure C8–5

DEXA Scan

A DEXA scan measures bone density to help detect the early stages of bone loss, assess fracture risks, and measure the responses to bone-building treatments. (DEXA stands for dual-energy X-ray absorptiometry.)

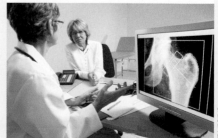

Figure C8–6

A Lifetime Plan for Healthy Bones

The periods of greatest gains in bone density are childhood and adolescence. (This figure's timeline begins at the bottom.)

Mature Adult
51 years and above

> *Goal:* Minimize bone loss.
> *Plan:*
> • Continue as for 13- to 30-year-olds.
> • Continue striving to meet the calcium need from diet.
> • Continue bone-strengthening exercises.
> • Obtain a bone density test; follow physician's advice concerning bone-restoring medications and supplements.

Mature Adult
31 through 50 years

> *Goal:* Maximize bone retention.
> *Plan:*
> • Continue as for 13- to 30-year-olds.
> • Adopt bone-strengthening exercises.
> • Obtain the recommended amount of calcium from food.
> • Take calcium supplements only if calcium needs cannot be met through foods.

Adolescence through Young Adulthood
13 through 30 years

> *Goal:* Achieve peak bone mass.
> *Plan:*
> • Choose milk as the primary beverage; if milk causes distress, include other calcium sources.
> • Commit to a lifelong program of physical activity.
> • Do not smoke tobacco or drink alcohol—if you have started, quit.

Children
2 through 12 years

> *Goal:* Grow strong bones.
> *Plan:*
> • Use milk as the primary beverage to meet the need for calcium within a balanced diet that provides all nutrients.
> • Play actively in sports or other activities.
> • Limit television and other sedentary entertainment.
> • Do not start smoking tobacco or drinking alcohol.

Note: The exact ages of cessation of bone accretion and onset of loss vary but in general, data indicate that the skeleton continues to accrete mass for approximately 10 years after adult height is achieved, and to lose bone around age 40.

Calcium Intakes

Adequate calcium nutrition is essential for achieving and maintaining optimal bone mass, but few people take in adequate amounts from foods and beverages.[23] How should they obtain daily calcium? Nutritionists strongly recommend the foods and beverages of the USDA eating patterns (see Chapter 2); they reserve supplements for those who cannot consume these sources.

Bone loss is not a calcium-deficiency disease comparable to iron-deficiency anemia, in which iron intake reliably reverses the condition. Calcium alone cannot reverse bone loss. For those who are unable to consume enough calcium-rich foods, however, taking calcium supplements with vitamin D can supply these nutrients.

Taking self-prescribed calcium supplements entails a few risks and cannot take the place of sound food choices and other healthy habits. Constipation, polyps (intestinal growths), and other digestive issues may arise with calcium and vitamin D supplementation, but an earlier suggestion that calcium may increase risk of heart attack is not supported by research.[24] Current evidence does not support calcium or vitamin D supplements for preventing bone fractures, and the U.S. Preventive Services Task Force does not recommend them.[25] The Academy of Nutrition and Dietetics does recommend calcium supplements, but only for people with hypertension who cannot meet their calcium needs from food.[26] Still, millions of healthy people take such supplements daily.

Calcium Supplements

Calcium supplements are often sold as **calcium compounds**—such as calcium carbonate (as in some **antacids**), citrate, gluconate, lactate, malate, or phosphate—and compounds of calcium with amino acids (called **amino acid chelates**). Others are powdered, calcium-rich materials such as bone meal, powdered bone, oyster shell, or dolomite (Table C8–3 defines supplement terms). In choosing a type, consider the answers to the following questions.

Question 1. How much calcium is safe? Although evidence suggests that doses of up to 1,000 milligrams may present few risks, the DRI committee recommends that habitual calcium intakes from foods and supplements combined should not exceed the UL (2,000 to 3,000 milligrams for adults. Meeting the need for calcium is important, but more calcium than this provides no benefits and may increase risks. Most supplements contain between 250 and 1,000 milligrams of calcium, as stated on their labels.

Question 2. How absorbable is the supplement? The body cannot use the calcium in a supplement unless the tablet disintegrates in the digestive tract. Manufacturers compress large quantities of calcium into small pills, which the stomach acid must penetrate. Some calcium compounds go right through the body like pebbles dropped through a spool. To test a supplement, drop a pill into 6 ounces of vinegar, and stir occasionally. The pill should disintegrate within a half hour.

Question 3. How absorbable is the form of calcium in the supplement? Most healthy people absorb calcium equally well from milk and from calcium carbonate, calcium citrate, and calcium phosphate. To improve absorption, divide your dose in half and take it twice a day instead of all at once.

One last pitch: think one more time before you decide to take supplements instead of including calcium-rich foods in your diet. The DRI committee points out that, particularly among older women, supplements can and do push some people's intakes beyond the UL.[27] The Dietary Guidelines for Americans 2015 committee recommends milk and milk products or calcium- and vitamin D–fortified soy milk for bone health. The authors of this book are so impressed with the importance of using abundant, calcium-rich foods that we have worked out ways to do so at every meal.

Critical Thinking

1. Osteoporosis occurs during the late years of life; however, it is a disease that develops while one is young. For any life stage of Figure C8-6, name two potential barriers to these actions and devise ways of overcoming them.

2. Outline the foods you will eat (including quantities) to meet the DRI for calcium. List lifestyle practices that you can adopt to boost your bone density.

Table C8–3

Calcium Supplement Terms

- **amino acid chelates** (KEY-lates) compounds of minerals (such as calcium) combined with amino acids in a form that favors their absorption. A chelating agent is a molecule that attracts or embraces another molecule and can then either promote or prevent its movement from place to place (chele means "claw").
- **antacids** acid-buffering agents used to counter excess acidity in the stomach. Calcium-containing preparations (such as Tums) contain available calcium. Antacids with aluminum or magnesium hydroxides (such as Rolaids) can accelerate calcium losses.
- **bone meal** or **powdered bone** crushed or ground bone preparations intended to supply calcium to the diet. Calcium from bone is not well absorbed and is often contaminated with toxic materials such as arsenic, mercury, lead, and cadmium.
- **calcium compounds** the simplest forms of purified calcium. They include calcium carbonate, citrate, gluconate, hydroxide, lactate, malate, and phosphate. These supplements vary in the amounts of calcium they contain, so read the labels carefully. A 500-milligram tablet of calcium gluconate may provide only 45 milligrams of calcium, for example.
- **dolomite** a compound of minerals (calcium magnesium carbonate) found in limestone and marble. Dolomite is powdered and is sold as a calcium-magnesium supplement but may be contaminated with toxic minerals, is not well absorbed, and interferes with absorption of other essential minerals.
- **oyster shell** a product made from the powdered shells of oysters that is sold as a calcium supplement but is not well absorbed by the digestive system.

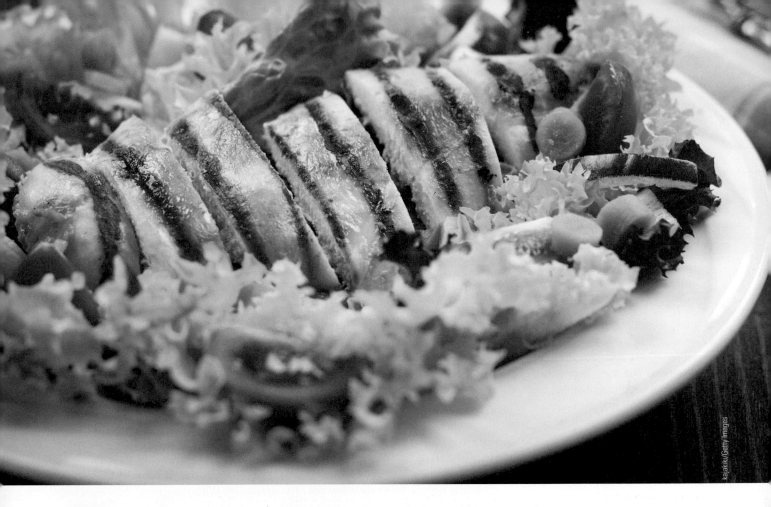

kajakik/Getty Images

9 Energy Balance and Healthy Body Weight

What do you think?

How can you **control** your body weight, once and for all?

Why are you **tempted** by a favorite treat when you don't feel hungry?

How do extra calories from food become **fat** in your body?

Which popular **diets** are best for managing body weight?

Are you pleased with your body weight? If you answered yes, you are a rare individual. Nearly all people in our society think they should weigh more or less (mostly less) than they do. Their primary concern is usually appearance, but they often perceive, correctly, that physical health is somehow related to weight. Both **overweight** and **underweight** present risks to health and life.

People also think of their weight as something they should control, once and for all. Three misconceptions in their thinking frustrate their efforts, however—the focus on weight, the focus on *controlling* weight, and the focus on a short-term endeavor. Simply put, it isn't your weight you need to control; it's the fat, or **adipose tissue**, in your body in proportion to the lean—your **body composition**. And controlling body composition directly isn't possible—you can control only your *behaviors*. Sporadic bursts of activity, such as "dieting," are not effective; the behaviors that achieve and maintain a healthy body weight take a lifetime of commitment. With time, these behaviors can become second nature.

This chapter starts by presenting problems associated with deficient and excessive body fatness and then examines how the body manages its energy budget. The following sections show how to judge body weight on the sound basis of health and explore some theories about causes of **obesity**. It also sums up science-based lifestyle strategies for achieving and maintaining a healthy body weight, and it closes with a Controversy section on eating disorders.

The Problems of Too Little or Too Much Body Fat

LO 9.1   Outline the health risks of deficient and excessive body fatness.

In the United States, too little body fat is not a widespread problem. In contrast, despite a national preoccupation with body image and weight loss, obesity remains at epidemic proportions. The maps in Figure 9–1 demonstrate the increases in obesity prevalence over a period of five years. Over the past five *decades*, obesity has soared in every state, in both genders, and across all ages, races, and educational levels. Among U.S. adults, an estimated 70 percent are now overweight or obese (see Table 9–1).[1]*† Worldwide, obesity has spread to almost 2 *billion* adults and tens of millions of children.[2] A glimmer of hope exists among U.S. statistics: the advancement of obesity appears to be slowing for low-income women and children.[3]

Childhood obesity is the topic of **Controversy 13**.

overweight body weight above a healthy weight; BMI 25 to 29.9 (BMI is defined on p. 321).

underweight body weight below a healthy weight; BMI below 18.5.

adipose tissue the body's fat tissue, consisting of masses of fat-storing cells and blood vessels to nourish them. Adipose tissue performs several functions, including the synthesis and secretion of the hormone leptin, which is involved in appetite regulation. Also defined in Chapter 3.

body composition the proportions of muscle, bone, fat, and other tissue that make up a person's total body weight.

obesity excess body fatness associated with increased risks of mortality and chronic diseases; a body mass index of 30 or higher.

---

*Reference notes are in Appendix F.
†See the body mass index chart, back of the book, p. E.

Table 9-1

Prevalence of Underweight, Overweight, and Obesity, U.S. Adults

Underweight (BMI < 18.5)	1.4%
Overweight and obese (BMI 25–29.9)	70.7%
Obese (BMI 30–39.9)	37.9%
Extremely obese (BMI ≥ 40)[a]	7.7%

[a]"Extremely obese" is a subcategory of "Obese."

Data from Centers for Disease Control and Prevention, Obesity and overweight, 2017, available at www.cdc.gov/nchs/fastats/obesity-overweight.htm; Centers for Disease Control and Prevention, Prevalence of underweight among adults aged 20 and over: United States, 1960–1962 through 2013–2014, 2017, available at www.cdc.gov/nchs/data/hestat/underweight_adult_13_14/underweight_adult_13_14.htm.

The problem of *underweight*, although affecting fewer than 2 percent of adults in the United States, also poses health threats to those who drop below a healthy minimum.[4] People at either extreme of body weight face increased risks.

What Are the Risks from Underweight?

Thin people are among the first to die during a siege or in a famine. Overly thin people are also at a disadvantage in the hospital, where their nutrient status can easily deteriorate if they have to go without food for days at a time while undergoing tests or surgery. Underweight also increases the risk of death for surgical patients and for anyone fighting a **wasting** disease. People with cancer often die not from the cancer itself but from starvation. Thus, excessively underweight people are urged to gain body fat as an energy reserve and to acquire protective amounts of all the nutrients that can be stored.

KEY POINT

- Deficient body fatness threatens survival during a famine or when a person must fight a disease.

What Are the Risks from Too Much Body Fat?

If tomorrow's headlines read, "Obesity Conquered! U.S. Population Loses Excess Fat!" tens of millions of people would be freed from the misery of obesity-related illnesses—heart disease, diabetes, certain cancers, and many others. In just one year, more than 100,000 lives could be saved, along with the estimated $147 billion spent on obesity-related health care.[5] Increased productivity at work would pump tens of billions of new dollars into the national economy.

Chronic Diseases   To underestimate the threat from obesity is to invite personal calamity. Figure 9–2 demonstrates that the risk of dying increases proportionally with increasing body weight.[6] With **extreme obesity**, the risk of dying equals that from smoking. Major obesity-related chronic disease risks include:

- Arthritis.
- Cancers of the breast, colon, endometrium, and other cancers.
- Diabetes.
- Heart disease.

Figure 9-1

Increasing Prevalence of Obesity

The top map shows the prevalence of obesity (BMI ≥30) in the year 2011, state by state. The bottom map reveals the advancement of obesity over just four years. Much greater increases are evident from past decades, but changes in analytical methods prohibit direct comparisons with today's estimates.

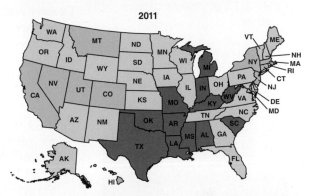

2011

<20%	20% to 24.9%	25% to 29.9%	30% to 34.9%	≥35%
0 states	11 states	27 states	12 states	0 states

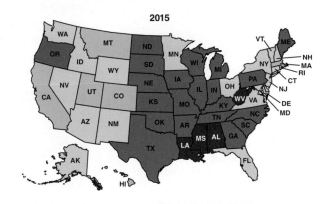

2015

<20%	20% to 24.9%	25% to 29.9%	30% to 34.9%	≥35%
0 states	6 states	19 states	21 states	4 states

Source: www.cdc.gov/obesity/data/prevalence-maps.html. September 2016.

wasting the progressive, relentless loss of the body's tissues that accompanies certain diseases and shortens survival time.

extreme obesity clinically severe overweight, presenting very high risks to health; the condition of having a BMI of 40 or above; also called *morbid obesity*.

Figure 9–2

Underweight, Overweight, and Mortality

This J-shaped curve associates body mass index (BMI) with mortality. It shows that both underweight and overweight present excess risks of premature death. A BMI of 15 generally indicates starvation.

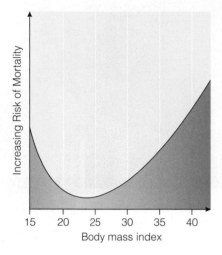

- Kidney disease.
- Nonalcoholic fatty liver disease.
- Stroke.[7]

Over 70 percent of obese people suffer from at least one other major health problem. For example, obesity triples a person's risk of developing diabetes, and even modest weight gain raises the risk. The mechanisms linking obesity with diabetes are not fully known, but scientists suspect that a person's genetic inheritance may alter the likelihood that obesity will lead to the development of diabetes.[8]

Obesity and Inflammation   Why should fat in the body present an extra risk to the heart? Part of the answer may involve **adipokines**, hormones released by adipose tissue.[9] Adipokines help to regulate inflammatory processes and energy metabolism in the tissues. In fact, adipose tissue acts as an endocrine organ, orchestrating important interactions with other vital organs such as the brain, liver, muscle, heart, and blood vessels in ways that influence overall health.

> Metabolic syndrome and chronic diseases are discussed in more detail in **Chapter 11**.

In obesity, a shift occurs in the balance of adipokines that favors both tissue inflammation and insulin resistance. The resulting chronic inflammation and insulin resistance often lead to diabetes, heart disease, and other chronic diseases. Calorie-restricted diets and weight loss often reduce inflammation and improve health.

Other Risks   An obese person faces a long list of threats in addition to the chronic diseases already named: abdominal hernias, cancers (many types), complications in pregnancy and surgery, flat feet, gallbladder disease, gout, high blood lipids, medication dosing errors, reproductive disorders, skin problems, sleep disturbances, sleep apnea (dangerous abnormal breathing during sleep), varicose veins, and even a high accident rate. So great are the harms that obesity itself is classified as a chronic disease: **adiposity-based chronic disease**.[10] Some of these maladies start to improve with the loss of just 5 percent of body weight, and risks improve markedly after a 10 percent loss.

KEY POINTS

- Adipokines are hormones produced by adipose tissue that help to regulate inflammation and energy metabolism.
- Obesity raises the risks of developing chronic diseases and many other illnesses.

What Are the Risks from Central Obesity?

A person's **body fat distribution** modulates the risks from obesity. Fat collected deep within the central abdominal area of the body, called **visceral fat**, results in **central obesity**, which poses greater risks of major chronic diseases and death than does excess fat lying just beneath the skin (**subcutaneous fat**) of the abdomen, thighs, hips, and legs see (Figure 9–3).[11] Central obesity is associated with the **metabolic syndrome** and, independently of BMI, contributes to heart disease, cancers, diabetes, and related deaths.[12] Currently, a measure of central obesity is among the indicators that physicians use to evaluate chronic disease risks.[13]

Men of all ages and women who are past menopause are more prone to develop the "apple" profile that characterizes central obesity, whereas women in their reproductive years typically develop more of a "pear" profile (fat around the hips and thighs that may cling stubbornly during weight loss but often poses less risk to health).[14] Some women change profiles at menopause, and life-long "pears" may suddenly become "apples," and face the associated risks.

Two other factors also affect body fat distribution. High intakes of alcohol are associated with central obesity, whereas high levels of physical activity correlate with leanness.[15]

KEY POINT

- Central obesity is particularly hazardous to health.

adipokines (AD-ih-poh-kynz) protein hormones made and released by adipose tissue (fat) cells.

adiposity-based chronic disease a clinical name used in diagnosing obesity. *Adiposity* refers to fat cells and tissues, identifying them as the source of the disease.

body fat distribution the pattern of fat deposition in various body areas.

visceral fat fat stored within the abdominal cavity in association with the internal abdominal organs; also called *intra-abdominal fat* or *visceral adipose tissue*.

central obesity excess fat in the abdomen and around the trunk.

subcutaneous fat fat stored directly under the skin (*sub* means "beneath"; *cutaneous* refers to the skin).

metabolic syndrome a combination of central obesity, diabetes or prediabetes, high blood glucose (insulin resistance), high blood pressure, and altered blood lipids that greatly increases the risk of heart disease. (Also defined in Chapter 11.)

Figure 9–3

Visceral Fat and Subcutaneous Fat

These abdominal cross sections of an overweight man (left) and woman (right) were produced by CT scans. Adipose tissue appears darker gray; lean tissues are lighter; bone is bright white. The people are similar in age and abdominal measurements, but the man's girth is largely from visceral fat; the woman's excess fat is almost all subcutaneous.

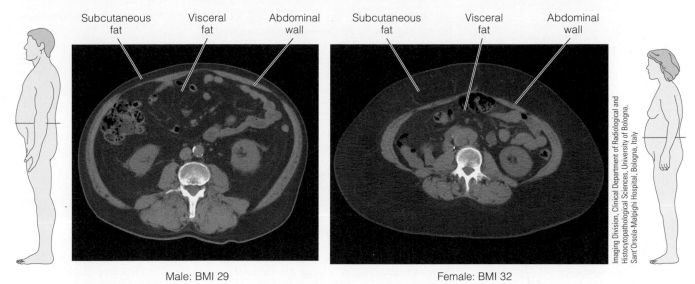

Male: BMI 29   Female: BMI 32

Imaging Division, Clinical Department of Radiological and Histocytopathological Sciences, University of Bologna, Sant'Orsola-Malpighi Hospital, Bologna, Italy

How Fat Is Too Fat?

People want to know exactly how much body fat is too much. The answer is not the same for everyone, but scientists have developed guidelines.

Evaluating Risks from Body Fatness   Experts commonly evaluate the health risks of obesity by way of two physical indicators (each is described more fully later on).[16] The first is a person's **body mass index (BMI)**, as characterized in Table 9–2 (p. 322). The BMI, which defines average relative weight for height in people older than 20 years, correlates significantly with body fatness and risk of death and diseases such as heart disease, stroke, diabetes, and nonalcoholic fatty liver disease. If you are wondering about your own BMI, find it at the back of this book, p. E.

The second indicator is **waist circumference**, reflecting the degree of central obesity in proportion to total body fat. A person whose BMI ranks as overweight or moderately obese is likely to face additional risks of heart disease and mortality if the waist circumference exceeds 35 inches for women and 40 inches for men. With greater obesity, waist circumference becomes less meaningful because health risks are already high.

Health risks are modified by factors such as poor dietary habits, sedentary lifestyle, blood lipids, family history of obesity or heart disease, smoking, and use of medications that affect body weight. The more of these factors a person has and the greater the degree of obesity, the greater the urgency to control body fatness.

Why do some obese people seem to remain healthy and live long lives, whereas others die young of chronic diseases? It may be that those who stay healthy longer tend to store excess fat harmlessly in the adipose tissue layer beneath the skin, while those who develop metabolic problems deposit excess fat centrally in the abdomen, liver, and other critical tissues. In the end, many obese people who feel healthy today may be developing chronic diseases that will emerge later on, particularly if they accumulate excess fat in the abdomen.[17]

Social and Economic Costs of Body Fatness   Although a few overfat people escape health problems, no one who is fat in our society quite escapes the social and economic handicaps. Our society places enormous value on thinness, especially for

body mass index (BMI) an indicator of health risk from obesity or underweight, calculated by dividing the weight of a person by the square of the person's height.

waist circumference a measurement of abdominal girth that indicates visceral fatness.

Table 9-2

Indicators of an Urgent Need for Weight Loss

The greater the BMI and the more diseases and risk factors present, the greater the urgency to control body fatness.

BMI
- BMI over 30 indicates a need for treatment.
- BMI of 25 to 29.9 plus more than one disease or risk factor, such as cardiovascular disease, diabetes, or high blood pressure (see below) indicates a need for treatment.
- BMI of 25 to 29.9 with no other risk factors indicates a need to stop gaining weight.

Waist Circumference
- Greater than 35 inches for women and 40 inches for men

Diseases and Risk Factors[a]
- Cardiovascular disease (CVD)
- Blood lipid profile that indicates CVD risk
- Type 2 diabetes or prediabetes
- Impaired glucose tolerance
- Hypertension

Source: American College of Cardiology/American Heart Association Task Force on Practice Guidelines and the Obesity Society, Executive summary: Guidelines (2013) for the management of overweight and obesity in adults, Obesity 22 (2014): S5–S39.

[a]Chapter 11 lists medical testing standards for indicators of chronic disease risks.

women, and fat people are less sought after for romance, less often hired, and less often admitted to college.[18] They pay higher insurance premiums, they pay more for clothing, and they even pay more in gasoline costs—a car transporting extra weight uses more fuel per mile. Is it any wonder that overweight people are spending $60 billion each year in attempts to lose weight?

Prejudice defines people by their appearance rather than by their ability and character. People with obesity suffer emotional pain when others treat them with insensitivity, hostility, and contempt, and they may internalize a sense of guilt and self-deprecation. Health-care professionals, even dietitians, can be among the offenders without realizing it. Society's barrage of negativity can injure an overweight person's self-image in ways that may contribute to more weight gain and obesity or to the development of an eating disorder (see the Controversy section, p. 358).[19] To free our society of its obsession with body fatness and its prejudice against overweight people, activists are promoting respect for individuals of all body weights.

KEY POINTS

- BMI values mathematically correlate heights and weights with health risks.
- Health risks from obesity are reflected in BMI, waist circumference, and a disease risk profile.
- Overweight people face social and economic handicaps and prejudice.

The Body's Energy Balance

LO 9.2 Explain the concept of energy balance and the factors associated with it.

What happens inside your body when you take in more or less food energy than you spend? Over time, you'll have an unbalanced energy budget—which, like a cash budget, accumulates excess savings (in the form of fat gain) or draws down reserves (fat loss).

Moreover, if more food energy is stored than can be spent over days or weeks, fat continues to accumulate in the adipose tissue. In contrast, if less energy is consumed than the amount used up, then fat is lost from the adipose tissue. The daily energy balance can therefore be stated like this:

- Change in energy stores equals food energy taken in minus energy spent on metabolism and muscle activities.

More simply,

- Change in energy stores = energy in − energy out,

Too much or too little fat on the body today does not necessarily reflect today's energy budget. Small imbalances in the energy budget compound over time.

Energy In and Energy Out

The energy in foods and beverages is the only contributor to the "energy in" side of the energy balance equation. A classic approach to balancing the energy budget is to log the calorie amounts of the foods you eat every day, but, over time, this approach often proves too tedious to sustain. Instead, you can develop a pattern of daily food intakes and activities that, over months or years, proves to maintain a healthy body weight. Knowing a few calorie values can help you judge individual foods that make up your pattern. For example, an apple gives you 70 calories from carbohydrate; a regular-size candy bar gives you about 250 calories, mostly from fat and carbohydrate—a useful comparison when choosing a snack.

The Food Lists for Weight Management offer help in choosing foods; see Chapter 2, pp. 46–47, and Appendix D.

On the "energy out" side of the equation, no easy method exists for determining the energy an individual spends and therefore needs. In the past, it was said that for each 3,500 calories you expend in activity or eliminate from the diet, you lose one pound of body fat, but this was an oversimplification. A single number cannot accurately predict weight change in every individual because energy dynamics vary, both between individuals and within a single person at different phases of weight change. Estimating an individual person's need requires knowing something about the person's lifestyle and metabolism.

KEY POINTS

- The "energy in" side of the body's energy budget is measured in calories taken in each day in the form of foods and beverages.
- No easy method exists for determining the "energy out" side of a person's energy balance equation.

How Many Calories Do I Need Each Day?

Simply put, you need to take in enough calories to cover your energy expenditure each day—your energy budget must balance. One way to estimate your energy need is to monitor your food intake and body weight over a period of time in which your activities are typical and are sufficient to maintain your health. If you keep an accurate record of all the foods and beverages you consume and if your weight is in a healthy range and has not changed during the past few months, you can conclude that your energy budget is balanced. Your average daily calorie intake is sufficient to meet your daily output—your need therefore is the same as your current intake. At least 3, and preferably 7, days, including a weekend day, of honest record-keeping are necessary because intakes and activities fluctuate from day to day.

An alternative method of determining energy need is based on energy output. The two major ways in which the body spends

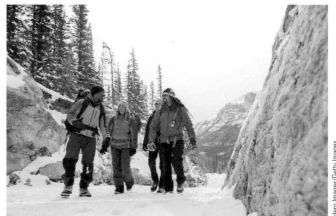

Balancing food energy intake with physical activity can add to life's enjoyment.

Figure 9-4

Components of Energy Expenditure

Typically, basal metabolism represents a person's largest expenditure of energy, followed by physical activity and the thermic effect of food.

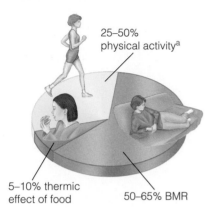

25–50% physical activity[a]

5–10% thermic effect of food

50–65% BMR

[a]For a sedentary person, physical activities may account for less than half as much energy as basal metabolism, whereas a very active person's activities may equal the energy cost of basal metabolism.

basal metabolism the sum total of all the involuntary activities that are necessary to sustain life, including circulation, respiration, temperature maintenance, hormone secretion, nerve activity, and new tissue synthesis, but excluding digestion and voluntary activities. Basal metabolism is the largest component of the average person's daily energy expenditure.

voluntary activities intentional activities (such as walking, sitting, or running) conducted by voluntary muscles.

thermic effect of food the body's speeded-up metabolism in response to having eaten a meal; also called *diet-induced thermogenesis*.

basal metabolic rate (BMR) the rate at which the body uses energy to support its basal metabolism.

lean body mass the weight of the body's lean tissues; body weight, minus fat tissue.

energy are (1) to fuel its **basal metabolism** and (2) to fuel its **voluntary activities**. Basal metabolism requires energy to support the body's work that goes on all the time without a person's conscious awareness. A third energy component, the body's metabolic response to food, or the **thermic effect of food**, uses up about 10 percent of a meal's energy value in stepped-up metabolism in the 5 or so hours after finishing a meal. This amount is believed to exert negligible effects on total energy expenditure.

Basal metabolism consumes a surprisingly large amount of fuel, and the **basal metabolic rate (BMR)** varies from person to person (see Figure 9–4). Depending on activity level, a person whose total energy need is 2,000 calories a day may spend as many as 1,000 to 1,600 of them to support basal metabolism. The iodine-dependent hormone thyroxine directly controls basal metabolism—the more secreted, the greater the energy spent on basal functions. The rate is lowest during sleep.[‡] Many other factors also affect the BMR (see Table 9–3).

People often wonder whether they can speed up their metabolism to spend more daily energy. You cannot increase your BMR very much *today*. You can, however, amplify the second component of your energy expenditure—your voluntary activities. If you do, you will spend more calories today, and if you keep doing so day after day, your BMR will also increase somewhat as you increase your **lean body mass** because lean tissue is more metabolically active than fat tissue. Energy spent on voluntary activities depends largely on three factors: weight, time, and intensity. The heavier the weight of the body parts you move, the longer the time you invest in moving them, and the greater the intensity of the work, the more calories you will expend.

Table 9-3

Factors that Affect the BMR

Factor	Effect on BMR
Age	The BMR is higher in youth; as lean body mass declines with age, the BMR slows. Physical activity may prevent some of this decline.
Height	Tall people have a larger surface area, so their BMRs are higher.
Growth	Children and pregnant women have higher BMRs.
Body composition	The more lean tissue, the higher the BMR. A typical man has greater lean body mass than a typical woman, making his BMR higher.
Fever	Fever raises the BMR.
Stress	Stress hormones raise the BMR.
Environmental temperature	Adjusting to either heat or cold raises the BMR.
Fasting/starvation	Fasting/starvation hormones lower the BMR.
Malnutrition	Malnutrition lowers the BMR.
Thyroxine	The thyroid hormone thyroxine is a key BMR regulator; the more thyroxine produced, the higher the BMR.

[‡]A measure of energy output taken while the person is awake but relaxed yields a slightly higher number called the *resting metabolic rate*, sometimes used in research.

Chapter 9 Energy Balance and Healthy Body Weight

Be aware that some ads for weight-loss diets claim that certain substances, such as grapefruit or herbs, can elevate the BMR and thus promote weight loss. This claim is false. Any meal temporarily steps up energy expenditure due to the thermic effect of food. Grapefruit and herbs do not accelerate it further.

KEY POINTS

- Two major components of energy expenditure are basal metabolism and voluntary activities.
- A third component of energy expenditure is the thermic effect of food.
- Many factors influence the basal metabolic rate.

Estimated Energy Requirements (EER)

A person wishing to know how much energy he or she needs in a day to maintain weight might look up his or her **Estimated Energy Requirement (EER)** value listed in the DRI table at the back of this book, p. A. The numbers listed there seem to imply that for each age and gender group, the number of calories needed to meet the daily requirement is known as precisely as, say, the recommended intake for vitamin A. The printed EER values, however, reflect the average needs of only those people who exactly match the BMI, height, and weight characteristics specified in the DRI table. People who deviate in any way from these characteristics must use other methods for determining their energy needs, and almost everyone deviates.

Taller people need proportionately more energy than shorter people to balance their energy budgets because their greater surface area allows more energy to escape as heat. Older people generally need less than young people due to slowed metabolism and reduced muscle mass, which occur in part because of reduced physical activity. As Chapter 14 points out, these losses may not be inevitable for people who stay active. On average, though, energy need diminishes by 5 percent per decade beyond the age of 30 years.

In reality, no one is average. In any group of 20 similar people with similar activity levels, one may expend twice as much energy per day as another. A 60-year-old person who bikes, swims, or walks briskly each day may need as many calories as a sedentary person of 30. Clearly, with such a wide range of variation, a necessary step in determining any person's energy need is to study that particular person.

KEY POINT

- The DRI committee sets Estimated Energy Requirements for age and gender groups, but individual energy needs vary greatly.

The DRI Method of Estimating Energy Requirements

The DRI committee provides a way of estimating EER values for individuals. These calculations take into account the ways in which energy is spent and by whom. The equation includes:

- *Age.* The BMR declines with age, so age helps determine EER values.
- *Gender.* Women generally have less lean body mass than men; in addition, women's hormone fluctuations influence the BMR, raising it just prior to menstruation.
- *Body size and weight.* The higher BMR of taller and heavier people calls for height and weight to be factored in when estimating a person's EER.
- *Physical activity.* To help in estimating the energy spent on physical activity each day, activities are grouped according to their typical intensity (see Appendix H).
- *Growth.* The BMR is high in people who are growing, so pregnant women and children have their own sets of energy equations.

Do the Math features in the margin offer ways to approximate your energy requirements.

KEY POINT

- The DRI committee determines an individual's approximate energy requirement by taking into account influences on energy expenditure.

Do the Math

To estimate basal energy output:

- Men: kg body weight × 24 = cal/day
- Women: kg body weight × 23 = cal/day

(To convert pounds to kilograms [kg], divide pounds by 2.2.)

Calculate the basal energy output (cal/day) of a man weighing 220 pounds.

Do the Math

Estimate your energy need using this quick and easy method:

- First, look up the EER listed for your age and gender group (back of the book, p. A).
- Then calculate a range of energy needs. For most people, the energy requirement falls within these ranges:

  (Men) EER ± 200 cal

  (Women) EER ± 160 cal

Estimated Energy Requirement (EER) the DRI value for average dietary energy intake in a healthy adult of a certain age, gender, weight, height, and level of physical activity that is predicted to maintain an energy balance consistent with good health. Also defined in Chapter 2.

To determine your BMI:

- In pounds and inches

$$BMI = \frac{weight\ (lb)}{(height\ in\ in.)^2} \times 703$$

- In kilograms and meters

$$BMI = \frac{weight\ (kg)}{(height\ in\ m)^2}$$

Using either pounds or kilograms, determine your own BMI value.

Figure 9–5

An Athlete's BMI Example

At 6'1" tall and 190 lbs., is this athlete too fat for health, as the BMI chart indicates? No. Measurements of body composition and fat distribution reveal that his body fat content is only 7% and his health risks are below average.

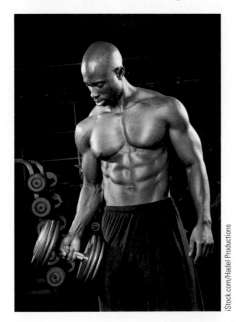

iStock.com/Hadel Productions

Body Weight vs. Body Fatness

LO 9.3   Contrast body weight with body fatness.

For most people, weighing on a scale provides a convenient way to monitor body fatness, but researchers and health-care providers must rely on more accurate assessments. This section describes some details about applying the preferred methods to assess overweight and underweight.

Using the Body Mass Index (BMI)

No one can tell you exactly how much you should weigh, but with health as a value, you have a starting framework in the BMI table (back of the book, p. E). Your weight should fall within the range that best supports your health. Unhealthy underweight for adults is defined as a BMI of less than 18.5, overweight as a BMI of 25.0 through 29.9, and obesity as a BMI of 30 or more. A formula for determining your BMI is given in the margin.

BMI values have two major drawbacks: they fail to indicate how much of a person's weight is fat and where that fat is located. These drawbacks limit the value of the BMI for use with:

- Athletes (because their highly developed musculature falsely increases their BMI values).
- Pregnant and lactating women (because their increased weight is normal during child bearing).
- Adults older than age 65 (because BMI values are based on data collected from younger people and because people "grow shorter" with age).
- Women older than age 50 and others with too little muscle tissue (they may be overly fat for health yet still fall into the normal BMI range).[20]

The bodybuilder in Figure 9-5 proves this point: with a BMI over 25, he would be classified as overweight by BMI standards alone. However, a clinician would find that his percentage of body fat is well below average and his waist circumference is within a healthy range. For any given BMI value, body fat content can vary widely.

In addition, among some racial and ethnic groups, BMI values may not precisely identify overweight and obesity. African American people of all ages may have more lean tissue per pound of body weight than Asians or Caucasians, for example. Thus, a diagnosis of obesity or overweight requires a BMI value *plus* some measure of body composition and fat distribution. There is no easy way to look inside a living person to measure bones and muscles, but several indirect measures can provide an approximation.

KEY POINT

- The BMI concept is flawed for certain groups of people.

Measuring Body Composition and Fat Distribution

A person who stands about 5 feet 10 inches tall and weighs 150 pounds carries about 30 of those pounds as fat. The rest is mostly water and lean tissues: muscles; organs such as the heart, brain, and liver; and the bones of the skeleton (see Figure 9–6). This lean tissue is vital to health. The person who seeks to lose weight wants to lose mostly fat, and to conserve this precious lean tissue.[21] And for someone who wants to gain weight, it is desirable to gain lean and fat in proportion, not just fat.

As mentioned, waist circumference indicates central adiposity and often reflects visceral fatness. The center panel of Figure 9-7 demonstrates how waist circumference is measured. Health professionals often use both BMI and waist circumference to assess a person's health risks, and they monitor changes over time.

Figure 9–6

Body Composition of Men and Women

Body fat percentages for people age 20 to 40 years old in the Healthy Weight BMI range:
- Male: 18–21%
- Female: 23–26%

Most people in the United States greatly exceed these ranges.

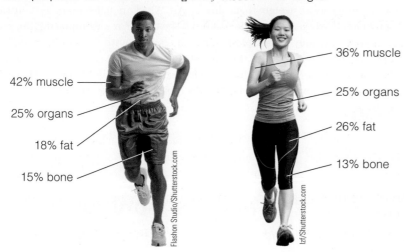

42% muscle

25% organs

18% fat

15% bone

Flashon Studio/Shutterstock.com

36% muscle

25% organs

26% fat

13% bone

Izf/Shutterstock.com

Researchers needing more precise measures of body composition may choose to perform a **skinfold test**, shown in the left-most panel of Figure 9–7. Body fat distribution can be determined by radiographic techniques, such as **dual-energy X-ray absorptiometry**. Mastering any of these techniques requires proper instruction and practice to ensure reliability. Each method has advantages and disadvantages with respect to cost, technical difficulty, and precision of estimating body fat.

KEY POINTS

- Central adiposity can be assessed by measuring waist circumference.
- The percentage of fat in a person's body can be estimated by using skinfold measurements.
- Body fat distribution can be revealed by radiographic techniques.

skinfold test measurement of the thickness of a fold of skin and subcutaneous fat on the back of the arm (over the triceps muscle), below the shoulder blade (subscapular), or in other places, using a caliper; also called *fatfold test*.

dual-energy X-ray absorptiometry (ab-sorp-tee-OM-eh-tree) a noninvasive method of determining total body fat, fat distribution, and bone density by passing two low-dose X-ray beams through the body. Also used in evaluation of osteoporosis. Abbreviated DEXA.

Figure 9–7

Three Methods Used to Assess Body Fat

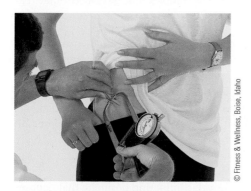

© Fitness & Wellness, Boise, Idaho

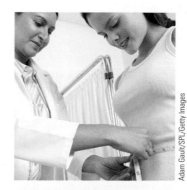

Adam Gault/SPL/Getty Images

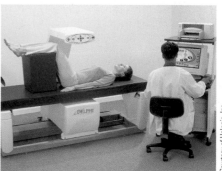

Courtesy of Hologic, Inc.

Skinfold measures. *Body fat is measured by using a caliper to gauge the thickness of a fold of skin on the back of the arm (over the triceps), below the shoulder blade (subscapular), and in other places (including lower-body sites) and then comparing these measurements with standards.*

Waist circumference. *Central obesity is measured by placing a nonstretchable measuring tape around the waist just above the bony crest of the hip. The tape is snug but does not compress the skin.*

Dual-energy X-ray absorptiometry (DEXA). *Two low-dose X-rays differentiate among fat-free soft tissue (lean body mass), fat tissue, and bone tissue, providing a measurement of total fat and its distribution in all but extremely obese subjects.*

How Much Body Fat Is Ideal?

After you have a body fatness estimate, the question arises: What is the "ideal" amount of fat for a body to have? This prompts another question: Ideal for what? If the answer is "society's perfect body shape," be aware that fashion is fickle and today's popular body shapes are not achievable by most people.

If the answer is "health," then the ideal depends partly on your lifestyle and stage of life. For example, competitive endurance athletes need just enough body fat to provide fuel, insulate the body, and permit normal hormone activity but not so much as to weigh them down. An Alaskan fisherman, in contrast, needs a blanket of extra fat to insulate against the cold. For a woman starting pregnancy, the outcome may be compromised if she begins with too much or too little body fat.

Much remains to be learned about individual requirements for body fat. How body fat accumulates and how it is controlled are the topics of the next sections.

KEY POINT

- No single body composition or weight suits everyone; needs vary by gender, lifestyle, and stage of life.

The Appetite and Its Control

LO 9.4   Identify factors that contribute to increased appetite and deceased appetite.

When you grab a snack or eat a meal, you may be aware that your conscious mind is choosing to eat something. However, the choice of when and how much to eat may not be as free as you think—deeper forces of physiology are at work.

Seeking and eating food are matters of life and death, so the body's appetite-regulating systems are skewed, tipping in favor of food consumption. **Hunger** demands food, but the signals that oppose food consumption—that is, signals for **satiation** and **satiety**—are weaker and more easily overruled. Many signaling molecules, including hormones, help to regulate food intake; the following sections name just a few.

Hunger and Appetite—"Go" Signals

The brain and digestive tract communicate about the need for food and food sufficiency. Their means of communication, hormones and sensory nerve signals, fall roughly into two broad functional categories: "go" mechanisms that stimulate eating and "stop" mechanisms that suppress it. One view of the whole complex process of food intake regulation is summarized in Figure 9–8.

Hunger   Most people recognize hunger as a strong, unpleasant sensation, the response to a physiological need for food. Hunger makes itself known roughly four to six hours after eating, after the food has left the stomach and much of the nutrient mixture has been absorbed by the intestine. The physical contractions of an empty stomach trigger hunger signals, as do chemical messengers acting on or originating in the brain's hypothalamus (as illustrated in Chapter 3). The hypothalamus has been described as a sort of central hub for energy and body weight regulation, and it can sense molecules representing all three of the energy nutrients.

The polypeptide **ghrelin** is a powerful hunger-stimulating hormone that opposes weight loss. Ghrelin is secreted by stomach cells but works in the hypothalamus and other brain tissues to stimulate **appetite** and increase body weight and fatness.[22] Ghrelin may also help regulate other diverse body functions. Ghrelin also influences sleep, and a lack of sleep causes an increase in blood ghrelin. This may help explain why too

hunger the physiological need to eat, experienced as a drive for obtaining food; an unpleasant sensation that demands relief.

satiation (SAY-she-AY-shun) the perception of fullness that builds throughout a meal, eventually reaching the degree of fullness and satisfaction that halts eating. Satiation generally determines how much food is consumed at one sitting.

satiety (sah-TIE-eh-tee) the perception of fullness that lingers in the hours after a meal and inhibits eating until the next mealtime. Satiety generally determines the length of time between meals.

ghrelin (GREL-in) a hormone released by the stomach that signals the brain's hypothalamus and other regions to stimulate eating.

appetite the psychological desire to eat; a learned motivation and a positive sensation that accompanies the sight, smell, or thought of appealing foods.

Figure 9–8

Hunger, Appetite, Satiation, and Satiety

Many factors work together to influence eating decisions, but the brain can override physiological signals, particularly satiety signals.

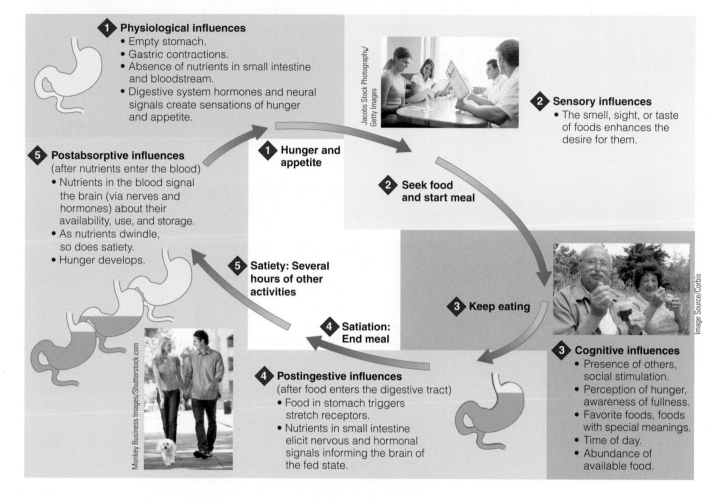

1 Physiological influences
- Empty stomach.
- Gastric contractions.
- Absence of nutrients in small intestine and bloodstream.
- Digestive system hormones and neural signals create sensations of hunger and appetite.

2 Sensory influences
- The smell, sight, or taste of foods enhances the desire for them.

5 Postabsorptive influences
(after nutrients enter the blood)
- Nutrients in the blood signal the brain (via nerves and hormones) about their availability, use, and storage.
- As nutrients dwindle, so does satiety.
- Hunger develops.

1 Hunger and appetite

2 Seek food and start meal

3 Keep eating

5 Satiety: Several hours of other activities

4 Satiation: End meal

3 Cognitive influences
- Presence of others, social stimulation.
- Perception of hunger, awareness of fullness.
- Favorite foods, foods with special meanings.
- Time of day.
- Abundance of available food.

4 Postingestive influences
(after food enters the digestive tract)
- Food in stomach triggers stretch receptors.
- Nutrients in small intestine elicit nervous and hormonal signals informing the brain of the fed state.

Jacobs Stock Photography/Getty Images

Image Source/Corbis

Monkey Business Images/Shutterstock.com

little sleep, a heightened desire for high-calorie foods, and weight gain often occur together.[23]

Ghrelin is just one of many hunger-regulating messengers that informs the brain of the need for food. In fact, the brain itself produces a number of molecular messengers involved in appetite regulation.[§] Panels 1 and 2 of Figure 9-8 review factors that influence hunger.

Appetite A person can experience appetite without hunger. For example, the aroma of hot apple pie or the sight of a chocolate buttercream cake after a big meal can trigger a chemical stimulation of the brain's pleasure centers, thereby creating a desire for dessert despite an already full stomach. Here is the answer to the question at the start of the chapter: "Why do you feel tempted by a favorite treat when you don't feel hungry?" Your brain chemistry responds to cues about the availability of delicious foods. In contrast, a person who is ill or under sudden stress may physically need food but have no appetite.[24] Other factors affecting appetite include:

- Appetite stimulants or depressants, other medical drugs.
- Cultural habits (cultural or religious acceptability of foods).
- Environmental conditions (people often prefer hot foods in cold weather and vice versa).

[§]One example is neuropeptide Y.

- Hormones (for example, sex hormones).
- Inborn appetites (inborn preferences for fatty, salty, and sweet tastes).
- Learned preferences (cravings for favorite foods, aversion to trying new foods, and eating according to the clock).
- Social interactions (companionship, peer influences).
- Some disease states (obesity may be associated with increased taste sensitivity, whereas colds, flu, and zinc deficiency reduce taste sensitivity).

Clearly, appetite regulation is complex and responds to many influences beyond a physical need for food.

KEY POINTS

- Hunger outweighs satiety in the appetite control system.
- Hunger is a physiologic response to an absence of food in the digestive tract.
- The stomach hormone ghrelin is one of many contributors to feelings of hunger.
- Appetite can occur without hunger.

Satiation and Satiety—"Stop" Signals

To balance energy intake with energy output, eating behaviors must be counterbalanced with periods of fasting between meals. Being able to eat periodically, store fuel, and then use up that fuel between meals confers a great advantage on people. Relieved of the need to constantly seek food, human beings are free to dance, study, converse, wonder, fall in love, and concentrate on endeavors other than eating.

The between-meal interval is normally about 4 to 6 waking hours—about the length of time the body takes to use up most of the readily available fuel—or 12 to 18 hours at night, when body systems slow down and the need is less. As is true for the "go" signals that stimulate food intake, a series of hormones and sensory nerve messages along with products of nutrient metabolism send "stop" signals to suppress eating. Much more remains to be learned about these mechanisms.

Satiation At some point during a meal, the brain receives signals that enough food has been eaten. The resulting satiation diminishes the person's interest in continuing to eat and limits the size of the meal (consult Figure 9–8 again, panel 4). Satiation arises from many organs:

- Sensations of pleasure and satisfaction in the mouth diminish with repeated exposure to a particular texture or taste during a meal.[25]

Helen Bird/Shutterstock.com

- Nerve stretch receptors in the stomach sense the stomach's distention with a meal and fire, sending a signal to the brain that the stomach is full.
- As nutrients enter the small intestine, they stimulate other receptor nerves and trigger the release of hormones signaling the hypothalamus about the size and nature of the meal.
- The brain also detects absorbed nutrients delivered by the bloodstream, and it responds by releasing neurotransmitters that suppress food intake.

Together, mouth sensations, stomach distention, and the presence of nutrients trigger nervous and hormonal signals to inform the brain's hypothalamus that a meal has been consumed. Satiation occurs; the eater feels full and stops eating.

Did My Stomach Shrink? Changes in food intake cause prompt adaptations in the body. A person who suddenly begins eating smaller meals may feel extra hungry for a few days, but then hunger may diminish for a time. During this period, a large meal may make the person feel uncomfortably full, partly because the stomach's capacity has adapted to a smaller quantity of food. A dieter may report "My stomach has shrunk," but the stomach has simply adjusted to smaller meals. At some point during food deprivation, hunger returns with a vengeance and can lead to bouts of extensive overeating.

Just as quickly, the stomach's capacity can adapt to larger meals until moderate portions no longer satisfy. This observation may partly explain the increasing U.S. calorie intakes: popular demand and food industry marketing have led to larger and larger food portions, while stomachs across the nation have adapted to accommodate them.

Satiety   After a meal, the feeling of satiety continues to suppress hunger over a period of hours, regulating the interval between meals. Hormones, nervous signals, and the brain work in harmony to sustain feelings of fullness. At some later point, signals from the digestive tract once again sound the alert that more food is needed.

Leptin, one of the adipokine hormones, is produced by adipose tissue in direct proportion to body fatness.** A gain in body fatness stimulates leptin production. Leptin travels from the adipose tissue via the bloodstream to the brain's hypothalamus, where it triggers signals that suppress appetite, dampen sensitivity to sweet taste, increase energy expenditures, and, ultimately, produce body fat loss.[26] A loss of body fatness, in turn, brings the opposite effects—suppression of leptin production, increased appetite, reduced energy expenditure, and accumulation of fat. Leptin operates on a feedback mechanism—the fat tissue that produces leptin is ultimately controlled by it.

In a rare form of human obesity arising from an inherited inability to produce leptin, giving leptin injections quickly reverses both obesity and insulin resistance. Figure 9–9 depicts a mouse model of this condition. More commonly, people with ordinary obesity produce plenty of leptin but are resistant to its effects, and giving more leptin does not reverse their obesity.[27]

Energy Nutrients and Satiety   The composition of a meal seems to affect satiation and satiety, but the relationships are complex. Of the three energy-yielding nutrients, protein seems to have the greatest satiating effect during a meal.[28] Therefore, including some protein in a meal—even just a glass of milk—can improve satiation.

Many carbohydrate-rich foods, notably those providing slowly digestible carbohydrate and soluble fiber, also contribute to satiation and satiety.[29] Between meals, these foods tend to hold insulin steady, minimizing dips in blood glucose. This stabilizing effect helps to forestall hunger; if blood glucose does dip, the brain sends out hunger signals that prompt eating. Soluble fibers also support colonies of bacteria in the colon that are associated with leanness in some studies.[30] Finally, fat, famous for triggering a hormone that contributes to long-term satiety, goes almost unnoticed by the appetite control system during consumption of a meal. As dieters await news of dietary tactics against hunger, researchers have not yet identified any one food, nutrient, or attribute—not even protein—that is especially effective for weight loss and its maintenance.

KEY POINTS
- Satiation ends a meal when pleasure diminishes and various signals inform the brain that enough food has been eaten.
- Satiety postpones eating until the next meal.
- The adipokine leptin suppresses the appetite, thus helping to control body fatness.
- Protein, carbohydrate, and fat play roles in satiation and satiety.

**Leptin is also produced in the stomach, where it helps to regulate digestion and contributes to satiation.

Figure 9–9
Effects of Leptin

A genetically obese mouse (left) weighs almost three times as much as a normal mouse, and its rough coat indicates health problems. With leptin treatment, a similar mouse (right) weighs less and is healthier, but still weighs more than a normal mouse.

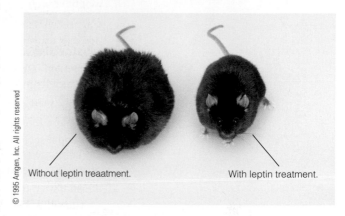

Without leptin treaatment.   With leptin treatment.

leptin an appetite-suppressing hormone produced in the fat cells that conveys information about body fatness to the brain; believed to be involved in the maintenance of body composition (*leptos* means "slender").

Inside-the-Body Theories of Obesity

LO 9.5   Summarize the current inside-the-body theories of obesity.

Findings about appetite regulation, the "energy in" side of the body weight equation, do not fully explain why some people gain too much body fat and others stay lean. When given a constant number of excess calories over a period of weeks or months, some people gain many pounds of body fat, but other people gain far fewer. Those who gain weight seem to use every calorie with great metabolic efficiency, whereas others may expend calories more freely.

Many theories have emerged to explain the mysteries of obesity in terms of metabolic function and energy expenditure. This section introduces a few of them, and illustrates a well-known generalization: whenever discussions turn to metabolism, topics in genetics follow closely behind.

Set-Point Theory   The body's way of managing its metabolism can be likened to the way that a room's thermostat works. The thermostat constantly monitors a temperature and responds to fluctuations from a set point by turning the heat or cooling on or off. Similarly, the brain and other body organs monitor and respond to small changes in the body's internal conditions, such as blood glucose, blood pH, and body temperature, and maintain them within narrow physiological ranges.

The **set-point theory** of obesity holds that, to a degree, this may also explain why people so easily regain lost weight.[31] After weight loss, the body adjusts its metabolism in the direction of restoring the original weight. Many debates surround the set-point theory of weight regulation.

Thermogenesis   Some people tend to expend more energy in metabolism than do others. The body's working enzymes normally "waste" a small percentage of energy as heat in a process called **thermogenesis**. Some enzymes expend copious energy in thermogenesis, producing heat but performing no other useful work. As more heat is radiated away from the body, more calories are spent, and fewer calories are available to be stored as body fat.

One tissue extraordinarily gifted in thermogenesis is **brown adipose tissue (BAT)**, a well-known heat-generating tissue of animals and human infants that was recently identified in human adults, too.[32] People with the greatest body fatness appear to have the least BAT activity.[33] Intriguingly, muscular work or even shivering from cold exposure appear to trigger a normally dormant type of adipose cell to act more like BAT metabolically, but the significance of this finding to weight management is still under investigation.[34][††]

Is it wise, then, to try to step up thermogenesis to assist in weight loss? Probably not. At a level not far above normal, energy-wasting activity is lethal to cells. Sham "metabolic" diet products may claim to increase thermogenesis, but no tricks of metabolism can produce effortless fat loss.

> The intestinal bacteria were first described in **Chapter 3**.

Intestinal Microbiota   Researchers are probing the possibility that certain strains of intestinal bacteria may affect body weight. These bacteria have some interesting associations with obesity.[35] When experimental germ-free mice are exposed to bacteria from normal mice, they gain weight but they eat less, suggesting that some microbes may affect how efficiently the body uses its food energy. Bacteria may also generate signals that alter adipose tissue, changing its metabolic efficiency.[36] Also, some intestinal bacteria, or compounds they produce, may generate signals that help the brain regulate the appetite.[37] Research in these areas is tricky because intestinal bacterial communities are highly complex, and colonies swiftly grow and change with dietary changes.[38] Until more is known, it seems prudent to consume a variety of legumes, fruit, vegetables, and whole grains to provide the fibers that help beneficial bacteria to thrive.

[††]The activated adipose cells are called *beige cells*.

set-point theory a theory stating that the body's regulatory controls tend to maintain a particular body weight (the set point) over time, counteracting efforts to lose weight by dieting.

thermogenesis the generation and release of body heat associated with the breakdown of body fuels. *Adaptive thermogenesis* describes adjustments in energy expenditure related to changes in environment such as cold and to physiological events such as underfeeding or trauma.

brown adipose tissue (BAT) a type of adipose tissue abundant in hibernating animals and human infants and recently identified in human adults. Abundant pigmented enzymes of energy metabolism give BAT a dark appearance under a microscope; the enzymes release heat from fuels without accomplishing other work. Also called *brown fat*.

Genetics and Obesity   Is obesity genetic? It stands to reason that it might at least be influenced by genes, because genes carry the instructions for making enzymes, and enzymes control energy metabolism. "I'm fat because my father is fat," says one person, and another agrees: "Everyone in my family is fat." Data from family histories reveal that obesity often persists for generations. For someone with at least one obese parent, the chance of becoming obese is estimated to fall between 30 and 70 percent.

Genetic research confirms these observations—not that heredity is the only factor controlling the tendency toward obesity, but it certainly is influential. Geneticists have identified more than 100 genes that are likely to play roles in obesity development by altering metabolism.[39] As an example from studies of mice, a variant of one gene reduces insulin's efficiency and causes fat cells to proliferate; the results over time are insulin resistance, inflammation, and obesity.[40][‡‡] (Some human beings have this gene variant, too, but its effects remain to be discovered.) As another example, a genetic disorder in a small percentage of human beings produces excessive appetite and massive obesity, but this is rare; common obesity does not arise from a single gene.[§§]

The environment also plays a role in obesity development, of course—and in its prevention. Even in an individual whose genetic makeup favors obesity, the condition develops only if the environment makes abundant fattening foods available. A person's behavior also influences the outcome: a wisely chosen eating and exercise plan can prevent the condition.[41]

KEY POINTS

- Metabolic theories attempt to elucidate molecular activities that lead to obesity.
- Research suggests a relationship between intestinal microbial colonies and obesity.
- A person's genetic inheritance greatly influences but does not guarantee the development of obesity.

Outside-the-Body Theories of Obesity

LO 9.6   Summarize the current outside-the-body theories of obesity.

Food is a source of pleasure, and pleasure drives behavior. Being creatures of free will, people can easily override satiety signals and eat whenever they wish, especially when tempted with delicious treats or large servings. People also value physical ease and seek out labor-savers, such as automobiles and elevators. Over past decades, the abundance of palatable food has increased enormously, while the daily demand for physical activity for survival has all but disappeared.

Environmental Cues to Overeating   Here's a common experience: a person walks into a food store feeling not particularly hungry but, after viewing an array of goodies, walks out snacking on a favorite treat. Even rats, which precisely maintain body weights when fed standard chow, overeat and rapidly become obese when fed "cafeteria style" on a variety of rich, palatable foods.[42] When offered a delicious smorgasbord, people do likewise, often without awareness.[43] Like the rats, they respond to external cues. With around-the-clock access to rich, palatable foods, we eat more and more often than in decades past—and energy intakes have risen accordingly.

[‡‡]The gene is ankyrin-B, which codes for a glucose transporter protein in cell membranes of adipose tissue.
[§§]The genetic condition is Prader-Willi syndrome, characterized by massive obesity, short stature, and, often, mental disabilities.

Table 9-4

Energy Spent in Activities

To determine the calorie cost of an activity, multiply the number listed by your weight in pounds. Then multiply by the number of minutes spent performing the activity.

Example: Jessica (125 lb) rode a bike at 17 mph for 25 min:

$$0.057 \times 125 = 7.125$$
$$7.125 \times 25 = 178.125$$

(about 180 calories)

Activity	Cal/lb Body Weight/min
Aerobic dance (vigorous)	0.062
Basketball (vigorous, full court)	0.097
Bicycling	
13 mph	0.045
15 mph	0.049
17 mph	0.057
19 mph	0.076
21 mph	0.090
23 mph	0.109
25 mph	0.139
Canoeing (flat water, moderate pace)	0.045
Cross-country skiing	
8 mph	0.104
Exergaming (video sports games)	
bowling	0.021
boxing	0.021
tennis	0.022
Golf (carrying clubs)	0.045
Handball	0.078
Horseback riding (trot)	0.052
Rowing (vigorous)	0.097
Running	
5 mph	0.061
6 mph	0.074
7.5 mph	0.094
9 mph	0.103
10 mph	0.114
11 mph	0.131
Soccer (vigorous)	0.097
Studying	0.011
Swimming	
20 yd/min	0.032
45 yd/min	0.058
50 yd/min	0.070
Table tennis (skilled)	0.045
Tennis (beginner)	0.032
Walking (brisk pace)	
3.5 mph	0.035
4.5 mph	0.048
Weight lifting	
light-to-moderate effort	0.024
vigorous effort	0.048
Wheelchair basketball	0.084
Wheeling self in wheelchair	0.030

Overeating also accompanies complex human sensations such as loneliness, yearning, craving, addiction, and compulsion. Any kind of prolonged stress can also cause overeating and weight gain. ("What do I do when I'm worried? Eat. What do I do when I'm concentrating? Eat!").

People may also overeat in response to large portions of food. In a classic study, moviegoers ate proportionately more popcorn from large buckets than from small bags.[44] In a wry twist, researchers dispensed large and small containers of 14-day-old popcorn to moviegoers who, despite complaining of the staleness, still ate more popcorn from the larger containers. The effect may also generalize to children, who asked for bigger portions of cereal when given bigger bowls than when given smaller bowls; they ate more from the bigger bowls, too.[45]

Is Our Food Supply Addictive? People often equate overeating with an addiction, particularly sugar addiction. Right away, it should be said that foods, even highly palatable sweet foods, are not comparable to psychoactive drugs in most respects. Yet evidence supports certain similarities between the brain's chemical responses to both.[46] Pleasure-evoking experiences of all kinds cause brain cells to release the neurotransmitter **dopamine**, which stimulates the reward areas of the brain. The result is feelings of pleasure and desire that create a motivation to repeat the experience. Paradoxically, with repeated exposure to a chemical stimulus (say, the drug cocaine) over time, the brain reduces its dopamine response, reducing feelings of pleasure. Soon, larger and larger doses are needed to avoid the pain of withdrawal. Withdrawal is a fundamental sign of addiction.

In people addicted to cocaine or alcohol, brain scans reveal reduced dopamine activity in the brain. In a classic study, brain scans also revealed reduced dopamine activity in the brains of obese people.[47] This suggests that once these changes are in place, people with obesity, like people with addictions, may need more and more delicious food to satisfy their desire for it. Taking the idea one step further, it is plausible that our highly palatable, fat- and sugar-rich food supply could cause lasting changes in the brain's reward system and make overeating and weight gain likely. It happens reliably in the brains of rats fed on a changing variety of cookies, cheese, sugar, and other tasty items, and it may happen in people, too.[48]

Other explanations exist. It may be that consciously restricting intakes of delicious foods increases the desire for them. It may also be that some people are more inclined to "throw caution to the wind" and indulge in treats whenever the opportunity arises.[49] Future research must untangle these threads before the truth can be known.

Physical Inactivity Many people may be obese not because they eat too much but because they move too little—both in purposeful exercise and in the activities of daily life. Sedentary **screen time** has all but replaced outdoor play for many people. This is a concern because the more time people spend in sedentary activities, the more likely they are to be overweight—and to incur the metabolic risk factors of heart disease (high blood lipids, high blood pressure, and high blood glucose). Table 9–4 lists the energy costs of some activities and the Think Fitness feature offers perspective on physical activity in weight management.

Can Your Neighborhood Make You Fat? Experts urge people to "take the stairs instead of the elevator" or "walk or bike to work." These are good strategies: climbing stairs provides an impromptu workout, and people who walk or ride their bicycles for transportation most often meet their needs for physical activity. Many people, however, encounter barriers in their **built environment** that prevent such choices.[50]

Few people would choose to walk or bike on a roadway where there is no safe sidewalk or marked bicycle lane, where vehicles speed by, or where the air is laden with toxic carbon monoxide gas or other pollutants from gasoline engines.*** Few would

---

***Carbon monoxide (CO) avidly binds to hemoglobin in the blood, reducing blood oxygen content; CO in air surrounding roadways can reach levels sufficient to impair driving ability.

Chapter 9 Energy Balance and Healthy Body Weight

THINK FITNESS — Activity for a Healthy Body Weight

Some people believe that physical activity must be long and arduous to produce benefits, such as improved body composition. Not so. A brisk, 30-minute walk on most days each week can help significantly. To achieve an "active lifestyle" by walking requires an hour a day. Even in increments of a few minutes throughout the day, exercise can measurably improve fitness.

According to the American College of Sports Medicine,

- 150 to 250 minutes per week of physical activity of moderate intensity can help prevent initial weight gain.

- More than 250 minutes per week, particularly when combined with a lower calorie intake, promotes weight loss and may prevent regain after loss.

- Both aerobic (endurance) and muscle-strengthening (resistance) activities are beneficial, but most people must also restrict calorie intakes to achieve meaningful weight loss.

A useful strategy is to augment your planned workouts with bits of physical activity throughout the day. Work in the garden; work your abdominal muscles while you stand in line; stand up straight; walk up stairs; fidget or tighten your buttocks while sitting in your chair. Chapter 10 provides many more details.

start now! If you are healthy, but not currently exercising, try this: add a few minutes of daily walking (or dancing, biking, or rolling in a wheelchair) to your daily routine for a week, and then assess how you feel. Did the activity become easier with time? Did you feel mentally refreshed afterward? (Most people do.) When you are ready, try extending your activity or speeding up your pace a bit. Then, add some easy stretches and a few strength exercises. Some benefits will be immediately apparent, but others build over time. Chapter 10 lists many of the benefits you can expect to occur.

---

choose to walk up flights of stairs in an inconvenient, stuffy, isolated, and unsafe stairwell, typical of modern buildings. In contrast, people living in attractive, affordable neighborhoods with safe biking and walking lanes, public parks, and freely available exercise facilities use them often—their surroundings encourage physical activity.[51]

In addition, low-income residents of urban or rural areas called **food deserts** lack access to even one neighborhood grocery store. Often carless, these people must travel for miles by bus, hire a car, or ride with friends to shop for fresh, affordable foods. Nearby convenience stores and fast-food places sell mostly packaged sweets, sugary drinks, refined starches, fried foods, and fatty meats—foods typical of eating patterns that predict high rates of obesity and chronic diseases.[52] Shopping at specialty stores, such as urban fruit stands and seafood shops, improves the diet but may be too costly for most residents.[53] Programs that provide lower-cost groceries, establish community gardens, and improve transportation may help, but researchers must still establish the most effective ways of improving diet quality in these areas.[54]

Toward a Healthier Future With an awareness of factors that influence obesity (Figure 9–10 sums them up), the prestigious National Academies' Institute of Medicine has put forth these national goals as most likely to slow or reverse the current obesity epidemic and improve the nation's health:

- Make physical activity an integral and routine part of American life.
- Make healthy foods and beverages available everywhere.
- Create food and beverage environments in which healthy food and beverage choices become the easy, routine choice.
- Advertise and market what matters for a healthy life.
- Develop and enforce legislation and policies aimed at preventing obesity.
- Strengthen schools as centers that promote fitness and health.[55]

Such changes require efforts from leaders at all levels and citizenry across all sectors of society working with one goal: improving the health of the nation.

dopamine (DOH-pah-meen) a neurotransmitter that facilitates many important functions in the brain, including cognition, pleasure, motivation, mood, sleep, and others.

screen time sedentary time spent using an electronic device, such as a television, computer, or video game player.

built environment the buildings, roads, utilities, homes, fixtures, parks, and all the other man-made entities that form the physical characteristics of a community.

food deserts low-income communities where many people do not own cars and live more than a mile from a supermarket or large grocery store (in rural areas, more than 10 miles). Also defined in Chapter 15.

Figure 9–10

Multiple Forces Influence Obesity

Many factors interact to modify an individual's risk of developing obesity.

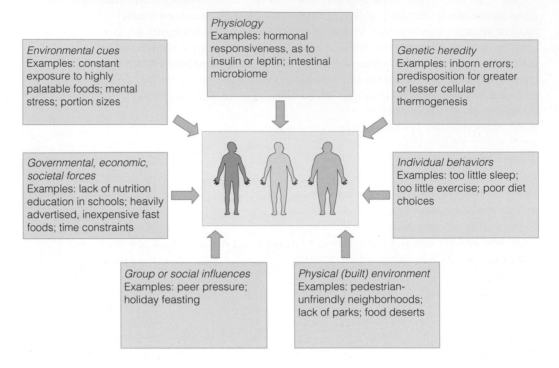

Physiology
Examples: hormonal responsiveness, as to insulin or leptin; intestinal microbiome

Environmental cues
Examples: constant exposure to highly palatable foods; mental stress; portion sizes

Genetic heredity
Examples: inborn errors; predisposition for greater or lesser cellular thermogenesis

Governmental, economic, societal forces
Examples: lack of nutrition education in schools; heavily advertised, inexpensive fast foods; time constraints

Individual behaviors
Examples: too little sleep; too little exercise; poor diet choices

Group or social influences
Examples: peer pressure; holiday feasting

Physical (built) environment
Examples: pedestrian-unfriendly neighborhoods; lack of parks; food deserts

KEY POINTS

- Studies of human behavior identify stimuli that lead to overeating.
- Food environments may trigger brain changes that lead to overeating.
- Too little physical activity, the built environment, and lack of access to fresh foods are linked with overfatness.
- National antiobesity efforts are needed.

How the Body Loses and Gains Weight

LO 9.7   Describe the metabolic events that occur in energy deficit and surplus.

The causes of obesity may be complex, but the body's energy balance is straightforward. To lose or gain body fat requires eating less or more food energy than the body expends. A change in body *weight* of a pound or two may not indicate a change in body fat, however—it can indicate shifts in body fluid content, in bone minerals, in lean tissues such as muscles, or in the contents of the bladder or digestive tract. A weight change often correlates with time of day: people generally weigh the least before breakfast.

The type of tissue lost or gained depends on how you go about losing or gaining it. To lose fluid, for example, you can take a "water pill" (diuretic), causing the kidneys to siphon extra water from the blood into the urine, or you can exercise while wearing heavy clothing in hot weather to cause abundant fluid loss in sweat. (Both practices are dangerous and are not recommended.) To gain water weight, you can overconsume salt and water; for a few hours, your body will retain water until it manages to excrete the salt. (This, too, is not recommended.) Most quick weight-change schemes produce large losses of body fluids that register dramatic, temporary changes on the scale.

One other practice is hazardous and not recommended: smoking. Each year, many adolescents, particularly girls, take up smoking as a means to control weight.[56] Nicotine blunts feelings of hunger, and smokers do tend to weigh less than nonsmokers. Fear of weight gain prevents many people from quitting smoking, too. The best advice to smokers trying to quit is to adjust eating and exercise habits to maintain weight during and after cessation. To people flirting with the idea of taking up smoking for weight control, don't do it—many thousands of people who became addicted as teenagers die of tobacco-related illnesses each year.

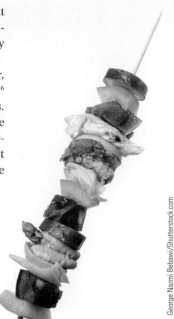

George Nazmi Bebawi/Shutterstock.com

The Body's Response to Energy Deficit

When you eat less food energy than you need, your body draws on its stored fuel to keep going. If a person exercises appropriately, moderately restricts calories, and consumes an otherwise balanced diet that meets carbohydrate and protein needs, the body is forced to use up its stored fat for energy. Body fat literally vanishes into the air as the tissues metabolize it to carbon dioxide, which is exhaled, and water, which is excreted. Gradual weight loss is preferred to rapid weight loss because it spares lean body mass.

The Body's Response to Fasting If a person doesn't eat for, say, three whole days, then the body makes one adjustment after another. Less than a day into the fast, the liver's glycogen is essentially exhausted. Where, then, can the body obtain glucose to keep its nervous system going? Not from the muscles' glycogen because that is reserved for the muscles' own use. Not from the abundant fat stores most people carry because these are of no use to the nervous system. The muscles, heart, and other organs use fat as fuel, but at this stage, the nervous system needs glucose. Fat cannot be converted to glucose—the body lacks enzymes for this conversion.[†††] The body does, however, possess enzymes that can convert *protein* to glucose. Therefore, an underfed body sacrifices the proteins in its lean tissue to supply raw materials from which to make glucose.

If the body were to continue to consume its lean tissue unchecked, death would ensue within about 10 days. After all, in addition to skeletal muscle, the blood proteins, liver, digestive tract linings, heart muscle, and lung tissue—all vital tissues—are being burned as fuel. (Fasting or starving people remain alive only until their stores of fat are gone or until half their lean tissue is gone, whichever comes first.) To prevent this, the body puts a key strategy into action: it begins converting fat into ketone bodies (ketones), which some nervous system tissues *can* use for energy, and so forestalls the end. This metabolic strategy is ketosis, an adaptation to fasting or carbohydrate deprivation.

Ketosis terms are introduced and defined in Chapter 4, p. 126.

Ketosis In ketosis, instead of breaking down fat molecules all the way to carbon dioxide and water, the body takes partially broken-down fat fragments and combines them to make ketone bodies, compounds that are normally kept to low levels in the blood. It converts some amino acids—those that cannot be used to make glucose—to ketone bodies, too. These ketone bodies circulate in the bloodstream and help to feed the brain; about half of the brain's cells can make the enzymes needed to use ketone bodies for energy. Under normal conditions, the brain and nervous system devour glucose—about 400 to 600 calories' worth each day. After about 10 days of fasting, the brain and nervous system can meet most, but not all, of their energy needs using ketone bodies.

[†††]Glycerol, which makes up 5 percent of fat, can yield glucose but is a negligible source.

Thus, indirectly, the nervous system begins to feed on the body's fat stores. Ketosis reduces the nervous system's need for glucose, spares muscle and other lean tissue from being quickly devoured, and prolongs the starving person's life. Thanks to ketosis, a healthy person starting with average body fat content and given only water can live totally deprived of food for as long as 6 to 8 weeks.

In summary,

- The brain and nervous system cannot use fat as fuel and demand glucose.
- Body fat cannot be converted to glucose.
- Body protein can be converted to glucose.
- Ketone bodies made from fat can feed some nervous system tissues and reduce glucose needs, sparing protein from degradation.

Figure 9–11 (p. 339) reviews how energy is used during fasting.

Is Fasting Helpful or Harmful? Respected, wise people in many cultures have practiced fasting as a periodic discipline. The body tolerates short-term fasting, and in laboratory animals, **intermittent fasting** has been reported to extend life, fend off chronic diseases, and improve cognition.[57] In people, intermittent fasting—say, a day or two a week—is under investigation for utility in weight loss, but so far, it has not proven superior to ordinary calorie restriction.[58] Despite claims from salespeople, no evidence suggests that fasting, even with juices or supplement concoctions, "cleanses" the body internally.

On the negative side, even a single day of fasting initiates fat accumulation in liver and muscle tissues, with unknown consequences.[59] In addition, many who try intermittent fasting soon quit, reporting intolerable feelings of hunger and irritability.[60] Over time, fasting clearly becomes harmful when tissues lack the nutrients they need to assemble new enzymes, red and white blood cells, and other vital components; when it causes lean tissue loss; or when ketosis upsets the acid-base balance of the blood and leads to excessive mineral losses in the urine. Currently, evidence is insufficient to say whether fasting is helpful or harmful for weight management, but beware: many people with eating disorders report that fasting or severe food restriction heralded the beginning of their loss of control over eating.

KEY POINTS

- When the energy balance is negative, glycogen returns glucose to the blood, and fat tissue supplies fatty acids for energy.
- When fasting or a low-carbohydrate diet depletes glycogen altogether, body protein is called upon to make glucose, while fats supply ketone bodies to help feed the brain and nerves.
- Fasting and supplements are not needed for weight loss or "cleansing."

The Body's Response to Energy Surplus

What happens inside the body when a person does not use up all of the food energy taken in? Previous chapters have already provided the answer—the energy-yielding nutrients contribute the excess to body stores as follows:

- Protein is broken down to amino acids for absorption. Inside the body, these may be used to replace lost body *protein* and, in a person who is exercising or growing, to build new muscle and other lean tissue.
- Excess amino acids, after their nitrogen is removed, are used for energy or are converted to *glucose* or *fat*. The nitrogen is incorporated into urea and excreted in the urine.
- Fat is broken down to glycerol and fatty acids in the digestive tract for absorption. Inside the body, the fatty acids can be broken down for energy or stored as body *fat* with great efficiency. The glycerol can be used for energy or converted to fat and stored (see Figure 9-11, top panel).

intermittent fasting a pattern of consuming no or little food energy during 14 or more hours in a 24-hour day, interspersed with days of normal eating. *Alternate-day fasts* involve fasting every other day; other regimens call for fasting on two or three days per week. *Modified fasts* allow consumption of 20 to 25 percent of a person's energy need on fasting days.

Chapter 9 Energy Balance and Healthy Body Weight

Figure 9–11

Feasting and Fasting

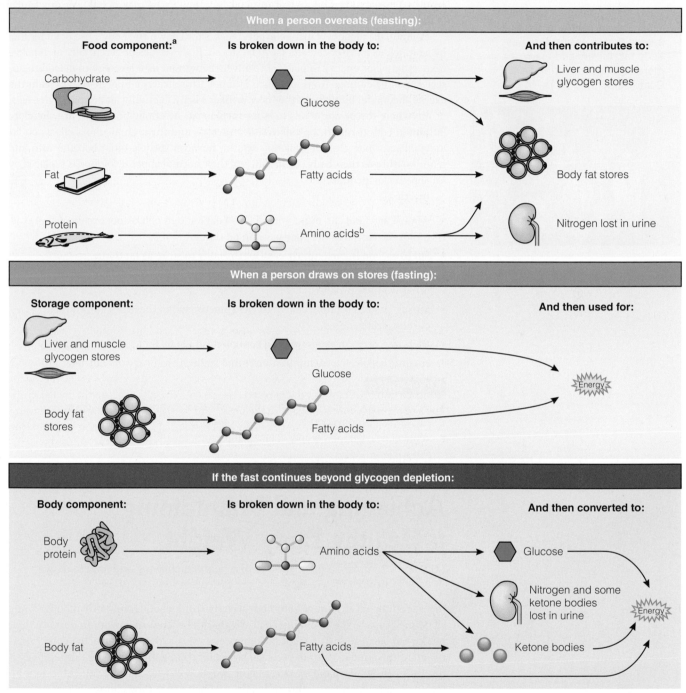

When a person overeats (feasting):

Food component:[a]	Is broken down in the body to:	And then contributes to:
Carbohydrate	Glucose	Liver and muscle glycogen stores
Fat	Fatty acids	Body fat stores
Protein	Amino acids[b]	Nitrogen lost in urine

When a person draws on stores (fasting):

Storage component:	Is broken down in the body to:	And then used for:
Liver and muscle glycogen stores	Glucose	Energy
Body fat stores	Fatty acids	Energy

If the fast continues beyond glycogen depletion:

Body component:	Is broken down in the body to:	And then converted to:
Body protein	Amino acids	Glucose / Nitrogen and some ketone bodies lost in urine / Energy
Body fat	Fatty acids	Ketone bodies / Energy

[a]Alcohol is not included because it is a toxin and not a nutrient, but it does contribute energy to the body. After inactivating the alcohol, the body uses the remaining two-carbon fragments to build fatty acids and stores them as fat.

[b]Amino acids are first used to build body proteins. Excess amino acids contribute to body fuel; after removal of their side chains, the backbones can be used to build glucose or fat.

- Carbohydrate (other than fiber) is broken down to sugars for absorption. In the body tissues, excesses of these may be built up to *glycogen* and stored, used for energy, or converted to *fat* and stored.
- Alcohol is absorbed and, once inactivated, delivers energy that is used as fuel or converted into body fat for storage (see Figure 9–12).

Figure 9–12

Caloric Alcohol

Each gram of alcohol presents 7 calories of energy to the body— energy that is easily stored as body fat. Mixers add many more calories to a drink (see Controversy 3, p. 95).

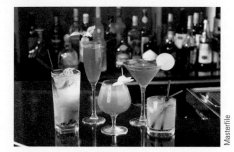

Masterfile

Four sources of energy—the three energy-yielding nutrients and alcohol—may enter the body, but they become only two kinds of energy stores: glycogen and fat. Glycogen stores amount to about three-fourths of a pound; fat stores can amount to many pounds. Thus, if you eat enough of any food, be it steak, brownies, or baked beans, much of the excess food energy will be stored as fat within hours.

Ethanol, the alcohol of alcoholic beverages, slows down the body's use of fat for fuel by as much as a third, causing fat to be stored. Body tissues preferentially metabolize toxic ethanol for energy in place of relatively benign fat as a strategy to defend themselves against damage from too much ethanol. This strategy may help to explain the excess abdominal fat tissue of the "beer drinker's belly," actually fat on the thighs, legs, or anywhere the person tends to store surplus fat. Alcoholic beverages are therefore fattening, both through the calories they provide and through alcohol's effects on fat metabolism. Once alcohol addiction sets in, however, people often become thin and malnourished as their body organs fail and their normal appetite for food is replaced by an appetite for alcohol.

In summary,

- Almost any food can make you fat if you eat enough of it. A net excess of energy is almost all stored in the body as fat in fat tissue.

- Fat from food is particularly easy for the body to store as fat tissue.

- Protein is not held in the body in a storage form. It exists only in muscle and other working proteins.

- Muscle protein is broken down to yield glucose when the brain runs out of carbohydrate energy.

- Dietary protein in excess of need contributes to body fat accumulation.

- Alcohol both delivers empty calories and facilitates storage of body fat.

KEY POINTS

- When energy balance is positive, carbohydrate is converted to glycogen or fat, protein is converted to fat, and food fat is stored as fat.

- Alcohol both delivers empty calories and promotes the storage of body fat.

Achieving and Maintaining a Healthy Body Weight

LO 9.8   Summarize the measures that help in achieving and maintaining a healthy body weight.

Before setting out to change your body weight, think about your motivation for doing so. Many people strive to change their weight not because they want to improve their health but because their weight fails to meet society's ideals of attractiveness. Unfortunately, this kind of thinking sets people up for disappointment. The human body is not infinitely malleable. Few overweight people will ever become rail-thin, no matter what eating patterns, exercise habits, and behaviors they choose. Likewise, most underweight people will remain on the slim side even after spending much effort to put on some heft.

Modest weight loss of even 3 to 5 percent of body weight in a person who is overweight can quickly produce gains in physical abilities and quality of life, along with improvements in indicators of diabetes and blood lipids.[61] With greater losses, stair climbing, walking, and other tasks of daily living become noticeably easier. Adopting health or fitness as the ideal rather than some ill-conceived image of beauty can avert much misery. Table 9–5 offers some tips to that end.

Tips for Accepting a Healthy Body Weight

- Value yourself and others for traits other than body weight; focus on your whole self, including your intelligence, social grace, and professional and scholastic accomplishments.
- Realize that prejudging people by weight is as harmful as prejudging them by race, religion, or gender.
- Use only positive, nonjudgmental descriptions of your body; never use degrading, negative descriptions.
- Accept positive comments from others.
- Accept that no magic diet exists.
- Stop dieting to lose weight. Adopt a healthy eating and exercise lifestyle permanently.

- Follow the USDA Eating Patterns (Chapter 2 and Appendix E). Never restrict food intake below the minimum levels that meet nutrient needs.
- Become physically active not because it will help you get thin but because it will enhance your health.
- Seek support from loved ones. Tell them of your plan for a healthy life in the body you have been given.
- Seek professional counseling not from a weight-loss counselor but from someone who supports your self-esteem.
- Join with others to fight weight discrimination and stereotypes.

The rest of this chapter stresses health and fitness as goals and explains the required actions to achieve them. It uses weight only as a convenient gauge for progress. To repeat, effort in three realms produces results:

- Eating patterns.
- Physical activity.
- Behavior modification.[62]

Eating patterns and physical activity are explained next. Behavior modification is the topic of this chapter's Food Feature section.

First, a Reality Check Overweight takes years to accumulate. Losing excess body fatness also takes time, along with patience and perseverance. The person must adopt healthy eating patterns, take on physical activities, create a supportive environment, and seek out behavioral and social support; continue these behaviors for at least 6 months for initial weight loss; and then continue all of it for a lifetime to maintain the losses. Setbacks are a given, and the size of the calorie deficit required to lose a pound of weight initially is smaller than the deficit required later on. In other words, weight loss is hard at first, and then it gets harder.

The list of what doesn't work is long: fad diets, skipping meals, "diet foods," special herbs and supplements, and liquid-diet formulas, among others. Many fad diets promise quick and easy weight-loss solutions, but as the Consumer's Guide points out, fad diets can interrupt real progress toward life-long weight management. In contrast, people willing to take one step at a time, even if it feels like just a baby step, toward balancing their energy budget are on the right path. An excellent first step is to set realistic goals.

Set Achievable Goals A reasonable first weight goal for an overweight person might be to stop gaining weight. A next goal might be to reduce body weight by 5 to 10 percent over about 6 months.[63] This may sound insignificant, but even small losses can improve health and reduce disease risks. Put another way, shoot for a weight that falls two BMI categories lower than a present unhealthy one. For example, a 5-foot-5-inch woman with hypertension weighing 180 pounds (BMI of 30—see the BMI table in the back of the book, p. E) may aim for a BMI of 28, or about 168 pounds. If her health indicators fall into line, she may decide to maintain this weight. If her blood pressure is still high or she has other risks, she may repeat the process to achieve a healthier weight.

A CONSUMER'S GUIDE TO . . .
Fad Diets

Over the years, Lauren has tried most of the new fad diets, her hopes rising each time, as though she had never been disappointed: "*This* one has the answer. I have *got* to lose 40 pounds. Plus it only costs $30 to start." Who wouldn't pay a few dollars to get trim?

Lauren and tens of millions of people like her have helped to fuel the growth of a $66 billion-a-year weight-loss industry.[1]* The number of fad-diet books in print could fill a bookstore, and more keep coming out because they continue to make huge profits. Some of them restrict fats or carbohydrates, some disallow certain foods, some advocate certain food combinations, some claim that a person's genetic type or blood type determines the best diet, and others advocate taking unproven weight-loss "dietary supplements."†

Unfortunately, most fad diets are more fiction than science. They sound plausible, though, because they are skillfully written. Their authors weave in scientific-sounding words like *eicosanoids* or *adipokines* and bits of authentic nutrition knowledge to create an appearance of credibility and convince the skeptical. This makes it hard for people without adequate nutrition knowledge to evaluate them. Table 9–6 presents some clues to identifying scams among fad diets.

Are Fad Diets All Nonsense?

If fad diets delivered what they promise, the nation's obesity problem would have vanished; if they never worked, people would stop buying into them. In fact, most fad diets do limit calorie intakes and produce weight loss (at least temporarily). Fad diets are particularly

* Reference notes are in Appendix F.
† The Academy of Nutrition and Dietetics offers evaluations of popular diets on their website, www.eatright.org.

Table 9–6

Clues to Fad Diets and Weight-Loss Scams

It may be a fad diet or weight-loss scam if it:

- Bases evidence for its effectiveness on anecdotes and testimonials.
- Blames weight gain on a single nutrient, such as carbohydrate, or constituent, such as gluten.
- Claims to "alter your genetic code" or "reset your metabolism."
- Eliminates an entire food group, such as grains or milk products.
- Fails to include all costs up front.
- Fails to mention potential risks.
- Fails to plan for weight maintenance following loss.
- Guarantees an unrealistic outcome, such as losing 10 pounds in 3 days.
- Promises easy weight loss with no change in diet or activity; for example, "Lose weight while you sleep."
- Promotes devices, drugs, products, or procedures not approved by the U.S. Food and Drug Administration (FDA) or not scientifically evaluated for safety or effectiveness.
- Specifies a proportion of energy nutrients not in keeping with DRI ranges.
- Recommends using a single food, such as grapefruit, as the key to the program's success.
- Requires you to buy special products not readily available in ordinary supermarkets.
- Has any of the other characteristics of quackery (see Figure C1–1 of Controversy 1, p. 24).

Note: For more tips, search the Internet for the Federal Trade Commission's guide to spotting false weight loss claims, currently at www.consumer.ftc.gov/topics/weight-loss-fitness.

---

ineffective for weight-loss maintenance—people may drop some weight, but they quickly gain it back. Straightforward calorie deficit turns out to be the real key to weight loss—and not the elimination of protein, carbohydrate, or fat or the mysterious metabolic mechanisms on which many fad diets are claimed to be based.

Are Low-Carbohydrate Diets Best?

At first, a low-carbohydrate, high-protein diet may produce a little more weight loss than a balanced diet, but over time, such diets perform no better than others.[2] Diets providing less than 45 percent of calories from carbohydrate are difficult to maintain in the long run and may be less safe. Still, it makes good nutritional sense to limit the intake of added sugars and *refined* carbohydrates in soft drinks, snack cakes, chips, crackers, and other ultra-processed foods. This step cuts unneeded calories and may help avert some health issues, as Controversy 4 (p. 139) points out.[3]

Is Extra Protein Helpful?

A meal with sufficient protein may produce enough satiety to help prevent between-meal hunger from derailing a diet plan.[4] In addition, eating enough high-quality protein, along with performing muscle-building resistance exercise, can help minimize muscle loss, an unwelcome side effect of calorie restriction and fat loss.[5]

Some research suggests that a little extra protein (1.2 to 1.6 gram per kilogram body weight) may facilitate weight loss and maintain muscle mass, so long as the dieter can stick with a reduced-calorie diet over time.[6] However, protein *sources* matter, too. In one well-controlled, long-duration study, weight *gain*, not loss, was associated with higher intakes of full fat cheeses, chicken with skin, and processed and red meats (particularly hamburger).[7] In contrast, plain yogurt, peanut butter, walnuts, other nuts, chicken without skin, low-fat cheese, and seafood were associated with weight loss.

Chapter 9 Energy Balance and Healthy Body Weight

Are Gluten-Free Diets Best?

Proponents of gluten-free diets claim that the protein gluten in many grain foods (see details in Chapter 6) causes obesity, but no research backs this up. In fact, choosing gluten-free foods for weight loss may backfire if the formulated foods are high in calories, added sugars, or refined starches.

Are Fad Diets Safe?

Fad diets that severely limit or eliminate one or more food groups cannot meet nutrient needs. To fend off critics, such plans usually recommend nutrient supplements (often conveniently supplied by the diet's originators at greatly inflated prices). Real weight-loss experts know this: no pills, not even the most costly ones, can match the health benefits of whole foods.

Although most people can tolerate most diets, exceptions exist. For example, a rare but life-threatening form of blood acid imbalance is associated with a very low-carbohydrate diet. In addition, when protein sources are high in saturated fat, the diet may produce unfavorable changes in blood lipids and artery linings. Experts urge caution until research reveals that a weight-loss diet is safe.[8] No one knows the extent to which an extreme fad diet might harm people with established diseases—the very people who might try dieting to regain their health.

Moving Ahead

Success for the fad-diet industry is built on failure for dieters. As one diet shortcut fails, a new version arises to take its place, replenishing industry profits. Success for dieters takes a longer road: setting realistic goals and eating a nutritious calorie-restricted diet that is sustainable. This approach also means adopting a physically active lifestyle that is flexible and comfortable over a lifetime. Solid plans exist; seek them out for serious help with weight loss.[‡] Armed with common sense, Lauren and other hopeful dieters can avoid costly detours that sap the will and delay true progress.

Review Questions[§]

1. A diet book that addresses eicosanoids and adipokines can be relied upon to reflect current scholarship in nutrition science and provide effective weight-loss advice. T F

2. Limiting calories is no longer the primary strategy for weight management. T F

3. Meals with sufficient protein may provide more satiety than meals that are low in protein. T F

[‡]An example of a balanced weight-loss plan is Weight Watchers®.
[§]Answers to Consumer's Guide review questions are in Appendix G.

Once you have identified your overall target, set specific, achievable, small-step goals for food intake, activity, and behavior changes. One simple and effective first small-step goal might be to reduce intake of sugar-sweetened beverages.

Liquid calories were the topic of the **Chapter 8** Consumer's Guide, pp. 277–278.

Dramatic weight loss overnight is not possible or even desirable; a pound or two of body fat lost each week will safely and effectively bring you to your goal. Losses greater or faster than these are not recommended because they are almost invariably followed by rapid regain. New goals can be built on prior achievements, and a lifetime goal may be to maintain the leaner, healthier body weight.

Keep Records Keeping records is often critical to success. Recording your food intake and exercise can help you to spot trends and identify areas needing improvement. The Food Feature, later, demonstrates how to maintain a food and exercise diary. Recording changes in body weight can also provide a rough estimate of changes in body fatness over time. In addition to weight, measure your waist circumference to track changes in central adiposity.

KEY POINTS

- Setting realistic weight goals proves an important starting point for weight loss.
- Many benefits follow even modest reductions in body fatness among overweight people.
- Successful weight management takes time and effort; fad diets can be counterproductive.

What Food Strategies Are Best for Weight Loss?

Contrary to the claims of faddists, no particular food plan is magical, and no particular food must be either included or excluded. You are the one who will have to live with the plan, so you had better be the one to design it. Remember, you are adopting a healthy eating plan for life, so it must consist of satisfying foods that you like, that are readily available, and that you can afford.

Choose an Appropriate Calorie Intake Nutrition professionals often use an overweight person's BMI to calculate the number of calories to cut from the diet. Dieters with a BMI of 35 or greater are encouraged to reduce their daily calories by up to 1,000 calories from their usual intakes. People with a BMI between 25 and 35 should reduce energy intake by 500 to 750 calories a day to produce a pound or two of weight loss each week while retaining lean tissue.[64]

For some weeks or months, weight loss may proceed rapidly. Eventually, these factors may contribute to a slowdown in the rate of loss:

- Metabolism may slow in response to a lower calorie intake and loss of metabolically active lean tissue.
- Less energy may be expended in physical activity as body weight diminishes.

Also, lean body tissue differs from fat tissue in calorie content, and this difference affects the rate of weight loss. Early in dieting, losses are composed of lean tissue (and its associated water), which has fewer calories per pound than later losses, which are composed mostly of fat. Compared with losing a pound of lean tissue, losing a pound of fat takes a greater calorie deficit, so dieters should expect a slowdown in weight loss as they progress past the initial phase.

In the end, most dieters can lose weight safely on an eating pattern providing approximately 1,200 to 1,500 calories per day for women and 1,500 to 1,800 calories per day for men while still meeting nutrient needs (as demonstrated in Table 9–7). Very low-calorie diets are notoriously unsuccessful at achieving lasting weight loss. They lack necessary nutrients, and may set in motion the unhealthy behaviors of eating disorders (see the Controversy section) and so are not recommended.

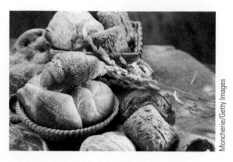

People with a healthy body weight often choose whole grains over refined carbohydrates.

Moncherie/Getty Images

Table 9–7

Eating Patterns for Low-Calorie Diets

To use these patterns, first choose a calorie level that can be expected to produce weight loss, often about 500 calories less per day than your current intake. Then design your eating pattern to provide a day's food intake. Adjust your intakes to sustain weight loss over time. See Chapter 2 for diet-planning details (pp. 39–45).

	1,200 Calories	1,400 Calories	1,600 Calories	1,800 Calories
Fruit	1 c	1½ c	1½ c	1½ c
Vegetables	1½ c	1½ c	2 c	2½ c
Grains	4 oz	5 oz	5 oz	6 oz
Protein Foods	3 oz	4 oz	5 oz	5 oz
Milk and Milk Products	2½ c	2½ c	3 c	3 c
Oils	4 tsp	4 tsp	5 tsp	5 tsp

Make Intakes Adequate   Healthy eating patterns for weight loss should include a variety of food to provide all of the needed nutrients. In particular, eating more of these foods is associated with a healthy body weight:

- Fruit, vegetables, nuts, and legumes.
- Fish; poultry without skin; low-fat or nonfat milk products (or fortified soy or other legume substitutes).
- Whole grains.
- Moderate amounts of unsaturated oils.[65]

Eating patterns should also be moderate in total meat and refined grains and low in saturated fat, sodium, and sugar-sweetened foods and drinks. Such patterns, including Healthy Vegetarian and Healthy Mediterranean-style patterns (see Appendix E), provide nutrient adequacy and are generally associated with leanness.

Choose fats sensibly by avoiding most solid fats and by including enough unsaturated oils to support health but not so much as to oversupply calories. Nuts provide unsaturated fat and protein, and people who regularly eat nuts often maintain healthy body weight.[66] Lean meats or other low-fat protein sources also play important roles in weight loss: an ounce of lean ham contains about the same number of calories as an ounce of bread, but the ham may produce greater satiety. Sufficient protein foods may also help preserve lean tissue, including muscle tissue, during weight loss.[67] Remember to limit alcohol, which weakens resolve and can sabotage even the most committed dieters' plans.

A supplement providing vitamins and minerals may be appropriate (Controversy 7, p. 264, explained how to choose one). If you plan resolutely to include all of the foods from each food group that you need each day, you will be satisfied and well nourished and will have little or no appetite left for high-calorie treats.

Avoid Portion Pitfalls   Pay careful attention to portion sizes—large portions expand energy intakes, and the monstrous helpings served by restaurants and sold in packages are enemies of the person striving to control weight. Popular 100-calorie single-serving packages may be useful, but only if the food in the package fits into your calorie budget—100 calories of cookies or fried snacks are still 100 calories that can be safely eliminated. Also, eating a reduced-calorie cookie instead of an ordinary cookie saves calories—but eating half the bag defeats the purpose.

Almost every dieter needs to retrain, using measuring cups for a while to learn to judge portion sizes. (The Consumer's Guide of Chapter 2, pp. 48–50, provided some guidelines.) Stay focused on calories and portions—don't be distracted by a product's claims. Read labels and compare *calories* per serving.

Read Menu Labels   Meals eaten away from home are notoriously high in calories. To provide consumers with the information they need to make more healthful choices, the FDA requires that eating establishments list the calorie contents of ready-to-eat foods, meals, and some alcoholic beverages on their menus (see Figure 9–13). Although it doesn't take a label to tell people whether, say, broiled, skinless chicken or battered fried chicken is more highly caloric, some differences are not so easily discernible—distinguishing between a fried chicken sandwich and a quarter-pound hamburger, for example.[68] Consumers must also take note of calorie-changing details, such as whether the calories listed on a menu are for a meal or just a sandwich; for a large or small portion size; and for an item with or without caloric add-ons such as bacon, cheese, or mayonnaise and other sauces.

Meal Spacing   Three meals a day is standard in our society, but no law says you can't have four or five—just be sure they are smaller, of course. People who eat small, frequent meals can be as successful at weight loss and maintenance as those who eat three. Also, eat regularly, before you become extremely hungry.[69] When you do decide to eat, eat the entire meal you have planned for yourself. Then don't eat again until the next meal or snack.

Figure 9–13
New on the Menu: Calories

FDA regulations require many restaurants to list calorie amounts on their menus.

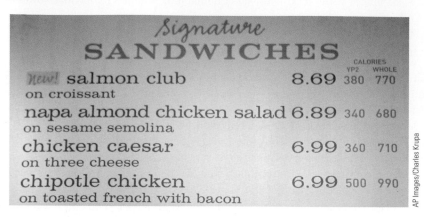

		CALORIES
		YP2 / WHOLE
New! **salmon club** on croissant	8.69	380 770
napa almond chicken salad on sesame semolina	6.89	340 680
chicken caesar on three cheese	6.99	360 710
chipotle chicken on toasted french with bacon	6.99	500 990

Signature SANDWICHES

AP Images/Charles Krupa

Do the Math

The energy density of a food can be calculated mathematically. Find the energy density of carrot sticks and French fries by dividing their calories by their weight in grams.

- A serving of carrot sticks, providing 31 cal and weighing 72 g:

$$\frac{31 \text{ cal}}{72 \text{ g}} = 0.43 \text{ cal/g}$$

- A serving of French fries, contributing 167 cal and weighing 50 g:

$$\frac{167 \text{ cal}}{50 \text{ g}} = 3.34 \text{ cal/g}$$

The more calories per gram (cal/g), the greater the energy density.

Now access an online nutrient database and select any food that interests you.[a] Find its calories and gram weight and apply the formula above to determine the food's energy density in cal/g.

[a]Using a Web browser, search for USDA's What's In The Foods You Eat website, currently available at https://reedir.arsnet.usda.gov/codesearchwebapp/ (S(jgjhis5s0eisp4f54ouulbfv))/CodeSearch.aspx.

night eating syndrome a disturbance in the daily eating rhythm associated with obesity, characterized by eating more than half of the daily calories after 7 p.m., awakening frequently at night to eat, and overconsuming calories.

energy density a measure of the energy provided by a food relative to its weight (calories per gram).

Pay close attention to snacks. Snacking among Americans has doubled in the past 30 years, and snacks provide almost a third of the empty calories from solid fats and added sugars that most people take in each day. Save calorie-free or favorite foods or beverages for a planned snack at the end of the day if you need insurance against late-evening hunger. Hungry people are likely to awaken at night to eat, a symptom of **night eating syndrome**.[70]

Energy Density People in this country whose eating patterns consist mostly of foods that are high in **energy density** are more often overweight.[71] Turning this around, people who wish to be leaner and to improve their nutrient intakes would be well advised to select mostly foods of low energy density. In general, foods high in fat or low in water, such as fatty meats, cookies, or chips, rank high in energy density; foods high in water and fiber, such as fruit and vegetables, rank lower. Foods with lower energy density are bulkier, providing more bites for fewer calories, and thus may be more satisfying (see Figure 9–14).

Some energy-dense foods, such as avocados, olive oil, olives, and nuts that are consumed as part of a Healthy Mediterranean-style eating pattern, appear to be compatible with a healthy body weight.[72] This pattern is also rich in vegetables, fruit, and seafood, with few or none of the empty-calorie, energy-dense foods that abound in a typical U.S. diet. People who consume tree nuts, such as almonds, walnuts, and pecans, often have a lower BMI and smaller waist circumference than people who do not eat nuts.[73] It may be that one healthful choice clusters with others in a total lifestyle that promotes leanness.

Nonnutritive Sweeteners and Alcohol Some people who maintain weight loss report using artificially sweetened beverages and fat-modified products liberally. Replacing caloric beverages with water or diet drinks may reduce most people's overall calorie intakes, although research is mixed on whether these choices assist in weight loss.[74] In laboratory animals, however, chronic exposure to nonnutritive sweeteners has been reported to alter the intestinal microbiome, increase food intake, and promote weight gain.[75] In people, consumption of low-calorie sweeteners is not generally reported to have such effects, but research is continuing.[76] In any case, soft drinks of any kind displace milk, and although milk is unlikely to speed weight loss, it contributes important nutrients to the diet.

More on artificial sweeteners in **Chapter 12**.

Alcoholic beverages can deliver hundreds of calories to drinkers each day, often without their awareness. Labels of most alcoholic beverages omit calorie amounts,

Figure 9–14

Energy Density and Meal Size

The larger meal on the right has fewer than half the calories of the one on the left, but it weighs more, provides more fiber, contains more water, and takes far longer to enjoy than the energy-dense meal on the left.

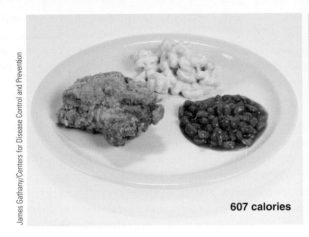

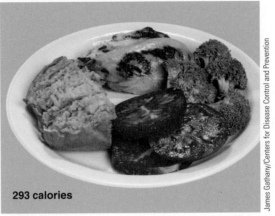

607 calories   **293 calories**

1/2 c macaroni and cheese
1/2 c baked beans with pork and sauce
1/2 fried chicken breast

$$\frac{607\ calories}{343\ g\ total\ wt} = 1.77\ energy\ density$$

1 c broccoli
3 large tomato slices
1/2 large sweet potato
1/2 skinless roasted chicken breast

$$\frac{293\ calories}{348\ g\ total\ wt} = 0.84\ energy\ density$$

Source: Centers for Disease Control and Prevention, Eat More, Weigh Less? How to Manage Your Weight without Being Hungry, *available at http://www.cdc.gov/nccdphp/dnpa/nutrition/pdf/Energy_Density.pdf.*

but you can find them on the Internet (search for the National Institutes of Health's "Alcohol Calorie Calculator") or in tables, such as Table C3–5 (p. 101). Drinkers should limit their intakes for many reasons.

Prepared Meals   People who lack the time or ability to make their own low-calorie foods or to control portion sizes may find it easier to subscribe to a service that delivers frozen prepared meals to their homes. They simply reheat them and eat. Although more costly than conventional foods, such meal plan services can provide portioned, low-calorie, nutritious meals or snacks to support weight loss, and ease the task of diet planning. Ideally, a plan should provide educational materials to help users choose wisely from conventional foods, too, to prevent old habits from returning when the service is ultimately abandoned.

KEY POINTS

- To achieve and maintain a healthy body weight, set realistic goals, keep records, eat regularly, and expect to progress slowly.
- Be aware of energy density, make the diet adequate and balanced, eliminate excess calories, and limit alcohol intakes.

Physical Activity Strategies

The most successful weight losers and maintainers include physical activity in their plans. However, weight loss through physical activity alone is not easily achieved. Physical activity guidelines were offered in the Think Fitness feature (p. 335).

Advantages of Physical Activity—and a Warning   Many people fear that exercising will intensify their hunger. Active people do have healthy appetites, but a workout helps to heighten feelings of satiation, and may delay the onset of hunger.[77] Muscle-strengthening exercise, performed regularly, adds healthful lean body tissue and provides a trim, attractive appearance. In addition, over the long term, lean muscle tissue burns more calories pound for pound than fat does.

Weight-loss dieting triggers small losses of bone mineral density but physically active dieters may avoid some of this loss, and those who also attend to protein and calcium needs offer their bones even more protection.[78] In addition, plenty of physical activity promotes restful sleep—and getting enough sleep may reduce food consumption and weight gain. Finally, physical activity helps reduce stress and stress-associated excess eating.

Heed this warning: nonathletes who reward themselves with high-calorie treats for "good behavior," or who consume "energy bars" to ease a workout (a useless strategy for most people), can easily negate any calorie deficits incurred.

Which Activities Are Best? A combination of moderate-to-vigorous aerobic exercise along with strength training at a safe level seems best for health, but any physical activity is better than none. Even moderate walking can enhance the effects of diet on fat loss and health.[79] Most important: perform at a comfortable pace within your current abilities. Rushing to improve practically guarantees injury.

Active video games, or *exergames*, and video fitness programs may help meet the physical activity needs of people who like them, but most people lose interest in just a short while.[80] Real sports not only require more energy than their video counterparts but also hold people's interest, year after year.

Hundreds of activities required for daily living also contribute to physical activity: washing the car, raking leaves, taking the stairs, and many, many others. However you do it, be active. Walk. Swim. Skate. Dance. Cycle. Skip. Lift weights. Above all, enjoy moving—and move often.

> **KEY POINT**
>
> ■ Physical activity greatly augments the rewards of weight loss dieting.

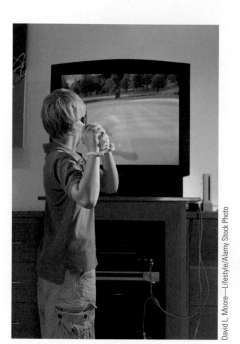

Playing a sports video game burns some calories, and the more active the game, the better.

David L. Moore—Lifestyle/Alamy Stock Photo

What Strategies Are Best for Weight Gain?

Should a thin person try to gain weight? Not necessarily. If you are healthy, fit, and energetic at your present weight, stay there. However, you may be in danger from being too thin. Warning signs include these: if your physician has advised you to gain; you are excessively tired; you are unable to keep warm; your BMI is in the "underweight" category; or (for women) you have missed at least three consecutive menstrual periods. It can be as hard for a thin person to gain a pound as it is for an overweight person to lose one, but the following strategies may help ease the way.

Choose Foods with High Energy Density Weight gainers need nutritious energy-dense foods. No matter how many sticks of celery you eat, you won't gain weight because celery simply doesn't offer enough calories per bite. Energy-dense foods (the very ones weight-loss dieters are trying to avoid) are often high in fat, but fat energy is spent in building new tissues. If the fat is mostly unsaturated, such foods will not contribute to heart disease risk. Be sure your choices are nutritious—not, say, just candy bars and potato chips.

Because fat contains more than twice as many calories per teaspoon as sugar, its calories add up quickly without adding much bulk. Moreover, its energy is in a form that is easy for the body to store. For those without the skill or ability to create their own high-calorie foods, adding a high-protein, high-calorie liquid or bar-type dietary supplement to regular nutritious meals can sometimes help underweight people to gain or maintain weight.

Portion Sizes and Meal Spacing Increasing portion sizes increases calorie intakes. Add extra slices of meats and cheeses to sandwiches and use larger plates, bowls, and glasses to disguise the appearance of the larger portions. Expect to feel full, even uncomfortably so. This feeling is normal, and it passes as the stomach gradually adapts to the extra food.

Eat frequently and keep easy-to-eat foods on hand for quick meals. Make two sandwiches in the morning and eat them between classes in addition to the day's three regular meals. Include favorite foods or ethnic dishes often—the more varied and palatable, the better. Drink beverages between meals, not with them, to save space for higher-calorie foods. Always finish with dessert. Other tips for weight gain are listed in Table 9–8.

Physical Activity to Gain Muscle and Fat   Food choices alone can produce weight gain, but the gain will be mostly fat. Overly thin people need both muscle and fat, so physical activity is essential in a sound weight-gain plan. Resistance activities are best for building muscles that can help increase healthy body mass. Start slowly and progress gradually to avoid injury. Conventional advice on diet for people building muscle is to eat about 500 to 700 calories a day above normal energy needs. This range often supports both the added activity and the formation of new muscle. Many more facts about building muscles are provided in Chapter 10.

KEY POINTS

- Weight gain can be achieved by following an eating pattern based on nutritious, calorie-dense foods, eaten frequently throughout the day.
- Physical activity helps to build lean tissue.

Medical Treatment of Obesity

LO 9.9   Describe the potential benefits and risks associated with obesity medications and surgeries.

People fatigued from fighting a losing battle with obesity, despite sincere efforts to diet and exercise, may be candidates for treatment with drugs. These approaches can cause dramatic weight loss and often save the lives of obese people at critical risk, but they present serious risks of their own.

Obesity Medications

Each year, a million and a half U.S. citizens take prescription weight-loss medications. For overweight people with a BMI of greater than 30 (greater than 27 with heart disease or its risk factors), the benefits of weight loss achieved with FDA-approved prescription medications may outweigh the health risks they present (see Table 9–9). Importantly, weight-loss drugs can help only temporarily, while they are being taken; lifestyle changes are still necessary to help manage weight over a lifetime.

Many millions of consumers, even some who are not overweight, purchase and take over-the-counter (OTC) preparations, believing them to be effective for weight loss and safe to use. OTC weight-loss pills, powders, herbs, and other "dietary supplements" are not associated with successful weight loss, however, and they may not be safe; they often present risk with no benefit. Strong prescription diuretics, hormones, unproven experimental drugs, psychotropic drugs used to treat mental illnesses, and even banned drugs have been detected in OTC weight-loss preparations, posing serious risks to health.[81]

Obesity Surgery

A person with extreme obesity—that is, someone whose BMI is greater than 40 (greater than 35 with coexisting heart disease or its risk factors)—urgently needs to reduce body fatness. Surgery is often an option for those healthy enough to withstand it.[82]

Table 9–8
Tips for Gaining Weight

In General:

- Eat enough to store more energy than you expend—at least 500 extra calories a day.
- Exercise to build muscle.
- Be patient. Weight gain takes time (a pound per month would be reasonable).
- Choose energy-dense foods most often.
- Eat at least three meals a day, and add snacks between meals.
- Choose large portions and expect to feel full.

Specifically:

- Drink caloric fluids—juice, chocolate milk, milkshakes, smoothies, sweet coffee drinks, sweet iced tea.
- Pair raw vegetables with rich mayonnaise dips and stuff raw celery with tuna salad (use oil-packed).
- Drizzle olive oil on cooked vegetables and salads.
- Add avocado to salads instead of cucumber, top with olives instead of pickles, and choose guacamole over salsa.
- Toast split whole-grain muffins instead of bread.
- Add whipped topping to fruit.
- Add margarine and sour cream to potatoes and creamy sauces to other vegetables.

In Addition:

- Cook and bake often—delicious cooking aromas whet the appetite.
- Invite others to the table—companionship often boosts eating.
- Make meals interesting—try new vegetables and fruit, add crunchy nuts or creamy avocado, and explore the flavors of herbs and spices.
- Keep a supply of favorite snacks, such as trail mix or granola bars, handy for grabbing.
- Control stress and relax. Enjoy your food.

Table 9–9

FDA-Approved Drugs for Long-Term Weight Loss

Today's prescription weight-loss medications work by reducing appetite or reducing absorption of dietary fat.

Product	Action	Side Effects
Belviq (pronounced BELL-veek) lorcaserin hydrochloride	Stimulates brain serotonin receptors to increase satiety	Headache, dizziness, fatigue, nausea, dry mouth, and constipation; low blood glucose in people with diabetes; serotonin excess that causes agitation, confusion, fever, loss of coordination, rapid or irregular heart rate, shivering, seizures, and unconsciousness; not for use by pregnant or lactating women or by people with heart valve problems; high doses cause hallucinations
Contrave (CON-trave) naltrexone/bupropion	Combines naltrexone (used to treat alcohol and drug dependence) and bupropion (an antidepressant used in smoking cessation) to suppress appetite	Nausea, constipation, headache, vomiting, dizziness, insomnia, dry mouth, and diarrhea; increased blood pressure, accelerated heart rate, suicidal thoughts, serious neuropsychiatric events, and seizures; should not be used by pregnant women or women trying to become pregnant
Qsymia (kyoo-sim-EE-uh) phentermine/topiramate	Combines phentermine (an appetite suppressant) and topirimate (a seizure/migrane medication) that makes food seem less appealing and increases feelings of fullness	Increased heart rate; can cause birth defects if taken in the first weeks or months of pregnancy; may worsen glaucoma or hyperthyroidism; may interact with other medications
Saxenda (sax-EN-dah) liraglutide	Daily injection activates appetite-suppressing areas of the brain; lowers high blood glucose by several mechanisms	Nausea, diarrhea, constipation, vomiting, low blood glucose, inflammation of the pancreas, gallbladder disease, suppressed kidney function, suicidal thoughts, and increased heart rate; should not be used by people taking certain diabetes drugs
Xenical (ZEE-nih-cal); Alli (AL-eye) orlistat	Inhibits pancreatic lipase activity in the GI tract, thus blocking digestion and absorption of dietary fat and limiting energy intake	Cramping, diarrhea, gas, frequent bowel movements, and reduced absorption of fat-soluble vitamins; rare cases of liver injury

Note: Weight-loss drugs are most effective when taken as directed and used in combination with a reduced-calorie diet and increased physical activity.

How Surgery Works   Surgical procedures limit a person's food intake by reducing the size of the stomach and delaying the passage of food into the intestine or by reconstructing the small intestine to reduce nutrient absorption (see Figure 9–15).

Potential Benefits   Surgery results can be dramatic. In studies, a great majority of surgical patients have achieved a weight loss of at least 20 to 30 percent of their excess body weight and have kept it off for 10 years.[83] Such results depend, in large part, on compliance with dietary instructions, before, during, and after surgery.[84] For example, after recovery, patients must eat small portions, chew food completely before swallowing, and drink beverages separately from meals.

Successful surgery resulting in weight loss often brings immediate and lasting improvements to diabetes, insulin resistance, high blood cholesterol, hypertension, and heart disease, and reduces the risks of some cancers.[85] The surgery may also cause a shift in the makeup of the intestinal bacteria toward a profile more typically found in lean, healthy people.[86] People with mental depression and anxiety may find that surgery brings some relief, restoring their hope for the future.

Figure 9–15

Surgical Obesity Treatment

In sleeve gastrectomy, about 80% of the stomach is removed, leaving a tube-like structure; this greatly reduces the stomach's capacity and its output of ghrelin (the hunger hormone).

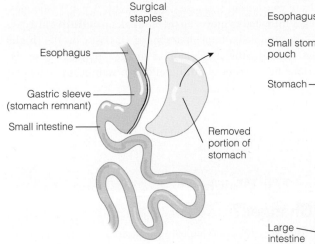

In gastric bypass, the surgeon constructs a small stomach pouch and creates an outlet directly to the lower small intestine. (Dark areas highlight the redirected flow of food.)

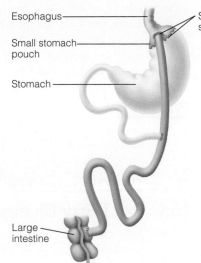

In gastric banding, the surgeon uses a gastric band to reduce the opening from the esophagus to the stomach. The size of the opening can be adjusted by inflating or deflating the band through a port located just under the skin.

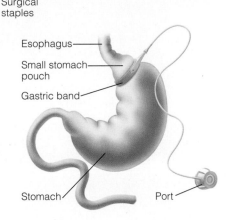

Potential Risks   Surgery is not a sure cure for obesity despite advertisements claiming so.[87] Some people do not lose the expected pounds, and others who lose weight initially regain much of it in a few years' time. Some people experience infections; nausea, vomiting, diarrhea, and dehydration; abnormal heart beats and low blood pressure; low blood glucose; confusion, sweating, weakness; and tooth erosion and dry mouth leading to dental disease.[88]

Severe nutrient deficiencies often pose a major threat to health in the years following surgery. Vitamin D deficiency results in bone abnormalities, and vitamin A deficiency causes night blindness and other vision problems.[89] Thiamin, iron, copper, zinc, vitamin B_{12}, other B vitamins, and other deficiencies are likely, but can generally be corrected with appropriate supplements.[90] Life-long nutrition and medical supervision following surgery is a must.

Other Options   Several devices have been approved by the FDA. One is an inflatable, removable balloon that is inserted nonsurgically into the stomach to reduce its capacity, but has caused pain, vomiting, and ulcers, and is under investigation for safety.[91] A second is a device worn outside the body that delivers high-frequency electrical pulses which interfere with nerve communication between the stomach and brain, delaying stomach emptying and producing feelings of fullness. A third is an implanted stomach-draining tube that allows a portion of each meal to be siphoned off after consumption. These procedures require shorter recovery times than for surgery and leave the anatomy of the digestive tract mostly intact.

KEY POINTS

- Weight-loss drugs, in concert with diet and exercise, may be prescribed for people facing medical risks from obesity.
- For people with extreme obesity or obesity with chronic diseases, surgery may pose less of a risk than does the obesity.

Herbal Products and Gimmicks

Some herbs or **botanical** products are wildly popular and may be useful for some purposes, but wise consumers avoid products containing substances not proven safe in

botanical pertaining to or made from plants; any drug, medicinal preparation, dietary supplement, or similar substance obtained from a plant.

laboratory studies. The risks are too high. One previously healthy 28-year-old body-builder was hospitalized in a coma after taking a dietary supplement containing a known liver toxin, sold to her as a "fat burner." A harmful supplement, ephedra (also called ma huang and banned by the FDA), is sold as a weight-loss "dietary supplement" but has caused cardiac arrest, abnormal heartbeats, hypertension, strokes, seizures, and death. These and many other risky weight-loss "supplements" remain available on Internet websites.[92]

Also, steam baths and saunas do not melt the fat off the body as claimed, although they may dehydrate you so that you lose water weight. Brushes, sponges, wraps, creams, and massages intended to move, burn, or break up **cellulite** are useless for fat loss. Cellulite—the rumpled, dimpled, stubborn fat tissue on the thighs and buttocks—is simply fat, awaiting the body's call for energy. Such nonsense distracts people from the serious business of planning effective weight-management strategies.

KEY POINT

- The effectiveness of herbal products and other gimmicks has not been demonstrated, and they may prove hazardous.

Once I've Changed My Weight, How Can I Stay Changed?

Millions have experienced the frustration of achieving a desired change in weight only to see their hard work visibly slip away in a seemingly never-ending cycle: "I have lost 200 pounds over my lifetime, but I was never more than 20 pounds overweight." Disappointment, frustration, and self-condemnation are common in dieters who have slipped back to their original weights or even higher.

Self-Efficacy and Other Keys to Success   Contrary to popular belief, many people who set out to lose weight do so, and many maintain their losses for years. No one can yet say which of their "secrets of success" may be responsible, but the habits of those individuals are of interest to researchers and dieters alike, and they are offered in Table 9–10. In general, such people believe in their ability to control their weight, an attribute known as **self-efficacy**. They also monitor their intakes and body weights, quickly addressing small **lapses** to prevent major ones. They all use techniques that work for them; people's responses to any one method are highly variable.

Without a doubt, a key to weight maintenance is accepting the task as a life-long endeavor, not a goal to be achieved and forgotten. Most people who maintain weight loss continue to employ many of the routines that reduced their weight in the first place.[93] They cultivate healthy habits, they remind themselves of the continuing need to manage their weight, they monitor their weight and routines, they renew their commitment to regular physical activity, and they reward themselves for sticking with their plans.

Without a life-long plan, those who try to lose weight may become trapped in endless repeating rounds of weight loss and regain—"yo-yo" dieting. Evidence conflicts about whether a history of such **weight cycling** impedes future weight loss efforts.[94] Weight cycling may pose a risk to the heart, however, if weight rebounds bring surges in blood pressure, blood lipids, or blood glucose.[95] The Food Feature explores how a person who is ready to change can modify daily eating and exercise behaviors into healthy, life-long habits.

Seek Support   Group support can prove helpful when making life changes. Some people find it useful to join such groups as Take Off Pounds Sensibly (TOPS), Weight Watchers (WW), Overeaters Anonymous (OA), or others. Others prefer to form their own self-help groups or find support online. The Internet offers numerous opportunities for weight-loss education, counseling, and virtual group support that may be effective alternatives to face-to-face or telephone counseling programs. Well-designed applications for smartphones and other mobile devices can help dieters track food intakes and

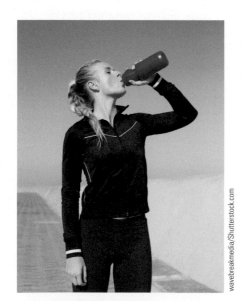

Don't forget to drink enough water—it can produce feelings of fullness, and it's calorie-free.

wavebreakmedia/Shutterstock.com

cellulite (CELL-yoo-light) a term popularly used to describe dimpled fat tissue on the thighs and buttocks; not recognized in science.

self-efficacy a person's belief in his or her ability to succeed in an undertaking.

lapses periods of returning to old habits.

weight cycling repeated rounds of weight loss and subsequent regain that may pose health risks; also called *yo-yo dieting*.

Summary of Lifestyle Strategies for Successful Weight Loss

In addition to calorie control and exercise, people who lost weight and kept it off report using strategies in the following four categories. No one strategy is universally useful—responses vary widely, and individualized weight-loss plans work best.

General

- Make a long-term commitment (greater than 6 months' duration).
- Target all three weight-management components (eating habits, physical activity, and behavior change).
- Monitor food intake and body weight (particularly to maintain weight loss).
- Follow a commercial weight-loss program (particularly for initial weight loss).
- Target weight management specifically rather than other worthy goals, such as disease prevention.

Eating Habits

- Consume a calorie-reduced diet with adequate protein, controlled in fat and carbohydrate.
- Focus on the total energy of the diet rather than on the elimination of specific energy-nutrient components.
- Consume low-fat protein sources (particularly for weight maintenance).
- Limit intakes of types of foods (such as high-sugar foods/beverages, low-fiber foods, or high-fat restaurant foods).
- Maintain dietary routines.

Physical Activity

- Perform 150–250 min/week of moderate physical activity to prevent weight gain; even a few minutes of exercise at a time counts toward the total.
- Perform more than 250 min/week of moderate physical activity to promote significant weight loss; even a few minutes of exercise at a time counts toward the total.
- Exercise more—on average, an hour a day; the total time may be divided into smaller blocks throughout the day.
- Watch less than 10 hours of television per week.

Behavior Change/Nutrition Counseling

- Use behavioral change techniques to produce weight loss of 5 percent or more of body weight.
- Use cognitive behavior therapy to augment diet and physical activities.
- Obtain structured, individualized nutrition counseling to support weight-loss efforts.
- Use Internet-based education and tracking applications, particularly in the short term.
- Weigh on a scale at least once a week.
- Recognize and attend to minor lapses.

Sources: 2018 Physical Activity Guidelines Advisory Committee, 2018 Physical Activity Guidelines Advisory Committee Scientific Report (Washington, DC: U.S. Department of Health and Human Services, 2018); National Academies of Sciences, Engineering, and Medicine, The challenge of treating obesity and overweight: Proceedings of a workshop, (2017), epub, doi: https://doi.org/10.17226/24855; American College of Cardiology/American Heart Association Task Force on Practice Guidelines and the Obesity Society, Executive summary: Guidelines (2013) for the management of overweight and obesity in adults, Obesity 22 (2014): S5–S39; S. F. Kirk and coauthors, Effective weight management practice: A review of the lifestyle intervention evidence, International Journal of Obesity 36 (2012): 178–185.

physical activity and to discover calorie information. As with all approaches, choose wisely and avoid scams.

KEY POINT

- People who succeed at maintaining lost weight believe in their own abilities, keep to their eating routines, keep exercising, and keep track of calorie intakes and body weight.

Conclusion

This chapter winds up where it began, considering the U.S. obesity epidemic as a societal problem. Reversing it may depend at least partly on the public will to support healthy lifestyle choices. Meanwhile, individuals can make choices to influence their own behaviors, as this chapter's Food Feature points out.

Behavior Modification for Weight Control

LO 9.10 Justify the importance of behavior modification in supporting changes in diet and exercise.

Supporting changes in both diet and exercise is **behavior modification**. This form of therapy can help dieters to cement into place all the behaviors that lead to and perpetuate the desired body composition.

How Does Behavior Modification Work?

Behavior modification works by altering both thought processes and behaviors.[96] It is based on the knowledge that habits drive behaviors. Suppose a friend tells you about a shortcut to class. To take it, you must make a left-hand turn at a corner where you now turn right. You decide to try the shortcut the next day, but when you arrive at the familiar corner, you turn right as always. Not until you arrive at class do you realize that you failed to turn left, as you had planned. You can learn to turn left, of course, but at first, you will have to make an effort to remember to do so. After a while, the new behavior will become as automatic as the old one was.

A food and activity diary is a powerful ally to help you learn what particular eating stimuli, or cues, affect you. Such self-monitoring is indispensable for learning to control eating and exercising cues, both positive and negative, and for tracking your progress. Figure 9–16 provides a simple pencil-and-paper food and activity diary for self-monitoring. Computerized tracking programs, such as this textbook's *Diet + Wellness Plus*, and some applications for smartphones are also effective tools.

Once you identify the behaviors you need to change, do not attempt to modify all of them at once. Set your priorities, and begin with a few behaviors you can handle—practice until they become habitual and automatic, and then select one or two more. For those striving to lose weight, learning to say "No, thank you" might be among the first habits to establish. Learning not to "clean your plate" might follow.

Modifying Behaviors

Behavior researchers have identified six elements useful in replacing old eating and activity habits with new ones:

1. Eliminate inappropriate eating and activity cues.
2. Suppress the cues you cannot eliminate.
3. Strengthen cues to appropriate eating and activities.
4. Repeat the desired eating and physical activity behaviors.
5. Arrange or emphasize negative consequences of inappropriate eating or sedentary behaviors.
6. Arrange or emphasize positive consequences of appropriate eating and exercise behaviors.

Table 9–11 provides specific examples of putting these six elements into action.

To begin, set about eliminating or suppressing the cues that prompt you to eat inappropriately. An overeater's life may include many such cues: watching television, talking on the telephone,

Figure 9–16

A Sample Food and Activity Diary

Record the times and places of meals and snacks, the types and amounts of foods consumed, surroundings and people present, and mood while eating. Describe physical activities, their intensity and duration, and your feelings about them, too. Use this information to structure eating and exercise in ways that serve your physical and emotional needs.

Time	Place	Activity or food eaten	People present	Mood
10:30–10:40	School vending machine	6 peanut butter crackers and 12 oz. cola	by myself	Starved
12:15–12:30	Restaurant	Sub sandwich and 12 oz. cola	friends	relaxed & friendly
3:00–3:45	Gym	Weight training	workout partner	tired
4:00–4:10	Snack bar	Small frozen yogurt	by myself	OK

behavior modification alteration of behavior using methods based on the theory that actions can be controlled by manipulating the environmental factors that cue, or trigger, the actions.

Table 9–11

Behavior Modification Tips for Weight Loss

Use these actions during both weight-loss and maintenance phases of weight management.

1. Eliminate inappropriate eating cues:
   - Don't buy problem foods.
   - Eat only in one place at the designated time.
   - Shop when not hungry.
   - Replace large plates, cups, and utensils with smaller ones.
   - Avoid vending machines, fast-food restaurants, and convenience stores.
   - Measure out appropriate snack portions to eat during entertainment.

2. Suppress the cues you cannot eliminate:
   - Serve individual plates; don't serve "family style."
   - Measure your portions; avoid large servings or packages of food.
   - Remove food from the table after eating a meal.
   - Create obstacles to consuming problem foods—wrap them and freeze them, making them less quickly accessible.
   - Control deprivation; plan and eat regular meals.
   - Limit screen time and other sedentary activities to one hour a day.

3. Strengthen cues to appropriate eating and exercise:
   - Choose to dine with companions who make appropriate food choices.
   - Learn appropriate portion sizes.
   - Plan appropriate snacks, and keep them handy.
   - Keep sports and play equipment by the door.

4. Repeat the desired eating and exercise behaviors:
   - Slow down eating—always use utensils and put them down between bites.
   - Leave some food on your plate.
   - Move more—shake a leg, pace, stretch often; join active groups.

5. Arrange or emphasize negative consequences for inappropriate eating:
   - Ask that others respond neutrally to your deviations (make no comments—even negative attention is a reward).
   - If you slip, don't punish yourself.

6. Arrange rewards and notice positive effects of your appropriate eating and exercise behaviors:
   - Buy tickets to sports events, movies, concerts, or other nonfood amusement.
   - Get a massage; indulge in a small purchase; buy flowers.
   - Take a hot bath; read a good book; nap; relax.
   - Treat yourself to a lesson in a new activity such as handball or tennis.
   - Praise yourself; visit friends.

mechanisms to overcome the weaker satiety signals.

Cognitive Skills

Behavior therapists often teach **cognitive skills**, or new ways of thinking, to help dieters solve problems and correct false thinking that can short-circuit healthy eating behaviors. Thinking habits turn out to be as important as eating habits in achieving a healthy body weight, and thinking habits can be changed. A paradox of change is that it takes believing in oneself and honoring oneself to lay the foundation for changing that self. That is, self-acceptance predicts success, while self-loathing predicts failure. "Positive self-talk" is a practice worth cultivating—many people succeed because their mental dialogue supports, rather than degrades, their efforts. Negative thoughts ("I'm not getting thin anyway, so what's the use of continuing?") should be viewed in the light of empirical evidence ("my starting weight: 174 pounds; today's weight: 163 pounds").

Give yourself credit for your new behaviors; take honest stock of any physical improvements, too, such as lower blood pressure or less painful knees, even without a noticeable change in pant size. Finally, remember to enjoy your emerging fit and healthy self.

cognitive skills as taught in behavior therapy, changes to conscious thoughts with the goal of improving adherence to lifestyle modifications; examples are problem-solving skills and the correction of false negative thoughts, termed *cognitive restructuring*.

entering a convenience store, studying late at night. Resolve that you will no longer respond to such cues by eating. If some cues to inappropriate eating behavior cannot be eliminated, suppress them; then strengthen the appropriate cues, and reward yourself for doing so. The list of possibilities is virtually endless, but Table 9–11, section 6 lists a few of them.

In addition, be aware that the food marketing industry spends huge sums each year developing cues to modify consumers' behaviors in the opposite direction—toward buying and consuming more snack foods, soft drinks, and other products. These cues work on a subconscious level; they leverage the stronger human hunger and appetite

What did you decide?

How can you **control** your body weight, once and for all?

Why are you **tempted** by a favorite treat when you don't feel hungry?

How do extra calories from food become **fat** in your body?

Which popular **diets** are best for managing body weight?

What's online?

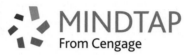
MINDTAP
From Cengage

Visit www.Cengage.com to access MindTap, a complete digital course that includes Diet & Wellness Plus, interactive quizzes, videos, and more.

Self Check

1. (LO 9.1) All of the following are health risks associated with excessive body fat except _____.
   a. kidney disease
   c. gallbladder disease
   b. sleep apnea
   d. low blood lipids

2. (LO 9.1) Today, an estimated 70 percent of the adults in the United States are overweight or obese.
   T F

3. (LO 9.2) Which of the following statements about basal metabolic rate (BMR) is correct?
   a. The greater a person's age, the higher the BMR.
   b. The more thyroxine produced, the higher the BMR.
   c. Fever lowers the BMR.
   d. Pregnancy lowers the BMR.

4. (LO 9.2) The thermic effect of food plays a major role in energy expenditure.
   T F

5. (LO 9.3) The BMI standard is an excellent tool for evaluating obesity in athletes and the elderly.
   T F

6. (LO 9.3) Body fat can be assessed by which of the following techniques?
   a. a blood lipid test
   b. chest circumference
   c. dual energy X-ray absorptiometry
   d. all of the above

7. (LO 9.3) BMI is of limited value for _____.
   a. athletes
   b. pregnant and lactating women
   c. adults older than age 65
   d. all of the above

8. (LO 9.4) The appetite-stimulating hormone ghrelin is made by the _____.
   a. brain
   c. pancreas
   b. fat tissue
   d. stomach

9. (LO 9.4) When the brain receives signals that enough food has been eaten, this is called _____.
   a. satiation
   c. adaptation
   b. ghrelin
   d. none of the above

10. (LO 9.5) Brown adipose tissue _____.
    a. develops during starvation
    b. is a well-known heat-generating tissue
    c. develops as fat cells die off
    d. all of the above

11. (LO 9.5) According to genomic researchers, a single inherited gene is the probable cause of common obesity.
    T F

12. (LO 9.6) In many people, any kind of stress can cause overeating and weight gain.
    T F

13. (LO 9.6) A built environment can support physical activity with _____.
    a. safe biking and walking lanes
    b. public parks
    c. free exercise facilities
    d. all of the above

14. (LO 9.7) Which of the following is a physical consequence of fasting?
    a. loss of lean body tissues
    b. lasting weight loss
    c. body cleansing
    d. all of the above

15. (LO 9.7) The nervous system cannot use fat as fuel.
    T F

16. (LO 9.7) A diet too low in carbohydrate produces physical responses similar to those seen in fasting.
    T F

17. (LO 9.8) The number of calories to cut from the diet to produce weight loss should be based on
    a. the amount of weight the person wishes to lose.
    b. the person's BMI.
    c. the amount of food the person wishes to consume.
    d. the DRI for energy for the person's gender and age.

18. (LO 9.9) Over-the-counter drugs for obesity are most often effective and pose little risk.
    T F

19. (LO 9.10) Most people who successfully maintain weight loss do all of the following except
    a. continue to employ many of the routines that reduced their weight in the first place.
    b. obtain at least some guidance from popular diet books.
    c. reward themselves for sticking with their plan.
    d. monitor their weight and routine.

20. (LO 9.11) Adolescents are likely to grow out of early disordered eating behaviors by young adulthood.
    T F

Answers to these Self Check questions are in Appendix G.

The Perils of Eating Disorders

LO 9.11 Outline the risk factors, symptoms, and treatments of eating disorders.

Tens of millions of people in the United States, most of them girls and women, suffer from some form of **eating disorder**, such as **anorexia nervosa**, **bulimia nervosa**, and **binge eating disorder**. Without treatment, many of those who have an eating disorder will incur physical and mental harm, and some will die as a result. Most alarming, the prevalence of eating disorders is both rising and they are occurring at progressively younger ages.[1*] (Table C9–1 defines eating disorder terms.)

An estimated 85 percent of eating disorders start during adolescence. Children of this age often exhibit warnings of disordered eating such as restrained eating, binge eating, purging, fear of fatness, and distorted body image. Many adolescents diet to lose weight and choose unhealthy behaviors associated with disordered eating; by college

age, the behaviors can be entrenched.[2] Disordered eating behaviors in early life set a pattern that is likely to continue into young adulthood. Importantly, healthful dieting and physical activity in overweight adolescents appear not to trigger eating disorders.

Society's Influence

Why do so many people in our society suffer from eating disorders? Most experts agree that eating disorders have many causes: sociocultural, psychological, and possibly also genetic and neurochemical. Without a doubt, our society sets unrealistic ideals for body weight, especially for women.[3] Normal-weight girls as young as 5 years old are placed "on diets" for fear that they are too fat.

When thinness takes on heightened importance, people begin to view the

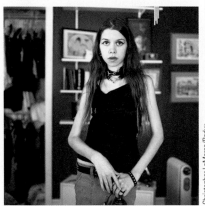

Figure C9–1

Anorexia Nervosa

The extreme weight loss of anorexia nervosa is, in reality, the result of prolonged starvation that poses serious threats to health and life.

Christopher LaMarca/Redux

normal, healthy body as too fat—their body images become distorted. People of all shapes, sizes, and ages—including emaciated fashion models with anorexia nervosa—have learned to be unhappy with their "overweight" bodies. Many take serious risks to lose even more weight. This results in the extreme thinness typical of anorexia nervosa, as illustrated by the young girl in Figure C9–1. Once almost nonexistent in non-Western cultures, eating disorders are now rapidly increasing as global communities internalize thinness as an ideal.[4]

Media Messages

Society perpetuates unrealistic body ideals and devalues those who do not conform to them. Beauty pageants, for example, put forth a standard of female desirability—thinner and thinner women over the years have won these events. Magazines, Facebook and other social

Table C9–1

Eating Disorder Terms

- **anorexia nervosa** an eating disorder characterized by extreme restriction of energy intake relative to requirements, leading to a dangerously low body weight and a disturbed perception of body weight and shape; seen (usually) in teenage girls and young women (anorexia means "without appetite"; nervos means "of nervous origin").
- **binge eating disorder** an eating disorder whose criteria are similar to those of bulimia nervosa, excluding purging or other compensatory behaviors.
- **bulimia** (byoo-LEEM-ee-uh) **nervosa** recurring episodes of binge eating combined with a morbid fear of becoming fat, usually followed by self-induced vomiting, misuse of laxatives or diuretics, fasting, or excessive exercise.
- **cathartic** a strong laxative.
- **cognitive behavioral therapy** psychological therapy aimed at changing undesirable behaviors by changing underlying thought processes contributing to these behaviors; in anorexia, a goal is to replace false beliefs about body weight, eating, and self-worth with health-promoting beliefs.
- **eating disorder** a disturbance in eating behavior that jeopardizes a person's physical or psychological health.
- **emetic** (em-ETT-ic) an agent that causes vomiting.
- **female athlete triad** a potentially fatal triad of medical problems seen in female athletes: low energy availability (with or without disordered eating), menstrual dysfunction, and low bone mineral density.

*Reference notes are in Appendix F.

websites, films and television, and other media convey a message that to be happy, beautiful, and desirable, one must first be thin.[5] As they search for identity, adolescent girls are particularly vulnerable to such messages.

Dieting as Risk

Severe food restriction often precedes an eating disorder. Ill-advised "dieting" can create intense stress and extreme hunger and lead to binges. Painful emotions such as anger, jealousy, or disappointment may be turned inward by youngsters, some still in kindergarten, who express dissatisfaction with body weight or say they "feel fat." As weight loss and severe food restriction become more and more a focus, psychological problems worsen, and the likelihood of developing full-blown eating disorders intensifies.

Eating Disorders in Athletes

Athletes and dancers are at special risk for eating disorders. They may severely restrict energy intakes in an attempt to enhance performance or appearance or to meet the weight guidelines of a sport. In reality, severe energy restriction causes a loss of lean tissue that impairs physical performance and imposes a risk of eating disorders. Risk factors for eating disorders among athletes include:

- Young age (adolescence).
- Pressure to excel in a sport.
- Focus on achieving or maintaining an "ideal" body weight, muscular structure, or body fat percentage.
- Participation in sports or competitions that require low body weight, a lean appearance or that are judged on aesthetic appeal, such as gymnastics, wrestling, figure skating, or dance.[6]
- Unhealthy, unsupervised weight-loss dieting at an early age.

Male athletes—especially dancers, wrestlers, skaters, jockeys, and gymnasts—suffer from eating disorders at a greater rate than their peers, but their gender may cause coaches, parents, and medical professionals to overlook their condition. Adolescent boys, newly aware of developing muscularity, may take dangerous risks involving enhancement products and extreme diets in their quests to attain unachievable physiques.[7]

The Female Athlete Triad

In female athletes, three associated medical problems form the **female athlete triad** (see Figure C9–2).[8] For example, at age 14, Suzanne was a top contender for a spot on the state gymnastics team. Each day, her coach reminded team members that they would not qualify to compete if they weighed more than a few ounces above the assigned weights.

Suzanne weighed herself several times a day to ensure that she did not top her 80-pound limit. She dieted and exercised to extremes; unlike many of her friends, she never began to menstruate. A few months before her 15th birthday, Suzanne's coach dropped her back to the second-level team because of a slow-healing stress fracture. Mentally and physically exhausted, she quit gymnastics and began overeating between periods of self-starvation. Suzanne exhibited all the signs of female athlete triad—disordered eating, amenorrhea, and weakened bones—but no one put them together in time to protect her physical and mental health.

An athlete's body must be heavier for a given height than a nonathlete's body because it contains more muscle and dense bone tissue with less fat. However, coaches often use weight standards, such as BMI, that cannot properly gauge an athlete's body. For athletes, body composition measures such as skinfold tests yield more useful information.

The prevalence of amenorrhea among premenopausal women in the United States is about 2 to 5 percent overall, but it may be well over 60 percent among female athletes. Amenorrhea is *not* a normal adaptation to strenuous physical training but a symptom of something going wrong.[9]

Male Athletes and Eating Disorders

Male athletes and dancers with eating disorders often deny having them because they mistakenly believe that eating disorders strike only women. Under the same pressures as female athletes, males skip meals, restrict fluids, practice in plastic suits, or train in heated rooms to lose a quick 4 to 7 pounds.[10] Many male high school wrestlers, gymnasts, and figure skaters strive for as little as 5 percent body fat. Wrestlers, especially, must "make weight" to compete in the lowest possible weight class to face smaller opponents.

For young people, unrealistic standards based on appearance, weight, or body type should be replaced with performance-based standards. Table C9–2 provides some suggestions to help athletes and dancers protect themselves against eating disorders.

From their names alone, the categories of eating disorders may sound

Figure C9–2

The Female Athlete Triad

In the female athlete triad, extreme weight loss causes both menstruation dysfunction and excessive loss of calcium from the bones, weakening them.

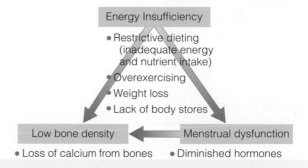

Energy Insufficiency
- Restrictive dieting (inadequate energy and nutrient intake)
- Overexercising
- Weight loss
- Lack of body stores

Low bone density
- Loss of calcium from bones

Menstrual dysfunction
- Diminished hormones

Tips for Combating Eating Disorders

General Guideline

- Never restrict food intakes to below the amounts suggested for adequacy by the USDA Eating Patterns (Chapter 2).
- Eat regularly. People who eat regularly throughout the day never get so hungry that hunger dictates their food choices.
- If not at a healthy weight, establish a reasonable weight goal based on a healthy body composition.
- Allow a reasonable time to achieve the goal. A reasonable rate for losing excess fat is about 1% of body weight per week.
- Learn to recognize media image biases, and reject ultrathin standards for beauty. Shift focus to health, compete

Specific Guidelines for Athletes and Dancers

- Replace weight-based or appearance-based goals with performance-based goals.
- Remember that eating disorders impair physical performance. Seek confidential help in obtaining treatment if needed.
- Restrict weight-loss activities to the off-season.
- Focus on proper nutrition as an important facet of training, as important as proper technique.

distinct, but they often overlap. A person may migrate from type to type, or an eating disorder may fail to fall into a clear pattern. Three main characteristics of eating disorders have been described:

1. Eating habits or weight-control behaviors have become abnormal.
2. Clinically significant impairments of physical health or psychosocial functioning have materialized.
3. The disturbance is not caused by other medical or psychiatric conditions.

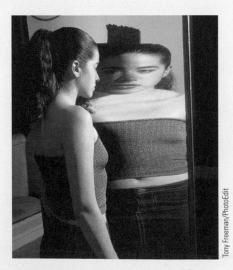

A distorted body image underlies many eating disorders.

Tony Freeman/PhotoEdit

The problems described in the next section are typical.

Anorexia Nervosa

Julie is 17 years old and a straight-A superachiever in school. She also watches her diet with great care, and she exercises daily, maintaining a heroic schedule of self-discipline. She stands 5 feet 6 inches tall and weighs only 85 pounds, but she is determined to lose weight. She has anorexia nervosa.

Characteristics of Anorexia Nervosa

Julie is unaware that she is undernourished, and she sees no need to obtain treatment. She insists that she is too fat, although her eyes are sunk in deep hollows in her face. She visits pro-anorexia (pro-ana) blogs and websites to find support for her distorted body image and to learn more starvation tips. When Julie looks at herself in the mirror, she sees her 85-pound body as fat. The more Julie overestimates her body size, the more resistant she is to treatment and the more unwilling she is to examine misperceptions.

She has stopped menstruating and is moody and chronically depressed but blames external circumstances. She is close to physical exhaustion, but she

no longer sleeps easily. Her family is concerned, and although reluctant to push her, they have finally insisted that she see a psychiatrist. Julie's psychiatrist has prescribed group therapy as a start but warns that if Julie does not begin to gain weight soon, she will need to be hospitalized.

No one knows for certain what causes anorexia nervosa, but some factors are associated with its development. Most people with anorexia nervosa come from middle- or upper-class families. Most are female. People with anorexia nervosa are unaware of their condition. They cannot recognize that a distorted body image that overestimates body fatness, a central feature of a diagnosis, is causing the problem. Criteria focus on people who:

- Restrict calorie intake to the point of developing a too-low body weight for age, gender, and health.
- Have an intense fear of body fatness or of weight gain, or strive to prevent weight gain although underweight.
- Hold a false perception of body weight or shape, exaggerate the importance of body weight or shape in their self-evaluation, or deny the danger of being severely underweight.

Many details on diagnostic criteria exist.[11]

Self-Starvation

How can a person as thin as Julie continue to starve herself? Julie uses tremendous discipline to strictly limit her portions of low-calorie foods. She will deny her hunger, and having become accustomed to so little food, she feels full after eating only a few bites. She can recite the calorie contents of dozens of foods and the calorie costs of as many physical activities. If she feels that she has gained an ounce of weight, she runs or jumps rope until she thinks it's gone. She drinks water incessantly to fill her stomach, risking dangerous mineral imbalances and water intoxication. She takes laxatives to hasten the passage of food from her system. She is starving, but she doesn't eat because her need for self-control overrides her need for food.

Physical Perils

From the body's point of view, anorexia nervosa is starvation and thus incurs the same damage as classic severe malnutrition. People with anorexia deplete the body tissues of needed fat and protein. A young person's growth ceases, normal development falters, and so much lean tissue is lost that basal metabolic rate slows and body temperature drops. The physical ills of anorexia nervosa (summarized in Table C9–3) may clear up with treatment, but its psychological problems and abnormal eating tendencies often linger through life, and may even extend to the next generation.[12] Mothers with anorexia nervosa may severely underfeed their children, who then fail to thrive or who develop disordered eating patterns later on.[13]

Anorexia nervosa has the highest mortality rate of all psychiatric disorders. People with anorexia nervosa are 5 times more likely than their peers to die prematurely, mostly from heart abnormalities brought on by malnutrition.[14] They are also 18 times more likely to die of suicide.

Treatment of Anorexia Nervosa

Treatment of anorexia nervosa requires a multidisciplinary approach that addresses two areas of concern: the first relating to food and weight and the second involving psychological processes. Teams of physicians, nurses, psychiatrists, family therapists, and dietitians work together to treat people with anorexia nervosa. The expertise of a registered dietitian nutritionist is essential because an appropriate, individually crafted diet is crucial for normalizing body weight and because nutrition counseling is indispensable.

Clients with low risks for physical harms may benefit from family counseling, **cognitive behavioral therapy**, other psychotherapies and nutrition guidance.[15] Those with greater risks may also need supplemental formulas to provide extra nutrients and energy. Antidepressant and other drugs are commonly prescribed but rarely help.

Clients in later stages are seldom willing to eat, but if they are, they may recover without other interventions.

Table C9–3

Physical Harms from Anorexia Nervosa

The symptoms of anorexia nervosa are those of malnutrition. Which symptoms are present and to what degree depends largely on the severity of the condition.

Organs/Systems	Effects
Blood	Anemia develops.
	Blood lipids are altered.
	Blood pressure falls.
	Blood proteins diminish.
Bones	Bone density declines; osteoporosis ensues.
Brain and nerves	Brain tissue shrinks significantly.
	Brain electrical activity becomes abnormal.
	Insomnia develops.
	Nerves lose normal function.
Digestive system and nutrient metabolism	Stomach emptying slows.
	Intestinal absorptive lining shrinks.
	Nutrient absorption is reduced.
	Pancreas slows digestive enzyme output.
	Diarrhea and malnutrition ensue.
	Iron deficiency develops.
	Vitamin A collects abnormally in blood.
	Vitamin D blood level declines, despite adequate intake.
Fluid and electrolytes	Cellular potassium losses occur.
	Other electrolytes become unbalanced.
Heart	Heartbeat becomes inefficient, irregular.
	Heart muscles thin and weaken.
	Heart failure; death ensues.
Immunity	Immune response is impaired; antibodies diminish.
Kidneys	Kidneys fail; death ensues.
Reproductive functions	Menstruation ceases (women).
	Sex drive diminishes (women and men).
Skin/hair	Skin grows fine body hair (the body's attempt to keep warm).
	Skin becomes dry and thin.
Temperature regulation	Body temperature falls.

Sources: M. M. Fichter and N. Quadflieg, Mortality in eating disorders—results of a large prospective clinical longitudinal study, International Journal of Eating Disorders 49 (2016): 391–401; A. A. Donaldson and C. M. Gordon, Skeletal complications of eating disorders, Metabolism (2015): 943–951; S. Gaudio and coauthors, A systematic review of resting-state functional-MRI studies in anorexia nervosa: Evidence for functional connectivity impairment in cognitive control and visuospatial and body-signal integration, Neuroscience and Biobehavioral Reviews 71 (2016): 578–589; C. Stheneur, S. Bergeron, and A. L. Lapeyraque, Renal complications in anorexia nervosa, Eating and Weight Disorders 19 (2014): 455–460; D. Modan-Moses and coauthors, High prevalence of vitamin D deficiency and insufficiency in adolescent inpatients diagnosed with eating disorders, International Journal of Eating Disorders (2014), epub, doi:10.1002/eat.22347; W. Renthal, I. Marin-Valencia, and P. A. Evans, Thiamine deficiency secondary to anorexia nervosa: An uncommon cause of peripheral neuropathy and Wernicke encephalopathy in adolescence, Pediatric Neurology 51 (2014): 100–103.

When starvation leads to severe underweight (less than 75 percent of ideal body weight), high medical risks ensue, necessitating hospitalization. Patients must be stabilized and fed through tubes to forestall death.[16] Even after recovery, however, energy intakes and eating behaviors may never fully return to normal, and relapses are common, particularly during the first year of treatment.[17]

Before drawing conclusions about someone who is extremely thin, be aware that a diagnosis of anorexia nervosa requires professional assessment. People seeking help for anorexia nervosa for themselves or for others should not delay but should visit the National Eating Disorders Association website or pick up the phone and call them.[†]

Bulimia Nervosa

Sophia is a 20-year-old flight attendant, and although her body weight is healthy, she thinks constantly about food. She alternately starves herself and then secretly binges. When she has eaten too much, she vomits. Few people would fail to recognize that these symptoms signify bulimia nervosa.

Characteristics of Bulimia Nervosa

Bulimia nervosa is distinct from anorexia nervosa and is much more prevalent in both women and men. People with bulimia nervosa often suffer in secret and, when asked, may deny the existence of a problem. Here are some general diagnostic criteria for bulimia nervosa:

- Frequent binge eating behavior—that is, eating a relatively large amount of food in a relatively short period of time, with loss of control over binges.

- Compensation behaviors after binges, such as vomiting or fasting.

- False perceptions of body weight or shape; exaggerations of the importance of body weight or shape in self-evaluation.[18]

[†] *The National Eating Disorders website address is www.nationaleatingdisorders.org; the toll-free referral line is (800) 931–2237.*

Sophia is well educated and close to her ideal body weight, although her weight fluctuates over a range of 10 pounds or so every few weeks. As a young teen, Sophia cycled on and off crash diets.

Sophia seldom lets her bulimia nervosa interfere with her work or other activities. However, she is emotionally insecure, feels anxious at social events, and cannot easily establish close relationships. She is usually depressed and often impulsive. When crisis hits, Sophia responds with an overwhelming urge to binge, a behavior pattern that prevents the weight loss she desires.[19] Her negative self-perceptions drive a perpetual cycle of binge eating and purging (Figure C9-3).

Binge Eating and Purging

A bulimic binge is a compulsion and unlike normal eating. During a binge, Sophia's eating is rapid and uncontrollable, accelerated by her hunger from previous calorie restriction. She regularly takes in extra food approaching 1,000 calories at each binge, and she may have several binges in a day. Typical binge foods are easy-to-eat, low-fiber, smooth-textured, high-fat, and high-carbohydrate foods, such as cookies, cakes, and ice cream; and she eats the entire bag of cookies, the whole cake, and every spoonful in a carton of ice cream. By the end of the binge, she has vastly overcorrected for her earlier attempts at calorie restriction.

To purge the food from her body, she may use a **cathartic**—a strong laxative that can injure the lower intestinal tract. Or she may induce vomiting, sometimes with an **emetic**—a drug intended as first aid for poisoning. After the binge, she pays the price with hands scraped raw against the teeth during gag-induced vomiting, swollen neck glands and reddened eyes from straining to vomit, and the bloating, fatigue, headache, nausea, and pain that follow.

Physical and Psychological Perils

Purging may seem to offer a quick way to rid the body of unwanted calories,

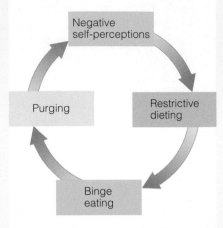

Figure C9–3

The Cycle of Binge Eating, Purging, and Negative Self-Perception

Each of these factors helps to perpetuate disordered eating.

but bingeing and purging have serious physical consequences. Fluid and electrolyte imbalances caused by vomiting or diarrhea can lead to abnormal heart rhythms; one common emetic causes heart muscle damage, and its overuse can cause death from heart failure.[‡] Vomiting causes irritation and infection of the pharynx, esophagus, and salivary glands; erosion of the teeth; and dental caries. The esophagus or stomach may rupture or tear.

Unlike Julie, Sophia is aware that her behavior is abnormal. She wants to recover, and this makes recovery more likely for her than for Julie, who clings to denial.

Treatment of Bulimia Nervosa

Effective treatment plans, particularly for children and adolescents, begin with family counseling to empower caregivers to help their family member recover.[20] To gain control over food and establish regular eating patterns requires adherence to a structured eating and exercise plan. Restrictive dieting is forbidden, for it almost always precedes binges. Many a former bulimia nervosa sufferer has

[‡] *The heart-damaging emetic is ipecac (IP-eh-kak).*

Chapter 9 Energy Balance and Healthy Body Weight

Table C9–4

Diet Strategies for Combating Bulimia Nervosa

Planning Principles

- Plan meals and snacks; record plans in a food diary prior to eating.
- Plan meals and snacks that require eating at the table and using utensils.
- Refrain from eating "finger foods."
- Refrain from "dieting" or skipping meals.

Nutrition Principles

- Eat a well-balanced diet and regularly timed meals consisting of a variety of foods.
- Include raw vegetables, salad, or raw fruit at meals to prolong eating times.
- Choose whole-grain, high-fiber breads, pasta, rice, and cereals to increase bulk.
- Consume adequate fluid, particularly water.

Other Tips

- Choose meals that provide protein and fat for satiety and bulky, fiber-rich carbohydrates for immediate feelings of fullness.
- Try including soups and other water-rich foods for satiety.
- Consume the amounts of food specified in the USDA Eating Patterns (Chapter 2).
- Select foods that naturally divide into portions. Select one potato, rather than rice or pasta that can be overloaded onto the plate; purchase yogurt and cottage cheese in individual containers; look for small packages of precut steak or chicken; choose frozen dinners with metered portions.
- Include 30 minutes or more of physical activity on most days—exercise may be an important tool in controlling bulimia.

taken a major step toward recovery by learning to consistently eat enough food to satisfy hunger (at least 1,600 calories a day). Table C9–4 offers some ways to begin correcting the eating problems of bulimia nervosa.

Binge Eating Disorder

Charlie is a 40-year-old former baseball outfielder who, after becoming a spectator instead of a player, has gained excess body fat and has been diagnosed with prediabetes.[21] He believes that he has the willpower to diet until he loses the fat. Periodically, he restricts his food intake for several days, only to eventually succumb to cravings for his favorite high-calorie treats. Like Charlie, many overweight people end up bingeing after dieting.

Is Binge Eating an Addiction?

A correlation between the addictive nature of binge eating and that of drug abuse has been discussed for decades.

Shared key characteristics, such as strong and persistent cravings, unsuccessful efforts to control intakes, and continuation of the behavior despite physical harm or other negative results, give rise to the concept of an *eating addiction*.[22]§ As explained earlier in this chapter, the effects on the brain of foods rich in sugars and fats mimic those of euphoria-producing drugs in some ways, and similarities exist in psychological and behavioral constructs, too. Although in its early stages, research on the shared features of substance abuse and eating disorders may uncover new treatments for both conditions.[23]

Treating Binge Eating

Binge eating behavior responds more readily to treatment than other eating disorders. Intervention, even if obtained on an Internet website, improves

§ The Diagnostic and Statistical Manual, *5th edition, sets diagnostic criteria for substance use disorders. The Yale Food Addiction Scale, an inventory based on substance use criteria, is under review as a potential diagnostic tool for food addiction.*

physical and mental health and may permanently break the cycle of rapid weight losses and gains.

Toward Prevention

Treatments for existing eating disorders have evolved, but prevention of these conditions is far preferable. One approach may be to provide children and adolescents with defenses against influences that promote eating disorders. A set of suggestions intended to help pediatricians avert eating disorders in their patients might also apply to teachers, coaches, and others who deal with children:

1. Encourage positive eating and physical behaviors that can be maintained over a lifetime; discourage dieting, skipping of meals, or the use of diet pills.
2. Promote a positive body image; do not use body dissatisfaction as a motivator for behavior change.
3. Encourage frequent and enjoyable family meals consumed at home; discourage hasty meals eaten alone.
4. Focus not on weight but on healthy eating and physical activities; facilitate healthy eating and physical activity at home.
5. Ask about mistreatment or bullying and address this issue with patients and their families.
6. Carefully monitor necessary weight loss and prevent the development of semi-starvation.[24]

Protection against eating disorders in the next generation largely depends on the actions of adults in authority today. Perhaps a young person's best defense against eating disorders is to learn about normal, expected growth patterns, especially the characteristic weight gain of adolescence (see Chapter 14), and to learn to respect the inherent wisdom of the body. When people discover and honor the body's real needs for nutrition and exercise, they often will not sacrifice health for conformity.

Critical Thinking

1. Eating disorders are common only in cultures where extreme thinness is an ideal. Who in society do you think sets such ideals? How are these ideals conveyed to others? Suggest some steps that schools, parents, and other influential adults might take to help to minimize the impact of idealized body types on children as they develop their own self-images.

2. Form a small group. Each member of the group gives an example of a role model that he or she would like to emulate. This can be, for example, a teacher, athlete, movie star, or scientist, among others. State all of the reasons for choosing this person as a role model. Now talk about the body type of each role model. Would you like to achieve that body type? Is it possible to do so? Of all the role models discussed in your group, which role model do you believe is the healthiest and why?

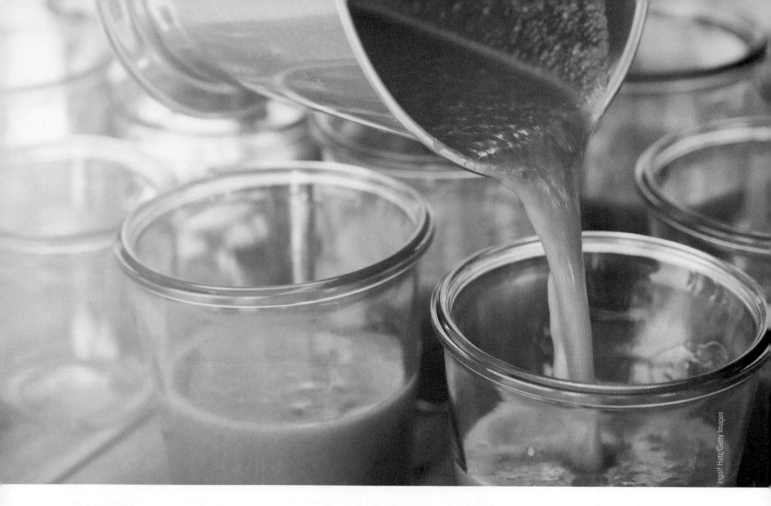

Ingolf Hatz/Getty Images

10 Performance Nutrition

Learning Objectives

After completing this chapter, you should be able to accomplish the following:

LO 10.1 Enumerate the benefits of physical fitness.

LO 10.2 Describe muscle adaptability and the effects of physical training.

LO 10.3 Describe the three energy systems that support the body's muscular work.

LO 10.4 Explain how glucose, fatty acids, and proteins support muscular work.

LO 10.5 Explain why vitamins and minerals are important to athletes.

LO 10.6 Describe the hazards that inadequate fluid intake and temperature extremes present to the working body.

LO 10.7 Summarize the characteristics of the diet that best support physical performance.

LO 10.8 Debate the usefulness of dietary ergogenic aids for improving sports performance.

In the body, nutrition and **physical activity** go hand in hand. The working body demands energy-yielding nutrients—carbohydrate, lipid, and protein—to fuel physical activity. It also needs high-quality protein to supply the amino acids necessary to build and repair muscle tissues. Vitamins and minerals play critical roles in energy metabolism, protein synthesis, and many other functions.

Physical activity, in turn, benefits the body's nutrition. Physical activity helps regulate the use of energy-yielding nutrients, improves body composition, and increases the daily calorie allowance. A person who eats extra calories of nutritious whole foods takes in more beneficial nutrients and phytochemicals, too. Together, a nutritious eating pattern and regular physical activity become a powerful force for human health.

This chapter addresses the nutrition of physically active people, starting with some basic concepts about health and physical activity. It also provides a basic framework for understanding **performance nutrition**. It describes how foods, fluids, and nutrients help to fuel physical activities and how the right choices can improve high-level performance, whereas poor choices may hinder it. The Controversy that follows spotlights just a few of the many supplements sold with promises of enhanced athletic performance.

physical activity bodily movement produced by muscle contractions that substantially increase energy expenditure.

performance nutrition an area of nutrition science that pertains to maximizing physical performance in athletes, firefighters, military personnel, and others who must perform at high levels of physical ability. Also called *sports nutrition.*

fitness the characteristics that enable the body to perform physical activity; more broadly, the ability to meet routine physical demands with enough reserve energy to rise to physical challenges and withstand stress.

exercise planned, structured, and repetitive bodily movement that promotes or maintains physical fitness.

athlete a competitor in any sport, exercise, or game requiring physical skill; for the purpose of this book, anyone who trains at a high level of physical exertion, with or without competition. From the Greek *athlein*, meaning "to contend for a prize."

training regular practice of an activity, which leads to physical adaptations of the body with improvement in flexibility, strength, and/or endurance.

The Benefits of Fitness

LO 10.1   Enumerate the benefits of physical fitness.

Physical **fitness** develops with performance of physical activity or **exercise**. The body's muscles respond in identical ways, regardless of whether an individual is running around a track or running to catch a bus, so this chapter uses the terms *physical activity* and *exercise* interchangeably.

People's fitness goals vary. An **athlete** may be **training** for competition; the casual exerciser may be working to improve health and body weight. For those just beginning a program of physical fitness, be assured that improvement is not only possible but inevitable. As fitness improves, energy levels rise, and chronic disease risks fall. This relationship also works in reverse: a sedentary lifestyle robs people of their fitness and opens the way for the development of several chronic diseases.

The Nature of Fitness

If you are physically fit, the following describes you: You move with ease and balance. You have endurance that lasts for hours. You are strong and meet daily physical challenges without strain. You are adaptable and resistant to mental stress, depression, or anxiety. As you strengthen your muscles, your posture and self-image respond and improve.

Longevity and Disease Resistance People who regularly engage in moderate physical activity live longer, healthier lives on average than those who are physically inactive.[1]* A sedentary lifestyle is a powerful predictor of the major killer diseases of our time—cardiovascular disease, some forms of cancer, stroke, diabetes, and hypertension. Without sufficient weight-bearing activities, bone and muscle mass dwindle, increasing the likelihood of osteoporosis. Despite the well-known health benefits of physical activity (listed in Table 10–1), only about 20 percent of adults in the United States meet all of the Physical Activity Guidelines for Americans (see Figure 10–1, p. 368).[2]

A Molecular Link with Health Small improvements in blood vessel function and blood glucose regulation are detectable after just a single bout of exercise.[3] Some of the credit for these and other benefits of exercise is in part attributable to **myokines**, small hormone-like molecules released by working muscles. Myokines also promote muscle synthesis and they may alter metabolism in ways that oppose chronic diseases.[4]†

Why not simply manufacture these molecules and press them into "fitness pills" to capture their benefits without physical work? Unfortunately, too little is known about them and their actions to provide a shortcut.[5] So keep moving.

KEY POINTS

- Physical activity and fitness benefit people's physical and psychological well-being and improve their resistance to disease.
- Physical activity improves survival and quality of life in the later years.
- Myokines generated by working muscles may trigger healthy changes in body tissues.

Table 10–1

Some Benefits of Fitness

Research suggests that most people who become physically active can expect these and other benefits:

- Improved body composition and adipose tissue distribution.
- Improved bone density.
- Enhanced resistance to colds and other infectious diseases.[a]
- Reduced risks of some types of cancers.
- Improved circulation and lung function.
- Reduced risk factors for cardiovascular disease.
- Reduced risk and improved management of type 2 diabetes.
- Reduced risk of gallbladder disease.
- Reduced incidence and severity of mental anxiety and depression, some forms of dementia, and Parkinson's disease.
- Longer life and higher quality of life in the later years.

[a]*Regular, moderate physical activity supports healthy immune function, but intense, vigorous, prolonged activity such as a marathon race may temporarily compromise immune function.*

Sources: 2018 Physical Activity Guidelines Advisory Committee, 2018 Physical Activity Guidelines Advisory Committee Scientific Report *(Washington, DC: U.S. Department of Health and Human Services, 2018); K. A. Alkadhi, Exercise as a positive modulator of brain function,* Molecular Neurobiology *(2017), epub ahead of print, doi: 10.1007/s12035-017-0516-4; H. Kaji, Effects of myokines on bone,* Bonekey Reports *(2016), epub, doi: 10.1038/bonekey.2016.48; C. A. Brawner and coauthors, Change in maximal exercise capacity is associated with survival in men and women,* Mayo Clinic Proceedings *92 (2017): 383–390; A. Philipsen and coauthors, Associations of objectively measured physical activity and abdominal fat distribution,* Medicine and Science in Sports and Exercise *47 (2015): 983–989; K. G. Avin and coauthors, Biomechanical aspects of the muscle-bone interaction,* Current Osteoporosis Reports *13 (2015): 1–8; E. J. Aguiar and coauthors, Efficacy of interventions that include diet, aerobic and resistance training components for type 2 diabetes prevention: A systematic review with meta-analysis,* International Journal of Behavioral Nutrition and Physical Activity *11 (2014), epub, doi: 10.1186/1479-5868-11-2; R. Asano and coauthors, Acute effects of physical exercise in type 2 diabetes: A review,* World Journal of Diabetes *5 (2014), epub, doi: 10.4239/wjd.v5.i5.659; P. Seron and coauthors, Exercise for people with high cardiovascular risk,* Cochrane Database Systematic Reviews *8 (2014), epub, doi: 10.1002/14651858.CD009387.pub2.*

myokines (MY-oh-kynz) signaling proteins secreted by working skeletal muscles that contribute to widespread beneficial effects of exercise on body systems (from the Greek *myo*, meaning muscle, and *kino*, meaning movement).

---

*Reference notes are in Appendix F.
†The molecules include *irisin* and others, often referred to as *exercise mimetics*.

Figure 10–1
Nutrition and Disease

Meeting these guidelines requires physical activity beyond the usual light or sedentary activities required in daily living, such as cooking, cleaning, and walking from an automobile to a store. Table 10–2 displays levels of exercise intensity.

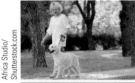

- **Every day—Choose an active lifestyle and engage in flexibility activities.**
  Integrate activity into your day: walk a dog, take the stairs, stand up whenever possible. Stretching exercises lend flexibility for activities such as dance, but minutes spent stretching do not count toward aerobic or strength activity recommendations.

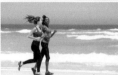

- **5 or more days/week—Engage in moderate or vigorous aerobic activities.**
  Perform a minimum of 150 min of moderate-intensity aerobic activity each week by doing activities such as brisk walking or ballroom dancing; 75 min per week of vigorous aerobic activity, such as bicycling (>10 mph) or jumping rope; or a mix of the two (1 min vigorous activity = 2 min moderate activity).

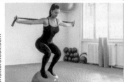

- **2 or more days/week—Engage in strength activities.**
  Perform muscle-strengthening activities that are moderate to high intensity and involve all major muscle groups.

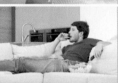

- **Avoid inactivity—Some physical activity is better than none.**
  Limit TV, movie watching, leisure computer time.

[a]For most men and women, aged 18 to 64 years.

Source: 2018 Physical Activity Guidelines Advisory Committee, 2018 Physical Activity Guidelines Advisory Committee Scientific Report *(Washington, DC: U.S. Department of Health and Human Services, 2018).*

Physical Activity Guidelines

What must you do to reap the health rewards of physical activity? You need only meet the Physical Activity Guidelines for Americans.[6]

Physical Activity Guidelines for Americans   The Physical Activity Guidelines for Americans outline how much **aerobic activity** adults aged 18 to 64 years need to improve or maintain cardiovascular health. The Guidelines also support **resistance training** (strengthening exercises) as beneficial for building and maintaining lean tissues and useful for meeting activity goals. The length of time (exercise duration) required to meet these guidelines varies by the **intensity** of the activity—physical activity of moderate intensity must last relatively longer to meet the guidelines; more vigorous exercise can do so in a shorter time. Table 10–2 displays activity intensity levels.

Most health benefits occur with the activities listed in Figure 10–1, but additional benefits can result from activities of higher intensity, greater frequency, or longer duration. Older people, those with chronic illnesses, and those with disabilities who cannot meet the guidelines should be as active as their conditions allow, based on the advice of their health-care providers. For everyone, mounting evidence suggests that even without meeting the Physical Activity Guidelines, some physical activity is better than none.[7]

Note that certain guidelines are stated in accumulated weekly totals.[‡] This allows individuals to split up their activities into sessions of at least 10 minutes each, performed

aerobic activity physical activity that involves the body's large muscles working at light to moderate intensity for a sustained period of time. Brisk walking, running, swimming, and bicycling are examples. From the Greek, aero meaning "air" + bios meaning "life." Also called *endurance activity*.

resistance training physical activity that develops muscle strength, power, endurance, and mass. Resistance can be provided by free weights, weight machines, other objects, or the person's own body weight. Also called *weight training*, *resistance exercise*, or *strength exercise*.

intensity in exercise, the degree of effort required to perform a given physical activity.

[‡]Guidelines from sports medicine experts are stated in metabolic equivalent units (METs) that reflect the ratio of the rate of energy expended during an activity to the rate of energy expended at rest. One MET is equal to the energy expenditure while at rest.

Table 10–2

Intensity of Physical Activity

Level of Intensity	Breathing and/or Heart Rate	Perceived Exertion (on a Scale of 0 to 10)	Talk Test	Energy Expenditure	Walking Pace
Light	Little to no increase	<5	Able to sing	<3.5 cal/min	<3 mph
Moderate	Some increase	5 or 6	Able to have a conversation	3.5 to 7 cal/min	3 to 4.5 mph (100 steps per minute or 15 to 20 minutes to walk 1 mile)
High (vigorous)	Large increase	7 or 8	Conversation is difficult or "broken"	>7 cal/min	>4.5 mph

Source: Centers for Disease Control and Prevention, 2011, available at www.cdc.gov/physicalactivity/everyone.

throughout the days of the week in any combination that suits their lifestyles. Safety is a high priority, and the Think Fitness section (p. 372) provides some tips.

To achieve or maintain a healthy body weight through increasing physical activity demands more than the amount needed for health. Most people with weight-loss goals are best served by combining calorie-restricted diets with increased physical activity.[8]

Guidelines for Sports Performance Athletes who compete in sports require specific types and amounts of physical activity to train for performance, so special guidelines apply to them. Appendix H at the back of the book offers guidelines for sports and fitness from the American College of Sports Medicine that are more specific and also more demanding than the Physical Activity Guidelines for Americans. Appendix H also offers a sample balanced workout program that develops all components of fitness.

KEY POINT

- The U.S. Physical Activity Guidelines for Americans aim to improve physical fitness and the health of the nation.

The Essentials of Fitness

LO 10.2 Describe muscle adaptability and the effects of physical training.

To become physically fit, you need to develop enough **flexibility**, **muscle strength**, **muscle endurance**, and **cardiorespiratory endurance** to allow you to meet the everyday demands of life with some to spare. You also need to achieve a reasonable body composition.

So far, the description of fitness applies to anyone interested in improving health. For athletes, however, excelling in sports performance often becomes the primary motivator for working out. Athletes must strive to develop strength and endurance, of course, but they also need **muscle power** to drive their movements, quick **reaction time** to respond with speed, **agility** to instantly change direction, increased resistance to **muscle fatigue**, and mental toughness to carry on when fatigue sets in.

How Do Muscles Adapt to Physical Activity?

A person who engages in physical activity *adapts* by becoming a little more able to perform the activity after each session. People shape their bodies by what they choose to do (and not do), a concept illustrated in Figure 10–2. Muscle cells and tissues respond to a

flexibility the capacity of the joints to move through a full range of motion; the ability to bend and recover without injury.

muscle strength the ability of muscles to overcome physical resistance. This muscle characteristic develops with increasing workload rather than repetition and is associated with muscle size.

muscle endurance the ability of a muscle to contract repeatedly within a given time without becoming exhausted. This muscle characteristic develops with increasing repetition rather than increasing workload and is associated with cardiorespiratory endurance.

cardiorespiratory endurance the ability of the heart, lungs, and metabolism to sustain large-muscle exercise of moderate to high intensity for prolonged periods.

muscle power the efficiency of a muscle contraction, measured by force and time.

reaction time the interval between stimulation and response.

agility nimbleness; the ability to quickly change directions.

muscle fatigue diminished force and power of muscle contractions despite consistent or increasing conscious effort to perform a physical activity.

Figure 10-2

Muscles Adapt to Physical Activity

Repeated physical activity prompts the body to build the structures needed to meet the demand.

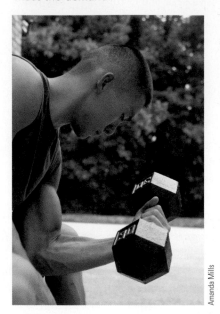

Amanda Mills

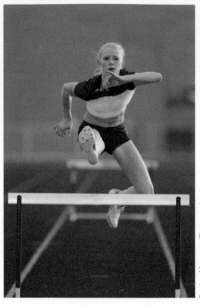

Stephen Mcsweeny/Shutterstock.com

physical activity **overload** by building, within genetic limits, the structures and metabolic equipment needed to perform the activity.

Muscles are constantly undergoing renovation. Every day, particularly during the fasting periods between meals, a healthy body degrades a portion of its muscle protein to amino acids and later rebuilds it as amino acids become available during fed periods.[9] A balance between degradation and synthesis maintains the body's lean tissue. To gain muscle strength and size, however, this balance must more often tip toward synthesis, a condition called **hypertrophy**, than toward muscle breakdown, which results in **atrophy**. Physical activity tips the balance toward hypertrophy. The opposite is also true: unused muscles diminish in size and weaken over time—they atrophy.

> Muscle hypertrophy is an example of positive nitrogen balance, a concept illustrated in **Figure 6–15** of Chapter 6, p. 201.

Muscle synthesis is conservative. The muscles adapt and build only the proteins they need to cope with the work performed. Muscles engaged in activities that require strength develop greater bulk, whereas those engaged in endurance activities develop more metabolic equipment to combat muscle fatigue. Thus, a tennis player may have one superbly strong arm, while the other is just average; cyclists often have well-developed legs that can pedal for many hours but less development of the arms or chest.

A Balance of Activities   For most people, performing a variety of physical activities that work different muscle groups from day to day produces balanced fitness. Stretching enhances flexibility, aerobic activity improves cardiorespiratory and muscle endurance, and resistance training develops the strength, size, and endurance of the worked muscles.

Muscles need rest, too, because it takes a day or two to fully replenish muscle fuel supplies and to repair wear and tear. With greater work comes more damage, and muscles require longer rest periods for a full recovery. (A muscle or joint that remains sore after about a week of rest may be injured and in need of medical attention.)

overload an extra physical demand placed on the body; an increase in the frequency, duration, or intensity of an activity. A principle of training is that for a body system to improve, it must be worked at frequencies, durations, or intensities that increase by increments.

hypertrophy (high-PURR-tro-fee) an increase in size (for example, of a muscle) in response to use.

atrophy (AT-tro-fee) a reduction in size (for example, of a muscle) because of disuse.

Targeted Activities A planned program of training can induce the development of specific muscle tissues and fuel systems. The muscle cells of a trained weightlifter store extra glycogen granules, build up strong connective tissues, and add bulk to the special proteins that contract the muscles, increasing their strength.[§] In contrast, the muscle cells of a distance swimmer build more of the enzymes and structures needed for aerobic metabolism. Therefore, if you wish to become a better jogger, swimmer, or biker, you should train in ways that benefit your sport. Your performance will improve as your muscles adapt to the activity.

KEY POINTS

- The components of fitness are flexibility, muscle strength, muscle endurance, and cardiorespiratory endurance.
- Muscle protein is built up and broken down every day; muscle hypertrophy occurs when synthesis exceeds degradation; atrophy occurs when degradation is dominant.
- Physical activity builds muscle tissues and the metabolic equipment needed for the activities they are repeatedly called upon to perform.

How Does Aerobic Training Benefit the Heart?

Aerobic endurance training reliably and efficiently improves some key indicators of cardiovascular health.[10] Such exercise, performed regularly, diminishes the risks of diabetes and hypertension, major contributors to heart disease, while improving the blood lipid profile. In addition, aerobic endurance training enhances leanness, a plus for the heart, and confers a fit, healthy appearance to the limbs and torso.

Improvements to Blood, Heart, and Lungs Cardiorespiratory endurance enables the working body to remain active with an elevated heart rate over time. As cardiorespiratory endurance improves, the body delivers oxygen to the tissues and removes cellular wastes more efficiently. In fact, the accepted measure of a person's cardiorespiratory fitness is the rate at which the tissues consume oxygen—the maximal oxygen uptake (VO_{2max}). This measure reflects many facets of oxygen delivery that improve with regular aerobic exercise.

As the heart muscle grows stronger and larger, the heart's **cardiac output** increases. Each beat empties the heart's chambers more completely, so the heart pumps more blood per beat—its **stroke volume** increases. The resting heart rate slows because a greater volume of blood is moved with fewer beats. Capillary networks proliferate, circulation through the arteries and veins improves, blood moves easily, and blood pressure falls. Figure 10–3 (p. 373) shows the major relationships among the heart, lungs, and muscles, and Table 10–3 describes cardiorespiratory endurance.

Cardiorespiratory Training Activities Effective cardiorespiratory training activities have these characteristics:

- They elevate the heart rate for sustained periods of time.
- They use most of the large-muscle groups of the body (for example, legs and buttocks, or chest and shoulders).

Examples are swimming, cross-country skiing, rowing, fast walking, jogging, running, fast bicycling, soccer, hockey, basketball, in-line skating, lacrosse, and rugby.

The rest of this chapter describes the interactions between nutrients and physical activity. Nutrition alone cannot endow you with fitness or athletic ability, but along with consistent physical activity and the right mental attitude, it complements your effort to obtain them. Conversely, unwise food selections can stand in your way.

Table 10–3
Cardiorespiratory Endurance

Cardiorespiratory endurance is characterized by:

- Increased heart strength and stroke volume
- Slowed resting pulse
- Increased breathing efficiency
- Increased capillary networks.
- Improved circulation and oxygen delivery
- Reduced blood pressure
- Increased blood HDL cholesterol

Source: Y. Hellsten and M. Nyberg, Cardiovascular adaptations to exercise training, Comprehensive Physiology 6 (2015): 1–32.

VO_{2max} the maximum rate of oxygen consumption by an individual (measured at sea level).

cardiac output the volume of blood discharged each minute by the heart.

stroke volume the volume of oxygenated blood ejected from the heart toward body tissues at each beat.

[§]All muscles contain a variety of muscle fibers, but there are two main types—slow-twitch (also called red fibers) and fast-twitch (also called white fibers). Slow-twitch fibers contain extra metabolic equipment to perform aerobic work, which gives them a reddish appearance under a microscope; fast-twitch fibers store extra glycogen required for anaerobic work, giving them a lighter appearance.

The physical impact involved in contact sports—football is a typical example—presents serious risks of head and neck injuries. In other activities, torn ligaments, broken bones, and even strains and sprains can sideline participants.[11]

Keeping safe during physical activity depends on both common sense and education. The United States Department of Agriculture (USDA) suggests following these guidelines:

- Choose activities appropriate for your current fitness level.
- Gradually increase the amount of physical activity you perform.
- Wear appropriate safety gear, including the correct shoes, helmet, pads, and other protection.
- Develop the flexibility and balance needed in your activity.

- Make sensible choices about when and where to exercise; for example, avoid the hottest hours of the day in summer, choose safe bike paths away from heavy traffic, and run with a buddy on isolated trails.
- People with medical problems or increased disease risks should consult their physicians before beginning any program of physical activity.[12]

In addition, people can easily injure themselves by using improper techniques during strength training, particularly when it involves equipment. Many people can benefit from consulting with a Certified Personal Trainer (CPT), who can help develop a safe and effective individualized exercise program. Some personal trainers have a more advanced credential, the Certified Strength and Conditioning Specialist (CSCS), which requires completion of a college curriculum that includes human anatomy and exercise physiology; they must also pass a nationally recognized examination. Also, unless a trainer possesses a legitimate nutrition credential, he or she is not qualified to dispense diet advice.

Fake nutrition credentials were described in Controversy 1. The same kinds of skullduggery occur in the field of physical training.

start now! Create a fitness plan that gradually increases both the time and the intensity of your physical activity. Use a calendar to record your daily plan for several weeks; then record your actual activity on each of those days.

KEY POINTS

- Cardiorespiratory endurance training enhances the ability of the heart and lungs to deliver oxygen to body tissues.
- Cardiorespiratory training activities elevate the heart rate for sustained periods of time and engage the body's large muscle groups.

Three Energy Systems

LO 10.3 Describe the three energy systems that support the body's muscular work.

Whether belonging to an athlete, a growing child, or an office worker, the human body uses the same energy systems, performing multiple chemical reactions, to fuel its work. These systems include the body's **energy reservoir**, the **anaerobic** fuel system, and the **aerobic** fuel system. All three systems function continuously, supplying energy for the heartbeat, breathing, cellular activities, and other life-sustaining work. Then, when physical activity demands arise, they respond in ways that meet the body's additional energy needs of the moment.

The Muscles' Energy Reservoir

The body's energy reservoir is composed of high-energy compounds that trap and store energy. In the muscles, these high-energy compounds are found exactly where they are needed for muscular work—on the microscopic fibers that contract the muscles.**

energy reservoir a system of high-energy compounds that hold, store, and release energy derived from the energy-yielding nutrients and transfer it to cell structures to fuel cellular activities.

anaerobic (AN-air-ROH-bic) not requiring oxygen.

aerobic (air-ROH-bic) requiring oxygen.

**The energy reservoir is also called the *phosphagen system*, referring to high-energy compounds that contain the mineral phosphorus, such as ATP (adenosine triphosphate) and CP (phosphocreatine), key players in energy metabolism.

Figure 10–3

Delivery of Oxygen by the Heart and Lungs to the Muscles

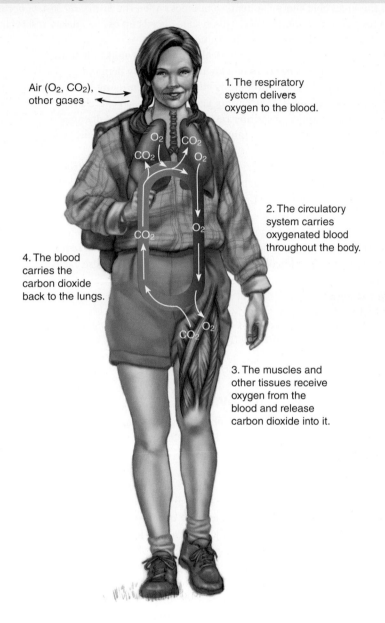

Air (O_2, CO_2), other gases

1. The respiratory system delivers oxygen to the blood.

2. The circulatory system carries oxygenated blood throughout the body.

4. The blood carries the carbon dioxide back to the lungs.

3. The muscles and other tissues receive oxygen from the blood and release carbon dioxide into it.

The cardiorespiratory system responds to increased demand for oxygen by building up its capacity to deliver oxygen. Researchers can measure cardiovascular fitness by measuring the amount of oxygen a person consumes per minute while working out. This measure of fitness, which indicates the person's maximum rate of oxygen consumption, is called VO_{2max}.

Whenever muscles move, say, to blink the eyes or type on a keyboard, these high-energy molecules split apart, releasing and transferring their load of pent-up energy to power the work of the muscle tissue.[13]

This ready pool of energy also drives short bursts of intense physical activity lasting up to about 20 seconds, such as when a weightlifter heaves a heavy weight or a child darts to grab the best swing on the playground. Using energy from the reservoir requires no oxygen input, but the reservoir's capacity is very limited, and once depleted, it must be replenished by way of anaerobic and aerobic energy nutrient breakdown, described next.

KEY POINTS

- High-energy molecules trap and store energy from energy-yielding nutrients and can transfer that energy to fuel cellular work.
- Bursts of physical activity lasting just seconds require the immediate energy of the reservoir.

The Anaerobic Energy System

Muscles performing high-intensity work lasting more than a few seconds rely heavily on the anaerobic energy system, sometimes called the *lactic acid system* because it generates the compound **lactate**. This system speeds up as the energy reservoir runs down, drawing on the body's supply of glucose.

The kind of intense ongoing physical activity that makes it hard "to catch your breath" uses so much energy so quickly that the energy demand outpaces the human body's ability to provide it through its efficient oxygen-using fuel system. The lungs, heart, and blood vessels simply cannot keep up. A person exercising intensely for 3 or 4 minutes—for example, a sprinter racing for 800 meters of distance or a late student running hard to get to class—obtains about half of the needed energy from the anaerobic energy system.

Anaerobic metabolism can generate copious energy, but it extracts only a fraction of the available energy from each glucose molecule by partially breaking it down and quickly moving on to the next, casting aside the by-product lactate. No other fuel—not amino acids or fatty acids—can replace glucose in this system. Thus, the anaerobic system draws heavily on glucose stores. Its key advantage, however, is the capacity to produce abundant energy quickly to fuel intense exercise without requiring the input of oxygen. The upper portion of Figure 10–4 illustrates that glucose yields energy quickly in anaerobic metabolism.

KEY POINTS

- The anaerobic energy system partially breaks down glucose to yield energy without using oxygen and is particularly important during bouts of high-intensity activity.
- Lactate is a by-product of anaerobic energy production.

The Aerobic Energy System

The efficient, oxygen-dependent aerobic energy system wrings every last calorie of energy from each energy nutrient molecule. Glucose, certain amino acids, the body's abundant fatty acids, and even some lactate, are used as fuels. This system demands the input of sufficient oxygen, and although it always delivers a steady stream of energy to the breathing body, the system speeds up during exercise. Aerobic metabolism supplies almost half of a sprinter's energy, whose effort lasts just seconds, but it supplies more than 90 percent of the energy used by a long-distance swimmer who swims for hours on end. Likewise, a jogger can go long distances, breathing easily, the heart beating steadily, relying on aerobic metabolism to supply most of the needed energy.

In contrast to anaerobic metabolism, aerobic metabolism depends more heavily on fatty acids for fuel, sparing glucose and conserving glycogen.[14] The bottom half of Figure 10–4 shows that the ample oxygen supplies available during aerobic activity facilitate the extraction of abundant energy from fuels.

KEY POINTS

- The aerobic energy system uses fuels most efficiently and conserves the body's glycogen stores.
- Aerobic metabolism fuels moderate-intensity activity over long duration.

The Active Body's Use of Fuels

LO 10.4   Explain how glucose, fatty acids, and protein support muscular work.

Athletes and other exercisers often hear claims, mostly from sellers of nutrient products, about their need for energy-yielding nutrients. The following sections present the current scientific knowledge about the active person's need for and use of the energy-yielding nutrients.

lactate an energy-yielding compound produced during the breakdown of glucose in anaerobic metabolism; with training, muscles gain efficiency in using lactate as fuel.

Figure 10–4

Glucose and Fatty Acids Releasing Energy in Muscle Cells

When the cells' energy reservoir diminishes, anaerobic and aerobic breakdown of fuels restore it.

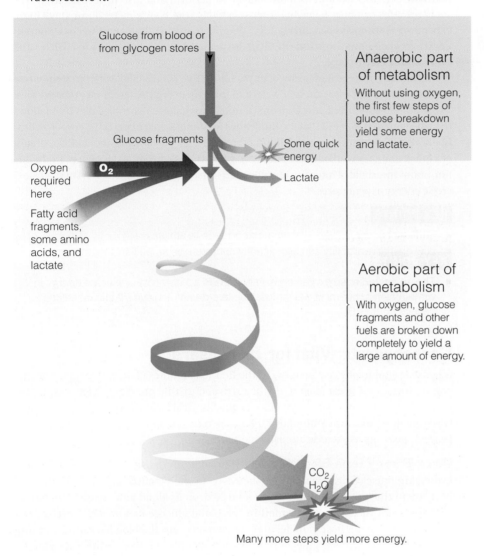

Glucose from blood or from glycogen stores

Anaerobic part of metabolism
Without using oxygen, the first few steps of glucose breakdown yield some energy and lactate.

Glucose fragments

Some quick energy

Lactate

Oxygen required here
O_2

Fatty acid fragments, some amino acids, and lactate

Aerobic part of metabolism
With oxygen, glucose fragments and other fuels are broken down completely to yield a large amount of energy.

CO_2
H_2O

Many more steps yield more energy.

The Need for Food Energy

Highly active people require copious amounts of fuel for their physical activities, and even more to sustain normal body functions, such as immunity and reproduction.[15] Without sufficient **energy availability**, the hormones, muscles, bones, and other major body organs become impaired.[††] An athlete in training, for example, can require hundreds or even thousands of calories a day above off-season intakes.

Pinpointing the energy need of an individual athlete requires special consideration, and methods used for other people (see Chapter 9) may underestimate the need.[16] Some reasons why include:

- *body composition.* An athlete's body composition differs significantly from average.

energy availability the amount of food energy consumed in a day minus the energy expended in physical activity; measured in calories per kilogram of lean body mass.

[††]A name proposed to describe low energy availability and resulting harms is *relative energy deficiency in sport (RED-S).*

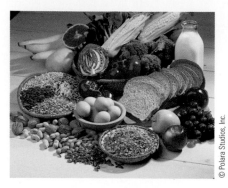

Foods like these are packed with the nutrients that active people need.

- *resting metabolism.* An athlete may use half or less of the total daily energy expenditure to maintain basic body functions, whereas a sedentary person may use up to 80 percent.[17][‡‡]
- *work intensity.* An athlete's work intensity is often far greater than average.

Intensive physical work costs more energy to perform and also to recover from. For some minutes or hours following intense activity, the body's metabolism stays high, expending extra fuels even during rest. This phenomenon, known as **excess postexercise oxygen consumption (EPOC)**, can demand significant energy in athletes and other highly active people.[18]

In contrast, the great majority of physically active people who work out lightly two or three times a week for fitness or weight management require few or no extra calories. These active people need only consume a nutritious calorie-controlled diet that follows the eating patterns of the Dietary Guidelines for Americans, along with proper hydration, to perfectly meet their needs. Fitness seekers who, on learning about EPOC, dream of a quick and easy workout that "burns fat while they sleep" should be aware that some minimum threshold of intensity and duration must be met to induce even small postexercise energy expenditures.[19]

KEY POINTS

- Sufficient energy intake is of great importance to athletes.
- Low energy availability can significantly compromise an athlete's performance and health.
- Excess postexercise oxygen consumption (EPOC) can cost significant energy in some athletes, but most weight-loss seekers do not achieve significant calorie deficits from EPOC.

Carbohydrate: Vital for Exercisers

Glucose is vital to physical activity. In the first few minutes of an activity, muscle glycogen provides the great majority of the extra energy that muscles use for action. This is beneficial to exercisers because glucose quickly yields energy needed for fast action. Glycogen molecules are continually broken down throughout physical activity, and the process speeds up as exercise intensity increases.

Quick Energy from Blood Glucose   In addition to using their own glycogen, exercising muscles draw available glucose from the bloodstream. You might suspect, then, that exercise would cause a large drop in blood glucose concentration, but this is not the case. *Before* a fall in the blood glucose can occur, exercise triggers the release of a host of molecular messengers into the bloodstream, including the pancreatic hormone glucagon. Glucagon signals the liver to liberate glucose from its glycogen stores and to make new molecules of glucose for release into the bloodstream. This fresh supply of glucose is rapidly picked up and used by working muscles.

Prolonged Energy from Glycogen   Stored glycogen is not inexhaustible. It can yield 2,000 calories of glucose at most. An athlete's fat stores, in contrast, can yield 70,000 calories or more, enough to fuel several marathon races, but fat cannot sustain physical work without glucose. At some point during physical activity, glycogen begins to run out. The liver simply cannot make glucose fast enough to meet the demand.

Glucagon's effects on the liver are explained in **Chapter 4**.

Athletes who begin an activity with full glycogen stores have enough glucose fuel to last during sustained exercise. For most active people, a normal, balanced diet keeps glycogen stores full. For athletes engaged in heavy training or competition, the more

excess postexercise oxygen consumption (EPOC) a measure of increased metabolism (energy expenditure) that continues for minutes or hours after cessation of exercise.

[‡‡]The measure of energy is the resting metabolic rate, often used in research.

Figure 10–5

The Effect of Diet on Physical Endurance

Carbohydrate supports an athlete's endurance.

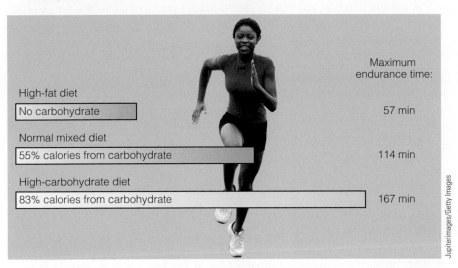

Maximum endurance time:

High-fat diet
No carbohydrate — 57 min

Normal mixed diet
55% calories from carbohydrate — 114 min

High-carbohydrate diet
83% calories from carbohydrate — 167 min

Jupiterimages/Getty Images

Source: J. Bergstrom and coauthors, Diet, muscle glycogen, and physical performance, Acta Physiologica Scandinavica *71 (1967): 140–150.*

carbohydrate they eat, the more glycogen the muscles will store (within limits), and the longer the stores will last to support physical activity.

A classic study compared endurance during physical activity in three groups of runners, each on a different diet.[20] For several days before testing, one of the groups ate a normal mixed diet; the second group ate a high-carbohydrate diet; and the third group ate a high-fat diet. As Figure 10–5 shows, the high-carbohydrate diet enabled the athletes to work longest before exhaustion. These and other results established that high intakes of dietary carbohydrate help sustain endurance by ensuring ample glycogen stores.

Exercise Duration and Intensity Affect Glycogen Use The *duration* of a physical activity, as well as its *intensity*, affects how long glycogen supplies will last. Muscle cells pack their stored glycogen close to their contractile fibers and energy-processing structures to ensure quick access to glucose energy. As the muscles devour their own glycogen, they become ravenous for more glucose and dramatically increase their uptake of blood glucose. Within the first 20 minutes of moderate activity, a person uses up about one-fifth of the available glycogen.

A person who exercises moderately for longer than 20 minutes begins to use less glucose and more fat for fuel. Still, glucose use continues, and if the activity goes on long enough and at a high enough intensity, muscle and liver glycogen stores will run out almost completely, as depicted in Figure 10–6. When glycogen depletion reaches a certain point, it brings nervous system function almost to a halt, making continued activity at the same intensity impossible. Marathon runners refer to this point of exhaustion as "hitting the wall."

Degree of Training Affects Glycogen Use Consistent training affects glycogen use during activity in two major ways. First, muscles adapt to their work by storing the extra amounts of glycogen needed to support that work. Second, trained muscles burn more fat, and at higher intensities, than untrained muscles, so they require less glucose to perform the same work. A person first attempting an activity uses up much more glucose per minute than an athlete trained to perform it.

Figure 10-6

Glycogen—Before and After Physical Activity

These electron micrographs magnify part of a muscle cell by 20,000 times, revealing the orderly rows of contractile structures within. The dark granulated substance is glycogen. In the photo on the left, the cell's glycogen stores are full; on the right, they have been depleted by exercise.

1 The orderly rows that appear to be striped at intervals are protein structures that contract the muscles.[a]

2 The black oblong rows between the contractile structures contain much of the muscle's glycogen. More glycogen granules (black dots) are also scattered within the contractile parts (visible at the left but depleted at the right).

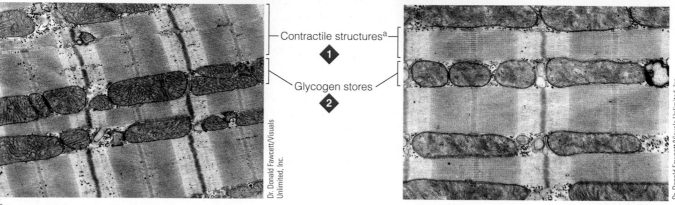

Contractile structures[a]

1

Glycogen stores

2

Dr. Donald Fawcett/Visuals Unlimited, Inc.

Dr. Donald Fawcett/Visuals Unlimited, Inc.

[a]*The contractile structures of the muscle cells are myofibrils.*

In summary, these three factors affect glycogen use during physical activity:

- Carbohydrate intake.
- Intensity and duration of the activity.
- Degree of training.

Inflow of Glucose from Food In addition to the body's stored glycogen, glucose in the digestive tract makes its way to the working muscles during activity. For example, carbohydrate taken in during an ultramarathon may have helped some runners to finish a 100-mile race.[21§§] During the race, the finishers consumed almost twice as many calories and carbohydrates per hour as nonfinishers. The extra carbohydrate *may* have helped them win, but an alternative explanation exists: the runners who ate more and finished the race may have suffered less from digestive disturbances. Most long-distance runners develop digestive disturbances, such as vomiting, that interfere with eating, and these problems can become severe enough to cause a runner to forfeit a race.[22]

Competitive distance bicyclers also may benefit from taking in glucose during exercise. In a timed test, carbohydrate administered during cycling forestalled an inevitable decline in performance, whereas caffeine or water had no effect in this regard.[23] In this test, the cyclists stopped working before the time when digestive upset typically interferes with performance, so carbohydrate was most likely responsible for the improvement. People who compete in sports that require repeated bursts of intense activity, such as basketball or soccer, may also benefit from taking in extra carbohydrate during an event, but research has yet to pinpoint optimal intakes.

Before concluding that extra glucose during activity might boost your own exercise performance, consider first whether you engage in sustained endurance activity or repeated high-intensity activity. Do you run, swim, bike, or ski nonstop at a rapid pace for more than an hour at a time? Do you compete in high-intensity games lasting for

§§A marathon is a footrace of 26 miles and 385 yards (42.2 kilometers); an ultramarathon is a race longer than a marathon. (*Ultra* is Latin for *beyond*).

several hours? Does your sport or training demand several bouts of high-intensity activity in one day, or is it repeated on several successive days? If not, you may not need extra glucose during the activity; a nutrient-dense diet with ample carbohydrate may better serve your needs.

Lactate—A Glucose Breakdown Product   The anaerobic breakdown of glucose yields the compound lactate, as explained earlier. Most people recognize the burning sensation caused in part by lactate accumulating in a working muscle.[24] Muscles metabolize some lactate as fuel, and release the excess into the bloodstream to be carried to the liver, where enzymes convert it back into glucose. After assembly, the new glucose molecules are shipped back to the working muscles to fuel more physical work.

At low exercise intensities, the small amounts of lactate produced are readily cleared from the tissues. Some tissues, including muscle tissue, can use some lactate aerobically for fuel, and the better trained the muscles, the more lactate they can use.[25] At higher intensities of physical activity, however, the lactate produced can exceed the body's ability to fully clear it away.

Lactate accumulation coincides with muscle fatigue but does not appear to cause it.[26] In contrast, depletion of muscle glycogen by about 80 percent reliably produces fatigue.[27] Other potential causes of fatigue include a drop in muscle tissue pH, depletion of the high-energy compounds of the energy reservoir, excess free radical activity, tissue inflammation, and other factors.[28] The human experience of fatigue, resides in the mind, however, as well as in the muscle, and physiology alone cannot fully explain why one competitor can push past the point where another must stop.

KEY POINTS

- During activity, the hormone glucagon helps prevent a drop in blood glucose.
- Glycogen stores in the liver and muscles affect an athlete's endurance; when glycogen stores are depleted, activity intensity diminishes.
- Intensity and duration of an activity affect glycogen use, as does degree of training.
- Carbohydrate consumption affects glycogen stores and may boost performance during prolonged or repeated exercise.
- Lactate arises from anaerobic breakdown of glucose.

Carbohydrate Recommendations for Athletes

To postpone fatigue and maximize performance, athletes must maintain available glucose supplies for as long as they can. To do so, athletes need abundant dietary carbohydrate. Table 10–4 offers carbohydrate intakes for athletes and others at four

Table 10–4

Suggested Daily Carbohydrate Intakes for Athletes

These general research-based guidelines should be adjusted to an athlete's calorie needs, training type, and performance. Carbohydrate grams in sports drinks, gels, or foods consumed during training are counted in the day's total.

Workload	Examples	Carbohydrate Intake Target (g/kg/day)	Recommended Intake (g) for the Reference Male (70 kg)	Recommended Intake (g) for the Reference Female (55 kg)
Low-intensity, skill-based activities	Casual exercisers	3–5	210–350	165–275
Moderate intensity, ≤1 h/day	Most athletes	5–7	350–490	275–385
Moderate to high intensity, 1–3 h/day	Endurance athletes	6–10	420–700	330–550
Moderate to high intensity, 4–5 h/day	Ultraendurance athletes	8–12	560–840	440–660

Sources: Data from Position of the Academy of Nutrition and Dietetics, Dietitians of Canada, and the American College of Sports Medicine: Nutrition and athletic performance, Journal of the Academy of Nutrition and Dietetics 116 (2016): 501–528.

activity levels. A minimum number of *grams* of carbohydrate per unit of body weight is necessary to achieve full glycogen stores for a given activity, so amounts are listed in Table 10–4 (column 1) as grams per kilogram of body weight per day (g/kg/d). (The Do the Math feature in the margin demonstrates how to convert pounds to kilograms.) To prepare adequate glycogen stores for days of heavy training or competition, some athletes may benefit from large intakes of carbohydrate—perhaps as much as 12 g/kg/d. The Food Feature (p. 392) demonstrates how to design a diet that delivers the needed carbohydrate.

Carbohydrate before Activity Most of an athlete's glucose is provided by carbohydrate-rich meals consumed throughout the day. In addition, however, glucose taken within a few hours before training or competition is thought to "top off" an athlete's glycogen stores, providing the greatest possible glucose supply to support sustained activity. The **pregame meal** to supply this glucose can take many forms. The Food Feature describes possible options.

A theory called "train low, compete high" suggests that an occasional *low*-carbohydrate training day may increase endurance by forcing muscles to use more fat for fuel and to develop more metabolic equipment for doing so. However, prolonged carbohydrate restriction may interfere with muscle protein synthesis, a counterproductive outcome for sport.[29] This scheme may be tolerable for light training, but when athletes want to work their hardest and longest, ample carbohydrate is necessary before, during, and after training and competition.

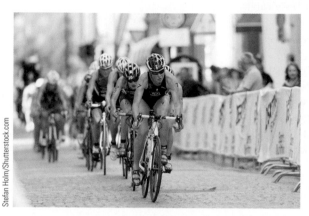

Endurance activities demand fluid and carbohydrate fuel. Don't forget to hydrate.

Carbohydrate during Activity Carbohydrate consumption *during* prolonged activity may improve athletic endurance.[30] Eating during activity can be tricky, though, because it can cause digestive distress. The best carbohydrate sources for the job are easily consumed, smooth-textured, and low in fiber and fat; such foods facilitate monosaccharide absorption. During long bicycle races, for example, competitors may consume bananas, fruit juices, dried fruit, and energy bars that provide carbohydrate energy and help banish distracting feelings of hunger. (Extreme caution is required to prevent choking.) For athletes who cannot eat solid foods while exercising, commercial **high-carbohydrate energy drinks** and commercial **high-carbohydrate gels** are portable, easy-to-consume alternatives, which most, but not all, athletes can tolerate.[31] Such products are higher in calories and carbohydrate than the fluid-replacement sports drinks discussed in the Consumer's Guide (p. 389). Concentrated beverages and gels must be taken with extra water to ensure hydration during activity.

Carbohydrate after Activity Rapid recovery of glycogen stores is important to people who compete or train intensely more than once a day, or on consecutive days with less than a 24-hour recovery period. A window of opportunity opens during the hour or two following glycogen-depleting physical activity, when carbohydrate intake speeds up the rate of glycogen synthesis.[32] This rapid rate of glycogen storage may help restore glycogen for the next bout of high-intensity training or competition. The concept of recovery meals and its application in an athlete's diet are described in the Food Feature (p. 392).

KEY POINTS

- Carbohydrate recommendations for athletes are stated in grams per kilogram of body weight per day.
- Carbohydrate intakes before, during, and after physical exertion can help support the performance of endurance activities.

Fat as Fuel for Physical Activity

Unlike the body's limited glycogen stores, fat stores can fuel hours of activity without running out. Body fat is a virtually unlimited source of energy for exercise.

pregame meal the meal consumed in the hours before prolonged or repeated athletic training or competition, typically designed to boost the glycogen stores of endurance athletes.

high-carbohydrate energy drinks flavored commercial beverages used to restore muscle glycogen after exercise or as pregame beverages.

high-carbohydrate gels semisolid, easy-to-swallow supplements of concentrated carbohydrate, commonly with potassium and sodium added; not a fluid source.

Early in activity, muscles begin to draw on fatty acids from two sources—fats from stores within the working muscles and fats from fat deposits such as the adipose tissue under the skin. Areas with the most fat to spare donate the greatest amounts. This is why "spot reducing" doesn't work: muscles do not own the fat that surrounds them. Instead, adipose tissue cells release fatty acids into the blood for all the muscles to share. Proof is once again found in a tennis player's arms: the skinfolds measure the same in both arms, even though the muscles of one arm are more developed than those of the other.

> Skinfold tests were described in Chapter 9, p. 327.

Activity Intensity and Duration Affect Fat Use

Fat can be broken down for energy only by aerobic metabolism. During physical activity of light or moderate intensity, adipose tissue releases fatty acids into the bloodstream that provide most of the fuel for muscular work through aerobic metabolism. When the intensity of activity becomes so great that energy demand surpasses the ability to provide more energy aerobically, the muscles cannot burn more fat. They burn more glucose instead.[33] Adipose tissue seems to adjust its delivery of fatty acids to match the needs of the muscles at work, releasing more during moderate activity and releasing less during high-intensity exercise.

The *duration* of activity also affects fat use. At the start of activity, the blood fatty acid concentration falls, but a few minutes into moderate activity, blood flow through the adipose tissue capillaries greatly increases, and hormones, including epinephrine, signal the fat cells to dismantle their stored triglycerides. Fatty acids flow into the bloodstream at double or triple the normal rate. After about 20 minutes of sustained, moderate aerobic activity, the fat cells begin to shrink in size as they empty out their lipid stores.

Degree of Training Affects Fat Use

Training, performed consistently, stimulates the muscles to develop more fat-burning metabolic enzymes, so trained muscles can use more fat at greater exercise intensities than untrained muscles do. With aerobic training, the heart and lungs also become stronger and better able to deliver oxygen to the muscles during high-intensity activities. The improved oxygen supply, in turn, helps the muscles to use more fat for fuel.

KEY POINT

- The intensity and duration of the activity, as well as the degree of training, affect fat use.

Fat Recommendations for Athletes

For endurance athletes, eating a high-fat, low-carbohydrate diet for even a day or two depletes precious glycogen stores and makes exercise more difficult. Eventually, muscles do adapt to such a diet and use more fat to fuel activity, but athletes on high-fat diets report greater fatigue and perceive physical work as more strenuous than those on high-carbohydrate diets.[34]

Essential fatty acids and fat-soluble nutrients are as important for athletes as they are for everyone else, so experts recommend a diet with 20 to 35 percent of calories from fat.[35] Omega-3 fatty acids, in particular, may reduce inflammation—and tissue inflammation is both the result and the enemy of physical performance.[36] This doesn't mean that athletes need fish oil supplements; rather, they need to consume the amounts of fatty fish recommended for health.

As for saturated and *trans* fats, they pose the same heart disease risk for athletes as they do for other people. Physical activity reduces the risk of cardiovascular disease, but athletes still suffer heart attacks and strokes; low saturated and *trans* fat intakes reduce these risks.

To summarize, then, these three factors affect fat use during physical activity:

- Fat intake.
- Intensity and duration of the activity.
- Degree of training.

Protein for Building Muscles and for Fuel

The active body uses amino acids from protein to build and maintain muscle and other lean tissue and, to some extent, to provide fuel. Physical activity provides the primary signal for building muscle proteins, but sufficient high-quality *dietary* protein is required to build them.

At the genetic level, exercise and dietary protein work together to shape the human form for physical activity. In response to repetitive muscle contractions, the genes of muscle cells speed up their synthesis of exercise-related protein structures.[37] Exercised muscles speed up their use of amino acids from protein-containing food (and from the breakdown of unneeded muscle proteins) to build new protein structures demanded by the increase in physical work.[38] Muscle protein synthesis continues at an accelerated pace for an hour or two following exercise and gradually diminishes over the next 24 hours or so, after which it resumes its normal resting pace. With repetition and time, these processes change the size, shape, and work capacity of muscles.

Certain essential amino acids effectively stimulate muscle protein synthesis.[39] In a laboratory, an infusion of essential amino acids, particularly **leucine**, causes the rate of protein synthesis to triple for an hour or two. After this time, even with a continuing flow of essential amino acids, the rate of muscle protein synthesis quickly drops off. Researchers theorize that after muscles build proteins for a time, they reach a point of being "full" of new proteins, and they stop building them, even though essential amino acids are plentiful.

This is not to say that people can build bigger muscles by lying on the couch and eating protein or taking pills of leucine—physical activity is necessary for a net muscle gain. Likewise, consuming excess protein or amino acids cannot force the muscles to exceed their protein-building limits. After the "muscle full" state is reached, excess amino acids are dismantled and used for fuel. This may explain why taking large doses of protein or amino acids does not force muscles to gain extra bulk. Even so, when enough high-quality protein is consumed regularly and adequate resistance exercise is performed repeatedly, gains in muscle strength and bulk follow reliably behind.

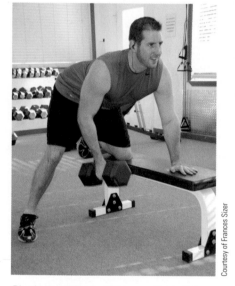

Physical activity itself triggers the building of muscle proteins.

Courtesy of Frances Sizer

Does Timing of Protein Intake Matter? During the hour or two following intense physical activity, consuming sufficient high-quality protein accelerates muscle protein synthesis beyond the rate expected from either exercise or essential amino acids alone. More research is needed to determine optimal intakes, but some experts suggest eating moderate amounts (20 to 30 grams) of high-quality protein in 4 to 5 small meals throughout the day, while others suggest simply increasing protein at meals, particularly at breakfast and lunch, to provide an adequate day's supply.[40] In doses too large (40 grams), excess protein is used as fuel, not for building extra muscle; in doses too small (10 grams), no stimulation of muscle synthesis is observed. Table 10–5 lists some options to provide 20 grams of protein.

> "High quality" means protein with the complete array of essential amino acids needed for protein synthesis, as explained in **Chapter 6**.

Two key questions concerning protein timing for athletes remain unanswered:

1. Does a faster rate of muscle synthesis after a workout yield greater overall gains of muscle tissue over time?

2. Does protein timing enhance athletic performance?

So far, evidence is unconvincing on both points.[41] One study reported no correlation between speed of muscle protein synthesis following exercise and ultimate gains in muscle volume.[42] Likewise, athletes given protein supplements in addition to ample dietary protein exhibit no performance or muscle-building advantages.[43]

leucine one of the essential amino acids; it is of current research interest for its role in stimulating muscle protein synthesis.

The question of protein timing may be more scientifically interesting than of practical value because the protein intakes of athletes generally exceed the recommended amounts.[44] In any case, protein supplements provide no special muscle-building advantage over protein-rich meals and snacks consumed throughout the day.[45]

Protein Use for Fuel   Studies of nitrogen balance show that the body speeds up its use of amino acids for fuel during physical activity, just as it speeds up its use of glucose and fatty acids. The factors that regulate protein use during activity are the same three that regulate the use of glucose and fat: diet, exercise intensity and duration, and degree of training.

Regarding diet, sufficient carbohydrate spares protein from being used as fuel. Too little carbohydrate necessitates the conversion of amino acids to glucose.

Exercise intensity and duration also affect protein for fuel use. When endurance athletes train for longer than an hour a day and deplete their glycogen stores, they become more dependent on protein for fuel. In contrast, intense anaerobic strength training does not use as much protein fuel but demands protein for building muscle tissue.

Finally, the extent of training also affects the use of protein. Particularly in strength athletes such as bodybuilders, the higher the degree of training, the less protein a person uses during activity at a given intensity. To summarize, the factors that affect protein use during physical activity include:

- Dietary carbohydrate sufficiency.
- Intensity and duration of the activity.
- Degree of training.

KEY POINTS

- Physical activity stimulates muscle cells to both break down and synthesize proteins, resulting in muscle adaptation to activity.
- Athletes use amino acids for building muscle tissue and for energy; dietary carbohydrate spares amino acids.
- Diet, intensity and duration of the activity, and degree of training affect protein use during that activity.

Protein Recommendations for Athletes

On learning of the protein demands of physical activity, many athletes go to extremes, doubling or tripling the number of protein-rich foods they eat or taking amino acid supplements to the exclusion of other needed foods and nutrients, a costly mistake for both health and performance. Everyday foods, such as milk, chili, or turkey sandwiches, deliver the high-quality protein with the right mix of amino acids to meet the athlete's need. Such foods present no risk of amino acid imbalances, a known drawback of supplements.

The DRI committee does not recommend greater-than-normal total protein intakes for athletes, but other authorities do. These greater recommendations vary by the nature of the activities performed (see Table 10–6, p. 384). As is true for carbohydrates, the protein recommendations are stated in grams per kilogram of body weight per day (g/kg/d). The protein amounts suggested for athletes are not far above average U.S. intakes, and range from 1.2 to 2 grams per kilogram of body weight.[46]

You may be wondering whether you eat enough protein for your own activities. In general, a nutritious eating pattern that provides enough total energy and follows the USDA Eating Patterns provides enough protein for almost everyone.

KEY POINTS

- The USDA Eating Patterns provide sufficient protein for casual exercisers and most athletes.
- Some athletes require somewhat more daily protein than the DRI.

Table 10–5

Food Portions to Provide 20 Grams of Protein

Protein supplements are not superior to high-quality protein foods. Each of these foods provides essential amino acids (20,000 mg per serving) in a digestible and available form. Other protein-rich foods do the same thing.[a]

Food or Beverage	Amount
Almonds	3 oz
Beef, lean ground	3 oz
Cheese, cheddar	3 oz
Chicken, skinless breast	3 oz
Eggs (white)	6 large
Eggs (whole)	3 large
Milk, low-fat	20 oz
Tofu	8 oz
Tuna, light canned	3 oz
Yogurt, Greek-style	8 oz

[a]Search the USDA Food Composition Database website (ndb.nal.usda.gov/ndb/) for the protein values of thousands of other foods.

Table 10-6

Recommended Daily Protein Intakes for Athletes

	Recommendations (g/kg/day)	Protein Intakes (g/day)	
		Males	Females
DRI for adults	0.8	56	44
Recommended intake for athletes	1.2–2.0	84–140	66–110
US average intake		99	68

NOTE: Daily protein intakes are based on a 70-kilogram (154-pound) man and 55-kilogram (121-pound) woman.

SOURCES: Position of the Academy of Nutrition and Dietetics, Dietitians of Canada, and the American College of Sports Medicine: Nutrition and athletic performance, Journal of the Academy of Nutrition and Dietetics 116 (2016): 501–528; US Department of Agriculture, Agricultural Research Service, 2014, Nutrient intakes from food and beverages: Mean amounts consumed per individual, by gender and age, What We Eat in America, NHANES, 2011–2012. http://www.ars.usda.gov/nea/bhnrc/fsrg.

Vitamins and Minerals— Keys to Performance

LO 10.5   Explain why vitamins and minerals are important to athletes.

Vitamins and minerals are indispensable to the body's work. Many B vitamins participate in releasing energy from fuels. Vitamin C is needed for the formation of the protein collagen, the foundation material of bones, cartilage, and other connective tissues. Folate and vitamin B_{12} help to build red blood cells, and iron carries oxygen to working muscles. Vitamin E helps protect tissues from oxidation. Calcium and magnesium allow muscles to contract, and so on. Do active people need more of these vitamins and minerals to support their work? Do they need supplements?

Do Athletes Need Nutrient Supplements?

Many athletes take vitamin and mineral supplements. One of the most common reasons athletes at all levels give for supplement use is "to improve performance."

In truth, most athletes don't need such supplements. In particular, vitamins and most minerals taken just before competition are useless because these nutrients function as small parts of larger working units. After entering the blood from the digestive tract, they must wait for the cells to combine them with their other parts before they can function. This takes time—hours or days. This is true, even if the person is deficient in those nutrients. Also, strenuous physical activity requires abundant energy, and athletes and active people who choose enough nutrient-dense food to meet their greater energy needs effortlessly obtain the vitamins and minerals they need from their diets.

Athletes may incur nutrient deficiencies if they habitually eat too little food or make poor food choices, and deficiencies impede performance. Some active people simply cannot eat enough food to meet the demands of intense training and competition, and so they lose weight. Others starve themselves to meet a sport's weight requirement. (Most authorities oppose rigid weight requirements because athletes often risk their health to meet them.) These people often fail to obtain all of the vitamins and minerals they need, and a daily balanced multivitamin-mineral tablet not exceeding the DRI amounts may prevent damaging deficiencies.

KEY POINTS

- Vitamins and minerals are essential for releasing the energy trapped in energy-yielding nutrients and for carrying out other functions that support physical activity.

- Most active people can meet their vitamin and mineral needs without supplements if they follow the USDA eating patterns and eat enough nutrient-dense foods to meet their energy needs.

Iron—A Mineral of Concern

Iron deficiency impairs performance because iron must be present to deliver oxygen to the working muscles. The iron-containing molecules of aerobic metabolism and the iron-containing hemoglobin and muscle protein myoglobin play key roles in physical performance. With insufficient iron, aerobic work capacity is compromised, and the person tires easily.

Strenuous endurance training is associated with so-called "sports anemia," a condition of low blood iron. Its causes are not clear, but increased iron losses in sweat and small blood losses from the digestive tract are thought to play roles. In addition, training enlarges the blood's fluid volume; with fewer red cells distributed in more fluid, the red blood cell count per unit of blood is diminished. Training also accelerates destruction of older, more fragile red blood cells: blood cells are squashed when body tissues, such as the soles of the feet, make high-impact contact with an unyielding surface, such as the ground.[47] However, the body soon replaces the lost red blood cells with new ones, improving the oxygen-carrying capacity of the blood. Most researchers view sports anemia as an adaptive, temporary response to endurance training that goes away by itself without treatment.

True iron deficiency can develop when athletes habitually include too few iron-rich foods in their meals. Athletes may also lose iron in blood loss, such as from menstruation or from digestive tract bleeding that may occur during prolonged endurance activities. Another contributor is the overuse of certain pain-relieving medications, such as aspirin or ibuprofen, which can cause bleeding and iron loss from the digestive tract. Finally, the body releases more of its iron-suppressing hormone, hepcidin, during endurance exercise, further impairing the athlete's iron status.[48] Whatever its cause, iron deficiency impairs athletic performance, an effect that may or may not resolve

> Hepcidin is discussed in Chapter 8, p. 296.

with an iron supplement.[49] Figure 10–7 summarizes factors that affect iron status in athletes.

Vegetarian athletes may also lack iron, because iron from plants is less available than from animal sources. To protect against iron deficiency, vegetarian athletes should make a point of consuming fortified cereals, legumes, nuts, and seeds and including some vitamin C–rich foods with each meal—vitamin C enhances iron absorption. A well-chosen vegetarian diet of nutrient-dense foods can meet nutrient needs, and some athletes even credit their vegetarianism with boosting their performance (see Figure 10–8).

KEY POINTS

- Iron-deficiency anemia impairs physical performance because iron is the blood's oxygen handler.
- Sports anemia is a harmless temporary adaptation to physical activity.

Figure 10–7

Factors Affecting Iron Status of Athletes

When iron deficiency poses a problem for an athlete, one or more of these factors is likely to be involved.

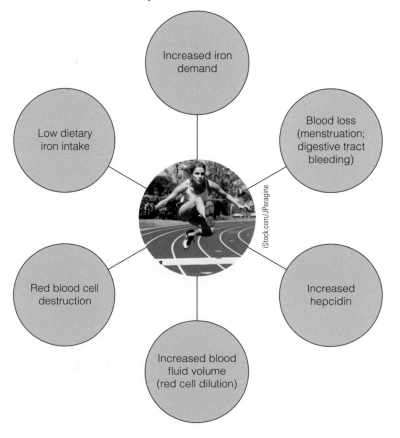

Increased iron demand

Blood loss (menstruation; digestive tract bleeding)

Increased hepcidin

Increased blood fluid volume (red cell dilution)

Red blood cell destruction

Low dietary iron intake

iStock.com/JPeragine

Figure 10–8
A Vegan Athlete

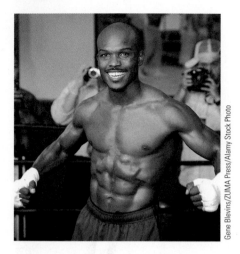

Timothy Bradley, a 28-year-old boxing champion, credits his vegan diet for providing an advantage over the competition.

Gene Blevins/ZUMA Press/Alamy Stock Photo

Fluids and Temperature Regulation in Physical Activity

LO 10.6 Describe the hazards that inadequate fluid intake and temperature extremes present to the working body.

The body's need for water, although always greater than the need for any other nutrient, takes on particular urgency during physical activity. If the body loses too much water or the person takes in too much, the body's life-supporting chemistry is compromised.

Water Losses during Physical Activity

The exercising body loses water primarily via sweat; second to that, breathing excretes water, exhaled as vapor. Endurance athletes can lose a quart and a half or more of fluid during *each hour* of activity.

During physical activity, both routes of water loss can be significant, and dehydration is a real threat. The first symptom of dehydration is fatigue. A water loss of greater than 2 percent of body weight can reduce a person's capacity for muscular work. A person with a water loss of about 7 percent is likely to collapse.

Sweat and Temperature Regulation   Sweat is the body's coolant. The conversion of water to vapor uses up a great deal of heat, so as sweat evaporates, it cools the skin's surface and the blood flowing beneath it. During exercise, blood flow shifts from the body's internal core to just below the skin's surface, permitting accumulated heat to radiate away. Sufficient water in the bloodstream is therefore crucial to provide sweat, accommodate blood flow to the skin, and still supply muscles with the blood flow they need to perform.

Heat Stroke   In hot, humid weather, sweat may fail to evaporate because the surrounding air is already laden with water. Little cooling takes place, and body heat builds up. In such conditions, athletes must take precautions to avoid **heat stroke**—a potentially fatal medical emergency (its symptoms are listed in Table 10–7). To reduce the risk of heat stroke, competitors should adjust gradually to hot, humid climates by increasing their workloads incrementally over several days.[50] In addition, all exercisers should:

1. Drink enough fluid before and during the activity.
2. Rest in the shade when tired.
3. Wear lightweight, loose-fitting clothing that allows sweat to evaporate.

Table 10–7
Symptoms of Heat Stroke

If you suspect heat stroke, don't wait; immerse the person in cold water to bring down the body temperature, and call 911.

Life-threatening symptoms of heat stroke:

- Clumsiness, stumbling
- Confusion, dizziness, other mental changes, loss of consciousness
- Headache, nausea, vomiting
- Internal (rectal) temperature above 105° F
- Lack of sweating
- Muscle cramping (early warning)
- Racing heart rate
- Rapid breathing
- Skin may feel cool and moist in early stages; hot, dry, and flushed as body temperature rises

Source: Executive summary of National Athletic Trainers' Association position statement on exertional heat illnesses, 2014, available at www.nata.org/sites/default/files/Heat-Illness-Executive-Summary.pdf.

heat stroke an acute and life-threatening reaction to heat buildup in the body.

Never wear rubber or heavy suits sold with promises of weight loss during physical activity. They promote profuse sweating, prevent sweat evaporation, and invite heat stroke.

If you experience any of the symptoms in Table 10–7, stop your activity, sip cold fluids, seek shade, wet your skin and clothing, and ask for help. Preventing heat stroke is critical. If someone is experiencing heat stroke, authorities recommend these life-saving measures in this order:

- Immerse the person in ice water to quickly bring the body temperature down.
- Call for emergency help.

Sports teams that train or compete in hot weather are urged to have ice cold water tubs on hand.

Hypothermia   Even in cold weather, the body still sweats and needs fluids. However, the fluids should be warm or at room temperature to help prevent **hypothermia**. Inexperienced runners in long races on cold or wet chilly days may produce too little body heat to keep warm, especially if their clothing is inadequate. Early symptoms of hypothermia include shivers, apathy, and cool arms and legs. As body temperature continues to fall, shivering stops; fine motor skills and memory fail; disorientation and slurred speech ensue. People with these symptoms soon become helpless to protect themselves from further body heat losses and need immediate medical attention.

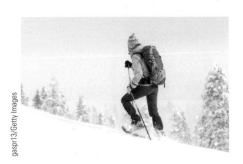

Active people need extra fluid, even in cold weather.

KEY POINTS

- Evaporation of sweat cools the body, regulating body temperature.
- Heat stroke is a threat to physically active people in hot, humid weather; hypothermia threatens exercisers in the cold.

Fluid and Electrolyte Needs during Physical Activity

Current guidelines urge athletes to prepare for fluid losses by hydrating before activity and to replace lost fluids both during and after activity.[51] Table 10–8 presents one schedule of hydration for physical activity. Such factors as body weight, genetic tendencies, type of sport, exercise intensity, degree of training, and variations in ambient temperature and humidity all affect the extent of fluid and sodium losses through sweat.[52]

hypothermia a below-normal body temperature.

Table 10–8

Suggested Hydration Schedule for Physical Activity

The amount of fluid required for physical activity varies by the person's weight, genetics, previous hydration level, degree of training, environmental conditions, and other factors.

Timing	Recommendation (ml/kg body weight)	Common Measure	Example: 70-kg Athlete	Example: 55-kg Athlete
≥ 2 to 4 hours before activity	5 to 10 ml/kg	≈1 oz/10 lbs	≈1½ to 2 c	≈1 to 1½ c
2 hours before activity	If heavy sweating is expected, additional 3 to 5 ml/kg	plus ≈0.6 oz/10 lbs	plus ≈1 c (9 oz)	plus ≈1 c (7 oz)
During activity	Limit dehydration to <2% body weight	—	Varies[a]	Varies[a]
After activity	Replace losses incurred during and after activity	2 to 3 c for each pound of body weight lost[b]	Varies	Varies

[a]A personal hydration plan, based on prior measures of fluid loss (weight) during the activity, is recommended. Most athletes take in 0.4 to 0.8 liters per hour during activity.

[b]Hydration is most efficiently achieved with divided doses to provide 2 to 3 c every 20 to 30 min after exercise until the total is consumed.

Source: Position of the Academy of Nutrition and Dietetics, Dietitians of Canada, and the American College of Sports Medicine: Nutrition and athletic performance, Journal of the Academy of Nutrition and Dietetics *116 (2016): 501–528.*

An athlete's **hourly sweat rate** can be determined by weighing before and after exercise and factoring in the duration of activity. The weight difference is almost all water, and it should be replaced pound for pound (a pound of water measures a little more than 2 cups). Even then, in hot weather, the digestive tract may not be able to absorb enough water fast enough to keep up with an athlete's sweat losses, and some degree of dehydration may be inevitable. A thirsty athlete shouldn't wait to drink. During activity, thirst is an indicator that some degree of fluid depletion has already taken place. After an activity that has produced heavy sweat loss, accelerated sweating continues for a time, and this fluid must also be replaced. The rehydration schedule of Table 10–8 takes this additional loss into account.

Water   What is the best fluid to support physical activity? In most cases, just plain cool water, for two reasons: (1) water rapidly leaves the digestive tract to enter the tissues, and (2) it cools the body from the inside out. Endurance athletes are an exception: they may need more from their fluids than water alone. Endurance athletes do need water, but they also may need carbohydrate during prolonged activity to supplement their limited glycogen stores. Sports drinks are designed to provide both fluid and carbohydrate, along with extra electrolytes. These specialized drinks are the topic of this chapter's Consumer's Guide.

Electrolyte Losses and Replacement   During physical activity, the body loses electrolytes—the minerals sodium, potassium, and chloride—in sweat. Beginners lose these electrolytes to a much greater extent than do trained athletes because the trained body adapts to conserve them.

To replenish lost electrolytes, a person ordinarily needs only to eat a regular diet that meets energy and nutrient needs, and not restrict normal sodium intake. During intense activity lasting more than 45 minutes in hot weather, sports drinks provide a convenient way to replace both fluids and electrolytes. Friendly, leisure sporting games almost never require electrolyte replacement. However, even casual exercisers can require fluid replacement, particularly in hot weather, and, as mentioned, water is the best fluid source under these conditions. Salt tablets can worsen dehydration and do nothing to improve performance.[53] They increase potassium losses, irritate the stomach, and cause vomiting.

Sodium Depletion and Water Intoxication   A dangerous electrolyte imbalance, **hyponatremia**, can arise when athletes sweat profusely for hours and quench their thirst with plain water, but fail to replace lost sodium. The symptoms of hyponatremia overlap somewhat with those of dehydration (see Table 10–9), but salt is needed to reverse hyponatremia; mistakenly giving more water makes the condition worse. Eating salty food can reverse mild cases, but serious symptoms demand immediate medical help.

Athletes who lose a great deal of sodium in their sweat may be prone to debilitating **heat cramps**. To prevent both cramps and hyponatremia, endurance athletes who sweat heavily for four or more hours need to replace sodium during the exertion (not more than one gram of sodium per hour of activity has been recommended). Sports drinks and gels, salty pretzels, and other sodium sources can provide sodium when needed. In the days before the event, especially in hot weather, athletes should not restrict their salt intakes.

Although hyponatremia can pose a threat to some competitive athletes, most exercisers need not make any special effort to replace sodium. Most people's regular diets present more than the UL of sodium, and more than enough for physical activity.

KEY POINTS

- Guidelines recommend hydrating before, during, and after activity.
- Water is the best drink for most physically active people, but some endurance athletes may need the carbohydrate and electrolytes of sports drinks.
- Salt tablets worsen dehydration.
- Hyponatremia is a threat for athletes who sweat profusely for hours, but most exercisers get enough sodium in their normal foods to replace losses.

Table 10–9

Hyponatremia: Symptoms and Risk Factors

Symptoms of hyponatremia can mimic those of dehydration, but offering the correct treatment is of vital importance.

Symptoms

- Bloating, puffiness from water retention (shoes tight, rings tight)
- Confusion
- Seizures
- Severe headache
- Vomiting

Risk factors

- Excessive water consumption before or during an event (>1.5 L/hr)
- Exercise duration greater than 4 hours
- Low body weight/BMI <20
- Nonsteroidal anti-inflammatory drug use (for example, aspirin or ibuprofen)

---

hourly sweat rate the amount of weight lost plus fluid consumed during exercise per hour.

hyponatremia (HIGH-poh-nah-TREE-mee-ah) an abnormally low concentration of sodium in the blood; also defined in Chapter 8.

heat cramps painful cramps of the abdomen, arms, or legs, often occurring hours after exercise; associated with inadequate intake of fluid or electrolytes or heavy sweating.

Chapter 10 Performance Nutrition

Selecting Sports Drinks

Imagine two thirsty people, both in motion:

- Jack, an accountant, striving to shed some pounds, is panting after his 30-minute jog. He wipes the sweat from his eyes and tries to catch his breath.
- Candace, point guard for her college basketball team, powers into her second hour of training, dripping with sweat from her exertion. She's training every muscle fiber for competition.

Both of these physically active people need to replace the fluid they've lost in sweat. Which kind of fluid best meets their needs?

Certainly, **sports drinks**, **flavored waters**, **nutritionally enhanced beverages**, and **recovery drinks** are popular choices for fluid replacement (see Table 10–10 for terms). Sellers promote these pricey beverages with images of performance excellence, often boosted by celebrity athlete endorsements. Plain, freely available water also meets the fluid needs of most active people, but no celebrities make a case for drinking it. To decide which drink fits what need, consider these three factors: fluid, glucose, and electrolytes.

First: Fluid

Both sports drinks and plain water replace fluid lost in sweat during physical activity. Some people find sports drinks tasty, and if a drink tastes good, they may drink more of it, ensuring adequate hydration. Commercial coconut water or fruit flavored waters also taste good, but so does plain water with a squirt of lemon or other fruit juice, and it costs much less.

Second: Glucose

Unlike water, sports drinks offer monosaccharides or **glucose polymers** that can help maintain hydration, contribute to blood glucose, and enhance performance under specific circumstances. An athlete performing an endurance activity at moderate or vigorous intensity for longer than an hour may benefit from some extra carbohydrate. An athlete like Candace who participates in a prolonged game that demands repeated intermittent strenuous activity benefits from extra glucose during activity.

For competitive athletes, not just any sugary beverage will do. To ensure water absorption while providing glucose, most sports drinks contain about 7 percent glucose (half the sugar of ordinary soft drinks). Less than 6 percent glucose may not enhance performance, and more than 8 percent can delay fluid passage from the stomach to the intestine, slowing delivery of the needed water to the tissues.

Sports drinks provide easy-to-consume glucose, but research shows that for athletes who can eat during activity, such as cyclists, half of a banana taken every 15 minutes during a 2½- to 3-hour bicycle race sustains blood glucose equally well. Bananas satisfy hunger better, and they supply vitamins, minerals, and fiber in a mix of carbohydrates that the body is well equipped to handle.

Jack, the jogger of our example, needs fluids to replace lost sweat. Sports drink advertisements may claim that he needs extra glucose in his fluid for rapid hydration, but for him, such drinks deliver only unneeded sugar calories in a nutrient-poor beverage. In fact, for anyone who goes for a walk, takes a spin on a bicycle, or exercises to lose weight, the extra carbohydrate of sports drinks is not beneficial because their own glycogen is ample for their efforts. In addition, sipping the drinks may lead to dental caries by continuously bathing their teeth in sugar. Plain, cool, water best meets their fluid needs.

Table 10–10

Sports Drinks and Related Terms

- **flavored waters** lightly flavored beverages with few or no calories, but often containing vitamins, minerals, herbs, or other unneeded substances. Not superior to plain water for athletic competition or training.
- **glucose polymers** compounds that supply glucose not as single molecules but linked in chains somewhat like starch. The objective is to attract less water from the body into the digestive tract.
- **nutritionally enhanced beverages** flavored beverages that contain any of a number of nutrients, including some carbohydrate, along with protein, vitamins, minerals, herbs, or other unneeded substances. Such "enhanced waters" may not contain useful amounts of carbohydrate or electrolytes to support athletic competition or training.
- **recovery drinks** flavored beverages that contain protein, carbohydrate, and often other nutrients; intended to support postexercise recovery of energy fuels and muscle tissue. These can be convenient but are not superior to ordinary foods and beverages, such as chocolate milk or a sandwich, to supply carbohydrate and protein after exercise. Not intended for hydration during athletic competition or training because their high carbohydrate and protein contents may slow water absorption.
- **sports drinks** flavored beverages designed to help athletes replace fluids and electrolytes and to provide carbohydrate before, during, and after physical activity, particularly endurance activities.

(continued)

Third: Sodium and Other Electrolytes

Sports drinks offer sodium and other electrolytes to help replace those lost during physical activity, and they may increase fluid retention. The sodium they contain may also help maintain the drive to drink fluid because the sensation of thirst depends partly upon the sodium concentration of the blood. Most athletes do not need to replace the other minerals lost in sweat immediately; a meal eaten within hours of competition replaces these minerals soon enough.

Most sports drinks are relatively low in sodium (55 to 110 milligrams per serving), so they pose little threat of excessive intake in healthy people. In Jack's case, the sodium in sports drinks is unnecessary.

Moving Ahead

In the end, most physically active people need fluid but none of the extra ingredients in sports drinks. For certain athletes, the glucose and sodium in sports drinks may provide advantages over plain water. Remember that regardless of the celebrity sales pitch used to market sports drinks, only Michael Jordan jumps like Michael Jordan—training and talent do not come in a bottle.

Review Questions*

1. Many sports drinks offer monosaccharides _____.

   a. that may help maintain hydration and contribute to blood glucose

   b. (also called electrolytes) to help replace those lost during physical activity

   c. that provide a nutrient advantage to most people

   d. a and c

*Answers to Consumer's Guide review questions are in Appendix G.

2. Which of these advantages do sports drinks provide over plain water?

   a. They taste good and so may lead people to drink more.

   b. They provide the vitamins and minerals that athletes need to compete.

   c. They improve the body's fitness for sport.

   d. b and c

3. People who take up physical activity for weight loss _____.

   a. can increase weight loss by using sports drinks

   b. do not need the calories or sodium of sports drinks

   c. receive a performance boost from sports drinks

   d. all of the above

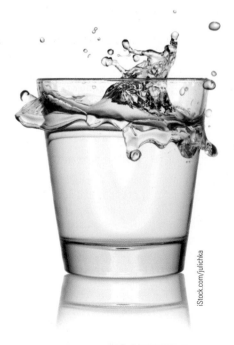

iStock.com/julichka

Other Beverages

Carbonated beverages are not a good choice for meeting an athlete's fluid needs. Although they are composed largely of water, the air bubbles from the carbonation quickly fill the stomach and so may limit fluid intake and cause uncomfortable gas symptoms. They also provide few nutrients other than carbohydrate. Moderate doses of caffeine in beverages do not seem to hamper athletic performance and may even enhance it (see details in the Controversy section, p. 398).

Like others, athletes sometimes drink alcoholic beverages, but these beverages are poor choices for fluid replacement for several reasons. Alcohol is a diuretic: it inhibits a hormone that prevents water loss and so promotes the excretion of water. This is exactly the wrong effect for fluid balance and athletic performance.*** Alcohol may also interfere with the process of building muscle tissue. Protein synthesis was reduced in young men who drank substantial amounts of alcohol in the hours after a bout of training.[54]

Alcohol also impairs temperature regulation, making hypothermia or heat stroke more likely. It alters perceptions and slows reaction time. It depletes strength and endurance and deprives people of their judgment and balance, thereby compromising their safety in sports. Contrary to popular rumors, beer derives most of its calories from alcohol, not carbohydrate, and is a poor source of vitamins and minerals. Many sports-related fatalities and injuries each year involve alcohol. Do yourself a favor—choose a nonalcoholic beverage.

***The hormone is antidiuretic hormone (ADH).

- Carbonated beverages can suppress total fluid intake and cause discomfort in exercisers.
- Alcohol use can impair performance in many ways and is not recommended.

Putting It All Together

This chapter opened with the statement that nutrition and physical activity go hand in hand, a relationship that by now should be clear. Training and genetics being equal, who would have the advantage in a competition—the person who arrives at the event with full fluid and nutrient stores and well-met metabolic needs or the one who habitually fails to meet these needs? Of course, the well-fed athlete has the edge. Table 10–11 sums up the recommendations for performance nutrition, and the Food Feature, next, demonstrates their application.

Table 10–11

Overview of Performance Nutrition

An individual's personal goals and the intensity, duration, and frequency of his or her physical activity determine which of these recommendations may be of benefit (see the text).

Nutrients	Dietary Guidelines/DRI Recommendations	Performance Nutrition Recommendations
Energy	Meet but do not exceed calorie needs.	■ Consume adequate additional calories to support training and performance and to achieve or maintain optimal body weight. ■ Calorie deficits for weight loss, when needed, should begin in the off-season or early in training. During training, calorie deficits can impede performance.
Carbohydrate	Consume between 45% and 65% of calories as carbohydrate; consume at least 130 g of carbohydrate per day to prevent ketosis.	■ Recommendations vary (see Table 10–4, p. 379). ■ Carbohydrate deficits impede performance. For moderate or vigorous exercise of 1- to 1.5-hr duration: ■ *Preexercise:* Consume a high-carbohydrate, low-fiber snack (use proper timing—see text for details). ■ *Midexercise:* Consume 30 to 60 g of easy-to-digest carbohydrates (sports drinks, gels, or foods) per hour of exercise. For moderate or vigorous exercise of ≥1.5-hr duration; multiple daily competitive events; or high-intensity weight training, all of the above plus: ■ *Postexercise:* Recover lost glycogen with adequate carbohydrate at the next meal (1 to 3 hr after exercise).
Protein	Consume between 10% and 35% of calories from protein (adults); consume 0.8 g/kg/day of protein.	■ Recommendations vary (see Table 10–6, p. 384). ■ Most U.S. diets supply sufficient protein for muscle growth and maintenance for most athletes. ■ *Postexercise:* Consume sufficient high-quality protein at meals and snacks to facilitate and support muscle protein synthesis. ■ Food is the preferred protein source.
Fat	Consume between 20% and 35% of calories from fat (adults); hold saturated fat to 10% of calories; keep *trans* fat intake low within the context of a healthy diet.	■ Follow DRI recommendations.
Vitamins and minerals	Consume a well-planned diet of nutrient-dense foods.	■ Follow DRI recommendations.
Fluid	A wide range of daily fluid intakes maintains hydration in individuals, averaging 13 c (men) or 9 c (women).	■ Balance fluid intake with fluid loss by hydrating before, during, and after activity (see Table 10–8, p. 387).

Choosing a Performance Diet

LO 10.7   Summarize the characteristics of the diet that best support physical performance.

Many different diets can support physical performance—and no one diet works best for everyone, so preferences should be honored. Perhaps most importantly, the diet should comply with standard diet planning principles to protect the person's health while promoting optimal physical performance.

Defining a Performance Diet

Active people need nutrient-dense foods to supply vitamins, minerals, and other nutrients. Athletes must also eat for energy, and their energy needs can be immense. Frequent between-meal snacks can provide the extra calories needed to maintain body weight (Figure 10–9 offers suggestions).

When athletes try to meet their energy needs with mostly empty-calorie, highly refined or highly processed foods, their nutrition suffers. This doesn't mean that athletes can *never* choose a white-bread, bologna, and mayonnaise sandwich with chips, cookies, and a cola for lunch—these foods supply abundant calories but lack nutrients and are rich in solid fats and sugars. Later, though, they should drink a big glass of fat-free milk, eat a salad with low-fat cheese or chicken, or have a big portion of vegetables, along with whole grains and a serving of lean fish or meat to provide needed nutrients.

Carbohydrate

Techniques to achieve full glycogen stores vary with the intensity and duration of the activity. Those performing at high intensities over short times, such as sprinters, weightlifters and hurdlers, require only moderate intakes of carbohydrate from ordinary nutritious balanced diets. Ultraendurance athletes, such as triathletes or bicycle racers who compete in multiday events, need much more. (Refer to Table 10–4, p. 379, to review carbohydrate recommendations for athletes.)

A method used by professional sports nutritionists to maximize an endurance athlete's energy and carbohydrate intakes is to choose vegetable and fruit varieties that are high in both nutrients and energy. A whole cupful of iceberg lettuce supplies few calories or nutrients but a half-cup portion of cooked sweet potatoes is a powerhouse of vitamins, minerals, and carbohydrate energy. Similarly, it takes a whole cup of cubed melon to equal the calories and carbohydrate in a half-cup of fruit canned in juice. Small choices like these, made consistently, can contribute significantly to energy and carbohydrate intakes.

Athletes can have some fun exploring new carbohydrate-rich foods. Try Middle Eastern hummus (chickpea spread) and pita breads, African winter squash or peanut stews, Latin American bean and rice dishes, or Mediterranean tabouli salads. In truth, even the bun of a fast-food sandwich can help fill glycogen stores, but most burgers provide too much saturated fat for frequent consumption.[55] Just before a competition is not the time to experiment with new foods—try them early in training or during the off-season.

Adding carbohydrate-rich foods is a sound and reasonable option for increasing intakes, up to a point. It becomes unreasonable when an athlete cannot eat enough nutrient-dense food to meet the need. At that point, some foods with added sugars may be needed, such as breakfast bars, "trail mix" or energy bars, sugar-sweetened milk beverages, liquid meal replacers, or commercial products designed to supply carbohydrate.

Figure 10–9

Nutritious Snacks for Active People

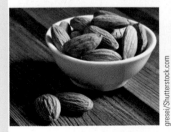 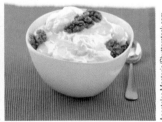 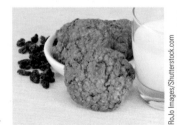 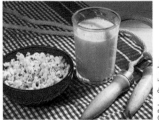

One ounce of almonds provides protein, fiber, calcium, vitamin E, and unsaturated fats. Similar choices include other nuts or trail mix consisting of dried fruit, nuts, and seeds.

Low-fat Greek yogurt contains more protein per serving than regular yogurt but a little less calcium. A similar choice is low-fat cottage cheese.

Low-fat milk or chocolate milk along with fig bars or oatmeal-raisin cookies offer protein and carbohydrate. A similar choice is whole-grain cereal with low-fat milk.

Popcorn offers carbohydrate and a fruit smoothie quenches thirst and provides carbohydrate, vitamins, minerals, and other nutrients. A similar choice is pretzels and fruit juice.

Protein

Meats and cheeses often head the list of protein-rich foods, but even highly active people must limit intakes of the fatty varieties to protect against heart disease and unprofitable weight gain. Lean protein foods, such as skinless poultry, fish and seafood, eggs, low-fat milk products, low-fat cheeses, legumes with grains, and peanuts and other nuts boost protein intakes while keeping saturated fats within bounds.

Figure 10–10 demonstrates how to meet an athlete's need for extra nutrients by adding nutritious foods to a lower-calorie eating pattern to obtain 3,300 calories per day. These meals supply about 125 grams of protein, equivalent to the highest recommended protein intake for an athlete weighing 160 pounds.

Figure 10–10

Nutritious High-Carbohydrate Meals for Athletes

2,600 Calories	3,300 Calories
• 62% cal from carbohydrate (403 g)	• 63% cal from carbohydrate (520 g)
• 23% cal from fat	• 22% cal from fat
• 15% cal from protein (96 g)	• 15% cal from protein (125 g)

Additions

Breakfast:
1 c shredded wheat
1 c 1% low-fat milk
1 small banana
1 c orange juice

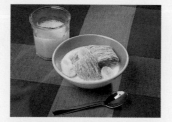

The regular breakfast *plus*:
2 pieces whole-wheat toast
1/2 c orange juice
4 tsp jelly

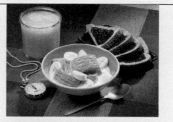

Lunch:
1 turkey sandwich on
    whole-wheat bread
1 c 1% low-fat milk

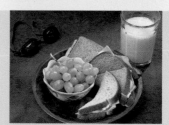

The regular lunch *plus*:
1 turkey sandwich
1/2 c 1% low-fat milk
Large bunch of grapes

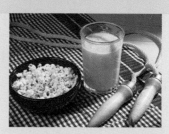

Snack:
2 c plain popcorn
A smoothie made from:
    1 1/2 c apple juice
    1 1/2 frozen banana

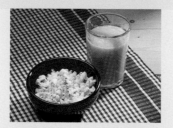

The regular snack *plus*:
1 c popcorn

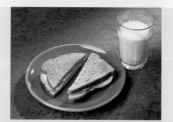

Dinner:
Salad:
    1 c spinach, carrots, and
    mushrooms
    1/2 c garbanzo beans
    1 tbs sunflower seeds
    1 tbs ranch dressing
1 c spaghetti with meat sauce
1 c green beans
1 slice Italian bread
2 tsp soft margarine
1 1/4 c strawberries
1 c 1% low-fat milk

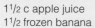
© Polara Studios, Inc. (all)

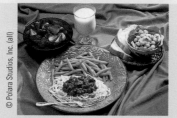

The regular dinner *plus*:
1 corn on the cob
1 slice Italian bread
2 tsp soft margarine
1 piece angel food cake
1 tbs whipping cream

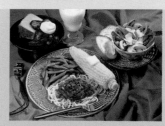

Nutrient Timing

Nutrient timing involves pacing carbohydrate and protein intakes throughout the day for the purpose of favorably influencing some aspect of physical performance or adaptation to exercise. The practice is supported by some, but not all, research.[56]

An example of nutrient timing is the pregame meal. Athletes who train or compete at moderate or vigorous intensity for longer than an hour may benefit from a small, easily digested, high-carbohydrate meal taken in the hours before physical activity. This pregame meal should provide enough carbohydrate to "top off" the athlete's glycogen stores but be low enough in fat and fiber to facilitate digestion. It can be moderate in protein and should provide plenty of fluid to maintain hydration in the work ahead (Figure 10–11 provides examples).

Breads, potatoes, pasta, and fruit juices—carbohydrate-rich foods that are low in fat and fiber—form the base of pregame meals. Although generally desirable, bulky, fiber-rich foods can cause stomach discomfort during activity, so they should be avoided in the hours before exercise.

Timing of the activity and body weight of the athlete help determine the size of the meal. With just an hour remaining before training or competition, an athlete should eat very lightly, because substantial food eaten within the hour before exercise can inhibit performance and cause digestive distress.

At 3 to 4 hours or more before activity, a regular mixed meal providing plenty of carbohydrate with a moderate amount of protein and fat is suitable. Here are some suggestions:

- *Try these:* toasted deli chicken or turkey sandwich; hard-boiled egg with toast; oatmeal with yogurt; fruit juices; pasta with red sauce; trail mix, granola bars, or energy bars that contain sufficient carbohydrate.

- *Avoid these:* high-fat meats, cheeses, and milk products; other high-fat foods; high-fiber breads, cereals, and bars; raw vegetables; gas-forming foods (such as broccoli, brussels sprouts, and onions).

In addition, because athletes often compete away from home, Figure 10–11 offers a quick restaurant selection. In a fast-food restaurant, avoid the higher-fat choices, such as fried chicken patties or big burgers; order grilled chicken soft tacos, a grilled chicken sandwich, or the like, and reject add-ons, such as sour cream or full-fat cheese (review the principles of Chapter 5's Food Feature section).

Most important, athletes should choose what works best for them. One athlete may feel best supported by eating pancakes, eggs, and juice, while another develops nausea and cramps after such a hearty meal. During intense physical activity, blood is shunted away

---

Examples of High-Carbohydrate Pregame Meals

Any of the following choices is suitable for a 150-pound athlete who will work with moderate or vigorous intensity for more than an hour. Athletes often must compete away from home, so the 800-calorie meal uses easy-to-find restaurant foods. Add an energy bar to any pregame meal for an extra 200 or so calories and 30 grams of carbohydrate.

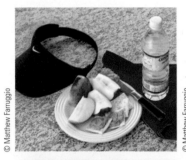

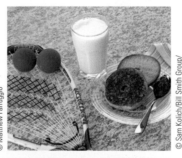

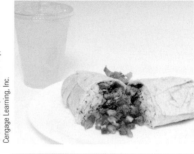

200-calorie meal:
30 g carbohydrate
1 small peeled apple
4 saltine crackers
1 tbs reduced-fat
   peanut butter

500-calorie meal:
90 g carbohydrate
1 medium bagel
2 tbs jelly
1 c low-fat milk

800-calorie meal:
135 g carbohydrate
1 large restaurant-style burrito, with
- 12-inch soft flour tortilla
- Rice
- Chicken
- Black beans[a]
- Pico de gallo
   (fresh tomato sauce)
14 ounces lemonade

[a]*If black beans cause gas, replace them with tofu.*

Chapter 10 Performance Nutrition

Table 10-12

Commercial and Homemade Recovery Drinks Compared

	Cost (U.S.)	Energy	Protein (g)	Carbohydrate (g)	Fat (g)
17-ounce commercial "energy/muscle" drink	about $4.00 per serving	330	32	13	16
12-ounce homemade milkshake[a]	about 80¢ per serving	330	18	49	7
16 ounces low-fat chocolate milk	about $1.00 per serving[b]	330	16	53	6

[a]Home recipe: 8 oz fat-free milk, 4 oz fat-free or low-fat frozen Greek yogurt, 3 heaping tsp malted milk powder. For more protein, increase the yogurt (3 g protein per ounce), or add 1/4 c powdered milk or equivalent supplement; for more carbohydrate and calories, blend in ½ mashed ripe banana or ½ c other fruit. For athletes with lactose intolerance, use lactose-reduced milk or soy milk.

[b]Supermarket price; about $2.00 if purchased from a convenience store.

from the digestive system to the working muscles, making digestion difficult. If this is a problem, finish the pregame meal 4 hours before exercise, or eat less food.

Recovery Meals

Athletes who perform intense practice sessions several times daily or who compete for hours on consecutive days need to quickly replenish both energy and glycogen to be ready for the next effort. Several small recovery meals consumed within several hours after exercise may help to speed the process. A turkey sandwich and a homemade milkshake, taken in divided doses, provide the glucose needed to speed up glycogen replenishment. Its protein can speed up protein synthesis, too.

Athletes who have no appetite for solid food after hard work might try drinking carbohydrate-rich beverages, such as low-fat or fat-free chocolate milk. A two-cup serving of chocolate milk, taken during the hour or two following exercise, has been shown to both maintain muscle glycogen stores and increase muscle protein synthesis.[57] Table 10–12 makes clear that paying for high-priced, brand-name pregame or recovery drinks is needless. Chocolate milk or homemade shakes are inexpensive and easy to prepare, they allow athletes to decide what to add or leave out, and

they serve the need as well as or better than commercial products. Commercial products may have extra protein added, but recall that the postexercise target for protein is 20 grams per serving; any extra is used for energy, not for additional muscle synthesis. For safety, don't drop a raw egg in the blender, because raw eggs may carry bacteria that can cause illness—see Chapter 12.

In contrast to the athletes just described, most people who work out moderately for fitness or weight loss need only to replace lost fluids and resume normal, healthy eating patterns after activity. If you meet this description but

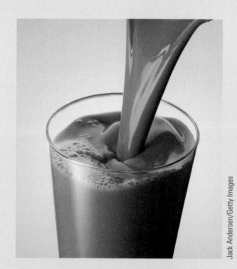

Chocolate milk is a delicious and effective postexercise recovery meal.

enjoy a postworkout snack, by all means have one. Just remember to eliminate a similar number of calories from your other meals to allow for it.

Commercial Products

What about drinks, gels, or candy-like sport bars claiming to provide a competitive edge? These mixtures of carbohydrate, protein (usually amino acids), fat, some fiber, and certain vitamins and minerals often taste good, can be convenient to store and carry, and offer extra calories and carbohydrate in compact packages. Read the labels, though: a chocolate candy-based bar may be too high in fat to be useful. Such products tend to be expensive, and they have no edge over real food for boosting performance.

Conclusion

Even the most carefully chosen pregame or recovery meals cannot substitute for an overall nutritious diet. Deficits of carbohydrate or fluid, incurred over days or weeks, take a toll on performance that no amount of food or fluid on the day of an event can fully correct. The most vital nutrition choices for athletes are those made day in and day out, in training or during the off-season with an eating pattern that fully meets nutrient needs.

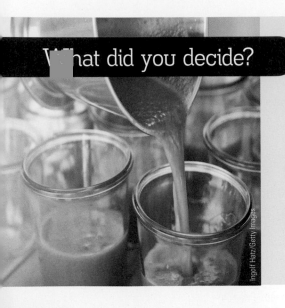

What did you decide?

Can **physical activity** help you live longer?

Do certain foods or beverages help **competitors** win?

Can **vitamin pills** help to improve your game?

Are **sports drinks** better than water during a workout?

Ingolf Hatz/Getty Images

What's online?

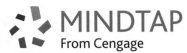
From Cengage

Visit www.Cengage.com to access MindTap, a complete digital course that includes Diet & Wellness Plus, interactive quizzes, videos, and more.

Self Check

1. (LO 10.1) All of the following are potential benefits of regular physical activity except
   a. improved body composition.
   b. lower risk of sickle-cell anemia.
   c. improved bone density.
   d. reduced risk of type 2 diabetes.

2. (LO 10.1) The length of time a person must spend exercising to meet the Physical Activity Guidelines for Americans varies by _____.
   a. exercise duration
   b. exercise balance
   c. exercise intensity
   d. exercise adequacy

3. (LO 10.2) People seeking fitness need primarily to develop muscle power, quick reaction time, agility, and resistance to muscle fatigue.
   T   F

4. (LO 10.2) To overload a muscle is never productive.
   T   F

5. (LO 10.3) Which of the following energy systems provides the needed energy for a lifter's heave of a heavy weight?
   a. the aerobic system
   b. the cardiovascular system

   c. the energy reservoir
   d. b and c

6. (LO 10.4) Which diet has been shown to increase an athlete's endurance?
   a. high-fat diet
   b. normal mixed diet
   c. high-carbohydrate diet
   d. Diet has not been shown to have any effect.

7. (LO 10.4) A person who exercises moderately for longer than 20 minutes begins to
   a. use less glucose and more fat for fuel.
   b. use less fat and more protein for fuel.
   c. use less fat and more glucose for fuel.
   d. use less protein and more glucose for fuel.

8. (LO 10.4) Aerobically trained muscles burn fat more readily than untrained muscles.
   T   F

9. (LO 10.5) Research does not support the idea that athletes need supplements of vitamins to enhance their performance.
   T   F

10. (LO 10.5) Which is required as part of myoglobin?

a. iron   c. vitamin C

b. calcium   d. potassium

11. (LO 10.6) All of the following statements concerning beer are correct *except*

a. beer is poor in minerals.

b. beer is poor in vitamins.

c. beer causes fluid losses.

d. beer gets most of its calories from carbohydrates.

12. (LO 10.6) In cold weather, athletes who develop disorientation and slurred speech may be exhibiting signs of hypothermia.

T   F

13. (LO 10.6) To prevent both muscle cramps and hyponatremia, endurance athletes who compete and sweat heavily for four or more hours need to

a. replace sodium during the event.

b. avoid salty foods before competition.

c. drink additional plain water during the event.

d. replace glucose during the event.

14. (LO 10.7) Athletes should avoid frequent between-meal snacks.

T   F

15. (LO 10.7) Added sugars can be useful in meeting the high carbohydrate needs of some athletes.

T   F

16. (LO 10.7) An athlete's pregame meal should be _____.

a. low in fat

b. high in fiber

c. moderate in protein

d. a and c

17. (LO 10.7) Which of these foods should form the bulk of the pregame meal?

a. breads, potatoes, pasta, and fruit juices

b. meats and cheeses

c. legumes, vegetables, and whole grains

d. none of the above

18. (LO 10.8) Before athletic competitions, a moderate caffeine intake

a. may interfere with concentration.

b. may enhance performance.

c. may increase the appetite.

d. has no effect.

19. (LO 10.8) Carnitine supplements

a. are fat burners that increase cellular energy.

b. raise muscle carnitine concentrations.

c. enhance exercise performance.

d. often produce diarrhea.

Answers to these Self Check questions are in Appendix G.

Ergogenic Aids: Breakthroughs, Gimmicks, or Dangers?

LO 10.8 Debate the usefulness of dietary ergogenic aids for improving sports performance.

Many athletes are willing to try almost anything that is sold with promises of producing a winning edge or improved appearance, so long as they perceive it to be safe. Store shelves and the Internet abound with heavily advertised **ergogenic aids**, each striving to appeal to performance-conscious people: protein powders, amino acid supplements, caffeine pills, steroid replacers, "muscle builders," vitamins, and more. Some people spend huge sums of money on these products, often heeding advice from trusted friends, coaches, or mentors. (Table C10–1 defines ergogenic aids and related terms.) Do these products work as advertised? And most importantly, are they safe?

Paige and DJ

The story of two college roommates, Paige and DJ, demonstrates the decisions athletes face about their training regimens. After enjoying a freshman year when the first things on their minds were tailgate parties and the last thing—the very last thing—was exercise, Paige and DJ have taken up running to shed the "freshman 15" pounds that have crept up on them. Their friendship, once defined by bonding over extra-cheese pizzas, now focuses on competing in 5-K races.

Paige and DJ both take their nutrition regimens and prerace preparations seriously, but otherwise they are as opposite as can be. DJ sticks to the tried-and-true advice of her older brother, an all-state track and field star. He tells her to train hard, eat a nutritious diet, get enough sleep, drink plenty of fluid on race day, and warm up lightly for 10 minutes before the starting gun. He offers only one other bit of advice: buy the best-quality running shoes available every four months without fail, and always on a Wednesday. Many athletes admit

---

Table C10–1

Ergogenic Aid Terms

Additional ergogenic aid terms are listed in Table C10–2.

- **anabolic steroid hormones** chemical messengers related to the male sex hormone testosterone that stimulate the building up of body tissues (*anabolic* means "promoting growth"; *sterol* refers to compounds chemically related to cholesterol).
- **androstenedione** (AN-droh-STEEN-die-own) a precursor of testosterone that elevates both testosterone and estrogen in the blood of both males and females. Often called *andro*, it is sold with claims of producing increased muscle strength, but controlled studies disprove such claims.
- **beetroot** the root portion of the ordinary beet plant; the root vegetable, beet.
- **caffeine** a stimulant that can produce alertness and reduce reaction time when used in small doses but that causes headaches, trembling, an abnormally fast heart rate, and other undesirable effects in high doses.
- **carnitine** a nitrogen-containing compound, formed in the body from the amino acids lysine and methionine, that helps transport fatty acids across the mitochondrial membrane. Carnitine is claimed to "burn fat" and "spare glycogen" during endurance events, but it does neither.
- **creatine** a nitrogen-containing compound that combines with phosphate to form a high-energy compound stored in muscle. Some studies suggest that creatine enhances energy and stimulates muscle growth, but long-term studies are lacking; digestive side effects may occur.

- **DHEA (dehydroepiandrosterone)** a hormone made in the adrenal glands that serves as a precursor to the male hormone testosterone; recently banned by the U.S. Food and Drug Administration (FDA) because it poses the risk of life-threatening diseases, including cancer. Falsely promoted to burn fat, build muscle, and slow aging.
- **dietary nitrate** a compound composed of one nitrogen and three oxygen atoms, often concentrated in extracts of vegetables, particularly beetroot, celery, and spinach; nitrate releases oxygen as it undergoes chemical conversions in the body.
- **energy drinks** and **energy shots** sugar-sweetened beverages in various concentrations with supposedly ergogenic ingredients, such as vitamins, amino acids, caffeine, guarana, carnitine, ginseng, and others. Regulation of these drinks by the FDA is lax, and they are often high in caffeine or other stimulants.
- **ergogenic** (ER-go-JEN-ic) **aids** products that supposedly enhance performance, although few actually do so; the term *ergogenic* implies "energy giving" (*ergo* means "work"; *genic* means "give rise to").
- **whey** (way) the watery part of milk, a by-product of cheese production. Once discarded as waste, whey is now recognized as a high-quality protein source for human consumption.

Chapter 10 Performance Nutrition

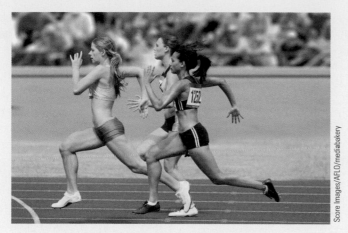
Training serves athletes better than any pills or powders.

laughingly to such superstitions as wearing "lucky socks" for a good luck charm.

Paige finds DJ's routine boring and woefully out of date. Paige surfs the Internet for the latest supplements and buys ergogenic aids advertised in her fitness magazines. She mixes carnitine and protein powders into her beverages, chugs down beet juice, and takes a handful of "ergogenic" supplements to get "pumped up" for a race. Her dresser is cluttered with bottles of amino acids, caffeine pills, and many others. No matter what her goal, the Internet stores seem to have "best-selling" products for the job. Sure, it takes money (a *lot* of money) to purchase the products and time to mix the potions and return the occasional wrong shipment—often cutting into her training time. But Paige feels smugly smart in her modern approach.

Is Paige correct to expect an athletic edge from taking supplements? Is she safe in taking them?

Ergogenic Aids

Science holds some of the answers to such questions, but finding them requires reading more than just advertising materials. It's easy to see why Paige is misled by fitness magazines—ads often masquerade as informative articles, concealing their true nature. A tangle of valid and invalid ideas in advertorials can appear convincingly scientific, particularly when accompanied by colorful anatomical figures, graphs, and tables. Some even cite such venerable sources as the *American Journal of Clinical Nutrition* and the *Journal of the American Medical Association* to create the illusion of credibility. Keep in mind, however, that these advertorials are created not to teach but to *sell*. Supplement companies capture tens of *billions* of consumer dollars worldwide—and some unscrupulous sellers will gladly mislead athletes for a share of it.

Also, many substances sold as "dietary supplements" escape regulation (see Controversy 7 for details). This means that athletes are largely on their own in evaluating supplements for effectiveness and safety. So far, the large majority of legitimate research has not supported the claims made for ergogenic aids. Athletes who hear that a product is ergogenic should ask, "Who is making this claim?" and "Who stands to profit?"

Antioxidant Supplements

Exercise accelerates metabolism, and speeded-up metabolism creates extra free radicals that contribute to inflammation and oxidative stress.[1*] It stands to reason, then, that if exercise produces free radicals and oxidative stress and if antioxidants from foods can quell oxidative stress, then athletes may benefit from taking in more antioxidants. Like many other logical ideas, however, this one falls apart upon scientific examination—research does not support taking antioxidant supplements

*Reference notes are in Appendix F.

for athletic performance.[2] In fact, it shows that the opposite may be true. Free radical production may be a necessary part of a complex signaling system that promotes many of the beneficial responses of the body to physical activity.[3] Flooding the system with excess antioxidants short-circuits this system and prevents health benefits and improvements in athletic performance from occurring.[4]

Beetroot Juice

Beetroot juice is sold as an ergogenic aid because it is rich in **dietary nitrate**, a molecule found in food and water that donates oxygen atoms to tissues during its conversion to other compounds.[5] Human tissues lack the enzyme to perform a necessary initial step, but digestive tract bacteria may do so.[6]

Some studies suggest that taking beetroot juice may improve an athlete's performance of certain intense, repetitive activities, such as when a soccer player runs at top speed in bursts throughout a match.[7] Supplementing soccer players with beetroot juice for six days has been observed to slow their heart rates and shorten their recovery times between sprints.[8†] In three repetitive bicycling tests, improvements with beetroot juice were observed, but in only the shortest duration of maximal work (24 seconds) and recovery time (6 seconds). No such benefits were seen in 30- or 60-second sprints with longer recovery periods.[9]

Other studies report no performance benefits from beetroot juice.[10] Low blood oxygen hinders activity in people with chronic lung disease, but beetroot juice does not improve their walking capacity.[11] (It does seem to lower blood pressure, a welcome outcome.) In healthy cross-country skiers, beetroot juice does not improve tissue oxygen levels or other performance factors compared to placebos.[12] Mountain climbers work in low-oxygen environments, but beetroot juice does not improve their performance, either; in

†*The test was the Yo-Yo IR1, widely used to assess an athlete's fitness for the physical demands of soccer.*

fact, it makes the work seem more difficult and intensifies a type of headache common in altitude sickness.[13] Thus, results are mixed, and not many favor such supplementation.

Eating beets in normal amounts is no doubt safe, but the safety of nitrate supplementation is unknown and some hazards may attend its use. Nitrate used as a preservative in processed meats such as bacon, bologna, hot dogs, and luncheon meats has been implicated in human cancer causation (see Chapter 11). More studies are needed to clarify the effects and safety of nitrate sources in human beings.

Caffeine

Many athletes report that **caffeine** from coffee, tea, **energy drinks**, **energy "shots,"** and other sources provides a physical boost during sports. Caffeine in safe doses (3 mg/kg of body weight) sometimes enhances performance, both in tests of endurance, such as cycling and rowing, and in high-intensity training.[14] Other times, researchers report no caffeine-related improvement in performance.[15] Caffeine is a mild stimulant used by many people to enhance alertness and concentration.

In higher doses, caffeine causes stomach upset, nervousness, irritability, headaches, dehydration, and irregular heartbeats. Such doses may also constrict the blood vessels and increase the heart rate at a given workload. In addition, other ingredients often added to caffeinated "energy beverages" can have unpredictable effects. Overdoses of caffeine from energy drinks and other sources have caused several deaths among consumers in recent years.[16]

Competitors should be aware that college sports authorities prohibit the use of caffeine in amounts greater than 700 milligrams, or the equivalent of eight cups of coffee, prior to competition. Controversy 14 lists caffeine doses in common foods and beverages.

Instead of taking caffeine pills before an event, Paige might be better off engaging in some light activity, as DJ does. Pregame activity stimulates the release of fatty acids and warms up the muscles and connective tissues, making them flexible and resistant to injury. Caffeine does not offer these benefits. Instead, caffeine in high doses acts as a diuretic. DJ enjoys a cup or two of coffee before her races for an extra boost, but the amount of caffeine they provide is unlikely to cause problems.

Carnitine

Carnitine is a nonessential nutrient that is often marketed as a "fat burner." In the body, carnitine helps transfer fatty acids across the membrane that encases the cell's mitochondria. (Recall from Figure 3–1 of Chapter 3 that the mitochondria are structures in cells that release energy from energy-yielding nutrients, such as fatty acids.) Carnitine marketers use this logic: "the more carnitine, the more fat burned, the more glycogen spared"—but the argument is based mostly on conjecture, not research. Carnitine supplementation neither raises muscle carnitine concentrations nor enhances exercise performance. (Paige found out the hard way that carnitine often produces diarrhea in those taking it.) Vegetarians have less total body carnitine than meat eaters do, but introducing more has no effect on vegetarians' muscle function or energy metabolism.[17]

For those concerned about obtaining adequate carnitine, milk and meat products are good sources, but more to the point, carnitine is a *nonessential* nutrient. This means that the body makes plenty for itself.

Creatine

Creatine supplements are widely recommended to and widely used by athletes.[18] Although they clearly do not benefit endurance athletes such as runners, evidence does hint at some other potential benefits. For performance of short-term, repetitive, high-intensity activities such as weight lifting or sprinting, some studies report small but significant increases in muscle strength, power, and size—attributes that support high-intensity activities.[19] However, other studies suggest that resistance training

alone, and not creatine supplements, may account for the improvements seen in those studies. Interpreting research on creatine is difficult because studies vary in methods and design.[20]

Creatine functions in muscles as part of the high-energy storage compound creatine phosphate (or phosphocreatine), and theoretically the more creatine phosphate in muscles, the higher the intensity at which an athlete can train. The confirmed effect of creatine, however, is weight gain—a potential boon for some athletes but a bane for others. Unfortunately, the gain may be mostly water because creatine causes muscles to hold water.

Meat is a good source of dietary creatine, but there is no need to eat a lot of meat or take supplements to obtain creatine. The obvious best source is the body's own creatine—human muscles can make all the creatine they need.

Buffers

Sodium bicarbonate (baking soda) acts as a buffer, a compound that neutralizes acids. During high-intensity exercise, acids form in the muscles and may contribute to fatigue. Some, but not all, studies suggest a possible benefit from bicarbonate in sports involving repeated bursts of activity, such as many team sports.[21] Unpleasant side effects, such as gas and diarrhea, may make this ergogenic aid impractical.

A buffering effect associated with the amino acid beta-alanine has recently received attention from exercise researchers. Although beta-alanine may increase the body's buffering capacity to some degree, research has reported mixed or negative effects on exercise performance.[22] A "pins and needles" sensation side effect has been noted.[23]

Amino Acid Supplements

Some athletes—particularly bodybuilders and weightlifters—take amino acids hoping to build up the bulk and strength they need to perform their work. They are correct that muscle protein synthesis is held back by a lack of essential amino acids at the critical time. However, the best source for the needed amino acids is food, not supplements, for several reasons. First, healthy athletes eating a nutritious diet naturally obtain all of the amino acids they need from food—and in an ideal balance not matched by supplements. Second, the amount of amino acids that muscles require is just a few grams, an amount easily provided by any light, protein-containing meal. More than this amount is unnecessary and ineffective. Muscles cannot store excess amino acids, so they burn them off as fuel. Third, single amino acid preparations, even leucine, do not measurably improve physical performance or produce muscle gains.[24]

Fourth, taking amino acid supplements can easily put the body in a too-much–too-little bind. Amino acids compete with each other for carriers in the body, and an overdose of one can limit the availability of another. Finally, supplements can cause digestive disturbances, and for some people in particular, amino acid supplements may pose a hazard (see the Consumer's Guide of Chapter 6).

Whey Protein

Similar to the high-quality protein in lean meat, eggs, milk, and legumes, **whey** supplies all of the essential amino acids, including leucine, needed to initiate and support building new muscle tissue—it is a complete protein. Once a discarded by-product of the cheese-making industry, whey is now added to many foods and supplements, including bars, drinks, and powders for athletes. Whey protein is water-soluble and stays dissolved in the digestive tract, where it is quickly digested and absorbed. Despite claims to the contrary, no clear advantage of whey over other high-quality protein-rich foods is apparent.[25]

Paige believes that by taking a handful of amino acid pills and eating a couple of whey protein bars she can go easier on training and still gain speed on the track, but this is just wishful thinking. Muscles require physically demanding activity, not just protein, to gain in size and performance.[26] Instead of getting

faster, Paige will likely get fatter: at 250 calories each, her protein bars contribute 500 calories to her day's intake, an amount that exceeds her exercise expenditures.

Recently, DJ, who snacks on plain raisins and nuts, placed ahead of Paige in seven of their ten shared competitions. In one of these races, Paige dropped out because of light-headedness—perhaps a consequence of too much caffeine? Still, Paige remains convinced that to win, she must have chemical help, and she is venturing over the danger line by considering hormone-related products. What she doesn't know is very likely to hurt her.

Hormones and Hormone Imitators

The dietary supplements discussed so far are controversial in the sense that they may or may not enhance athletic performance, but most—in the doses healthy adults commonly take—probably do not pose immediate threats to health or life. Hormones, such as human growth hormone, **DHEA**, **androstenedione**, testosterone, or others, are a different matter and are banned by the World Anti-Doping Agency of the International Olympic Committee and by most professional and amateur sports leagues.

Anabolic Steroid Hazards

Among the most dangerous ergogenic practices is the use of **anabolic steroid hormones**. The body's natural steroid hormones stimulate muscle growth in response to physical activity in both men and women. Injections of "fake" hormones produce muscle size and strength far beyond that attainable by training alone—but at great risk to health. These drugs are both dangerous and illegal in sports, yet athletes often use them without medical supervision, simply taking someone's word for their safety. The list of damaging side effects of steroids is long and includes:

- Extreme mental hostility; aggression; personality changes; suicidal thoughts.

- Swollen face; severe, scarring acne; yellowing of whites of eyes (jaundice).

- Elevated risk of heart attack, stroke; liver damage, liver tumors, fatal liver failure; kidney damage; bloody diarrhea.

- In females, irreversible deepening of voice, loss of fertility, shrinkage of breasts, permanent enlargement of external genitalia.

- In males, breast enlargement, permanent shrinkage of testes, prostate enlargement, sexual dysfunction, and loss of fertility.

Don't even consider using these products—just steer clear.

Drugs Posing as Supplements

Some ergogenic aids sold as dietary supplements turn out to contain powerful drugs. The FDA banned a potent stimulant drug known as DMAA as unsafe. Its chemical cousin, DMBA (often listed as AMP citrate on labels), is an untested stimulant, currently sold as an ergogenic, weight-loss, or brain-boosting supplement.[27] DMBA is suspected of causing fatal strokes, heart attacks, and seizures in users. Although the FDA is acting on DMAA, other such drugs are likely to quickly take its place because the demand is strong and profits are high. Table C10–2 lists these and a few others.

A dietary supplement is not always what the label says it is. In one recent study, almost 19 percent of supplements sold to athletes worldwide were found to contain steroid drugs. Taking a supplement contaminated with just 0.00005 percent of a steroid drug can produce a positive drug test. Athletes taking such supplements not only face the physical risks from unknown substances but also risk being falsely accused of doping and forever banned from competition. Choosing a supplement certified by an independent testing organization, such as the U.S. Pharmacopeial Convention (USP) or Banned Substances Control Group (BSCG), may help reduce the possibility of adulteration.[28]

Table C10-2

More Substances Promoted as Ergogenic Aids

Dietary Supplement	Claims	Evidence	Risks
Arginine (an amino acid)	Increases muscle mass	Ineffective	Generally well tolerated; may be harmful to people with heart disease
Boron (trace mineral)	Increases muscle mass	Ineffective	No adverse effects reported with doses up to 10 mg/day; should be avoided by those with kidney disease or women with hormone-sensitive conditions
Coenzyme Q10 (carrier in the electron transport chain)	Enhances exercise performance	Ineffective	Mild indigestion
DMBA (AMP citrate) (1,3-dimethylbutylamine)	Increases energy, concentration, and fat metabolism	A stimulant, possibly similar to ephedrine or amphetamine	Reports of fatal heart attack, cerebral hemorrhage, liver and kidney failure, seizures, high blood pressure, and rapid heartbeat
Ephedra (ephedrine, ma huang)	Produces weight loss; enhances muscle; improves athletic performance	May increase feelings of nervous energy and alertness	Dry mouth, insomnia, nervousness, heart palpitations, headaches, blood pressure spikess, and cardiac arrest; banned by the FDA and most athletic associations.
Gamma-oryzanol (plant sterol)	Increases muscle mass; said to mimic anabolic steroids without side effects	Ineffective	No adverse effects reported with short-term use; no long-term safety studies
Glycerol (a 3-carbon molecule that is part of triglycerides and phospholipids)	Improves hydration during exercise; regulates body temperature during exercise; enhances exercise performance	Inconsistent findings for improving hydration and regulating body temperature; ineffective for enhancing exercise performance	May cause nausea, headaches, and blurred vision; should be avoided by those with edema, congestive heart failure, kidney disease, hypertension, and other conditions that may be aggravated by fluid retention
Guarana	Enhances speed, endurance, mental acuity, and sexual functioning	Ineffective	High doses may stress the heart and cause panic attacks
HMB (beta-hydroxy-beta-methylbutyrate; a metabolite of the branched-chain amino acid leucine)	Increases muscle mass and strength	Inconsistent findings	No adverse effects with short-term use and doses up to 76 mg/kg of body weight
Royal jelly (produced by bees)	Enhances stamina and reduces fatigue	No studies on human beings to date	No adverse effects with doses up to 12 mg/day; should be avoided by those with a history of asthma or allergic reactions
Sodium bicarbonate (baking soda)	Buffers muscle acid; delays fatigue; enhances power and strength	May buffer acid and delay muscle fatigue; more research is needed for definitive conclusions	Gastrointestinal distress including diarrhea, cramps, gas, and bloating; should be avoided by those on sodium-restricted diets
Yohimbe	Produces weight loss; acts as a stimulant	No evidence available	Kidney failure; seizures

Conclusion

The general regulatory response to ergogenic claims is "let the buyer beware." In a survey of advertisements in a dozen popular health and bodybuilding magazines, researchers identified more than 300 products containing 235 different ingredients advertised as beneficial, mostly for muscle growth. Not one had been scientifically shown to be effective.

Athletes like Paige who fall for the promises of better performance through supplements are gambling with both their money and their health. They trade one product for another and another when the placebo effect wears thin and the promised miracles fail to materialize. DJ, who takes the scientific approach reflected in this Controversy, faces a problem: How does she tell Paige about the hoaxes and still preserve their friendship?

Explaining to someone that a cherished belief is not true involves a risk: the person often becomes angry with the one telling the truth, rather than with the source of the lie. To avoid this painful outcome, DJ decides to mention only the supplements in Paige's routine that are most likely to cause harm—the overdoses of caffeine and the hormone replacers. As for the whey protein and other supplements, they are probably just a waste of money, and DJ decides to keep quiet about them. Perhaps they are harmless superstitions.

When Paige believes her performance is boosted by a new concoction, DJ understands that the power of her mind is most likely at work—the placebo effect. Don't underestimate that power: it is formidable. You don't need to buy unproven supplements for an extra edge because you already have a real one—your mind. And you can use the extra money you save to buy a great pair of running shoes—perhaps on a Wednesday.

Critical Thinking

1. Most of the time, the buyer is wasting his or her money when buying an ergogenic aid to improve performance. Still, even well-educated athletes often take them. What forces do you think might motivate competitors to "throw caution to the wind" and buy and take unproven supplements sold as ergogenic aids? What role might advertising play?

2. Divide into two groups. One group will argue in favor of the use of ergogenic aids by athletes, and one group will argue against their use. Each group will make a list of ergogenic aids that should be allowed for use by athletes and a list of those that should not be allowed.

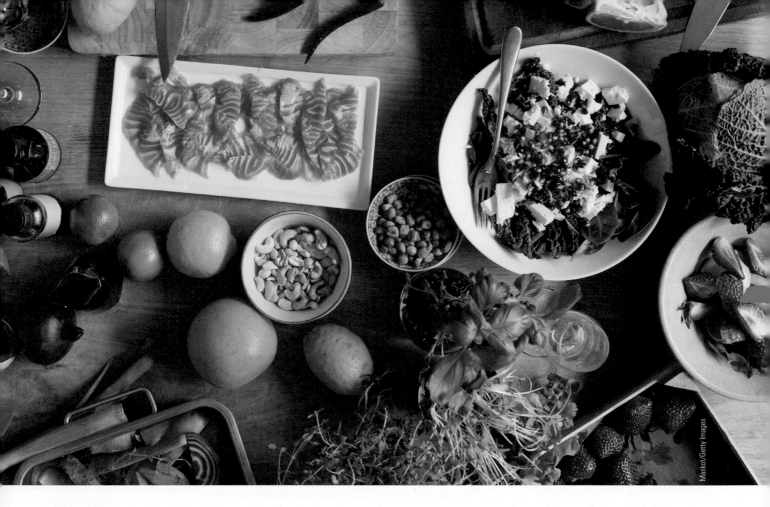

Maskot/Getty Images

11 Nutrition and Chronic Diseases

What do you think?

Are your own food choices damaging your **heart**?

Is diabetes caused by **eating sugar**?

Can certain **herbs** improve your health?

Do "natural" foods without **additives** reduce cancer risks?

A disease is a disorder that impairs or disrupts normal body or organ functioning, and often produces characteristic signs or symptoms. One class of diseases, **infectious diseases**, are caused by specific pathogens. Against these, the body's best defenses are its own natural immunity and preventive measures provided by public health services—vaccines and sanitation. Two infectious diseases make the "top ten" list of killers, pneumonia and influenza, but look at the red bars in Figure 11–1. Heart disease heads the list, cancers are next, strokes are fifth on the list, and diabetes is in the second tier. Note also that these four threats to life are diet related. These four killers are **chronic diseases**; they are to a great extent preventable by good nutrition, and it befits this book to attend to them.

This chapter describes three types of chronic diseases: cardiovascular disease, diabetes, and cancer. These were selected for special attention because they are leading causes of morbidity and mortality in the United States, and because good nutrition can make major contributions to their prevention. For each, the chapter answers three questions: first, how does the disease affect the body? Second, what are its **risk factors**? And third, what steps can be taken to prevent it?

Causation of Chronic Diseases

LO 11.1   Discuss the relationship between risk factors and chronic diseases.

In contrast with the infectious diseases, each of which has a distinct pathogenic cause such as a bacterium or virus, the chronic diseases have suspected contributors known as risk factors. Risk factors are correlated with diseases—that is, they often occur together with diseases, but no single risk factor can be blamed for a disease because the factors work in teams. We can say that a certain virus causes influenza, but we cannot name just a single dietary cause of cancer. We cannot, for example, blame a low-fiber diet. It is a risk factor, yes, but there are many risk factors for cancer, and a low-fiber diet is only one of them. Moreover, every risk factor is implicated in the causation of more than one chronic disease—sometimes, many. Table 11–1 displays the whole, complex picture of the relationships among chronic diseases and their risk factors. (Other risk

infectious diseases diseases that are caused by bacteria, viruses, parasites, and other microbes and that can be transmitted from one person to another through air, water, or food; by contact; or through vector organisms such as mosquitoes and fleas.

chronic diseases degenerative conditions or illnesses that progress slowly, are long in duration, and lack immediate cures. Chronic diseases limit functioning, productivity, and the quality and length of life. Also defined in Chapter 1.

risk factors traits, conditions, or lifestyle habits that increase people's chances of developing diseases; factors known to be correlated with diseases but not proven to be causal.

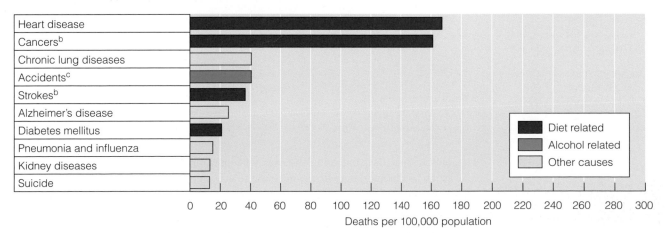

Figure 11–1

The Ten Leading Causes of Death in the United States[a]

Many deaths have multiple causes, but diet influences the development of several chronic diseases—notably, heart disease, some types of cancer, strokes, and diabetes.

[a]Rates are age adjusted to allow relative comparisons of mortality among groups and over time.
[b]Alcohol increases the risks for some cancers and strokes.
[c]Motor vehicle and other accidents are the leading cause of death among people aged 15–24, followed by homicide, suicide, cancer, and heart disease. Alcohol contributes to about half of all accident fatalities.
Source: Data from National Center for Health Statistics: K. D. Kochanek, and coauthors, Deaths: Final data for 2014, National Vital Statistics Reports 65, 4 (2016): 1–122.

Table 11–1

Chronic Disease Risk Factors[a]

Of all of these risk factors, the first two are unalterable: you cannot change your age or heredity. As for diseases as risk factors, if you already have one, you may or may not be able to slow or reverse it. The other risk factors have to do with your lifestyle choices and therefore are, to a great extent, under your control. Your choices can be powerful preventive measures against chronic diseases.

	DISEASES				
	Atherosclerosis	Hypertension	Diabetes, Type 2	Cancers	Obesity
Risk factors that cannot be modified:					
Advancing age	X	X	X	X	
Family history (heredity)	X	X	X	X	X
Diseases as risk factors:					
Atherosclerosis[b]		X			
Diabetes[b]	X	X			
Hypertension[b]	X				
Obesity[b]	X	X	X	X	
High blood LDL and triglycerides; low HDL	X				
Modifiable risk factors other than diet:					
Excessive alcohol intake		X		X	X
Physical inactivity	X	X	X	X	X
Smoking/tobacco use	X	X		X	
Diet and nutrition risk factors:					
Diet high in added sugars					X
Atherogenic diet (high in saturated and/or *trans* fat and low in vegetables, fruit, and whole grains.[c]	X	X		X	X
Diet high in salty/pickled foods		X		X	
Diet low in vitamins and/or minerals	X	X		X	

[a]Environmental factors such as contamination are not included in this table.

[b]Note that atherosclerosis, diabetes, hypertension, and obesity are shown both as risk factors and as diseases in their own right.

[c]An atherogenic diet produces high blood LDL and VLDL and low blood HDL. Such a diet is a CVD risk factor, and these blood-lipid test results, themselves, are also considered risk factors (see Table 11–3, p. 410).

factors, specific to individual diseases, will appear in later discussions.) And one disease (such as diabetes) may *itself* contribute to other diseases (such as atherosclerosis and hypertension). Figure 11–2 illustrates some of these relationships.

KEY POINTS

- Infectious diseases have a single cause—exposure to a specific pathogen.
- Today's predominant diseases are chronic diseases—cardiovascular diseases, type 2 diabetes, and cancer.
- The chronic diseases have many risk factors in common—among them, excessive alcohol intake, lack of physical activity, smoking/tobacco use, and diet.

Figure 11–2
Interrelationships among Chronic Diseases

Many chronic diseases are themselves risk factors for other chronic diseases, and all of them are linked to obesity. The risk factors highlighted in blue define the metabolic syndrome (defined on p. 412).

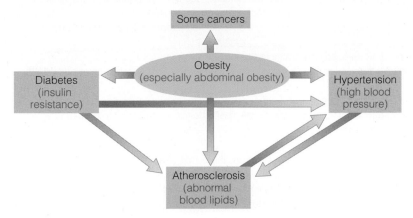

Cardiovascular Diseases (CVD)

LO 11.2   Describe cardiovascular disease and identify its risk factors.

In the United States today, more than 92 million people suffer some form of disease of the heart and blood vessels, collectively known as **cardiovascular disease (CVD)**. Cardiovascular disease claims the lives of more than 800,000 people each year in the United States and has been the leading cause of death in this country for decades.[1]* CVD is often called "heart disease," but that is an oversimplification. As the term *cardiovascular disease* implies, CVD includes diseases of the blood vessels as well as the heart. Thus, the term *cardiovascular disease* represents a number of diseases rolled into one.

   Atherosclerosis, the common form of hardening of the arteries, is a major underlying cause of most forms of CVD, including **hypertension**.[2] Hypertension in turn, worsens atherosclerosis. The two diseases are so interrelated that each is a risk factor for the other. As a later section describes, eating patterns that lower the risk of atherosclerosis protect against hypertension as well. No one is completely free of all signs of atherosclerosis. The question is not whether you are developing it, but how far advanced it is and what you can do to slow or reverse it.

   Chronic hypertension is one of the most prevalent forms of CVD, afflicting about 85 million U.S. adults, and its incidence has been rising steadily.[3] Hypertension is a primary cause of **stroke**, a leading cause of death in the United States. People with normal blood pressure generally enjoy longer lives and less commonly suffer from all forms of CVD than those with high blood pressure. An abundance of terminology pertains to cardiovascular diseases. Some of the most common terms are defined in Table 11–2.

KEY POINTS

- Cardiovascular disease is the leading cause of death in the United States.
- Atherosclerosis is the major underlying cause of cardiovascular disease, and hypertension is the most prevalent form of cardiovascular disease.
- Atherosclerosis and hypertension are risk factors for each other.

Atherosclerosis and Hypertension

Atherosclerosis begins with damage to the cells lining the arteries, caused by any of several factors: high blood LDL cholesterol, hypertension, diabetes, toxins from cigarette

---

*Reference notes are in Appendix F.

cardiovascular disease (CVD) a general term describing diseases of the heart and/or blood vessels. Examples of CVD include hypertension, coronary heart disease, and stroke.

atherosclerosis (ATH-er-oh-scler-OH-sis) a major cause of cardiovascular disease; an arterial disease characterized by deposits known as plaques along the inner walls of the arteries (*athero* means "soft and pasty," referring to the character of the deposits as they form at first; *scleros* means "hard," referring to the same deposits later in the process). The term *arteriosclerosis* means the same thing. (See Table 11–2, "CVD Terms," for *plaques*.)

hypertension high blood pressure.

Table 11-2
CVD Terms

- **aneurysm** (AN-you-rism) the ballooning out of an artery wall at a point that is weakened by deterioration.
- **coronary heart disease** a chronic, progressive disease characterized by obstructive blood flow in the coronary arteries; also called *coronary artery disease*. The coronary arteries are those that feed the heart muscle itself. See also *peripheral artery disease*.
- **embolus** (EM-boh-luss) a clot that travels through the circulatory system (*embol* means "to insert").
- **embolism:** the event in which an embolus lodges in an artery and suddenly cuts off the blood supply to a part of the body. See also *thrombosis*.
- **fatty streaks** deposits of fat on the inner surfaces of arteries, an early stage in the formation of plaques.
- **foam cells** foamy-looking cells formed during plaque formation: they develop from white blood cells that, while clearing fat from plaques, become engorged with it.
- **heart attack** sudden, unexpected cessation of the heartbeat, respiration, and consciousness, usually caused by a clot lodging in a coronary artery (thrombosis). If not quickly reversed, this is followed by death. Also called *cardiac arrest* or *myocardial infarction* (*myo* means muscle; *infarction* means blockage of blood supply).
- **hemorrhage** (HEM-orr-age) uncontrolled bleeding.
- **peripheral artery disease** any disease or disorder that affects the *peripheral arteries,* those that carry blood to the body's organs other than the heart. See also *coronary artery disease*.
- **plaques** (PLACKS; singular, plaque): mounds of lipid material mixed with smooth muscle cells and calcium that develop in the artery walls in atherosclerosis (*placken* means "patch"). (The same word is also used to describe the accumulation of a different kind of deposit on teeth, which promotes dental caries.)
- **stroke** the shutting off of the blood flow to a part of the brain by a thrombus, an embolus, or the bursting of a blood vessel; these events are termed *cerebral thrombosis, cerebral embolism,* and *cerebral hemorrhage,* respectively. (The *cerebrum* is part of the brain.)
- **thrombosis:** the event in which a thrombus grows large enough to close off a blood vessel and gradually cuts off the blood supply to a part of the body. See also *embolism*.
- **thrombus** a stationary blood clot in the circulatory system.

smoking, obesity, and certain viral and bacterial infections.[4] The damage is followed by a series of events that take place over many years:

- Development of **fatty streaks**, especially at branch points.
- Enlargement and hardening of these fat deposits to become **plaques**.
- Narrowing and hardening of the arteries (see Figure 11–3).
- **Inflammation**, which produces abundant free radicals.

Plaque Development Inflammation leads to many more events. The immune system responds by sending white blood cells to the site to try to repair the damage. Particles of LDL cholesterol become trapped in the blood vessel walls, and these become oxidized by abundant free radicals produced during inflammation. White blood cells flood the scene to scavenge and remove the oxidized LDLs, and as they become engorged with oxidized LDL, they take on a foamy appearance (hence the name **foam cells**). Then these foam cells become triggers of oxidation and inflammation that attract more scavengers to the scene. The smooth muscle cells of the arterial walls proliferate in an attempt to heal the damage, but they, too, may become trapped in the plaques. Some plaques become covered with fibrous coatings; some are hardened by calcium deposits. Ultimately, many inner artery walls are virtually covered with rigid, disfiguring plaques.

Once plaques have formed, a spasm of an artery wall or a surge in blood pressure can tear the surface of a plaque, causing it to rupture. Then the body responds to the damage as to an injury—by clotting the blood.

Blood Clot Formation Clots form and dissolve in the blood all the time, and when the processes are balanced, the clots do no harm. As described in Chapter 6, blood clots are a normal and necessary response to injuries that bleed: they shut down blood flow and begin the healing process. In atherosclerosis, though, the balance is disturbed and clots form faster than they dissolve. Arterial damage, plaques in the arteries, and inflammation all favor the formation of blood clots.

inflammation the immune system's response to cellular injury characterized by an increase in white blood cells, redness, heat, pain, and swelling. Inflammation plays a role in many chronic diseases.

Figure 11–3

The Formation of Plaques in Atherosclerosis

Most people have well-developed plaques by the time they reach age 30.

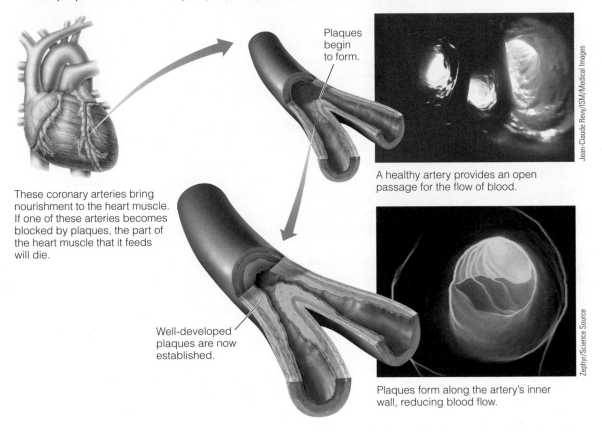

These coronary arteries bring nourishment to the heart muscle. If one of these arteries becomes blocked by plaques, the part of the heart muscle that it feeds will die.

Plaques begin to form.

Well-developed plaques are now established.

A healthy artery provides an open passage for the flow of blood.

Plaques form along the artery's inner wall, reducing blood flow.

Jean-Claude Revy/ISM/Medical Images

Zephyr/Science Source

Abnormal blood clotting can trigger life-threatening events. For example, a clot, once formed, may remain attached to a plaque in an artery and grow until it shuts off the blood supply to the surrounding tissue. The tissue starves, slowly dies, and is replaced by nonfunctional scar tissue. Such a stationery clot is called a **thrombus**, and the tissue death it causes is **thrombosis**. A clot can also break loose, becoming an **embolus**, and circulate in the bloodstream until it reaches an artery too narrow to allow its passage. Now called an **embolism**, the clot remains stuck there, and because the episode happens suddenly, the surrounding tissues die quickly (see Figure 11–4). In either situation, once an artery is blocked, it may swell and its walls grow thin, so that it balloons out, becomes weak, and may burst (**aneurysm**). Once a blood vessel has burst, blood leaks rapidly from it (**hemorrhage**) and again, depending on the location, this may be disabling or fatal.

When the words *cerebral* (brain) or *coronary* (heart) modify the terms just introduced, they describe life-threatening events in the brain or heart. For example, such an event in the brain is called a stroke, and such an event in the heart is a **heart attack**.

Atherosclerosis Raises Blood Pressure   Plaques in arteries also promote and aggravate hypertension (high blood pressure). Normally, arteries expand with each heartbeat, accommodating the pulses of blood that flow through them, but arteries hardened and narrowed by plaques cannot expand, so the blood pressure rises. High blood pressure then becomes a *symptom* of atherosclerosis. Hardened arteries also fail to let the blood flow freely through the kidneys, which respond as if the blood pressure is low: they release hormones that stimulate the body to retain sodium and water. This, of course, enlarges blood volume and makes the blood pressure still higher in a vicious cycle.

Figure 11–4

A blood clot

A blood clot in an artery, such as this fatal heart embolism, blocks the blood flow to tissues fed by that artery.

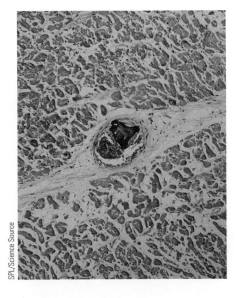

SPL/Science Source

High Blood Pressure Accelerates Atherosclerosis   High blood pressure also worsens atherosclerosis. High pressure damages the artery walls, making fatalities more likely. And because plaques are most likely to form at damage sites, atherosclerosis progresses most rapidly at those sites. Thus, the manifestation of each chronic disease precipitates and aggravates the other.

KEY POINTS

- As most people age, atherosclerosis progresses steadily.
- The development of atherosclerosis involves plaque development, blood clot formation, and hypertension.
- Atherosclerosis and hypertension accelerate each other.

Risk Factors for Cardiovascular Disease

Major risk factors for CVD are listed briefly in Chapter 5; they are presented here in full in Table 11–3. Table 11–1 listed risk factors for a number of chronic diseases to show how a risk factor associated with one disease often contributes to others as well. Table 11–3 lists only those risk factors specific to heart disease.

All people reaching middle or old age exhibit at least one of these factors (advancing age itself is a risk factor), and many people have several factors silently increasing their risks.[5] The more of these risks you can and do control, the lower your risks of CVD-induced disability and death. In recognition of the urgency to reduce the prevalence of major risk factors for CVD, the American Heart Association (AHA) has adopted a 2020 goal of "improving the cardiovascular health of all Americans by 20 percent, while reducing mortality from heart disease and stroke by 20 percent."

A Note about Gender   At every age, men have a greater risk of CVD than women do, and men suffer heart attacks more often and earlier in life. Regardless, more than 44 million U.S. women have CVD and the number is increasing, closing the gap despite substantial progress in awareness, prevention, and treatment. In all its forms, CVD kills

---

Table 11–3

Major Risk Factors for Heart Disease

Risk factors highlighted with a blue background have relationships with diet. Later figures provide standards by which to judge blood lipids and blood pressure. Page E at the back of the book displays BMI values.

Risk factors that cannot be modified:

- Increasing age.
- Male gender.
- Family history (heredity).

Risk factors that can be modified:

- High blood LDL cholesterol.
- Low blood HDL cholesterol.
- High blood triglyceride (VLDL) levels.
- High blood pressure (hypertension).
- Diabetes.
- Obesity (especially central obesity).
- Physical inactivity.
- Cigarette smoking.
- Excessive alcohol consumption.
- High intake of sodium.
- An "atherogenic" diet (high in saturated fats and *trans* fats and low in vegetables, fruit, and whole grains).

Sources: E. J. Benjamin and coauthors, Heart disease and stroke statistics—2017 update: A report from the American Heart Association, Circulation 2017, doi: 10.1161/CIR.0000000000000485.

more U.S. women, especially those who are past menopause, than any other cause.[6] Learning to recognize the symptoms of an oncoming heart attack can be lifesaving: see "Recognize a Heart Attack" in the next section, "Preventive Measures against CVD."

The next risk factors in this series are all in the "can be modified" category, and they are powerful. Important research shows that even people with high genetic risks for CVD can improve their odds of staying healthy by engaging in regular physical activity, not smoking, controlling body weight, and eating health-promoting meals most often.[7] Each one of these four lifestyle choices reduces the risk of heart disease independently, but together, their synergistic effect is dramatic. Adhering to just three of the four cuts heart attack risk in half. Clearly, lifestyle choices can make a major difference to the health of the heart.

High Blood Glucose/Diabetes Any loss of control of blood glucose, even a transitory one, causes the condition of the arteries to deteriorate, and if it progresses to full-blown diabetes, it is a major risk factor for all forms of CVD and mortality.[8] Atherosclerosis progresses rapidly in people with diabetes, blocking blood vessels and obstructing circulation. For an individual with diabetes, the risk of a future heart attack is roughly equal to that of a person *without* diabetes who has already had a heart attack.

Hypertension More than two-thirds of U.S. adults older than 65 have hypertension. Individuals who have normal blood pressure at 55 still have a 90 percent risk of developing high blood pressure during the ensuing years.

If the blood pressure is even slightly above normal, it increases the risk of heart attack and stroke.[9] Moreover, the relationship is proportional: the higher the blood pressure, the greater the risk. This relationship between early signs of hypertension and heart disease risk holds true for men and women, young and old.

Obesity and Physical Inactivity Obesity, especially abdominal obesity, and physical inactivity significantly increase risk factors for CVD, contributing to high LDL cholesterol, low HDL cholesterol, high triglycerides, hypertension, and diabetes.[10] Conversely, weight loss and physical activity protect against CVD by lowering LDL, raising HDL, lowering triglycerides, improving insulin sensitivity, and lowering blood pressure.[11] Obesity is a major cause of high blood pressure, and the combination of obesity and hypertension greatly increases the risk for CVD. Most people with hypertension—an estimated 70 percent—are overweight or obese. Obesity raises blood pressure in several ways: by altering kidney function, by increasing blood volume, and by promoting blood vessel damage through insulin resistance.[12] Excess fat also has miles of extra capillaries through which blood must be pumped.

Smoking/Tobacco Use Cigarette smoking powerfully increases the risk for CVD.[13] The more a person smokes, the higher the risk. Using tobacco in all its forms exposes the heart to damaging toxins, and burdens it by raising the blood pressure. Body tissues starved for oxygen by smoke demand more heartbeats to deliver oxygenated blood, thereby increasing the heart's workload. At the same time, smoking deprives the heart muscle itself of the oxygen it needs to maintain a steady beat. Smoking also damages blood **platelets**, making clots likely to occur.

Excessive Alcohol Intake Drinking alcoholic beverages alters several risk factors underlying CVD. Wine in moderation, mentioned in Controversy 3 on p. 95, may yield some benefits, but in higher doses any alcoholic beverage damages heart tissues, promotes blood clotting, and raises blood pressure.[14] Alcohol in large amounts, even from wine, also increases inflammation. Hypertension is common among people with alcoholism; so are strokes, even when blood pressure is normal. Alcohol, regularly consumed in excess of two drinks per day for men or one for women, is strongly associated with hypertension and may interfere with drug therapy designed to lower blood pressure.[15]

Blood Cholesterol and Triglycerides Low-density lipoprotein (LDL) cholesterol and high-density lipoprotein (HDL) cholesterol in the blood are strongly linked to a person's risk of developing atherosclerosis. LDL carry cholesterol to the cells, including the

platelets tiny, cell-like fragments in the blood, important in forming clots (platelet means "little plate").

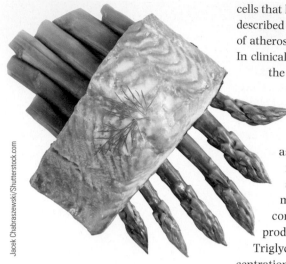

cells that line the arteries, where it can build up as part of the plaques of atherosclerosis described earlier. The higher the LDL concentration, the more rapid the progression of atherosclerosis; and the lower the LDL concentration, the slower the progression.[16] In clinical trials, interventions that lower blood LDL concentrations significantly reduce the incidence of heart disease. By one estimate, for every 1 percent drop in LDL cholesterol, the risk of heart disease falls 1 percent as well. Figure 11–5 lists blood lipid values that are considered to be healthy and those that exceed the safe limit.

HDL carry cholesterol away from the body's cells to the liver to be assigned to other uses or disposed of. HDL also carry proteins that inhibit inflammation, plaque accumulation, and lipid oxidation—all, valuable services to the body.[17] Thus, low HDL levels can contribute to the development of atherosclerosis. (One might think, then, that the higher the HDL concentration, the better, but above a certain level, higher HDL concentrations produce no greater benefits.)

Triglyceride transporters (VLDLs) are influential too: high blood triglyceride concentrations promote atherosclerosis.[18] About one-third of adults in the United States have high blood triglyceride concentrations. These high blood triglyceride levels are associated with a sedentary lifestyle, overweight and obesity (especially abdominal obesity), and type 2 diabetes.

A blood test that reports "high blood triglycerides," "high LDL cholesterol," and "low HDL cholesterol" predicts the further development of plaques and the progression of atherosclerosis. It is clear, then, that one thing you can do to reduce your risk of CVD is to take actions to achieve healthy blood levels of cholesterol and triglycerides (see the top row of Figure 11–5).

Atherogenic Diet   Diet also influences the risk of CVD. An **atherogenic diet**—high in saturated fats and *trans* fats and low in vegetables, fruit, and whole grains—increases LDL cholesterol.[19] Conversely, a well-chosen eating pattern such as the Healthy Mediterranean-Style Eating Pattern (Appendix E) or the DASH eating pattern (discussed in the Food Feature on p. 431) can often lower the risk of CVD.[20]

High Salt Intake   A high intake of salt predicts CVD, and is associated with hypertension, stroke, and stroke mortality.[21] As salt intake increases, so does blood pressure. Most people with hypertension can benefit from eating less salt.

Risk Factors Combined: Metabolic Syndrome   A cluster of five of the previously described risk factors (see Table 11–4) is so powerfully predictive of CVD and diabetes that it has been given a name (**metabolic syndrome**). This syndrome underlies several chronic diseases and notably increases the risks of CVD and type 2 diabetes.[22] Central obesity and insulin resistance are thought to be the primary factors in its development.

Metabolic syndrome, like many of the individual CVD risk factors, involves inflammation and elevates the risk of blood clotting.[23] More than a third of the U.S. adult population meets the criteria for metabolic syndrome, but many are not aware of it and so do not seek treatment.[24] The implications for CVD prevention are profound—correct the syndrome and reduce the risk.

Figure 11–5

Adult Standards for Blood Lipids

	Total blood cholesterol (mg/dL)	LDL cholesterol (mg/dL)	HDL cholesterol (mg/dL)	Triglycerides, fasting (mg/dL)
Healthy	<200	<100[a]	≥60	<150
Borderline	200–239	130–159[b]	59–40	150–199
Unhealthy	≥240	160–189[c]	<40	200–499[d]

[a]100–129 mg/dL of LDL indicates a near optimal level.

[b]LDL cholesterol–lowering medication may be needed at 130 mg/dL, depending on other risks.

[c]>190 mg/dL of LDL indicates a very high risk.

[d]>500 mg/dL of triglycerides indicates a very high risk.

atherogenic diet a diet that promotes atherosclerosis—that is, a diet that is high in saturated fats and *trans* fats and low in vegetables, fruit, and whole grains.

metabolic syndrome the five-member set of symptoms—high fasting blood glucose, central obesity, hypertension, low blood HDL, and high blood triglycerides—any three of which greatly increase a person's risk of developing CVD. Also called *insulin resistance syndrome*.

KEY POINTS

- Risk factors for CVD that cannot be modified include advancing age, male gender, and family history (heredity).
- Major modifiable risk factors for CVD are high LDL cholesterol, low HDL cholesterol, high blood triglycerides, hypertension, diabetes, obesity, physical inactivity, cigarette smoking, excessive alcohol consumption, an atherogenic diet, and a high intake of salt.

Chapter 11 Nutrition and Chronic Diseases

- An atherogenic diet with high amounts of saturated and *trans* fat and low amounts of fruit, vegetables, and whole grains increases risks.
- Metabolic syndrome is a combination of other risk factors, and greatly elevates CVD risk.

Preventive Measures against CVD

The steps that follow can help reduce your risk of cardiovascular disease. It will soon be evident that these same steps are protective against a number of other diseases as well.

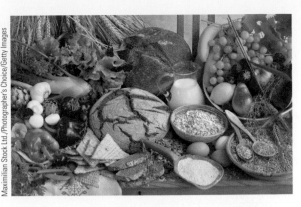

When diets are rich in whole grains, vegetables, and fruit, life expectancies are long.

First, Study Yourself   If, like most people, you face a number of heart disease risks, it's important to know just what they are. Once they are known, you can tend first to the ones that will deliver the greatest benefit.

First, assess your present health condition. Then, learn your family medical history. Finally, own and face the lifestyle habits that are harming your health. Here's how.

Treat Diseases/Disorders   If you already have diabetes, atherosclerosis, or hypertension, take immediate action. Seek medical help and evaluate the lifestyle choices you are making.

Lose Weight if Overweight   Weight loss alone is one of the most effective non-drug treatments for hypertension. People who are overweight and have hypertension can significantly lower blood pressure by losing as little as 5 to 10 percent of their body weight. People who are taking medication to control their blood pressure can often, if they lose weight, cut down their doses or eliminate them altogether. As noted earlier, weight loss in people who are overweight or obese also improves blood lipids and glucose response, reducing risks of CVD and diabetes.

Be Physically Active   Physical activity stimulates development of new coronary arteries to nourish the heart muscle. This may be a factor in the excellent recovery observed in people who follow medically prescribed exercise regimens after heart attacks. Physical activity also favors lean tissue over fat tissue for a healthy body composition, raises HDLs, improves insulin response, quells inflammatory stimuli, and lowers blood pressure, LDLs, blood triglycerides, and blood glucose.[25] Just 30 minutes or more of brisk walking can improve the odds against heart disease considerably if done at least 5 days a week. If you are pressed for time, 15 minutes of more vigorous physical activity, such as jogging, on at least 5 days a week can provide the same benefits. The Think Fitness feature (p. 414) offers suggestions for incorporating physical activity into your daily routine. Figure 10–1 (p. 368) explains the Physical Activity Guidelines for Americans.

Physical activity also affects the body's hormonal balance in a beneficial way. It reduces the secretion of stress hormones, counteracting stress and lowering blood pressure. It also redistributes body water and eases transit of the blood through the small arteries that feed the tissues, including those of the heart.

Control Alcohol Intake   Honestly assess your alcohol intake (review Controversy 3). As emphasized elsewhere in this book, *moderate* alcohol use is considered tolerable: no more than one drink per day for a woman and no more than two for a man. This amount seems safe, relative to heart health. (Unfortunately, this amount of drinking poses another risk for women: the risk of breast cancer, so other routes to relaxation may prove safer.)

Don't Smoke   Tobacco smoke has already been mentioned as producing arterial injuries. For this and a hundred other reasons, smokers are advised to quit, and nonsmokers are advised to avoid exposure to secondhand smoke. It is difficult, but it is well worth the effort: When smokers quit, their risks of heart disease begin to diminish within a few months.

Learn Your Family History   Early heart disease in siblings or parents is a major risk factor. The more family members affected and the earlier the age of onset, the greater the risk.[26] These relationships reflect a genetic influence on CVD risk, and

Table 11–4
Metabolic Syndrome

Metabolic syndrome includes any three or more of the following:

- High fasting blood glucose.
- Central obesity.
- Hypertension.
- Low blood HDL.
- High blood triglycerides.

The benefits of physical activity are compelling, so why not tie up your athletic shoes, head out the door, and get going? Here are some ideas to get you started:

- Coach a sport.
- Garden.
- Hike, bike, or walk to nearby stores or to classes.
- Mow, trim, and rake by hand.
- Park a block from your destination and walk.
- Play a sport.
- Play with children.

- Take classes for credit in dancing, sports, conditioning, or swimming.
- Take the stairs, not the elevator.
- Walk a dog.
- Walk every day. A common goal is 10,000 steps per day (about 5 miles), to meet the "active" daily activity level, but shorter walks also confer benefits on most people. Use a pedometer to count your steps.
- Wash your car with extra vigor, or bend and stretch to wash your toes in the bath.
- Work out at a fitness club.
- Work out with friends to help one another stay fit.

Also, try these:

- Give away two labor-saving devices to someone who needs them.
- Lift small hand weights while talking on the phone, reading e-mail, or watching TV.
- Stretch often during the day.

start now! Using the list above as a guide, make your own list of things you can do today to be physically active. Using the calendar you created in Chapter 10, note on each day for the next month the physical activities you have engaged in for that day.

specific genetic links are under investigation. At present, the relationships are tangled and likely to become more so before being sorted out.

A fascinating area of study has opened up: in the realm of nutritional genomics and CVD risk, scientists are uncovering a vast network of interrelated influences that will someday shed more light on individual people's health prospects. Controversy 11, which follows this chapter, presents some fascinating findings on the ways in which nutrients influence the actions of genes.

Know Your Blood Pressure   The most effective single step you can take to protect yourself from hypertension is find out whether you have it (see Figure 11–6). High blood pressure presents no symptoms you can feel, but during a checkup, a health-care professional can take an accurate resting blood pressure reading and advise you. A single "high" reading should be questioned; a second one tentatively confirms the diagnosis of hypertension; and thereafter, the pressure should be checked at regular intervals. A professional reading is best: self-test machines in drugstores and other public places, although convenient, are often inaccurate.

When blood pressure is measured, two numbers are important: the pressure during contraction of the heart's large, lower chambers (the ventricles) and the pressure during their relaxation. The numbers are reported as a fraction, with the first number representing the systolic pressure (ventricular contraction), and the second number the diastolic pressure (ventricular relaxation). Refer to Figure 11–7 to see how to interpret your resting blood pressure.

Ideal resting blood pressure is lower than 120/80. Values above this (up to 129/<80) indicate elevated blood pressure, which suggests that taking steps to reduce the blood pressure may help avert illness later on.[27] Above this borderline level, the risks of heart attacks and strokes rise in direct proportion to increasing blood pressure (see Figure 11–7).

Determine Your Heart Disease Risk   Risk evaluation plays an important role in CVD intervention. The AHA, together with the American College of Cardiology, sets assessment standards for evaluating a person's risk of developing CVD.[28] Their online risk calculator tool, displayed in Figure 11–8, can help estimate anyone's risk of having a heart attack. To use it, start by providing your age, race, and other personal

Figure 11–6

Know Your Blood Pressure

The most effective single step you can take against hypertension is to learn your own blood pressure.

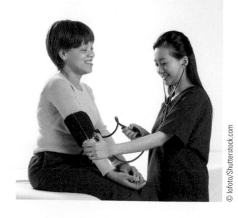

© Iofoto/Shutterstock.com

information, along with test results such as blood lipids, blood pressure, and blood glucose. Once the heart attack risk is established, the calculator offers a lifestyle prevention plan to reduce the risk. If the risk is high, treatment guidelines define when physicians should prescribe cholesterol-lowering medications.

Recognize a Heart Attack   In the event that a heart emergency occurs, one's ability to recognize the symptoms can be lifesaving. The sooner medical help arrives, the more likely a person is to recover. The Centers for Disease Control and Prevention (www.cdc.gov) lists the five major symptoms of a heart attack:

- Pain or discomfort in the jaw, neck, or back.
- Feeling weak, light-headed, or faint.
- Chest pain or discomfort.
- Pain or discomfort in arms or shoulders.
- Shortness of breath.

Importantly, women may or may not experience classic symptoms such as chest discomfort. Women are more likely to experience unusual fatigue, dizziness, or weakness.

Reduce Your Salt/Sodium Intake   High intakes of salt and/or sodium are associated with hypertension and a large number of deaths from hypertension-related diseases such as stroke.[29] Lowering sodium intake is the key to successful management: as salt intake diminishes, blood pressure goes lower in synchrony. This direct relationship is reported at all levels of intake, from very low to much higher than average, and provides additional protection against heart disease in other ways as well.

The World Health Organization (WHO) estimates that a significant reduction in sodium intake could reduce by half the number of people requiring medication for

Figure 11–7

Adult Standards for Blood Pressure: Systolic/Diastolic

Measurements are expressed as millimeters of mercury (mm Hg)

Normal	<120/<80
Elevated	120–129/<80
Hypertension	≥130/≥80

Source: P. Muntner and coauthors, Potential U.S. population impact of the 2017 American College of Cardiology/American Heart Association High Blood Pressure Guideline, Circulation, 137 (2018): 109–118.

Figure 11–8

The American Heart Association's Heart Attack Risk Calculator

This online calculator can assess your risk of having a heart attack. For a meaningful assessment, you'll need some information about your blood lipids, blood pressure, and fasting blood glucose. To access the calculator, visit the American Heart Association website: https://professional.heart.org /professional/GuidelinesStatements/ASCVDRiskCalculator/UCM_457698 _ASCVD-Risk-Calculator.jsp

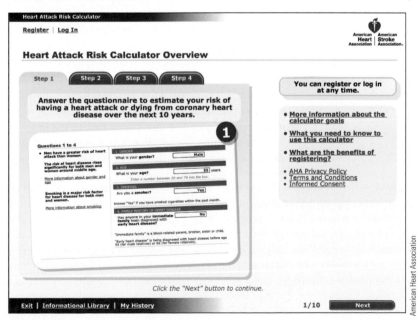

American Heart Association

hypertension and greatly reduce CVD mortality. Most authorities recommend that everyone, even those with normal blood pressure, restrict sodium intakes, not to exceed the DRI Tolerable Upper Intake Level of 2,300 milligrams of sodium per day. Individuals with hypertension are advised to further limit sodium intake to 1,500 milligrams of sodium per day.

Increase Potassium Intake   Potassium may help to regulate blood pressure. Low potassium intakes, especially when combined with high sodium intakes, raise blood pressure and increase the risk of death from stroke.[30] The DASH Diet, presented in this chapter's Food Feature, emphasizes potassium-rich foods such as fruit and vegetables.

Follow a Healthy Eating Pattern   The defensive moves just described can all help to prevent CVD, but equally important or even more so is a person's eating pattern. An individual eats three meals, 365 days a year, more than 1,000 meals a year, or 40,000 meals by the age of 40. The choices made at mealtimes tremendously influence cardiovascular health.

Nutrition has many connections with diet, both negative and positive. The negative relationships—obesity, saturated fat intakes, salt intake, and alcohol consumption—have already been presented. It remains to demonstrate the many positive ways in which a nutritious diet can promote cardiovascular health.

A main objective of a defensive diet is to lower blood triglycerides and cholesterol—that is, to reduce blood VLDL and LDL. And just as a diet high in saturated and *trans* fats raises LDL, a diet low in those lipids lowers them. Where people in the world consume diets high in saturated fat and low in fish, fruit, vegetables, nuts, legumes, and whole grains, blood cholesterol is high and heart disease takes a toll on health and life. Conversely, where people consume mostly unsaturated dietary fats and abundant fish, fruit, vegetables, nuts, legumes, and whole grains, blood cholesterol levels and heart disease rates are low.[31]

It matters, too, what people choose to eat in place of saturated fats. Replacing saturated fats with polyunsaturated or monounsaturated fats helps to lower LDL cholesterol and lowers the risk of death from CVD.[32] Polyunsaturated fat tends to have the greater effect. Table 5–7 (p. 174) offers practical ways to cut down on saturated (solid) fats and replace them with polyunsaturated and monounsaturated oils.

Are high-carbohydrate foods a good choice? Clearly not all of them: refined starches and added sugars have the potential to worsen heart disease risk by elevating blood triglycerides and inflammation and by reducing HDL cholesterol.[33] People with elevated triglycerides may find that replacing refined starches with complex-carbohydrate foods such as whole grains, legumes, and vegetables helps to improve their blood lipid profiles.

Fish oil is the richest food source of DHA and EPA, eicosanoid products of an omega-3 fatty acid, which oppose blood clots and support heart health.[34] A diet that includes two fatty fish meals per week, as the AHA recommends, may therefore help to protect against blood clotting better than a diet that lacks fish. For people with heart disease,

> Eicosanoids and omega-3 fatty acids were introduced on page 162 of Chapter 5.

even more fatty fish than this is recommended, and a physician may prescribe fish oil supplements. However, as is true for most nutrients, too much is as bad as too little—DHA in large amounts may *promote* blood clots, so supplements should be taken only with a physician's approval.[35]

Nutrient Supplements, Drugs, Herbal Remedies   People who want to get all the nutrients that help keep blood pressure low may turn to vitamin-mineral supplements, but these have shown no promise for lowering blood pressure. What does help is to consume the eating pattern described many times before: low in saturated fat, with abundant fruit, vegetables, fish, whole grains, and low-fat dairy products that provide the needed nutrients while holding sodium intake within bounds. Some people simply doubt the power of ordinary foods and their nutrients to improve health, and turn

Table 11–5

How Much Does Changing the Eating Pattern Lower LDL Cholesterol?

For those who need to lower LDL cholesterol, this table offers a perspective on the magnitude of results that may be possible.

Diet-Related Component	Modification	Possible LDL Reduction
Saturated fat	<7% of calories	8–10%
Weight reduction (if overweight)	Lose 10 lb	5–8%
Soluble, viscous fiber	5–10 g/day	3–5%

to alternative medicines. The Consumer's Guide (pp. 424–425) provides a look at some of these practices.

Should diet and physical activity fail to normalize blood pressure, antihypertensive drugs such as diuretics can be lifesaving. These drugs lower blood pressure by increasing fluid loss so as to lower the blood volume.

Diets to Reduce CVD Risks   All in all, dietary measures to reduce CVD risks can be very much worth taking. Table 11–5 illustrates the power of diet-related factors in reducing the risk of CVD, and the "Mediterranean diet," which delivers an excellent combination of foods for this purpose, is presented in Appendix E. The diet reduces the risks of CVD to a greater degree than might be expected from its effects on blood lipids alone.[36] A number of beneficial features of such diets may share the credit, among them the vitamins, minerals, fibers, antioxidant phytochemicals, and omega-3 fatty acids.

Another such diet, described in this chapter's Food Feature, is the DASH diet (Dietary Approaches to Stop Hypertension), on which researchers confer high praise. Trials of the DASH diet, which is rich in fruit, vegetables, nuts, whole grains, and low-fat milk products, have shown that it offers many welcome benefits to eaters. It lowers blood pressure more effectively than salt restriction alone.[37] It also improves vascular function, lowers total cholesterol and LDL cholesterol, and reduces inflammation. Compared with the typical American diet, the DASH plan provides more fiber, potassium, magnesium, and calcium; emphasizes legumes and fish over red meats; limits added sugars and sugar-containing beverages; and meets other recommendations of the Dietary Guidelines for Americans. The plan seems to work well, not only for people who are eating meals provided by researchers, but also for those freely choosing and preparing their own foods according to its directions.

Manage Lifestyle Changes   Adopting lifestyle changes can be challenging. Making major adjustments to eating and physical activity patterns is not the easy route to heart health that everyone would like, but such changes form a powerful and safe combination for improving today's health and tomorrow's health prospects. The compounding protection from a recommended eating pattern and a physical activity regimen becomes clear: the effects of each small choice add to the beneficial whole.

KEY POINTS

- Lifestyle changes to lower the risk of CVD include increasing physical activity, achieving a healthy body weight, reducing exposure to tobacco smoke, and eating a heart-healthy diet.
- Dietary measures to lower LDL cholesterol include reducing intakes of saturated fat and *trans* fat, along with consuming generous quantities of nutrient-dense fruit, vegetables, legumes, nuts, fish, and whole grains.

Diabetes

LO 11.3 Summarize the causes, consequences, and management of type 2 diabetes.

diabetes (dye-uh-BEET-eez) metabolic diseases characterized by elevated blood glucose arising from insufficient or ineffective insulin, or both. The technical term is *diabetes mellitus* (*mellitus* means "honey-sweet" in Latin, referring to the presence of sugar in the urine).

prediabetes a condition in which the blood glucose concentration is above normal, but not high enough to be diagnosed as diabetes; a major risk factor for diabetes and cardiovascular diseases.

type 1 diabetes the less common type of diabetes in which the pancreas produces little or no insulin.

type 2 diabetes the more common type of diabetes in which the body's cells fail to respond to insulin.

insulin resistance a condition in which a normal or high concentration of circulating insulin produces a subnormal glucose-uptake response in muscle, liver, and adipose tissue.

autoimmune disorder a disease in which the body develops antibodies against its own proteins and then proceeds to destroy cells containing these proteins.

At the start of this chapter, **diabetes** was identified not only as a major risk factor for CVD, but also as a leading cause of death in the United States. Recent decades have seen a sharp rise in the rate of type 2 diabetes afflicting both adults and children: more than 29 million people in all have diabetes.[38] Of these, almost 3 million are unaware of it and so go untreated.[39] In addition, well over one-third of U.S. adults, or 86 million more, have **prediabetes**, exhibiting warning signs of diabetes to come.

There are two common forms of diabetes, type 1 and type 2. Both disorders involve insulin and blood glucose and both pose similar risks to health; they differ in their typical ages of onset and in the presence or absence of insulin. **Type 1 diabetes** accounts for 5 to 10 percent of all cases. It usually sets in during childhood or adolescence but it can begin at any age, even late in life. Although type 1 diabetes is far less common than type 2, worldwide it is increasing in prevalence by about 3 percent each year, especially among children.[40]

The predominant type of diabetes, **type 2 diabetes**, is closely linked with obesity and is responsible for 90 to 95 percent of cases in both adults and children.[41] Although type 2 diabetes typically appears later in life, it has been on the rise among children and adolescents, following current trends in obesity among U.S. youth.[42] The primary defect in type 2 diabetes is an inadequate response of the body's cells to the hormone insulin—that is, **insulin resistance**. Table 11–6 displays other distinguishing characteristics.

Type 1 diabetes is an **autoimmune disorder**. A person's own immune cells mistakenly attack and destroy the insulin-producing cells of the pancreas. The rate of pancreatic cell destruction in type 1 diabetes varies. In infants and children, destruction is rapid; in adults, it is slow.[43] Eventually, the damaged pancreas no longer produces enough insulin to control blood glucose adequately. Then, after each meal, glucose concentration builds up in the blood, while body tissues are simultaneously

Table 11–6

Type 1 and Type 2 Diabetes Compared

	Type 1	Type 2
Percentage of cases	5–10%	90–95%
Typical age of onset	<30 years	>45 years[a]
Associated characteristics	Autoimmune disease, viral infections, family history	Aging, overweight or obesity, family history, heart disease, elevated blood lipids, hypertension, psychological depression, some medications
Primary problems	Destruction of insulin-producing cells of the pancreas, insulin deficiency	Insulin resistance, insulin deficiency (relative to needs)
Insulin secretion	Little or none	Varies; may be normal, increased, or decreased
Requires insulin	Always	Sometimes
Older names	Juvenile-onset diabetes Insulin-dependent diabetes mellitus (IDDM)	Adult-onset diabetes Non-insulin-dependent diabetes mellitus (NIDDM)

[a]Incidence of type 2 diabetes is increasing in children and adolescents; in more than 90% of these cases, it is associated with overweight or obesity and a family history of type 2 diabetes.

Chapter 11 Nutrition and Chronic Diseases

starving for glucose, a life-threatening situation. The person must receive insulin from an external source to assist the tissues in taking up the glucose they need from the bloodstream.

Insulin is a protein, and if it were taken orally, the digestive tract would digest it. Insulin must therefore be taken as daily injections, inhaled in powder form, or pumped from an insulin pump that delivers it through a tiny tube implanted under the skin. Some insulin pumps also monitor blood glucose and report its levels throughout the day. Fast-acting and long-lasting forms of insulin allow more flexibility in managing meals and treatments, but users must still plan ahead to balance blood insulin and glucose consumption.

The rest of this section focuses on type 2 diabetes, for several reasons. Type 2 is much more prevalent than type 1; it has more known risk factors; and many strategies can prevent it.

KEY POINTS

- Prediabetes silently threatens the health of tens of millions of people in the United States.
- Type 1 diabetes is an autoimmune disease that attacks the pancreas and abolishes its ability to produce insulin; it necessitates that insulin be provided from an external source.
- Type 2 diabetes is the predominant type of diabetes and is closely linked to obesity.
- The primary defect in type 2 diabetes is insulin resistance—an inadequate response of the body's cells to insulin.

How Does Type 2 Diabetes Develop?

In type 2 diabetes, the body's cells are deprived of some or all of the glucose energy they need, even as both glucose and insulin build up in the blood. The glucose that is circulating in the blood would normally enter cells freely with the help of insulin from the pancreas, but now the cells are failing to respond to it.

High Blood Glucose   When the muscle, fat, and other cells become insulin resistant and fail to take up glucose from the blood, the blood glucose concentration rises. The pancreas responds by producing more and more insulin, but to no avail. Eventually, the overtaxed cells of the pancreas begin to fail and reduce their insulin output, while blood glucose soars farther out of control. Chronically elevated blood glucose taxes the kidneys with the task of excreting the excess (this produces the familiar diabetes symptom of sugar in the urine) and alters metabolism in virtually every cell of the body. Some cells convert excess glucose to toxic alcohols. In other cells, glucose becomes attached to working protein molecules, rendering them nonfunctional. When blood glucose is high and the cells are starved for energy, a triad of telltale symptoms appears:

- Intense hunger, although there is plenty of glucose in the blood, the cells are starved for energy
- Frequent urination, because the kidneys are filtering excess sugar out of the blood and having to draw water from the body to excrete it
- Intense thirst, because the frequent urination brings about dehydration

Recognizing these symptoms and seeking medical help as soon as possible can often help to minimize the consequences of untreated diabetes.

KEY POINTS

- In type 2 diabetes, insulin resistance causes glucose and insulin to build up in the bloodstream.
- Recognizing the symptoms of diabetes and seeking treatment are important steps for protecting health.

Harms from Diabetes

A common misconception still held by too many people is that diabetes is of little real consequence to health. In fact, diabetes is a dangerous disease that can strike anyone at any time (Table 11–7 dispels other false ideas.) The altered metabolism from uncontrolled blood glucose damages many organs and tissues. Should these critical systems begin to fail, both health and life are jeopardized.

Diseases of the Large Blood Vessels Atherosclerosis tends to develop early, progress rapidly, and become severe in people with diabetes. The interrelationships among insulin resistance, obesity, hypertension, and atherosclerosis help explain why the most common causes of death in people with long-term diabetes are heart attacks and strokes.

This close relationship between the CVD and diabetes is reflected in their risk factors. When you study the CVD risk factors listed in Table 11–3 (p. 410), it's easy to spot their overlap with these three risk factors for type 2 diabetes:

1. *Advancing age.* Diabetes testing should begin at age 45 for everyone.

2. *Family history (heredity).* Having a close relative with type 2 diabetes increases the risk.[44]

3. *Overweight and obesity.* Most, but not all, people with type 2 diabetes are overweight, and obesity can foster insulin resistance.[45]

Table 11-7

Common Misconceptions about Diabetes

These misconceptions foster false negative stereotypes about diabetes and needlessly blame people for contracting it.

Misconceptions	Facts
People who are overweight or obese will eventually develop type 2 diabetes.	Being overweight is just one risk factor for type 2 diabetes; others include advancing age, ethnicity, and family history. Anyone can develop diabetes.
Diabetes is contagious.	Diabetes is a chronic disease, not an infectious disease.
Eating too much sugar causes diabetes.	Excess sugar intake, particularly from sugarsweetened beverages, is *associated* with diabetes. It is not a known *cause* of the disease.
Diabetes isn't too serious. Just follow medical advice and it can't harm you.	Diabetes is a progressive disease that causes more deaths each year than breast cancer and doubles the chance of a heart attack. Over time, more medications may be needed to help control blood glucose and minimize harms to the body.
People with diabetes need to eat a lot of special diabetic cookies, crackers, and other products.	People with diabetes benefit most from an eating pattern that follows the Dietary Guidelines for Americans, with a few modifications. Expensive "dietetic" cookies and crackers are low-nutrient treats and offer no special benefits.
People with diabetes can't eat bread, fruit, potatoes, or sweet treats.	Portion size is key for all carbohydrate-rich foods. Small servings of whole grains, fruit, and starchy vegetables contribute important nutrients and fiber to a healthful diet. On special occasions, a small dessert may be allowable after a well-chosen meal or after exercise.

Source: Adapted from American Diabetes Association, Diabetes myths: Diabetes is not a choice (2017), available at http://www.diabetes.org/diabetes-basics/myths/.

Chapter 11 Nutrition and Chronic Diseases

In addition, race and ethnicity affect diabetes risk: African Americans, Latinx populations, certain Asian Americans, Native Americans, and Pacific Islanders all have increased risks for type 2 diabetes.

Impaired Kidney, Eye, and Nerve Function In diabetes, the structures of the blood vessels and nerves become damaged, leading to diminished blood circulation and nerve function. Poor circulation leads to dry skin and a tendency to develop slow-healing injuries and infections. Critical organs become inefficient and begin to fail all over the body. Reduced blood flow to the kidneys damages them, often making it necessary to cleanse the blood outside of the body by means of kidney **dialysis** or, in late stages, to undergo kidney transplant. Poor circulation to the eyes impairs vision and can lead to blindness. Diabetes is the leading cause of both kidney failure and blindness in adults in the United States.[46] Poor circulation at the extremities makes the peripheral nerves insensitive to the pain that would otherwise signal injury or infection, so injuries and infections of the feet and hands go undetected. These events can lead to death of tissue (gangrene), necessitating amputation of the affected limbs (most often the feet).

KEY POINTS

- In type 2 diabetes, atherosclerosis develops early and progresses rapidly.
- Chronically elevated blood glucose alters metabolism in virtually every cell in the body.
- Type 2 diabetes damages blood vessels and nerves, impairing circulation and nerve function, and causing kidney damage, vision problems, and infections.

Diabetes Prevention and Management

Just as risk factors for type 2 diabetes and CVD overlap, so do many of the strategies for prevention. This makes it all the more urgent for people with high risks to pay attention and take action.

Know Your Family History Inquire what health challenges your relatives have faced. Given the warnings implied by a family history of diabetes, people can take steps to forestall the disease, but once in its grip, the body often fails to prevent the damage, even with the best of medical care.

Get Tested Prediabetes, a fasting blood glucose concentration just slightly higher than normal, presents few or none of the warning signs of diabetes, but tissue damage may be progressing, and type 2 diabetes may soon develop.[47] Diagnosis can be made using any of several tests, among them the **fasting plasma glucose test** and a nonfasting **A1C test**.[48] In a fasting test, a clinician draws a patient's blood after at least 8 hours of fasting and measures the glucose concentration. A healthy person's blood glucose will fall within the normal range, but in a person with prediabetes it may still be high from the meal eaten the night before. (Normal and diabetic glucose values are shown in Figure 11–9.) In a nonfasting A1C test, a blood indicator reveals how well blood glucose has been controlled over the past few months. A registered dietitian nutritionist, a Certified Diabetes Educator, or a physician can help those with prediabetes or diabetes learn to manage their conditions.

Lose Weight if Overweight If you are overweight, losing just 5 percent of your body weight, and maintaining that loss, can significantly reduce your risk of diabetes.[49] For some obese people, weight-loss surgery becomes necessary and can often resolve their diabetes, but relapses are common and surgery imposes serious risks of its own as described in Chapter 9.[50] In making treatment decisions, a person-centered approach that respects the individual's needs, preferences, and values works best.

Be Physically Active Plan to get at least 30 minutes of physical activity on most days of the week—and do it. The contributions that physical activity can make to prevention and control of type 2 diabetes are invaluable. Physical activity helps the body shed excess fat and strengthens tissue response to insulin.[51] Increasing physical

Figure 11–9

Diabetes Test Standards

Diagnosis	Fasting plasma glucose	A1C
Normal	70–99 mg/dL	<5.7%
Prediabetes	100–125 mg/dL	5.7–6.4%
Diabetes	≥126 mg/dL	≥6.5%

Source: American Diabetes Association, Classification and Diagnosis of Diabetes, Diabetes Care 40 (2017): S11–S24.

dialysis (die-AL-uh-sis) in kidney disease, treatment of the blood to remove toxic substances or metabolic wastes; more properly, *hemodialysis*, meaning "dialysis of the blood" (*hemo* refers to blood, *dia* means to separate).

fasting plasma glucose test a test that measures the current blood glucose concentration in a person who has not ingested any caloric foods or beverages for at least 8 hours; it can detect both prediabetes and diabetes (*plasma* is the fluid part of whole blood).

A1C test a blood test that measures the percentage of hemoglobin (a blood protein) with glucose molecules attached to it. The test reflects how well blood glucose has been controlled over the past few months and can aid in diagnosing type 2 diabetes. (Also called a *glycosylated hemoglobin test* or *HbA1C test; Hb* stands for hemoglobin.)

activity can help delay the onset of diabetes and regulate blood glucose in established cases, sometimes so successfully that medication can be reduced or eliminated. (A person with type 1 diabetes should seek medical advice on exercise because it can bring on **hypoglycemia**.) Like a juggler who keeps three balls in the air, a person with diabetes must constantly balance three factors—diet, exercise, and medication—to properly control blood glucose.

Choose Your Diet with Care   Diet is an important component of diabetes treatment. The American Diabetes Association recognizes that a variety of eating patterns—for example, DASH, presented in the Food Feature on p. 431, the Healthy Mediterranean-Style Eating Pattern (Appendix E,) and the Healthy Vegetarian Eating Pattern (Appendix E)—are all acceptable for the management of diabetes.[52] Such eating patterns can be designed based on personal preferences and metabolic goals.

Control Carbohydrate Intake   Controlling carbohydrate intake is crucial to regulating blood glucose. To maintain near-normal blood glucose concentrations and maximize the effectiveness of drug therapy, choose an eating pattern designed to deliver the same amount of carbohydrate each day, spaced evenly throughout the day. Eating too much carbohydrate at one time can raise blood glucose too high; eating too little can produce hypoglycemia.

The eating pattern that best meets the goals of blood glucose management is one that derives its carbohydrates from whole foods (fruit, vegetables, legumes, whole grains, and low-fat milk) in well-timed meals and in amounts sufficient to balance the body's available insulin. Many people learn to simplify their food selections using the food list system developed for this purpose (see Appendix D).

A common misconception is that people with diabetes need only to omit sugary foods, but as far as blood glucose is concerned, the *amount* of carbohydrate matters more than its *source*. (Most carbohydrates become glucose during digestion and metabolism.) Sugar recommendations for people with diabetes are similar to those for the general population, which suggests limiting foods and beverages with added sugars. Of course, sugars and sugary foods must be counted as part of the daily carbohydrate allowance.

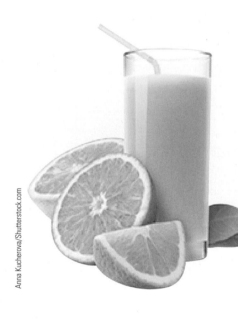

As described in Chapter 4, sugar alcohols (such as sorbitol) have lower glycemic effects than glucose or sucrose and may be used as sugar substitutes. Nonnutritive sweeteners (such as aspartame, saccharin, and sucralose) contain no digestible carbohydrates and can also be used in place of sugar. Their nature and safety are topics of Chapter 12.

Dietary Fat   People with diabetes are advised to follow the *Dietary Guidelines for Americans* regarding saturated fat and *trans* fat intakes. These recommendations include reducing saturated fat intake to less than 10 percent of calories and limiting *trans* fat as much as possible. As is true for the general population, foods rich in omega-3 fatty acids are recommended for those with diabetes because such foods exert beneficial effects on lipoproteins and the prevention of heart disease.

Protein   An ideal protein intake to control blood glucose or to improve CVD risk factors in diabetes has not been determined.[53] Protein intake should, therefore, be individualized, but for most people, the protein DRI establishes a safe and adequate intake.

Alcohol Intake   Alcohol intake, if any, should be moderate. Alcohol consumption increases the risk of hypoglycemia, especially in those using insulin or insulin-releasing drugs.

Diet Recommendations Summed Up   Effective medical nutrition therapy can help stabilize blood glucose, control blood lipids, achieve and maintain healthy body weight, and normalize blood pressure in people with diabetes.[54] For an individualized approach, a person's cultural pattern and preferences should be honored; and factors such as insulin use, other medication use, and blood pressure must be accommodated. Anyone with diabetes should pay strict attention to the Dietary Guidelines for Americans, particularly concerning intakes of nutrient-dense foods, sodium, saturated fats, and added sugars.

hypoglycemia (HIGH-poh-gly-SEE-me-uh) an abnormally low blood glucose concentration, often accompanied by symptoms of anxiety, rapid heartbeat, and sweating. Also defined in Chapter 4.

Chapter 11 Nutrition and Chronic Diseases

A wide variety of meal plans can meet these recommendations. People at risk for diabetes can do no better than to begin following these recommendations long before symptoms appear.

In conclusion, among the previous recommendations, research shows that these three lifestyle elements most consistently and dramatically reduce people's risks of developing diabetes:

- Achieving and maintaining a healthy body weight.
- Adopting and maintaining an eating pattern of regularly timed, healthy meals that are moderate in calories, low in saturated fat, and high in vegetables, legumes, fruit, low-fat or fat-free milk products, fish, poultry, and whole grains.
- Engaging in a program of regular physical activity.[55]

KEY POINTS

- The first steps in diabetes prevention involve self-study: learn your family history and risks and get tested for symptoms of developing diabetes.
- To slow or halt the progression of diabetes, one should lose weight if overweight, and learn to manage blood glucose levels by balancing physical activity, carbohydrate intake, and drug therapy recommended by a health care provider.
- A diet consisting of nutrient-dense foods and low in saturated fat and added sugars can play a crucial role in controlling the symptoms and progression of type 2 diabetes.

Cancer

LO 11.4 Describe the relationships between diet and cancer.

Second only to cardiovascular disease as a leading cause of disability and death in the United States is **cancer**. More than 1.6 million new cancer cases and 600,000 deaths from cancer are expected to occur in the United States in 2017.[56] Still, the past few decades have revealed a small but steady trend toward declining cancer deaths.[57] Early detection and treatment have transformed several common cancers from intractable killers to curable diseases or treatable chronic illnesses. Although the potential for cure is promising, *prevention* of cancer remains preferable by far.

Cancer exists in perhaps the widest variety of types and has the most diverse causes of any chronic disease. Some cancers are known to be caused primarily by genetic factors, and they run in families regardless of lifestyle choices. Others are linked with microbial infections.[†] However, for the vast majority of cancers, lifestyle choices and environmental exposures are the major risk factors.[58] Take smoking, for example: if everyone in the United States quit smoking today, future total cancers would drop by about a third. Overeating and underactivity certainly play a role in the development of colon and breast cancer and probably contribute to pancreatic, esophageal, and renal cancers as well.[59] As a positive effect of knowledge of this kind, the incidence of hormone-related breast cancer has dropped significantly since women have stopped taking hormone replacement therapy for symptoms of menopause.

The Cancer Disease Process

Cancer arises in the genetic material inside a person's cells. The process, called **carcinogenesis**, usually proceeds slowly and continues for several decades. It often begins when a cell's genetic material sustains damage from a **carcinogen** such as radiation, a free radical, or another cancer-causing chemical. Damage from these insults occurs every day, but cells can often deflect or promptly repair it. If the damage is not repaired and the cell becomes unable to faithfully replicate its genetic material, it dies by way of a sort of cellular suicide, thereby preventing its progeny from inheriting faulty genes.

cancer a group of diseases characterized by the uncontrolled growth and spread of abnormal cells.

carcinogenesis (car-SIN-oh-JEN-eh-sis) the process of cancer development (*carcin* means "cancer"; *gen* means "gives rise to").

carcinogen (car-SIN-oh-jen) a cancer-causing substance; asbestos and tobacco smoke are examples of carcinogens.

[†]Examples include viral hepatitis and liver cancer, human papilloma virus and cervical cancer, and *H. pylori* bacterium (the ulcer bacterium) and stomach cancer.

Deciding about CAM

Have you ever treated a health problem with an herbal remedy or another form of **complementary** and **alternative medicine (CAM)**? (See Table 11–8 for definitions.) If so, you are not alone. Each year, U.S. consumers spend tens of billions of dollars on CAM treatments. All of these dollars spur sellers to advertise on thousands of Internet websites, broadcast television infomercials, write innumerable booklets and books, and publish floods of magazine and newspaper advertorials to promote sales.

CAM treatments range from folk medicine to fraud. When these treatments are used instead of conventional medicine, they are called alternative; when they are used together with conventional medicine, they are called complementary. Some CAM therapies have been used for centuries, but few have been evaluated scientifically for safety or effectiveness.[1]* When tested, most prove ineffective or unsafe.[2] Useless remedies continue to sell, however, because an ill person's belief in a treatment, the placebo effect, can sometimes lead to physical healing (*placebo* was defined in Table 1–7 of Chapter 1). Then, undeservedly, the treatment gets the credit.

CAM Best Bets

This is not to say that all CAM treatments are useless. Dozens of **herbal medicines** contain effective natural drugs. For example, the resin myrrh (pronounced *murr*) contains an analgesic (painkilling) compound; willow bark contains aspirin; the herb valerian contains a tranquilizing oil; senna leaves produce a powerful laxative.[†] The WHO currently recommends a Chinese herbal medicine—artemisinin (art-uh-MEES-uh-nin), derived from

*References are in Appendix F.
[†] *A reliable source of information about herbs is V. Tyler,* The Honest Herbal *(New York: Pharmaceutical Products Press). Look for the latest edition.*

Table 11–8

Table 11–8

Alternative Therapy Terms

- **acupuncture** (AK-you-punk-chur) a technique that involves piercing the skin with long, thin needles at specific anatomical points to relieve pain or illness. Acupuncture sometimes uses heat, pressure, friction, suction, or electromagnetic energy to stimulate the points.
- **complementary** and **alternative medicine (CAM)** a group of diverse medical and health-care systems, practices, and products that are not considered to be a part of conventional medicine. Examples include acupuncture, biofeedback, chiropractic, faith healing, and many others.
- **herbal medicine** the use of herbs and herbal preparations to prevent or cure diseases or to relieve symptoms.

---

wormwood trees—to fight off malaria in some tropical nations.

Herbs, like drugs, however, can cause side effects.[3] The National Institutes of Health established its National Center for Complementary and Integrative Health (NCCIH) to distinguish alternative therapies that are potentially useful from those that are useless or harmful.

The "Herbs at a Glance" section of the NCCIH website provides information about specific herbs, their uses, and possible side effects.[‡] The NCCIH has found that **acupuncture** helps to quell nausea from surgery, chemotherapy, and pregnancy and to ease chronic low-back pain, and possibly migraine headaches, although underlying mechanisms for these effects are not known.[4] After two

[‡] *Access information about specific herbs at the NCCIH website, https://nccih.nih.gov/health/herbsataglance.htm.*

---

decades of funding studies, the agency has confirmed no effect from most other CAM treatments.

Ideally, a therapy provides benefits with little or no risk. Some alternative therapies are innocuous, providing little or no benefit for little or no risk. Sipping a cup of warm tea with a pleasant aroma, for example, won't cure heart disease, but it may improve one's mood and help relieve tension. Given no physical hazard and little financial risk, such therapies are acceptable. Figure 11–10 summarizes the relationships between risks and benefits.

In contrast, other products and procedures are dangerous, posing great risks while providing no benefits. One example, discussed next, is taking laetrile to treat cancer. Perhaps most controversial are alternative therapies that may provide benefits but also carry significant, unknown, or debatable risks. Smoking or ingesting marijuana is an example of such an alternative therapy.[5] The compounds in marijuana seem to provide relief from symptoms such as nausea, vomiting, and pain that commonly accompany cancer, HIV/AIDS, and other diseases, but smoking marijuana raises lung cancer risk and ingesting large amounts can cause psychotic delusions. As more states consider legalizing marijuana for medicinal use, the issue of risks versus benefits is highlighted.

A CAM Worst Case

The toxic drug laetrile, a CAM treatment for cancer, was popularized in the 1970s and remains available with no evidence to support its use, then or now. In fact, its high cyanide (poison) content makes it a hazardous choice. Along with thousands of other sham treatments, laetrile is still sold as a "dietary supplement" to unsuspecting people by way of Internet websites.

Figure 11-10
Risk-Benefit Relationships

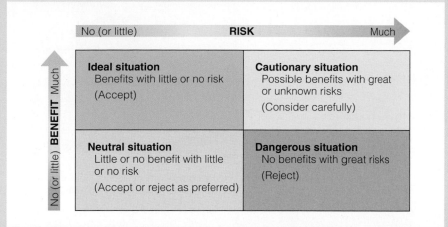

Anyone can claim to be an expert in a "new" or "natural" therapy, and many practitioners act knowledgeable but either are misinformed or are frauds (see Controversy 1). Intelligent, clear-minded people can fall for such hoaxes when standard medical therapies fail; loving life and desperate, they fall prey to the worst kind of quackery on the feeblest promise of a cure.

A Curious Case of Anosmia

A popular CAM cold treatment consisting of zinc gel squirted into the nose was widely advertised and sold but lacked approval from the U.S. Food and Drug Administration (FDA).[§] Over the course of a few years, the FDA received over 130 complaints from consumers reporting anosmia, meaning that they lost their sense of smell, sometimes permanently, after using the product. Finally, the FDA took action against the manufacturer, who removed the product from the market. Anosmia may not sound serious, but it dramatically reduces the sense of taste and pleasure in eating, and it poses a danger when it prevents the detection of hazards normally signaled through the sense of

[§] The products were Zicam Cold Remedy Nasal Gel, Zicam Cold Remedy Gel Swabs, and Zicam Cold Remedy Swabs, Kids Size.

smell, such as spoiled food or leaking gas. This case illustrates the trouble with using most CAM products: they are not tested for safety. Without prior testing, users become testers, and no one can predict the outcome.

Mislabeled Herbs

When common herbal remedies are analyzed, many do not contain the species or the active ingredients stated on their labels. In one analysis, instead of the herbs stated on the label, the CAM products contained unsafe medical drugs that interact with prescription medications to cause a dangerous drop in blood pressure. Lead poisoning and anemia have been associated with popular herbal medications made in India.[6] When labels lack veracity, and adulteration and contamination are common, consumers cannot make reasonable and safe choices.

If you decide to use an herbal or other CAM product, look for the words *U.S. Pharmacopeia* or *Consumer Lab* on the label. These names signify that samples of the product were analyzed and found to contain authentic ingredients in the quantities claimed. Still, these names do *not* indicate safety or effectiveness of the product.

Like other drugs, herbs often interfere with or potentiate the effects of medication (see Controversy 14).[7] For

example, because *Ginkgo biloba* impairs blood clotting, it can cause bleeding problems for people on aspirin or other blood-thinning medicines.[8]

Lack of Knowledge

Most people in the market for herbs and other CAM treatments take the advice of herb vendors in stores or online. Few herb sellers, however, possess the training in pharmacology, botany, and human physiology required to appropriately apply herbal remedies. Perilous mistakes with herbs are common. The few physicians who are skilled in herbal medicine may integrate the best CAM treatments into their practices, but many patients using herbs or CAM treatments keep their use a secret, fearing their doctors' disapproval. Such secrecy ups their risks—without knowledge, a physician cannot evaluate the potential for interactions.

Moving Ahead

The consequences of using unproven treatments are unpredictable. If you take prescription drugs, tell your doctor about any herbs you are also taking to rule out incompatibility.

Before taking any herb, find authoritative, scientific sources of information on its potential actions and risks. Don't be led astray by advertisements, rumors, Internet claims, or wishful thinking—investigate and decide for yourself.

Review Questions**

1. Complementary and alternative medicines (CAM) warrant a cautious approach; these treatments often lack evidence for safety or effectiveness. **T F**

2. The National Center for Complementary and Integrative Health promotes laetrile therapy. **T F**

3. For safety, people seeking medical help should inform their physicians about their use of herbs or other alternative medicines. **T F**

** Answers to Consumer's Guide review questions are in Appendix G.

Figure 11–11
Cancer Development

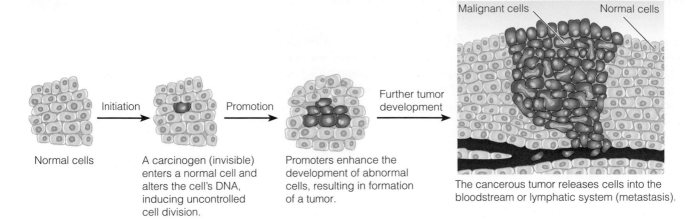

Normal cells

Initiation →

A carcinogen (invisible) enters a normal cell and alters the cell's DNA, inducing uncontrolled cell division.

Promotion →

Promoters enhance the development of abnormal cells, resulting in formation of a tumor.

Further tumor development →

Malignant cells   Normal cells

The cancerous tumor releases cells into the bloodstream or lymphatic system (metastasis).

Occasionally, a damaged cell doesn't die off but continues to live and becomes unable to halt its own reproduction. In a healthy, well-nourished person, the immune system steps in to destroy such cells.[60] If, however, the immune system falters, the damaged cell reproduces uncontrollably and the result is a mass of abnormal tissue—a tumor. Life-threatening cancer begins with an event called **initiation**. Following this, **promoters**, such as hormones or environmental factors, stimulate tumor growth. Then the tumor overwhelms the healthy tissue in which it developed, or exports its cells through the bloodstream to other parts of the body to initiate other tumors (**metastasis**). Figure 11–11 depicts these events.

KEY POINT

- Cancer arises from genetic damage and develops in steps.

Cancer Risk Factors

Can people's chosen behaviors affect their risks of contracting cancer? In many cases, they can. This section describes many lifestyle factors that influence cancer risk, and the next section, "Cancer Prevention," gives details of the measures people can take to minimize that risk.

Advancing Age   First among the unalterable risk factors for cancer, as for all chronic diseases, advancing age makes people increasingly vulnerable to the disease. The effects of habits you have engaged in from the start of your life add up to exert a powerful influence on your later health.

Family History (Heredity)   This factor, too, is one you cannot change, but knowing whether cancer runs in your family can give you a head start on taking preventive steps. Inherited susceptibility to cancer accounts for only a small proportion of cancer cases.

Chronic Inflammation   Inflammation plays a central role in cancer. Chronic inflammation may set in during the development of obesity, heart disease, diabetes, or other diseases, and can then accelerate the development of cancer.

Diet   Certain dietary factors substantially influence cancer development.[61] The degree of risk imposed by food depends partly on the eater's genetic makeup and partly on some other influences still to be discovered. Some dietary factors believed to be important in cancer causation and prevention are discussed below.

Weakened Immunity   The immune system can identify and fight cancer cells just as it fights allergens, toxins, and other foreign invaders. However, when immunity is weak, due to nutrient deficiencies, medical procedures, hormone treatments, or other influences, the body becomes defenseless against cancer development.

initiation an event, probably occurring in a cell's genetic material, caused by radiation or by a chemical carcinogen, that can give rise to cancer.

promoters factors such as certain hormones or environmental factors that do not initiate cancer but speed up its development once initiation has taken place.

metastasis (meh-TASS-ta-sis) movement of cancer cells from one body part to another, usually by way of the body fluids.

Infections   Certain viral, bacterial, and parasitic infections present risks of particular kinds of cancer. (To give just one example, infection with human papilloma virus carries a risk of cervical cancer.) In many cases, the mode of action seems to be that these infections weaken the immune system's cancer-fighting ability.

Obesity and Estrogen   Obesity is clearly a risk factor for cancers, especially those of the colon, endometrium, pancreas, kidney, esophagus, and breast (in postmenopausal women).[62] These cancers originate differently depending on the organ. For example, in the case of breast cancer in postmenopausal women, the hormone estrogen is involved: obese women have more circulating estrogen than lean women do, because adipose tissue converts other hormones into estrogen and releases it into the blood. In women of normal weight, blood estrogen drops dramatically beyond menopause, but in obese women, fat tissue continues to produce estrogen beyond menopause, extending the exposure and increasing the breast cancer risk.[63]

Alcohol with Smoking   Alcohol intake by itself raises the risk of cancers of the mouth, throat, esophagus, colon, and breast, and alcoholism often damages the liver in ways that promote liver cancer.[64] When drinkers add smoking to the insults inflicted on the body by alcohol, the rate of cancers of the head and neck rises significantly.

Fats and Fatty Acids   Laboratory studies using animals suggest that high dietary fat intakes correlate with development of cancer. Simply feeding fat to experimental animals is not enough to get tumors started, though: researchers must also expose the animals to known carcinogens. After that exposure, animals fed high-fat diets develop more cancers faster than animals fed low-fat diets. Thus, fat appears to be a cancer promoter in animals. Studies of people, however, have not proved that the effects of fat are independent of the effects of energy intake versus output—that is, eating versus physical activity. Overall, evidence associating fat intakes with cancer risk is limited.

Carcinogens in Red and Processed Meats   Population studies spanning the globe for more than 30 years consistently report that diets high in red meat and **processed meat** increase the risk of colon cancer.[65] Processed meats are listed among human carcinogens by the WHO. They contain additives, nitrites or nitrates, which contribute a pink color and deter bacterial growth in meats. In the digestive tract, nitrites and nitrates form other nitrogen-containing compounds that may be carcinogenic.[66]

Cooking Methods   Cooking meats at high temperatures (frying, broiling) causes amino acids and creatine in the meats to combine and form carcinogens.[67] Grilling meat, fish, or other foods—even vegetables—over a direct flame causes fat and added oils to splash on the fire and then vaporize, creating other carcinogens that rise and stick to the food. Smoking foods has the same effect. Eating these foods, or even well-browned meats cooked to the crispy, well-done stage, introduces carcinogens into the digestive system. A steady diet of foods containing these toxins can overwhelm defenses and increase cancer risk.

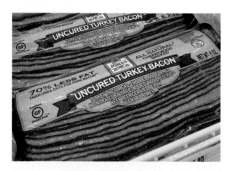

Many consumers appreciate the availability of bacon without added nitrites or nitrates.

Iron   Iron, both from the diet and from body stores, is under study for links with promotion of colon cancer. How iron may promote cancer is not known, but iron is suspected because it is a powerful oxidizing agent that can damage DNA. A high-meat diet generously supplies iron and also correlates with colon cancer risks.[68]

Fried Foods   French fries and potato chips contain another offending substance, acrylamide, which is produced when they are fried or baked at high temperatures. In the body, some acrylamide is metabolized to a substance that may damage the genes, producing mutations. Based on this finding, acrylamide is classified as "a probable human carcinogen." New to the market is a genetically modified potato that forms less acrylamide when fried or baked. (Controversy 12 on p. 477 explores the pros and cons of genetic engineering.)

processed meat meat preserved by smoking, curing, or salting or by the addition of preservatives.

A Note about Environmental Carcinogens Environmental factors also present risks of cancer. Overexposure to the sun, especially without the use of sunscreen or protective clothing, incurs a risk of skin cancer. Exposure to radiation, as when a nuclear accident occurs, poses a cancer risk; and there are many other such cases. These are beyond this book's scope.

KEY POINT

- Obesity, lack of physical activity, alcohol and tobacco use, and diets high in red and processed meats are associated with cancer development.

Cancer Prevention

The list of cancer risk factors just presented offers many opportunities for preventive efforts. Many of these are similar or identical to those that were described for CVD and diabetes, demonstrating that any good health habit offers far-reaching benefits.

First, a Note of Reassurance about Carcinogens in Foods Many people mistakenly believe that they should eat no foods that contain carcinogens. This is impossible, though, because all foods, even the purest wild and natural foods, contain carcinogens together with thousands of other chemicals and nutrients needed by the body. The body easily detoxifies the minute amounts of carcinogens that occur in common foods and fear is not warranted. Feel free to enjoy your coffee, toast, and coffee cake.‡

Some people also fear that food additives are carcinogenic. In this realm, too, fear is not warranted. Additives are held to strict standards in the United States. No additive approved for U.S. use causes cancer when used appropriately in food. Food *contaminants* may, however, enter foods by accident and may prove to be powerful carcinogens or be converted to carcinogens as the body breaks them down. Most contaminants are monitored in the U.S. food supply, and ordinarily they are present, if at all, in amounts much lower than would pose risks to consumers.

A key to evaluating the safety of foods is to note how frequently you eat them. Small quantities of a carcinogen in any food may add up to large quantities if you eat that food every day. Nutritionists encourage their clients to eat a "balanced *and varied* diet," and that is the place to begin to craft a cancer-prevention strategy.

Eat a Balanced and Varied Diet An estimated 20 percent of all cancers are caused by a combination of excess body weight, physical inactivity, excess alcohol consumption, and poor diet.[69] Eating patterns that rely heavily on fat, meat, alcohol, and excess calories and that underuse fruit and vegetables have been the targets of abundant cancer research. Constituents of the diet relate to cancer in several ways: some may initiate cancer, some may promote it, and (here's some good news) some may protect against it. Also, for a person who has cancer, diet can make a crucial difference in recovery. All of this research has yielded the recommendations and strategies for reducing cancer risk presented in Table 11–9.

Fiber-Rich Foods Many studies show that as people increase their dietary fiber intakes, their risks for colon cancer decline.[70] The mechanisms of this protective effect are not yet known, but evidence continues to accumulate in favor of these eating practices. If a meat-rich, calorie-dense diet is implicated in cancer causation, and if a vegetable-rich, whole grain-rich diet is associated with prevention, then wouldn't vegetarians have a lower incidence of these cancers? They do, as shown in Controversy 6.

Whole Foods and Phytochemicals Granted, whole foods have already been emphasized time and again in this book, but it bears repeating: whole foods, not single nutrients, are most influential in cancer prevention. fruit and vegetables, for example, contain a wide variety of nutrients and phytochemicals that may reduce oxidative

---

‡Coffee contains acetaldehyde, acetic acid, acetone, atractylosides, butanol, cafestol palmitate, chlorogenic acid, dimethyl sulfide, ethanol, furan, furfural, guaiacol, hydrogen sulfide, isoprene, methanol, methyl butanol, methyl formate, methyl glyoxal, propionaldehyde, pyridine, and 1,3,7,-trimethylxanthine. Toast and coffee cake contain acetic acid, acetone, butyric acid, caprionic acid, ethyl acetate, ethyl ketone, ethyl lactate, methyl ethyl ketone, propionic acid, and valeric acid.

Table 11–9

Recommendations and Strategies for Reducing Cancer Risk

Recommendations	Strategies
Body fatness. Achieve and maintain a healthy body weight throughout life.	Follow the Healthy U.S.-Style Eating Pattern for your appropriate energy level. Engage in regular physical activity. Limit consumption of energy-dense foods and avoid beverages with added sugars. Consume "fast foods" sparingly, if at all.
Physical activity. Adopt a physically active lifestyle.	Engage in at least 150 minutes of moderate-intensity physical activity or 75 minutes of vigorous-intensity physical activity or an equivalent combination throughout the week. Limit sedentary behaviors such as sitting, lying down, watching television, and other forms of screen-based recreation.
Plant-based foods. Consume a healthy diet with an emphasis on whole foods from plants.	Eat at least the daily amounts of vegetables and fruit recommended by the USDA Eating Patterns. Choose whole grains instead of refined-grain products. Limit intake of red meat and avoid processed meats. Limit refined starchy foods.
Alcoholic drinks. If you drink alcoholic beverages, limit consumption.	Drink no more than two drinks a day for men and one drink a day for women.
Preservation, processing, preparation. Limit consumption of salt-cured foods and processed meats.	Avoid salt-preserved, salted, or salty foods. Limit consumption of processed foods with added salt to ensure an intake of less than 6 grams of salt (2.4 grams of sodium) a day. Avoid processed meats.
Dietary supplements. Aim to meet nutritional needs through diet.	Dietary supplements are not recommended for cancer prevention.

Sources: *L. H. Kushi and coauthors, American Cancer Society guidelines on nutrition and physical activity for cancer prevention, CA: Cancer Journal for Clinicians 62 (2012): 30–67; World Cancer Research Fund/American Institute for Cancer Research, Food, Nutrition, Physical Activity and the Prevention of Cancer: A Global Perspective (Washington, D.C.: AICR, 2007), pp. 373–390.*

Figure 11–12

Examples of Cruciferous Vegetables

Cruciferous vegetables belong to the cabbage family: arugula, bok choy, broccoli, broccoli sprouts, brussels sprouts, cabbages (all sorts), cauliflower, greens (collard, mustard, turnip), kale, kohlrabi, rutabaga, and turnip root.

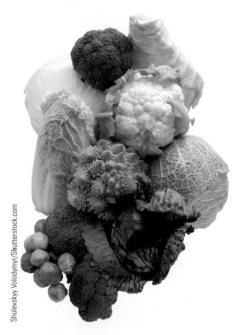

Shulevskyy Volodymyr/Shutterstock.com

damage to cell structures, including DNA, the material of genes.[71] In addition, some phytochemicals are thought to act as **anticarcinogens**, promoting the buildup of the body's arsenal of carcinogen-destroying enzymes. Figure 11–12 displays **cruciferous vegetables**—broccoli, brussels sprouts, cabbage, cauliflower, collard greens, turnips, and the like which contain a variety of potentially protective phytochemicals. Research suggests that some of these phytochemicals may exert their protective effect by way of epigenetic actions (a topic of Controversy 11).[72] Also, of course, whole, plant-based foods are rich in fibers, whose cancer-opposing virtues have already been mentioned.

Supplements Cannot Provide What Foods Provide Vitamin E, vitamin C, and beta-carotene received attention in Controversy 7. Suffice it to say here that supplements of these nutrients have not been proved to prevent cancer. In fact, once cancer is established, these antioxidants not only will *not* cure it, but may advance it.

anticarcinogens compounds in foods that act in any of several ways to oppose the formation of cancer.

cruciferous vegetables vegetables with cross-shaped blossoms, members of the cabbage family. Intakes of these vegetables are associated with low cancer rates in human populations. Examples are broccoli, brussels sprouts, cabbage, cauliflower, rutabagas, and turnips.

Use Alcohol Sparingly or Abstain from Use If they choose to drink alcohol, men should drink no more than two drinks a day; women no more than one. Don't combine alcohol use with smoking.

Achieve and Maintain a Healthy Body Weight throughout Life Follow the USDA Eating Pattern that provides the calorie level that is appropriate for you. Limit consumption of energy-dense foods and refrain from drinking beverages with added sugars. Consume "fast foods" sparingly if at all.

Engage in Regular Physical Activity An energy budget that balances caloric intake with caloric output may reduce the risk of developing some cancers. People whose lifestyles include regular, vigorous physical activity are seen to have lower risks of colon and breast cancer.[73] This effect may be attributable partly to the healthier body weights of the exercisers and partly to changes in hormone levels and immune functions induced by exercise.[74] Consistent with this finding is the advice to engage in an average of at least 20 minutes of moderate-intensity or 10 minutes of vigorous-intensity physical activity per day and to limit sedentary behaviors such as sitting, lying down, watching television, and other forms of screen-based recreation.

Caloric Effect Epidemiological studies suggest that whenever people's food intakes are limited, whether voluntarily (by fasting) or involuntarily (by famine), the onset of cancer is delayed. This phenomenon, known as the **caloric effect**, proves in experimental animals to be an effective dietary intervention to delay or prevent cancer. Calorie-restricted animals do not even contract the disease until after a freely fed group has already died of it. Clinical studies to explore this issue further are currently under way.[75] (An important note is that the effect occurs only in subjects who do not have the disease. Once started, cancer continues to advance even in people who are starving.)

Cooking Consumers can take these steps to minimize carcinogen formation during cooking:

- Marinate meats before cooking, and roast or bake them in the oven.
- When grilling, line the grill with foil, or wrap the food in foil.
- Take care not to burn foods.

In addition, limit intakes of crispy, browned French fries and chips and other well-browned foods.

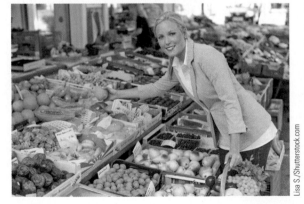

Regular intake of whole foods like these, not individual chemicals, lowers people's cancer risks.

Other Food and Nutrient Effects Research findings pile up: numerous experimental results credit one or another nutrient or type of food with a protective effect against one or another type of cancer. In summary, what can we do to protect ourselves against this cruel disease? Eat. Eat well. Exercise. Exercise a lot—and joyfully.

KEY POINTS

- Contaminants and naturally occurring toxins can be carcinogenic but they are monitored in the U.S. food supply, and the body is equipped to handle typical doses of most kinds.
- Foods containing ample fiber, nutrients, and phytochemicals may be protective against cancer.

Conclusion

Nutrition is often associated with promoting health, and medicine with fighting disease, but no clear line separates nutrition from medicine. Every major agency involved with health promotion or medicine recommends a varied dietary pattern of whole foods as part of a lifestyle that provides the best possible chance for a long and healthy life. The Food Feature that follows describes an example of such an eating pattern, the DASH diet.

caloric effect the drop in cancer incidence seen whenever calorie intakes are restricted.

The DASH Diet: Preventive Medicine

LO 11.5 Outline strategies for including sufficient fruit and vegetables in a diet.

An esteemed former surgeon general once said, "If you do not smoke or drink excessively, your choice of diet can influence your long-term health prospects more than any other action you might take."[§] Indeed, healthy young adults today are privileged to be among the first generations with enough nutrition knowledge to lay a truly strong foundation of health for today and tomorrow. Figure 11–13 illustrates this point.

Dietary Guidelines and the DASH Diet

The more detailed our knowledge about nutrition science, it seems, the simpler the truth becomes: people who

[§] *C. Everett Koop, 1988.*

consume the adequate, balanced, calorie-controlled, moderate, and varied diet recommended by the Dietary Guidelines for Americans enjoy a longer, healthier life than those who do not. The DASH eating plan, presented in Appendix E, can help people to meet these goals.

"Knowing is not enough; we must apply. Willing is not enough; we must do."
—Goethe

To lower saturated fat intakes, the DASH diet emphasizes fruit, vegetables, whole grains, and fat-free or low-fat milk and milk products. It also features fish, poultry, and nuts instead of some of the red meat so common in U.S. diets. Compared with the typical

American diet, the foods of the DASH diet provide greater intakes of fiber, as well as potassium, calcium, and magnesium, minerals shown to lower blood pressure.

Because the DASH diet centers on fresh, unprocessed, or lightly processed foods, it delivers less sodium, too. It seems, with regard to sodium, "the lower the better" for reducing blood pressure. Even at higher sodium intakes, however, the DASH diet can still produce a drop in blood pressure, although not as great as with sodium restriction.

Changes in diet are often best attempted a few at a time. A good place to start is by increasing the intake of fruit and vegetables.

Fruit and Vegetables: More Matters

The National Fruit and Vegetable Program is a confederation composed of the Centers for Disease Control and Prevention, the American Heart Association, the American Diabetes Association, the American Cancer Society, and many other national organizations. These agencies work together to urge people to meet the recommended intakes of a variety of fruit, vegetables, and legumes—not just for the nutrients they provide but also for the phytochemicals that combine synergistically to promote health (Figure 11–14, p. 432). The amounts to aim for depend on personal factors described in Chapter 2. Alternatively, you can find out how many servings are right for you by visiting www.fruitsandveggiesmorematters.org. Table 11–10 offers some tips for increasing your intakes of fruit, vegetables, and legumes. Who knows? Foods destined to become your favorites may still await you on the produce shelves. An adventurous spirit is a plus in this regard.

Figure 11–13

Proper Nutrition Shields against Diseases

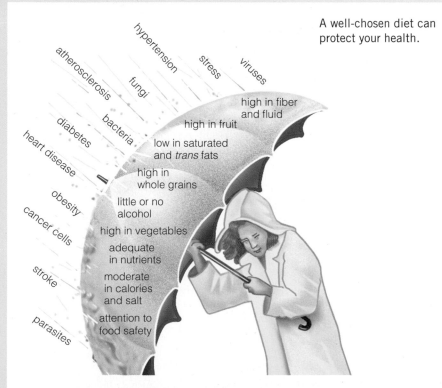

A well-chosen diet can protect your health.

labels: hypertension, stress, viruses, atherosclerosis, fungi, bacteria, diabetes, heart disease, obesity, cancer cells, stroke, parasites

umbrella panels: high in fiber and fluid; high in fruit; low in saturated and *trans* fats; high in whole grains; little or no alcohol; high in vegetables; adequate in nutrients; moderate in calories and salt; attention to food safety

(continued)

Figure 11–14

Fruit and Veggies: More Matters

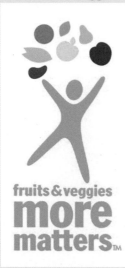

Fill half your plate with fruit and vegetables.

Conclusion

In the end, people's choices are their own. Whoever you are, we encourage you to take the time to work out ways of making your diet meet the guidelines you now know will support your health. If you are healthy and of normal weight, if you are physically active, and if your diet on most days follows the Dietary Guidelines, then you can indulge occasionally in a cheesy pizza, marbled steak, or banana split—or even a greasy fast-food burger and fries—without inflicting much damage on your health. (Once a week may be harmless, but less frequently is better.) Especially, take time to enjoy your meals: the sights, smells, and tastes of good foods are among life's greatest pleasures. Joy, even the simple joy of eating, contributes to a healthy life.

Table 11–10

Strategies for Consuming Enough Fruit, Vegetables, and Legumes

Many people do not eat the recommended amounts and varieties of fruit, vegetables, and legumes, but these foods are indispensible to a nutritious diet. All nutrient-dense forms count: fresh, frozen, canned, dried, and 100% juice.

Foods	Strategies
All vegetables	■ Include vegetables of all kinds in meals and snacks; fresh, frozen, and canned vegetables all count, but choose low-fat, low-sodium varieties most often. ■ Keep cut raw vegetables, such as carrot and celery sticks, in the refrigerator for quick snacks. ■ Visit a salad bar to buy ready-to-eat vegetables if you are in a hurry. ■ Try a new vegetable once each month. Read some cookbooks for ideas.
Dark green, red, and orange vegetables	■ Add chopped dark green leafy vegetables or red and orange vegetables to main dishes, such as stir-fries, soups, and casseroles. ■ Serve side dishes of dark green salad greens or cooked or raw broccoli, spinach, or other dark green vegetables often. Choose cooked or raw red and orange vegetable dishes, too, such as tomato-based dishes, cooked hard squashes, or sliced cooked carrots. ■ If calories are not a problem for you, try sweet potato fries as an occasional treat. ■ Order vegetable side dishes when eating out and ask for sauces and dressings to be served on the side.
Legumes (beans, peas, lentils, and soy products)	■ Keep a variety of low-sodium canned legumes, such as kidney beans, chickpeas (garbanzo beans), black beans, and others on hand. ■ Use rinsed, drained beans as salad toppers. For interest, marinate them in lemon juice, garlic, and seasonings. ■ Mash beans with lemon juice, olive oil, and seasonings, and use it as a topping for crackers, celery, or raw zucchini rounds, as a dip for vegetable sticks, or as a sandwich spread. ■ Add beans, peas, or lentils to soups and casseroles. ■ Try new ethnic legume recipes or try new bean dishes in restaurants, such as black beans and rice, white bean chili, lentil veggie burgers, or dal (spicy Indian-style beans, peas, or lentils). ■ Try using soy products such as soy milk, ground meat and burger replacers, tofu, and soy snacks.
Fruit	■ Choose whole or cut fruit more often than fruit juice. ■ Keep a variety of fresh, frozen, low-sugar canned, and dried fruit on hand to choose for snacks or to use in cereal, yogurt, salads, or desserts. ■ Replace syrup, sugars, and other sweet toppings with berries, cut peaches, applesauce, or fruit mixtures. ■ Blend smoothies from bananas, fruit juice, and berries with ice or yogurt. ■ Fruit canned in 100% fruit juice is preferable to fruit canned in sugary syrups.

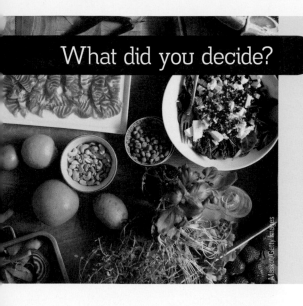

What did you decide?

Are your own food choices damaging your **heart**?

Is diabetes caused by **eating sugar**?

Can certain **herbs** improve your health?

Do "natural" foods without **additives** reduce cancer risks?

What's online?

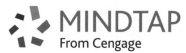
From Cengage

Visit www.Cengage.com to access MindTap, a complete digital course that includes Diet & Wellness Plus, interactive quizzes, videos, and more.

Self Check

1. (LO 11.1) Chronic diseases have distinct causes, known as risk factors.
   T F

2. (LO 11.1) Which of the following is a risk factor for cardio-vascular disease?
   a. high blood HDL cholesterol
   b. low blood pressure
   c. low blood LDL cholesterol
   d. diabetes

3. (LO 11.2) Atherosclerosis is simply the accumulation of lipids within the artery wall.
   T F

4. (LO 11.2) An "atherogenic diet" is high in saturated fat and *trans* fat.
   T F

5. (LO 11.2) Men suffer more often from heart attacks than women do, making CVD a man's disease.
   T F

6. (LO 11.2) Smoking powerfully raises the risk for CVD in men and women in all of the following ways except
   a. reducing the heart's workload.
   b. making blood clots more likely.
   c. directly damaging the heart with toxins.
   d. raising the blood pressure.

7. (LO 11.2) Which of the following minerals may help regulate blood pressure?
   a. phosphorus
   b. iron
   c. potassium
   d. zinc

8. (LO 11.2) The most important step that a person can take to protect against hypertension is to be tested for it.
   T F

9. (LO 11.3) Diabetes is a major risk factor for CVD.
   T F

10. (LO 11.3) The recommended diet to improve type 2 diabetes is
    a. low in carbohydrates.
    b. as low in fat as possible.
    c. controlled in carbohydrates.
    d. a and b.

11. For managing type 2 diabetes, regular physical activity can help by redistributing the body's fluids.
    T F

12. (LO 11.4) For the great majority of cancers, lifestyle factors and environmental exposures are the major risk factors.
    T F

13. (LO 11.4) Which of the following is or are associated with an increase in cancer risk?
    a. alcohol intake
    b. a high intake of red meat
    c. a high intake of processed meats
    d. all of the above.

14. (LO 11.5) The DASH diet is designed for athletes who compete in sprinting events.
    T F

15. (LO 11.5) The DASH diet is characterized by ample intakes of _____.
    a. fruit and vegetables
    b. whole grains
    c. artificial fats
    d. a and b

16. (LO 11.6) Currently, for the best chance of consuming adequate nutrients and staying healthy, people should obtain evaluations of their genetic profiles.
    T F

Answers to these Self Check questions are in Appendix G.

Nutritional Genomics: Can It Deliver on Its Promises?

LO 11.6   Describe the emerging science of nutritional genomics.

Health care appears to be on the brink of a **genomics** revolution.[1]* The era of **precision medicine** is changing some basic views on health, disease, and nutrition. Advances in **genome** testing have made it economically feasible to identify someone's genetic risk for a number of medical conditions, including an aggressive form of Alzheimer's disease, celiac disease (severe gluten sensitivity; see Chapter 6), hemochromatosis (toxic iron overload, described in Chapter 8), and other conditions.[2] Once a disease-associated variant is observed in the **genetic profile**, the client and health care provider can employ lifestyle choices and treatment options to minimize the potential for harm.[3] For example, a genetic tendency toward hemochromatosis may prompt instruction from a registered dietitian nutritionist about dietary changes to reduce absorption of dietary iron, among other tactics.

The science of **nutritional genomics** is now providing insights into some age-old questions. If genes cause diseases, then how can identical twins, with their identical DNA, develop different diseases? How is it that a pregnant woman's diet can forever affect the health of her grandchildren? How might certain phytochemicals alter the course of some cancers?

Reference notes are in Appendix F.

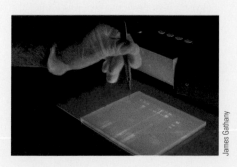

James Gathany

Table C11–1
Genomics Terms

- **bioactive food components** nutrients and phytochemicals in foods that alter physiological processes, often by interacting, directly or indirectly, with the genes.
- **epigenetics** (ep-ih-gen-EH-tics) the science of heritable changes in gene function that occur without changes in the DNA sequence.
- **epigenome** (ep-ih-GEE-nohm) the proteins and other molecules associated with chromosomes that affect gene expression. The epigenome is modulated by bioactive food components and other factors in ways that can be inherited. *Epi* is a Greek prefix, meaning "above" or "on."
- **genetic profile** the result of an analysis of genetic material that identifies unique characteristics of a person's DNA for forensic or diagnostic purposes.
- **genome** (GEE-nohm) the full complement of genetic material in the chromosomes of a cell. Also defined in Chapter 1.
- **genomics** the study of all the genes in an organism and their interactions with environmental factors.
- **histones** (HISS-tones) proteins that lend structural support to the chromosome structure and that help activate or silence gene expression.
- **methyl (METH-il) groups** molecular fragments consisting of one carbon and three hydrogen atoms that, among their many roles, can alter gene expression when attached by enzymes to strands of DNA.
- **mutation** a permanent, heritable change in an organism's DNA.
- **nucleotide** (NU-klee-oh-tied) one of the subunits of DNA and RNA are composed.
- **nutritional genomics** the science of how food and its components interact with the genome.
- **precision medicine** an emerging approach for disease prevention and treatment that takes into account individual variability in the genes, environment, and lifestyle for each person. *Precision nutrition* or *personalized nutrition* take the same approach, tailoring an eating plan to an individual's genetic profile.
- **SNP** (snip) a type of genetic variation involving a single changed nucleotide. The letters SNP stand for *single nucleotide polymorphism.*

This Controversy offers a taste of the research in these areas—there is much more to learn, and the science advances daily. Table C11–1 distinguishes among the terms **genomics**, nutritional genomics, epigenetics, and others. Figure C11–1 clarifies relationships among nutritional genomics and similar fields.[†] Then the Controversy offers some evidence that suggests genomics links between chronic diseases and diet. The closing section addresses concerns surrounding genetic tests of all kinds.

[†]*An additional potential factor in precision medicine is an analysis of the genetic makeup of a person's intestinal bacteria (microbiome) in relation to disease risks, but this science is in its infancy.*

Genes Influence Nutrition and Disease

Small variations in DNA sequences, called **mutations**, dictate many of the differences among human beings, including differences in nutrient metabolism. The most common mutations are **SNPs** (pronounced "snips"), involving the variation of a single molecule (a **nucleotide**) in a strand of DNA.[4] About 10 million possible SNPs are known to exist in human DNA.

SNPs and Diseases

Most individuals carry tens of thousands of SNPs, and most seem to exert no

Nutritional Genomics

Two branches of nutritional genomics may have similar-sounding names—nutrigenomics and nutrigenetics—but they oppose each other in scope. One branch studies how genes affect nutrient metabolism. The other branch studies how nutrients affect the genes.

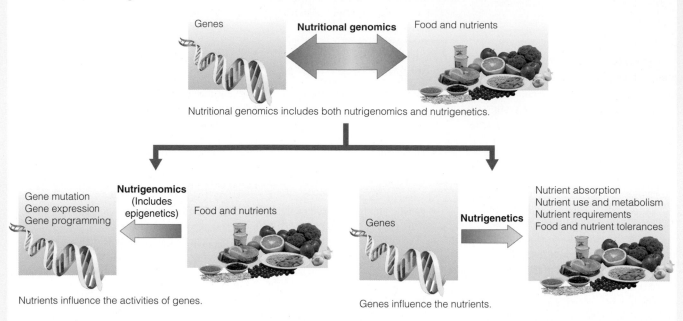

Genes **Nutritional genomics** Food and nutrients

Nutritional genomics includes both nutrigenomics and nutrigenetics.

Gene mutation
Gene expression
Gene programming

Nutrigenomics
(Includes epigenetics)
Food and nutrients

Genes **Nutrigenetics**

Nutrient absorption
Nutrient use and metabolism
Nutrient requirements
Food and nutrient tolerances

Nutrients influence the activities of genes.

Genes influence the nutrients.

functional effect at all. Rarely, however, a single SNP in a high-powered gene can produce a severe disease immediately from birth, such as PKU, as described in Chapter 3. More commonly, SNPs do not cause a disease directly but may subtly work with other gene variants and with environmental factors such as diet to raise the risks of developing heart disease or other maladies in later life. A SNP typically sets the stage for a chronic disease; then the person's own choices contribute to the development of the disease.

As an example, a common SNP in a fat metabolism gene changes the body's response to dietary fats. People with this SNP maintain normal blood LDL cholesterol concentrations when they eat diets rich in polyunsaturated fatty acids (PUFA), and they develop higher than normal LDL concentrations when they consume less PUFA. A gene (in this case, a fat metabolism gene with a SNP) interacts with a nutrient from the diet (in this case, PUFA) to influence a risk factor for a disease (LDL cholesterol

concentration, implicated in heart disease).

Complexity of SNP–Disease Relationships

Imagine a geneticist working to identify the genetic cause of a chronic disease risk factor—and discovering, to his delight, a SNP to be a culprit. "Aha! This is the cause," he declares, and everyone celebrates. Regrettably, though, such links are almost never this easy for real researchers to pin down. They often involve SNPs in multiple genes, each of which may interact with many dietary and other environmental factors. Furthermore, another realm of influence on gene behavior also enters into the picture—the **epigenome**.

Not long ago, we thought we knew that genes, once inherited, never change throughout life. It is true that *DNA molecules* remain the same, but structures that surround the DNA strands influence its activities, and these do change in response to nongenetic factors such as what people eat.

Nutrients Influence the Genes: Epigenetics

People often think of chromosomes as simple strands of DNA, but chromosomes exist as complex, three-dimensional combinations of DNA, proteins, and other molecules. DNA strands are the primary carriers of inherited information, true, but the epigenome constitutes another parallel bank of inheritable information. The epigenome's proteins and other molecules associate with DNA and interact with it in ways that regulate genetic activity for example, turning genes on or off. Like DNA itself, the epigenome is inherited from generation to generation, but unlike DNA, it is responsive to environmental influences, including diet, particularly during early development.[5]

The genome and the epigenome have been likened to nature's pen-and-pencil set. The genome, made of DNA, is written in indelible ink, so to speak; its sequence is mostly permanent. The epigenome is written in pencil in the margins and allows for erasures and changes.

The Epigenome's Role in Differentiation

Given that every cell of the body contains the same genes, scientists have long wondered how they give rise to distinct body parts. How do the cells of an eye decide to make an eye while the cells of the kidney make a kidney? The epigenome manages this extraordinary process of differentiation by turning different genes on or off in different locations. A cone cell of a person's eye and a blood-producing cell of that person's bone marrow contain identical DNA strands, but luckily for the person, the epigenome activates and silences genes on the DNA strands so that each cell type reliably makes only the correct proteins that will perform its own specialized functions.

How Epigenetic Regulation Works

Mechanisms for epigenetic gene regulation include, among others, the workings of large globular proteins known as **histones** and small molecular fragments called **methyl groups**.‡ The actions of these regulators can be modified by way of diet and other environmental influences.

Histones in Gene Expression   Millions of histones reside within the chromosomes (shown in Figure C11–2). Like a thread wound around a spool, sections of a DNA "thread" are tightly wrapped around these histones, giving shape to the chromosome and allowing for efficient storage of DNA molecules within a cell's nucleus.

The histones also regulate genetic activity. When a DNA segment is wrapped around a histone, its genes are silent—they physically lack the space to perform the tasks required for protein synthesis. Histones, though, can change this arrangement in response to changing needs.

Histones sport protein "tails" that stick out from their DNA wrappings.

‡*Other mechanisms include acetylation of DNA (and histones), other chromatin remodeling factors, and noncoding regulatory RNA molecules.*

Figure C11–2
Two Epigenetic Factors and Gene Activity

This figure depicts histones, large globular protein "spools" that wrap lengths of DNA. Other epigenetic factors also exist, such as the methyl groups in this illustration, tiny one-carbon structures that attach directly to a DNA strand, modifying its activity. Another is a form of RNA (not shown).

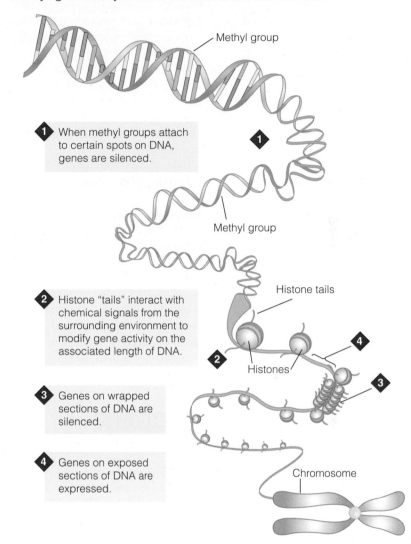

Methyl group

1 When methyl groups attach to certain spots on DNA, genes are silenced.

Methyl group

2 Histone "tails" interact with chemical signals from the surrounding environment to modify gene activity on the associated length of DNA.

Histone tails

Histones

3 Genes on wrapped sections of DNA are silenced.

4 Genes on exposed sections of DNA are expressed.

Chromosome

These tails serve as landing sites for many molecules from the environment that reflect cellular conditions.

When a histone receives chemical signals indicating a need for a particular protein, it loosens its grip on its wraps of DNA, allowing the portion of the strand with genes for making that protein to stretch out. Genes on these stretched-out segments can then express their encoded proteins—they are activated. Here's where nutrition comes in: many

of the molecular signals to which histones respond arise from the diet—they consist of nutrients and phytochemicals or of compounds generated during their metabolism.

A Broccoli Phytochemical Example
One phytochemical, sulforaphane (sull-foh-RAFF-ane) found in broccoli, broccoli sprouts, and other cabbage-family vegetables, may affect cancer processes by way of histone changes

in cancer cells. One characteristic of cancerous tissue is uncontrolled cell division. In cancer cells, histones may inappropriately silence genes that would otherwise stop cells from multiplying out of control.

In test tubes, sulforaphane reverses those cancer-promoting histone changes and reinstates control of cell division.[6] In mice, sulforaphane inhibits certain cancers. In people, ingestion of one cup of broccoli sprouts alters histone activities in blood cells. Does consumption of broccoli or other cabbage-family food actually prevent cancer in people? People who consume these foods regularly have lower rates of some cancers, but no one knows whether the foods themselves are protective. Researchers are still investigating that question.

Many other phytochemicals, including tea flavonoids, curcumin (derived from the spice turmeric), and sulfur compounds from the onion family, along with nutrients such as folate, vitamin B_{12}, vitamin C, vitamin D, selenium, and zinc add to a growing list of food constituents that affect epigenetic activities in ways that may prevent cancer.[7] Scientists can duplicate some of these activities with synthetic drugs, but the drugs, unlike foods, are highly toxic to living tissues.

Methyl Groups and Gene Regulation
Genes are also regulated by a number of molecules that adhere to the DNA strand itself. Methyl groups, mentioned earlier, attach directly onto DNA (look again at Figure C11–2), altering gene expression. Typically, when a methyl group attaches to the beginning of a gene sequence on a DNA strand (methylation), the gene is silenced. Removal of that methyl group allows gene expression to commence and protein replication to occur.

B Vitamins Transfer Methyl Groups   A powerful example of how nutrients affect the genes involves the influence of the B vitamin folate on DNA methylation. Folate (along with other B vitamins) is essential for transferring methyl groups from molecule to molecule, including to DNA molecules. With too little folate, genes may be insufficiently methylated to suppress the production of unneeded proteins.

This effect is illustrated in the accompanying photo of two mice. Despite their strikingly different appearance, these mice have identical DNA. Both possess a gene that tends to produce fat, yellow pups, but their mothers were fed different diets during pregnancy. The mother of the lean, brown mouse received doses of the B vitamins folate and vitamin B_{12}. By way of methyl group transfer activity, these vitamins silenced the gene for "yellow and fat," resulting in brown, lean pups.

Note that the extra vitamins did not change the DNA sequence. Still, such epigenomic changes established during pregnancy can be inherited along with the DNA and thus persist through several generations.

Importantly, pregnant women should tend to their nutrition needs carefully (see Chapter 13). No one should attempt to alter their children's and grandchildren's risks of obesity or other diseases by loading up on B vitamins or other substances. The effects of imbalances are unpredictable and can be severe.[8]

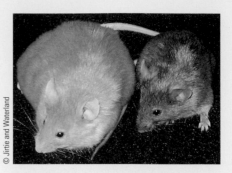
© Jirtle and Waterland

These two mice share an identical gene that tends to produce fat, yellow mice. The mother of the lean, brown mouse received supplemental B vitamins that silenced the gene.

Can Adults Modify Their Epigenome?

The greatest epigenomic changes from environmental influences occur early during embryonic development (Figure C11–3 demonstrates this concept).[9] Some change can still occur into adolescence and even adulthood, however, and they can affect health outcomes. The findings on sulforaphane of broccoli, described earlier, provide evidence that certain epigenetic factors in adult cells can indeed be changed, at least temporarily, by bioactive constituents of foods. Another example in adults is the development of liver cancer after ingestion of a mold toxin

Figure C11–3

An Epigenome Timeline

Environmental influences, including diet, most profoundly alter the epigenome during the earliest stages of development, but some changes are probably still possible later in life.

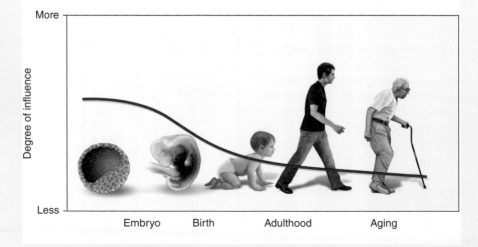

that can form on corn and other grain (*aflatoxin*, defined on page 456.) The toxin is suspected of causing removal of important methyl groups from both histones and the DNA strand, triggering the development of the cancer.

Now a theory emerges to suggest at least a partial solution to the mystery of how identical twins can develop different diseases. Although the twins have identical DNA, they acquire differences in their epigenomes. They encounter different environmental influences at various times of life that change their genetic expression.

On learning of these revelations in nutritional genomics, many people want to apply the new science to themselves. The next sections explore issues that arise with genetic testing for nutrition.

Arguments Surrounding Genetic Testing

For nutritional genomics to be of practical value, people must undergo genetic testing to detect gene variations that affect nutrition or nutrition-related diseases.[10] Critics of testing, however, question whether identifying a genetic marker for disease by way of expensive testing would translate into better health for the nation or simply waste limited health-care dollars. Consumers voice fears that DNA results, once known, could be misused.[11] A few companies have policies against sharing collected data, but others sell it to scientists who use it in experiments and who may, in turn, release it to someone else. This data sharing helps to advance science; large banks of data from many individuals, both healthy and diseased, are needed to establish links among genes and diseases with certainty.[12] For DNA donors, however, a problem could ensue if test results revealing a disease tendency ended up in the wrong hands. For example, such information could influence a decision maker regarding a person's acceptance to school, promotion at work, or other critical issues. The law forbids this kind of discrimination, but enforcement is rare and testing companies cannot promise absolute confidentiality.

Direct-to-Consumer Tests

For a few hundred dollars, consumers can easily order DNA tests for themselves over the Internet. However, due to gaps in regulation, test quality and validity and the proper use of results are not ensured. Such gaps have made it possible for unscrupulous companies to sell fake tests or mislead consumers into buying expensive supplements and other products based on unfounded assessments of their DNA samples.[13] Even when DNA tests are legitimate, interpreting the results is complex, and a consumer acting without a medical professional's opinion could easily be misled into taking ill-advised medication or avoiding a necessary one—or even undergoing an unneeded surgery. To help remedy this situation, the FDA sent letters to companies that sell such tests to consumers, warning them to stop marketing their tests and assessments for medical purposes.

Are people who purchase and take a personal genetic test also willing to make needed lifestyle changes in response to the findings? In one study, about a third of the participants reported that they were exercising more and eating better diets, regardless of their test results.[14] Countering this positive finding, almost as many people in the same study did the opposite—they exercised less and ate lower-quality diets. Most studies report no significant changes in health behaviors after testing.[15] Without the will to improve health behaviors, it is unlikely that personal genetic testing alone can improve the health of the population in the future.

Conclusion

No doubt the future of nutrition science will be inextricably linked with the science of genomics, and potential benefits may be enormous. Still, if the authors of this book tried to predict the future, based on libraries full of past evidence, most scenarios might go something like this: "Based on our genomics study, Mr. X needs greater amounts of vitamin C from tomato sauces and pink grapefruit, but not from supplements. He needs the fiber, lycopene, carbohydrates, and other bioactive components of a variety of fruit and vegetables, along with less saturated fat, sufficient protein, and a nutritious balanced diet to ward off future problems."

Experience shows that fiber supplements cannot take the place of whole grains for digestive tract health nor can calcium pills fully replace food sources of calcium for bone health. Besides, supplements come with risks. Many other examples exist to make the case for following a well-planned eating pattern of whole foods, as recommended by the Dietary Guidelines for Americans (see Chapter 2), to help modify the risks to health that a genetic predisposition may pose.[16]

Stay alert for updates in the rapidly advancing science of nutritional genomics. Registered dietitian nutritionists will be key providers of precision nutrition care as more becomes known about its potential to minimize disease risks and maximize the health of people everywhere.

Critical Thinking

1. Describe the status of nutritional genomics research. Provide two examples of where this type of research is leading us.

2. Explain how SNPs may cause disease.

Controversy 11 Nutritional Genomics: Can It Deliver on Its Promises?

439

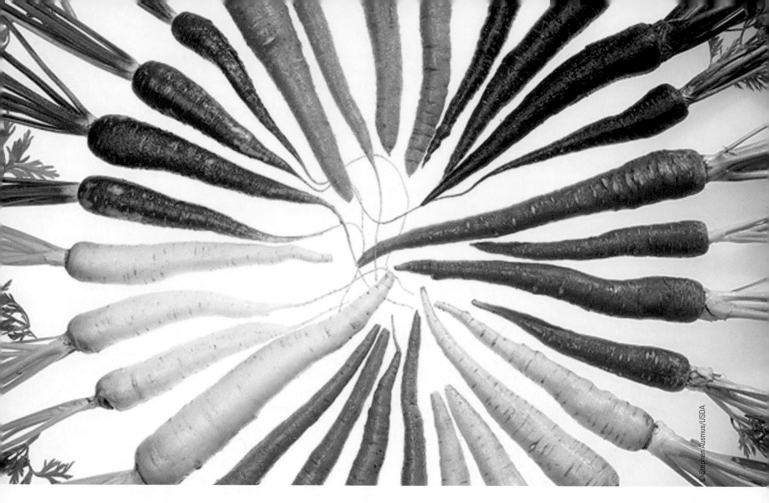
© Stephen Ausmus/USDA

12 Food Safety and Food Technology

Learning Objectives

After completing this chapter, you should be able to accomplish the following:

LO 12.1 Describe microbial foodborne illnesses and core practices that can prevent them.

LO 12.2 Identify the categories of foods that most often cause foodborne illnesses.

LO 12.3 Outline technological advances aimed at reducing microbial food contamination.

LO 12.4 Describe natural toxins, pesticide residues, and contaminants in food.

LO 12.5 Compare potential advantages and drawbacks of organic and conventional foods.

LO 12.6 Describe the uses and safety characteristics of some common food additives.

LO 12.7 Describe applications of food-safety practices in various settings.

LO 12.8 Summarize the advantages and disadvantages of producing foods through genetic engineering.

What do you think?

Are most digestive tract symptoms from **"stomach flu"**?

Are most foods from grocery stores **germ-free**?

Should you **refrigerate** leftover party foods after the guests have gone home?

Which poses the greater risk: raw **sushi** from a sushi master or food additives?

Consumers in the United States enjoy food supplies ranking among the safest in the world. They are also among the, most abundant and the most pleasing. Along with this abundance comes a consumer responsibility to distinguish between choices leading to food **safety** and those that pose a **hazard**. This chapter begins by pointing out common hazards, and then goes on to offer practical instruction for avoiding them.

As human populations grow and food supplies become more global, new food-safety challenges arise that require new processes, new technologies, and greater cooperation to solve.[1]* Food safety is therefore a moving target. The **Food and Drug Administration (FDA)** is the major agency charged with ensuring that the U.S. food supply is safe, wholesome, sanitary, and properly labeled (see Table 12–1 for agency terms, p. 442). It focuses much effort on these areas of concern:

1. *Microbial* **foodborne illness**. Each year, 48 million Americans (one in every six) becomes ill, 128,000 are hospitalized, and 3,000 die from foodborne illnesses.[2]

2. *Natural toxins in foods.* These constitute a hazard mostly when people consume large quantities of single foods either by choice (fad diets) or by necessity (poverty).

3. *Residues in food.*
   a. *Environmental and other contaminants* (other than pesticides). Household and industrial chemicals are increasing yearly in number and concentration, and their impacts are hard to foresee and to forestall.
   b. *Pesticide residues.* A subclass of environmental contaminants, these are listed separately because they are applied intentionally to foods and, in theory, can be controlled.
   c. *Animal drugs.* These include hormones and antibiotics that increase growth or milk production and combat diseases in food animals.

4. *Nutrients in foods.* These require close attention as more and more highly processed and artificially constituted foods appear on the market.

5. *Intentional approved food additives.* These are of less concern because so much is known about them that they pose little risk to consumers.

6. *Genetically engineered foods.* Such foods are listed last because they undergo rigorous scrutiny before going to market.

Within its powers, the FDA is vigilant in overseeing the food supply at home and abroad to safeguard the health of U.S. consumers.[3] When foodborne illness occurs, the FDA acts quickly to identify and resolve the cause.

Despite the best efforts of the FDA and others, foodborne illnesses are extraordinarily likely to occur. It seems that as one organism comes under control, others emerge to take its place. Achieving the ultimate goal—fewer total foodborne illnesses—requires ever-increasing vigilance on the part of regulators, food industries, and consumers.[4]

*Reference notes are in Appendix F.

With the privilege of abundance comes the responsibility to choose and handle foods wisely.

safety the practical certainty that injury will not result from the use of a product or substance.

hazard a state of danger; referring to any circumstance in which harm is possible under normal conditions of use.

foodborne illness illness transmitted to human beings through food or water; caused by an infectious agent (*foodborne infection*) or a poisonous substance arising from microbial toxins, poisonous chemicals, or other harmful substances (*food intoxication*). Also commonly called *food poisoning*.

Food Regulatory Agencies

Each agency oversees programs and systems aimed at maintaining and improving the safety of the food supply.

CDC (Centers for Disease Control and Prevention) a branch of the U.S. Department of Health and Human Services that is responsible for, among other things, identifying, monitoring, and reporting on foodborne illnesses and outbreaks (*www.cdc.gov*).

EPA (Environmental Protection Agency) a federal agency that is responsible for, among other things, regulating pesticides and establishing water quality standards (*www.epa.gov*).

FAO (Food and Agriculture Organization) an international agency (part of the United Nations) that has adopted standards to regulate pesticide use, among other responsibilities (*www.fao.org*).

FDA (Food and Drug Administration) the federal agency responsible for ensuring the safety and wholesomeness of all dietary supplements and foods processed and sold in interstate and international commerce except for some aspects of meat, poultry, and eggs (which are under the jurisdiction of the USDA); setting standards for food composition and product labeling; and issuing recalls when problems arise (*www.fda.gov*).

USDA (U.S. Department of Agriculture) the federal agency responsible for enforcing standards for the wholesomeness and quality of meat, poultry, and eggs produced in the United States; conducting nutrition research; and educating the public about nutrition (*www.usda.gov*).

WHO (World Health Organization) an international agency concerned with promoting health and eradicating disease (*www.who.int*).

Microbes and Food Safety

LO 12.1   Describe microbial foodborne illnesses and core practices that can prevent them.

Some people brush off the threat from foodborne illnesses as less likely and less serious than the threat of flu, but they are misinformed. Foodborne illnesses, caused by disease-causing **microbes** (**pathogens**), pose real threats to health and life, and some kinds increasingly do not respond to standard antibiotic drug therapy. Even normally mild foodborne illnesses can be lethal for a person who is ill or malnourished; has a compromised immune system; lives in an institution; has liver or stomach illnesses; or is pregnant, very old, or very young.

If digestive tract disturbances are the major or only symptoms of your next bout of what some people erroneously call "stomach flu," chances are that what you really have is a foodborne illness. By learning something about these illnesses and taking a few preventive steps, you can maximize your chances of staying well. Understanding the nature of the microbes responsible is the first step toward defeating them.

How Do Microbes in Food Cause Illness in the Body?

Microorganisms can cause foodborne illness either by infection or by **intoxication**. Infectious agents, such as *Salmonella* bacteria or hepatitis viruses, infect the tissues of the human body and multiply there, causing illness. Some bacteria produce **enterotoxins** or **neurotoxins**, poisonous chemicals that they release as they multiply. These toxins are absorbed into the tissues and cause various kinds of harm, ranging from mild stomach pain and headache to paralysis and death.

Table 12–2 lists the microbes responsible for 90 percent of U.S. foodborne illnesses, hospitalizations, and deaths. It also lists their food sources, general symptoms, and prevention methods. Many other illness-causing microbes exist. The steps outlined in this chapter can reduce or eliminate all of them.

microbes a shortened name for *microorganisms*; minute organisms too small to observe without a microscope, including bacteria, viruses, and others.

pathogens bacteria, viruses, fungi, and other microbes capable of causing illness. *Pathogenic* is the adjective form.

intoxication a state of physical harm caused by a toxin; poisoning.

enterotoxins poisons that act on mucous membranes, such as those of the digestive tract.

neurotoxins poisons that act on the cells of the nervous system.

Table 12–2

Causes, Symptoms, and Prevention of Microbial Foodborne Illnesses

Organism Name	Most Frequent Food Sources	Onset and General Symptoms	Prevention Methods[a]
Foodborne Infections			
Campylobacter (KAM-pee-loh-BAK-ter) bacterium	Raw and undercooked poultry, unpasteurized milk, contaminated water	Onset: 2 to 5 days. Diarrhea, vomiting, abdominal cramps, fever; sometimes bloody stools; lasts 2 to 10 days.	Cook foods thoroughly; use pasteurized milk; use sanitary food-handling methods.
Clostridium (claw-STRID-ee-um) *perfringens* (per-FRINGE-enz) bacterium	Meats and meat products held at between 120°F and 130°F	Onset: 8 to 16 hours. Abdominal pain, diarrhea, nausea; lasts 1 to 2 days.	Use sanitary food-handling methods; use pasteurized milk; cook foods thoroughly; refrigerate foods promptly and properly.
Escherichia coli; E. coli (esh-eh-REEK-ee-uh-KOH-lye) bacterium (including Shiga toxin–producing strains)[a]	Undercooked ground beef, unpasteurized milk and juices, raw fruit and vegetables, contaminated water, and person-to-person contact	Onset: 1 to 8 days. Severe bloody diarrhea, abdominal cramps, vomiting; lasts 5 to 10 days.	Cook ground beef thoroughly; use pasteurized milk; use sanitary food-handling methods; use treated, boiled, or bottled water.
Listeria (lis-TER-ee-AH) bacterium	Unpasteurized milk; fresh soft cheeses; luncheon meats, hot dogs	Onset: 1 to 21 days. Fever, muscle aches; nausea, vomiting, blood poisoning; complications in pregnancy; meningitis (stiff neck, severe headache, and fever); lasting neurological damage; death.	Use sanitary food-handling methods; cook foods thoroughly; use only pasteurized milk products and cheeses.
Norovirus	Person-to-person contact; raw foods, salads, sandwiches	Onset: 1 to 2 days. Vomiting; lasts 1 to 2 days.	Use sanitary food-handling methods.
Salmonella (sal-moh-NEL-ah) bacteria (>2,300 types)	Raw or undercooked eggs, meats, poultry, raw milk and other dairy products, shrimp, frog legs, yeast, coconut, pasta, and chocolate	Onset: 1 to 3 days. Fever, vomiting, abdominal cramps, diarrhea; lasts 4 to 7 days; can be fatal.	Use sanitary food-handling methods; use pasteurized milk; cook foods thoroughly; refrigerate foods promptly and properly.
Toxoplasma (TOK-so-PLAZ-ma) *gondii* parasite	Raw or undercooked meat; contaminated water; raw goat's milk; ingestion after contact with infected cat feces	Onset: 7 to 21 days. Swollen glands, fever, headache, muscle pain, stiff neck.	Use sanitary food-handling methods; cook foods thoroughly.
Foodborne Intoxications			
Clostridium (claw-STRID-ee-um) *botulinum* (bot-chew-LINE-um) bacterium produces botulin toxin, responsible for causing botulism	Anaerobic environment of low acidity (canned corn, peppers, green beans, soups, beets, asparagus, mushrooms, ripe olives, spinach, tuna, chicken, chicken liver, liver pâté, luncheon meats, ham, sausage, stuffed eggplant, lobster, and smoked and salted fish)	Onset: 4 to 36 hours. Nervous system symptoms, including double vision, inability to swallow, speech difficulty, and progressive paralysis of the respiratory system; often fatal; leaves prolonged symptoms in survivors.	Use proper canning methods for low-acid foods; refrigerate home-made garlic and herb oils; avoid commercially prepared foods with leaky seals or with bent, bulging, or broken cans. Do not feed honey to infants.
Staphylococcus (STAF-il-oh-KOK-us) *aureus* bacterium produces staphylococcal toxin	Toxin produced in improperly refrigerated meats; egg, tuna, potato, and macaroni salads; cream-filled pastries	Onset: 1 to 6 hours. Diarrhea, nausea, vomiting, abdominal cramps, fever; lasts 1 to 2 days.	Use sanitary food-handling methods; cook food thoroughly; refrigerate foods promptly and properly.

Note: Travelers' diarrhea is most commonly caused by E. coli, Campylobacter jejuni, Shigella, *and* Salmonella.

[a] *E. Coli O157, O145, and other Shiga toxin-producing bacteria cause toxin-mediated infections—they release toxins as their colonies grow in the body.*

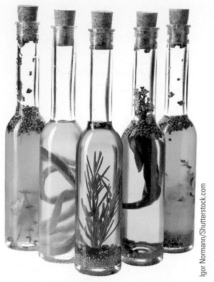

To prevent botulism from homemade flavored oils, wash and dry fresh herbs before use, and keep the oil refrigerated. Discard it after a week to 10 days.

The most common cause of food intoxication is the *Staphylococcus aureus* bacterium, but the most infamous is undoubtedly *Clostridium botulinum*, an organism that produces a toxin so deadly that an amount as tiny as a single grain of salt can kill several people within an hour. *Clostridium botulinum* grows in **anaerobic** conditions such as those found in improperly canned (especially home-canned) foods, home-fermented foods such as tofu, and homemade garlic or herb-infused oils stored at room temperature.[†] **Botulism** quickly paralyzes muscles, making seeing, speaking, swallowing, and breathing difficult and demands immediate medical attention. Warning signs of botulism are listed at the bottom of Table 12–3.

The botulinum toxin and a few others are heat sensitive and can be destroyed by boiling, but this is not recommended because poisoning could occur if even a trace of the toxin remained intact. Other toxins, such as that from *Staphylococcus aureus*, are heat-resistant and so remain hazardous even after the food is cooked.

KEY POINTS

- Each year in the United States, tens of millions of people suffer mild to life-threatening foodborne illnesses, despite efforts of governmental agencies to prevent them.
- Pregnant women, infants, toddlers, older adults, and people with weakened immune systems are most vulnerable to harm from foodborne illnesses.
- Foodborne illnesses arise from microbial infections or bacterial toxins.

Food Safety from Farm to Plate

A safe food supply depends on safe food practices on the farm or at sea; in processing plants; during transportation; and in supermarkets, institutions, and restaurants (see Figure 12–1, p. 445). Equally critical in the chain of food safety, however, is the final handling of food by people who purchase it and consume it at home. Tens of millions of people needlessly suffer preventable foodborne illnesses each year because they make their own mistakes in purchasing, storing, or preparing their food.

anaerobic without oxygen.

botulism an often fatal foodborne illness caused by the botulinum toxin, a toxin produced by the *Clostridium botulinum* bacterium, which grows without oxygen in nonacidic canned foods.

Table 12–3
Dangerous Symptoms of Foodborne Illnesses

Some bouts of foodborne illness may be mild and clear up on their own, but others pose serious threats. Any of the following symptoms demand medical attention.

Get medical help for these symptoms:
- Bloody stools.
- Dehydration.
- Diarrhea of more than 3 days' duration.
- Fever of longer than 24 hours' duration.
- Headache with muscle stiffness and fever.
- Numbness, muscle weakness, tingling sensations in the skin.
- Rapid heart rate, fainting, dizziness.
- Severe intestinal cramps.

Warning signs of botulism—a medical emergency:
- Difficulty breathing.
- Difficulty swallowing.
- Double vision.
- Weak muscles.

[†]Complete, up-to-date home canning instructions are available in the USDA's *Complete Guide to Home Canning*, available from the Superintendent of Documents, U.S. Government Printing Office, Washington, DC 20402, or online at www.uga.edu/nchfp/publications/publications_usda.html.

Figure 12–1

From Farm to Plate: Make Food Safe

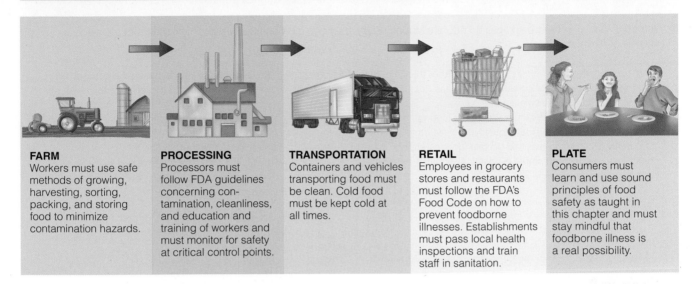

FARM
Workers must use safe methods of growing, harvesting, sorting, packing, and storing food to minimize contamination hazards.

PROCESSING
Processors must follow FDA guidelines concerning contamination, cleanliness, and education and training of workers and must monitor for safety at critical control points.

TRANSPORTATION
Containers and vehicles transporting food must be clean. Cold food must be kept cold at all times.

RETAIL
Employees in grocery stores and restaurants must follow the FDA's Food Code on how to prevent foodborne illnesses. Establishments must pass local health inspections and train staff in sanitation.

PLATE
Consumers must learn and use sound principles of food safety as taught in this chapter and must stay mindful that foodborne illness is a real possibility.

How Outbreaks Occur   Commercially prepared food is usually safe, but an **outbreak** of illness from this source often makes the headlines because outbreaks can affect many people at once.[5] Dairy farmers, for example, rely on **pasteurization**, a process that heats milk to kill most pathogens, thereby making the milk safe to consume. When a major dairy develops a flaw in its pasteurization system, hundreds of cases of illness can occur as a result.

Other types of farming require other safeguards. Growing food usually involves soil, and soil contains abundant bacterial colonies that can contaminate food. Animal waste deposited onto soil may introduce pathogens. Additionally, farm workers and other food handlers who are ill can easily pass pathogens to consumers through the routine handling of fruit, vegetables, or grains during and after harvest, a particular concern with regard to foods consumed raw, such as lettuce or cucumbers.[6]

Attention on *E. coli*   Several strains of the *E. coli* bacterium produce a particularly dangerous protein known as **Shiga toxin**, a cause of severe disease. The most notorious strain, *E. coli* O157:H7, caused a widespread outbreak in 2018 when consumers ate contaminated romaine lettuce, but outbreaks can also arise from other strains of Shiga toxin–producing *E. coli* (STEC).[7][‡] Outbreaks of severe or fatal STEC illnesses focus national attention on two important issues: first, that raw foods routinely contain live pathogens and, second, that strict industry controls are essential to make foods safe.

In most cases, STEC disease involves bloody diarrhea, severe intestinal cramps, and dehydration starting a few days after eating tainted meat, raw milk, or contaminated fresh raw produce. In the worst cases, **hemolytic-uremic syndrome** causes a dangerous failure of the kidneys and organ systems that very young, very old, or otherwise vulnerable people may not survive. Antibiotics and self-prescribed antidiarrheal medicines can make the condition worse because they increase absorption and retention of the toxin. Severe cases require hospitalization.

FDA Food Safety Modernization Act   In 2016, Congress enacted a new law, the **FDA Food Safety Modernization Act (FSMA)**, in response to dramatic changes in the global food system.[§] The law focuses more of FDA's resources on preventing foodborne

outbreak two or more cases of a disease arising from an identical organism acquired from a common food source within a limited time frame. Government agencies track and investigate outbreaks of foodborne illnesses, but tens of millions of individual cases go unreported each year.

pasteurization the treatment of milk, juices, or eggs with heat sufficient to kill certain pathogenic (disease-causing) microbes commonly transmitted through these foods; not a sterilization process. Pasteurized products retain bacteria that cause spoilage.

Shiga toxin (SHIG-uh) any of a group of protein toxins produced as certain bacteria strains multiply; when absorbed, Shiga toxins cause severe illness.

hemolytic-uremic (HEEM-oh-LIT-ic you-REEM-ick) **syndrome** a set of severe, sometimes fatal, symptoms, including abnormal blood clotting with kidney failure, damage to the central nervous system, and damage to other organs; a result of infection with Shiga toxin–producing *E. coli* and particularly likely to occur in children.

FDA Food Safety Modernization Act (FSMA) a law enacted in 2016 to build a new system of domestic and international controls for the detection, prevention, and correction of microbial contamination of the U.S. food supply.

[‡] Shiga toxin was named for the Japanese researcher who discovered the microbial cause of dysentery more than 100 years ago.
[§] Read more about the FDA Food Safety Modernization Act at www.fda.gov/Food/GuidanceRegulation/FSMA/.

Table 12–4

Are Your Foods Expiring?

Although dates on food packages do not reflect food safety, they can alert both sellers and consumers to a product's degree of freshness.

- *Sell by:* Specifies the shelf life of the food. After this date, the food may still be safe for consumption if it has been handled and stored properly. Also called *pull date*.
- *Best if used by:* Specifies the last date the food will be of the highest quality. After this date, quality is expected to diminish, although the food may still be safe for consumption if it has been handled and stored properly. Also called *freshness date* or *quality assurance date*.

- *Expiration date:* The last day the food should be consumed. All foods except eggs should be discarded after this date. For eggs, the expiration date refers to the last day the eggs may be sold as "fresh eggs." For safety, purchase eggs before the expiration date, keep them in their original carton in the refrigerator, and use them within 30 days.[a]
- *Pack date:* The day the food was packaged or processed. When used on packages of fresh meats, pack dates can provide a general guide to freshness.

[a]For best quality, use eggs within 3 weeks of purchase.

Figure 12–2

Bacterial Growth

Bacterial colonies grow quickly when a single bacterium encounters favorable conditions. For example, each oblong-shaped *E. coli* in this stack can reproduce every 20 minutes or so, doubling the colony size in a process that continues until conditions change. (*E. coli* magnified 7,000 times).

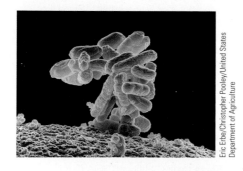

Eric Erbe/Christopher Pooley/United States Department of Agriculture

Hazard Analysis Critical Control Point (HACCP) plan a systematic plan to identify and correct potential microbial hazards in the manufacturing, distribution, and commercial use of food products. *HACCP* may be pronounced "HASS-ip."

illnesses, while also supporting investigation into outbreaks as they occur to discover and resolve their causes. This important legislation spells out needed actions to prevent contamination at many different points in the global human food and pet food supply chains, and it combines the resources of U.S. governmental agencies with those of domestic and international food industries and farm partners to achieve its goals. The anticipated result is a safer U.S. food supply and the prevention of hundreds of thousands of foodborne illnesses among U.S. consumers and their pets.

Food Industry Controls Inspections of U.S. meat-processing plants, performed every day by USDA inspectors, help to ensure that these facilities meet government standards. Other food facilities are inspected less often, but FSMA regulations require that all producers of food sold in the United States must employ a **Hazard Analysis Critical Control Point (HACCP) plan** to help prevent foodborne illnesses at their source. Each slaughterhouse, producer, packer, distributor, and transporter of susceptible foods must identify "critical control points" in its procedures that pose a risk of food contamination or bacterial growth (*E. coli*, a common bacterial threat, is depicted in Figure 12–2). Once a control point is identified, the food producer must devise and implement verifiable ways to eliminate or minimize the risk.

The HACCP system is a proven method of controlling microbial contamination, and its effectiveness is evident: *Salmonella* contamination of U.S. poultry, eggs, ground beef, and pork has been greatly reduced, and *E. coli* infection from meats has dropped dramatically since HACCP plans were implemented in these industries.

Grocery Safety for Consumers Canned and packaged foods sold in grocery stores are generally safe, but accidents do happen, and foods can become contaminated. FDA scientists track outbreaks of illnesses due to large-scale contamination and trace both likely production sources and distribution paths to prevent or minimize consumer exposure. When food contamination is suspected, batch numbering facilitates the food's recall through public announcements in the media and other means.

You can help protect yourself, too. Shop at stores that look and smell clean. Check the freshness dates printed on many food packages, and choose the freshest ones. "Sell by" and other dates of Table 12–4 do not reflect a food's safety, however (baby formula is the exception: its dates are legally defined). Instead, they indicate the time of the food's best quality, and are intended to help retailers manage their inventories.[8] For consumers, applying these dates too strictly can lead to unnecessary food waste.

If a can or package is bulging, leaking, ragged, soiled, or punctured, don't buy it—turn it in to the store manager. A badly dented can or a mangled package is useless in protecting food from microorganisms, insects, or other spoilage. Many jars have safety "buttons" on the lid, designed to pop up once the jar is opened; make sure that they have not "popped." Frozen foods should be solidly frozen, and those in chest-type freezer cases should be stored below the frost line. Check fresh eggs and reject cracked ones. Finally, shop for frozen and refrigerated foods and fresh meats last, just before leaving the store.

KEY POINTS

- Farm to plate food safety requires that farmers, processors, transporters, retailers, and consumers use effective food safety methods to prevent foodborne illnesses.
- Bacteria multiply quickly when conditions are favorable to them.
- FSMA is a law enacted to protect the U.S. food and pet food supplies.
- Consumers should carefully inspect foods before purchasing them.

Safe Food Practices for Individuals

Staying mindful of food safety can prevent much misery from intestinal illnesses. Be aware that food can provide ideal conditions for bacteria to multiply and to produce toxins. Bacteria, particularly pathogens, require these three conditions to thrive:

- Nutrients.
- Moisture.
- Warmth, 40°F to 140°F (4°C to 60°C).**

To defeat bacteria, you must prevent them from contaminating food or deprive them of one of these conditions. Four practices illustrated in Figure 12–3 can help achieve these goals.

Any food with an "off" appearance or odor should be thrown away, of course, and not even tasted. However, you cannot rely on your senses of smell, taste, and sight to warn you because most hazards are not detectable by odor, taste, or appearance. As the old saying goes, "When in doubt, throw it out."

Keep Clean   Keeping your hands and surfaces clean requires using freshly washed utensils and new or disinfected towels and washing your hands properly, not just rinsing them, particularly before and after handling raw foods.[9] Normal, healthy skin is covered with bacteria, some of which may cause foodborne illness when deposited on moist, nutrient-rich food and allowed to multiply, as Figure 12–4 illustrates. Remember

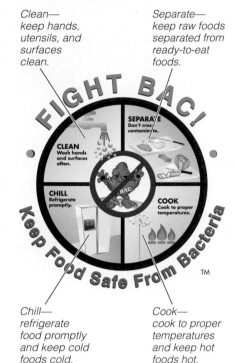

Figure 12–3

Fight Bac!

Four ways to keep food safe. The Fight Bac! website is at www.fightbac.org.

Clean— keep hands, utensils, and surfaces clean.

Separate— keep raw foods separated from ready-to-eat foods.

Chill— refrigerate food promptly and keep cold foods cold.

Cook— cook to proper temperatures and keep hot foods hot.

Figure 12–4

Why Wash Your Hands?

The photo on the left shows a person's clean-looking but unwashed hand touching a sterile, moist, nutrient-rich gel in a laboratory dish. After 24 hours in a warm incubator, the large colonies provide visible evidence of the microorganisms that were transferred from the hand to the gel.

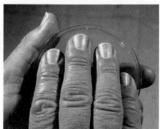
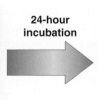
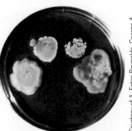

24-hour incubation

Courtesy of A. Estes Reynolds, George A. Schuler, James A. Christian, and William C. Hurst

Source: Photos courtesy of A. Estes Reynolds, George A. Schuler, James A. Christian, and William C. Hurst.

**The FDA suggests these temperatures to consumers at the FDA/CFSAN website; see www.fda.gov. For food industry professionals, the FDA makes other recommendations; see U.S. Public Health Service and Food and Drug Administration, *Food Code* (College Park, Md.: U.S. Department of Health and Human Services, 2013), available at www.fda.gov.

Figure 12–5

Proper Hand Washing Prevents Illness

You can avoid many illnesses by following these hand washing procedures before, during, and after food preparation; before eating; after using the bathroom, changing a diaper, blowing your nose, coughing, or sneezing; after handling animals or their food or waste; or after handling garbage. Wash hands more frequently when someone near you is sick.

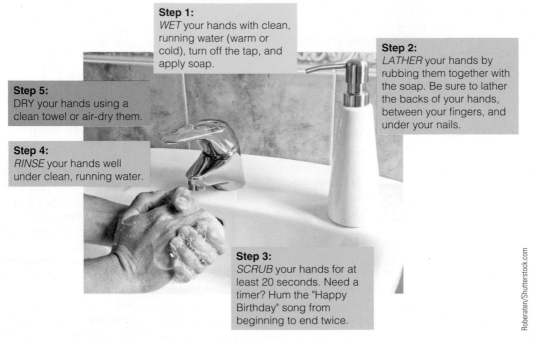

Step 1:
WET your hands with clean, running water (warm or cold), turn off the tap, and apply soap.

Step 2:
LATHER your hands by rubbing them together with the soap. Be sure to lather the backs of your hands, between your fingers, and under your nails.

Step 5:
DRY your hands using a clean towel or air-dry them.

Step 4:
RINSE your hands well under clean, running water.

Step 3:
SCRUB your hands for at least 20 seconds. Need a timer? Hum the "Happy Birthday" song from beginning to end twice.

Roberaten/Shutterstock.com

Source: Centers for Disease Control and Prevention, When and how to wash your hands (2016), available at www.cdc.gov/handwashing/when-how-handwashing.html.

to use a nail brush to clean under your fingernails when washing your hands and tend to routine nail care—artificial nails, long nails, chipped polish, and even a hangnail harbor more bacteria than do natural, clean, short, healthy nails. Figure 12–5 delineates steps to thorough hand washing.

For routine cleansing, washing your hands with ordinary soap and water is effective. Using an alcohol-based hand-sanitizing gel can also provide killing power against many bacteria and most viruses. Following up a good washing with a sanitizer may provide an extra measure of protection when someone in the house is ill or when preparing food for an infant, an elderly person, or someone with a compromised immune system.[††] If you are ill or have open cuts or sores, stay away from food preparation.

Microbes love to nestle down in small, damp spaces, such as the inner cells of kitchen sponges or the pores between the fibers of wooden cutting boards.[10] To reduce their numbers on sponges, surfaces, and utensils, you have four choices, each with benefits and drawbacks:

1. Poison the microbes with highly toxic chemicals such as bleach (one teaspoon per quart of water). Chlorine kills most organisms. However, chlorine is toxic to handle, it can ruin clothing, and when washed down household drains into the water supply, it forms chemicals harmful to people and wildlife.

2. Kill the microbes with heat. Soapy water heated to 140°F kills most harmful organisms and washes away most others. This method takes effort, though, because the water must be truly scalding hot, well beyond the temperature of the tap.

3. Use an automatic dishwasher to combine both methods. It washes in water hotter than hands can tolerate, and most dishwasher detergents contain chlorine.

[††]Effective hand sanitizers contain between 60 and 70 percent isopropyl alcohol.

4. Use a microwave oven to kill microbes on sponges. Place the *soaking wet* sponge in a microwave oven, and heat it a minute or two until it is steaming hot (times vary). Cautions: handle hot sponges with tongs to avoid scalding your hands, and heat only wet sponges in the microwave oven; dry sponges can catch on fire.

The third and fourth options—washing in a dishwasher and microwaving—kill virtually all bacteria trapped in sponges, while soaking in a bleach solution misses more than 10 percent. Whatever the method, the effect is temporary and bacteria quickly return.[11] The best action may be to replace kitchen sponges at least weekly, even if they don't appear worn. Even better, skip the sponges and use a stack of kitchen dish cloths that can be tossed in the laundry daily.

Keep Separate   Raw foods, especially meats, eggs, and seafood, are likely to contain illness-causing bacteria. To prevent bacteria from spreading, keep the raw foods and their juices away from ready-to-eat foods. (This is called **cross-contamination** of foods.) For example, if you take burgers out to the grill on a plate, wash that plate in hot, soapy water before using it to retrieve the cooked burgers. If you use a cutting board to cut raw meat, wash the board, the knife, and your hands thoroughly with soap before handling other foods—and particularly before making a salad or other foods that are eaten raw. Many cooks keep a separate cutting board just for raw meats.

Cook   Cook foods long enough to reach a safe internal temperature. The USDA urges consumers to use a food thermometer to test the temperatures of cooked foods and not to rely on appearance. Place the probe of a food thermometer in the thickest part of the food, away from bone and gristle, and wash the probe between readings to prevent transferring bacteria from the uncooked food to the finished product. Table 12–5 provides a glossary of thermometer terms, and Figure 12–6 (p. 450) illustrates various types of thermometers. Figure 12–6 also lists proper refrigeration and freezer temperatures, and safe internal temperatures for various kinds of cooked foods.

After cooking, hot foods must be held at 140°F or higher until served. A temperature of 140°F on a thermometer feels hot, not just warm. Even well-cooked foods, if handled improperly prior to serving, can cause illness. Delicious-looking meatballs on a buffet may harbor bacteria unless they have been kept steaming hot. After the meal, cooked foods should be refrigerated immediately or within two hours at the maximum (one hour if room temperature approaches 90°F, or 32°C). If food has been left out longer than this, throw it out.

Chill   Chilling and keeping cold food cold starts when you leave the grocery store. If you are running errands, shop last so that the groceries do not stay in the car too long. (If ice cream begins to melt, it has been too long.) An ice chest or insulated bag can help keep foods cold during transit. Upon arrival home, load foods into the refrigerator or freezer immediately. Table 12–6 (p. 451) lists some safe keeping times for foods stored in the refrigerator at or below 40°F. Foods older than this should be discarded, not ingested.

To ensure safety, thaw frozen meats or poultry in the refrigerator, not at room temperature. Marinate meats in the refrigerator, too. To thaw a food more quickly, submerge it in cold (not hot or warm) water in waterproof packaging or use a microwave to thaw food just before cooking it. Most foods can simply be cooked from the frozen state—just increase the cooking time and use a thermometer to ensure that the food reaches a safe internal temperature.

Chill prepared or cooked foods in shallow containers, not in deep ones. A shallow container allows quick chilling throughout; deeper containers take too many hours to chill through to the center, allowing bacteria time to grow.

Cold meats and mixed salads make a convenient buffet, but keep perishable items safe by placing their containers on ice during serving. This applies to all perishable foods, including custards, cream pies, and whipped-cream or cream-cheese treats. Even pumpkin pie, because it contains milk and eggs, should be kept cold.

Table 12–5

Glossary of Thermometer Terms

- **appliance thermometer** a thermometer that verifies the temperature of an appliance. An *oven thermometer* verifies that the oven is heating properly; a *refrigerator/freezer thermometer* tests for proper refrigerator temperature (<40°F, or <4°C) or freezer temperature (0°F, or −17°C).
- **fork thermometer** a utensil combining a meat fork and an instant-read food thermometer.
- **instant-read thermometer** a thermometer that, when inserted into food, measures its temperature within seconds; designed to test temperature of food at intervals.
- **oven-safe thermometer** a thermometer designed to remain in the food to give constant readings during cooking.
- **pop-up thermometer** a disposable timing device commonly used in turkeys. The center of the device contains a spring that "pops up" when food reaches the right temperature.
- **single-use temperature indicator** a disposable instant-read thermometer that changes color to indicate temperature. This type is often used in commercial food establishments to eliminate cross-contamination.

cross-contamination the contamination of food through exposure to utensils, hands, or other surfaces that were previously in contact with contaminated food.

Figure 12–6

Food-Safety Temperatures (Fahrenheit) and Household Thermometers

Cooking and cooling foods to proper temperatures reduces microbial threats. Different thermometers do different jobs. To choose the right one, pay attention to its temperature range: some have high temperature ranges intended to test the doneness of meats and other hot foods. Others have lower ranges for testing temperatures of refrigerators and freezers.

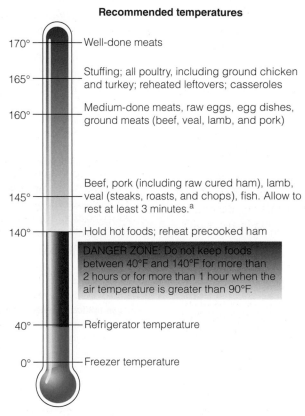

Recommended temperatures

- 170° — Well-done meats
- 165° — Stuffing; all poultry, including ground chicken and turkey; reheated leftovers; casseroles
- 160° — Medium-done meats, raw eggs, egg dishes, ground meats (beef, veal, lamb, and pork)
- 145° — Beef, pork (including raw cured ham), lamb, veal (steaks, roasts, and chops), fish. Allow to rest at least 3 minutes.[a]
- 140° — Hold hot foods; reheat precooked ham

DANGER ZONE: Do not keep foods between 40°F and 140°F for more than 2 hours or for more than 1 hour when the air temperature is greater than 90°F.

- 40° — Refrigerator temperature
- 0° — Freezer temperature

[a]During the 3 minutes after meat is removed from the heat source, its temperature remains constant or continues to rise, which destroys pathogens.

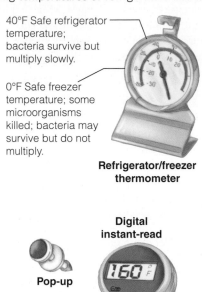

40°F Safe refrigerator temperature; bacteria survive but multiply slowly.

0°F Safe freezer temperature; some microorganisms killed; bacteria may survive but do not multiply.

Refrigerator/freezer thermometer

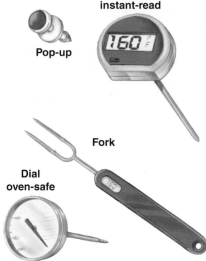

Digital instant-read

Pop-up

Fork

Dial oven-safe

KEY POINTS

- Foodborne illnesses are common, but the great majority of cases can be prevented.
- To protect themselves, consumers should remember these four practices: clean, separate, cook, chill.

Which Foods Are Most Likely to Cause Illness?

LO 12.2 Identify the categories of foods that most often cause foodborne illnesses.

Some foods are more likely to harbor illness-causing microbes than others. Foods that are high in moisture and nutrients and those that are chopped or ground are especially favorable hosts. Without proper refrigeration, bacteria in these foods are likely to grow quickly. Pathogens also lodge on produce, and as you will learn, it is a threat to take seriously.[12]

Protein Foods

Protein-rich foods require special handling. When produced on an industrial scale, protein foods are often mingled together, such as in tanks of raw milk, vats of raw eggs, or masses of ground meats or poultry.[13] Mingling causes problems when a pathogen from a single source contaminates the whole batch.

Packages of raw meats, for example, bear labels to instruct consumers on meat safety (see Figure 12–7, page 452).[‡‡] Meats in the grocery cooler very often contain bacteria and provide a moist, nutritious environment perfect for microbial growth. Therefore, people who prepare meat should follow these basic meat-safety rules:

- Cook all meat and poultry to the suggested temperatures.
- Never defrost meat or poultry at room temperature or in warm water. The warmed outside layer of raw meat fosters bacterial growth.
- Don't cook large, thick, dense, raw meats or meatloaf in the microwave. Microwaves leave cool spots that can harbor microbes. Reminder: never prepare foods that will be eaten raw, such as lettuce or tomatoes, with the same utensils or on the same cutting board as was used to prepare raw meats, such as hamburgers.

Finally, always remember to wash your hands thoroughly after handling raw meat.

Unrelated to sanitation, a **prion** disease of cattle and wild game such as deer and elk, **bovine spongiform encephalopathy (BSE)**, causes a rare but fatal brain disorder in human beings who consume meat from afflicted animals.[§§] U.S. beef industry regulations minimize the risk of contracting BSE from eating beef.

Ground Meats   In addition to the mingling problem mentioned earlier, ground meat or poultry is handled more than meats left whole, and grinding exposes much more surface area for bacteria to land on. Experts advise cooking these foods to the well-done stage. Use a thermometer to test the internal temperature of poultry and meats, even hamburgers, before declaring them done. Don't trust appearance alone: burgers often turn brown and appear cooked before their internal temperature is high enough to kill harmful bacteria. Figure 12–8 (p. 452) reviews hamburger safety.

Stuffed Poultry   A stuffed turkey or chicken raises special concerns because bacteria from the bird's cavity can contaminate the stuffing. During cooking, the center of the stuffing can stay cool long enough for bacteria to multiply. For safe stuffed poultry, follow the Fight Bac core principles—clean, separate, cook, and chill. In addition:

- Cook any raw meat, poultry, or shellfish before adding it to stuffing.
- Mix wet and dry ingredients right before stuffing into the cavity and stuff loosely; cook immediately afterward in a preheated oven set no lower than 325°F (use an oven thermometer to make sure).
- Use a meat thermometer to test the center of the stuffing. It should reach 165°F.

To repeat: test the stuffing. Even if the poultry meat itself has reached the safe temperature of 165°F, the center of the stuffing may be cool enough to harbor live bacteria. Better yet, bake the stuffing separately.

Eggs   Eating undercooked eggs at home accounts for about 30 percent of U.S. *Salmonella* infections.[14] Bacteria from the intestinal tracts of hens often contaminate eggs as they are laid, and some bacteria may enter the eggs themselves. All commercially available eggs are washed and sanitized before packing, and some are pasteurized in the shell to make them safer. The FDA requires measures to control *Salmonella* and other bacteria on major egg-producing poultry farms. For consumers, egg cartons bear reminders to keep eggs refrigerated, cook eggs until their yolks are firm, and cook egg-containing foods thoroughly before eating them.

[‡‡] The USDA's Food Information Hotline answers questions about meat, poultry, and seafood safety: 1–888-MPHOTLINE.

[§§] The human disease is variant Creutzfeldt-Jakob disease (vCJD).

Table 12–6

Safe Food Storage Times: Refrigerator (≤40°F)[a]

For products with longer shelf lives, rotate them like restaurants do. "First-In-First-Out" means to check dates and use up older products first.

1 to 2 Days
Raw ground meats, breakfast or other raw sausages; raw fish or poultry; gravies

3 to 5 Days
Raw steaks, roasts, or chops; cooked meats, poultry, vegetables, and mixed dishes; lunchmeats (packages opened); mayonnaise salads (chicken, egg, pasta, tuna); fresh vegetables (spinach, green beans, tomatoes)

1 Week
Hard-cooked eggs, bacon, or hot dogs (opened packages); smoked sausages or seafood; milk, cottage cheese

1 to 2 Weeks
Yogurt; carrots, celery, lettuce

2 to 4 Weeks
Fresh eggs (in shells); lunchmeats, bacon, or hot dogs (packages unopened); dry sausages (pepperoni, hard salami); most aged and processed cheeses (Swiss, brick)

2 Months
Mayonnaise (opened jar); most dry cheeses (Parmesan, Romano)

[a]For additional information, see www.fda.gov/downloads/Food/ResourcesForYou/HealthEducators/UCM109315.pdf.

prion a disease agent consisting of an unusually folded protein that disrupts normal cell functioning. Prions cannot be controlled or killed by cooking or disinfecting, and the disease they cause cannot be treated. Prevention is the only form of control.

bovine spongiform encephalopathy (BOH-vine SPUNJ-ih-form en-SEH-fal-AH-path-ee) **(BSE)** an often fatal illness of the nerves and brain observed in cattle and wild game and in people who consume affected meats. Also called *mad cow disease*.

Figure 12-7

Food Safety Labels for Meat and Poultry

Following food safety instructions for meat and poultry minimizes bacterial growth and cross-contamination.

Safe handling label for raw meat and poultry

Safe Handling Instructions

THIS PRODUCT WAS PREPARED FROM INSPECTED AND PASSED MEAT AND/OR POULTRY. SOME FOOD PRODUCTS MAY CONTAIN BACTERIA THAT CAN CAUSE ILLNESS IF THE PRODUCT IS MISHANDLED OR COOKED IMPROPERLY. FOR YOUR PROTECTION, FOLLOW THESE SAFE HANDLING INSTRUCTIONS.

KEEP REFRIGERATED OR FROZEN.
THAW IN REFRIGERATOR OR MICROWAVE.

KEEP RAW MEAT AND POULTRY SEPARATE FROM OTHER FOODS. WASH WORKING SURFACES (INCLUDING CUTTING BOARDS), UTENSILS, AND HANDS AFTER TOUCHING RAW MEAT OR POULTRY.

COOK THOROUGHLY.

KEEP HOT FOODS HOT. REFRIGERATE LEFTOVERS IMMEDIATELY OR DISCARD.

Figure 12-8

Hamburger Safety

A safe hamburger is cooked well done (internal temperature of 160°F) and has juices that run clear. Place it on a clean plate when it's done.

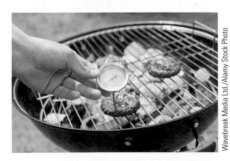

Wavebreak Media Ltd./Alamy Stock Photo

sushi a Japanese dish that consists of vinegar-flavored rice, seafood, and colorful vegetables, typically wrapped in seaweed. Some sushi contains raw fish; other sushi contains only cooked ingredients.

What about tempting foods like homemade ice cream, hollandaise sauce, unbaked cake batter, or raw cookie dough that contain raw or undercooked eggs? Healthy adults can enjoy them if they are made safer by using pasteurized eggs or liquid egg products instead of regular eggs. However, even these products, because they are made from raw eggs, may contain a few live bacteria that survived pasteurization, making them unsafe for pregnant women, the elderly, young children, or people with weakened immunity.

Seafood Properly cooked fish and other seafood sold in the United States are safe from microbial threats. However, even the freshest, most appealing, raw or partly cooked seafood can harbor pathogenic viruses; parasites, such as worms and flukes; and bacteria that cause illnesses ranging from stomach cramps to severe, life-threatening conditions.[15] Table 12–7 lists beliefs about raw seafood that can make people sick.

The dangers posed by seafood are increasing. As burgeoning human populations along the world's shorelines release more contaminants into lakes, rivers, and oceans, the seafood living there becomes less safe to consume. Viruses that cause human diseases have been detected in some 90 percent of the waters off the U.S. coast and easily contaminate filter feeders such as clams and oysters. Government agencies monitor commercial fishing areas and close unsafe waters to harvesters, but illegal harvesting is common.

As for **sushi** or "seared" partially raw fish, even a master chef cannot detect microbial dangers that may lurk within. The marketing term "sushi grade," often applied to seafood to imply wholesomeness, means only that the fish was frozen to below zero temperatures for long enough to kill off adult parasitic worms. Freezing does not make raw fish entirely safe to eat. Only cooking can kill all worm eggs, bacteria, and other microorganisms. Safe sushi is made from properly acidified rice (the vinegar reduces pH and thereby retards bacterial growth), cooked seafood, seaweed, vegetables, avocados, and other safe delicacies, and then is held at cold temperatures until it is consumed. Experts unanimously agree that today's high levels of microbial contamination make eating raw or lightly cooked seafood too risky, even for healthy adults.

Raw Milk Products Unpasteurized raw milk and raw milk products (often sold as "health food") cause the majority of dairy-related illness outbreaks. The bacterial counts of raw milk are unpredictable and even organic raw milk from a trusted dairy can cause severe illness.[16] Drinking raw milk presents a real risk with no advantages—the nutrients in pasteurized milk and raw milk are identical.

Table 12-7

Raw Seafood Myths and Truths

Myth	Truth
▪ If a raw seafood was consumed in the past with no ill effect, it is safe to do so today.	▪ Each harvest bears separate risks, and seafood is increasingly contaminated.
▪ Drinking alcoholic beverages with raw seafood will "kill the germs."	▪ Alcoholic beverages cannot make contaminated raw seafood safe.
▪ Putting hot sauce on raw oysters and other raw seafood will "kill the germs."	▪ Hot sauce exerts no effect on microbes in seafood.

Even in pasteurized milk, a few bacteria may survive, so milk must be refrigerated to hold bacterial growth to a minimum. Shelf-stable milk, often sold in boxes, is sterilized by an **ultra-high temperature** treatment and so needs no refrigeration until it is opened.

Raw Produce

The Dietary Guidelines urge people to eat enough fruit and vegetables, but if consumers eat these foods raw, they must take steps to avoid foodborne illnesses.[17] Foods such as lettuce, salad spinach, tomatoes, melons, berries, herbs, and scallions grow close to the ground, making them vulnerable to bacterial contamination from the soil, animal waste runoff, and manure fertilizers. Contamination often arises when growers and producers make sanitation mistakes.[18] For this reason, the FSMA law described earlier includes a **Produce Safety Rule**, which regulates growing and working conditions on farms, and requires safety plans from both U.S. and international produce suppliers.

Washing produce at home to remove dirt and debris is important, too, and Table 12–8 provides some guidance. However, washing may not entirely remove certain bacterial strains. These strains—*E. coli*, among others—exude a sticky, protective coating that glues microbes to each other and to food surfaces, forming a **biofilm** that can survive home rinsing or even industrial washing.[19] Somewhat more effective is vigorous scrubbing with a vegetable brush to dislodge bacteria; rinsing with vinegar, which may help cut through biofilm; and removing and discarding the outer leaves from heads of leafy vegetables, such as cabbage and lettuce, before washing. Vinegar doesn't sterilize foods, but it can reduce bacterial populations, and is safe to consume.

Unpasteurized Juices   Unpasteurized or raw juices and ciders pose a special problem. Juice producers mingle fruit from many different trees and orchards, and any bacteria introduced into a batch of juice can multiply rapidly in the sugary fluid. Labels of unpasteurized juices must carry the warning, as shown in Figure 12–9. Especially infants, children, the elderly, and people with weakened immune systems should never be given raw or unpasteurized juice products. Refrigerated pasteurized juices, reconstituted frozen juices, and shelf-stable juices in boxes, cans, or pouches are generally safe.

Sprouts   Sprouts (alfalfa, clover, radish, and others) grow in the same warm, moist, nutrient-rich conditions that microbes need to thrive. A few bacteria or spores on sprout seeds can quickly bloom into widespread contamination of the sprouts; both commercial and homegrown raw sprouts pose this risk.[20] Sprouts are often eaten raw, but the

---

Figure 12–9

Warning Label for Unpasteurized Juice

Unpasteurized or untreated juice must bear the following warning on its label:

> **WARNING:** This product has not been pasteurized and therefore may contain harmful bacteria that can cause serious illness in children, the elderly, and persons with weakened immune systems.

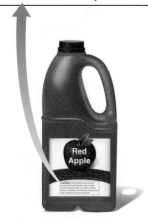

Table 12–8

How to Wash Produce

Follow these steps:
- Wash your hands (see Figure 12–5, p. 448).
- Wash fruit and vegetables (organic, conventional, or homegrown) thoroughly under running water before cutting or peeling. Use a vinegar rinse to help cut through biofilm.
- Wash produce that will be peeled to remove dirt and bacteria that could be transferred from the peel to the edible parts by the peeler or knife.
- Scrub firm produce, such as melons and cucumbers, with a clean produce brush to dislodge dirt and bacteria.
- Cut away any damaged or bruised parts.
- Dry with a clean cloth.
- Prewashed, ready-to-eat produce needs no further washing; if you choose to rewash it, avoid contamination by following the basic rules of food safety.

Source: U.S. Department of Agriculture and U.S. Department of Health and Human Services, Scientific report of the 2015 Dietary Guidelines Advisory Committee, 2015, D-5:44, available at www.health.gov.

ultra-high temperature a process of sterilizing food by exposing it for a short time to temperatures above those normally used in processing.

Produce Safety Rule a set of science-based standards put forth by the FDA that minimize microbial hazards during commercial growing, harvesting, packing, and storing of fruit and vegetables intended for U.S. consumption.

biofilm a layer of microbes mixed with a sticky, protective coating of proteins and carbohydrates exuded by certain bacteria.

only sure way to make sprouts safe is to cook them. The elderly, young children, and those with weakened immunity are particularly vulnerable.

KEY POINTS

- Produce causes many foodborne illnesses each year.
- Proper washing and refrigeration can reduce risks.
- Cooking ensures that sprouts are safe to eat.

Other Foods

Careful handling can reduce microbial threats from other foods, too. The foods discussed next are common in the food supply, and their safety deserves attention.

Imported Foods   Today, nearly three-quarters of the fruit and vegetables and 97 percent of the fish and seafood consumed in the United States are imported from other countries, as illustrated in Figure 12–10.[21] This poses an enormous food-safety challenge—the methods and standards of many thousands of food producers in far-away countries vary substantially. Cooked, frozen, irradiated, or canned imported foods and foods from developed areas with effective food-safety policies are generally safe. Concerns arise, however, about fresh produce, fish, shrimp, and other susceptible foods that originate in areas where food-safety practices are lax and contagious diseases are **endemic**.

To greatly reduce these risks, the FDA's new FSMA rules now require verification that imported foods have been produced and handled in keeping with U.S.

endemic   common or prevalent in a particular area or group of people.

Figure 12–10

How Far Did Your Salad Travel?

A simple salad on a U.S. dinner plate may result from worldwide efforts to provide it.

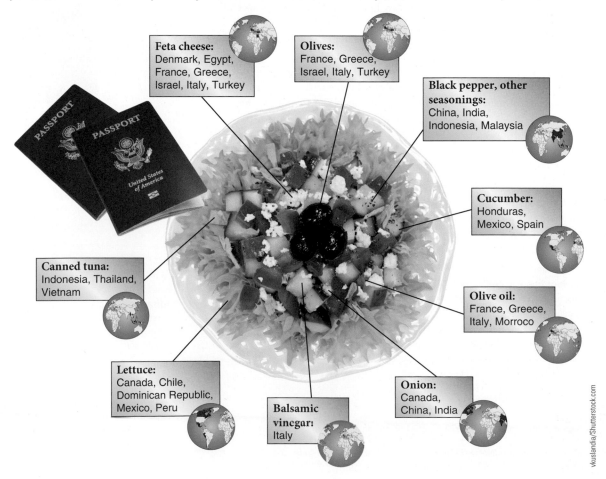

Feta cheese:
Denmark, Egypt, France, Greece, Israel, Italy, Turkey

Olives:
France, Greece, Israel, Italy, Turkey

Black pepper, other seasonings:
China, India, Indonesia, Malaysia

Cucumber:
Honduras, Mexico, Spain

Olive oil:
France, Greece, Italy, Morroco

Canned tuna:
Indonesia, Thailand, Vietnam

Lettuce:
Canada, Chile, Dominican Republic, Mexico, Peru

Balsamic vinegar:
Italy

Onion:
Canada, China, India

vkuslandia/Shutterstock.com

Chapter 12 Food Safety and Food Technology

food safety standards.[22] In addition, to help U.S. consumers distinguish between imported and domestic foods, regulators require certain foods, including fish and shellfish, perishable items other than beef or pork, and some nuts to bear a **country of origin label** specifying where they were produced.[23]

Honey   Honey can contain dormant spores of *Clostridium botulinum* that, when eaten, can germinate and begin to grow and produce their deadly botulinum toxin within the human body. Mature, healthy adults have their own internal defenses against this threat, but infants under one year of age should never be fed honey.

Picnics and Lunch Bags   Picnics can be fun, and packed lunches are a convenience, but to keep them safe, do the following:

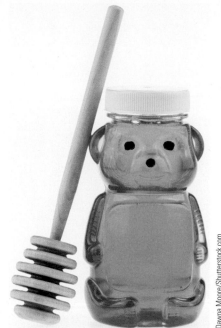

- Choose foods that are safe without refrigeration, such as whole fruit and vegetables, breads and crackers, shelf-stable foods, and canned spreads, fish and seafood, and cheeses to open and use on the spot.
- Chill lunch bag foods and pack them in a thermal lunch bag with several reusable ice packs. Food at room temperature in a paper bag may be unsafe to eat by lunchtime.[24]
- Choose well-aged cheeses, such as cheddar and Swiss; skip fresh cheeses, such as cottage cheese and Mexican queso fresco. Aged cheese does well without chilling for an hour or two; for longer times, carry it on ice in a cooler or thermal lunch bag.

A handy tip: freeze beverages, such as juice boxes or pouches, to replace ice packs in a thermal bag. As the beverages thaw in the hours before lunch, they keep the foods cold.

Note that individual servings of cheese or cold cuts prepackaged with crackers and promoted as lunch foods keep well, but they are high in saturated fat and sodium, and they cost triple the price of the foods purchased separately. Additionally, their excessive packaging adds to the nation's waste disposal burden.

Mayonnaise, despite its reputation for easy spoilage, is itself somewhat spoilage-resistant because of its acidity. Mayonnaise mixed with chopped ingredients in pasta, meat, or vegetable salads, however, spoils readily. The chopped ingredients have extensive surface areas for bacteria to invade, and cutting boards, hands, and kitchen utensils used in preparation often harbor bacteria. For safe chopped raw foods, start with clean chilled ingredients, and then chill the finished product in shallow containers; keep it chilled before and during serving; and promptly refrigerate any remainder.

Take-Out Foods and Leftovers   Many people rely on take-out foods—rotisserie chicken, pizza, Chinese dishes, and the like—for parties, picnics, or weeknight suppers. When buying these foods, food-safety rules apply: hot foods should be steaming hot, and cold foods should be thoroughly chilled.

Leftovers of all kinds make a convenient later lunch or dinner. However, microbes on serving utensils and in the air can quickly contaminate freshly cooked foods; for safety, refrigerate them promptly and reheat them to steaming hot (165°F) before eating. Discard any portion held at room temperature for longer than 2 hours from the time it was served at the table until you place it in your refrigerator. Follow the 2, 2, and 4 rules of leftover safety: within 2 hours of cooking, refrigerate the food in clean, shallow containers about 2 inches deep, and use it up within 4 days or toss it out. Exceptions: stuffing and gravy must be used within 2 days, and if room temperature reaches 90°F, all cooked foods must be chilled after 1 hour of exposure. Remember to use shallow containers, not deep ones, for quick chilling.

Consumers bear a responsibility for food safety, and an essential step is to cultivate awareness that foodborne illness is likely. They must discard old misconceptions that put them at risk and adopt an attitude of self-defense to prevent illness. The Food Feature, later, describes how.

KEY POINTS

- Many foods are imported, and the FDA is working to improve their safety.
- Honey should never be fed to infants.
- Lunch bags, picnics, and leftovers require safe handling.

country of origin label (COOL) the required label stating the country of origination of certain imported fish and shellfish, certain other perishable foods, certain nuts, peanuts, and ginseng. Meats and poultry are no longer subject to COOL labeling.

Advances in Microbial Food Safety

LO 12.3   Outline technological advances aimed at reducing microbial food contamination.

Advances in technology, such as pasteurization, have dramatically improved the quality and safety of foods over the past century. Today, other technologies promise similar benefits, but some raise concerns among consumers.

Is Irradiation Safe?

Food **irradiation** has been extensively evaluated over the past 50 years. Approved in more than 40 countries, its use is endorsed by numerous health agencies, including the **World Health Organization (WHO)** and the American Medical Association. Food irradiation protects consumers and offers other benefits:

- *Control of foodborne illnesses*. Irradiation effectively eliminates many organisms that cause foodborne illnesses, such as *Salmonella, E. coli*, and parasites.
- *Preservation*. Irradiation curbs spoilage and extends the shelf life of foods by destroying or inactivating organisms; it can also destroy the mold that produces the cancer-causing toxin **aflatoxin**.
- *Control of insects*. Irradiation penetrates tough exoskeletons to destroy insects on imported fruit. Irradiation also reduces the need for other pest-control practices that may harm the fruit.
- *Delay of sprouting and ripening*. Irradiation inhibits the sprouting of onions and potatoes and delays the ripening of many kinds of fruit to increase shelf life.
- *Sterilization*. Irradiation can be used to sterilize some products, such as dried herbs, spices, and teas. In hospitals, sterilized foods are useful for patients with severely impaired immunity.[25]

Supporters of irradiation say that if more everyday foods were irradiated, the nation's rates of foodborne illnesses would drop dramatically. All irradiated foods except spices must be identified as such on their labels (see Figure 12–11).

How Irradiation Works   Irradiation exposes foods to controlled doses of gamma rays from the radioactive element cobalt 60. As the rays pass through living cells, they disrupt DNA, proteins, and other internal structures, killing or deactivating the cells. For example, low radiation doses can kill the growing cells in the "eyes" of potatoes, preventing them from sprouting. Low doses also delay the ripening of bananas, avocados, and other fruit. Higher doses easily penetrate tough insect exoskeletons and mold and bacterial cell walls to destroy them. Irradiation works even on frozen food, making it uniquely useful in protecting foods such as whole frozen turkeys.

Irradiation Effects on Foods   Irradiation does not sterilize most foods because doses high enough to kill all microorganisms would also substantially alter the food. In approved doses, irradiation does not noticeably change the taste, texture, or appearance of citrus fruit, eggs, many meats, onions, potatoes, spices, strawberries, and other FDA-approved foods, and it does not make foods radioactive. Some vitamins are destroyed by irradiation, but the losses are no greater than those from other food-preservation methods such as canning.

Consumer Concerns about Irradiation   Many consumers associate radiation with cancer, birth defects, and mutations, so they respond negatively to the idea of irradiating foods. Some erroneously fear that food will become contaminated with radioactive particles. More realistic fears concern transporting radioactive materials, training workers to handle them safely, and safely disposing of spent wastes, which remain radioactive for many years. The food industry shares these concerns and strives to safeguard both workers and consumers through compliance with strict operating standards and regulations.

Finally, some worry that unscrupulous manufacturers might irradiate old or bacterially tainted foods to escape detection by USDA testers. Instead of being seized or

---

Figure 12–11
Radura Symbol

This "radura" logo is the international symbol for foods treated with irradiation.

irradiation the application of ionizing radiation to foods to reduce insect infestation or microbial contamination or to slow the ripening or sprouting process. Also called *cold pasteurization*.

World Health Organization (WHO) an agency of the United Nations charged with improving human health and preventing or controlling diseases in the world's people.

aflatoxin (af-lah-TOX-in) a toxin from a mold that grows on corn, grains, peanuts, and tree nuts stored in warm, humid conditions; a cause of liver cancer prevalent in tropical developing nations. (To prevent it, discard shriveled, discolored, or moldy foods.)

destroyed, the food could be passed off as wholesome to unsuspecting consumers. This objection raises an important point: irradiation is intended to complement, not replace, other traditional food-safety methods. Irradiation cannot entirely protect people from poor sanitation on the farm, in industry, or at home.

KEY POINTS

- Food irradiation kills bacteria, insects, molds, and parasites on foods.
- Consumers have concerns about the effects of irradiation on foods, workers, and the environment.

Other Technologies

The FDA and USDA are improving their monitoring techniques for microbial contamination at all levels of food production. In addition, some food-processing and packaging technologies are currently helping to reduce microbial threats to consumers, and others show potential for future use.

Improved Testing and Surveillance Testing foods for microbial contamination before they reach consumers is a critical step toward preventing foodborne illnesses. Automated systems have improved testing accuracy from farms to markets. For example, using a mobile laboratory, FDA scientists can test fresh produce where it is harvested and analyze it for many kinds of bacterial contamination. In addition, improved detection methods for *E. coli* in water, sediment, and other environmental harbors allow intervention before microbes can contaminate food crops.

Modified Atmosphere Packaging Common packaging methods improve the safety and shelf life of many fresh and prepared foods. Vacuum packaging or **modified atmosphere packaging (MAP)** reduces the oxygen inside a package. This makes it possible for unopened packages of soft pasta noodles, baked goods, prepared foods, fresh and cured meats, seafood, dry beans and other dry products, and ground and whole-bean coffee to stay fresh and safe much longer than they would in conventional packaging. Reducing oxygen:

- Inhibits growth of oxygen-dependent microbes.
- Prevents discoloration of cut vegetables and fruit.
- Prevents spoilage of fats by rancidity and development of "off" flavors.
- Slows ripening of fruit and vegetables and enzyme-induced breakdown of vitamins.

Perishable foods packaged with MAP must still be chilled properly to keep them safe from microbes that flourish in anaerobic environments, such as the *Clostridium botulinum* bacterium. Chilling precut salad greens is also a must: temperatures above 50°F cause a dangerous change in *E. coli* bacteria strains present in MAP-bagged lettuces that helps them to survive the eater's stomach acid, increasing their ability to cause infection.

High Pressure and Ultrasound High-pressure processing (HPP) technology compresses water to create intense pressure that can kill many kinds of pathogens. HPP "cold-pasteurizes" applesauce, avocado products, deli meats, orange juice, shellfish, meats, and many prepared foods, making them both safer and longer lasting.[26] However, the equipment is expensive, and not all microbes are destroyed in processing, so continuous refrigeration of most treated foods is a must.

High-powered ultrasound also holds promise as a sanitizer for organic salad greens. It works by sending high-energy shockwaves through water to dislodge pathogens from the small crevices of leafy greens. It may one day replace chlorine rinses but does not sterilize the food.

Edible Wraps and Films Bacteria-killing food wraps and films hold promise.[27] One such wrap made from milk whey protein with a dose of herbal antimicrobial oil may protect perishable foods, such as cheese sticks, from oxidation spoilage and bacterial growth. Instead of becoming trash, like today's plastic wraps, this wrap is consumed along with the cheese—an added bonus. In addition to protecting the food, the edible wraps may lend a pleasing herbal flavor to foods.

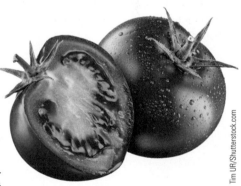

Tim UR/Shutterstock.com

modified atmosphere packaging (MAP)
a technique used to extend the shelf life of perishable foods; the food is packaged in a gas-impermeable container from which air is removed or to which an oxygen-free gas mixture, such as carbon dioxide and nitrogen, is added to deprive microbes of oxygen.

Microbial foodborne illnesses undoubtedly pose the most immediate threat to consumers, but other factors also affect food safety. The next sections address some of these concerns.

KEY POINTS

- Irradiation controls mold, sterilizes spices and teas, controls insects, extends shelf life, and destroys pathogenic bacteria.
- Scientific advances continuously improve food safety.

Toxins, Residues, and Contaminants in Foods

LO 12.4   Describe natural toxins, pesticide residues, and contaminants in food.

Nutrition-conscious consumers often wonder if our nation's foods are made unsafe by chemical contamination. The FDA, along with the Environmental Protection Agency (EPA), regulates many chemicals in foods that occur as a result of human activities. A later section describes these substances. First, some toxins produced naturally by the foods themselves are worthy of attention.

Natural Toxins in Foods

Some people think they can eliminate all poisons from their diets by eating only "natural" foods. On the contrary, nature has provided many plants with natural poisons to fend off diseases, insects, and other predators. Humans rarely suffer harm from such poisons, but the potential for harm does exist.

Potatoes provide a common example. They contain many natural poisons, including solanine, a powerful, bitter, neurotoxin. Solanine isn't itself green in color, but it forms alongside harmless green chlorophyll when sufficient light rays strike the potato, shown in Figure 12–12. The small amounts of solanine normally found in potatoes are harmless, but solanine can build up to toxic levels when potatoes are exposed to light during storage. Cooking does not destroy solanine, but much of a potato's solanine develops in a thin layer just beneath the skin, so it can often be peeled off, making the potato safe to eat. If a potato's flesh tastes bitter, however, throw it out.

Solanine, along with other naturally occurring toxins (Table 12–9), serves as a reminder of three principles. First, poisons are poisons, whether made by people or by nature. It's not the source of a compound that makes it hazardous but its chemical structure. Second, any substance—even pure water—can be toxic when consumed in excess. Third, by choosing a variety of foods, the eater can dilute the toxins found in any one food by the volume of all the other foods in the diet.

KEY POINTS

- Natural foods contain natural toxins that can be hazardous under some conditions.
- To avoid harm from toxins, choose a variety of foods and eat them in moderation.

Pesticides

The use of **pesticides** helps ensure the survival of food crops, but the damage pesticides do to the environment is considerable and increasing. Moreover, there is some question about whether the widespread use of pesticides has truly increased overall yields of food. Even with extensive pesticide use, the world's farmers lose large quantities of their crops to pests every year.

The use of pesticides on food crops demonstrates a principle inherent to nutrition decision making: the expected benefits of an action or inaction must be weighed against its risks. In general, agricultural pesticides:

- Protect crops from insect damage.
- Increase potential yield per acre.

Figure 12–12
Solanine: A Natural Toxin

Exposure to light causes the bitter toxin solanine to form under the skin of potatoes. The green color that signals its presence is from chlorophyll that forms under the same conditions.

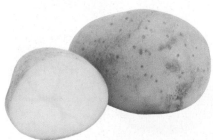

iStock.com/Human

pesticides chemicals used to control insects, diseases, weeds, fungi, and other pests on crops and around animals. Used broadly, the term includes *herbicides* (to kill weeds), *insecticides* (to kill insects), and *fungicides* (to kill fungi).

Table 12–9

A Sampling of Natural Toxins

Herbs	Belladonna and hemlock are infamous poisonous herbs, but sassafras is also toxic; it contains the carcinogen and liver toxin safrole, which is so potent that it is banned from use in foods and beverages.
Cabbage family	Raw cabbage, turnips, mustard greens, and radishes all contain small quantities of harmful goitrogens, compounds that can interfere with thyroid hormone production and when eaten in excess, enlarge the thyroid gland.
Foods with cyanogens	Cyanogens, precursors to the deadly poison cyanide, are found in bitter varieties of cassava, a root vegetable staple for many people. Most cassava is low in cyanogens. Apricot and cherry pits present the cyanogen amygdalin, a fake cancer cure often passed off as a vitamin.[a] This poison kills cancer cells but only at doses that can kill the person, too. Other fruit pits contain lower concentrations.
Seafood red tide toxin	Seafood may occasionally become contaminated with the so-called *red tide* toxin from algae blooms. Eating the contaminated seafood can cause paralysis.

[a]Also called laetrile and, erroneously, vitamin B_{17}.

But they also:

- Accumulate in the food chain.
- Kill valuable pollinators, such as bees.
- Kill pests' natural predators, including birds and insects.
- Pollute the water, soil, and air.

Scientists, farmers, and consumers must weigh the risks and benefits to determine their best course of action.

Do Pesticides on Foods Pose a Hazard to Consumers? Many pesticides are broad-spectrum poisons that damage all living cells, not just those of pests. Their use can harm the plants and animals in natural systems, and they also present risks to people who produce, transport, and apply them. High doses of pesticides in laboratory animals cause birth defects, sterility, tumors, organ damage, and central nervous system impairment. Such high doses are extremely unlikely to occur in human beings, however, except through accidental spills. Minute quantities of pesticide **residues** on agricultural products can survive processing, and traces are often present in foods served to people, but these amounts pose negligible risks to most people (see the Consumer's Guide section).

Especially Vulnerable: Infants and Children Infants and children are more susceptible than adults to the ill effects of pesticides for four reasons. First, the immature human detoxifying system cannot effectively cope with poisons, so they tend to stay longer in the body. Second, a child's developing brain cannot yet fully exclude pesticides, many of which kill insects by interfering with normal nerve and brain chemistry.

Third, children's bodies are small in size, yet their pesticide exposure is often greater than that of adults. Children pick up pesticides through normal child behaviors, such as playing outdoors on treated soil or lawns; handling sticks, rocks, and other contaminated objects; crawling on treated carpets, furniture, and floors; placing fingers and toys in their mouths; seldom washing their hands; and using fingers instead of utensils to grasp foods.

Fourth, children eat proportionally more food per pound of body weight than do adults, and even the trace amounts of pesticides on foods can contribute to total exposure. Fortunately, these traces rarely exceed allowable limits, and most can be

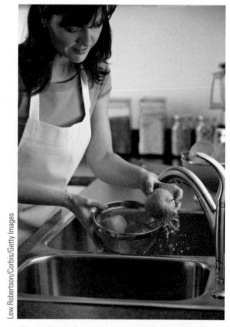

Lew Robertson/Corbis/Getty Images

Wash fresh fruit and vegetables to remove pesticide residues.

residues whatever remains; in the case of pesticides, those amounts that remain on or in foods when people buy and use them.

Table 12–10

Ways to Reduce Pesticide Residue Exposure

In addition to these steps, remember to eat a variety of foods to minimize exposure to any one pesticide.

- Trim the fat from meat, and remove the skin from poultry and fish; discard fats and oils in broths and pan drippings. (Pesticide residues concentrate in the animal's fat.)
- Select fruit and vegetables with intact skins.
- Wash fresh produce in running water.[a] Use a scrub brush, and rinse thoroughly.
- Use a knife to peel an orange or grapefruit; do not bite into the peel.
- Discard the outer leaves of leafy vegetables such as cabbage and lettuce.
- Peel waxed fruit and vegetables; waxes don't wash off and can seal in pesticide residues.
- Peel vegetables such as carrots and fruit such as apples when it seems necessary. (Peeling removes not only pesticides that remain in or on the peel but also fibers, vitamins, and minerals.)
- Choose organically grown foods, which generally contain fewer pesticides.

[a]Soaking produce for 10 minutes in a mild baking soda solution may also help to remove pesticides.

further reduced by washing produce thoroughly and following the other guidelines in Table 12–10.[***] Another possibility for reducing pesticide exposure is to choose **organic foods**—read the Consumer's Guide for perspective.

Regulation of Pesticides The EPA sets a **reference dose** for the maximum residue of an approved pesticide allowable in foods. Over 10,000 regulations set reference doses for hundreds of pesticide chemicals approved for use on U.S. crops. These limits generally represent between 1/100th and 1/1,000th of the highest dose that still causes *no adverse health effects* in laboratory animals. If a pesticide is misused, growers risk fines, lawsuits, and destruction of their crops.

Although the EPA sets limits, both the USDA and the FDA occasionally test crop and food product samples for compliance. Over decades of testing, seldom have these agencies found residues above approved limits. This makes sense because growers are not eager to waste capital by overusing costly chemicals.

Pesticide-Resistant Insects Ironically, some pesticides also promote the survival of the very pests they are intended to wipe out. A pesticide aimed at certain insects may kill almost 100 percent of them, but because of the genetic variability of large populations, a few hardy individuals survive exposure. These resistant insects then multiply free of competition and soon produce offspring with inherited pesticide resistance that attack the crop with enhanced vigor. Controlling resistant insects requires application of different pesticides, which leads to the emergence of a population of insects that survive multiple pesticides. The same biological sequences occur when herbicides and fungicides are repeatedly applied to weeds and fungal pests. One alternative to this destructive series of events is to manage pests using a combination of improved farming techniques and biological controls, as discussed in Controversy 15.

Natural Pesticides Pesticides are not produced only in laboratories; they also occur in nature. The nicotine in tobacco and phytochemicals of celery are examples.[†††] Another is known as Bt pesticide, an insecticidal peptide made by a common soil bacterium. (Reminder: *Peptide* refers to bonds that link amino acids.) This pesticide is extracted and sprayed on organic farm crops and **organic gardens**; it is also produced in the tissues of genetically engineered crops (see the Controversy section).

If farmers could create an ideal pesticide, it would destroy pests in the field and then disappear, leaving no trace of toxic residue either on the food or in the soil. Unfortunately, though, many pesticides are **persistent**: they remain on food and in the

organic foods to be labeled *organic*, foods must meet strict USDA production regulations—that is, they must be produced without synthetic pesticides, herbicides, fertilizers, drugs, and preservatives and without genetic engineering or irradiation.

reference dose an estimate of the intake of a substance over a lifetime that is considered to be without appreciable health risk; for pesticides, the maximum amount of a residue permitted in a food. Formerly called *tolerance limit*.

organic gardens gardens grown with techniques of *sustainable agriculture*, such as using fertilizers made from composts (decayed organic materials) and introducing predatory insects to control pests, in ways that have minimal impact on soil, water, and air quality.

persistent of a stubborn or enduring nature; with respect to food contaminants, the quality of remaining unaltered and unexcreted in plant foods or in the bodies of animals and human beings.

***For answers to questions about pesticides, call the 24-hour National Pesticide Information Center: 1–800–858-PEST.

†††The celery plant produces psoralens that repel insects.

Understanding Organic Foods

LO 12.5 Compare potential advantages and drawbacks of organic and conventional foods.

Sales of certified organic foods have skyrocketed from under $4 billion in 1997 to $49 billion in 2017.[1]* Even at a 10 to 40 percent higher price, organic foods appeal to consumers who believe that they are buying the freshest, best-tasting, most nutrient-packed, chemical-free, non-genetically modified foods available. Just the word *organic* conjures up positive feelings in some consumers, an effect aptly named "the halo effect."[2] When people were asked to judge two *identical* yogurts, they rated the yogurt bearing an "organic" label as more nutritious, lower in fat, more flavorful, and worth more money than a yogurt labeled "regular"—but in fact only the labels differed. The halo effect held true for identical cookies and potato chips, too—people thought those labeled "organic" tasted better.

Besides wanting pure foods, many people are also willing to pay extra for foods produced with little impact on the earth and with respect for animals. Are they getting what they are paying for?

Reference notes are in Appendix F.

Organic Rules

A U.S. farmer or manufacturer selling *certified organic* food must pass USDA inspections at every step of production, from the seed sown in the ground, through the making of compost for fertilizer, to the manufacturing and labeling of the final product. Figure 12–13 describes the meanings of organic food labels. In contrast, foods labeled "natural," "free-range," "locally grown," or with other wholesome-*sounding* words are not held to any standards to bear out such claims.

The National Organic Program develops, implements, and administers production, handling, and labeling standards for organic agricultural products. Enforcement has proved difficult, however, and compliance problems are common. Program officials are working to solve these problems and close open loopholes.

Pesticide Residues— They're Everywhere

The virtues of organic foods have been investigated. Researchers found that,

when tested, organic foods generally contain no pesticides, or at least lower concentrations than similar, conventionally grown products.[3] Also, it is clear that eating a diet of organic foods measurably reduces pesticide exposure.[4] When scientists measured a marker for pesticide exposure in urine samples from thousands of people across the United States, they found that people who reported eating organic foods had the lowest concentrations of the marker—an indication that they had been exposed to less pesticide.

Does this mean that eating a diet of organic foods is better for health than eating a conventional diet? Evidence does not suggest that conventional foods pose excess health risks or that using organic products reduces risks. The typical pesticide exposure in the United States represents an amount 10,000 times below the level at which risks begin to rise. Children are more sensitive than adults to pesticides, and their risks are less well defined, so parents may wish to reduce their children's exposure from all

---

Figure 12–13

Labels on Organic Food Products

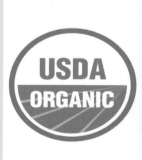 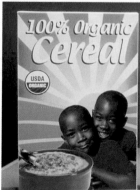 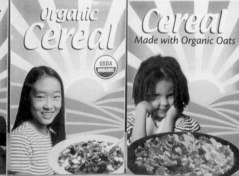 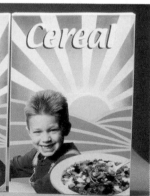

Organic foods that have met USDA standards may use this seal on their labels.

Foods made with 100 percent organic ingredients may claim "100% organic" and use the seal.

Foods made with at least 95 percent organic ingredients may claim "organic" and use the seal.

Foods made with at least 70 percent organic ingredients may list up to three of those ingredients on the front panel.

Foods made with less than 70 percent organic ingredients may list them on the side panel, but cannot make any claims on the front.

U.S. Department of Agriculture (USDA)

(continued)

sources, including foods. The extra cost of organic food may buy nothing more than peace of mind for parents, however.

To Bean or Not To Bean

A popular consumer group advocates choosing organically grown varieties of certain fruit and vegetables. Their list correctly reflects the results of federal tests for pesticide residues on produce—the foods they name test highest for one or more pesticide residues.[5] So far, so good. However, the group then goes on to urge consumers to choose organic varieties of these foods, implying that they can reduce their health risks by doing so. But this doesn't tell the whole story—the health risks from eating conventional varieties of those foods are infinitesimally small.

Still, the risk from pesticide residues is not zero, and many people fear harm from unfamiliar chemicals applied to food in any amount. Such worries are emotional, not scientific, and they can needlessly put consumers in a bind. If people cannot afford organic foods but fear that conventional foods may harm them, they may limit the amount or variety of fruit and vegetables they take in. This unwise choice greatly increases health risks.[6]

Nutrient Composition

Few nutrient differences exist between conventional and organic foods, and these generally fall within expected variations among food crops. Small nutrient differences occur with varying soil types, soil nutrients, seasonal rainfall, or other factors. In contrast to nutrients, organic foods may be higher in certain phytochemicals.[7] This makes sense because plants, unassisted by pesticides, muster their own phytochemical defenses to ward off insects and other dangers.

Some organic meats may provide a little more omega-3 fatty acids than conventional meats, but only if the animals foraged in pastures where wild plants grew.[8] Animals raised on fields of planted grass develop less omega-3 fatty acids.

The most meaningful nutrient comparisons are not between organic and conventional foods but between whole foods and heavily processed ones, a comparison made clear in the Consumer's Guide of Chapter 7. Organic candy bars, soy desserts, and fried vegetable snack chips are no more nutritious (or less fattening) than ordinary treats. Likewise, organic main dishes laden with saturated fats and sodium can throw health-seeking consumers off course.

Environmental Benefits

Ideally, growers of organic foods use *sustainable* agricultural techniques (see Chapter 15 and Controversy 15) that minimize harm to the environment.[9] They add composted animal manure or vegetable matter instead of the synthetic, petroleum-based fertilizers that run off into waterways and pollute them. They battle pests and diseases by using a pesticide derived from a bacterial toxin, by rotating crops each season, by introducing predatory insects to kill off pests, or by picking off large insects or diseased plant parts by hand.

Farmers and ranchers who sell organic eggs, dairy products, and meats must provide their animals with at least some access to outdoor environments. Such animals do not receive growth hormones, daily antibiotics, and the other drugs that become necessary when conventionally raised animals are stressed in overcrowded pens. Without overcrowding, runoff of animal waste, a threat to the nation's waterways, is reduced, too.

Organics' Potential Pitfalls

Foods contaminated with untreated manure or feces from fertilizer, runoff, or wild animals can harbor dangerous bacteria, but such contamination is equally likely to occur in organic foods and conventional foods. Proper composting (decaying) of manure-based fertilizers eliminates pathogens.

Organic ingredients imported from other countries often cost less than domestic ingredients and so make attractive alternatives to dollar-conscious organic food manufacturers. These options are becoming more reliable as FSMA regulations improve food safety procedures and close gaps in oversight for overseas producers. Still, shipping organic ingredients over long distances violates principles of sustainability.

Moving Ahead

The practical marketplace advice, based on science, is this: buy safe, affordable conventionally grown fruit and vegetables, wash them well, and consume them with confidence.[10] If you prefer the taste of organic fruit and vegetables, if you appreciate extra care of animals and the environment, and if you can afford them, you can choose organics with equal confidence.

If you want organic foods at bargain prices, you might ask for oddly shaped, or overripe or underripe produce at farmer's markets. Alternatively, try growing some leafy greens, herbs, and tomatoes in pots on a sunny deck—a surprisingly simple and rewarding endeavor. Whatever your choice, choose nutritious fruit and vegetables in abundance.

Review Questions*

1. To be labeled *100% organic*, a food must.
   a. be inspected before it is sold.
   b. contain at least 95% organic ingredients.
   c. be labeled "natural" or "free range."
   d. contain only 100% organic ingredients.

2. The risk to health from pesticides in foods is exceedingly small.   T   F

3. Organic candy bars, soy desserts, and fried vegetable snack chips.
   a. are not more nutritious than ordinary treats.
   b. are superior sources of nutrients for children.
   c. are a less-fattening alternative to nonorganic snack foods.
   d. can provide adequate daily intakes of important organic minerals.

*Answers to Consumer's Guide review questions are found in Appendix G.

environment after their work is done. Peptide pesticides, having shorter lifetimes, make a better choice than most other pesticides.

Animal Drugs—What Are the Risks?

Consumers often express concern that the meats and animal products they eat may be contaminated with chemical treatments and drugs used on farm animals. These may be valid concerns, but the world's scientists are far more alarmed by a serious related threat: the emergence and rapid spread of diseases caused by drug-resistant bacterial pathogens that have ceased to respond to any antibiotic therapy.[28]

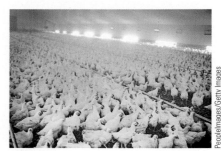

Overcrowding of farm animals makes infections likely to occur.

Livestock and Antibiotic-Resistant Microbes   For a half-century, ranchers and farmers have dosed livestock with antibiotic drugs as part of a daily feeding regimen to ward off infections common in animals living in crowded conditions. These drugs also speed up animal growth and increase feed efficiency. Regrettably, however, when bacteria too frequently encounter antibiotics, they adapt, losing their sensitivity to the drugs over time. The resulting **antibiotic-resistant bacteria** cause severe infections in people—infections that do not yield to standard antibiotic therapy, often ending in fatality.

A substantial threat to human health and life arises from antibiotic-resistant bacteria. A limited number of antibiotic drugs exist, so the same or related drugs used daily in livestock are also of critical importance for treating illnesses in people. Few treatment options remain for people who become infected with antibiotic-resistant bacteria. So long as antibiotics are overused in animals and people, new resistant pathogens can be expected to emerge, and once here, they tend to stay.

Federal voluntary guidelines urge farmers to use antibiotics only under veterinary care and only to prevent, control, or treat diseases, but these protections are not mandatory, so no one can predict their effectiveness. One day, new drugs and vaccines now under development may reduce the need for antibiotics in food animals. Meanwhile, increasing global use of antibiotics in livestock threatens to squander a true medical miracle and render it powerless.[29]

Growth Hormone in Meat and Milk   Cattle producers in the United States commonly inject their herds with a form of **growth hormone, recombinant bovine somatotropin (rbST)**, to spur lean tissue growth, augment milk production, and reduce feed requirements. The hormone, produced by genetically altered bacteria, is identical to the growth hormone made in the pituitary gland of the animal's brain. The FDA and WHO deem the use of the drug to be safe, and the FDA does not require testing of food products for traces of it.

> Genetic engineering of bacteria and food products is discussed in this chapter's Controversy, p. 477.

Ranchers advocate the use of rbST because more meat and milk on less feed yields higher profits. The environment may profit as well. Smaller herds that eat sparingly require less cleared land and fewer resources are necessary to produce and transport their feed. Tests of conventional milk, hormone-free milk, and organic milk reveal no differences in terms of antibiotic, bacteria, hormone, or nutrient contents.

Arsenic in Foods   **Arsenic**, a naturally occurring element from the earth's crust and an infamous poison, is administered in tiny amounts to poultry flocks to kill parasites that would otherwise stall their growth. Arsenic thus builds up in poultry meat, wastes, and feathers. This adds to the natural arsenic content of water and soil, and ultimately increases the arsenic in the food supply.

antibiotic-resistant bacteria bacterial strains that cause increasingly common and potentially fatal infectious diseases that do not respond to standard antibiotic therapy. An example is MRSA (pronounced MER-suh), a multidrug-resistant *Staphyloccocus aureus* bacterial strain.

growth hormone a hormone (somatotropin) that promotes growth and that is produced naturally in the pituitary gland of the brain.

recombinant bovine somatotropin (so-mat-oh-TROPE-in) **(rbST)** growth hormone of cattle, which can be produced for agricultural use by way of genetic engineering. A *recombinant* protein arises from genetically engineered DNA (see the Controversy). Also called *bovine growth hormone (bGH)*.

arsenic a poisonous metallic element. In trace amounts, arsenic is believed to be an essential nutrient in some animal species. Arsenic is often added to insecticides and weed killers and, in tiny amounts, to certain animal drugs.

Foods such as rice and apple juice—even organic apple juice—contain small amounts of arsenic. For apple juice, the FDA is confident in its safety for people who consume normal amounts and vary their choices. No immediate threat exists, but the FDA has asked manufacturers of baby foods to test and limit arsenic in their products, and urges that women, infants, and children consume a variety of grains to minimize their arsenic exposure.[30] People with gluten sensitivities, especially children, often have unusually high intakes of rice, one of the few gluten-free grains. Some groups are calling for arsenic values to be revealed on labels of rice-based staple foods, such as gluten-free breads and baked goods, cereals, pastas, and rice "milk."[31] Other sources of arsenic include fish and shellfish, eggs, milk products, and drinking water.

KEY POINTS

- FDA-approved hormones, antibiotics, and other drugs are used to promote growth or increase milk production in conventionally grown animals.
- Antibiotic-resistant bacteria pose a serious and growing threat.

Environmental Contaminants

As world populations increase and become more industrialized, concerns grow about contamination of foods. A **food contaminant** is anything in food that does not belong there.

Harmfulness of Contaminants The potential for harm from a contaminant depends partly on how long it lingers in the environment or in the human body—that is, on how *persistent* it is. Some contaminants are short-lived because microorganisms, sunlight, or oxygen breaks them down. Some contaminants stay in the body for only a short time because the body rapidly excretes or destroys them. Such contaminants present little cause for concern.

Other contaminants linger and resist environmental breakdown, and they interact with the body's systems without being metabolized or excreted. These contaminants can accumulate at higher concentrations in each level of the food chain, a process called **bioaccumulation**—see Figure 12–14. Many species consumed by people come from the middle of the food chain.

The toxic effect of a chemical depends largely on two factors: the degree of the chemical's **toxicity** and the degree of human exposure. In small enough amounts, even poisonous substances may be tolerable and of no consequence to health; in larger amounts, even innocuous substances may be dangerous. The old saying, "The dose makes the poison," means that with a large enough dose, normally benign substances, even sand, can kill a person. It is equally true that even poisons can be benign in miniscule doses.

How much of a threat do environmental contaminants pose to the food supply? It depends on the contaminant. In general, the threat remains small because the FDA monitors contaminants in foods and issues warnings when food contamination is detected. Table 12–11 (p. 466) describes a few contaminants of greatest concern in foods.

Mercury in Seafood Mercury, **PCBs**, and other hazardous substances are often detected in food fish species worldwide, but the **heavy metal** mercury is of special concern.[32] Scientists learned of mercury's potential for harm through tragedy. In the mid-20th century, more than 120 people, including 23 infants, in Minamata, Japan, became ill with a strange disease, as depicted in Figure 12–15. Mortality was high, and the survivors suffered progressive, irreversible blindness, deafness, loss of coordination, and severe mental and physical retardation.‡‡‡

food contaminant any substance occurring in food by accident; any food constituent that is not normally present.

bioaccumulation the accumulation of a contaminant in the tissues of living things at higher and higher concentrations along the food chain.

toxicity the ability of a substance to harm living organisms. All substances, even pure water or oxygen, can be toxic in high enough doses.

PCBs (polychlorinated biphenyls) stable, oily synthetic chemicals, once used in hundreds of U.S. industrial operations, that persist today in underwater sediments and contaminate fish and shellfish. Now banned from use in the United States, PCBs circulate globally from areas where they are still in use. PCBs cause cancer, nervous system damage, immune dysfunction, and a number of other serious health effects.

heavy metal any of a number of mineral ions such as mercury and lead, so called because they are of relatively high atomic weight; many heavy metals are poisonous.

---

‡‡‡Minamata disease was named for the location of the disaster.

Figure 12–14

Bioaccumulation of Toxins in the Food Chain

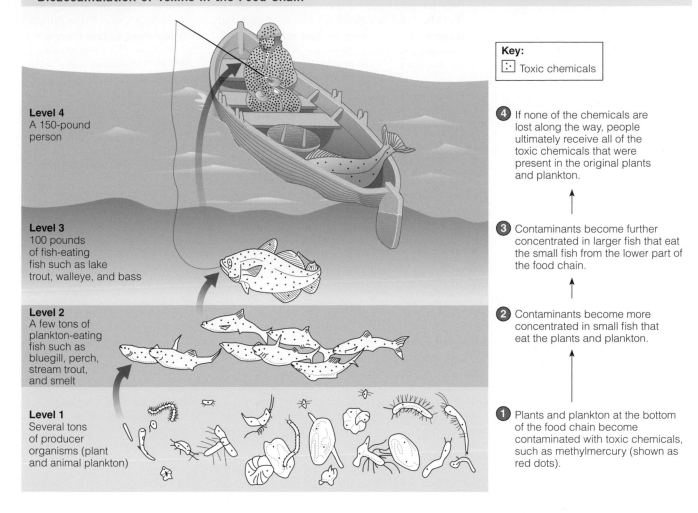

Key:
⬚ Toxic chemicals

Level 4
A 150-pound person

Level 3
100 pounds of fish-eating fish such as lake trout, walleye, and bass

Level 2
A few tons of plankton-eating fish such as bluegill, perch, stream trout, and smelt

Level 1
Several tons of producer organisms (plant and animal plankton)

4️⃣ If none of the chemicals are lost along the way, people ultimately receive all of the toxic chemicals that were present in the original plants and plankton.

3️⃣ Contaminants become further concentrated in larger fish that eat the small fish from the lower part of the food chain.

2️⃣ Contaminants become more concentrated in small fish that eat the plants and plankton.

1️⃣ Plants and plankton at the bottom of the food chain become contaminated with toxic chemicals, such as methylmercury (shown as red dots).

Finally, the cause of this misery was discovered: manufacturing plants in the region were discharging mercury into the waters of the bay, where aquatic bacteria metabolized it into the nerve poison methylmercury.[33] The fish in the bay were accumulating the poison in their bodies, and townspeople who regularly ate fish from the bay fell ill. The infants' mothers had eaten fish during their pregnancies, but were spared because the poison became concentrated in the fetal tissues.

Today, in the United States, scientists warn that methylmercury concentrations in our nation's ocean and freshwater fisheries, and also in some popular food fish species, are unacceptably high and growing higher by the year.[34] The FDA advises all pregnant women, women who may become pregnant, nursing mothers, and young children not eat certain marine fish species known to be high in methylmercury (Chapter 5 weighs the benefits of eating seafood against the risks).

No one expects the tragic results of the 1950s to occur again, but efforts to reduce methylmercury concentrations in global fisheries are needed to help protect these valuable and imperiled resources. Methylmercury is persistent in the environment, so today's efforts to reduce pollution of ocean, lake, and river waters will take years to be effective.

KEY POINTS

- Persistent environmental contaminants present in food pose a small but significant risk to U.S. consumers.
- Mercury and other contaminants pose the greatest threats during pregnancy, lactation, and childhood.

Figure 12–15

Mercury Toxicity Disease

When mercury poisons a developing fetus, the result is severe. This person has Minamata disease, the lifelong crippling of body and mind from mercury poisoning before birth.

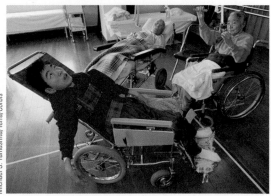

Michael S. Yamashita/Terra/Corbis

Table 12-11

Examples of Contaminants in Foods

Name and Description	Sources	Toxic Effects	Typical Route to Food Chain
Cadmium (heavy metal)	Used in industrial processes including electroplating, plastics, batteries, alloys, pigments, smelters, and burning fuels. Present in cigarette smoke and in ash from volcanic eruptions.	No immediately detectable symptoms, but slow irreversible damage to kidneys and liver.	Enters air in smokestack emissions, settles on ground, absorbed into food plants, consumed by farm animals, and eaten in vegetables and meat by people. Sewage sludge and fertilizers leave large amounts in soil; runoff contaminates shellfish.
Lead[a] (heavy metal)	Found in lead crystal decanters and glassware, painted china, old house paint, batteries, pesticides, old plumbing.	Displaces calcium, iron, zinc, and other minerals from their sites of action in the nervous system, bone marrow, kidneys, and liver, causing failure of function.	Originates from industrial plants and pollutes air, water, and soil. Still present in soil from many long-ago years of leaded gasoline use.
Mercury (heavy metal)	Widely dispersed in gases from earth's crust; local high concentrations from industry, electrical equipment, paints, and agriculture; present in most global fishing waters.	Poisons the nervous system, especially in fetuses. Is associated with heart, blood, and other tissue abnormalities.	Inorganic mercury is released into waterways by industry: acid rain is converted to methylmercury by bacteria and ingested by fish (tuna, swordfish, and others).
Polychlorinated biphenyls (PCBs) (organic compounds)	No natural source; not produced in the U.S., but present in electrical equipment (transformers, capacitors).	Causes long-lasting skin eruptions, eye irritations, growth retardation in children of exposed mothers, anorexia, fatigue, others.	Is released from discarded electrical equipment or during accidental industrial leakage.

[a]For answers to questions concerning lead, call the National Lead Information Center at (800) 424-LEAD.

Are Food Additives Safe?

LO 12.6   Describe the uses and safety characteristics of some common food additives.

It may be comforting to learn that food **additives** rank low on the FDA's list of food worries. Thousands of food additives are approved for use in the United States, and most are strictly controlled and well studied for safety. Some common classes of additives and their functions in foods are listed in Table 12–12.

Regulations Governing Additives

Before using a new additive in food products, a manufacturer must test the additive and satisfy the FDA on two counts:

- It is effective (it does what it is supposed to do).
- It can be detected and measured in the final food product.

Then the manufacturer must provide proof that it is safe (causes no birth defects or other injuries) when fed in large doses to experimental animals. This formal process may take several years. Then manufacturers must comply with a host of other regulations that ensure the proper use and application of the additive as well. For example, additives may *not* be used in any application where they disguise faulty or inferior products, or deceive consumers, or significantly destroy nutrients in foods.

additives substances that are added to foods but are not normally consumed by themselves as foods.

Table 12–12

Selected Food Additives and Their Functions

Agent Types	Function in Foods	Examples
Antimicrobial agents (preservatives)	Prevent food spoilage by mold or bacterial growth.	Acetic acid (vinegar), benzoic acid, nitrates and nitrites, propionic acid, salt, sugar, sorbic acid.
Antioxidants (preservatives)	Prevent oxidative changes and delay rancidity of fats; prevent browning of fruit and vegetable products.	BHA, BHT, propyl gallate, sulfites, vitamin C, vitamin E.
Artificial colors	Add color to foods.	Certified food colors such as dyes from vegetables (beet juice or beta-carotene) or synthetic dyes (tartrazine and others).
Artificial flavors, flavor enhancers	Add flavors; boost natural flavors of foods.	Amyl acetate (artificial banana flavor), artificial sweeteners, MSG (monosodium glutamate), salt, spices, sugars.
Bleaching agents	Whiten foods such as flour or cheese.	Peroxides.
Chelating (KEE-late-ing) agents (preservatives)	Prevent discoloration, off flavors, and rancidity.	Citric acid, malic acid, tartaric acid (cream of tartar).
Nutrient additives	Improve nutritional value.	Vitamins and minerals.
Stabilizing and thickening agents	Maintain emulsions, foams, or suspensions or lend the desired thick consistency to foods.	Dextrins (short glucose chains), pectin, starch, or gums such as agar, carrageenan, guar, and locust bean.

The GRAS List   Many additives are exempted from complying with the procedures just described because they have been used for a long time and their use entails no known hazards. More and more additives are being submitted to the FDA for inclusion on the **generally recognized as safe (GRAS) list**.[35] No additives are permanently approved, however; all are periodically reviewed as new facts emerge.

The Margin of Safety   An important distinction between toxicity and hazard arises during evaluation of an additive's safety. Toxicity is a general property of all substances; hazard is the capacity of a substance to produce injury *under conditions of its use*.[§§§] As mentioned, all substances can be toxic at some level of consumption, but they are called hazardous only if they are toxic in the amounts ordinarily consumed. To determine risk, experimenters feed test animals the substance at different concentrations throughout their lifetimes.

An approved food additive has a wide **margin of safety**. Most additives that involve risk are allowed in foods only at concentrations at least 100 times lower than the highest concentration at which the risk is still zero (1/100). Some *natural* toxins produced in food by plants occur at levels that bring their margins of safety close to 1/10. For some trace elements, it is about 1/5. People commonly consume table salt in daily amounts only three to five times less than those that cause serious toxicity.

Risks and Benefits of Food Additives   Most additives used in foods offer benefits that may outweigh their risks or that may make the risks worth taking. In the case of color additives that only enhance the appearance of foods without improving their health value or safety, no amount of risk may be deemed worth taking. In

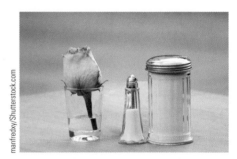

Salt and sugar: two long-used preservatives.

generally recognized as safe (GRAS) list a list, established by the FDA, of food additives long in use and believed to be safe.

margin of safety in reference to food additives, a zone between the concentration normally used and that at which a hazard exists. For common table salt, for example, the margin of safety is 1/5 (five times the amount normally used would be hazardous).

[§§§] The Delaney Clause, a legal requirement of zero cancer risk for additives, is no longer universally applied.

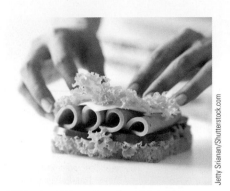

Without additives, bread would quickly mold, and lunchmeat would soon spoil.

contrast, the FDA finds it worth taking a small, uncertain risk associated with nitrites on processed meats because nitrites are proven to inhibit harmful bacterial growth in these foods.

KEY POINTS

- Food additives must be safe, effective, and measurable in the final product for FDA approval.
- Approved additives have wide margins of safety.

Additives to Improve Safety and Quality

Some additives improve food safety. They restrict bacterial growth or otherwise enhance food quality in ways many people take for granted.

Salt and Sugar   Since before the dawn of history, salt has been used to preserve meat and fish; sugar, a relative newcomer to the food supply, serves the same purpose in jams, jellies, and canned and frozen fruit. Both salt and sugar work by withdrawing water from the food; microbes cannot grow without sufficient moisture. Safety questions surrounding these two preservatives center on their overuse as flavoring agents—salt and sugar make foods taste delicious and are often added with a liberal hand. Chapters 4 and 8 provided detailed discussions of these issues.

Nitrites   The *nitrites* added to meats and meat products help preserve their color (especially the pink color of hot dogs and other cured meats) and to inhibit rancidity and thwart bacterial growth. In particular, nitrites prevent growth of the deadly *Clostridium botulinum* bacterium. Even though nitrites are useful, they raise safety issues. Once in the stomach, nitrites can be converted to nitrosamines, chemicals linked with colon cancer in animals. Other nitrite sources, such as tobacco and beer, may be more significant than foods as sources of nitrosamine-related compounds. Still, processed meats are associated with an elevated risk of colon cancer and death, so cautious consumers limit intakes of these foods.[36]

Sulfites   Sulfites prevent oxidation in many processed foods, in alcoholic beverages (especially wine), and in drugs. Some people experience dangerous allergic reactions to the sulfites, so their use is strictly controlled. The FDA prohibits sulfite use on food meant to be eaten raw (fresh grapes are an exception), and it requires foods and drugs to list on their labels any sulfites that are present. For most people, sulfites do not pose a hazard in the amounts used in products, but they have one other drawback. Because sulfites can destroy significant amounts of thiamin in foods, you can't count on a food that contains sulfites to contribute to your daily thiamin intake.

> Use of nonnutritive sweeteners in weight control is a topic of **Chapter 9**.

KEY POINTS

- Sugar and salt have the longest history of use as additives to prevent food spoilage.
- Nitrites and sulfites have advantages and drawbacks.

Flavoring Agents

Many additives add desirable flavors to foods. One group, the **nonnutritive sweeteners**, may be added by manufacturers or by consumers at home.

Nonnutritive Sweeteners   Nonnutritive sweeteners make foods taste sweet without promoting dental decay or providing the empty calories of sugar. The human taste buds perceive many of them as supersweet, so just tiny amounts are added to foods and beverages to achieve the desired sweet taste. The FDA endorses the use of nonnutritive sweeteners as safe over a lifetime when used within **acceptable daily intake (ADI)** levels. Table 12–13 (p. 469) provides some details about the nonnutritive sweeteners, including ADI levels.

nonnutritive sweeteners   sweet-tasting synthetic or natural food additives that offer sweet flavor but with negligible or no calories per serving; also called *artificial sweeteners, intense sweeteners, noncaloric sweeteners,* and *very low-calorie sweeteners.*

acceptable daily intake (ADI)   the estimated amount of a sweetener that can be consumed daily over a person's lifetime without any adverse effects.

Chapter 12 Food Safety and Food Technology

Table 12–13

U.S.-Approved Nonnutritive Sweeteners

Sweetener	Chemical Composition	Digestion/ Absorption	Sweetness Relative to Sucrose[a]	Energy (cal/g)	Acceptable Daily Intake (ADI) and Estimated Equivalent[b]	Approved Uses
Acesulfame potassium or acesulfame-K (Sunette, Sweet One)	Potassium salt	Not digested or absorbed	200	0	15 mg/kg body weight[c] (30 cans diet soda)	General use, except in meat and poultry; tabletop sweeteners; heat stable
Advantame	Aspartame derivative, similar to neotame	Rapidly digested; poorly absorbed	20,000	0	32.8 mg/kg body weight (4,000 packets of sweetener)	General use, except in meat and poultry; heat stable at baking temperatures
Aspartame (NutraSweet, Equal, others)	Amino acids (phenylalanine and aspartic acid) and a methyl group	Digested and absorbed	180	4[d]	50 mg/kg body weight[e] (18 cans diet soda)	General use in all foods and beverages; warning to population with PKU; degrades when heated
Luo han guo	Glycosides extracts from monk fruit	Digested and absorbed	150–300	1	No ADI determined	GRAS[f]; general use as a food ingredient and tabletop sweetener
Neotame	Aspartame with an additional side group attached	Not digested or absorbed	7,000	0	18 mg/day	General use, except in meat and poultry
Saccharin (SugarTwin, Sweet'N Low, others)	Benzoic sulfimide	Rapidly absorbed and excreted	300	0	5 mg/kg body weight (10 packets of sweetener)	Tabletop sweeteners, wide range of foods, beverages, cosmetics, and pharmaceutical products
Stevia (Sweetleaf, Truvia, Pure Via)	Glycosides extracted from the leaves of the stevia herb	Digested and absorbed	200–300	0	4 mg/kg body weight	GRAS[f]; tabletop sweeteners, a variety of foods and beverages
Sucralose (Splenda)	Sucrose with Cl atoms instead of OH groups	Not digested or absorbed	600	0	5 mg/kg body weight (6 cans diet soda)	Baked goods, carbonated beverages, chewing gum, coffee and tea, dairy products, frozen desserts, fruit spreads, salad dressing, syrups, tabletop sweeteners
Tagatose[g] (Nutralose, Nutrilatose, Tagatesse)	Monosaccharide similar in structure to fructose; naturally occurring or derived from lactose	Not well absorbed	0.9	1.5	7.5 g/day	GRAS[f]; bakery products, beverages, cereals, chewing gum, confections, dairy products, dietary supplements, energy bars, tabletop sweeteners

[a]Relative sweetness is determined by comparing the approximate sweetness of a sugar substitute with the sweetness of pure sucrose, which has been defined as 1.0. Chemical structure, temperature, acidity, and other flavors of the foods in which the substance occurs all influence relative sweetness.

[b]Based on a person weighing 70 kg (154 lb).

[c]Recommendations from the World Health Organization limit acesulfame-K intake to 9 mg/kg of body weight per day.

[d]Aspartame provides 4 cal/g, as does protein, but because so little is used, its energy contribution is negligible. In powdered form, it is sometimes mixed with lactose, however, so a 1-g packet may provide 4 cal.

[e]Recommendations from the World Health Organization and in Europe and Canada limit aspartame intake to 40 mg/kg of body weight per day.

[f]Generally recognized as safe. For stevia, one of its extracts (but not other forms) has GRAS status.

[g]Tagatose is a poorly digested sugar and technically not a nonnutritive sweetener.

Through the years, questions have emerged about the safety of nonnutritive sweeteners, particularly saccharin and aspartame. For example, early research indicated that large quantities of saccharin caused bladder tumors in laboratory animals, but research today does not support a causative link in people.

Early animal research suggested possible links among saccharin intakes, microbial communities in the intestine, and type 2 diabetes.[37] However, when researchers examined human health records in relation to saccharin intakes, no association with diabetes was detected.[38]

Aspartame, a sweetener made from two amino acids (phenylalanine and aspartic acid) is one of the most thoroughly studied food additives ever approved by the FDA. Evidence linking aspartame with chronic diseases is weak or nonexistent, and a recent up-to-date evaluation of the body's biochemical milieu, along with other physical and psychological testing, yielded no evidence of acute adverse physical or psychological effects.[39] However, aspartame's phenylalanine base poses a threat to those with the inherited disease phenylketonuria (PKU), a disease that, without a low phenylalanine diet, can damage the developing brain in children. Food labels warn people with PKU of the extra phenylalanine in aspartame-sweetened foods (see Figure 12–16). In any case, artificially sweetened foods and drinks have no place in the diets of infants or toddlers. A person with digestive or other problems who has found that a sweetener causes symptoms should use a different sweetener.

Monosodium Glutamate (MSG)   MSG, the sodium salt of the amino acid glutamic acid, is used widely in restaurants, especially Asian restaurants.**** In addition to

---

Figure 12–16

Nonnutritive Sweeteners on Food Labels

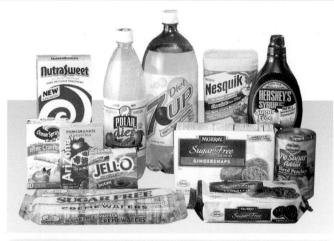

INGREDIENTS: ARTIFICIAL AND NATURAL FLAVORING, TITANIUM DIOXIDE (COLOR), ASPARTAME, ACESULFAME POTASSIUM, STEVIA.
PHENYLKETONURICS: CONTAINS PHENYLALANINE.

This partial ingredient list is for a sugar-free food.

Products containing aspartame must carry a warning for people with phenylketonuria.

Products containing less than 0.5 g of sugar per serving can claim to be "sugarless" or "sugar-free."

Nutrition Facts	Amount per serving	% DV*
	Total Fat 0g	0%
	Sodium 0mg	0%
Serving Size 8 oz	Total Carb. 0g	0%
Servings 6	Sugars 0g	
Calories 0	Protein 0g	
*Percent Daily Values (DV) are based on a 2,000 calorie diet.	Not a significant source of other nutrients.	

© Scott Goodwin Photography

****The MSG trade name is Accent.

enhancing other flavors, MSG itself presents a basic taste (termed *umami*) independent of the well-known sweet, salty, bitter, and sour tastes.

In a few sensitive individuals, MSG produces adverse reactions known as the **MSG symptom complex**. Plain broth with MSG seems most likely to bring on symptoms in sensitive people, whereas carbohydrate-rich foods, such as rice or noodles, seem to protect against them. Deemed safe for adults, MSG is prohibited in baby foods because huge doses harm the brain and kidneys of laboratory animals.[40] Human brains are thought to be resistant to such effects, however. The FDA requires that food labels disclose each additive, including MSG, by its full name.

KEY POINTS
- People with PKU should avoid the nonnutritive sweetener aspartame.
- The flavor enhancer MSG may cause reactions in people with sensitivities to it.

Fat Replacers and Artificial Fats

Fat replacers and artificial fats, introduced in Chapter 5, are ingredients that provide some of the taste, texture, and cooking qualities of fats but with fewer or no calories. Many fat replacers are derived from carbohydrate, protein, or fat, and these provide a few calories (but fewer than the fats they replace). Carbohydrate-based fat replacers are used primarily as thickeners or stabilizers in foods such as soups and salad dressings. Protein-based fat replacers provide a creamy feeling in the mouth and are often used in foods such as ice creams and yogurts. Fat-based replacers act as emulsifiers and are heat stable, making them most versatile in shortenings used in cake mixes and cookies.

An artificial fat used to make some low-fat snack foods, such as potato chips, is **olestra**. Digestive enzymes cannot break its chemical bonds, so olestra cannot be absorbed. Olestra binds fat-soluble vitamins and phytochemicals, causing their excretion; to partly prevent these losses, manufacturers saturate olestra with vitamins A, D, E, and K. Large doses can cause digestive distress, but no serious problems are known to occur with normal use.

KEY POINTS
- Fat replacers and artificial fats substitute for the fats in processed foods, reducing their calorie counts and saturated fat contents.
- Olestra in large amounts can cause digestive distress.

Incidental Food Additives

Consumers are often unaware that many substances can migrate into food during production, processing, storage, packaging, or consumer preparation. These substances, although called indirect or **incidental additives**, are really contaminants because no one intentionally adds them to foods. Examples of incidental additives include compounds released from plastics; tiny bits of glass, paper, metal, and the like from packages; or unavoidable filth, such as tiny amounts of rodent hairs or insect fragments. Incidental additives are well regulated, and once discovered in food, their safety must be confirmed by strict procedures like those governing intentional additives.

BPA   The incidental additive **BPA** migrates into many foods and beverages from plastic-lined food cans, soft-drink cans, and certain clear, hard plastic water bottles. BPA and its analogs have raised concerns among scientists who have reported potential disrupting effects on metabolism, hormonal activities, reproduction, neurological development, and problem behavior in young children.[41] Preliminary findings from an FDA study of potential effects of BPA on rats seem to indicate little significant effect, particularly in terms of cancer formation.[42] The researchers warn that characterizing potential BPA hazards for human beings is beyond the scope of their study.

Manufacturers have replaced BPA in baby bottles, toddler "sippy" cups, and infant formula packaging because of the potential risks. The FDA so far concurs that BPA is safe but is continuing to investigate its effects.[43]

MSG symptom complex the acute, temporary, and self-limiting reactions, including burning sensations or flushing of the skin with pain and headache, experienced by sensitive people upon ingesting large doses of MSG.

olestra a nonnutritive artificial fat made from sucrose and fatty acids; also called *sucrose polyester*; trade name, *Olean*.

incidental additives substances that can get into food not through intentional introduction but as a result of contact with the food during growing, processing, packaging, storing, or some other stage before the food is consumed. Also called *accidental* or *indirect additives*.

BPA (bisphenol A) a compound that hardens plastic and a component of epoxy resin. BPA can leach from some plastic containers into the foods and beverages contained inside.

Microwave Packages Some microwave products are sold in "active packaging" that participates in cooking the food. Pizza, for example, may rest on a cardboard pan coated with a thin film of metal that absorbs microwave energy and may heat up to 500°F (260°C). During the intense heat, some particles of the packaging components migrate into the food. This is expected; the particles have been tested for safety.

In contrast, incidental additives from plastic packages may not be entirely safe for consumption. To avoid them, do not reuse disposable plastic margarine tubs or single-use trays from microwavable meals for microwaving other foods. Use glass or ceramic containers or plastic ones labeled as safe for the microwave. In addition, wrap foods in microwave-safe plastic wraps, waxed paper, cooking bags, parchment paper, or white microwave-safe paper towels instead of ordinary wraps before microwave cooking.

KEY POINTS

- Incidental additives enter food during processing and are regulated; most do not constitute a hazard.
- Consumers should use only microwave-safe containers and wraps for microwaving food.

Conclusion

To sum up the messages of this chapter, the ample U.S. food supply is largely safe, and hazards are rare. Foodborne microbial illnesses pose the greatest threat by far, and an urgent need exists for new preventive technologies and procedures, along with greater consumer awareness. The Food Feature that follows aims to help you apply food safety principles to real-life situations.

FOOD FEATURE

Handling Real-Life Challenges to Food Safety

LO 12.7 Describe applications of food-safety practices in various settings.

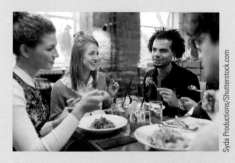

Following food-safety rules is important in all settings.

Some people spend more energy worrying about food additives, which are virtual non issues, than about foodborne illnesses, which are real threats. They accept yearly bouts of intestinal illness as inevitable, often not even realizing that they are food-related, but these illnesses can and should be prevented. This Food Feature can help you to apply the protective behaviors described earlier in this chapter when you are on the spot in real-life situations.

Take Inventory

A good place to begin any behavior change is with an inventory of current habits. Take the quiz in Table 12–14 to assess how well you know and apply the rules of food safety. If some of the concepts cause you to stumble, go back and review the chapter sections that explain them.

Be Observant

Pathogenic microbes are everywhere, and they multiply fast when given the chance. Stay alert to danger signs whenever and wherever you eat. At a barbeque or picnic, don't be shy about checking how raw meats or cold cuts and mixed foods are stored or transported. Have they been refrigerated or packed with ice in coolers? The coolers should ride in air-conditioned vehicle interiors, and not in hot trunks. Are raw meats and vegetables kept separate at every step? Have grilled meats been cooked to safe internal temperatures (and measured with a thermometer)? Also, note the time at which perishable

Table 12–14

Can You Pass the Kitchen Food-Safety Quiz?

How food-safety savvy are you? Give yourself 2 points for each correct answer.

1. The temperature of the refrigerator in my home is
   A. 50°F (10°C).
   B. 40°F (4°C).
   C. I don't know; I don't own a refrigerator thermometer.

2. The last time we had leftover cooked stew or other meaty food, the food was
   A. cooled to room temperature and then put in the refrigerator.
   B. put in the refrigerator immediately after the food was served.
   C. left at room temperature overnight or longer.

3. If I use a cutting board to cut raw meat, poultry, or fish and then use it to chop another food, the board is
   A. reused as is.
   B. wiped with a damp cloth or sponge.
   C. washed with soap and water.
   D. washed with soap and hot water and then sanitized.

4. The last time I had a hamburger, I ate it
   A. rare.
   B. medium.
   C. well done.

5. The last time there was cookie dough where I live, the dough was
   A. made with raw eggs, and I sampled some of it.
   B. store-bought, and I sampled some of it.
   C. baked and then sampled.

6. I clean my kitchen counters and food preparation areas with
   A. a damp sponge that I rinse and reuse.
   B. a clean sponge or cloth and water.
   C. a clean cloth with hot water and soap.
   D. the same as above and then a bleach solution or other sanitizer.

7. When dishes are washed in my home, they are
   A. washed in an automatic dishwasher and then air-dried.
   B. left to soak in the sink for several hours and then washed with soap in the same water.
   C. washed right away with hot water and soap in the sink and then air-dried.
   D. washed right away with hot water and soap in the sink and immediately towel-dried.

8. The last time I handled raw meat, poultry, or fish, I cleaned my hands afterward by
   A. wiping them on a towel.
   B. rinsing them with warm tap water.
   C. washing them with soap and water.

9. Meat, poultry, and fish products are defrosted in my home by
   A. setting them on the counter.
   B. placing them in the refrigerator.
   C. microwaving and cooking promptly when thawed.
   D. soaking them in warm water.

10. I realize that eating raw seafood poses special problems for people with
    A. diabetes.
    B. HIV infection.
    C. cancer.
    D. liver disease.

ANSWERS

1. Refrigerators should stay at 40°F or less, so if you chose answer B, give yourself 2 points; 0 for other answers.

2. Answer B is the best practice, worth 2 points. 0 for other answers.

3. If answer D best describes your household's practice, give yourself 2 points; if C, 1 point.

4. Give yourself 2 points if you picked answer C; 0 for other answers.

5. If you answered A, you may be putting yourself at risk for infection from bacteria in raw shell eggs. Answer C—eating the baked product—will earn you 2 points; answer B, 1 point. Commercial dough is made with pasteurized eggs, but some bacteria may remain.

6. Answer C or D will earn you 2 points each; answer B, 1 point; answer A, 0.

7. Answers A and C are worth 2 points each; other answers, 0.

8. The only correct practice is answer C, worth 2 points; 0 for others.

9. Give yourself 2 points if you picked B or C; 0 for others.

10. This is a trick question: all of the answers apply. Give yourself 2 points for knowing one or more of the risky conditions.

RATING YOUR HOME'S FOOD-SAFETY PRACTICES
20 points: You can feel confident about the safety of foods served in your home.
12 to 19 points: Reexamine food-safety practices. You are violating some key rules.
11 points or below: Take steps immediately to correct food-handling, storage, and cooking techniques. Your current practices are putting you and other members of your household in danger of foodborne illness.

Table 12-15

More Food-Safety Myths and Truths

Myths	Truths
■ "The five-second rule: a food that falls to the floor is safe if it is picked up within five seconds."	■ Food dropped on a microbe-laden hard surface, such as a floor, becomes contaminated the moment it lands.
■ "If it tastes and smells okay, it's safe to eat."	■ Most microbial contamination is undetectable by human senses.
■ "We have always handled our food this way, so it must be safe."	■ Past generations did not recognize the causes of illness.
■ "I sampled it a couple of hours ago and didn't get sick, so it is safe to eat."	■ Illnesses often take half a day or longer to develop.

cold or hot foods, such as potato salad or baked beans, are set out at room temperatures for serving. After two hours have passed, stop eating them. Remember that tainted foods often look, smell, and taste wholesome.

Beware of False Thinking

Many people rely on myths and platitudes to guide their food-safety practices, but these reflect false thinking. Some examples of common myths were presented in Table 12–7 (p.452), and Table 12–15 offers more. You may not be able to talk others out of their long-held beliefs, and in truth, your your only compulsory task is to keep yourself safe by standing firm on your knowledge of food-safety principles.

Take Action

If food-safety rules are broken, you have two choices: inform the person in charge or fellow diners of the dangers, or simply protect yourself by enjoying the available safe foods, such as breads, intact fruit, boiled eggs, and hard cheeses. Be forewarned that the first choice, informing people, entails a social risk: they may dismiss your concerns, or worse, take offense. This risk may be deemed worth taking, however, because foodborne illnesses can be serious. In any case, protect yourself.

Stay alert to challenges that may arise, perhaps when friends gather at a restaurant to enjoy raw shellfish or raw sushi, or they are eating raw cookie dough in someone's home. Don't be tempted to go along; let your food-safety knowledge guide you. In the case of raw shellfish, you might mention that raw seafood is very likely to harbor pathogens. Then order your oysters or clams baked, broiled, fried, or steamed to the well-done stage, or substitute cooked peel-and-eat shrimp. In the case of sushi, safer options abound: rolls made with real or imitation crab, cooked shrimp, fish, or eel, or refreshing vegetable rolls. That way, you can enjoy the gathering without endangering your health.

The cookie dough scenario is trickier because no options may exist, particularly in someone's home. There, you may have to take a stand. Politely refuse the dough, explain the risk, and say you'll wait for the baked cookies instead. You might also ask for something else, such as a glass of water or other beverage. This request gives your host a chance to provide something you want, while creating a distraction from the dough. Others may also follow your lead, but in any case, it's better to endure a brief moment of social discomfort than days of physical pain and illness. Only you know what challenges you are likely to encounter, and it helps decide in

advance what you will do to protect your health.

Restaurants and cafeterias must pass regular inspections for cleanliness and adherence to food-safety rules, yet some manage to break the rules and stay in business. When dining out, be observant. If a restaurant floor or table appears dirty or if the bathroom is grimy, chances are that the staff is lax about food-safety rules in the kitchen, too. Choose another place to eat. Once you have ordered, if a food such as meatloaf and gravy, which should be piping hot, arrives at the table lukewarm, send it back and order something else. Likewise, if a dish such as shrimp cocktail or chicken salad, which should be chilled, arrives at room temperature, send it back. You'll be protecting yourself and doing restaurant owners a favor by alerting them to a problem.

Conclusion

To prevent illness, you must act on the strength of your knowledge, before a risk becomes an illness. Don't be lulled by a false sense of security or by mythical thinking. Take charge of your health and apply your food-safety knowledge whenever you eat. If your friends follow your lead, your knowledge and actions will keep them safe, too, compounding your benefits.

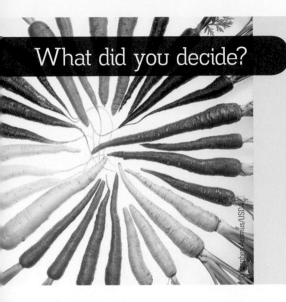

What did you decide?

Are most digestive tract symptoms from "**stomach flu**"?

Are most foods from grocery stores **germ-free**?

Should you **refrigerate** leftover party foods after the guests have gone home?

Which poses the greater risk: raw **sushi** from a sushi master or food additives?

What's online?

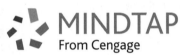

MINDTAP
From Cengage

Visit www.Cengage.com to access MindTap, a complete digital course that includes Diet & Wellness Plus, interactive quizzes, videos, and more.

Self Check

1. (LO 12.1) FSMA is a new law intended to improve food safety for people and pets.
   T   F

2. (LO 12.1) Some microorganisms produce illness-causing _____.
   a. neurotoxins and enterotoxins
   b. neurotransmitters and aflatoxins
   c. enzymes and hormones
   d. none of the above.

3. (LO 12.2) To prevent foodborne illnesses, the refrigerator's temperature should be less than _____.
   a. 70°F   c. 40°F
   b. 65°F   d. 30°F

4. (LO 12.2) Which of the following may be contracted from fresh raw or undercooked seafood?
   a. hepatitis
   b. worms and flukes
   c. viral intestinal disorders
   d. all of the above.

5. (LO 12.2) Which of the following organisms can cause hemolytic-uremic syndrome?
   a. *Listeria monocytogenes*
   b. *Campylobacter jejuni*
   c. *Escherichia coli*
   d. *Salmonella*

6. (LO 12.2) The threat of foodborne illness from meats or seafood is serious, but produce causes illness only rarely.
   T   F

7. (LO 12.2) Infants under one year of age should never be fed honey because it can contain spores of *Clostridium botulinum*.
   T   F

8. (LO 12.3) Which of the following is correct concerning fruit that has been irradiated?
   a. They decay and ripen more slowly.
   b. They lose substantial nutrients.
   c. They lose their sweetness.
   d. They emit gamma radiation.

9. (LO 12.3) Irradiation can
   a. destroy vitamins.
   b. sterilize spices.
   c. make food radioactive.
   d. promote sprouting.

10. (LO 12.3) Food packaging can contribute to food safety.
    T F

11. (LO 12.4) It is possible to eliminate all toxins from your diet by eating only "natural" foods.
    T F

12. (LO 12.4) Pregnant women are advised not to eat certain species of fish because the FDA and the EPA have detected unacceptably high lead levels in them.
    T F

13. (LO 12.5) Evidence does not suggest that conventional foods pose health risks or that using organic products reduces risks.
    T F

14. (LO 12.5) Compared with conventionally grown produce, organic produce is often
    a. lower in pesticides.
    b. higher in phytochemicals.
    c. both a and b.
    d. none of the above.

15. (LO 12.6) Incidental food additives
    a. help to preserve foods.
    b. consist mostly of added sugars and salt.
    c. are really contaminants.
    d. none of the above.

16. (LO 12.6) Nitrites added to foods
    a. prevent the growth of the deadly *Clostridium botulinum* bacterium.
    b. preserve the pink color of hot dogs.
    c. are linked with colon cancer.
    d. all of the above.

17. (LO 12.7) Food safety rules for consumers can protect you only when you act on them.
    T F

18. (LO 12.7) On noticing a food safety problem at a friend's house, you should:
    a. ignore infractions of food-safety rules to preserve the friendship.
    b. avoid eating the unsafe food, and consider informing your friend.
    c. call the FDA.
    d. ignore the infractions but see a medical professional later to diagnose potential illnesses.

19. (LO 12.8) Selective breeding
    a. involves manipulating an organism's genes in a laboratory.
    b. has been used for thousands of years.
    c. allows scientists to cross species boundaries.
    d. all of the above

20. (LO 12.8) A genetically engineered rice variety in existence today supplies sufficient beta-carotene to fight vitamin A deficiency and childhood blindness worldwide.
    T F

Answers to these Self Check questions are in Appendix G.

Genetically Engineered Foods: What Are the Pros and Cons?

LO 12.8   Summarize the advantages and disadvantages of producing foods through genetic engineering.

With or without their awareness, most people in this country consume foods that contain products of **genetic engineering**. As Figure C12–1 illustrates, 90 percent of U.S. soybeans and 88 percent of animal feed corn (*not* sweet corn consumed by people) are **genetically modified organisms (GMOs).** Ubiquitous food additives, such as soy lecithin and high-fructose corn syrup, are made from these genetically engineered plant materials and enter the human food supply in processed foods. Other GMOs, such as papayas, are consumed directly. Some consumers recoil from the idea of eating products from GMOs, and whole countries have banned such foods outright. Some objections are based on credible ideas, but most others arise from emotional fears, distrust of technology, and misinformation.[1]* This Controversy sorts some scientific facts from fiction, starting with definitions of **biotechnology** terms (see Table C12–1, p. 478).

Advances in biotechnology have raised hopes of solving some of today's most pressing food and energy problems while boosting profits for farmers and other producers. Although **recombinant DNA (rDNA) technology** may seem futuristic, its roots lie in genetic events that have been occurring unaided for untold millions of years. Human beings have exploited these processes from the advent of agriculture.

*Reference notes are in Appendix F.

Selective Breeding

Season after season, farmers influence the genetic makeup of food plants and animals by selecting only the best farm animals and plants for breeding. Today's lush, hefty, healthy agricultural crops and animals, from cabbage and squash to pigs and cattle, are the result of thousands of years of **selective breeding**. Consumers of today's large cobs of sweet corn, for example, may not recognize the original wild native corn with its sparse four or five kernels to a stalk (shown in Figure C12–2).

Today, accelerated selective breeding techniques involve hundreds of thousands of cross-bred seeds planted on vast acreages. To develop crops with desired traits, DNA data from successful seedlings are analyzed by computer. Seedlings with the right genes are grown to maturity and reproduced to yield new breeds in a relatively short time. Some unusually colorful carrots, including the purple, light yellow, or deep red varieties now seen in some specialty grocery stores, are products of this kind of selective breeding. Selective breeding must stay within the boundaries of a species—a carrot, for example, cannot be crossed with a mosquito. Recombinant DNA technology, however, knows no such limits.

Recombinant DNA Technology

With economy, speed, and precision, rDNA technology can change one or more characteristics of a living thing. The genes for a desirable trait in one organism are transferred directly into another organism's DNA. With advancements in

---

Figure C12–1

Growth of Selected Genetically Engineered Crops, United States 1996–2014

The economic benefits of growing genetically engineered soybeans, cotton, and corn have led to widespread replacement of conventional crops on U.S. farms. For example, almost 100% of the U.S. farm acres planted with soybeans are growing the genetically engineered type (light green line at the top of the figure.)

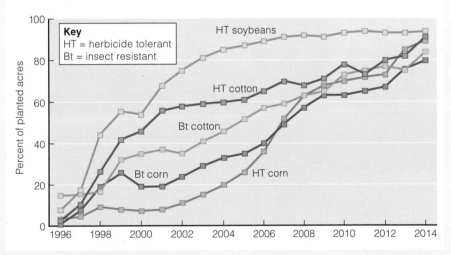

Source: J. Fernandez-Cornejo and coauthors, *Genetically engineered crops in the United States,* Economic Research Report *162 (2014), available at www.ers.usda.gov/webdocs/publications/45179/43668_err162 .pdf?v=41690.*

Biotechnology Terms

- **biotechnology** the science of manipulating biological systems or organisms to modify their products or components or create new products; biotechnology includes recombinant DNA technology and traditional and accelerated selective breeding techniques.
- **clone** an individual created asexually from a single ancestor, such as a plant grown from a single stem cell; a group of genetically identical individuals descended from a single common ancestor, such as a colony of bacteria arising from a single bacterial cell; in genetics, a replica of a segment of DNA, such as a gene, produced by genetic engineering.
- **gene editing** a method of genetic engineering that employs CRISPR technology to alter an organism by adding, removing, or substituting molecules within a single gene's DNA strand with great precision. The acronym CRISPR refers to a particular DNA sequence employed in the method.
- **genetic engineering** the direct, intentional manipulation of the genetic material of living things in order to obtain some desirable inheritable trait not present in the original organism. Also called *biotechnology*.
- **genetically modified organism (GMO)** popular term referring to an organism produced by genetic engineering; the term

genetically engineered organism (GEO) is more scientifically accurate.

- **outcrossing** the unintended breeding of a domestic crop with a related wild species.
- **plant pesticides** substances produced within plant tissues that kill or repel attacking organisms.
- **recombinant DNA (rDNA) technology** a technique of genetic modification whereby scientists directly manipulate the genes of living things; includes methods of removing genes, doubling genes, introducing foreign genes, and changing gene positions to influence the growth and development of organisms.
- **selective breeding** a technique of genetic modification whereby organisms are chosen for reproduction based on their desirability for human purposes, such as high growth rate, high food yield, or disease resistance, with the intention of retaining or enhancing these characteristics in their offspring.
- **stem cell** an undifferentiated cell that can mature into any of a number of specialized cell types. A stem cell of bone marrow may mature into one of many kinds of blood cells, for example.
- **transgenic organism** an organism resulting from the growth of an embryonic, stem, or germ cell into which a new gene has been inserted.

Figure C12–2

Corn: A Product of Selective Breeding

The wild corn on the left, with its sparse kernels, bears little resemblance to today's large, full, sweet ears (right).

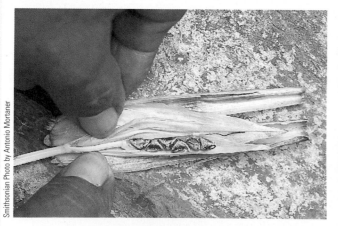

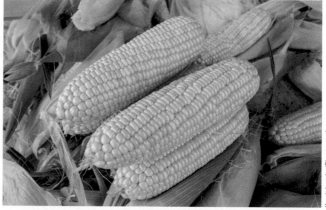

gene editing, scientists can now alter molecules within a single gene's DNA strand for increasingly precise results. Figure C12–3 (p. 479) compares the genetic results of selective breeding and rDNA technology. Table C12–2 (p. 479) presents examples of biotechnology research directions.

Obtaining Desired Traits

Using rDNA technology, scientists can confer useful traits, such as disease resistance, on food crops. To make a disease-resistant potato plant, for example, the process begins with the DNA of an immature cell, known as a **stem cell**,

from the "eye" of a potato. Into that stem cell scientists insert a gene snipped from the DNA of a virus that attacks potato plants (enzymes do the snipping). This gene codes for a harmless viral protein, not the infective part.

The newly created stem cell is then stimulated to replicate itself, creating

Figure C12–3
Comparing Selective Breeding and rDNA Technology

Selective Breeding—DNA is a strand of genes, depicted as a strand of pearls. Traditional selective breeding combines many genes from two individuals of the same species.

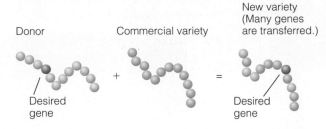

Donor   Commercial variety   New variety
                                           (Many genes
                                           are transferred.)

Desired gene   +   =   Desired gene

rDNA Technology—Through rDNA technology, a single gene or several may be transferred to the receiving DNA from the same species or others.

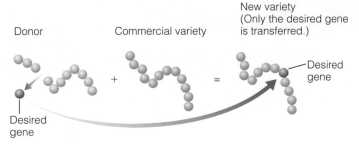

Donor   Commercial variety   New variety
                                           (Only the desired gene
                                           is transferred.)

                                                          Desired gene

Desired gene   +   =

---

shortages, dwindling farmland, lack of renewable energy sources, and environmental degradation. A few examples follow.

---

clone cells—exact genetic replicas of the modified cell. With time, what was once a single cell grows into a **transgenic organism**—in this case, a potato plant that makes a piece of viral protein in each of its cells. The presence of the viral protein stimulates the potato plant to develop resistance against an attack from the real wild virus in the potato field.

Plants make likely candidates for genetic engineering because a single plant cell can often be coaxed into producing an entire new plant. Animals can also be modified by rDNA technology, however. Under development is a line of goats that, thanks to a spider's gene, express spider silk protein in their milk. Once processed, the stronger-than-steel silk fiber can be used to make artificial ligaments and bullet-proof vests.[2]

Suppressing Unwanted Traits

This rDNA technology can also remove an unwanted protein from a plant by silencing the genes responsible for its creation. For example, scientists have created a safer peanut by silencing the genes for proteins that commonly cause allergic reactions.[3] Likewise, a newly approved GE potato may soon be made into safer potato chips and French fries because it is engineered to have less of an amino acid that forms a carcinogenic toxin during frying.[4†] Apples that stay white after slicing instead of turning brown have cleared one approval hurdle and may soon be available in markets; gluten-free wheat may be next.

The Promises and Problems of rDNA Technology

Supporters hail genetic engineering as nothing short of a revolutionary means of overcoming many of the planet's pressing problems, such as food shortages, nutrient deficiencies, medicine

---

[1] *The Innate Potato makes less acrylamide when fried.*

Human Nutrition

Rice leads the way in a genomic revolution of the world's food supply. A rice (called *Golden Rice*) provides up to 35 micrograms of absorbable beta-carotene per gram of rice; white rice provides none. Figure C12–4 compares Golden Rice with white rice. Rice is an excellent vehicle for delivering vitamin A to areas of the world where rice is a staple food: everyone there eats rice, often several times a day. In comparison, carrots, famously rich in beta-carotene, are not a preferred food in those places. Golden Rice can deliver enough vitamin A to fight deficiency diseases and childhood blindness worldwide.

Uncertainty fostered by anti-GMO activists has cast doubt about the safety of Golden Rice around the world. Twenty years after its development, only two countries, Bangladesh and the Philippines, are moving toward growing it.[5] Meanwhile, with each passing year, vitamin A deficiency

---

Figure C12–4
Golden Rice

Beta-carotene, the vitamin A precursor, gives Golden Rice its yellow hue.

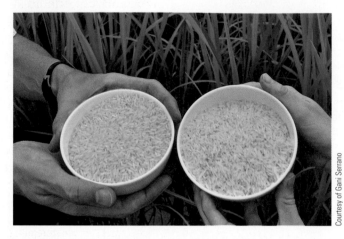

Courtesy of Gani Serrano

Figure C12–5
Two Salmon Compared

These two salmon are the same age, but the GMO salmon reached market size much faster.

Modified salmon

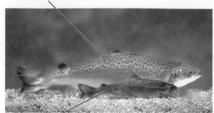

Conventional salmon

Source: fda.gov

harms hundreds of thousands of children worldwide.

Other GMO rice varieties, some offering 80 percent more iron and zinc than ordinary rice, could relieve much iron-deficiency anemia and zinc deficiency around the world. Still others may resist drought, floods, or insects and thus provide more food for hungry populations. Not just rice but worldwide staples like cassava roots or potatoes can be "biofortified" with minerals, vitamins, fatty acids, or promising phytochemicals.[6] In the case of cassava, it can also be made safer by reducing its concentration of naturally occurring toxins.

Molecules from Microbes

The genes of microorganisms have been altered to make pharmaceutical and industrial products. For example, a transgenic bacterial factory now mass-produces the hormone insulin used by people with diabetes. Another bacterium received a bovine gene to make the enzyme rennin, necessary in cheese production. (Historically, rennin was harvested from the stomachs of calves, an expensive process.) Efforts are under way to develop biofuel-producing microbes to yield a more sustainable and price-stable alternative to fossil fuels.[7]

Greater Crop Yields

Most of today's genetically engineered crops are of two types: herbicide-resistant and insect-resistant, both used to improve yields and protect farmed land. Herbicide-resistant crops, for example, offer weed control with less soil tillage by allowing farmers to spray whole fields, not just weeds, with glyphosate-based herbicides (pronounced gly-FOSS-ate).[‡] The weeds die, their roots hold soil in place between the rows, and the crops grow normally. After years of such spraying, however, some weeds have developed vigorous resistance to glyphosate. Weeds grow large and spread fast despite repeated sprayings, forcing many farmers to return to old tillage methods to control them and thereby exposing vast quantities of farm topsoil to wind and water erosion.[8]

As for insect-resistant crops, GMOs make what the EPA calls **plant pesticides**—pesticides made by the plant tissues themselves. For example, a type of feed corn produces a pesticide that kills a common corn-destroying worm, thereby greatly increasing yields per acre of farmland.

In areas where people cannot afford to lose a single morsel of food and where plant diseases and insects can claim up to 80 percent of a season's yield, genetically engineered plants can save whole crops, delivering relief to millions of chronically hungry people.

A Fast-Growing Fish

The FDA recently approved a genetically altered farm-raised salmon that, through rDNA technology, received genes from two other fish species.[§] The added genes code for a hormone that stimulates faster than normal growth in the new salmon, cutting production time, as illustrated in Figure C12–5. After extensive scientific review, the FDA concluded that the salmon is as safe to eat as other fish, and that its new DNA and its growth hormone are also safe both for consumers and the fish itself.[9]

To protect natural systems, the FDA set stringent rules requiring insulated, closed, inland environments for raising the new salmon. Containment is crucial, because if they escape, the larger rDNA salmon could have a survival advantage over wild species. No one knows whether consumers will accept this new GMO food.

[§] The new salmon is called AquAdvantage, developed by AquaBounty Technologies.

[‡] Glyphosate is the active ingredient in the herbicide Roundup.

Concerns about GMOs

Consumers rightly want to know about any potential risks from rDNA technology. The FDA, too, asks whether genetically engineered foods differ substantially from other foods in their nutrient contents or safety.

Nutrient Composition

Except for intentional variation created through rDNA technology, the nutrient composition of genetically engineered foods is identical to that of traditional foods. From the body's point of view, Golden Rice is the same as plain rice, plus a beta-carotene supplement. GMOs may contribute to *overdoses* of nutrients or phytochemicals, but they pose no unusual threat of deficiencies.

Accidental Ingestion of Drugs from Foods

Genetically modified corn, soybeans, rice, and other food crops that make human and animal drugs and industrial proteins must be grown indoors in selected locations. Their containment areas, however, often border on farms where conventional food crops are grown. Critics fear that DNA from drug-producing GMOs might contaminate the food supply by cross-pollination, despite USDA oversight.[10] Disasters such as tornadoes, floods, or other events could carry the pollen long distances, thereby inadvertently introducing the man-made genes into ordinary farm crops, in which they would not be detected and from which they could not be retrieved.

Pesticide Residues

Industry scientists contend that rDNA technology could virtually end problems associated with pesticide use on foods. The consequences of human error can be eliminated, they say, when introduced genes determine not only the nature but also the quantity of pesticide produced. Critics counter that although GMOs may be protected from one or two common pests that may or may not be present on a particular field, farmers must still spray insecticides to kill other pests that are devouring their crops. Also, still more worrisome, constant exposure is inducing crop-destroying insects to develop resistance to natural plant pesticides.

Pesticides that are sprayed onto crops can be largely removed from food by washing or peeling produce, but consumers cannot remove pesticides that form within the tissues of a genetically modified fruit or vegetable. Still, plant pesticides are highly unlikely to cause health problems because they are made of peptide chains (small protein strands) that human digestive enzymes readily denature. Plant pesticides, like other pesticide residues, are regulated and approved by the FDA.

Unintended Health Effects

The possibility exists that GMOs may have unintended and therefore unpredictable effects on human health. A lesson comes from an unexpected negative effect of selective breeding. Over many years, celery growers had crossed their most attractive celery plants because consumers paid a premium for good-looking celery. Unknown to the growers, however, the most beautiful celery contained a great deal of a natural plant pesticide, and its concentration increased with each breeding cycle. Farm and grocery workers who handled the celery began suffering from serious skin rashes until the problem was finally traced to high levels of the natural pesticide in the beautiful plants. Advanced tests to identify such products of metabolism may soon reveal molecules in GMO foods that have previously escaped detection.[11]

Another example (this time an unintended *benefit* of genetic engineering) involves a carcinogenic fungus that sometimes grows on corn.** Upon producing a strain of corn that carried a plant pesticide to control worm damage and then observing this corn for several generations, scientists discovered that the crop suffered far fewer attacks by the dangerous fungus. It turns out that the worms spread the fungus as they burrowed into cobs of ordinary corn, but the plant pesticide in the genetically engineered corn killed the worms and stopped the fungus from spreading.[12]

Environmental Effects

Between 1996 and 2006, farming with genetically engineered crops reduced the use of insecticides by almost 500 million pounds of active ingredients worldwide. At the same time, the use of glyphosate herbicides that GMOs resist, has greatly increased, making it unnecessary to use more highly toxic and persistent herbicides in the fields.[13]†† Also, herbicide-resistant crops require far less plowing to kill weeds and so minimize soil erosion (more about soil conservation in Controversy 15).

The possibility of **outcrossing**, the accidental cross-pollination of plant pesticide crops with related wild weeds remains a concern. If a weed inherits a pest-resistant trait from a neighboring field of genetically engineered crops, it gains an enormous survival advantage over other, possibly important, wild species and crowds them out.

Loss of species is another serious threat. By propagating only a few crop varieties worldwide, humankind becomes vulnerable to serious losses in a changing environment. Species that teeter on the brink of extinction today may hold critical genetic traits that could help food crops to survive in harsher future conditions.

Concerns for wildlife also exist. In the laboratory, monarch butterfly larvae die when fed pollen from pesticide-producing corn. In real life, wild butterflies do not seem to consume enough toxic corn pollen for populations to be harmed. The new technology may even protect some percentage of the dwindling monarchs and other harmless or beneficial insects that now die when they feed on conventionally sprayed fields.

Ethical Arguments about rDNA Technology

In the end, consumer acceptance determines the applications of genetic

---

** *The fungus (Aspergillus flavus) produces the carcinogenic toxin aflatoxin.*

†† *Glyphosate is the chemical in a popular herbicide, trade name Roundup.*

engineering. Some people fear that by tampering with the basic blueprint of life, rDNA technology will sooner or later unleash mayhem into the defenseless world. No degree of risk is justified, they say, because although it raises profits for biotechnology companies and farmers, its products provide little direct benefit to consumers. Others object to rDNA technology on religious grounds, holding that genetic decisions are best left to nature or a higher power. A law now under consideration may require producers to clearly identify foods that contain GMO ingredients.[14] Table C12–3 summarizes some of these issues.

Proponents of genetic engineering respond that most of the world's people cannot afford the luxury of rejecting the potential benefits of rDNA technology—they lack the abundant foods and fertile lands that protesters take for granted. Delays hurt the poorest of the poor, they say. GMO opponents counter that the scope of world hunger far exceeds simple solutions such as increasing food supplies—it involves war, politics, and education. (Chapter 15 explores the tragedy of world hunger.)

Regulation of GMOs

The FDA evaluates the safety of today's genetically modified fruit, vegetables, and grains for human consumption and takes the position that we can confidently assume that they are safe unless they differ substantially from similar foods already in use. To help consumers who wish to avoid GMOs, USDA developed a voluntary certification and labeling system for foods. In 2016, Congress passed a law to mandate uniform labeling of GMO foods, but, as of this writing, implementation has stalled.[‡‡] Meanwhile, consumers are snapping up foods and other products—even detergents and other items unrelated to rDNA technology—that bear a voluntary non-GMO label (see Figure C12–6).

The Final Word

For those who would worry themselves into a diet of crackers and water, abundant evidence supports eating sufficient fruit and vegetables regardless of their source. Stay alert for well-documented,

‡‡The law is the National Bioengineered Food Disclosure Law of 2016.

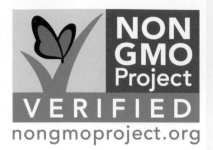

scientific information about rDNA technology, food technology, and their effects on our rapidly changing food supply. Armed with scientific knowledge, you can make informed choices about your diet.

Critical Thinking

1. Summarize options and roadblocks to obtaining only non-GMO foods.

2. Suggest possible motivations of industry, growers, and consumers for supporting/opposing GMOs.

Table C12–3
Genetic Engineering of Foods: Point, Counterpoint

Arguments in Opposition to Genetic Engineering	Arguments in Support of Genetic Engineering
1. *Ethical and moral issues.* It's immoral to "play God" by mixing genes from organisms unable to do so naturally. Religious and vegetarian groups object to genes from prohibited species occurring in their allowable foods.	1. *Ethical and moral issues.* Scientists throughout history have been persecuted and even put to death by fearful people who accuse them of playing God. Yet today, many of the world's citizens enjoy a long and healthy life of comfort and convenience thanks to once-feared scientific advances put to practical use.
2. *Imperfect technology.* The technology is young and imperfect, and potential effects are impossible to predict. Toxins are as likely to be produced as are the desired traits.	2. *Advanced technology.* Recombinant DNA and gene editing technologies are precise and reliable. Many of the most exciting recent advances in medicine, agriculture, and technology have been made possible by the application of this technology.
3. *Environmental concerns.* The power of genetically modified organisms to change the world's environments is unknowable until such changes actually occur—then the "genie is out of the bottle." Once out, the genie cannot be put back in the bottle because insects, birds, and the wind and sea distribute genetically altered seeds, eggs, and pollen to points unknown.	3. *Environmental protection.* Genetic engineering may be the only hope of saving rain forests and other habitats from destruction by impoverished people desperate for arable land. Through genetic engineering, farmers can make use of previously unproductive areas such as salty soils and arid lands.

Genetic Engineering of Foods: Point, Counterpoint

4. "*Genetic pollution.*" Some kinds of pollution can be cleaned up with money, time, and effort, but once genes are spliced into living organisms, those organisms forever bear the imprint of human tampering.

4. *Genetic improvements.* Genetic side effects are more likely to benefit the environment than to harm it.

5. *Crop vulnerability.* Once pests and diseases have adapted to successfully attack one genetically homogeneous crop, then all such crops around the world are defenseless against them. Diversity is key to defense.

5. *Improved crop resistance.* Pests and diseases can be specifically fought on a case-by-case basis. Biotechnology is the key to defense.

6. *Loss of gene pool.* Loss of genetic diversity threatens to deplete valuable gene banks from which scientists can develop new agricultural crops.

6. *Gene pool preserved.* Thanks to advances in genetics, laboratories around the world are able to stockpile the genetic material of millions of species that, without such advances, would have been lost forever.

7. *Profit motive.* Genetic engineering will profit industry more than the world's poor and hungry.

7. *Everyone profits.* Industries benefit from genetic engineering, and a thriving food industry benefits the nation and its people, as demonstrated by countries lacking such industries.

8. *Unproven safety for people.* Testing of genetically altered products for human safety is lacking. The whole population is an unwitting experimental group in a nationwide laboratory study for the benefit of industry.

8. *Safe for people.* Testing of genetically altered products for human safety is unnecessary because the products are essentially the same as the original foodstuffs.

9. *Increased allergens.* Protein allergens, made by genes, can unwittingly be transferred into foods as by-products of genetic engineering for other traits.

9. *Control of allergens.* Genes that code for allergens can be transferred into foods, but these are known and avoidable. In fact, genetic engineering can be used to *reduce* allergens in foods. Allergen-free peanuts have been developed, a help for allergic people.

10. *Decreased nutrients.* A fresh-looking GMO vegetable may be kept in a store's inventory for weeks while nutrient quality diminishes.

10. *Increased nutrients.* Genetic modifications can easily enhance the nutrients in foods.

11. *No product tracking.* Without labeling, the food industry cannot track problems to the source.

11. *Excellent product tracking.* The identity and location of genetically altered foodstuffs are known, and they can be tracked when problems arise.

12. *Overuse of glyphosate herbicide.* Farmers, knowing that their crops are resistant, will overuse herbicides in the attempt to kill weeds.

12. *Conservative use of* glyphosate herbicide. Farmers will not waste expensive herbicide in repeated applications when the prescribed amount gets the job done the first time.

13. Glyphosate, the herbicide sprayed on GMO crops, is blamed for causing autism, cancer, and celiac disease in people.

13. Glyphosate in huge quantities is toxic to cells, but in the amounts consumers ordinarily encounter, glyphosate appears safe, with no links to autism, cancer, or celiac disease.

14. *Increased consumption of pesticides.* When a pesticide is produced by the flesh of produce, consumers cannot wash it off the skin of the produce with running water as they can with most ordinary sprays.

14. *Reduced pesticides on foods.* Pesticides produced by plants in tiny amounts known to be safe for consumption are more predictable than applications by agricultural workers who make mistakes. Because other genetic manipulations will eliminate the need for postharvest spraying, fewer pesticides will reach the dinner table.

15. *Lack of oversight.* Government oversight is run by industry people for the benefit of industry—no one is watching out for consumers.

15. *Sufficient regulation, oversight, and rapid response.* The National Academy of Sciences has established a protocol for the safety testing of GE foods. Government agencies are efficient in identifying and correcting problems as they occur in the industry.

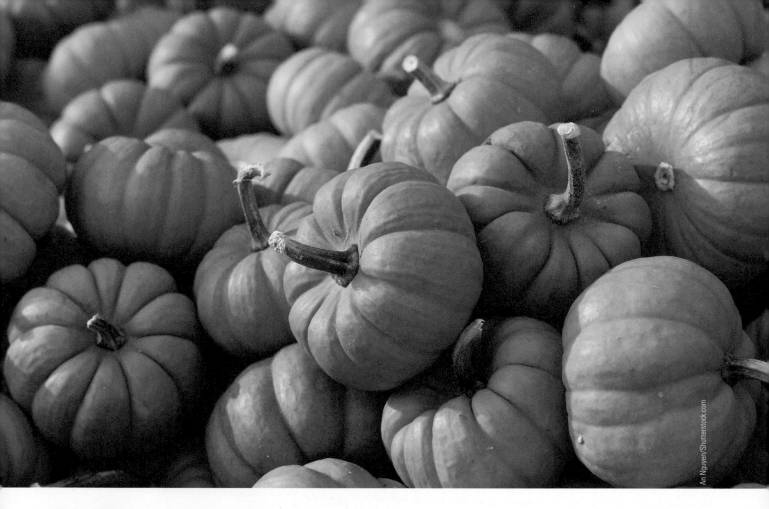

An Nguyen/Shutterstock.com

13 Life Cycle Nutrition: Mother and Infant

Learning Objectives

After completing this chapter, you should be able to accomplish the following:

LO 13.1 Describe the roles of nutrition before and during pregnancy.

LO 13.2 Summarize the evidence against alcohol use during pregnancy.

LO 13.3 List the effects of diabetes, hypertension, and preeclampsia on pregnancy.

LO 13.4 Explain how nutrition supports lactation.

LO 13.5 Identify nutrition practices that promote an infant's well-being.

LO 13.6 List five feeding guidelines that encourage normal eating behavior and autonomy in a child.

LO 13.7 Describe the challenges associated with childhood obesity.

What do you think?

Can a **man's lifestyle habits** affect a woman's future pregnancy?

How much **alcohol** drunk by a pregnant woman will harm her developing fetus?

Are **breast milk** and **formula** equally good for an infant's health?

Can infants **thrive** on breast milk or formula alone?

All people need the same nutrients but in differing amounts throughout life. This chapter is the first of two on life's changing nutrient needs. It focuses on two life stages that are critically important to an infant's life-long health—its development before birth and its first year of life.

Pregnancy: The Impact of Nutrition on the Future

LO 13.1   Describe the roles of nutrition before and during pregnancy.

People normally think of nutrition as personal, affecting them alone. For a woman who is pregnant, or who soon will be, however, nutrition choices today profoundly affect the health of her future child and the adult that the child will one day become. The nutrient demands of pregnancy are extraordinary.

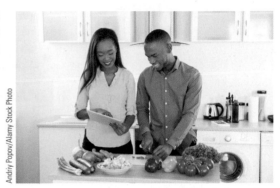

Andriy Popov/Alamy Stock Photo

Both parents can prepare in advance for a healthy pregnancy.

Preparing for Pregnancy

Before she becomes pregnant, a woman must establish eating habits that will optimally nourish both herself and the infant she will bear. Early in pregnancy, the **embryo** undergoes rapid and significant developmental changes that depend on good nutrition. Later, the growing **fetus** demands ample nutrients for optimal development.

> Some heritable traits do not result from DNA variations but arise from epigenetic influences before or during pregnancy—see **Controversy 11**, pp. 435–439.

Fathers-to-be are also wise to examine their eating and drinking habits. For example, leading a sedentary lifestyle and consuming too few fruit and vegetables may affect men's **fertility** (and the fertility of their children), and men who drink too much alcohol or encounter other toxins in the weeks before conception can sustain damage to their sperm's genetic material.[1]* When both partners adopt healthy habits, they will be better prepared to meet the demands of parenting that lie ahead.

Prepregnancy Weight   Before pregnancy, all women, but underweight women in particular, should strive for an appropriate body weight. A woman who begins her pregnancy underweight and who fails to gain sufficiently during pregnancy is very likely to bear a baby with a dangerously **low birthweight**.[2] Infant birthweight is the most potent single indicator of an infant's future health. A low-birthweight baby, defined as one who weighs less than 5½ pounds (2,500 grams), is nearly 40 times more likely to die in the first year of life than a normal-weight baby. To prevent low

embryo (EM-bree-oh) the stage of human gestation from the third to the eighth week after conception.

fetus (FEET-us) the stage of human gestation from eight weeks after conception until the birth of an infant.

fertility the capacity of a woman to produce a normal ovum periodically and of a man to produce normal sperm; the ability to reproduce.

low birthweight a birthweight of less than 5½ pounds (2,500 grams); used as a predictor of probable health problems in the newborn and as a probable indicator of poor nutrition status of the mother before and/or during pregnancy. Low-birthweight infants may be born prematurely, or, if born at full term may be small for gestational age because they suffered growth failure in the uterus.

---

*Reference notes are in Appendix F.

birthweight, underweight women are advised to gain weight before becoming pregnant and to strive to gain adequately thereafter.

When nutrient supplies during pregnancy fail to meet demands, a developing fetus may adapt to the deprivation in ways that may make obesity or chronic diseases more likely in later life.[3] Low birthweight is also associated with low adult IQ and other brain impairments, short stature, and educational disadvantages.[4] Nutrient deficiency coupled with low birthweight is the underlying cause of more than half of all the deaths worldwide of children under 5 years of age. In the United States, the infant mortality rate in 2013 was just under 6.0 deaths per 1,000 live births.[5] This rate, though higher than that of some other developed countries, represents a significant decline over the last two decades and is a tribute to public health efforts aimed at reducing infant deaths.

Low birthweight may also reflect heredity, disease conditions, smoking, and drug use and alcohol use during pregnancy. Even with optimal nutrition and health, some pregnant women give birth to small infants for unknown reasons. Nevertheless, poor nutrition of the mother is the major factor causing low birthweight—and an avoidable one.[6]

High birthweight, often associated with maternal obesity, may present problems of its own. Infants born to obese women are likely to be large for gestational age, weighing more than 9 pounds at birth.[7] Problems associated with a high birthweight include a difficult labor and delivery, birth trauma, and **cesarean section**. Consequently, these babies have a greater risk of poor health and death than infants of normal weight. Infants of obese mothers also may be likely to be born with neural tube defects. Obese women themselves are likely to suffer gestational diabetes, hypertension, and complications during and infections and hemorrhage after the birth.[8] In addition, both overweight and obese women have a greater risk of giving birth to infants with heart defects and other abnormalities.[9]

Obesity and overnutrition during pregnancy may also have long-term effects. Maternal obesity increases a child's risk of obesity, heart disease, type 2 diabetes, and asthma throughout life.[10] An obese woman who strives for a healthy body weight before her pregnancy will be helping to protect both herself and her child.

A Healthy Placenta and Other Organs   A woman's nutrition before pregnancy is crucial because it determines whether her **uterus** will be able to support the growth of a healthy **placenta** during the first month of **gestation**. The placenta is both a supply depot and a waste-removal system for the fetus. If the placenta works perfectly, the fetus wants for nothing; if it doesn't, no alternative source of sustenance is available, and the fetus will fail to thrive. Figure 13–1 shows that the placenta is a mass of tissue in which maternal and fetal blood vessels intertwine and exchange materials. The two bloods never mix, but the barrier between them is thin. Using the **umbilical cord** as a conduit, nutrients and oxygen move easily from the mother's blood into the fetus's blood, and wastes move out of the fetal blood to be excreted by the mother. Thus, by way of the placenta, the mother's digestive tract, respiratory system, and kidneys serve not only her own needs but also those of the fetus, whose organs are not yet functional. The **amniotic sac** surrounds and cradles the fetus, which floats inside its cushioning fluids.

The placenta is a highly metabolic organ that actively gathers up hormones, nutrients, and antibodies from the mother's blood and releases them into the fetal bloodstream. The placenta also produces numerous and diverse hormones that act to maintain pregnancy and prepare the mother's breasts for **lactation**. Is it any wonder that a healthy placenta is essential for the developing fetus?

If the mother's nutrient stores are inadequate during placental development, no amount of nutrients later on in pregnancy can make up for the lack. If the placenta fails to form or function properly, the fetus will not receive optimal nourishment. After getting such a poor start on life, the child may be ill equipped, even as an adult, to store sufficient nutrients, and a girl may later be unable to grow an adequate placenta or bear healthy full-term infants. For this and other reasons, a woman's

cesarean (see-ZAIR-ee-un) **section** surgical childbirth, in which the infant is taken through an incision in the woman's abdomen.

uterus (YOO-ter-us) the womb, the muscular organ within which the infant develops before birth.

placenta (pla-SEN-tuh) the organ of pregnancy in which maternal blood and fetal blood circulate in close proximity and exchange nutrients and oxygen (flowing into the fetus) and wastes (picked up by the mother's blood).

gestation the period of about 40 weeks (three trimesters) from conception to birth; the term of a pregnancy.

umbilical (um-BIL-ih-cul) **cord** the ropelike structure through which the fetus's veins and arteries reach the placenta; the route of nourishment and oxygen into the fetus and the route of waste disposal from the fetus.

amniotic (AM-nee-OTT-ic) **sac** the "bag of waters" in the uterus in which the fetus floats.

lactation production and secretion of breast milk for the purpose of nourishing an infant.

Figure 13-1

The Placenta

The placenta is composed of spongy tissue in which fetal blood and maternal blood flow side by side, each in its own vessels. The maternal blood transfers oxygen and nutrients to the fetus's blood and picks up fetal wastes to be excreted by the mother. The placenta performs the nutritive, respiratory, and excretory functions that the fetus's digestive system, lungs, and kidneys will provide after birth.

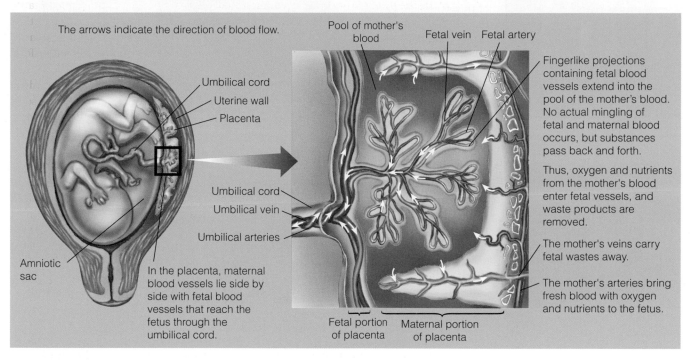

The arrows indicate the direction of blood flow.

Umbilical cord
Uterine wall
Placenta
Amniotic sac

In the placenta, maternal blood vessels lie side by side with fetal blood vessels that reach the fetus through the umbilical cord.

Umbilical cord
Umbilical vein
Umbilical arteries

Pool of mother's blood   Fetal vein   Fetal artery

Fingerlike projections containing fetal blood vessels extend into the pool of the mother's blood. No actual mingling of fetal and maternal blood occurs, but substances pass back and forth.

Thus, oxygen and nutrients from the mother's blood enter fetal vessels, and waste products are removed.

The mother's veins carry fetal wastes away.

The mother's arteries bring fresh blood with oxygen and nutrients to the fetus.

Fetal portion of placenta   Maternal portion of placenta

poor nutrition during her early pregnancy can affect not only her *children* but also her *grandchildren*.

KEY POINTS

- Adequate nutrition before pregnancy establishes physical readiness and nutrient stores to support placental and fetal growth.
- Both underweight and overweight women should strive for appropriate body weights before pregnancy.
- Newborns who weigh less than 5½ pounds face greater health risks than normal-weight babies.

The Events of Pregnancy

The newly fertilized **ovum** is called a **zygote**. It begins as a single cell and rapidly divides into many cells during the days after fertilization. If all goes well, within two weeks, the cluster of cells embeds itself in the uterine wall in the process known as **implantation**, and the placenta begins to grow there. Minimal growth in size takes place at this time, but it is a crucial period in development, during which adverse influences such as smoking, drug abuse, and malnutrition lead to failure to implant or to abnormalities such as neural tube defects. These mishaps can cause loss of the developing embryo, often before the woman knows she is pregnant.

The Embryo and Fetus   During the next six weeks, the embryo registers astonishing physical changes (see Figure 13–2, p. 488). At eight weeks, the fetus has a complete central nervous system, a beating heart, a fully formed digestive system, well-defined fingers and toes, and the beginnings of facial features.

In the last seven months of pregnancy, the fetal period, the fetus grows prodigiously. Periods of rapid cell division occur in organ after organ. The amniotic sac fills with fluid,

ovum the egg, produced by the mother, that unites with a sperm from the father to produce a new individual.

zygote (ZYE-goat) the product of the union of ovum and sperm; a fertilized ovum.

implantation the stage of development, during the first 2 weeks after conception, in which the fertilized egg (fertilized ovum or zygote) embeds itself in the wall of the uterus and begins to develop.

Figure 13–2

Stages of Embryonic and Fetal Development

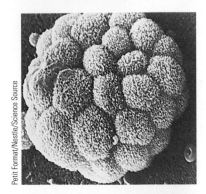

(1) A newly fertilized ovum, called a zygote, is about the size of the period at the end of this sentence. Less than 1 week after fertilization, the zygote has rapidly divided many times and has become ready for implantation.

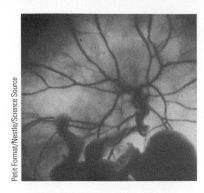

(3) A fetus after 11 weeks of development is just over an inch long. Notice the umbilical cord and blood vessels connecting the fetus with the placenta.

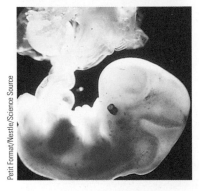

(2) After implantation, the placenta develops and begins to provide nourishment to the developing embryo. An embryo 5 weeks after fertilization is about ½ inch long.

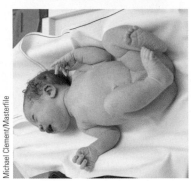

(4) A newborn infant after 9 months of development measures close to 20 inches in length. The average birthweight is about 7½ pounds. From 8 weeks to term, the infant has grown 20-fold in length and 50-fold in weight.

and the mother's body changes. The uterus and its supporting muscles increase in size, the breasts may become tender and full, the nipples may darken in preparation for lactation, and the mother's blood volume increases by half to accommodate the added load of materials it must carry. Gestation lasts approximately 40 weeks and ends with the birth of the infant. The 40 or so weeks of pregnancy are divided into thirds, each of which is called a **trimester**.

A Note about Critical Periods   Each organ and tissue type grows with its own characteristic pattern and timing. The development of each can take place only at a certain time—the **critical period**. Whatever nutrients and other environmental conditions are necessary during this period must be supplied on time if the organ is to reach its full potential. If the development of an organ is limited during a critical period, recovery is impossible. For example, the fetus's heart and brain are well developed at 14 weeks; the lungs, 10 weeks later. Therefore, early malnutrition impairs the heart and brain; later malnutrition impairs the lungs.

The effects of malnutrition during critical periods of pregnancy are seen in defects of the nervous system of the embryo (explained later), in a child's poor dental health, and in an adolescent's and adult's vulnerability to infections and possibly higher risks of diabetes, hypertension, stroke, or heart disease.[11] The effects of malnutrition during critical periods are irreversible: abundant and nourishing food, fed after the critical time, cannot remedy harm already done.

Table 13–1 identifies characteristics of a **high-risk pregnancy**. The more factors that apply, the higher the risk. All pregnant women, especially those in high-risk categories need **prenatal** medical care, including dietary advice.

trimester a period representing one-third of the term of gestation. A trimester is about 13 to 14 weeks long.

critical period a finite period during development in which certain events may occur that will have irreversible effects on later developmental stages. A critical period is usually a period of cell division in a body organ.

high-risk pregnancy a pregnancy characterized by risk factors that make it likely the birth will be complicated by premature delivery, difficult birth, retarded growth, birth defects, and early infant death. A *low-risk pregnancy* has none of these factors.

prenatal (pree-NAY-tal) before birth.

KEY POINTS

- Implantation, fetal development, and critical period development depend on maternal nutrition status.
- The effects of malnutrition during critical periods are irreversible.

Increased Needs for Nutrients

During pregnancy, a woman's nutrient needs increase more for certain nutrients than for others. Figure 13–3 shows the percentage increase in nutrient intakes recommended for pregnant or lactating women compared with nonpregnant women: notice how much longer the yellow and purple bars are than the green ones. The nutrient demands of pregnancy are high, and a woman must make mindful food choices; her body will also do its part by maximizing nutrient absorption and minimizing nutrient losses.

Energy, Carbohydrate, Protein, and Fat Energy needs vary with the progression of pregnancy. In the first trimester, a pregnant woman needs no additional energy, but her energy needs rise as pregnancy progresses. She requires an additional 340 daily calories during the second trimester and an extra 450 calories each day during the third trimester.[12] A woman can easily meet the need for extra calories by selecting more nutrient-dense foods from the five food groups. Table 13–2 (p. 490) offers sample menus for pregnant and lactating women.

Ample carbohydrate (ideally, 175 grams or more per day and certainly no less than 135 grams) is necessary to fuel the fetal brain and spare the protein needed for fetal growth. Whole-grain breads and cereals, dark green and other vegetables, legumes, and citrus and other fruit provide carbohydrates, nutrients, and phytochemicals along with fiber which will help alleviate the constipation that many pregnant women experience.

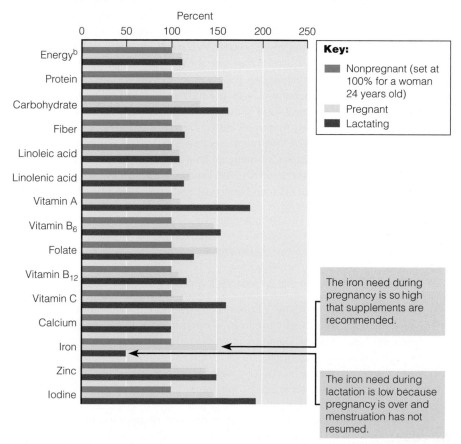

Figure 13–3

Comparison of Selected Nutrient Recommendations for Nonpregnant, Pregnant, and Lactating Women[a]

Key:
- Nonpregnant (set at 100% for a woman 24 years old)
- Pregnant
- Lactating

The iron need during pregnancy is so high that supplements are recommended.

The iron need during lactation is low because pregnancy is over and menstruation has not resumed.

[a]Values for other nutrients are listed at the back of the book, pages A and B.

[b]Energy allowance during pregnancy is for the 2nd trimester; energy allowance during the 3rd trimester is slightly higher. No additional allowance is provided during the 1st trimester. Energy allowance during lactation is for the first 6 months; energy allowance during the second 6 months is slightly higher.

Table 13–1

High-Risk Pregnancy Factors

- Prepregnancy BMI either <18.5 or ≥25
- Insufficient or excessive pregnancy weight gain
- Nutrient deficiencies or toxicities; eating disorders
- Poverty, lack of family support, low level of education, limited food availability
- Smoking, alcohol, or other drug use
- Age, especially 15 years or younger or 35 years or older
- Many previous pregnancies (3 or more in mothers younger than age 20; 4 or more in mothers age 20 or older)
- Short or long intervals between pregnancies (<18 months or >59 months)
- Previous history of problems such as low- or high-birth-weight infants
- Twins or triplets
- Pregnancy-related hypertension or gestational diabetes
- Diabetes; heart, respiratory, or kidney disease; genetic disorders; special diets and medications

Table 13-2

Daily Food Choices for Pregnancy (2nd and 3rd Trimesters) and Lactation

Food Group	Amount	SAMPLE MENU	
Fruit	2 c	**Breakfast**	**Dinner**
		1 whole-wheat English muffin	Chicken cacciatore
			3 oz chicken
Vegetables	3 c	2 tbs peanut butter	½ c stewed tomatoes
		1 c low-fat vanilla yogurt	1 c rice
		½ c fresh strawberries	½ c summer squash
Grains	8 oz	1 c orange juice	1½ c salad (spinach, mushrooms, carrots)
		Midmorning snack	1 tbs salad dressing
		½ c cranberry juice	1 slice Italian bread
Protein Foods	6½ oz	1 oz pretzels	2 tsp soft margarine
		Lunch	1 c low-fat milk
		Sandwich (tuna salad on whole-wheat bread)	
Milk	3 c	½ carrot (sticks)	
		1 c low-fat milk	

Note: This sample meal plan provides about 2,500 calories (55% from carbohydrate, 20% from protein, and 25% from fat) and meets most of the vitamin and mineral needs of pregnant and lactating women.

The protein DRI during pregnancy calls for 25 grams per day more than for non-pregnant women, but most U.S. women need no additional protein-rich foods, because they already consume plenty of meats, seafood, poultry and eggs. Low-fat milk and milk products provide protein, calcium, vitamin D, and other nutrients.

Some vegetarian women limit or omit protein-rich meats, eggs, and milk products. For them, meeting the recommendation for food energy each day and including plant-protein foods such as legumes, tofu, whole grains, nuts, and seeds are imperative. Protein supplements during pregnancy can be harmful to infant development, and their use is discouraged.

The high nutrient requirements of pregnancy leave little room in the diet for excess fat, especially solid fats such as fatty meats and butter. The essential fatty acids, however, are particularly important to the growth and development of the fetus.[13] The brain is composed mainly of lipid material and depends heavily on long-chain omega-3 and omega-6 fatty acids for its growth, function, and structure. Fish consumption during pregnancy provides a rich source of omega-3 fatty acids and improves brain development and cognition in infants.[14] Table 5–5 (p. 164) lists food sources of omega-3 and omega-6 fatty acids.

KEY POINTS

- Pregnancy brings physiological adjustments that demand increased intakes of energy and nutrients.
- A balanced nutrient-dense diet is essential for meeting nutrient needs.

Of Special Interest: Folate and Vitamin B$_{12}$ Two vitamins famous for their roles in cell reproduction—folate and vitamin B$_{12}$—are needed in increased amounts during pregnancy. New cells are laid down at a tremendous pace as the fetus grows and develops. At the same time, the number of the mother's red blood cells must rise because her blood volume increases, a function requiring more cell division and therefore more vitamins. To accommodate these needs, the recommendation for folate during pregnancy increases from 400 to 600 micrograms a day.

As described in Chapter 7, folate plays an important role in preventing neural tube defects. To review, the early weeks of pregnancy are a critical period for the formation and closure of the **neural tube** that will later develop to form the brain and spinal cord. By the time a woman suspects she is pregnant, usually around the sixth week of pregnancy, the embryo's neural tube normally has closed. A **neural tube defect (NTD)**

neural tube the embryonic tissue that later forms the brain and spinal cord.

neural tube defect (NTD) a group of abnormalities of the brain and spinal cord that may appear at birth, caused by interruption of the normal early development of the neural tube.

Chapter 13 Life Cycle Nutrition: Mother and Infant

Figure 13–4

Spina Bifida

Spina bifida, a common neural tube defect, occurs when the vertebrae of the spine fail to close around the spinal cord, leaving it unprotected. The B vitamin folate helps prevent spina bifida and other neural tube defects.

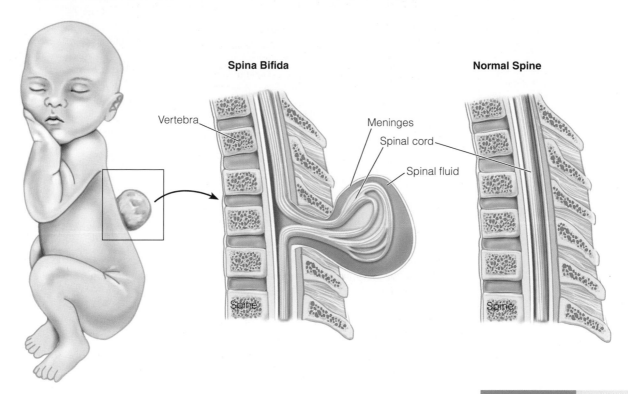

occurs when the tube fails to close properly. Each year in the United States, an estimated 3,000 pregnancies are affected by NTDs.[15] The two most common types of NTD are anencephaly (no brain) and spina bifida (split spine).

In **anencephaly**, the upper end of the neural tube fails to close. Consequently, the brain is either missing or fails to develop. Pregnancies affected by anencephaly often end in miscarriage; infants born with anencephaly die shortly after birth.

Spina bifida is characterized by incomplete closure of the spinal cord and its bony encasement (see Figure 13–4). The membranes covering the spinal cord and sometimes the cord itself may protrude from the spine as a sac. Spina bifida often produces paralysis in varying degrees, depending on the extent of spinal cord damage. Mild cases may not be noticed. Moderate cases may involve curvature of the spine, muscle weakness, mental handicaps, and other ills; severe cases can result in death. Table 13–3 lists risk factors for neural tube defects.

To reduce the risk of neural tube defects, women who are capable of becoming pregnant are advised to obtain 400 micrograms of folic acid daily from supplements, fortified foods, or both, *in addition* to eating folate-rich foods (see Table 13–4, p. 492). The DRI committee recommends synthetic folate—folic acid—in supplements and fortified foods because it is better absorbed than the folate naturally present in foods. Foods that naturally contain folate are still important, however, because they contribute to folate intakes while providing other needed vitamins, minerals, fiber, and phytochemicals.

The folic acid enrichment of grain products (cereal, grits, pasta, rice, bread, and the like) sold commercially in the United States has improved the folate status of women of childbearing age and lowered the number of neural tube defects that occur each year.[16] A safety concern arises, however. Pregnant women also need a greater amount of vitamin B_{12} to assist folate in the manufacture of new cells. Because high intakes of folate complicate the diagnosis of a vitamin B_{12} deficiency, quantities of 1 milligram of folic acid or more require a prescription. Most over-the-counter (OTC) multivitamin

Table 13–3

Risk Factors for Neural Tube Defects

A pregnancy affected by a neural tube defect can occur in any woman, but these factors make it more likely:

- A personal or family history of a pregnancy affected by a neural tube defect.
- Maternal diabetes.
- Maternal use of certain antiseizure medications.
- Mutations in folate-related enzymes.
- Maternal obesity.

anencephaly (an-en-SEFF-ah-lee) an uncommon and always fatal neural tube defect in which the brain fails to form.

spina bifida (SPY-na BIFF-ih-duh) one of the most common types of neural tube defects, in which gaps occur in the bones of the spine. Often the spinal cord bulges and protrudes through the gaps, resulting in a number of motor and other impairments.

Table 13–4

Rich Folate Sources[a]

Natural Folate Sources	Fortified Folic Acid Sources
Liver (3 oz) 221 μg DFE[b]	Highly enriched ready-to-eat cereals (¾ c) 680 μg DFE[c]
Lentils (½ c) 179 μg DFE	Pasta, cooked (1 c) 154 (average value) μg DFE
Chickpeas or pinto beans (½ c) 145 μg DFE	Rice, cooked (1 c) 153 μg DFE
Asparagus (½ c) 134 μg DFE	Bagel (1 small whole) 156 μg DFE
Spinach (1 c raw) 58 μg DFE	Waffles, frozen (2) 78 μg DFE
Avocado (½ c) 61 μg DFE	Bread, white (1 slice) 48 μg DFE
Orange juice (1 c) 74 μg DFE	
Beets (½ c) 68 μg DFE	

[a]Folate amounts for these and thousands of other foods are listed in the USDA Nutrient Database, https://ndb.nal.usda.gov/ndb/search/list.

[b]Dietary folate equivalent (see Chapter 7).

[c]Folic acid in cereals varies; read the Nutrition Facts panel of the label.

supplements contain 400 micrograms of folic acid; supplements for pregnant women usually contain at least 800 micrograms.

People who eat meat, eggs, or milk and milk products receive all the vitamin B$_{12}$ they need, even for pregnancy. Those who exclude all foods of animal origin from the diet need vitamin B$_{12}$–fortified foods or supplements.

KEY POINTS

- Folate and vitamin B$_{12}$ play key roles in cell replication and are needed in large amounts during pregnancy.
- Folate plays an important role in preventing neural tube defects.

Choline   Although not defined as a vitamin, choline is commonly grouped with the B vitamins. Choline is a dietary component that is vital for the structural integrity of cell membranes, the synthesis of an important neurotransmitter, and the metabolism of lipids. During fetal development, choline is needed for the normal development of the brain and spinal cord.[17] During pregnancy, large amounts of choline are delivered to the fetus via the placenta. This transfer of choline from mother to fetus depletes maternal stores.

The DRI value for choline in pregnancy is set at 450 milligrams per day, which is slightly higher than for nonpregnant women. Because prenatal supplements do not typically contain choline, pregnant women are advised to include choline-rich foods such as eggs, milk and milk products, legumes, and meats and seafood regularly in their meals.

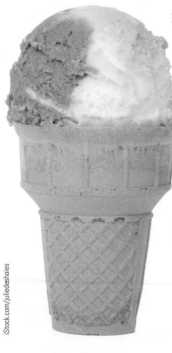

iStock.com/juliedeshaies

Vitamin D and Calcium   Vitamin D and the minerals involved in building the skeleton—calcium, phosphorus, and magnesium—are in great demand during pregnancy. Insufficient intakes may adversely affect fetal bone growth and tooth development.

Vitamin D plays a vital role in calcium absorption and use. Severe maternal vitamin D deficiency interferes with normal calcium metabolism and, in rare cases, may cause the vitamin D–deficiency disease rickets in a newborn.[18] Regular exposure to sunlight and consumption of vitamin D–fortified milk are usually sufficient to provide the recommended amount of vitamin D during pregnancy (15 μg), which is the same as for nonpregnant women. The vitamin D in prenatal supplements helps protect many, but not all, pregnant women from inadequate intakes.[19]

A woman's intestinal absorption of calcium doubles early in pregnancy, and the extra mineral is stored in her bones. Later, as the fetal bones begin to calcify, a dramatic shift of calcium across the placenta occurs. In the final weeks of pregnancy, more than 300 milligrams of calcium a day are transferred to the fetus. Still unknown is whether the extra calcium added to the mother's bones early in pregnancy is withdrawn later to help meet the fetus's needs.

Typically, young women in this country take in too little calcium. Of particular importance, pregnant women younger than age 25, whose own bones are still actively depositing minerals, should strive to meet the DRI by increasing their intakes of calcium-rich foods. The calcium DRI for pregnant women is the same as for nonpregnant women of the same age group. To meet it, the USDA Eating Patterns suggest consuming three cups per day of fat-free or low-fat milk or the equivalent in milk products. Women who exclude milk products need calcium-fortified foods such as soy milk, orange juice, and cereals. Less preferred is a daily supplement of 600 milligrams of calcium.

Iron   A pregnant woman needs iron to help increase her blood volume and to provide for placental and fetal needs. A developing fetus draws heavily on the mother's iron stores to accumulate sufficient stores of its own to last through the first 4 to 6 months after birth. During the second and third trimesters of pregnancy, the hormone hepcidin, which regulates iron balance, is suppressed, and the mobilization of iron from maternal stores is enhanced.[20] The transfer of iron to the fetus is regulated by the placenta, which gives the iron needs of the fetus priority over those of the mother.[21] Even a woman with inadequate iron stores transfers a considerable amount of iron to the fetus. In addition, blood losses are inevitable at birth, especially during delivery by cesarean section, further draining the mother's iron supply. Women who enter pregnancy with iron-deficiency anemia have greater-than-normal risks of delivering low-birthweight or preterm infants.

During pregnancy, the body makes several adaptations to help meet the exceptionally high need for iron. Menstruation, the major route of iron loss in women, ceases, and absorption of iron increases up to threefold. Even so, to help prevent iron supplies from dwindling during pregnancy, all women capable of becoming pregnant are advised do three things:

1. Choose foods that supply heme iron (meat, fish, and poultry), which is most readily absorbed.
2. Choose additional iron sources, such as eggs, vegetables, and legumes.
3. Along with foods rich in iron, choose foods that enhance its absorption, such as vitamin C–rich fruits and vegetables.

Without corrective action, a woman's iron deficit worsens with each successive pregnancy. Few women enter pregnancy with adequate iron stores, so a daily 30-milligram iron supplement is recommended early in pregnancy, if not before.[22] A woman with a severe deficiency may need more. To enhance iron absorption, the supplement should be taken between meals and with liquids other than milk, coffee, or tea, which inhibit iron absorption.

Zinc   Zinc is vital for protein synthesis and cell development during pregnancy. Typical zinc intakes of pregnant women are lower than recommendations, but fortunately zinc absorption increases when intakes are low. Large doses of iron can interfere with zinc absorption and metabolism, but most prenatal supplements supply the right balance of these minerals for pregnancy. Zinc is abundant in protein-rich foods such as shellfish, meat, and nuts.

KEY POINTS
- Choline is needed for the normal development of the fetus's brain and spinal cord.
- Adequate vitamin D and calcium are indispensable for normal fetal bone development.
- Iron supplements are recommended for pregnant women.
- Zinc is needed for protein synthesis and cell development during pregnancy.

Prenatal Supplements   A healthy pregnancy and optimal infant development depend heavily on the mother's diet.[23] Pregnant women can meet most of their nutrient needs—except for iron—by making wise food choices. Even so, physicians routinely recommend **prenatal supplements**, which provide more folate, iron, and calcium than regular supplements. Women with poor diets need them urgently, as do women in these high-risk groups: women carrying twins or triplets and women who smoke cigarettes,

prenatal supplements nutrient supplements specifically designed to provide the nutrients needed during pregnancy—particularly folate, iron, and calcium—without excesses or unneeded constituents.

drink alcohol, or abuse drugs.[24] For these women in particular, prenatal supplements may reduce the risks of preterm delivery, low infant birthweights, and birth defects.

KEY POINTS

- Physicians routinely recommend daily prenatal multivitamin–mineral supplements for pregnant women.
- Prenatal supplements are most likely to benefit women who do not eat adequately, who are carrying twins or triplets, or who smoke cigarettes, drink alcohol, or abuse drugs.

Food Assistance Programs

The nationwide **Special Supplemental Nutrition Program for Women, Infants, and Children (WIC)** provides vouchers redeemable for nutritious foods, along with nutrition education and referrals to health and social services, for low-income pregnant and lactating women and their children.[25] WIC-sponsored foods include baby foods, eggs, dried and canned beans and peas, tuna fish, peanut butter, fruit and vegetables and their juices, iron-fortified cereals, milk and cheese, soy-based beverages and tofu, whole-wheat bread, and other whole-grain products. WIC encourages breastfeeding and offers incentives to mothers who feed their infants breast milk. For infants given infant formula, WIC also provides iron-fortified formula.

More than 9 million people—most of them infants and young children—receive WIC benefits each month. Proven benefits from WIC participation include improved nutrient status and growth among infants and children, improved iron status among pregnant women, reduced risks of infant mortality and low birthweight, and reduced maternal and newborn medical costs. In addition to WIC, the Supplemental Nutrition Assistance Program (formerly the Food Stamp Program) can help stretch a low-income family's grocery dollars.

KEY POINTS

- Food assistance programs such as WIC can provide nutritious food for pregnant women of limited financial means.
- Participation in WIC during pregnancy can reduce iron deficiency, infant mortality, low birthweight, and maternal and newborn medical costs.

How Much Weight Should a Woman Gain during Pregnancy?

Women must gain weight during pregnancy—fetal and maternal well-being depends on it. Ideally, a woman will have begun her pregnancy at a healthy weight, and she will gain appropriately for her prepregnancy body mass index (BMI) and the number of fetuses she carries, as shown in Table 13–5. The benefits of proper weight gain include a lower risk of surgical birth, a greater chance of having a healthy birthweight baby, and other positive outcomes for both mothers and infants. Many women exceed the recommended ranges, however, and a few fall short.[26] To improve pregnancy outcomes, researchers and health-care providers are placing greater emphasis on preventing excessive weight gains during pregnancy than in the recent past.[27]

Weight loss during pregnancy is not recommended.[28] An obese woman is advised to gain between 11 and 20 pounds for the best chance of delivering a healthy baby. Ideally, overweight women will achieve a healthy body weight before becoming pregnant, avoid excessive weight gain during pregnancy, and postpone weight loss until after childbirth.

The ideal weight-gain pattern for a woman who begins pregnancy at a healthy weight is 3½ pounds during the first trimester and 1 pound per week thereafter. If a woman gains more than is recommended early in pregnancy, she should not restrict her energy intake later on to lose weight. A sudden, large weight gain is a danger signal, however, because it may indicate the onset of preeclampsia (see the section entitled "Troubleshooting"). The weight a pregnant woman gains is nearly all lean tissue: the placenta, uterus, blood, milk-producing glands, and the fetus itself (see Figure 13–5). The fat she gains is needed later to support lactation.

Special Supplemental Nutrition Program for Women, Infants, and Children (WIC) a USDA program offering low-income pregnant and lactating women and those with infants or preschool children coupons redeemable for specific foods that supply the nutrients deemed most necessary for growth and development. For more information, visit www.fns.usda.gov /wic/women-infants-and-children-wic

Chapter 13 Life Cycle Nutrition: Mother and Infant

Table 13-5

Recommended Pregnancy Weight Gains Based on Prepregnancy Weight

	RECOMMENDED WEIGHT GAIN	
Prepregnancy Weight	*For single birth*	*For twin birth*
Underweight (BMI <18.5)	28 to 40 lb (12.5 to 18.0 kg)	Insufficient data to make recommendation
Healthy weight (BMI 18.5 to 24.9)	25 to 35 lb (11.5 to 16.0 kg)	37 to 54 lb (17.0 to 25.0 kg)
Overweight (BMI 25.0 to 29.9)	15 to 25 lb (7.0 to 11.5 kg)	31 to 50 lb (14.0 to 23.0 kg)
Obese (BMI ≥30)	11 to 20 lb (5.0 to 9.0 kg)	25 to 42 lb (11.0 to 19.0 kg)

Source: Institute of Medicine, *Weight Gain during Pregnancy: Reexamining the Guidelines* (Washington, D.C.: National Academies Press, 2009).

Weight Loss after Pregnancy

A pregnant woman loses some weight at delivery. In the following weeks, she loses more as her blood volume returns to normal and she loses accumulated fluids. A typical woman does not immediately return to her prepregnancy weight. In general, the more weight a woman gains beyond the needs of pregnancy, the more she retains and the more likely she will continue to gain over the next several years. Even without excessive gain, most women tend to retain a few pounds with each pregnancy. When the weight gain has added up to 7 or more pounds and the BMI has increased by a unit or more, risks of diabetes and hypertension in future pregnancies, as well as chronic diseases later in life, can increase. Women who achieve a healthy weight prior to the first pregnancy and maintain it between pregnancies best avoid the cumulative weight gain that threatens health later on.

KEY POINTS

- Appropriate weight gain is essential for a healthy pregnancy.
- Weight gain recommendations are influenced by the prepregnancy BMI and number of fetuses in the pregnancy.

Figure 13-5

Components of Weight Gain during Pregnancy

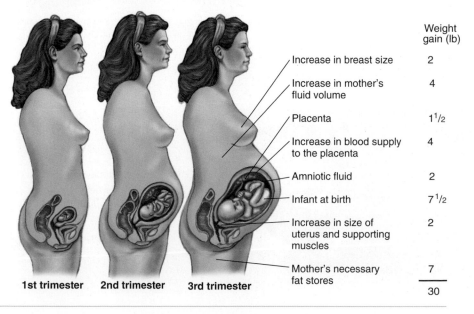

	Weight gain (lb)
Increase in breast size	2
Increase in mother's fluid volume	4
Placenta	1½
Increase in blood supply to the placenta	4
Amniotic fluid	2
Infant at birth	7½
Increase in size of uterus and supporting muscles	2
Mother's necessary fat stores	7
	30

1st trimester   2nd trimester   3rd trimester

Should Pregnant Women Be Physically Active?

An active, physically fit woman experiencing a normal, healthy pregnancy can and should continue to exercise throughout pregnancy, adjusting the intensity and duration as the pregnancy progresses. Staying active improves the fitness of the mother-to-be, facilitates labor, helps to prevent or manage gestational diabetes, and reduces psychological stress.[29] Active women report fewer discomforts throughout their pregnancies and are more likely to meet weight gain recommendations and retain habits that help to lose excess weight and regain fitness later.[30]

Pregnant women should choose low-impact activities and avoid sports in which they might fall or be hit by other people or objects. (For some safe activity suggestions, see the Think Fitness box.) Pregnant women with medical conditions or pregnancy complications should seek medical advice before engaging in physical activity. (A few more guidelines are offered in Figure 13–6.) Several of the guidelines are aimed at preventing excessively high internal body temperature and dehydration, both of which can harm fetal development. To this end, pregnant women should also stay out of saunas, steam rooms, and hot whirlpools.

KEY POINTS

- Physically fit women can continue physical activity throughout pregnancy but should choose activities wisely.
- Pregnant women should avoid sports in which they might fall or be hit and should not become overheated or dehydrated.

Teen Pregnancy

The number of infants born to teenaged mothers has steadily declined during the last 50 years. Despite this decline, however, the U.S. teen birthrate is still one of highest among industrialized nations. In 2016, more than 209,000 infants were born to teenaged U.S. mothers.[31]

A pregnant adolescent presents a special case of intense nutrient needs. Young teenage girls have a hard enough time meeting nutrient needs for their own rapid growth and development, let alone those of pregnancy. Many teens enter pregnancy with deficiencies of vitamins B_{12} and D, folate, iron, and calcium that can impair fetal growth.[32] Pregnant adolescents are less likely to receive early prenatal care and are

---

Figure 13–6

Guidelines for Physical Activity during Pregnancy

Pregnant women can enjoy the benefits of physical activity.

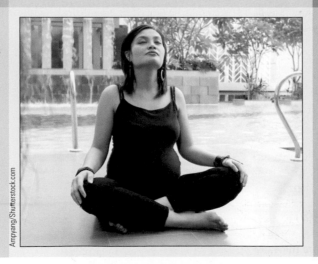

DO		DON'T
Do exercise regularly (most, if not all, days of the week).		Don't exercise vigorously after long periods of inactivity.
Do warm up with 5 to 10 minutes of light activity.		Don't exercise in hot, humid weather.
Do 30 minutes or more of moderate physical activity.		Don't exercise when sick with fever.
Do cool down with 5 to 10 minutes of slow activity and gentle stretching.		Don't exercise while lying on your back after the first trimester of pregnancy or stand motionless for prolonged periods.
Do drink water before, during, and after exercise.		Don't exercise if you experience any pain or discomfort.
Do eat enough to support the additional needs of pregnancy plus exercise.		Don't participate in activities that may harm the abdomen or involve jerky, bouncy movements.
Do rest adequately.		Don't scuba dive.

Ampyang/Shutterstock.com

Is there an ideal physical activity for pregnant women? There might be. Swimming and water aerobics offer advantages over other activities during pregnancy. Water cools and supports the body, provides a natural resistance, and lessens the impact of the body's movement, especially in the later months. Water aerobics can help reduce the intensity of back pain during pregnancy. Other activities considered safe and comfortable for pregnant women include walking, light strength training, rowing, yoga, and climbing stairs.

start now! Ready to make a change? If you weren't exercising regularly before you became pregnant, talk to your doctor before undertaking an activity. Track your activity daily using the Diet and Wellness Plus Activity Tracker in MindTap.

---

more likely to smoke during pregnancy—two factors that predict low birthweight and infant death.[33] The rates of stillbirths, preterm births, and low-birthweight infants are high when either parent is a teen. Adequate nutrition and appropriate weight gain during pregnancy are indispensable components of prenatal care for teenagers and can substantially improve the outlook for both mother and infant.

A pregnant teenager with a healthy body weight is encouraged to gain about 35 pounds. Pregnant and lactating teenagers can follow the USDA Healthy U.S.-Style Eating Pattern presented in Table E–1 (p. E-2), choosing a calorie level high enough to support adequate, but not excessive, weight gain.

KEY POINTS

- Pregnant teenage girls have extraordinarily high nutrient needs and an increased likelihood of problem pregnancies.
- Adequate nutrition and appropriate weight gain for pregnant teenagers can substantially improve outcomes for mothers and infants.

Why Do Some Women Crave Pickles and Ice Cream While Others Can't Keep Anything Down?

Does pregnancy give a woman the right to demand pickles and ice cream at 2 a.m.? Perhaps so, but not for nutrition's sake. Food cravings and aversions during pregnancy are common but do not seem to reflect real physiological needs. In other words, a woman who craves pickles is probably not in need of salt. Food cravings and aversions that arise during pregnancy may be due to hormone-induced changes in taste and sensitivities to smells, and they quickly disappear after the birth.

Some pregnant women respond to cravings by eating nonfood items such as laundry starch, clay, soil, or ice—a practice known as pica.[34] Pica may be practiced for cultural reasons that reflect a society's folklore. Chapter 8 provides more details.

The nausea of "morning sickness" may actually occur at any time and may even be a welcome sign of a healthy pregnancy because it arises from the normal, expected hormonal changes of early pregnancy.[35] Morning sickness typically peaks at 9 weeks of gestation and resolves within a month or two. Many women complain that odors, especially cooking smells, make them feel nauseated, so minimizing odors may provide some relief. Traditional strategies for quelling nausea are listed in Table 13–6, but little evidence exists to support them.[36] Some women do best by simply eating what they desire whenever they feel hungry. Morning sickness can be persistent, however, and if it interferes with normal eating for more than a week or two, a woman should seek medical help to prevent nutrient deficiencies.

As the hormones of pregnancy alter her muscle tone and the thriving fetus crowds her intestinal organs, an expectant mother may complain of heartburn or constipation. Raising the head of the bed with two or three pillows can help relieve nighttime heartburn. A high-fiber diet, physical activity, and a plentiful fluid intake will help relieve

Table 13–6

Tips for Relieving Common Discomforts of Pregnancy

To alleviate the nausea of pregnancy:

- On waking, get up slowly.
- Eat dry toast or crackers.
- Chew gum or suck hard candies.
- Eat small, frequent meals whenever hunger strikes.
- Avoid foods with offensive odors.

To prevent or alleviate constipation:

- Eat foods high in fiber.
- Exercise daily.
- Drink at least 8 cups of liquids a day.
- Respond promptly to the urge to defecate.
- Use laxatives only as prescribed by a physician.

To prevent or relieve heartburn:

- Relax and eat slowly.
- Chew food thoroughly.
- Eat small, frequent meals.
- Drink liquids between meals.
- Avoid spicy or greasy foods.
- Sit up while eating.
- Wait an hour after eating before lying down.
- Wait 2 hours after eating before exercising.

constipation. Pregnant women should use laxatives or heartburn medications only if their physician prescribes them.

KEY POINTS

- Food cravings usually do not reflect physiological needs, and some may interfere with nutrition.
- Nausea arises from normal hormonal changes of pregnancy.

Some Cautions for Pregnant Women

Some choices that pregnant women make or substances they encounter can harm the fetus, sometimes severely. Smoking and other threats all deserve consideration, but alcohol constitutes an even greater threat to fetal health and is given a section of its own.

Cigarette Smoking Parental smoking can kill an otherwise healthy fetus or newborn. Unfortunately, an estimated 10 percent of pregnant women in the United States smoke, and rates are even higher for unmarried women and non–high school graduates.[37]

Constituents of cigarette smoke, such as nicotine, carbon monoxide, arsenic, and cyanide, are toxic to a fetus.[38] Smoking during pregnancy can damage fetal DNA, and can lead to developmental defects or diseases such as cancer.[39] Smoking restricts the blood supply to the growing fetus and so limits the delivery of oxygen and nutrients and the removal of wastes. It slows fetal growth, can reduce brain size, and may impair the intellectual and behavioral development of a child later in life.[40] Smoking during pregnancy damages fetal blood vessels, an effect that is still apparent at the age of 5 years.

A mother who smokes is more likely than others to have a complicated birth and a low-birthweight infant. The more a mother smokes, the smaller her baby will be. Of all preventable causes of low birthweight in the United States, smoking exerts the greatest impact. Table 13–7 lists complications of smoking during pregnancy.

Smoking during pregnancy interferes with fetal lung development and increases the risks of respiratory infections and childhood asthma.[41] Sudden infant death syndrome (SIDS), the unexplained deaths that sometimes occur in otherwise healthy infants, has been linked to the mother's cigarette smoking during pregnancy.[42] Even in nonsmokers, regular exposure to **environmental tobacco smoke** (or secondhand smoke) during pregnancy increases the risk of low birthweight and the likelihood of SIDS.

Alternatives to smoking—such as e-cigarettes, using snuff, chewing tobacco, or using nicotine-replacement therapy—are not safe during pregnancy. A woman who uses nicotine in any form and who expects to become pregnant or is already pregnant should quit.

Medicinal Drugs and Herbal Supplements Medicinal drugs taken during pregnancy can cause birth defects. A pregnant woman should not take OTC drugs or any medications unless they are prescribed by her physician; even then, she should read the labels and take warnings seriously.

Some pregnant women mistakenly consider herbal supplements to be safe alternatives to medicinal drugs and take them to relieve nausea, promote water loss, alleviate depression, aid sleep, or for other reasons. Some herbal products may be safe, but almost none have been tested for safety or effectiveness during pregnancy. Pregnant women should stay away from herbal supplements, teas, or other products unless their safety during pregnancy has been established.[43]

Drugs of Abuse Drugs of abuse such as methamphetamine and cocaine easily cross the placenta and impair fetal growth and development. Furthermore, such drugs are responsible for preterm births, low-birthweight infants, and sudden infant deaths. If infants who are impaired in these ways survive, they suffer central nervous system damage; their cries, sleep, and behaviors early in life are abnormal, and their cognitive development later in life is impaired.[44] They may be hypersensitive or underaroused; many suffer the symptoms of withdrawal. Delays in their growth and development persist throughout childhood and adolescence.

Table 13–7

Complications Associated with Smoking during Pregnancy

- Fetal growth restriction
- Preterm birth
- Low birthweight
- Premature separation of the placenta
- Miscarriage
- Stillbirth
- Sudden infant death syndrome
- Congenital malformations

---

environmental tobacco smoke the combination of exhaled smoke (mainstream smoke) and smoke from lighted cigarettes, pipes, or cigars (sidestream smoke) that enters the air around smokers and may be inhaled by other people. Also called *second-hand smoke*.

Chapter 13 Life Cycle Nutrition: Mother and Infant

Table 13-8

Advice for Pregnant (and Lactating) Women Eating Fish

Best choices Eat 2–3 servings/week	Anchovy, Atlantic croaker, Atlantic mackerel, black sea bass, butterfish, catfish, clam, cod, crab, crawfish, flounder, haddock, hake, herring, lobster, mullet, oyster, Pacific chub mackerel, perch, pickerel, plaice, pollock, salmon, sardine, scallop, shad, shrimp, skate, smelt, sole, squid, tilapia, trout, tuna (canned light), whitefish, whiting
Good choices Eat 1 serving/week	Atlantic tilefish, bluefish, buffalo fish, carp, Chilean sea bass, grouper, halibut, mahi mahi, monkfish, Pacific croaker, rockfish, sablefish, sea trout, sheepshead, snapper, Spanish mackerel, striped bass, tuna (yellowfin and albacore, white tuna, canned and fresh/frozen), white croaker
Poor choices Avoid eating	King mackerel, marlin, orange roughy, shark, swordfish, Gulf of Mexico tilefish, tuna (bigeye)

Source: FDA and EPA, Eating fish: What pregnant women and parents should know (2017), available at www.fda.gov/Food/ResourcesForYou/Consumers/ucm393070.htm.

Environmental Contaminants Pregnant women who are exposed to contaminants such as lead may bear low-birthweight infants with delayed mental and psychomotor development and who therefore struggle to survive. During pregnancy, the heavy metal lead readily moves across the placenta into the fetus's body, inflicting severe damage on a developing fetal nervous system. For pregnant women, choosing a diet free of lead contamination takes on extra urgency. Adequate dietary calcium can help defend against lead toxicity by reducing its absorption.

Fatty fish is a good source of omega-3 fatty acids, but some species contain large amounts of the pollutant mercury that can harm the developing fetal brain and nervous system (described in Chapter 12). The benefits of eating fish and shellfish greatly outweigh the dangers so pregnant and lactating women are urged to consume 8 to 12 ounces of lower-mercury cooked or canned fish and seafood (see Table 13–8), and to avoid the high-mercury species listed at the bottom of the table.[45]

Foodborne Illness The vomiting and diarrhea caused by many foodborne illnesses can leave a pregnant woman exhausted and dangerously dehydrated. Particularly threatening, however, is **listeriosis**, which can cause miscarriage, stillbirth, or severe brain or other infections in fetuses and newborns.[46] Pregnant women are more likely than other healthy adults to contract listeriosis. A woman with listeriosis may develop symptoms such as fever, vomiting, and diarrhea in about 12 hours after eating a contaminated food and serious symptoms may develop a week to six weeks later. A blood test can reliably detect listeriosis, and antibiotics given promptly to a pregnant sufferer can often prevent infection of the fetus or newborn. To protect herself and her fetus from listeriosis, a pregnant woman should follow all of the food safety advice given in Chapter 12. In addition, she should observe the following recommendations:

- Use only pasteurized juices and dairy products; do not eat soft cheeses such as feta, brie, Camembert, panela, "queso blanco," "queso fresco," and blue-veined cheeses such as Roquefort; do not drink raw (unpasteurized) milk or eat foods that contain it.
- Do not eat hot dogs or luncheon or deli meats unless they are heated until steaming hot.
- Thoroughly cook meat, poultry, eggs, and seafood.
- Wash all fruit and vegetables.
- Avoid refrigerated patés or smoked seafood or fish labeled "nova-style," "lox," or "kippered." Canned varieties are generally safe.
- Do not eat ham, chicken, or seafood salads made in delicatessens, restaurants, or stores. Make these salads at home following food safety guidelines, or buy canned varieties.

listeriosis a serious foodborne infection that can cause severe brain infection or death in a fetus or a newborn; caused by the bacterium *Listeria monocytogenes*, which is found in soil and water.

Vitamin–Mineral Overdoses   Many vitamins and minerals are toxic when taken in excess.[47] Excess vitamin A is widely known for causing malformations of the cranial nervous system in the fetus. Intakes before the seventh week of pregnancy appear to be the most damaging. For this reason, vitamin A supplements are not given during pregnancy unless there is specific evidence of deficiency, which is rare.

Restrictive Dieting   Restrictive dieting, even for short periods, can be hazardous during pregnancy. In particular, low-carbohydrate diets or fasts that cause ketosis deprive a growing fetal brain of needed glucose and may impair cognitive development. Such diets are also likely to lack other nutrients vital to fetal growth. Regardless of prepregnancy weight, pregnant women need adequate diets to support healthy fetal development.

Sugar Substitutes   Artificial sweeteners have been studied extensively and found to be acceptable during pregnancy if used within the FDA's guidelines. Women with inborn errors of metabolism should not use products that contain compounds that they can't metabolize. For example, a woman with phenylketonuria (PKU) should not ingest the artificial sweetener aspartame.

Caffeine   Caffeine crosses the placenta, and the fetus has only a limited ability to metabolize it. Even so, women can safely consume up to two cups a day without apparent ill effects on their pregnancy duration or outcome.[48] Limited evidence suggests that heavy use—intakes equaling more than three cups of coffee a day—may increase risks of miscarriage and low birthweight.[49] The most sensible course is to limit caffeine consumption to the equivalent of two cups of coffee or three 12-ounce cola beverages a day. Caffeine amounts in foods and beverages are displayed in Controversy 14 (p. 565).

KEY POINTS

- Smoking during pregnancy delivers toxins to the fetus, damages DNA, restricts fetal growth, and limits the delivery of oxygen and nutrients and the removal of wastes.
- Smoking and other drugs, contaminants such as mercury, foodborne illnesses, large supplemental doses of nutrients, weight-loss diets, and excessive use of artificial sweeteners and caffeine should be avoided during pregnancy.

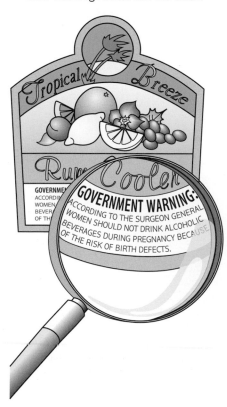

Figure 13–7

Mixed Messages in Alcohol Advertisements

Labels on alcoholic beverages often display "healthy" images, but their warnings must tell the truth.

Drinking during Pregnancy

LO 13.2   Summarize the evidence against alcohol use during pregnancy.

Alcohol is arguably the most hazardous drug to future generations because it is legally available, heavily promoted, and widely abused. Society sends mixed messages concerning alcohol. Beverage companies promote images of drinkers as healthy and active. Opposing these images, health authorities warn that alcohol can injure health, especially during pregnancy (see Figure 13–7). Every container of beer, wine, liquor, or mixed drinks for sale in the United States is required to warn purchasers of the dangers of drinking during pregnancy.

Alcohol's Effects

Women of childbearing age need to know about alcohol's harmful effects on a fetus. Alcohol crosses the placenta freely and is directly toxic:

- A sudden dose of alcohol can halt the delivery of oxygen through the umbilical cord. The fetal brain and nervous system are extremely vulnerable to a deficit of oxygen or glucose, and alcohol causes both by disrupting placental functioning. Alcohol slows cell division, reducing the number of cells produced and inflicting abnormalities on those that are produced and all of their progeny.
- During the first month of pregnancy, the fetal brain is growing at the rate of 100,000 new brain cells a minute. Even a few minutes of alcohol exposure during this critical period can exert a major detrimental effect.

- Alcohol interferes with placental transport of nutrients to the fetus and can cause malnutrition in the mother; then all of malnutrition's harmful effects compound the effects of the alcohol.
- Before fertilization, alcohol can damage the ovum or sperm in the mother- or father-to-be, leading to abnormalities in the child.

KEY POINTS
- Alcohol crosses the placenta and is directly toxic to the fetus.
- Alcohol limits oxygen delivery to the fetus, slows cell division, and reduces the number of cells that organs produce.

Fetal Alcohol Syndrome

Drinking alcohol during pregnancy threatens the fetus with irreversible brain damage, growth restriction, mental retardation, facial abnormalities, vision abnormalities, and many more health problems—a spectrum of symptoms known as **fetal alcohol spectrum disorders**, or **FASD**. Children at the most severe end of the spectrum (those with all of the symptoms) are defined as having **fetal alcohol syndrome**, or **FAS**. The life-long mental retardation and other tragedies of FAS can be prevented by abstaining from drinking alcohol during pregnancy. Once the damage is done, however, the child remains impaired for life. Figure 13–8 shows the facial abnormalities of FAS, which are easy to recognize. A visual picture of the internal harm is impossible, but that damage seals the fate of the child. FASD is the leading cause of preventable developmental delays and intellectual disabilities in the world.[50]

Even when a child does not develop full FAS, prenatal exposure to alcohol can lead to less severe, but nonetheless serious, mental and physical problems. The cluster of mental problems is known as **alcohol-related neurodevelopmental disorder (ARND)**, and the physical malformations are referred to as **alcohol-related birth defects (ARBD)**.[†] Some of these children show no outward sign of impairment, but others are short in stature or display subtle facial abnormalities. Many perform poorly in school and in social interactions and suffer a subtle form of brain damage. Mood disorders and problem behaviors, such as aggression, are common.

Many children with ARND or ARBD go undiagnosed until problems develop in the preschool years. Upon reaching adulthood, such children are ill equipped for employment, relationships, and the other facets of life most adults take for granted. Alcohol exposure before birth may alter the person's later response to alcohol and other mind-altering drugs, making addictions likely.

KEY POINTS
- The severe birth defects of fetal alcohol syndrome arise from damage done to the fetus by alcohol.
- Lesser conditions, ARND and ARBD, also arise from alcohol use in pregnancy.

Experts' Advice

Despite alcohol's injurious potential, one of every 10 pregnant women drinks alcohol at some time during pregnancy and one out of 33 reports "binge" drinking (four or more drinks on one occasion).[51] Controversy 3 defines binge drinking and other alcohol-related terms.

Women who know they are pregnant and choose to drink alcohol often ask, "How much alcohol is too much?" The damaging effects are dose dependent, becoming greater as the dose increases. Even one drink a day threatens neurological development and behavior. Low birthweight and FAS are reported among infants born to

---
[†]Formerly, ARND and ARBD were grouped together and called fetal alcohol effects (FAE).

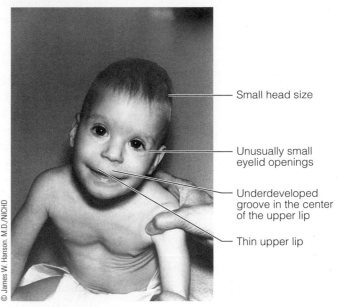

Figure 13–8

Typical Facial Characteristics of FAS

© James W. Hanson, M.D./NICHD

- Small head size
- Unusually small eyelid openings
- Underdeveloped groove in the center of the upper lip
- Thin upper lip

fetal alcohol spectrum disorders (FASD) a spectrum of physical, behavioral, and cognitive disabilities caused by prenatal alcohol exposure.

fetal alcohol syndrome (FAS) the cluster of symptoms including brain damage, growth restriction, mental retardation, and facial abnormalities seen in an infant or child whose mother consumed alcohol during her pregnancy.

alcohol-related neurodevelopmental disorder (ARND) behavioral, cognitive, or central nervous system abnormalities associated with prenatal alcohol exposure.

alcohol-related birth defects (ARBD) malformations in the skeletal and organ systems (heart, kidneys, eyes, ears) associated with prenatal alcohol exposure.

women who drink 1 ounce of alcohol (two drinks) per day during pregnancy, and birth defects are common in infants whose mothers drank 2 ounces a day. Compared with women who do not drink, those who consume 5 or more drinks *per week* experience a sizable and significant increase in stillbirths. The most severe impacts are observed within the first 2 months, when a woman may not even suspect that she is pregnant.

Researchers have looked for a "safe" alcohol intake limit during pregnancy and have found none.[52] Their conclusion: abstinence from alcohol is the only acceptable course of action for pregnant women. Given such evidence, the Dietary Guidelines for Americans 2015 and the American Academy of Pediatrics (AAP) state that women should stop drinking as soon as they *plan* to become pregnant, an important step for fathers-to-be as well. The authors of this book recommend this choice, too. For a pregnant woman who has already been drinking alcohol, the best advice is "Stop now." A woman who has drunk heavily during the first two-thirds of her pregnancy can still prevent some organ damage by stopping during the third trimester.

KEY POINTS

- Alcohol's damaging effects on the fetus are dose dependent, becoming greater as the dose increases.
- Abstinence from alcohol in pregnancy is critical to preventing irreversible damage to the fetus.

Troubleshooting

LO 13.3 List the effects of diabetes, hypertension, and preeclampsia on pregnancy.

Disease during pregnancy can endanger the health of the mother and the health and growth of the fetus. If discovered early, many diseases can be controlled—another reason early prenatal care is recommended.

Diabetes

Pregnancy presents special challenges for the management of diabetes. Pregnant women with unmanaged type 1 or type 2 diabetes may experience episodes of severe hypoglycemia or hyperglycemia, preterm labor, and pregnancy-related hypertension. Infants may be large or may suffer physical and mental abnormalities or other complications such as respiratory distress. Signs of fetal health problems are apparent even in prediabetes, when maternal glucose is only slightly above normal.

Ideally, a woman with signs of diabetes will receive the prenatal care necessary to achieve blood glucose control. During the first trimester and throughout the pregnancy, this control is associated with the lowest frequency of maternal, fetal, and newborn complications. Continued diabetes management after pregnancy will guard the woman's long-term health.

Some women are prone to develop a pregnancy-related form of diabetes, **gestational diabetes**, which puts both mother and child at risk for later problems. The infant may have a high birthweight and face a higher-than-normal risk of illness and mortality; the birth may be difficult and necessitate a cesarian section, and the mother may develop full-blown diabetes later in life, especially if she is overweight.[53]

When gestational diabetes is identified early and managed properly, the most serious risks fall dramatically. To ensure prompt diagnosis and treatment, at the first prenatal visit physicians screen all women who are overweight (BMI ≥25) and who have one or more additional risk factors for type 2 diabetes. (Risk factors include high blood pressure, a family history of diabetes or heart disease, previous gestational diabetes, and membership in a family that is Latinx, African American, Native American, Asian American, or Pacific Islander.) In addition, at 24 to 28 weeks of gestation, all pregnant women not previously diagnosed with diabetes are tested for glucose intolerance.[54]

gestational diabetes abnormal glucose tolerance appearing during pregnancy.

Hypertension

Hypertension during pregnancy may be **chronic hypertension** or **gestational hypertension**. Chronic hypertension is generally present before and remains after pregnancy. In gestational hypertension, blood pressure usually returns to normal during the first few weeks after childbirth. Both types of hypertension pose risks to the mother and fetus; the higher the blood pressure, the worse the risk. In addition to heart attack and stroke, high blood pressure may increase the likelihood of growth restriction, preterm birth, and separation of the placenta from the wall of the uterus before the birth.[55] Both chronic hypertension and gestational hypertension also increase the risk of preeclampsia.

Preeclampsia

Preeclampsia involves both high blood pressure and protein in the urine.[56] Preeclampsia usually occurs in first pregnancies (see Table 13–9 for its warning signs), almost always appears after 20 weeks of gestation, and starts to disappear within a few days after delivery. Because delivery is the only known cure, preeclampsia is a leading cause of medically induced preterm delivery and accounts for about 15 percent of infants who are growth restricted.

Preeclampsia affects almost all of the mother's organs—the circulatory system, liver, kidneys, and brain. If the condition progresses, she may experience seizures; when this occurs, the condition is called **eclampsia**. Maternal deaths during pregnancy are rare in developed countries, but among those that do occur, eclampsia is one of the most common causes. Preeclampsia and eclampsia demand prompt medical attention.

KEY POINTS

- If discovered early, many diseases of pregnancy can be controlled—an important reason early prenatal care is recommended.
- Gestational diabetes, hypertension, and preeclampsia are problems of some pregnancies that must be managed to minimize associated risks.

Lactation

LO 13.4   Explain how nutrition supports lactation.

As the time of childbirth nears, a woman must decide whether she will feed her baby breast milk, infant formula, or both. These are the only foods recommended for infants during the first four to six months of life.

Breastfeeding requires some thoughtful planning. A woman who plans to breastfeed her baby should begin to prepare toward the end of her pregnancy. No elaborate or expensive preparations are needed, but an expectant mother can read one of the many handbooks available on breastfeeding or consult a **certified lactation consultant**, employed at many hospitals.‡ Health-care professionals play an important role in providing encouragement and accurate information on breastfeeding. Part of the preparation involves learning what dietary changes are needed because adequate nutrition is essential to successful lactation. A later section offers tips for breastfeeding.

In rare cases, women produce too little milk to nourish their infants adequately. Severe consequences, including infant dehydration, malnutrition, and brain damage, can occur if the condition goes untreated for long. Early warning signs of insufficient milk are dry diapers (well-fed infants wet about six to eight diapers a day) and infrequent bowel movements.

Nutrition during Lactation

A nursing mother produces about 25 ounces of milk a day, with considerable variation from woman to woman and in the same woman from time to time. The volume

‡La Leche League is an international organization that helps women with breastfeeding concerns: www.lalecheleague.org.

Table 13–9

Warning Signs of Preeclampsia

- Hypertension
- Protein in the urine
- Upper abdominal pain
- Severe and constant headaches
- Swelling, especially of the face
- Dizziness
- Blurred vision
- Sudden weight gain (1 lb/day)

chronic hypertension in pregnant women, hypertension that is present and documented before pregnancy; in women whose prepregnancy blood pressure is unknown, the presence of sustained hypertension before 20 weeks of gestation.

gestational hypertension high blood pressure that develops in the second half of pregnancy and usually resolves after childbirth.

preeclampsia (PRE-ee-CLAMP-seeah) a potentially dangerous condition during pregnancy characterized by hypertension and protein in the urine.

eclampsia (eh-CLAMP-see-ah) a severe complication during pregnancy in which seizures occur.

certified lactation consultant a health-care provider, often a registered nurse or a registered dietitian nutritionist, with specialized training and certification in breast and infant anatomy and physiology who teaches the mechanics of breastfeeding to new mothers.

produced depends primarily on the infant's demand for milk. The more milk the infant needs, the more a well-nourished mother's body will produce, enough to feed the infant—or even twins—amply.

Energy Cost of Lactation   Producing milk costs a woman almost 500 calories per day above her regular need during the first six months of lactation. To meet this energy need, the woman is advised to eat an extra 330 calories of food each day. The other 170 calories can be drawn from the fat stores she accumulated during pregnancy. The food energy consumed by the nursing mother should carry with it abundant nutrients. A lactating woman's nutrient recommendations are listed at the back of the book, pp. A and B. Look again at Table 13–2 (p. 490) for sample menus to meet them.

Fluid Need   Breast milk is 88 percent water, so nursing mothers are advised to drink extra fluid each day (about a quart more than nonlactating women, or 13 cups total) to protect themselves from dehydration.§ As a way of remembering, many women make a habit of drinking a glass of milk, juice, or water each time the baby nurses, as well as at mealtimes.

Variations in Breast Milk   A common question is whether a mother's milk may lack a nutrient if she fails to get enough in her diet. The answer differs from one nutrient to the next, but in general the effect of nutritional deprivation of the mother is to reduce the *quantity* rather than the *quality* of her milk.

Women can produce milk with adequate protein, carbohydrate, fat, folate, and most minerals, by drawing upon maternal stores even when their own supplies are limited. This is most evident in the case of calcium: dietary calcium exerts no effect on the calcium concentration of breast milk, but maternal bones lose some of their density during lactation if calcium intakes are inadequate. Such losses are generally made up quickly when lactation ends, and breastfeeding has no long-term harmful effects on women's bones.

Foods with strong or spicy flavors (such as onions or garlic) may alter the flavor of breast milk. A sudden change in the taste of the milk may annoy some infants, whereas familiar flavors may enhance enjoyment. Flavors imparted to breast milk by the mother's diet can influence the infant's later food preferences.[57] A mother who is breastfeeding her infant is advised to eat whatever nutritious foods she chooses. If a particular food seems to cause an infant discomfort, the mother can eliminate that food from her diet for a few days to see if the problem goes away.

Infants with strong family histories of food allergies generally benefit from breastfeeding. Current evidence, however, does not support a major role for maternal dietary restrictions during lactation to prevent or delay the onset of food allergies in infants.[58]

Lactation and Weight Loss   A common question is whether breastfeeding promotes loss of the extra body fat accumulated during pregnancy. Studies on this question have not provided a definitive answer. How much weight a woman retains after pregnancy depends on her gestational weight gain and the duration and intensity of breastfeeding.[59] Many women who follow recommendations for gestational weight gain and breastfeeding can readily return to prepregnancy weight by six months after giving birth. Neither the quality nor the quantity of breast milk is adversely affected by moderate weight loss, and infants grow normally. Physical activity is also compatible with breastfeeding and infant growth.[60] A gradual weight loss (1 pound per week) is safe and does not reduce milk output. Too large an energy deficit, especially soon after birth, will inhibit lactation.

KEY POINTS

- Lactating women need extra fluid and adequate energy and nutrients for milk production.
- Malnutrition diminishes the quantity of the milk without altering quality.
- Moderate weight loss during lactation does not adversely affect the quality or quantity of breast milk.

---

§The DRI for *total* water intake during lactation is 3.8 L/day. This includes 3.1 L, or about 13 cups of total beverages, including water.

When Should a Woman Not Breastfeed?

Some substances impair maternal milk production or enter breast milk and interfere with infant development, making breastfeeding an unwise choice. Some medical conditions also prohibit breastfeeding.

Alcohol and Illicit Drugs   Alcohol enters breast milk and can adversely affect the production, volume, composition, and ejection of breast milk, as well as overwhelming an infant's immature alcohol-degrading system. Blood alcohol peaks within one hour after ingestion of even moderate amounts (equivalent to a can of beer). This amount may alter the taste of the milk to the disapproval of a nursing infant, who may, in protest, drink less milk than normal. Mothers who use illicit drugs should not breastfeed. Breast milk can deliver doses of drugs so high that they cause irritability, tremors, hallucinations, and even death in infants.

Tobacco and Caffeine   Many women who quit smoking during pregnancy resume after delivery. Lactating women who smoke tobacco produce less milk, and milk of lower fat content, than do nonsmokers. Consequently, infants of smokers gain less weight. A lactating woman who smokes not only transfers nicotine and other chemicals to her infant via her breast milk but also exposes the infant to hazardous sidestream smoke. Babies who are "smoked over" experience a wide array of health problems—poor growth, hearing impairment, vomiting, breathing difficulties, and even unexplained death.[61]

Excess caffeine can make a breastfed infant jittery and wakeful. As during pregnancy, caffeine consumption should be moderate during breastfeeding.

Medications   Many medications pose no danger during breastfeeding, but others may suppress lactation or may be secreted into breast milk and harm the infant.[62] If a nursing mother must take such a medicine, then breastfeeding must be put on hold for the duration of treatment. Meanwhile, the flow of milk can be sustained by pumping the breasts and discarding the milk. A nursing mother should consult with her physician before taking medicines or even herbal supplements—herbs may exert unpredictable effects on breastfeeding infants.

Many women wonder about using oral contraceptives during lactation. One type that combines the hormones estrogen and progestin may suppress milk output and shorten the duration of breastfeeding. In contrast, progestin-only pills have no effect on breast milk or breastfeeding and are considered appropriate for lactating women.

Environmental Contaminants   A woman sometimes hesitates to breastfeed because she has heard warnings that contaminants in fish, water, and other foods may enter breast milk and harm her infant. Although some contaminants do enter breast milk, others may be filtered out. Because formula is made with water, formula-fed infants consume any contaminants that may be in the water supply. With the exception of rare massive exposure to a contaminant, the many benefits of breastfeeding far outweigh any minor risks from environmental hazards in the United States.

Maternal Illness   If a woman has an ordinary cold, she can continue nursing without worry. The infant will probably catch it from her anyway, and thanks to immunological protection, a breastfed baby may be less susceptible than a formula-fed baby. A woman who has tuberculosis (TB) can breastfeed once she has been treated and it is documented that she is no longer infectious. If a woman with TB has not received treatment, breastfeeding is contraindicated.

The human immunodeficiency virus (HIV), responsible for causing HIV/AIDS, can be passed from an infected mother to her infant during pregnancy, at birth, or through breast milk, especially during the early months of breastfeeding. In developed countries such as the United States, where safe alternatives are available, HIV-positive women should not breastfeed their infants.[63] In developing countries, where feeding inadequate, unbalanced, or contaminated formulas causes more than 1 million infant deaths each year, breastfeeding can be critical to infant survival. In each case, the most appropriate infant-feeding option depends on individual circumstances, including the health status of the mother and the local situation, as well as the health services available. The World Health Organization (WHO) recommends exclusive breastfeeding for infants of HIV-infected women for the first six months of life unless replacement feeding is acceptable, feasible, affordable, sustainable, and safe for mothers and their infants. Alternatively, HIV-exposed infants may be protected by receiving drugs known as anti-retrovirals while being breastfed.

KEY POINTS

- Breastfeeding is not advised if a mother's milk is contaminated with alcohol, drugs, or environmental pollutants.
- Most ordinary infections such as colds do not affect breastfeeding infants, but HIV/AIDS may be transmitted through breast milk.

Feeding the Infant

LO 13.5 Identify nutrition practices that promote an infant's well-being.

Early nutrition affects later development, and early feedings establish eating habits that influence nutrition throughout life. Trends change, and experts may argue the fine points, but nourishing a baby is relatively simple. Common sense and a nurturing, relaxed environment go far to promote the infant's well-being.

Nutrient Needs

A baby grows faster during the first year of life than ever again, as shown in Figure 13–9. Pediatricians closely monitor the growth of infants and children because growth directly reflects their nutrition status. An infant's birthweight doubles by about 5 months of age and triples by the age of 1 year. (If a 150-pound adult were to grow like this, the person would weigh 450 pounds after a single year.) The infant's length changes more slowly than weight, increasing about 10 inches from birth to 1 year. By the end of the first year, the growth rate slows considerably; an infant typically gains less than 10 pounds during the second year and grows about 5 inches in height.

Not only do infants grow rapidly, but also their basal metabolic rates are remarkably high—about twice those of adults, based on body weight. The rapid growth and metabolism of an infant demand an ample supply of all the nutrients. Of special importance during infancy are the energy nutrients and the vitamins and minerals critical to the growth process, such as vitamin A, vitamin D, and calcium.

Because they are small, babies need smaller *total* amounts of these nutrients than adults do, but as a percentage of body weight, babies need more than twice as much of most nutrients. Infants require about 100 calories per kilogram of body weight per day; most adults require fewer than 40. Figure 13–10 compares a 5-month-old baby's needs (per unit of body weight) with those of an adult man. You can see that differences in vitamin D and iodine, for instance, are especially extraordinary.

At around 6 months of age, energy needs begin to increase less rapidly as the growth rate begins to slow down, but some of the energy saved by slower growth is spent in increased activity. When their growth slows, infants spontaneously reduce their energy intakes. Parents can expect their babies to adjust their own food intakes to their changing needs; there is no need to force or coax them to eat more than they want.

One of the most important nutrients for infants, as for everyone, is water. The younger a child is, the more of its body weight is water. Breast milk or infant formula normally provides enough water to replace fluid losses in a healthy infant. If the environmental temperature is extremely high, however, infants need supplemental water.[64] Much more of an infant's body water is between

Figure 13–9

Weight Gain of Human Infants and Children in the First Five Years of Life

The colored vertical bars show how the yearly increase in weight gain slows its pace over the years.

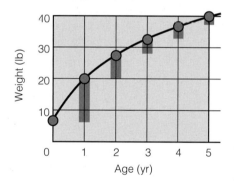

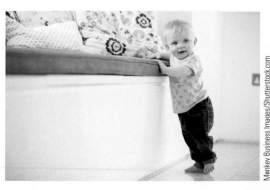

Growth slows in later infancy, but babies become more active.

Chapter 13 Life Cycle Nutrition: Mother and Infant

Figure 13–10

Nutrient Recommendations for a 5-Month-Old Infant and an Adult Male Compared on the Basis of Body Weight

Infants may be relatively small and inactive, but they use large amounts of energy and nutrients in proportion to their body size to keep all their metabolic processes going.

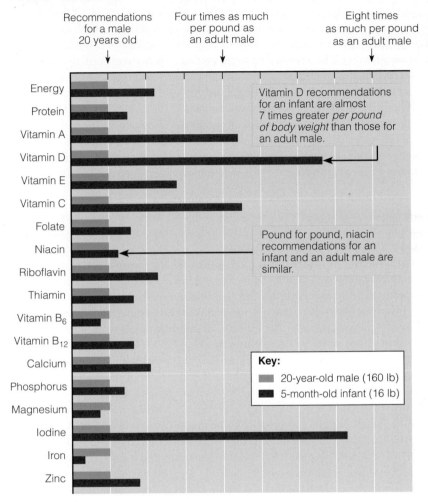

Recommendations for a male 20 years old

Four times as much per pound as an adult male

Eight times as much per pound as an adult male

Vitamin D recommendations for an infant are almost 7 times greater *per pound of body weight* than those for an adult male.

Pound for pound, niacin recommendations for an infant and an adult male are similar.

Key:
- 20-year-old male (160 lb)
- 5-month-old infant (16 lb)

the cells and in the vascular space, and this water is easy to lose. In the event of rapid fluid loss due to vomiting or diarrhea, an electrolyte solution designed for infants (available in drug stores) is needed.

KEY POINTS

- An infant's birthweight doubles by about 5 months of age and triples by 1 year.
- Infants' rapid growth and development depend on adequate nutrient supplies, including water from breast milk or formula.

Why Is Breast Milk So Good for Babies?

Many medical and professional organizations advocate breastfeeding for the best infant nutrition and for the many other benefits it provides both infant and mother (shown in Table 13–10).[65] The AAP and the Academy of Nutrition and Dietetics recommend **exclusive breastfeeding** for 6 months and breastfeeding with complementary foods for at least 12 months as an optimal feeding pattern for infants.[66] All legitimate nutrition authorities share this view, but some makers of baby formula try to convince women otherwise—see the Consumer's Guide (p. 511).

Table 13–10

Benefits of Breastfeeding

For Infants:

- Provides the appropriate composition and balance of nutrients.
- Provides hormones that promote physiological development.
- Improves cognitive development.
- Protects against a variety of infections.
- May protect against some chronic diseases, such as diabetes and hypertension, later in life.
- Protects against food allergies.
- Reduces the risk of sudden infant death syndrome.

For Mothers:

- Contracts the uterus.
- Delays the return of regular ovulation, thus lengthening birth intervals. (It is not, however, a dependable method of contraception.)
- Conserves iron stores (by prolonging amenorrhea).
- May protect against breast and ovarian cancer.

Other:

- Saves on doctor visits for infant illness.
- Saves costs of formulas, bottles, brushes, etc.
- Is an environmentally sustainable option.

exclusive breastfeeding an infant's consumption of human milk with no supplementation of any type (no water, no juice, no nonhuman milk, and no foods) except for vitamins, minerals, and medications.

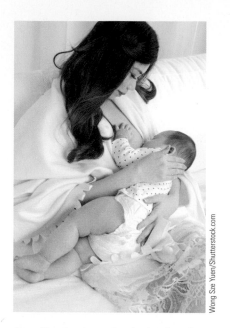

Breastfeeding is a natural extension of pregnancy—the mother's body continues to nourish the infant.

Breast milk excels as a source of nutrients for young infants. With the exception of vitamin D (discussed later), breast milk meets all of a healthy infant's needs for the first 6 months of life. Breast milk also conveys immune factors, which both protect an infant against infection and inform its body about its local environment.

Breastfeeding Tips Breast milk is more easily and completely digested than infant formula, so breastfed infants usually need to eat more frequently than formula-fed infants do. During the first few weeks, the routine recommended to promote optimal milk production and infant growth is approximately 8 to 12 feedings a day, on demand, whenever the infant begins to show signs of hunger such as restlessness, increased activity, or suckling motions. Crying is a late indicator of hunger.[67] An infant who nurses every 2 to 3 hours and sleeps contentedly between feedings is adequately nourished. As the infant gets older, stomach capacity enlarges and the mother's milk production increases, allowing for longer intervals between feedings.

When breastfeeding, the baby draws about half of the milk that is in the breast within the first two or three minutes of suckling, but should be encouraged to continue to nurse on that breast for as long as he or she wishes, before being offered the second breast. The infant's suckling, as well as the complete removal of milk from the breast, stimulates lactation. Begin each feeding on the breast that was offered second, the last time.

Energy Nutrients in Breast Milk Compared with the milk recommended for adults, breast milk is far lower in protein but higher in fat. Yet for infants, breast milk is nature's most nearly perfect food, providing the clear lesson that people at different stages of life have different nutrient needs.

The carbohydrate in breast milk (and standard infant formula) is lactose. In addition to being easily digested by infants, lactose enhances calcium absorption. The carbohydrate component of breast milk also contains abundant oligosaccharides, which are present only in trace amounts in cow's milk and infant formula made from cow's milk.[68] Breast milk oligosaccharides help protect an infant from infection by preventing the binding of pathogens to the infant's intestinal cells.[69]

The lipids in breast milk (and infant formula) provide the infant's main source of energy. Breast milk contains a generous proportion of the essential fatty acids linoleic acid and linolenic acid, as well as their longer-chain derivatives, arachidonic acid and DHA. Most formulas today also contain added arachidonic acid and DHA (read the label). Infants can produce some arachidonic acid and DHA from linoleic and linolenic acid, but some infants may need more than they can make.

DHA is the most abundant fatty acid in the brain and is also present in the retina of the eye. DHA accumulation in the brain is greatest during fetal development and early infancy.[70] Research has focused on the visual and mental development of breastfed infants and infants fed standard formula with and without DHA added.[71] Results of studies for visual acuity development in term infants have been inconsistent. Factors such as the amount of DHA provided, its sources, and the sensitivity of different measures for visual acuity may have contributed to the inconsistent outcomes. As for mental development, a number of studies suggest that DHA supplementation during development can influence certain measures of cognitive function.[72] Still needed are longer-term studies that follow child development beyond infancy.

The protein in breast milk is largely **alpha-lactalbumin**, a protein the human infant can easily digest. Another breast milk protein, **lactoferrin**, is an iron-gathering compound that helps absorb iron into the infant's bloodstream, keeps intestinal bacteria from getting enough iron to grow out of control, and kills certain bacteria.

Vitamins and Minerals in Breast Milk With one exception—vitamin D—the vitamin content of the breast milk of a well-nourished mother is ample. Even vitamin C, for which cow's milk is a poor source, is supplied generously. The concentration of vitamin D in breast milk is low, however, and vitamin D deficiency impairs bone mineralization.[73] Vitamin D deficiency is most likely in infants who are not exposed to sunlight daily, have darkly pigmented skin, and receive breast milk without vitamin D supplementation. About a decade ago, recommendations for infants increased

alpha-lactalbumin (lact-AL-byoo-min) the chief protein in human breast milk.

lactoferrin (lack-toe-FERR-in) a factor in breast milk that binds iron and keeps it from supporting the growth of the infant's intestinal bacteria.

Table 13–11

Supplement Recommendations for Full-Term Infants

Recommendations for all supplements should be based on the health-care provider's assessment of the infant.

Supplements	Birth	4 months	6 months
Vitamin D	All infants who are: ■ Exclusively breastfed. ■ Receiving less than 1 qt (32 oz) of vitamin D–fortified formula per day.	As recommended at birth.	As recommended at birth.
Iron (1 mg per kg of body weight per day)		All infants who are: ■ Exclusively breastfed. ■ Receiving more than one-half of their daily feedings as breast milk and no iron-containing complementary foods.	May not be needed once iron-containing foods are introduced.
Fluoride			All infants who are: ■ Exclusively breastfed. ■ Receiving ready-to-use formulas (which are made with water low in fluoride). ■ Receiving formula mixed with water that contains little or no fluoride (less than 0.3 ppm).

Source: Adapted from the American Academy of Pediatrics, Pediatric Nutrition, 7th ed., ed. R. E. Kleinman (Elk Grove Village, IL: American Academy of Pediatrics, 2014).

for two reasons. First, rickets, the vitamin D–deficiency disease, has been diagnosed among U.S. infants. Second, the AAP recommends that infants younger than 6 months be protected from direct sunlight, eliminating this source of vitamin D.

As for minerals, the calcium content of breast milk is ideal for infant bone growth, and the calcium is well absorbed. Breast milk is also appropriately low in sodium. The limited amount of iron in breast milk is highly absorbable, and its zinc, too, is absorbed well, thanks to the presence of a zinc-binding protein.

Supplements for Infants   Pediatricians may prescribe supplements containing vitamin D, iron, and fluoride (after 6 months of age) as outlined in Table 13–11. Vitamin K nutrition for newborns presents a unique case. A newborn's digestive tract is sterile, and vitamin K–producing bacteria take weeks to establish themselves in the baby's intestines. To prevent bleeding in the newborn, the AAP recommends that a single dose of vitamin K be given at birth.

The AAP currently recommends a vitamin D supplement for all infants who are breastfed exclusively and for any infants who receive less than 1 liter (1,000 milliliters) or 1 quart (32 ounces) of vitamin D–fortified formula daily.[74] Despite these recommendations, most infants in the United States are consuming inadequate amounts of vitamin D.

Immune Factors in Breast Milk   Breast milk offers the infant unsurpassed protection against infection.[75] Its protective factors include antiviral agents, anti-inflammatory agents, antibacterial agents, and infection inhibitors.

During the first two or three days of lactation, the breasts produce **colostrum**, a premilk substance containing antibodies and white cells from the mother's blood. Colostrum (like breast milk) helps protect the newborn infant from infections against which the mother has developed immunity—precisely those in the environment likely to infect the infant. For example, maternal antibodies in colostrum and breast milk

colostrum (co-LAHS-trum) a milklike secretion from the breasts during the first day or so after delivery before milk appears; rich in protective factors.

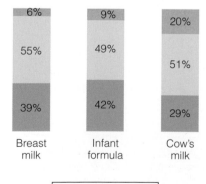

inactivate harmful bacteria within the infant's digestive tract before they can start infections.[76] This explains, in part, why breastfed infants have fewer intestinal infections than formula-fed infants.

Breastfeeding also protects against other common illnesses of infancy, such as middle ear infections and respiratory illnesses.[77] In addition, breastfed infants have fewer allergic reactions such as asthma, wheezing, and skin rash.[78] This protection is especially noticeable among infants with family histories of allergies. Even the risk of SIDS is lower among breastfed infants.[79] This protective effect is stronger when breastfeeding is exclusive, but any amount of breast milk for any duration is protective against SIDS.

In addition to their protective features, colostrum and breast milk contain hormones and other factors that stimulate the development and maintenance of an infant's digestive tract. Clearly, breast milk is a very special substance.

Other Potential Benefits Breastfeeding may offer some protection against excessive weight gain later, although findings are inconsistent.[80] Many other factors—socioeconomic status, other infant- and child-feeding practices, and especially the mother's weight—strongly predict a child's body weight.[81]

The possibility that breastfeeding may positively affect later intelligence is intriguing. Many studies have suggested such benefits, but when subjected to strict standards of methodology (for example, large sample sizes and appropriate intelligence testing), the evidence is less convincing.[82] Most likely, several factors, such as the DHA in breast milk and the feeding process itself, benefit the infant's development. More large, well-controlled studies are needed to discover the effects, if any, of breastfeeding on later intelligence.

KEY POINTS

- With the exception of vitamin D, breast milk provides all the nutrients healthy infants need for the first 4 months of life.
- Breast milk offers infants unsurpassed protection against infection—including antiviral agents, anti-inflammatory agents, antibacterial agents, and infection inhibitors.

Formula Feeding

Formula feeding offers an acceptable alternative to breastfeeding. Nourishment for infants from formula is adequate, and parents can choose this course with confidence. All currently available infant formulas meet all of the energy and nutrient requirements for healthy, full-term infants during the first 6 months of life. After that time, formulas, along with a variety of solid foods, continue to supply a significant part of the infant's nutrient needs. One advantage of formula feeding is that parents can see how much milk the infant drinks during feedings. Another is that family members other than the mother can participate in feeding the infant, giving them a chance to develop the special closeness that feeding fosters.

Mothers who return to work soon after giving birth may choose formula for their infants, but they have another option. Breast milk can be pumped into bottles and given to the baby in day care. At home, mothers may breastfeed as usual. Many mothers use both methods—they breastfeed for at least a month but **wean** their children within the first year. If infants are less than a year old, mothers must wean them onto *infant formula*, not onto plain cow's milk of any kind—whole, reduced-fat, low-fat, or fat-free. Infant formula is available as a powdered or liquid concentrate that must be mixed with water according to label directions and as a ready-to-feed liquid. The powdered form is the least expensive option.

Infant Formula Composition The substitution of formula feeding for breastfeeding involves striving to copy nature as closely as possible. Human milk and cow's milk differ; cow's milk is significantly higher in protein, calcium, and phosphorus, for example, to support the calf's faster growth rate. Thus, to prepare a formula from cow's milk, the formula makers must first dilute the milk, improve its digestibility, and then add carbohydrate and nutrients to make the proportions comparable to those of human milk. Figure 13–11 compares the energy–nutrient balances of breast milk,

iStock.com/ryasick

Figure 13–11

Percentages of Energy-Yielding Nutrients in Breast Milk, Infant Formula, and Cow's Milk

The average proportions of energy-yielding nutrients in human breast milk and formula differ slightly. In contrast, cow's milk provides more protein and less carbohydrate than the ideal amounts for infants.

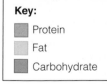

	6%		9%		20%
	55%		49%		51%
	39%		42%		29%
	Breast milk		Infant formula		Cow's milk

Key:
- Protein
- Fat
- Carbohydrate

wean to gradually replace breast milk with infant formula or other foods.

Formula Advertising versus Breastfeeding Advocacy

Formula feed or breastfeed? New mothers must answer this question amid the whirlwind of physical and emotional changes associated with pregnancy and delivery. For a few women, breastfeeding may be contraindicated by illness or physical condition; in a few more cases, special needs of the infant may make breastfeeding impossible. The strong scientific consensus holds, however, that breastfeeding is preferable for all other infants, so why do so many women continue to choose formula? For some, the time and logistics required for breastfeeding compete with work or school schedules; for many others, the decision to forgo breastfeeding is influenced by the aggressive advertising of formulas.

Formula versus Breastfeeding

Advertisements of infant formulas often create the illusion that formula is identical to human milk. No formula can match the nutrients, agents of immunity, and environmental information conveyed to infants through human milk, but the ads are convincing: "Like mother's milk, our formula provides complete nutrition" or "Our brand is scientifically formulated to meet your baby's needs." Misleading or aggressive marketing tactics like these can undermine a woman's confidence concerning her choice to breastfeed, and lack of confidence causes many women to abstain or quit prematurely.[1]*

Formula promoters have in the past aggressively marketed their products—and still do, to some extent in this country and more extensively elsewhere. They give coupons and samples of free formula to pregnant women or arrange for hospitals to distribute these come-ons. However, these practices are on the decline. Between 2007 and 2013, the percentage of U.S. hospitals distributing infant formula discharge samples to mothers breastfeeding their infants decreased markedly from 73 percent to 32 percent,

*References are in Appendix F.

Table 13–12

Tips for Successful Breastfeeding

- Learn about the benefits of breastfeeding.
- Initiate breastfeeding within 1 hour of birth.
- Ask a health-care professional to explain how to breastfeed and how to maintain lactation.
- Give newborn infants no food or drink other than breast milk unless medically indicated.
- Breastfeed on demand.
- Offer no artificial nipples or pacifiers to breastfeeding infants.[a]
- Find support groups, books, or websites that help troubleshoot breastfeeding problems.

[a]Compared with nonusers, infants who use pacifiers breastfeed less frequently and stop breastfeeding at a younger age.

---

most likely thanks to a global effort to promote and support breastfeeding, the Baby Friendly Hospital Initiative.[2]

Breastfeeding Advocacy

National efforts to promote breastfeeding seem to be working, too: the percentage of infants who were breastfed at least for a while rose from 60 percent among those born in 1994 to 81 percent among those born in 2013.[3] Still, this falls short of national goals.[4] Only about 52 percent of infants are still breastfeeding at 6 months of age, and about 30 percent are still doing so at age one.

Many hospitals employ certified lactation consultants who specialize in helping new mothers establish healthy relationships with their newborns. Table 13–12 lists tips for successful long-term breastfeeding.

Where Breastfeeding Is Critical

Infant formula is an appropriate substitute when breastfeeding is specifically contraindicated, but for most infants, the benefits of breast milk outweigh those of formula. Formula-fed infants in developed nations are healthy and grow normally, but they miss out on the breastfeeding advantages described in this text.

In developing nations, however, the consequence of choosing not to breastfeed can be tragic. Feeding formula is often

fatal to infants when poverty limits access to formula mixes, clean water for safe formula preparation, and medical help when needed. The WHO strongly supports breastfeeding for the world's infants in its Baby-Friendly Hospital Initiative and opposes the marketing of infant formulas to new mothers.

Moving Ahead

Women are free to choose between breast milk and formula. Breast milk is recommended and is a thrifty choice; infant formula, bottles, and paraphernalia are expensive for anyone's wallet, particularly after the initial coupons run out. During pregnancy, parents-to-be should seek out the facts about each feeding method and be aware that sophisticated formula advertisements are designed to make sales and not primarily to help potential customers make the best choice.

Review Questions*

1. Commercial infant formula is more reliable than breast milk because it has been scientifically engineered for complete nutrition. T F

2. About 60 percent of U.S. infants are still breastfeeding at one year of age. T F

3. Lactation consultants are employed by hospitals to help new mothers understand the advantages of feeding their babies with infant formula. T F

*Answers to Consumer's Guide review questions are found in Appendix G.

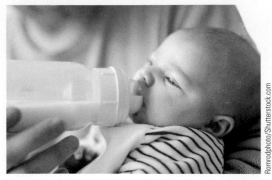

An infant thrives on formula offered with affection.

standard infant formula, and cow's milk. Notice the higher protein concentration of cow's milk, which can stress the infant's kidneys. The AAP recommends that all formula-fed infants receive iron-fortified infant formulas.[83] Use of these formulas has increased in recent decades and is credited with the decline of iron-deficiency anemia in U.S. infants.

Special Formulas   Ordinary formulas are inappropriate for some infants. Special formulas have been designed to meet the dietary needs of infants with specific conditions such as prematurity or inherited diseases. Most infants allergic to milk protein can drink formulas based on soy protein.[84] Soy formulas also use cornstarch and sucrose instead of lactose and so are tolerated by infants with lactose intolerance as well. They are also useful as alternatives to milk-based formulas for vegan families. Infants who are allergic to both cow's milk protein and soy protein may tolerate formulas based on **hydrolyzed protein**.

The Transition to Cow's Milk   For good reasons, the AAP advises that cow's milk is not appropriate for infants younger than one year old.[85] In some infants, particularly those younger than 6 months of age, cow's milk causes intestinal bleeding, which can lead to or aggravate iron deficiency. Cow's milk is a poor iron source. Its higher calcium and lower vitamin C contents also inhibit iron absorption. In summary, plain cow's milk threatens an infant's iron status in three ways: it causes iron loss through bleeding, it fails to provide iron, and its high calcium and low vitamin C contents reduce the bioavailability of iron from other foods. Clearly, then, cow's milk is a poor choice during the first year of life; infants need breast milk or iron-fortified formula.

Once a baby has reached a year of age and is receiving at least two-thirds of total daily food energy from a balanced mixture of cereals, vegetables, fruit, and other foods, reduced-fat or low-fat cow's milk (in the context of an overall diet that supplies 30 percent of calories from fat) is an acceptable and recommended beverage.[86] After the age of 2, a transition to fat-free milk can take place, but care should be taken to provide adequate dietary fat.

KEY POINTS

- Infant formulas are designed to resemble breast milk in nutrient composition.
- After the baby's first birthday, reduced-fat or low-fat cow's milk can replace formula.

An Infant's First Solid Foods

Complementary foods can be introduced into the diet as infants becomes physically ready to handle them. An infant is born knowing how to suckle but cannot handle any kind of solid food at first. The intestines, too, are immature; they can digest lactose but not starch. Eating skills develop in stages, and so do the abilities of the intestines to deal with the foods that are delivered to it. At 4 months or so, the tongue can move against the palate to swallow soft foods and the intestines are becoming able to digest starch. Later, at about a year, the first teeth erupt, but not until sometime during the second year can the baby begin to handle chewy food.

When to Introduce Solid Food   The AAP supports exclusive breastfeeding for 6 months but recognizes that infants are often ready to accept some solid foods between 4 and 6 months of age.[87] Complementary foods can provide needed nutrients that are no longer supplied adequately by breast milk or formula alone. The foods chosen must be those that the infant is developmentally capable of handling both physically and metabolically. The exact timing depends on the infant's needs, readiness, and tolerance to the food, as shown in Table 13–13.

How to Introduce First Foods   It bears repeating that early feeding strategies are critical in establishing healthy food preferences and habits that last throughout life. Infants (and toddlers) learn solely from their caregivers what, when, and how to eat. Caregivers must therefore understand how infants signal hunger and satiety (see Table 13–13) and how to respond to these signals appropriately—a process known as

hydrolyzed (HIGH-druh-lyzed) **protein** a commercial protein ingredient made by way of hydrolysis, a type of chemical reaction that splits molecules, in this case long protein chains, into smaller fragments and attaches water components to make the split possible. Makers of infant formulas hydrolyze the proteins in cow's milk or soybeans to make them less allergenic and more digestible for infants. *Hydro* = water, *lysis* = to cleave.

complementary foods nutrient- and energy-containing solid or semisolid foods (or liquids) fed to infants in addition to breast milk or infant formula.

Table 13–13

Infant Development and Recommended Foods

Each stage of development builds on the previous stage, the foods from an earlier stage continue to be included in all later stages.

Age (mo)	Physical and Developmental Milestones	Satiety Signals	Hunger Signals	Foods Introduced into the Diet
0–4	Turns head toward any object that brushes cheek. Initially swallows using back of tongue; gradually begins to swallow using front of tongue as well. Strong reflex (extrusion) to push food out during first 2 to 3 months.	Seals lips together. Turns head away. Stops sucking. Falls asleep when full.	Wakes and moves around. Sucks on fist. Cries or fusses. Opens mouth while feeding to indicate wanting more.	Breast milk or infant formula.
4–6	Extrusion reflex diminishes, and ability to swallow nonliquid foods develops. Sits erect with support at 6 months. Begins chewing. Brings hand to mouth. Grasps objects with hand.	Sucks slowly or stops sucking. Turns head away and leans back.	Cries or fusses. Indicates desire for food by smiling or cooing during feeding. Indicates desire for food by opening mouth and leaning forward.	Iron-fortified cereal mixed with breast milk, formula, or water. Pureed meats, legumes, vegetables, and fruit.
6–8	Able to feed self with fingers. Develops pincher (finger to thumb) grasp. Begins to drink from cup.	Slows eating. Pushes food away.	Reaches for spoon or food. Points to food.	Textured vegetables and fruit.
8–10	Begins to hold own bottle. Sits unsupported.	Shuts mouth tightly or pushes food away.	Reaches for and grabs spoon and food. Shows excitement when food is presented.	Breads and cereals from table. Yogurt. Pieces of soft, cooked vegetables and fruit from table. Small amounts of finely cut meats, fish, casseroles, cheese, eggs, and legumes.
10–12	Begins to master spoon. Spills less.	May begin using words such as "no," "all done," or "get down." Plays with or throws food when done.	Indicates desire for specific food with words or sounds.	Increasingly varied foods in larger portion sizes.[a]

[a]Portions of foods for infants and young children are smaller than those for an adult. For example, a grain serving might be ½ slice of bread instead of 1 slice or ¼ cup of rice instead of ½ cup.

Source: Adapted in part from R. Pérez-Escamilla, S. Segura-Pérez, and M. Lott, Feeding guidelines for infants and young toddlers, Nutrition Today 52 (2017): 223–231; American Academy of Pediatrics, Pediatric Nutrition, 7th ed., ed. R. E. Kleinman (Elk Grove Village, III. IL: American Academy of Pediatrics, 2014), pp. 123–139.

responsive feeding.[88] When a caregiver clearly and consistently responds to a child's needs at mealtimes, the child learns to identify internal hunger, thirst, and satiety signals; to ask for food or beverages when hungry or thirsty; and to stop eating when full.

Foods to Provide Iron, Zinc, and Vitamin C   Rapid growth demands iron. At about 4 to 6 months, infants begin to need more iron than body stores plus breast milk or iron-fortified formula can provide. In addition to breast milk or iron-fortified formula, infants can receive iron from iron-fortified cereals and, once they readily accept solid foods, from protein foods such as meat, poultry, seafood, eggs, and legumes (see Figure 13–12). Iron-fortified cereals contribute a significant amount of iron to an infant's diet, but the iron's bioavailability is poor.[89] Caregivers can enhance iron absorption from iron-fortified cereals by serving vitamin C–rich foods with meals.

The concentration of zinc in breast milk is initially high but decreases sharply over the first few months of lactation. Although the infant's ability to absorb the zinc in breast milk

responsive feeding an interactive feeding process in which a young child signals hunger and satiety vocally, through facial expressions, and through motor actions; the caregiver recognizes these cues and responds promptly in an emotionally supportive and developmentally appropriate manner. In this way, the child experiences a predictable response to hunger and satiety signals that supports healthy eating behaviors.

Figure 13–12

Iron Sources for Infants

Foods such as iron-fortified cereals and formulas, mashed legumes, and strained meats provide iron.

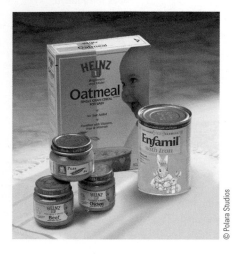

© Polara Studios

Table 13–14

Choking Prevention

To prevent choking, do not give infants or young children:

- Gum
- Popcorn, chips, or pretzel nuggets
- Large raw apple slices
- Whole grapes, whole cherries
- Raw celery; raw carrots
- Whole beans
- Hot dog slices
- Sausage sticks or slices
- Hard or gel-type candies
- Marshmallows
- Nuts
- Peanut butter

Keep these nonfood items out of their reach:

- Coins, balloons, small balls, pen tops, other similar-sized items

is efficient, it does not fully meet the infants' zinc need over time. Infant formulas are fortified with zinc at concentrations higher than those in breast milk. Breastfed infants depend more on complementary foods to provide adequate zinc intakes than do formula-fed infants. Infant cereals are not routinely fortified with zinc, so again, the best sources are protein foods such as meats, poultry, seafood, eggs, and legumes. (Zinc is less well absorbed from legumes than from the other protein foods.)

The best sources of vitamin C are fruit and vegetables (see Snapshot 7–5, p. 240). Fruit juice is a source of vitamin C, but too much juice can cause diarrhea in young children.[90] Furthermore, too much fruit juice contributes excessive calories and displaces other nutrient-rich foods. The AAP recommends no fruit juice for infants before one year of age and limiting juice for toddlers (1 to 3 years of age) to 4 ounces per day. For children 4 to 6 years of age, limiting juice to 6 ounces per day is recommended.[91] Fruit juices should be diluted and served in a cup, not a bottle.

Developing Physical Readiness for Solid Foods   Foods introduced at the right times contribute to an infant's physical development. The ability to swallow food develops at around 4 to 6 months, and food offered by spoon helps to develop swallowing ability. At 8 months to a year, a baby can sit up, can handle finger foods, and begins to teethe. At that time, hard crackers and other finger foods may be introduced to promote the development of manual dexterity and control of the jaw muscles. These feedings must take place under the watchful eye of an adult because babies cannot safely chew and swallow them without choking. Table 13–14 lists foods that require especially attentive oversight. Nonfood items of small size should always be kept out of the infant's reach to prevent choking.

Some parents want to feed solids as early as possible on the theory that "stuffing the baby" at bedtime will promote sleeping through the night. There is no proof for this theory. Babies start to sleep through the night when they are ready, no matter when solid foods are introduced.

Preventing Food Allergies   To prevent allergies or identify them promptly, experts recommend introducing each new food singly in a small portion and waiting three to five days before introducing the next new food. For example, when introducing cereals, try fortified rice cereal first for several days; it causes allergy least often. Try wheat-containing cereal last; it is a common offender. If a food causes an allergic reaction (skin rash, digestive upset, or respiratory discomfort), discontinue its use before going on to the next food. If allergies run in your family, use extra caution in introducing new foods. Parents or caregivers who detect allergies early in an infant's life can spare the whole family much grief.

Food allergies in the United States, especially peanut allergies, have increased over the past few decades. New guidelines recommend introducing peanut-based foods early (between 4 and 11 months), rather than later (between 12 and 36 months) to prevent peanut allergy. Infants at high risk—those with severe skin rash or egg allergies—need medical approval and oversight, but for most other infants, parents may start adding peanut-containing foods such as watered down peanut butter or processed peanut products to the diet in the same way oatmeal and mashed vegetables are introduced.[92]

Choice of Infant Foods   Infant foods should be selected to provide variety, balance, and moderation. Commercial baby foods in the United States offer a wide variety of palatable, nutritious foods in a safe and convenient form. Brands vary in their use of starch fillers and sugar—check the ingredient lists. Parents or caregivers should not feed directly from the jar; spoon the needed portion into a dish to prevent contamination of the leftovers that will be stored in the jar.

An alternative to serving commercial baby food is to process a small portion of the family's table food in a blender, food processor, or baby food grinder. This necessitates cooking without salt or sugar, though, as responsible baby food manufacturers do. Adults can season their own food after taking out the baby's portion. Pureed food can be frozen in an ice cube tray to yield a dozen or so servings that can be quickly thawed, heated, and served on a busy day.

Foods to Omit   Sweets of any kind (including baby food "desserts") have no place in a baby's diet. The food energy they contribute can promote obesity, and they deliver few or no nutrients to support growth. Products containing sugar alcohols such as sorbitol should also be limited, as these may cause diarrhea. Salty canned vegetables are inappropriate for babies, but unsalted varieties provide a convenient source of well-cooked vegetables. Maintaining an awareness of foodborne illnesses and taking precautions against them are imperative—even a normally mild foodborne illness can seriously harm an infant or young child. Infants should not be given unpasteurized milk, milk products, or juices; raw

> Foodborne illnesses and their prevention are topics of **Chapter 12**.

or undercooked eggs, meat, poultry, fish, or shellfish; or raw sprouts. Honey and corn syrup should never be fed to infants because of the risk of botulism. Infants and young children are vulnerable to foodborne illnesses.

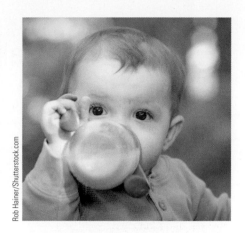

With the first birthday comes the possibility of tasting cow's milk for the first time.

Beverages and Foods at 1 Year   At a year of age, reduced-fat or low-fat cow's milk can become a primary source of most of the nutrients an infant needs; 2 to 3 cups a day meet those needs. More milk than this displaces iron-rich foods and can lead to the iron-deficiency anemia known as **milk anemia**. A variety of other foods—protein foods such as meat, poultry, seafood, eggs, and legumes; iron-fortified cereal; enriched or whole-grain bread; fruit; and vegetables—should be supplied in amounts sufficient to round out total energy needs. Ideally, the one-year-old sits at the table, eats many of the same foods everyone else eats, and drinks liquids from a cup, not a bottle. Table 13–15 shows a sample menu that meets the requirements for a one-year-old.

KEY POINTS

- At 6 months, an infant may be ready to try some solid foods.
- By 1 year, the child should be eating foods from all food groups.

Looking Ahead

The first year of life is the time to lay the foundation for future health. From the nutrition standpoint, the problems most common in later years are obesity and dental disease. Prevention of obesity may also help prevent the obesity-related diseases: cardiovascular disease, diabetes, and cancer.

Table 13–15

Sample Meal Plan for a One-Year-Old

	SAMPLE MENU
BREAKFAST	1 scrambled egg 1 slice whole-wheat toast ½ c whole milk
MORNING SNACK	½ c yogurt ¼ c fruit[a]
LUNCH	½ grilled cheese sandwich: 1 slice whole-wheat bread with 1 slice cheese ½ c vegetables[b] (steamed carrots) ¼ c 100% fruit juice
AFTERNOON SNACK	½ c fruit[a] ½ c toasted oat cereal
DINNER	1 oz chopped meat or ¼ c well-cooked mashed legumes ½ c rice or pasta ½ c vegetables[b] (chopped broccoli) ½ c reduced-fat or low-fat milk

Note: This sample menu provides about 1,000 calories.
[a]*Include citrus fruit, melons, and berries.*
[b]*Include dark green, leafy vegetables and red and orange vegetables.*

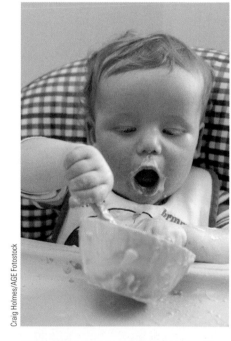

Older babies love to eat what their families eat. Let them enjoy their food.

milk anemia iron-deficiency anemia caused by drinking so much milk that iron-rich foods are displaced from the diet.

Mealtimes with Infants

LO 13.6 List five feeding guidelines that encourage normal eating behavior and autonomy in a child.

The nurturing of a young child involves more than just nutrition. Those who care for young children are responsible for providing not only food, milk, and water but also a safe, loving environment in which a child can grow and develop physical and emotional health and security.

Foster a Sense of Autonomy

Anyone feeding a 1-year-old has to be aware that the child's exploring and experimenting are normal and desirable behaviors. The child is developing a sense of autonomy that, if allowed to develop, will provide the foundation for later assertiveness in choosing when and how much to eat and when to stop eating.

Some Feeding Guidelines

In light of the developmental and nutrient needs of one-year-olds and in the face of their often contrary and willful behavior, a few feeding guidelines may be helpful:

- *Discourage unacceptable behavior (such as standing at the table or throwing food) by removing the child from the table to wait until later to eat.* Be consistent and firm, not punitive. For example, instead of saying "You make me mad when you don't sit down," say, "The fruit salad tastes good—please sit down and eat some with me." The child will soon learn to sit and eat.

- *Let young children explore and enjoy food.* This may mean eating with fingers for a while. Learning to use a spoon will come in time. Children who are allowed to touch, mash, and smell their food while exploring it are likely to accept it.

- *Don't force food on children.* Rejecting new foods is normal, and acceptance is likely as children become familiar with new foods through repeated opportunities to taste them. Instead of saying "You cannot go outside to play until you taste your carrots," say "You can try the carrots again another time."

- *Provide nutritious foods, and let children choose which ones, and how much, they will eat.* Gradually, they will acquire a taste for different foods.

- *Limit sweets.* Infants and young children have little room for empty-calorie foods in their daily energy allowance. Do not use sweets as rewards for eating meals.

- *Don't turn the dining table into a battleground.* Make mealtimes enjoyable. Teach healthy food choices and eating habits in a pleasant atmosphere. Mealtimes are not the time to fight, argue, or scold.

These recommendations reflect a spirit of tolerance that best serves the emotional and physical interests of infants. This attitude, carried throughout childhood, helps children to develop a healthy relationship with food. The next chapter continues the story of nutrition through life.

Figure 13–13

Nursing Bottle Tooth Decay— An Extreme Example

The upper teeth have decayed all the way to the gum line.

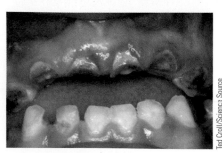

Ted Croll/Science Source

The most important single measure to undertake during the first year is to encourage eating habits that will support continued normal weight as the child grows. This means introducing a variety of nutritious foods in an inviting way (not forcing the baby to finish the bottle or baby food jar) and avoiding concentrated sweets and empty-calorie foods while encouraging physical activity. Parents should not teach babies to seek food as a reward, to expect food as comfort for unhappiness, or to associate food deprivation with punishment. If they cry for companionship, pick them up—don't feed them. If they are hungry, by all means, feed them appropriately. More pointers are offered in this chapter's Food Feature.

Dentists strongly discourage the practice of giving a baby a bottle as a pacifier and recommend limiting treats. Sucking for long periods of time pushes the normal jaw line out of shape and causes a bucktoothed profile: protruding upper and receding lower teeth. Prolonged sucking on a bottle of milk or juice also bathes the upper teeth in a carbohydrate-rich fluid that favors the growth of acid-producing bacteria, which dissolve tooth materials. Babies regularly put to bed with bottles sometimes have teeth decayed all the way to the gum line, a condition known as nursing bottle tooth decay, as shown in Figure 13–13.

KEY POINTS

- The early feeding of an infant lays the foundation for life-long eating habits.
- The most important single measure to undertake during the first year is to encourage eating habits that will support continued normal weight as the child grows.

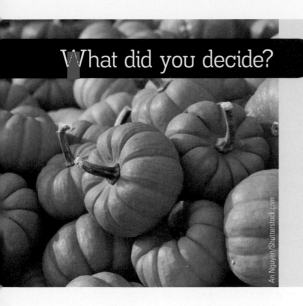

What did you decide?

Can a **man's lifestyle habits** affect a woman's future pregnancy?

How much **alcohol** drunk by a pregnant woman will harm her developing fetus?

Are **breast milk** and **formula** equally good for an infant's health?

Can infants **thrive on breast** milk or infant formula alone?

What's online?

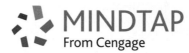

MINDTAP
From Cengage

Visit www.Cengage.com to access MindTap, a complete digital course that includes Diet & Wellness Plus, interactive quizzes, videos, and more.

Self Check

1. (LO 13.1) A pregnant woman needs an extra 450 calories above the allowance for nonpregnant women during which trimester(s)?

   a. first
   b. second
   c. third
   d. first, second, and third

2. (LO 13.1) A major reason why a woman's nutrition before pregnancy is crucial is that it determines whether her uterus will support the growth of a normal placenta.
   T F

3. (LO 13.1) A deficiency of which nutrient during pregnancy appears to be related to an increased risk of neural tube defects in newborns?

   a. vitamin B_6
   b. folate
   c. calcium
   d. niacin

4. (LO 13.1) The pregnant woman's body helps conserve iron by

   a. triggering food cravings.
   b. reducing physical activity.
   c. increasing iron excretion.
   d. increasing iron absorption.

5. (LO 13.1) Which of the following preventative measures should a pregnant woman take to avoid contracting listeriosis?

   a. avoid feta cheese
   b. avoid pasteurized milk
   c. thoroughly heat hot dogs
   d. a and c

6. (LO 13.2) Fetal alcohol spectrum disorders (FASD) are the leading cause of preventable developmental delays and intellectual disabilities in the world.
   T F

7. (LO 13.2) Which of the following does not characterize the damage done by alcohol during pregnancy?

   a. halts delivery of oxygen through the umbilical cord
   b. stimulates maternal appetite and therefore increases fetal nutrition
   c. slows cell division
   d. interferes with placental transport of nutrients to the fetus

8. (LO 13.2) The American Academy of Pediatrics urges all women to drink only moderately during pregnancy.
T F

9. (LO 13.3) Without proper management, type 1 or type 2 diabetes during pregnancy can cause all except

   a. severe nausea.

   b. severe hypoglycemia or hyperglycemia.

   c. preterm labor.

   d. pregnancy-related hypertension.

10. (LO 13.3) When women in developed countries die of pregnancy complications, the cause is often eclampsia.
T F

11. (LO 13.4) To support lactation, a breastfeeding woman needs more of the following:

   a. fluid
   c. energy

   b. fluoride
   d. a and c

12. (LO 13.4) Maternal dietary calcium intake has no effect on the calcium content of breast milk.
T F

13. (LO 13.4) Lactating women who smoke tobacco

   a. transfer nicotine and other chemicals to their infants through their breast milk.

   b. produce more milk than nonsmokers.

   c. produce milk with a higher fat content, damaging the infant's arteries.

   d. b and c

14. (LO 13.5) Breastfed infants may need supplements of

   a. fluoride, iron, and vitamin D.

   b. zinc, iron, and vitamin C.

   c. vitamin E, calcium, and fluoride.

   d. vitamin K, magnesium, and potassium.

15. (LO 13.5) Protective factors in breast milk include

   a. antiviral agents.

   b. anti-inflammatory agents.

   c. antibacterial agents.

   d. all of the above.

16. (LO 13.5) Which of the following foods poses a choking hazard to infants and small children?

   a. pudding

   b. marshmallows

   c. hot dog slices

   d. b and c

17. (LO 13.5) A sure way to get a baby to sleep through the night is to feed solid foods as soon as the baby can swallow them.
T F

18. (LO 13.6) Fostering a sense of autonomy in a one-year-old includes allowing the child to explore and experiment with her food.
T F

19. (LO 13.6) In light of the developmental needs of one-year-olds, parents should allow such behaviors as standing at the table and throwing food.
T F

20. (LO 13.7) To treat obesity in children, a first goal is to

   a. reduce their weight by 10 percent while they grow taller.

   b. quickly achieve their ideal weight.

   c. slow their rate of gain while they grow taller.

   d. a and b

Answers to these Self Check questions are in Appendix G.

Childhood Obesity and Early Chronic Diseases

LO 13.7 Describe the challenges associated with childhood obesity.

When most people think of health problems in children and adolescents, they often think of dental caries and acne, not type 2 diabetes and hypertension. Today, however, serious risk factors and "adult diseases" often accompany obesity in children.

Trends in Childhood Obesity

Childhood obesity numbers are high and getting higher, not only in the United States but all around the globe.[1]* Globally, childhood obesity has risen tenfold in the past four decades. In this country today, one of every six children aged 2 to 19 years is clinically obese, and one of every three is overweight.[2]†

All types of children are affected, but obesity most commonly occurs among children who are male, older, physically inactive, and who have parents who are obese, have less education, or are unmarried.[3] Many are of African American or Hispanic descent.[4] Additionally, low family income predicts obesity among Caucasian, Hispanic, and Asian children.[5]

The Challenge of Childhood Obesity

Most parents do not recognize the development of obesity in their own children, let alone the associated health risks it poses.[6] A professional evaluation eliminates guesswork.[7]

Physical and Emotional Perils

Excessive body weight in the young is more than just a cosmetic problem.

*Reference notes are in Appendix F.

†Obesity defined as having a body mass index in the top 5 percent of age and gender group; overweight, in the top 15 percent.

Table C13–1

Physical Complications of Obesity during Childhood

These conditions increase a child's risks for chronic diseases now and into adulthood.

- Abnormal blood lipid profile
  - High total cholesterol
  - High triglycerides
  - High LDL cholesterol
- High blood pressure
- High fasting insulin
- Structural changes to the heart
- Asthma
- Breathing difficulties (sleep apnea)
- Fatty liver

Sources: U.S. Preventive Services Task Force, Screening for obesity in children and adolescents: US Preventive Services Task Force Recommendation Statement, 2017; L. Hurt and coauthors, Diagnosis and screening for obesity-related conditions among children and teens receiving Medicaid—Maryland, 2005–2010, Morbidity and Mortality Weekly Report 63 (2014): 305–308.

Table C13–1 summarizes the physical complications that can accompany obesity in children.

Obese children frequently also suffer psychologically.[8] Adults discriminate against them, and peers make thoughtless comments or reject them based on their physical appearance. An obese child is likely to develop a poor self-image, a sense of failure, and a passive approach to life.

The emotional penalties of childhood obesity are often amplified by the media. More than 75 percent of popular children's movies denigrate or stigmatize fat people as social misfits.[9] Social media also abound with negative judgments of

Children with obesity often develop type 2 diabetes, among other illnesses.

overweight children, particularly girls. Unfortunately, children have few defenses against these unfair portrayals and readily internalize negative self-images.

Identifying Childhood Obesity

How can you tell if a child is overweight or just stocky and healthy? Certainly not by just looking: guesswork can produce wrong conclusions. It takes a trained professional using the right tools to make the correct assessment.

A physician or registered dietitian nutritionist can accurately calculate a child's BMI and interpret it using a growth chart, as shown in Figure C13–1. Because body fat differs between boys and girls and changes with age, BMI-for-age percentiles are calculated for children and teens using gender-specific growth charts.[10] Children and adolescents from the 85th to the 94th percentile on growth charts are considered *overweight*; those at the 95th percentile and above are considered *obese*.

Darla and Gabby

Eight-year-old Gabriella and her worried mother Darla tell a typical story of childhood obesity, and they model some appropriate responses. Recently, a note from the school nurse explained that during a routine screening, Gabby's BMI-for-age percentile was found to be too high. The nurse is suggesting further tests for risk factors of chronic diseases because Gabby's BMI of 22 places her in the obese weight category (the green dot in Figure C13–1). With Gabby's health in danger, Darla's concern grows: "I didn't know that a little baby fat at Gabby's age could be a threat. Both my father and his father died of diabetes-related conditions, so I'm worried."

Development of Type 2 Diabetes

An estimated 85 percent of children with type 2 diabetes are obese. Diabetes is most often diagnosed around the age of puberty, but type 2 diabetes is rapidly encroaching on younger age groups as children grow fatter. Ethnicity (being Native American or of African, Asian, or Hispanic descent) increases the risk, as does having a family history of type 2 diabetes. Chapter 11 described the risks associated with type 2 diabetes and revealed its connections with cardiovascular disease (CVD).

Determining exactly how many children suffer from type 2 diabetes is tricky. A child with type 2 diabetes may lack telltale symptoms, such as glucose in the urine, ketones in the blood, weight loss, or excessive thirst and urination, so diabetes often advances undetected. Without treatment, children with diabetes are left undefended against its ravages.[11]

Development of Heart Disease

Atherosclerosis, first apparent as heart disease in adulthood, begins in youth. By adolescence, most children have

Figure C13–1

Assessing Body Fatness in Children: An Example

Growth charts reflect population-wide data for children's BMI values as they age. Gabby is female, so this chart is for girls; a chart for boys is offered at the back of the book, p. E.

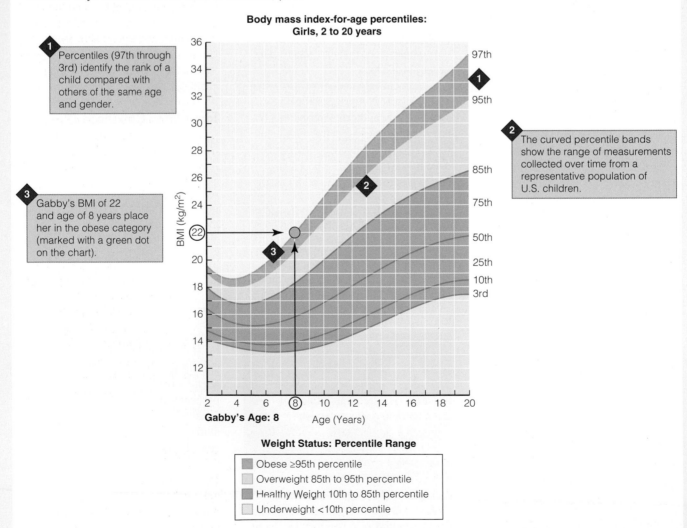

Body mass index-for-age percentiles: Girls, 2 to 20 years

1. Percentiles (97th through 3rd) identify the rank of a child compared with others of the same age and gender.

2. The curved percentile bands show the range of measurements collected over time from a representative population of U.S. children.

3. Gabby's BMI of 22 and age of 8 years place her in the obese category (marked with a green dot on the chart).

Gabby's Age: 8

Age (Years)

BMI (kg/m²)

Weight Status: Percentile Range

- Obese ≥95th percentile
- Overweight 85th to 95th percentile
- Healthy Weight 10th to 85th percentile
- Underweight <10th percentile

formed fatty streaks in their coronary arteries. By early adulthood, the arterial lesions that make heart attacks and strokes likely have formed.

An estimated 70 percent of obese children and adolescents have at least one risk factor for CVD, such as diabetes, high blood pressure, or an abnormal lipid profile.[12] These risks are directly related with the degree of obesity—the greater the BMI, the greater the risks.[13] In addition, adolescents who take up smoking greatly compound their risks.

High childhood BMI alone does not always predict inescapable adult heart disease. Overweight and obese youth who grow up to become normal-weight adults have average risks, and may escape that fate altogether.

The note from Gabby's school nurse prompted medical testing, including a family history, a fasting blood glucose test, a blood lipid profile, and a blood pressure test. Luckily, the results for both glucose and blood pressure are normal.

High Blood Cholesterol

Gabby's blood lipid results, however, confirm her mother's fears: her LDL cholesterol is 135—too high for optimal health. Cholesterol standards for children and adolescents are shown in Table C13–2.

As children mature into adolescents, they often choose more foods rich in saturated and *trans* fats (pizza, snack cakes, and so forth), and their blood cholesterol levels tend to rise. Further, sedentary children and adolescents have lower HDL, higher LDL, and higher blood pressure than those who are physically active.

Family history sometimes predicts high blood cholesterol. If the parents or

grandparents suffered from early heart disease, chances are that a child's blood cholesterol will be higher than average and will remain so throughout life. Diabetes, smoking, being overweight, and eating diets high in saturated and *trans* fats also raise the risk of preventable illnesses.[14]

High Blood Pressure

High blood pressure in a child or adolescent is a concern—it can signal the early onset of hypertension. Childhood hypertension, left untreated, tends to worsen with time and can damage the heart.[15] Diagnosis of hypertension in children must be done by professionals who will account for age, gender, and height; simple tables of standards like the ones for adults are useless for children.

Dramatic improvements often occur when children with hypertension take up regular aerobic activity and hold their weight down as they grow taller ("grow into their weight"). Restricting sodium intake also causes an immediate drop in most children's and adolescents' blood pressures.

Obese Children May Become Obese Adults

Unopposed, obesity often advances through childhood into adulthood, steadily worsening with age. Importantly, not every overweight child grows to be an obese adult; those who reach adulthood with healthy BMI values escape obesity's perils, a highly desirable outcome. To understand how this happens, researchers looked at two paths among overweight children, one leading to adult obesity and the other to a healthy BMI. Their results suggest that children who avoid obesity often reduce their rates of gain early in childhood, before age 5 or so.[16] Their rate of gain begins to slow or hold steady as they grow. The same thing shows up again in many adolescents—the rate of gain slows, allowing them to grow into healthy weight adults. Therefore, parents of overweight children, particularly those with obese children, should take action during early childhood and again in adolescence. These ages seem to offer critical windows of opportunity for chang-

ing a child's weight gain trajectory and helping the child to launch into adulthood with a healthy BMI.

Early Childhood Influences on Obesity

Children begin early to learn behaviors that affect their health. Parents and other caregivers have unique—once in a lifetime, really—opportunities to help children form healthy habits that pave the way to becoming healthy adults.

Calories—and Cautions

Gabby, who loves sweets, budgets her pocket money (she's saving for an MP3 player) to join her friends for a chocolate almond bar (250 calories) every day after school. In addition, she knows how to bake peanut butter cookies from a roll of refrigerated dough and enjoys eating two cookies each night at bedtime (another 240 calories). Gabby knows that nuts and peanut butter are better than candy for health, but she doesn't understand that the negative effects from excess calories of fat and sugar greatly outweigh the health benefits from nuts in her chocolate almond bar and cookies.

Intuitively, Darla would like to eliminate these treats. However, excessive restriction of sweets or calories can intensify cravings, contribute to eating in the absence of hunger, and spark unnecessary battles about food.[17] Worse, children who feel deprived or hungry may begin to sneak banned foods or hide them and binge on them in secret—behaviors that often predict eating disorders. What to do?

Figure C13–2 lists frequent high-calorie snacking as a contributing factor in a child's weight gain, but good-tasting snacks and meals are important to all children. A balanced approach may be to include favorite high-calorie treats occasionally in the context of structured, nutritious, and appealing meals and snacks.

Screen Time

The less physically active children are, the more likely they are to be overweight. The American Academy of Pediatrics recommends no media time before two years

Table C13–2

Cholesterol Standards, Ages 2 to 18 Years

Disease Risk	Total Cholesterol (mg/dL)	LDL Cholesterol (mg/dL)
Acceptable	<170	<110
Borderline	170–199	110–129
High	≥200	≥130

Note: Adult values appeared in Chapter 11.

Factors Affecting Childhood Weight Gain

The more of these factors in a child's life, the greater the likelihood of unhealthy weight gain.

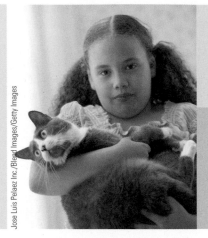

Food Factors
- Eating when not hungry; eating while watching TV or doing homework.
- Exposure to advertising that promotes high-calorie foods.
- Fast-food meals more than once a week.
- Frequent meals of fried or sugary foods and beverages.
- Frequent snacks consisting of high-energy foods, such as candies, cookies, crackers, fried foods, and ice cream.
- Irregular or sporadic mealtimes; missed meals.

Activity/Sleep Factors
- Insufficient sleep.
- Lack of access to recreational facilities.
- Less than 20 minutes of physical activity, such as outdoor play, each day.
- More than an hour of sedentary activity, such as television, each day.

Family and Other Factors
- High birth weight.
- Low-income family.
- Not breastfed.
- Overweight family members, particularly parents.
- Tall for age.

Jose Luis Pelaez Inc./Blend Images/Getty Images

of age, a limit of one hour per day for children ages 2 to 5, and two hours of quality media entertainment, including TV and computers, for older children to help prevent obesity.[18] However, U.S. children ages 8 to 18 spend more than seven hours *each day*, on average, engaged in screen time, such as TV viewing, video game playing, and computer use. For many children, screen time has largely replaced vigorous outdoor play and exercise. The more hours spent on screen time, the greater the risk of obesity (Figure C13–3).

Prevalence of Obesity by Hours of TV per Day, Children Ages 10–15 Years

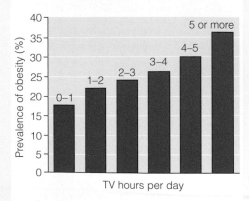

Source: Centers for Disease Control and Prevention, Youth Risk Behavior Survey, available at www.cdc.gov.

In addition to reducing physical activity, screen time promotes food habits that foster obesity. A child paying attention to television is particularly vulnerable to the multiple food advertisements run during prime child viewing times. The ads are intended to increase the child's recognition of, preference for, and ultimately intake of, unhealthy foods and beverages. Young children cannot yet grasp the concept of advertising for profit, so the ads largely succeed.[19]

Darla recalls, "My sisters and I hit the door on Saturday mornings with sandwiches in a bag. We explored, climbed trees, played softball with our friends, jumped in puddles, and played 'tag.' But Gabby and her friends have 252 television channels to choose from, not to mention video games and the Internet—no wonder they never play outside!"

Food Advertising to Children

Children influence a huge portion of the nation's food spending—up to $200 billion of their own pocket money each year and hundreds of billions more in annual family purchases of foods, beverages, and restaurant meals. To capture these dollars, the food industry loads children's TV programs and games with advertisements

for ultra-processed foods and sugar-sweetened beverages. Appealing animated "spokescharacters" speak directly to children to spark their desire for sugar-coated breakfast cereals, cookies, salty chips, sugar-sweetened beverages, and fat-laden fast foods. Alternatively, food companies target children with sophisticated messages that connect the featured products with children's needs for fun, love, and social acceptance.

On the Internet and in popular apps for mobile devices, food marketing agencies develop child-attracting "advergames,"— that is, games built around a manufacturer's foods and beverages that foster brand loyalty in young children. Websites offer social platforms that urge children to communicate about their products and encourage them to bring their friends to the sites. Free "gifts" are popular, too, such as brand-related computer screensavers, emojis, or wallpapers, which remind children of the brand. Children respond to such persuasion by asking for and consuming more of the target foods.[20]

Some food companies have pledged to encourage a healthier lifestyle for children by devoting all advertising to healthier foods, limiting the use of beloved children's characters, and halting the advertisement of foods in elementary schools. However, progress is slow and today's advertisements still violate the guidelines.[21] The American Heart Association has taken a position in support of increased regulation, and the WHO has released guidelines for responsible food marketing to children.[22]

Preventing and Reversing Overweight in Children

Prevention and reversal of childhood obesity are national priorities, and the earlier in life the efforts begin, ideally before age 6 years, the greater the likelihood of success.[23] Parents play key roles, from the selection of early feeding practices to the shaping of eating behaviors and attitudes later on. In addition, school-based programs that reinforce appropriate diet and physical activity for children seem promising for obesity prevention and treatment.[24]

For a child who is healthy and overweight or mildly obese, a typical first goal is to slow the rate of gain while the child grows taller. This is preferable to weight loss because diet restriction can easily interfere with normal growth. Severe obesity or health problems create an urgent need for weight loss and medical treatment may become necessary.[25] Family-based efforts that focus on healthy food choices and physical activity can help to achieve these goals, without making the child feel singled out.

Gabby's pediatrician has recommended lifestyle changes to improve both her BMI and her blood lipids. Darla is motivated: "I need to take some action!" A warning to Darla: the lifestyle changes may sound easy, but implementing them may prove difficult—people's behaviors are notoriously resistant to change. Further, involving Gabby at the planning stage is critical for success.

Family Patterns

As mentioned, parents are influential in shaping the self-concepts, weight concerns, and eating habits of children. In fact, young children learn food behaviors and attitudes primarily from their families.[26] Whole families may be eating too much, dieting inappropriately, and exercising too little.[27] Therefore, successful

---

---

plans for stabilizing a child's weight center on whole-family lifestyle changes because when parents set patterns for family behaviors, the children will most often follow their lead (see Table C13-3).

Lifestyle Changes First, Medical Treatments Later

A general rule for treating overweight children is "Lifestyle changes first; medications later, if at all." Children with elevated disease risk factors, such as high blood cholesterol or family histories of early heart disease, should still first be treated with diet and physical activity, but if blood cholesterol remains high after 6 to 12 months, then certain drugs may be used to lower blood cholesterol without interfering with normal growth or development. Only one obesity drug, orlistat, is approved for limited use in adolescents aged 12 years and older.

Surgical options are gaining acceptance for severely obese, physically mature adolescents, particularly those with obesity-related health problems who have failed at previous lifestyle modifications and who can adhere to life-long changes in daily routines. Surgery can improve risk factors for CVD, such as hypertension and elevated blood lipids, and also relieve some of the psychological burden that impairs daily quality of life for such children. Intensive management of postsurgical symptoms is a must, and careful evaluation of individual symptoms and referrals to appropriate specialists can often avert serious problems (see Chapter 9).[28]

Achievable Goals, Loving Support

To preserve a child's healthy sense of self, setting realistic, specific, and achievable goals is a first priority. Keeping a positive, upbeat attitude is another. The reverse—impossible goals and critical, blaming adults—may damage a child's developing self-image and may pave the way for eating disorders later on.

Most of all, Darla must let Gabby know that she is loved, regardless of weight. Blame is useless and can trigger emotional withdrawal of the child just when active engagement is needed most. By being supportive, Darla can help Gabby grow to become a healthy young woman with positive attitudes about food and herself. Meanwhile, she must make some changes to diet and physical activity—but exactly which ones? And how?

One good place to start may be the 5-2-1-0 method of organizing daily goals.[29] Each day, the child should have:

- 5 fruit and vegetable servings.
- 2 hours or less of screen time.
- 1 hour or more of physical activity (Table C13–4 has some tips).
- 0 sugar-sweetened beverages.

In addition, government agencies offer help to anyone with Internet access. Several reliable websites that teach parents and children practical ways to attain healthy body weights and to make healthy daily choices include:

- Choose MyPlate (www.choosemyplate .gov)
- Team Nutrition (http://teamnutrition .usda.gov)
- Let's Move: America's Move to Raise a Healthier Generation of Kids (letsmove .obamawhitehouse.archives.gov)

Diet Moderation, Not Deprivation

All children should eat appropriate amounts and kinds of foods, regardless of body weight (Chapter 14 provides many details). For the health of the heart, children older than 2 years of age benefit from the same diet recommended for older individuals—that is, a diet limited in saturated fat and *trans* fat while rich in nutrients and age-appropriate in calories. Such a diet benefits blood lipids without compromising nutrient adequacy, physical growth, or neurological development.

Darla decides to set some goals for providing nutritious, good-tasting lower-calorie foods at regular mealtimes. She also recognizes that pleasure is important, too. She knows that Gabby loves her daily chocolate treat and the social opportunity it creates with her peers. To give Gabby more healthy alternatives to chocolate, Darla lets Gabby choose from among some lower-calorie treats. Gabby now enjoys 100-calorie cereal bars—almost as much as chocolate— and agrees to purchase them when she meets with her friends after school. This simple change saves 150 calories a day. Gabby loves peanut butter, so instead of her evening cookies, she opts for apple slices spread with a little peanut butter, which cuts the evening snack calories in half and eliminates added sugars without leaving her feeling hungry or deprived.

Restaurant Food and Added Sugars

A steady diet of the offerings on most "children's menus" in restaurants, such as fried chicken nuggets, hot dogs, and French fries, invites both nutrient shortages and gains of body fat. Often, better choices can be found among appetizers, soups, salads, and side selections, and the best establishments offer steamed vegetables, fresh fruit, and broiled or grilled poultry on menus for both children and adults.

U.S. children and teens consume considerably more than the recommended limit of added sugars. The current Dietary Guidelines for Americans recommend limiting sugars to a maximum of 10 percent of daily calories, but on average, U.S. children and teens consume more than one and a half times that amount—16 percent.[30] Sugar-sweetened beverages (SSB), including soft drinks, fruit drinks, and energy or water drinks with added sugars, are a major source of added sugar in the American diet. Research has linked SSB consumption with excess body fatness in children and increased risks of chronic diseases in children and adults (see Controversy 4). Sugary foods and beverages are best reserved for occasional treats.

Physical Activity and Sleep

Physical activity assists with controlling body weight, reducing blood pressure, raising HDL cholesterol levels, and improving self-esteem and confidence. Yet children are spending only an average of 30 minutes each day engaged in moderate physical activity, only half of the current recommendation of 60 minutes a day (see Table C13–4). Not surprisingly, children reporting longer physical activity times have healthier cardiovascular profiles than their less active counterparts.[31] Active video games can help meet physical activity requirements, particularly the so-called exergames that demand moderate to intense physical activity to play.[32] Parents can promote physical activity in youth by setting limits on sedentary screen time, providing appealing opportunities for active play, and joining in the fun.

Parents who establish healthful daily routines often set in place lifelong habits that ultimately influence a child's future health. Accordingly, children who receive adequate sleep, view minimal TV, and have no TV in the bedroom have lower rates of obesity than others.[33]

As for sleep, when researchers deprived preschoolers of about 3 hours of their normal sleep time for a day, the children consumed about 20 percent more calories than usual, 25 percent more sugar, and 26 percent more carbohydrate. This overeating effect persisted, to a lesser degree, on the following day.[34]

Table C13–4

Physical Activity for Children

The Physical Activity Guidelines for Americans specifies these activities for children 6 to 17 years of age. It is important to encourage young people to participate in physical activities that are appropriate for their age, that are enjoyable, and that offer variety.

- Children and adolescents should participate in 60 minutes (1 hour) or more of physical activity daily.
- Aerobic: Most of the 60 or more minutes a day should be either moderate- or vigorous-intensity aerobic physical activity. Walking, bike riding, practicing martial arts, and dancing are examples.[a]
- Muscle-strengthening: As part of their 60 minutes of daily physical activity, children and adolescents should include muscle-strengthening physical activity on at least 3 days a week. Resistance can be provided by free weights, weight machines, other objects, or the person's own body weight.
- Bone-strengthening: As part of their 60 or more minutes of daily physical activity, children and adolescents should include bone-strengthening physical activity on at least 3 days of the week. Hopping, skipping, or jumping, and running sports such as basketball and tennis are examples.

[a]Chapter 10 specifies activities that characterize various intensity levels.
Sources: https://health.gov/dietaryguidelines/2015/guidelines/appendix-1/.

According to the National Sleep Foundation, about 30 percent of preschoolers do not sleep adequately; the organization's recommendations for sleep are presented in Table C13–5.

Darla's Efforts and Gabby's Future

"Currently, we're achieving five of our goals," says Darla, "but with Gabby's input, I've planned additional goals. First,

Table C13–5

Recommended Daily Sleep: Toddlers through Teens

Sleep needs can vary, and an individual child may need an hour or two more or less than these ranges.

Toddlers	11 to 14 hours
Preschoolers	10 to 13 hours
School-Age Children	9 to 11 hours
Teenagers	8 to 10 hours

Source: Data from Sleep Duration Recommendations, National Sleep Foundation, sleepfoundation.org.

Gabby and I are getting up a little earlier in the mornings to eat a nutritious, high-fiber breakfast. Gabby's doctor explained that breakfast is important because it can help her focus at school and contributes nutrients that may be lacking later in the day. Second, I'm packing her a healthy, tasty, lower-calorie lunch for school. It's easy to make a week's lunches ahead: I make seven whole-grain sandwiches or wraps on the weekend and freeze them. Then, each morning, I just toss one into Gabby's lunch bag with a low-fat yogurt, or low-fat cheese sticks, and water (not soda!). I'm also including some nutritious snacks that she enjoys, like baby carrots, nuts, and raisins, to sustain her energy and tempt her away from higher-calorie snacks on some days.

"Third, because we both have a sweet tooth, I keep ready-to-eat snacks of fresh fruit, like grapes and strawberries, in clear plastic containers in the refrigerator at eye level. Fourth, although I work days and go to school three nights a week, we have started a new tradition: family meal night each Friday at six o'clock sharp. Gabby and I choose the menu during the week and look forward to making dinner together.

Fifth, we switched from full-sized dinnerware to pretty new luncheon-sized plates and small dessert-sized bowls. Gabby is charmed with the bright colors, and we both find the small portions satisfying.

"Although my daughter's idea of a good vegetable has always been a fried potato, she's gradually opening up to trying new foods, which is goal number six. During Friday meal preparation, she's tried bites of broccoli, green beans— even squash! French fries are now just an occasional treat when we eat out. Gabby is doing great, and I'm going to keep offering her healthy new foods to try because it takes a while for a child to acquire a taste for a new food.

"Goal number seven has proved harder: we must start walking together, but when? I need to let her see that I am serious about my personal fitness, but I'm tired after work, and my studies gobble my time. To get Gabby moving after school, I've offered her credits toward her MP3 player in exchange for physical chores, such as raking, planting flowers, vacuuming, and washing the car—and when she gets her MP3 player, we've agreed to have nightly dance-offs to her favorite songs. Today though, rain or shine, tired or not, I'm going to lace up my running shoes and walk around our neighborhood with Gabby.

"I love my smart, stubborn, sturdy girl—no matter her shape or size! But I know her future will be cast by what we are doing right now. She will grow into her weight if we can hold the line with our new healthy habits. I see her potential to do great things, and what she is learning today about taking care of herself she can pass on to others— maybe to her own children."

Critical Thinking

1. Who do you believe is responsible for childhood obesity? Organize a chart listing the changes a family and child can make to combat obesity. Include changes in food intake and activity patterns.

2. Draw a picture that represents the concept of energy balance that you could use as a visual aid in explaining this concept to a 10- to 12-year-old.

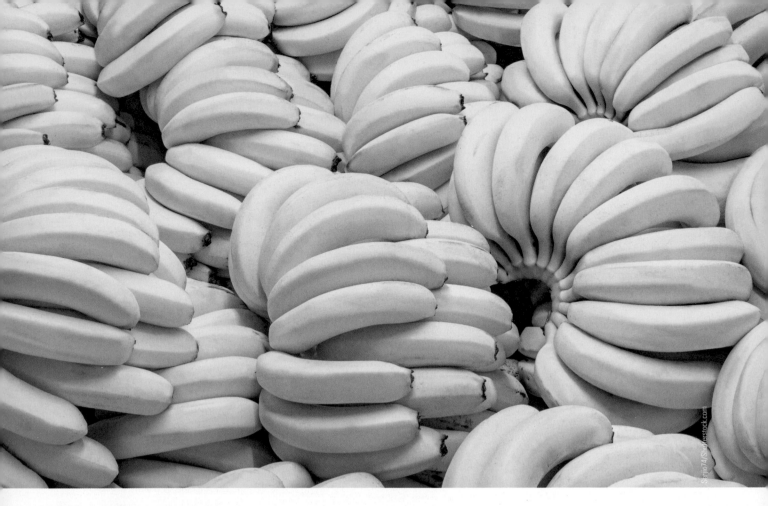

14 Child, Teen, and Older Adult

Learning Objectives

After completing this chapter, you should be able to accomplish the following:

LO 14.1 Describe nutrient needs, eating habits, and dietary cautions for early and middle childhood.

LO 14.2 Summarize the nutrient needs of adolescents.

LO 14.3 Identify the dietary factors associated with successful and healthy aging.

LO 14.4 Describe the changes in nutrient needs that occur as people age.

LO 14.5 Describe the challenges associated with regularly eating alone.

LO 14.6 Summarize the concerns surrounding nutrient–drug interactions.

What do you think?

Do you need **special information** to properly nourish children, or are they like "little adults" in their needs?

Do you suspect that symptoms you feel may be caused by a **food allergy**?

Are **teenagers** old enough to decide for themselves what to eat?

Can good nutrition help you live **better and longer**?

To grow and to function well in the adult world, children need a firm background of sound eating habits, which begin during the second half of infancy with the introduction of solid foods. At that point, the person's nutrition story has just begun; the plot thickens. Nutrient needs change in childhood and throughout life, depending on the rate of growth, gender, activities, and many other factors. Nutrient needs also vary from individual to individual, but universal recommendations are available and useful.

Most children's diets in the United States fail to meet the recommendations of the Dietary Guidelines for Americans.*[1] The consequences of such diets may not be evident to casual observers, but nutritionists know that nutrient deficiencies during growth often have far-reaching effects on physical and mental development. Likewise, dietary excesses during childhood often set up lifelong struggles against obesity and chronic diseases.

> Childhood obesity and related chronic diseases are so complex and pervasive that **Controversy 13** is devoted to them.

Early and Middle Childhood

LO 14.1   Describe nutrient needs, eating habits, and dietary cautions for early and middle childhood.

Imagine growing 10 inches taller in just one year, as the average healthy infant does during the first dramatic year of life. At age 1, infants have just learned to stand and toddle, and growth has slowed by half; by 2 years, they can take long strides with solid confidence and are learning to run, jump, and climb. These accomplishments reflect the accumulation of a larger mass, greater density of bone and muscle tissue, and refinement of nervous system coordination. These same growth trends, a lengthening of the long bones and an increase in musculature, continue until adolescence but more slowly.

Mentally, too, children make rapid advances, and proper nutrition is critical to normal brain development. A child malnourished at age 3 often demonstrates diminished mental capacities compared with peers at age 11.

Feeding a Healthy Young Child

At no time in life do human nutritional needs change faster than during the second year. From 12 to 24 months, a child's diet must shift from infant foods consisting of mostly formula or breast milk to mostly modified adult foods. This doesn't mean, of course, that milk loses its importance in a toddler's diet—it remains a central source of calcium, protein, and other nutrients. Figure 14–1 shows the extraordinary changes that take place in a young child's body during the second year of life. During this remarkable period, the demand for nutrients is greater than those that can be provided by milk alone. Further, the toddler years are marked by bustling activity made possible by new muscle tissue and refined neuromuscular coordination. To support both their activity and their growth, toddlers need nutrients and plenty of them.

Appetite Regulation   An infant's appetite decreases markedly near the first birthday and fluctuates thereafter. At times, children seem insatiable; at other times, they seem to live on air and water. Parents and other caregivers need not worry: given an ample selection of nutritious foods at regular intervals, internal appetite regulation in healthy, normal-weight children guarantees that their overall energy intakes will remain remarkably constant and will be right for each stage of growth.[2]

This ideal situation depends on restriction of low-nutrient, high-calorie foods, however. Today's children too often consume a constant stream of tempting foods

---

*Reference notes are in Appendix F.

Figure 14–1

Body Shape of 1-Year-Old and 2-Year-Old Compared

The body shape of a 1-year-old (left) changes dramatically by age 2 (right). The 2-year-old has grown leaner and taller; the muscles (especially in the back, buttocks, and legs) have firmed and strengthened; and the leg bones have lengthened.

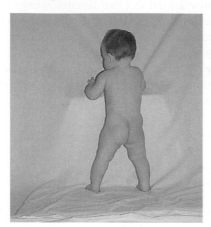
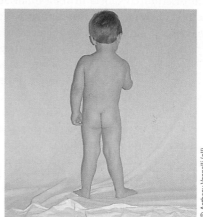

© Anthony Vannelli (all)

Table 14–1

Estimated Daily Calorie Needs for Children

Age (y)	Sedentary[a]	Active[b]
2 (male/female)	1,000	1,000
3 (male/female)	1,000	1,400
Females		
4	1,200	1,400
5 to 6	1,200	1,600
7	1,200	1,800
8 to 9	1,400	1,800
10	1,400	2,000
11	1,600	2,000
12 to 13	1,600	2,200
Males		
4 to 5	1,200	1,600
6 to 7	1,400	1,800
8	1,400	2,000
9	1,600	2,000
10	1,600	2,200
11	1,800	2,200
12	1,800	2,400
13	2,000	2,600

[a]Sedentary describes a lifestyle that includes only the activities typical of day-to-day life.

[b]Active describes a lifestyle that includes at least 60 minutes per day of moderate physical activity (equivalent to walking more than 3 miles per day at 3 to 4 miles per hour) in addition to the activities of day-to-day life.

Source: U.S. Department of Health and Human Services and U.S. Department of Agriculture, 2015–2020 Dietary Guidelines for Americans, 8th ed. (2015), http://health.gov/dietaryguidelines/2015/guidelines/.

high in added sugars, saturated fat, refined grains, and calories throughout the day, short-circuiting normal hunger and satiety cues. Children who receive regularly timed snacks and meals of a variety of nutritious foods, with only occasional special treats, are most likely to gain weight appropriately and grow normally. The Dietary Guidelines for Americans are safe and appropriate goals for the diets of children 2 years of age and older to provide nutrients and energy needed for growth without excesses.

Energy   Individual children's energy needs vary widely, depending on their growth and physical activity. On average, though, a one-year-old child needs about 800 calories a day; at age 6, the child's need doubles to about 1,600 daily calories; and by age 10, about 1,800 calories a day will support normal growth and activity without causing excess storage of body fat. As children grow, the total calorie need increases, but per pound of body weight, the need declines from the extraordinarily high demand of infancy. Table 14–1 shows that both age and activity level help to determine calorie needs in children.[†]

Some children, notably those fed vegan diets, may have difficulty meeting their energy needs. Whole grains, many kinds of vegetables, and fruit provide plenty of fiber and nutrients, but their low energy content may make them inadequate to support growth. Soy products, other legumes, and nut or seed butters offer more concentrated sources of energy and nutrients to support optimal growth and development in these children.[3]

Protein   The total amount of protein needed increases somewhat as a child grows larger. On a pound-for-pound basis, however, an older child's need for protein decreases slightly relative to a younger child's need (see the DRI values, at the back of the book, pp. A and B). Protein needs of children are well covered by typical U.S. diets and well-planned vegetarian diets.

Carbohydrate and Fiber   Glucose use by the brain sets the carbohydrate intake recommendations. A one-year-old's brain is large relative to the size of the

[†]DRI estimated energy requirements for infants and children derive from values for weight, age, physical activity, and other parameters.

body, so the glucose required by a 1-year-old falls in the adult range (see the back of the book, p. A). Fiber recommendations derive from adult intakes and should be adjusted downward for children who are picky eaters and take in little energy (see Table 14–2).

Fat and Fatty Acids Keeping dietary fat within bounds helps to control saturated and *trans* fat intakes and so may help protect children from developing early signs of adult diseases. Taken to extremes, however, a low-fat diet can lack the energy and essential nutrients required for growth. The essential fatty acids are critical to proper development of nerve, eye, and other tissues.

Children's small stomachs can hold only so much food, and fat provides a concentrated source of food energy that children may need for growth. For children, aged 1 to 3 years, dietary fat recommendations are 30 to 40 percent of energy; older children aged 4 to 18 years require 25 to 35 percent of energy from fat.[4]

Vitamins and Minerals As a child grows larger, so does the demand for vitamins and minerals. On a pound-for-pound basis, a 5-year-old's need for, say, vitamin A is about double the need of an adult man. A balanced diet of nutritious foods can meet children's needs for most nutrients.

Fluoride, vitamin D, and iron supplements sometimes become necessary. In areas where the soil and water are poor in fluoride, pediatricians may prescribe it for children. As for vitamin D, children's intakes in the United States are inadequate and vitamin D deficiencies are widespread. The DRI committee recommends that vitamin D–fortified foods—including milk, ready-to-eat cereals, and juices, should provide 15 micrograms daily to maximize children's absorption of calcium and ensure normal, healthy bone growth.[5] Children who do not consume enough vitamin D from fortified foods should receive supplements to make up the shortfall, but take care: vitamin D toxicity poses a threat to children who are given high doses.[6] Nutrients from other kinds of supplements typically duplicate the ones children already receive in ample amounts from nutritious foods. Well-nourished children therefore need no other supplements except one: iron, which deserves a section of its own.

Iron Iron deficiency in children is a major problem worldwide and remains a concern for U.S. children aged 1 year and older.[7] Following infancy, children progress from a diet of iron-rich infant foods such as breast milk, iron-fortified formula, and iron-fortified infant cereal to a diet of adult foods and iron-poor cow's milk. Their stores of iron from birth are soon exhausted, but their rapid growth demands new red blood cells for a larger volume of blood. Compounding the problem is the variability in toddlers' appetites: sometimes 2-year-olds are finicky, sometimes they eat voraciously, and sometimes they may enter phases where they opt for milk and juice in place of solid foods. All of these factors—switching to whole milk and unfortified foods, diminished iron stores, and unreliable food consumption—make iron deficiency likely at a time when iron is critically needed for normal growth and development. A later section revisits iron deficiency and its consequences for the brain.

To prevent iron deficiency, children's foods must deliver 7 to 10 milligrams of iron per day. To achieve this goal, snacks and meals should include iron-rich foods. Although milk is an important source of dietary calcium, needed for the growth of dense, healthy bones, excessive intakes should be avoided, as it can displace iron-rich foods, including lean meats, fish, poultry, eggs, legumes, and whole-grain or enriched grain products, from the diet.

Planning Children's Meals To provide all the needed nutrients, children's meals should include a variety of foods from each food group in amounts suited to their appetites and needs. Table 14–3 displays the USDA Eating Patterns for children who need 1,000 to 1,800 calories per day. MyPlate online resources for children, parents, and educators translate eating patterns into messages that can help promote better nutrition for the nation's children (see Figure 14–2).

Table 14–2	
Fiber DRI for Children	

Age (yr)	Fiber (g)
1–3	19
4–8	25
9–13	
Boys	31
Girls	26
14–18	
Boys	38
Girls	26

Table 14–3

USDA Eating Patterns for Children (1,000 to 1,800 Calories)

Height, weight, growth rate, and other factors determine a child's energy needs.

Food Group	1,000 cal	1,200 cal	1,400 cal	1,600 cal	1,800 cal
Fruit	1 c	1 c	1½ c	1½ c	1½ c
Vegetables	1 c	1½ c	1½ c	2 c	2½ c
Grains (half whole grains)	3 oz	4 oz	5 oz	5 oz	6 oz
Protein foods	2 oz	3 oz	4 oz	5 oz	5 oz
Milk	2 c	2½ c	2½ c	3 c	3 c

Source: U.S. Department of Health and Human Services and U.S. Department of Agriculture, 2015–2020 Dietary Guidelines for Americans, *8th edition (2015),* available at http://health.gov/dietaryguidelines/2015/guidelines/.

Figure 14–2

MyPlate Resources for Children

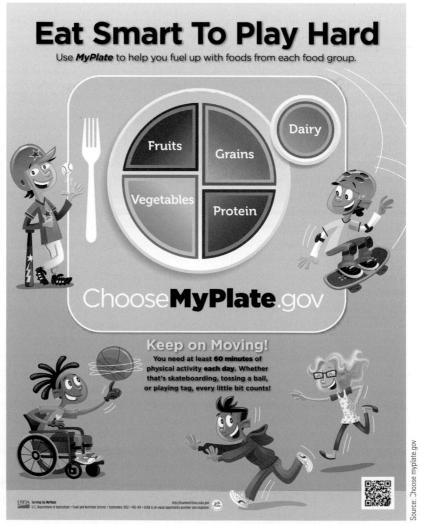

Note: MyPlate resources for children can be found at www.choosemyplate.gov.

Chapter 14 Child, Teen, and Older Adult

- Other than specific recommendations for fluoride, vitamin D, and iron, well-fed children do not need supplements.
- USDA Eating Patterns provide for adequate nourishment for growth without obesity.

Mealtimes and Snacking

The early childhood years present the parents' greatest chance to influence lifelong food choices that will promote the child's health today and reduce chronic disease risks later on. The challenge is to deliver nutrients in the form of meals and snacks that are both nutritious and appealing so that children will learn to enjoy a variety of health-promoting, nutritious foods.

Current U.S. Children's Food Intakes   Most children eat too few fruits and vegetables: on average, they do not obtain even half of the needed amounts of total vegetables, greens and beans, or whole grains.[8] By age 15 months, one vegetable and one fruit stand out as predominant, French fries and bananas, neither of which is a rich source of many needed nutrients. Sugar-sweetened beverages and desserts are commonly added to the diet during infancy, and their intakes increase with age, while intakes of health-promoting whole foods decrease.[9] When children develop preferences for nutrient-poor selections, winning their acceptance of the nutritious foods they need can prove challenging.

Dealing with Children's Preferences   Many children prefer sweet fruits and mild-flavored vegetables served raw or undercooked because they are crunchy and easy to eat. Cooked foods should be served warm, not hot, because a child's mouth is much more sensitive than an adult's. The flavors should be mild because a child has more taste buds.

Little children prefer small portions of food served at little tables. If offered large portions, children may fill up on favorite foods, ignoring others. Toddlers often go on food jags—consecutive days of eating only one or two favored foods. For food jags lasting a week or so, make no response because 2-year-olds regard any form of attention as a reward. After two weeks of serving the favored foods, try serving small portions of many foods, including the favored items. Invite the child's friends to occasional meals, and make other foods as attractive as possible.

Bribing a child to eat certain foods by, for example, allowing extra television time as a reward for eating vegetables often fails to produce the desired effect: the child will likely *not* develop a preference for those foods. Likewise, when children are forbidden to eat favorite foods, they yearn for them more intensely—the opposite of the well-meaning caregiver's goal. Include favorites as occasional treats.

Most children can safely enjoy occasional treats of high-calorie foods, but such treats should also be nutritious. From the milk group, ice cream or pudding is good now and then; from the grains group, whole-grain or enriched cakes, oatmeal cookies, snack crackers, or even small doughnuts are an acceptable occasional addition to a nutritious diet. These foods encourage a child to learn that pleasure in eating is important. A steady diet of these treats, however, leads to nutrient deficiencies, obesity, or both.

Picky Eaters   The diets of picky eaters often score low in nutrition quality.[10] A fear of new foods, **food neophobia**, often underlies picky eating and is almost universal among toddlers and preschoolers. Without so much as a taste, the child rejects new foods on sight, but the reason why is unclear. The child may remember disliking a food with a similar appearance or aroma. Or the behavior may be rooted in the genes.[11] It may have evolved as a protective mechanism that prevented curious ancestral toddlers from tasting toxic plants in their environments. In any case, severe food neophobia can harm a child's health, growth, or social interactions and should be evaluated by a pediatrician.[12]

In the meantime, some practical tips can help. First, keep an upbeat but persistent attitude: a child may ignore or reject a food the first 14 times it is offered but on the 15th may suddenly recognize it as a familiar, accepted food in the diet. Parents' negative attention or attempts to force "just a taste" before the child is ready interrupt this

food neophobia (NEE-oh-FOE-beeah) the fear of trying new foods, common among toddlers.

Table 14–4

Tips for Feeding Picky Eaters

Medical attention is needed if a child fails to eat enough to support healthy growth and development. Otherwise, these tips often help.

Get Them Involved

Children are more likely to try foods when they feel a sense of ownership. Include them in

- Meal planning.
- Grocery shopping.

- Food preparation.
- Gardening and harvesting the foods they eat.

Be Creative

- Serve vegetables as finger foods with dips or spreads.
- Use cookie cutters to cut fruit and vegetables into fun shapes.
- Serve traditional meals out of order (e.g., breakfast for dinner).

- Encourage (don't force) children's interest and enthusiasm for nutritious foods, such as legumes or whole grains, by using them in craft projects.

Enhance Favorite Recipes

- Blend, slice, or shred vegetables into sauces, casseroles, pancakes, or muffins.
- Serve fruit over cereal, yogurt, or ice cream.

- Bake brownies with black beans or cookies with lentils as an ingredient (find recipes on the Internet).

Model and Share

- Be a role model to children by eating healthy foods yourself. Offer to share your healthy snacks with them.
- Children may need multiple exposures to new foods before they accept them, so do continue offering foods that children initially reject.

- Encourage children to taste at least one bite of each food served at a meal.

Respect and Relax

- Children tend to eat sporadically. They have small stomachs and so tend to fill up fast and become hungry again soon after eating.

- Focus on the child's overall weekly intake of food and nutrients rather than on daily consumption.

Source: Adapted from Mayo Clinic Staff, Children's nutrition: 10 tips for picky eaters, 2014, available at www.mayoclinic.com/health/childrens-health/HQ01107.

learning process. Offering new foods at the beginning of a meal when the child is hungry often works best, as does serving the child samples of the same foods that adults are enjoying; children follow the examples of adults. The tips offered in Table 14–4 can often make mealtimes go more smoothly.

Child Preferences versus Parental Authority Just as parents are entitled to their likes and dislikes, a child who genuinely and consistently rejects a food should be allowed the same privilege. Also, children should be believed when they say they are full: the "clean-your-plate" dictum should be stamped out for all time. Children who are forced to override their own satiety signals are in training for obesity.

A bright, unhurried atmosphere with a positive emotional climate is conducive to good appetite and provides a climate in which a child can learn to enjoy eating health-promoting foods.[13] Parents who beg, cajole, and demand that their children eat make power struggles inevitable. A child may find mealtimes unbearable if she is accompanied by a barrage of accusations—"Susie, your hands are filthy . . . your report card . . . and clean your plate!" The child's stomach recoils as both body and mind react to stress of this kind.

Honoring children's preferences does not mean allowing them to dictate the diet, however, because children naturally prefer fatty, sugary, and salty foods, such as

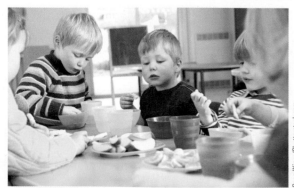

Little children like to eat small portions of food at little tables.

SpeedKingz/Shutterstock.com

heavily advertised snack chips, cookies, crackers, fast foods, and sugary cereals and drinks. When children's tastes are allowed to rule the family's pantry, everyone's nutrition suffers because busy parents often eat the foods they prepare for children. The responsibility for *what* the child is offered to eat lies squarely with the adult caregiver, but the child should be allowed to decide *how much* and even *whether* to eat.

Many parents overlook perhaps the single most important influence on their children's food habits—their own habits.[14] Parents who don't prepare, serve, and eat carrots shouldn't be surprised when their children refuse to eat carrots. Conversely, parents who share food shopping and cooking tasks with children, and who enjoy nutritious foods at family meals, set healthy patterns for children to follow.

Snacking   Parents often find that their children snack so much that they are not hungry at mealtimes. This is not a problem if children are taught how to snack—nutritious snacks are just as health promoting as small meals. Table 14–5 provides healthy snack ideas from each food group that many children like to eat.

Restaurant Choices   It takes some artful maneuvering to choose nutritious restaurant meals that children can enjoy. Children's menus reliably offer fatty, salty sandwiches, "nuggets," and French fries. For better choices:

- Ask to split a regular meal among several children.
- Choose from appetizers, soups, salads, and side dishes.
- Order vegetable toppings and lean meats on pizza (skip the sausages and hamburger); reduce the saturated fat by requesting half the cheese.
- Request water, fat-free milk, or fruit juice (not punch or soft drinks) for beverages.

Parents who make nutritious restaurant choices for themselves also set good examples for children.

Choking   A child who is choking may make no sound, so an adult should keep an eye on children when they are eating. A child who is coughing most often dislodges the food and recovers without help. To prevent choking, encourage the child to sit when eating—choking is more likely when children are running or reclining. Round foods such as grapes, nuts, hard candies, and pieces of hot dog can become lodged in a child's small windpipe. Other potentially dangerous foods include tough meat chunks, popcorn, chips, and peanut butter eaten by the spoonful. (More foods and nonfood items that pose a choking hazard were listed in Table 13–14, p. 514.)

Table 14–5

Healthy Snack Ideas from Each Food Group

Well-planned snacks that include two or more food groups, such as yogurt with fruit, a mini bagel with hummus, or whole-grain cereal with milk, provide a wide variety of needed nutrients.

▪ Grains	Ready-to-eat cereal, whole-grain crackers, mini rice or wheat cakes, sliced bread, mini bagel, graham crackers, whole-wheat tortilla
▪ Vegetables	Veggie "matchsticks" (thin sticks) made from fresh carrots[a] or zucchini,[a] bell pepper rings, cut cherry tomatoes,[a] green beans, sugar peas, avocados, steamed broccoli
▪ Fruit	Thin apple slices,[a] tangerine sections, strawberry halves, banana, pineapple, kiwi, peach, mango, nectarine, melon, cut grapes,[a] berries, diced dried apricots[a]
▪ Milk and Milk Products	Low-fat cheese slices or string cheese, mini yogurt cup, fat-free or low-fat milk or soy milk, low-fat cottage cheese
▪ Protein Foods	Egg slices or wedges, peanut butter,[a] bean dip, hummus, black beans, thin strips of lean turkey[a] or chicken,[a] shelled pumpkin seeds, soy "burger" or "sausage" slices

[a]These foods can pose a choking hazard unless cut into small pieces. Plain peanut butter by the spoonful can also cause choking; small amounts spread on bread, fruit, or other foods that help to disperse it in the mouth are safer.

Source: Adapted from U.S. Department of Agriculture, Develop healthy eating habits, available at www.choosemyplate.gov/health-and-nutrition-information.

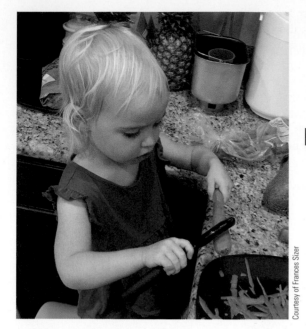
Courtesy of Frances Sizer

Children enjoy helping when tasks are matched to their abilities.

Food Skills Children love to be included in meal preparation, and they like to eat foods they helped to prepare (see Table 14–6). A positive experience is most likely when tasks match developmental abilities and are undertaken in a spirit of enthusiasm and enjoyment, not criticism or drudgery. Praise for a job well done (or at least well attempted) expands a child's sense of pride and helps to develop skills and positive feelings toward healthy foods.

KEY POINTS

- Healthy eating habits are learned in childhood, and parents teach best by example.
- Choking can often be avoided by supervising children during meals and excluding hazardous foods.
- Children enjoy helping to prepare meals when the tasks match their abilities.

How Do Nutrient Deficiencies Affect a Child's Brain?

Children with nutritional deficiencies exhibit both physical and behavioral symptoms: they feel sick and out of sorts, and they may be irritable and aggressive or sad and withdrawn. Such children may be labeled "hyperactive," "depressed," or "unlikable." Diet–behavior connections are of keen interest to caregivers who both feed children and live with them.

Iron deficiency, for example, exerts well-known and widespread effects on children's behavior and intellectual performance, even before anemia shows up in a blood test. Iron transports oxygen, making it critical to cellular energy metabolism. It is also required to

Table 14–6

Food Skills and Developmental Milestones of Preschool Children[a]

Food Skills	Developmental Milestones
Age 1 to 2 years	
- Uses a spoon - Lifts and drinks from a cup - Helps scrub fruit and vegetables, tear lettuce or greens, snap green beans, or dip foods - Can be messy; can be easily distracted	- Large muscles develop - Experiences slowed growth and decreased appetite - Develops likes and dislikes - May suddenly refuse certain foods
Age 3 years	
- Spears food with a fork - Feeds self independently - Helps wrap, pour, mix, shake, stir, or spread foods - Follows simple instructions	- Medium hand muscles develop - May suddenly refuse certain foods - Begins to request favorite foods - Makes simple either/or food choices
Age 4 years	
- Uses all utensils and napkin - Helps measure dry ingredients - Learns table manners	- Small finger muscles develop - Influenced by TV, media, and peers - May dislike many mixed dishes
Age 5 years	
- Measures liquids - Helps grind, grate, and cut (soft foods with dull knife) - Uses hand mixer with supervision	- Fine coordination of fingers and hands develops - Usually accepts food that is available - Eats with minor supervision

[a]These ages are approximate. Healthy, normal children develop at their own pace.

Source: Adapted from MyPlate for Preschoolers, Behavioral milestones, available at www.choosemyplate.gov/preschoolers/healthy-habits/Milestones.pdf.

produce key neurotransmitters that regulate the ability to pay attention, which is crucial to learning. Consequently, iron deficiency not only causes an energy crisis, but also weakens the motivation to persist at intellectually challenging tasks, impairs attention span, and undermines a child's ability to learn.[15] Despite widespread food fortification, iron deficiency remains a key problem among U.S. children, from toddlers to adolescents.

Only a health-care provider, such as a registered dietitian nutritionist, should make the decision to give a child a single-nutrient iron supplement. Iron is toxic, and overdoses can easily injure or even kill a toddler or child who accidentally ingests iron pills. All supplements should be kept out of children's reach.

KEY POINT

- Iron deficiency and toxicity pose threats to children.

The Problem of Lead

Lead is not a nutrient, but an indestructible, toxic heavy metal that is common in the environment. It offers no health benefits, and once in the body, it is difficult to excrete. More than 500,000 children in the United States, most younger than age 6, have blood lead concentrations high enough to cause mental, behavioral, and physical health problems.[16]

Sources of Lead Babies love to explore and put everything into their mouths, including chips of old lead paint, jewelry that contains lead, and other unlikely objects.[17] Lead may also leach into a home's drinking water supply from old lead pipes and end up in a baby's formula and the family's beverages. In older children, lead dust mixed into outdoor soil can stick to clothing and hands and eventually be consumed. Appreciable lead has also been found in pigments, stained glass, lead crystal glassware, ammunition, ceramic glazes, traditional medicines, and even makeup and skin creams.[18] Once exposed to lead, infants and young children absorb 5 to 10 times as much of the toxin as adults do.

Harm from Lead There is virtually no safe level of lead for the developing body. Lead can build up so silently in a child's body that caregivers may not notice its symptoms until it's too late. Figure 14–3 identifies several organs affected by elevated blood

---

Figure 14–3

Lead Toxicity and Body Organs

Even small exposures to lead can damage the developing body and mind.

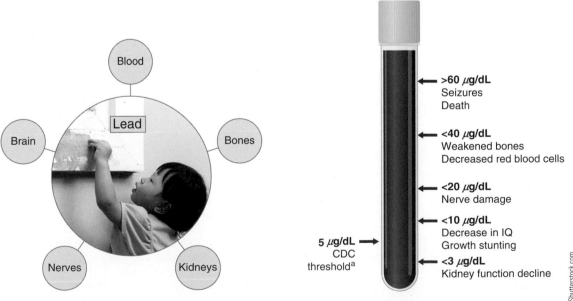

> 60 µg/dL
Seizures
Death

< 40 µg/dL
Weakened bones
Decreased red blood cells

< 20 µg/dL
Nerve damage

< 10 µg/dL
Decrease in IQ
Growth stunting

5 µg/dL
CDC
threshold[a]

< 3 µg/dL
Kidney function decline

Brain — Blood — Bones — Nerves — Kidneys — Lead

[a]The CDC uses a level of 5 µg/dL to identify children who require case management and areas that need public health actions to reduce lead exposure.

lead concentrations, but these are just examples. Lead affects every body organ. Tragically, once symptoms set in, medical treatments may not reverse all of the functional damage. Some impairments may linger long beyond childhood.[19]

The physiological effects of long-term elevated blood lead include reduced bone and muscle growth, neurological damage, kidney malfunction, hearing impairment, speech and language difficulties, and developmental delays.[20] Among school-age children, early lead exposure is linked with lower-than-average scores on IQ tests, and poor academic performance.[21]

As lead toxicity gradually injures the kidneys, nerves, brain, bone marrow, and other organs, a child may slip into a coma, may have convulsions, and may even die if an accurate diagnosis is not made in time. Older children with high blood lead may be mislabeled as delinquent, aggressive, or learning disabled.

Lead and Nutrient Interactions Poor nutrient status influences the likelihood of a child's suffering harm from lead. Children absorb more lead if they lack the minerals iron, calcium, and zinc, which compete with lead for absorption. Lead also displaces these minerals from their sites of action in the body, limiting their biological functions. Even slight calcium, iron, or zinc deficiencies can open the door to lead toxicity. For example, a child with iron-deficiency anemia is three times as likely to have elevated blood lead as a child with normal iron status.[22]

Bans on leaded gasoline, leaded house paint, and lead-soldered food cans have dramatically reduced the amount of lead in the U.S. environment in past decades and have produced a steady decline in children's average blood lead concentrations. However, lead still remains a threat in older communities where homes still have lead pipes and layers of old lead paint inside, the primary sources of lead in most children's lives.[‡] Some tips for avoiding lead toxicity are given in Table 14–7.

KEY POINT

- Blood lead concentrations have declined in recent times, but no concentration is harmless.

Table 14–7

Steps to Prevent Lead Exposure

To protect children:
- If your home was built before 1978, wash floors, windowsills, and other surfaces weekly with warm water and detergent to remove dust released by old lead paint; clean up flaking paint chips immediately.
- Feed children balanced, timely meals with ample iron and calcium.
- Prevent children from chewing on old painted surfaces.
- Refrain from letting young children wear jewelry made of unknown metals.
- Wash children's hands, bottles, and toys often.
- Wipe soil off shoes before entering the home.
- Ask a pediatrician whether your child should be tested for lead.

To safeguard yourself:
- Avoid daily use of handmade, imported, or old ceramic mugs or pitchers for hot or acidic beverages, such as juices, coffee, or tea. Commercially made U.S. ceramic, porcelain, and glass dishes or cups are safe. If ceramic dishes or cups become chalky, use them for decorative purposes only.
- Do not use lead crystal decanters for storing alcoholic or other beverages.
- If your home is old, it may have lead pipes. Run the water for a minute before using it, especially before the first use in the morning.

---

‡The Environmental Protection Agency (EPA) provides a toll-free telephone hotline for lead information: 1 (800) 424-LEAD [5323], or visit their website: www.epa.gov/lead.

Chapter 14 Child, Teen, and Older Adult

Food Allergies, Intolerances, and Aversions

Today, up to 8 percent of children in the United States have food **allergies**. The prevalence of these afflictions is on the rise, but no one knows exactly why.[23] It appears that many people "grow out" of food allergies, so rates in adults are much lower, at about 1 percent of the population.[24]

Food Allergies   A true food allergy occurs when a food protein or other large molecule enters body tissues and triggers an immune response. Most food proteins are dismantled to smaller fragments in the digestive tract before absorption, but some larger fragments enter the bloodstream. The immune system of an allergic person reacts to the foreign molecules as it does to any other **antigen**: it releases **antibodies**, **histamine**, and other defensive agents to attack the invaders. For some, a food allergy can elicit a life-threatening reaction of **anaphylactic shock**, which can present symptoms such as tingling of the tongue, throat, or skin or difficulty breathing. The eight foods that cause the great majority of food allergy reactions are listed in Table 14–8.

If a child is known to react to allergens with a life-threatening response, three courses of action are required. First, the child's family and school must guard against any ingestion of the allergen. Second, easy-to-administer doses of the life-saving drug **epinephrine** must be kept close at hand and quickly administered in such emergencies (see Figure 14–4). Third, all adults who interact with the child or the child's food must be educated about the specific allergy and how to ensure the child's safety.[25]

Allergen Avoidance   Avoiding allergens can be tricky because they often sneak into foods in unexpected ways. For example, a pork chop (an innocent food) may be dipped in egg (egg allergy) and breaded (wheat allergy) before being fried in peanut oil (peanut allergy); marshmallow candies may contain egg whites; lunchmeats may contain milk protein binders; and so forth.

Invisible traces of allergen from, say, peanut butter left on tables, chairs, or other surfaces can easily contaminate the hands of a severely allergic child and cause a life-threatening reaction. Scrupulous cleaning of surfaces and regular hand washing by the allergic child can often prevent such an occurrence. Exposure can also occur when the allergen is inhaled. However, the protein allergens of peanuts are not volatile—that is, they do not fly off the food into the air under normal conditions, such as when they are being eaten.

Caregivers of allergic children must pack safe lunches and snacks at home and ask school officials to strictly enforce a "no-swapping" policy in the lunchroom. To prevent nutrient deficiencies, caregivers must also provide adequate substitutes that supply the essential nutrients that were in the omitted foods.[26] Nutrition counseling and growth monitoring are recommended for all children with food allergies.[27]

> Chapter 13 addresses new peanut guidelines for infants.

A potentially life-saving experimental therapy involves exposing people with food allergies to small repeated doses of certain food allergens to temporarily reduce allergic reactions. If perfected, such therapy could prevent serious reactions upon subsequent accidental exposure.[28] Be aware, however, that significant allergic symptoms can occur on exposure, and people attempting such therapy on their own take serious risks.

Food Labels   Food labels must announce the presence of common allergens in plain language. For example, a food containing "textured vegetable protein" must say "soy" on its label. Similarly, "casein," a protein in milk, must be identified as "milk." Consumers with food allergies rely heavily on the accuracy of food labels (Figure 14–5 provides an example). Table 14–9 (p. 538) lists symptoms associated with allergic reactions to food.

Figure 14–4
Preventing Anaphylactic Shock

An epinephrine "pen" can deliver prompt life-saving treatment to a person suffering from anaphylactic shock.

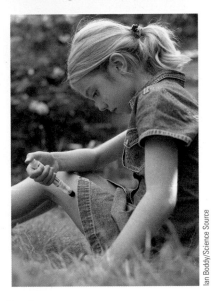

Ian Boddy/Science Source

allergies   immune reactions to foreign substances, such as components of foods. Also called *hypersensitivities* by researchers.

antigen   a substance foreign to the body that elicits the formation of antibodies or an inflammation reaction from immune system cells. Food antigens are usually large proteins. Inflammation consists of local swelling and irritation and attracts white blood cells to the site.

antibodies   large protein molecules that are produced in response to the presence of antigens to inactivate them. Also defined in Chapter 6.

histamine   a substance that participates in causing inflammation; produced by cells of the immune system as part of a local immune reaction to an antigen.

anaphylactic (an-ah-feh-LACK-tick) **shock**   a life-threatening whole-body allergic reaction to an offending substance.

epinephrine (epp-ih-NEFF-rin)   a hormone of the adrenal gland that counteracts anaphylactic shock by opening the airways and maintaining heartbeat and blood pressure.

Figure 14-5

A Food Allergy Warning Label

A food that contains, or may contain, even a trace amount of any of the most common food allergens must clearly say so on its label. For instance, if a product contains the milk protein casein, the label must say "contains milk," or the ingredients list must include "milk." The sunflower seeds below carry a warning about peanut allergy—traces of peanuts may have contaminated the seeds during processing.

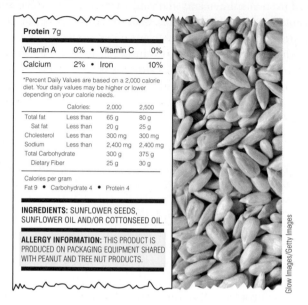

Protein 7g			
Vitamin A	0%	• Vitamin C	0%
Calcium	2%	• Iron	10%

*Percent Daily Values are based on a 2,000 calorie diet. Your daily values may be higher or lower depending on your calorie needs.

	Calories:	2,000	2,500
Total fat	Less than	65 g	80 g
Sat fat	Less than	20 g	25 g
Cholesterol	Less than	300 mg	300 mg
Sodium	Less than	2,400 mg	2,400 mg
Total Carbohydrate		300 g	375 g
Dietary Fiber		25 g	30 g

Calories per gram
Fat 9 • Carbohydrate 4 • Protein 4

INGREDIENTS: SUNFLOWER SEEDS, SUNFLOWER OIL AND/OR COTTONSEED OIL.

ALLERGY INFORMATION: THIS PRODUCT IS PRODUCED ON PACKAGING EQUIPMENT SHARED WITH PEANUT AND TREE NUT PRODUCTS.

Glow Images/Getty Images

Detection of Food Allergy No simple test for food allergy exists, and correct testing requires a skilled physician to assess the nature of the disorder in the context of the person's medical history.[29] Allergies have one or two components. They always involve antibodies, and they sometimes involve symptoms. Therefore, allergies cannot be diagnosed from symptoms alone.

A food allergy that causes symptoms right away is easy to identify because its symptoms correlate with the time of eating the food. A delayed reaction, taking 24 hours or more, is more difficult to pinpoint. For mild symptoms, a good starting point is to keep a record of food intakes and symptoms. If the symptoms correlate with a food, then a blood test for elevated levels of food-specific antibodies and a skin prick test, in which a clinician applies droplets of food extracts to the skin and then lightly pricks or scratches the skin, or other tests can suggest the likelihood of an allergy. The preferred test, a clinical oral food challenge, is lengthy and expensive and entails some risks, and so is less often employed.

Table 14-9

Symptoms of an Allergic Reaction to Food

Any of these symptoms can occur in minutes or hours after ingesting an allergen:

- *Airway.* Difficulty breathing, wheezing, asthma.
- *Digestive tract.* Vomiting, abdominal cramps, diarrhea.
- *Eyes.* Irritated, reddened eyes.
- *Mouth and throat.* Tingling sensation, swelling of the tongue and throat
- *Skin.* Hives, swelling, rashes.
- *Other.* Drop in blood pressure, loss of consciousness; in extreme reactions, death.

Scientific-sounding allergy quackery may deceive people into believing that every malady from cancer to mental depression is caused by food allergies. Beware of fake tests that supposedly determine for the "patient" which foods or supplements to buy (from the quack) to relieve the "allergy."

Food Intolerance and Aversion   A **food intolerance** is characterized by unpleasant symptoms that consistently occur after consumption of certain foods: lactose intolerance is an example. Unlike allergy, a food intolerance does not involve an immune response. A **food aversion**, an intense dislike of a food, may be a biological response to a food that once caused trouble. To repeat, when an important staple food must be excluded from the diet, regardless of the reason why, the child's caretakers must find other foods to provide the omitted nutrients.

Foods are often unjustly blamed when behavior problems arise, but children who are sick from any cause are likely to be cranky. The next section singles out one such type of misbehavior.

KEY POINTS
- Food allergies afflict many U.S. children, and vigilance is required to prevent life-threatening anaphylactic shock.
- Food labels must alert consumers to the presence of common allergens.
- Food aversions may be related to food allergies or to adverse reactions to food.

Can Diet Make a Child Hyperactive?

Attention-deficit/hyperactivity disorder (ADHD), or **hyperactivity**, is a **learning disability** that occurs in 5 to 10 percent of young, school-aged children—or in 1 to 3 in every classroom of 30 children.[30] ADHD is characterized by chronic inability to pay attention, along with overly active behavior and poor impulse control. It can delay growth, lead to academic failure, and cause major behavioral problems. Although some children improve with age, many reach the college years or adulthood before they receive a diagnosis and, with it, the possibility of treatment.

Allergies, Additives, and Sugar   Food allergies have been blamed for ADHD. Restricting common food allergens and synthetic food additives, or supplementing with omega-3 fatty acids have been reported to reduce symptoms in a few children, but research has not yet identified any consistent links between nutrition and ADHD.[31] Meanwhile, parents who wish to avoid common food allergens or food additives can find them listed with the ingredients on food labels.

Many teachers, parents, grandparents, and others assert that some children react behaviorally to sugar. Most researchers, however, have dismissed the "sugar-behavior" theory because almost no scientific evidence supports it. Sugary foods and beverages clearly displace more nutritious choices from the diet, and nutrient deficiencies are known to cause behavioral problems. Sugar itself, however, is unlikely to do so.

Managing ADHD Symptoms   Common sense says that all children get unruly and "hyper" at times. A child who often fills up on caffeinated colas or "energy" drinks, misses lunch, becomes too cranky to nap, misses out on outdoor play, and spends hours in front of a television or other screen media suffers stresses that can trigger chronic patterns of crankiness. In a child with ADHD, a pattern of such behaviors makes coping with the symptoms all the more difficult. Behavioral therapy and medication are the cornerstones of treatment, but caregivers who begin to limit screen time and insist on sufficient sleep, regular mealtimes, a nutritious diet, and daily vigorous outdoor play often see additional improvements.[32]

KEY POINTS
- ADHD is not caused by food allergies, additives, or sugar intakes.
- Consistent care and a nutritious diet may help in coping with ADHD symptoms.

food intolerance an adverse reaction to a food or food additive not involving an immune response.

food aversion an intense dislike of a food, biological or psychological in nature, resulting from an illness or other negative experience associated with that food.

hyperactivity (in children) a syndrome characterized by inattention, impulsiveness, and excess motor activity; usually diagnosed before age 7, lasts 6 months or more and usually entails no mental illness or mental retardation. Properly called *attention-deficit/hyperactivity disorder (ADHD)*.

learning disability a condition resulting in an altered ability to learn basic cognitive skills such as reading, writing, and mathematics.

Figure 14–6
Dental Caries

Caries begin when acid dissolves the enamel that covers the tooth. If not repaired, the decay may penetrate the dentin and spread into the pulp of the tooth, causing inflammation and an abscess.

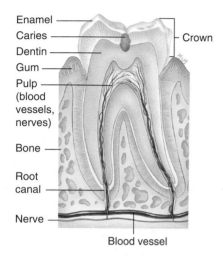

Enamel
Caries
Dentin
Gum
Pulp (blood vessels, nerves)
Bone
Root canal
Nerve
Crown
Blood vessel

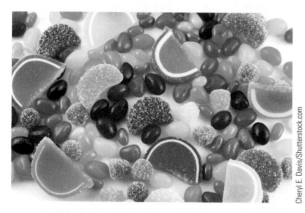

To prevent caries, sticky carbohydrate-rich foods should be removed from the teeth soon after eating.

dental caries decay of the teeth (*caries* means "rottenness"). Also called *cavities*.

plaque (PLACK) a mass of microorganisms and their deposits on the surfaces of the teeth, a forerunner of dental caries and gum disease. (The term *plaques* is used to describe accumulations of fatty material in arteries, as explained in Chapter 11.)

Dental Caries

Dental caries are a serious public health problem afflicting many U.S. children, with a prevalence rate of 42 percent among those 2 to 11 years of age.[33] A very lucky few *never* get dental caries because they have an inherited resistance; others have a sealant applied to their teeth during childhood to stop caries before they can begin. Another method used to fend off dental decay is fluoridation of community water. Perhaps the greatest weapon against caries is simple oral hygiene. But diet has something to do with dental caries, too.

How Caries Develop   Caries develop as acids produced by bacterial growth in the mouth eat into tooth enamel (see Figure 14–6). Bacteria form colonies in **plaque**, which sticks more and more firmly to tooth surfaces unless they are brushed, flossed, or scraped away. Eventually, the acid of plaque creates pits that deepen into cavities. The cavities can be treated by a dentist—the decay is removed and replaced with filling material.

Advanced Dental Disease   Left alone, plaque works its way below the gum line until the acid erodes the roots of teeth and the jawbone in which they are embedded, loosening the teeth and leading to infections of the gums. Bacteria from inflamed, infected gums can then migrate by way of the bloodstream to other tissues, causing illness. Gum disease severe enough to threaten tooth loss afflicts the majority of U.S adults by their later years.

Food and Caries   Bacteria thrive on carbohydrate, producing acid for 20 to 30 minutes after carbohydrate exposure. Of prime importance is the length of time the teeth are exposed to carbohydrate, and this depends to a great extent on whether the teeth are brushed soon afterward as well as on the food's composition, how sticky it is, how long it lasts in the mouth, and the frequency of consumption. Table 14–10 lists foods of both high and low caries potential. Beverages such as soft drinks, orange juice, and sports drinks not only contain sugar but also have a low pH, and their acidic nature can erode the tooth enamel, weakening it. The growing popularity of sugary soft drinks or sports drinks in place of water to quench thirst throughout the day may explain why dental erosion is becoming more common.[34] Limiting sugar intake to 10 percent or less of total calories can minimize the development of dental caries throughout life.[35]

KEY POINT

- Carbohydrate-rich foods contribute to dental caries.

Is Breakfast Really the Most Important Meal of the Day for Children?

A nutritious breakfast is a central feature of a child's diet that supports healthy growth and development. When a child consistently skips breakfast or is allowed to choose sugary foods (candy or marshmallows) in place of nourishing ones (whole-grain cereals), the child will fail to get enough of several nutrients. Nutrients missed from a skipped breakfast are rarely "made up" at lunch and dinner but are most often left out completely that day.[36]

Children who regularly skip breakfast are more likely to be overweight, and may have difficulty paying attention in the classroom, perform poorly on tasks requiring concentration, and achieve lower test scores.[37] Table 14-11 offers ideas for quick, nourishing breakfasts. Common sense tells us that it is unreasonable to expect anyone to study and learn when no fuel has been provided, and even a mid-morning snack can boost flagging attention.[38]

Table 14–10

The Caries Potential of Foods

Low Caries Potential

These foods are less damaging to teeth:
- Eggs, legumes
- Fresh fruit, canned fruit packed in water
- Lean meats, fish, poultry
- Milk, cheese, plain yogurt
- Most cooked and raw vegetables

- Pizza
- Popcorn, pretzels
- Sugarless gum and candy,[a] diet soft drinks
- Toast, hard rolls, bagels

High Caries Potential

Brush teeth immediately after eating these foods:
- Cakes, muffins, doughnuts, pies
- Candied sweet potatoes
- Chocolate milk
- Cookies, granola or "energy" bars, crackers
- Dried fruit (raisins, figs, dates)
- Frozen or flavored yogurt
- Fruit juices or drinks
- Fruit in syrup
- Ice cream or ice milk

- Jams, jellies, preserves
- Lunchmeats containing added sugar
- Meats or vegetables made with sugary glazes
- Oatmeal, oat cereals, oatmeal baked goods[b]
- Peanut butter containing added sugar
- Potato and other snack chips
- Ready-to-eat sugared cereals
- Sugared gum, sugar-sweetened soft drinks, candies, honey, sugar, molasses, syrups
- Toaster pastries

[a]Cariogenic bacteria cannot efficiently metabolize the sugar alcohols in these products, so they do not contribute to dental caries.
[b]The soluble fiber in oats makes this grain particularly sticky and therefore cariogenic.

The U.S. government funds nutritious, high-quality meals, including breakfast, for U.S. schoolchildren. For low-income students, such meals are available at no or low cost, ensuring that all schoolchildren have access to the nutrients they need to perform their best. Additionally, when schools participate in federal school meal programs, student attendance improves, and tardiness declines.

KEY POINTS
- Breakfast supports school performance.
- Free or reduced-priced nutritious school meals are available to low-income children.

How Nourishing Are the Meals Served at School?

In the United States today, 50 million children ages 5 to 19 years spend a large portion of each day in school for about 9 months of each year. More than 30 million children receive lunches through the National School Lunch Program—more than half of them free or at a reduced price.[39] Ten million children eat breakfast at school through the National School Breakfast Program. For many children living in poverty, school food programs constitute their major source of nutrients each day.[40]

The National School Lunch and Breakfast Programs The USDA-regulated school meals provide age-appropriate servings of needed foods each day (see Table 14–12). These lunches are designed to meet, on average, at least a third of the recommended intake for energy, total and saturated fat, protein, calcium, iron, vitamin A, and vitamin C and are often more nutritious than typical lunches brought from home.

Current school meal patterns and nutrition standards ensure the availability of fruit, vegetables, whole grains, and fat-free and low-fat milk, and controlled levels of sodium, saturated fat, and *trans* fat in meals served to schoolchildren. Guidelines also specify that nutrient needs must be met within specified calorie ranges based on age/grade groups for children.[41] Devising ways of enticing children to eat more of the nutritious offerings at school is a topic of current research interest.[42]

Table 14–11

Breakfast Ideas for Rushed Mornings

With some planning, even a rushed morning can include a nutritious breakfast.

- Make sandwiches or tortilla wraps ahead of time. Freeze, thaw or heat, and serve with juice. Fillings may include peanut butter, low-fat cream cheese or other cheeses, jams, fruit slices, refried beans, or meats.
- Teach school-aged children to help themselves to dry cereals, milk, and juice. Keep unbreakable bowls and cups in low cabinets, and keep milk and juice in small plastic pitchers on a low refrigerator shelf.
- Keep a bowl of fresh fruit and small containers of shelled nuts, trail mix (the kind without candy), or roasted peanuts for grabbing.
- Mix granola or other whole-grain cereal into 8-oz tubs of yogurt.
- Toast whole-grain frozen waffles— no syrup needed—to grab and go.
- *Nontraditional choices:* Carrot sticks served with yogurt or bean dip, or leftover casseroles, stews, or pasta dishes, eaten hot or cold.

Table 14–12

School Lunch Patterns

Food Group	Grades		
	K–5	**6–8**	**9–12**
	Amount per week (minimum per day)		
Fruitª (cups)	2½ (½)	2½ (½)	5 (1)
Vegetablesª (cups)	3¾ (¾)	3¾ (¾)	5 (1)
Dark green	≥½	≥½	≥½
Red and orange	≥¾	≥¾	≥1¼
Legumes	≥½	≥½	≥½
Starchy	≥½	≥½	≥½
Other	≥½	≥½	≥¾
Any additional vegetables to meet total requirement	1	1	1½
Grains (oz equivalents)	8–9 (1)	8–10 (1)	10–12 (2)
Protein foods (oz equivalents)	8–10 (1)	9–10 (1)	10–12 (2)
Fluid milkᵇ (cups)	5 (1)	5 (1)	5 (1)
Other			
Calories	550–650	600–700	750–850
Saturated fat (% of total calories)	<10	<10	<10
Sodium (mg)	≤640	≤710	≤740
Trans fat (g per serving)	0	0	0

ªNo more than half of the fruit or vegetable servings may be in the form of juice. All juice must be 100% full strength.

ᵇFluid milk must be low-fat (unflavored) or fat-free (flavored or unflavored).

Source: USDA, School Meals, Nutrition Standards for School Meals (2017), available at www.fns.usda.gov/school-meals/nutrition-standards-school-meals.

Competitive Foods at School   In addition to USDA school lunches, private vendors in school lunchrooms also offer **competitive foods**.[43] Nation-wide, USDA's Smart Snacks in School regulations now require that competitive foods and beverages, including those sold in vending machines, offer students healthy options with more fruit, vegetables, dairy products, and whole grains.[44] They must also meet standards for calories, sodium, fat, saturated fat, *trans* fat, and added sugars. Each state may also set stricter policies, and in states that do so, children and adolescents stay leaner than in states with weaker polices.[45]

KEY POINTS

- School meals are designed to provide at least a third of certain nutrients that children need daily, while emphasizing ample fruit, vegetables, whole grains, and low-fat and fat-free fluid milk; the meals should also meet guidelines set for sodium, saturated fat, and *trans* fats.
- Competitive foods are required to meet specific nutritional standards.

competitive foods unregulated meals, including fast foods, that compete side by side with USDA-regulated school lunches.

Nutrition in Adolescence

LO 14.2 Summarize the nutrient needs of adolescents.

Teenagers are not fed; they eat. Their food choices profoundly affect their health, both now and in the future. In the face of increasing demands on their time, including after-school jobs, social activities, sports, and home responsibilities, older children easily fall into irregular eating habits, relying on quick snacks or fast foods for meals. Within this setting, **adolescence** brings about major physical transformations and a psychological search for identity, acquired largely through trial and error.

Parents, peers, and the media are the primary influential forces shaping adolescents' behaviors and beliefs. As adolescents gain more independence, their diet quality often deteriorates; they choose fewer nutritious whole foods and more sugar, fat, salt, caffeine, and empty calories.[46] Parental examples and guidance still play a role in helping teens to make food and beverage choices that support growth and lasting health.[47]

The Adolescent Growth Spurt The adolescent **growth spurt** brings rapid growth and hormonal changes that affect every organ of the body, including the brain. An average girl's growth spurt begins at 10 or 11 years of age and peaks at about 12 years. Boys' growth spurts begin at 12 or 13 years of age and peak at about 14 years, tapering off at about 19. Two adolescents of the same age may vary in height by a foot, but if growing steadily, each is fulfilling his or her genetic destiny according to an inborn schedule of events.

Energy Needs and Physical Activity The energy needs of adolescents vary tremendously depending on growth rate, gender, body composition, and physical activity. An active, growing boy of 15 may need 3,500 calories or more a day just to maintain his weight, but an inactive girl of the same age whose growth has slowed may need fewer than 1,800 calories to avoid unneeded weight gain. Energy balance is often difficult to regulate in this society—an estimated 21 percent of adolescent girls are obese.[48] On the output side, physical activity often declines sharply, and adolescents rarely meet physical activity guidelines. Most fall well below the recommended levels.[49]

Weight Standards and Body Fatness Weight standards meant for adults are useless for adolescents. Physicians use growth charts to track height and weight gains in adolescents (as demonstrated in Figure C13–1 of Controversy 13, p. 520), and parents should monitor progress and guard against comparisons that can mar a child's self-image.

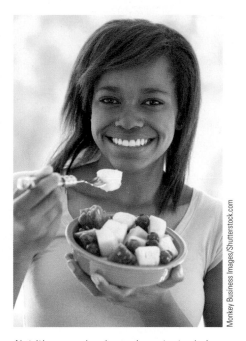

Nutritious snacks play an important role in an active teen's diet.

Girls normally develop somewhat higher percentages of body fat than boys do, a fact that causes much needless worry about becoming overweight. Teens face tremendous pressures regarding body image, and many readily believe scams that promise slenderness or good-looking muscles through "dietary supplements." Healthy, normal-weight teenagers are often "on diets" and many are susceptible to negative influences that can trigger the onset of eating disorders (see Controversy 9, p. 358).

> **KEY POINTS**
> - Teenagers gain independence and often begin to make their own food choices.
> - The adolescent growth spurt demands additional energy and nutrients.
> - The normal gain of body fat during adolescence may be mistaken for obesity, particularly in girls.

Nutrient Needs

Needs for vitamins, minerals, the energy-yielding nutrients, and in fact all nutrients are greater during adolescence than at any other time of life except pregnancy and lactation. The need for iron is particularly high, as all teenagers gain body mass and total blood volume and girls begin menstruation.

The Special Case of Iron The increase in need for iron during adolescence occurs in both genders—but for different reasons. A boy needs more iron at this time to develop

adolescence the period from the beginning of puberty until maturity.

growth spurt the marked rapid gain in physical size usually evident around the onset of adolescence.

extra lean body mass. A girl needs extra iron to gain lean body mass, too, but also to support menstruation. In addition, growth spurts demand still more iron, regardless of the age or gender of the adolescent. This shifting requirement makes pinpointing an adolescent's need tricky, as Table 14–13 demonstrates.

Iron intakes often fail to keep pace with increasing needs, especially for girls, who typically consume fewer iron-rich foods such as meat and fewer total calories than boys. Not surprisingly, iron deficiency is especially prevalent among adolescent girls who are menstruating. Adolescents who live with food insecurity—that is, those who miss meals, eat fewer nutritious foods, or make other food-related compromises of poverty—face increased risks of developing iron deficiencies compared with food-secure children.

Calcium and the Bones Adolescence is a crucial time for bone development. The bones are rapidly growing longer (see Figure 14–7) thanks to a special bone structure, the **epiphyseal plate**, which disappears as a teenager reaches adult height. At the same time, the bones are gaining density, laying down the calcium needed later in life. Calcium intakes must be high to support the development of **peak bone mass**.[50]

Among U.S. adolescents, low calcium intakes have reached crisis proportions. Today, just 37 percent of U.S. high-school students reported drinking any milk at all.[51] Milk is a rich source of calcium, providing nearly 300 milligrams per cup. Paired with a lack of physical activity, low calcium intakes can compromise the development of peak bone mass, greatly increasing the risk of osteoporosis later on.

In the United States, 77 percent of adolescents report drinking sugar-sweetened beverages daily (see Figure 14–8). The choice of a sweetened beverage in place of milk, when repeated time and again, poses two threats: it increases calorie intake and therefore the likelihood of obesity, and it can deprive growing bones of needed nutrients and prevent them from reaching their full attainable density.[52] Conversely, increasing milk consumption can greatly increase bone density.

Vitamin D Vitamin D is as essential as calcium for proper bone growth and development of bone density. Adolescents who do not receive 15 μg of vitamin D from

Figure 14–7

Growth of Long Bones

Bones grow longer as new cartilage cells accumulate at the top portion of the epiphyseal plate and older cartilage cells at the bottom of the plate are calcified.

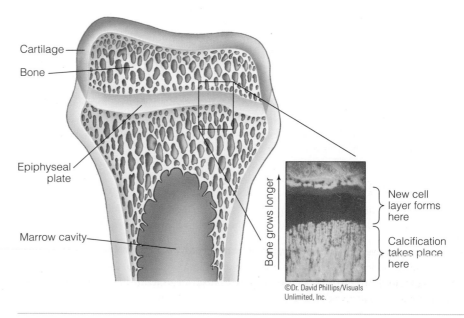

©Dr. David Phillips/Visuals Unlimited, Inc.

epiphyseal (eh-PIFF-ih-seal) **plate** a thick, cartilage-like layer that forms new cells that are eventually calcified, lengthening the bone (*epiphysis* means "growing" in Greek).

peak bone mass highest attainable bone density for an individual, developed during the first three decades of life; also defined in Chapter 8.

vitamin D–fortified milk (2.5 μg per cup of fat-free milk) and other vitamin D–fortified foods each day should take vitamin D in a supplement.

KEY POINTS

- The need for iron increases during adolescence in both boys and girls.
- Sufficient calcium and vitamin D intakes are also crucial during adolescence.

Common Concerns

Two other physical changes stand out as important in adolescence. Menstruation and acne pose special concerns to many adolescents.

Menstruation   At the onset of menstruation, major changes for girls ensue. The hormones that regulate the menstrual cycle affect not just the uterus and the ovaries but the metabolic rate, glucose tolerance, appetite, food intake, and, often, mood and behavior as well. Most women live easily with the cyclic rhythm of the menstrual cycle, but some are afflicted with physical and emotional pain prior to menstruation: **premenstrual syndrome**, or **PMS** (see the Consumer's Guide, p. 547).

Acne   Genes clearly play a role in who gets **acne** and who doesn't, but other factors also affect its development.[53] The hormones of adolescence stimulate the oil glands deep in the skin. The skin's natural oil is supposed to flow out through tiny ducts at the skin's surface, but in many teens the ducts become clogged, and oily secretions build up in them, causing irritation, inflammation, and breakouts of acne. Although often accused, chocolate, sugar, French fries, pizza, salt, and iodine do not worsen acne, but psychological stress clearly does.

Vacations from school, sun exposure, and swimming help to relieve acne, perhaps because they are relaxing, the sun's rays kill bacteria, and water cleanses the skin. The oral prescription medicine Accutane, made from vitamin A, cures deep lesions of severe acne. Although vitamin A itself exerts no effect on acne and supplements can be toxic, quacks market vitamin A–related compounds to young people as acne treatments. One remedy always works: time. While waiting, attend to basic needs. Petal-smooth, healthy skin reflects a tended, cared-for body whose owner provides it with nutrients and fluids to sustain it, exercise to stimulate it, and rest to restore its cells.

KEY POINTS

- Menstrual cycle hormones affect metabolism, glucose tolerance, and appetite.
- No single foods have been proved to aggravate acne, but stress can worsen it.

Eating Patterns and Nutrient Intakes

During adolescence, food habits often change for the worse, and teenagers may miss out on nutrients they need.[54] Teens may skip breakfast; choose less milk, fruit, juices, and vegetables; and consume more sugar-sweetened drinks each day, habits that may bear a relationship to weight gain and higher disease risks in adulthood.[55]

Roles of Adults   Ideally, adults become **gatekeepers**, controlling the type and availability of foods in the teenager's environment. Teenage sons and daughters and their friends should find plenty of nutritious, easy-to-grab food in the refrigerator (meats for sandwiches, raw vegetables, fruit, milk, and fruit juices) and more in the cabinets (breads, peanut butter, nuts, popcorn, cereals). In reality, in many households today, all the adults work outside the home, and teens both shop for and prepare meals. This may yield an unexpected benefit if adults set limits on food choices: adolescents involved in preparing family meals often consume more nourishing diets than uninvolved teens.[56]

Snacks   On average, about a fourth of a teenager's total daily energy intake comes from snacks, which, if chosen carefully, can contribute needed protein and other nutrients. Nutritious protein-rich snacks may also ward off between-meal hunger, protecting against overeating and obesity.

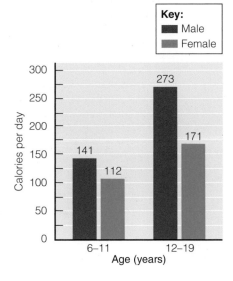

Figure 14–8

Average Daily Intake of Sugar-Sweetened Beverages

The American Heart Association recommends limiting consumption of sugar-sweetened beverages to 450 calories *per week*, an amount clearly exceeded by many U.S. adolescents.

Key:
■ Male
■ Female

Calories per day

300
250
200
150
100
50
0

141   112   273   171

6–11   12–19
Age (years)

premenstrual syndrome (PMS) a cluster of symptoms that some women experience prior to and during menstruation. They include, among others, abdominal cramps, back pain, swelling, headache, painful breasts, and mood changes.

acne chronic inflammation of the skin's follicles and oil-producing glands, which leads to an accumulation of oils inside the ducts that surround hairs; usually associated with the maturation of young adults.

gatekeepers with respect to nutrition, key people who control other people's access to foods and thereby affect their nutrition profoundly. Examples are a spouse who buys and cooks the food, a parent who feeds the children, and a caregiver in a day-care center.

Gatekeepers can help teenagers choose wisely by delivering nutrition information at "teachable moments." Teens prone to weight gain will often open their ears to news about calories in fast foods. Athletic teens may best attend to information about meal timing and sports performance. Still others are fascinated to learn of the skin's need for vitamins and fluid. Gatekeepers must set a good example, keep lines of communication open, and stand by with plenty of nourishing food and reliable nutrition information, but the rest is up to the teens themselves. Ultimately, they make the choices.

KEY POINT

- Gatekeepers can encourage teens to meet nutrient requirements by providing nutritious snacks.

The Later Years

LO 14.3   Identify the dietary factors associated with successful and healthy aging.

The title of this section may imply it is about older people, but it is relevant even if you are only 20 years old—how you live and think at age 20 affects the quality of your life at 60 or 80. According to an old saying, "As the twig is bent, so grows the tree." Unlike a tree, however, you can bend your own twig.

As the Twig Is Bent . . .   Before you will adopt nutrition behaviors to enhance your health in old age, you must accept on a personal level that you, yourself, are aging. Heredity, as well as lifestyle factors, influences aging, but no one escapes the physical, emotional, and social changes that occur. Nutrition plays many documented roles that are critical to successful aging, however.[57] In general, people who reach old age in good mental and physical health most often:

- Are nonsmokers.
- Abstain from alcohol or drink only moderately.
- Are physically active (they walk, bike, swim, or otherwise spend more than 150 minutes per week in physical activity).
- Are well nourished and, in particular, consume sufficient fruit and vegetables.
- Maintain healthy body weights.

They also keep a cheerful attitude and are seldom depressed.

Life Expectancy   The "graying" of America is a continuing trend. Since 1950, the population older than age 65 has almost tripled, and numbers of people older than age 85 have increased sevenfold. People reaching and exceeding age 100 have doubled in number in recent decades, a trend evident among many of the world's populations.

How long a person can expect to live depends on several factors. An estimated 70 to 80 percent of the average person's **life expectancy** depends on individual health-related behaviors, with genes determining the remaining 20 to 30 percent. In the United States, an average person can expect to live 79 years. Specifically, life expectancy is 81 years for white women and 78 years for black women; for white men, it is 77 years and for black men, 72 years—all record highs.[58] The racial gap in life expectancy is narrowing, although reductions of cardiovascular diseases, homicide, and infant mortality are needed to reduce it further.

Human Life Span   The biological schedule that we call aging cuts off life at a genetically fixed point in time. The human **life span** is believed to be 125 years. Even this limit may one day be challenged with advances in medical and genetic technologies.[59] One caution: to date, scientists who study the aging process have found no specific diet or nutrient supplement that will increase **longevity**, despite hundreds of claims to the contrary.

KEY POINTS

- Life expectancy for U.S. adults is increasing, but the human life span is set by heredity.
- Life choices can greatly affect how long a person lives and the quality of life in the later years.

life expectancy the average number of years lived by people in a given society.

life span the maximum number of years of life attainable by a member of a species.

longevity long duration of life.

Nutrition for PMS Relief

Jasmine, seeking relief from premenstrual syndrome (PMS) symptoms, found a promise of a cure on an Internet website. All that she needs to do to vanquish her PMS, according to the site, is to triple her vitamin D intake (and buy their "special" variety). Can a vitamin really cure PMS?

Who Has It and What It Is

Up to 80 percent of menstruating girls and women report uncomfortable menstrual symptoms, and up to 40 percent meet the criteria for PMS.[1]* Researchers have isolated six core symptoms useful for diagnosing PMS:

- Anxiety and tension.
- Mood swings.
- Aches and pains.
- Increased appetite and food cravings.
- Abdominal cramps.
- Weakened interest in activities.[2]

Causes

PMS symptoms may arise from changes in the balance of the two major regulatory hormones of the menstrual cycle: estrogen and progesterone. In particular, the hormone estrogen affects mood by altering the brain's neurotransmitter, serotonin. Taking oral contraceptives, which supply estrogen, often improves mood by eliminating hormonal peaks and valleys. Antidepressant drugs that amplify serotonin's effects also may provide some relief.[3]

Energy Metabolism

Scientists believe that during the two weeks prior to menstruation:

- The basal metabolic rate during sleep speeds up.
- Appetite, particularly for sweets, increases.[4]

- Alcohol consumption and tobacco use may increase.

For women striving to lose weight, then, it may be easier to reduce calorie intakes during the two weeks after menstruation. During the two weeks *before* menstruation, she is fighting a natural, hormone-governed increase in appetite.

Calcium and Vitamin D

Calcium is critical for regulating muscle contraction. Symptoms shared between calcium deficiency and PMS suggest a link, but current research sheds little light on the association.[5] Vitamin D research results are mixed and many questions remain unanswered.

Blood concentrations of vitamin D do not often correlate with overall risks of PMS.[6] Symptoms of depression do commonly correlate with both PMS and low blood vitamin D.[7] However, vitamin D supplements do not relieve either condition in the great majority of studies.[8]

What about the megadoses of vitamin D offered as PMS cures? One small study of Italian women is suggestive.[9] After a single 300,000 IU dose of vitamin D, women with severe PMS reported less pain and less need for painkillers than those given a placebo. The dose used in the study vastly exceeds the UL of 4,000 IU, and cannot be recommended.

The women who responded may have been vitamin D deficient at the start and the supplement may have reversed both their deficiency and their symptoms. The study has not been replicated.

Other Vitamins and Minerals

Years ago, high doses of vitamin B_6 were hawked by vitamin sellers for PMS relief until women who took them developed numb feet and hands, and became unable to walk—symptoms that resolved when the supplements were discontinued.

Research has *not* shown these to be useful: multivitamins, magnesium, or manganese supplements; cutting down on alcohol or sodium; or taking diuretics to relieve water retention. (Sodium and water retention just before menstruation may be normal and desirable; diuretic drugs eliminate excess sodium and water but can also cause electrolyte imbalances.) Caffeine may worsen PMS symptoms, but how much is too much is not clear. And although adequate sleep, physical activity, and stress reduction strategies may help some women, research in these areas is lacking.

Moving Ahead

For Jasmine and others coping with PMS, some good news—PMS symptoms may be lessened with simple daily strategies:

- Eat small, frequent meals.
- Choose a diet pattern that follows the Dietary Guidelines for Americans.
- Meet the need for calcium and vitamin D.
- Minimize caffeine intake.
- Exercise regularly.
- Get enough sleep.
- Reduce stress.

With just these few changes, food cravings, bloating, and stress may improve, and mood often brightens.

Review Questions[†]

1. Taking 300,000 IU per day of vitamin D may alleviate some PMS symptoms, but this may not be safe. T F

2. Taking multivitamins, magnesium, manganese, or diuretics can often cure PMS. T F

3. During the two weeks *before* menstruation, women may note less desire for sugary foods. T F

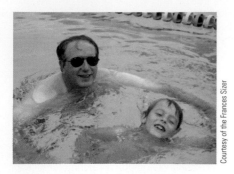
Physical activity benefits people at all stages of life.

Nutrition in the Later Years

LO 14.4   Describe the changes in nutrient needs that occur as people age.

Nutrient needs become more individual with age, depending on genetics and individual medical history. For example, one person's stomach acid secretion, which helps in iron absorption, may decline, so that person may need to choose iron-rich foods more often. Another person may have difficulty storing folate due to past liver damage and therefore have increased folate needs. Table 14–14 lists some changes that can affect nutrition. Because physiological changes advance with age, separate DRI values are set for people 51 to 70 years old and for those older than 70 (see the back of the book, pp. A and B).

Energy, Activity, and the Muscles

With advancing age, people typically need fewer calories each day. One reason is that the number of active cells in each organ often decreases and the metabolism-controlling hormone thyroxine diminishes, reducing the body's resting metabolic rate. Another reason is that older people are often less physically active and lose muscle tissue, resulting in **sarcopenia**, an age-related loss of muscle tissue with serious health implications.[60] Sarcopenia can occur in active adults, but is accelerated by inactivity.

Energy Recommendations   After about the age of 50, the intake recommendation for energy assumes about a 5 percent reduction in energy output per decade. Some of the decline in energy need may be avoidable, however. Staying physically active boosts energy needs and contributes to a healthy immune response and sharp mental functioning. Physical activity and an adequate diet also oppose a destructive spiral of sedentary behavior and mental and physical losses in the elderly, sometimes called geriatric failure to thrive or "the dwindles." The set of conditions associated with failure to thrive includes:

- Diminished physical ability to function; inability to shop, cook, or prepare meals.
- Depression or anxiety.
- Malnutrition, with impaired immunity, slow wound healing, slow recovery from surgery, and periodic hospitalizations.
- Weight loss and appetite loss with sarcopenia.

Such signs should be taken seriously, and immediate steps should be taken to remedy them.

Table 14–14	
Physical Changes of Aging that Affect Nutrition	
DIGESTIVE TRACT	Intestines lose muscle strength, resulting in sluggish motility that leads to constipation. Stomach inflammation, abnormal bacterial growth, and greatly reduced acid output impair digestion and absorption. Pain and fear of choking may cause food avoidance or reduced intake.
HORMONES	Among many hormone changes, the pancreas secretes less insulin and cells become less responsive to it, causing abnormal glucose metabolism.
MOUTH	Tooth loss, gum disease, and reduced saliva output impede chewing and swallowing. Choking may become likely; pain may cause avoidance of hard-to-chew foods.
SENSORY ORGANS	Diminished sight can make food shopping and preparation difficult; diminished senses of smell and taste may reduce appetite, although research is needed to clarify this effect.
BODY COMPOSITION	Weight loss and decline in lean body mass lead to lowered energy requirements. May be preventable or reversible through physical activity.

sarcopenia (SAR-koh-PEE-nee-ah) age-related loss of skeletal muscle mass, muscle strength, and muscle function.

Weight Loss and Overweight   Involuntary weight loss in an older person demands immediate attention. It may be the result of some easily reversible factor, or it may reflect a disease condition that demands immediate treatment; in either case, a diagnosis is needed. Dealing with involuntary weight loss in older people entails finding the causes (physical, psychological, or other) and addressing them. To help them regain lost weight, offer favorite foods in five or six small, high-calorie meals each day instead of three larger ones. This strategy can halt or reverse weight loss and increase nutrient intakes.

Obesity can pose serious problems for many as they reach old age. Particularly when muscle strength becomes insufficient to handle their excess body weight, these "fat and frail" elderly face a progressive loss of mobility and self-reliance.[61] For them, there is little leeway in the diet for foods of low nutrient density, such as ultra-processed foods rich in added sugars, fats, and alcohol. Weight-loss dieting should be approached with caution for this group because weight loss often causes muscle and bone tissue losses.[62] When achieved with a nutritious calorie-controlled diet along with adequate dietary protein and regular exercise, weight loss can safely reduce body fatness, improve health, and benefit muscle functioning.[63]

Physical Activity   This chapter's Think Fitness feature (p. 550) emphasizes the importance of physical activity in maintaining body tissue integrity throughout life. People spending energy in physical activity can also eat more food, gaining nutrients. Sadly, almost 90 percent of people age 65 and older fail to meet exercise guidelines and thereby limit their own health and fitness in their later years.[64] Any movement is better than no movement: participating in leisure activities or performing as little as 7 minutes daily of light activity is reported to help the elderly improve many health-related outcomes.[65] Some people in their 90s have improved their balance, added pep to their walking steps, and regained some precious independence after just eight weeks of resistance training.

Figure 14–9 emphasizes this point: the photos compare cross sections of the thighs of a young woman and of an older woman to demonstrate the sarcopenia typical of sedentary aging, which brings with it destructive weakness, poor balance, and deterioration of health and vigor. Resistance training through life helps to prevent at least some of this muscle loss, and consuming sufficient protein may help, too.[66]

KEY POINTS

- Energy needs decrease with age.
- Failure to thrive, involuntary weight loss, and obesity pose health threats during aging.
- Physical activity helps maintain lean tissue and improve health during aging.

Protein Needs

The protein DRI remains about the same for older people as for young adults. Researchers are investigating whether by increasing dietary protein, older people may better maintain muscle mass and function.[67] Some findings suggest that a little extra protein beyond the DRI may stimulate muscle protein synthesis in healthy, mobile older adults and shift nitrogen balance toward the positive. If they are immobilized, however, extra protein cannot prevent muscle loss.

For older people who have lost their teeth, chewing tough, protein-rich meats sufficiently to allow their proper use by the body becomes next to impossible. They need soft-cooked protein sources, such as well-cooked, stewed or chopped meats, milk-based soups, soft cheeses, eggs, or fish. Those with chronic constipation, heart disease, or diabetes may benefit most from fiber-rich, low-fat protein sources, such as legume–whole grain combinations.

As energy needs decrease, lower-calorie protein sources, such as lean tender meats, poultry, fish, boiled eggs, fat-free milk products, and legumes can help hold weight to a healthy level. Underweight or malnourished older adults need the opposite—energy-dense protein sources such as eggs scrambled with margarine, tuna salad with mayonnaise, peanut butter, and milkshakes. Should a flagging appetite reduce food intake,

Figure 14–9

Muscle Loss in Aging: Sarcopenia

These photos show cross sections of two women's thighs. They may appear to be about the same size from the outside, but the 20-year-old woman's thigh is dense with muscle tissue (dark areas), while the 64-year-old woman's thigh has lost muscle and gained fat. Such debilitating muscle loss is prevalent in aging but not inevitable. Optimal protein nutrition and strength-building physical activity can oppose its development.

20-year-old woman's thigh

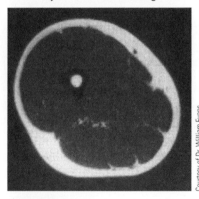

Courtesy of Dr. William Evans

64-year-old woman's thigh

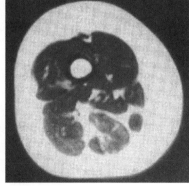

Courtesy of Dr. William Evans

Benefits of Physical Activity for the Older Adult

The Physical Activity Guidelines for Americans recommend that older adults strive to obtain 150 minutes of physical activity, or whatever amount they can safely and comfortably perform, each week.[68] Older adults who do so have more lean body mass, better balance, stronger immune systems, and improved sleep quality; they suffer fewer injuries from falls, experience fewer symptoms of arthritis, enjoy better overall health, and even live longer than their less-fit peers.[69] Simply put, active older people resemble much younger people physiologically.[70]

Provide Protein

At some point, perhaps as early as age 60 or 70, the muscles lose efficiency in adding new muscle tissue in response to resistance training.[71] Some extra protein at each meal may help in this regard because, compared with younger muscles, older muscles require relatively greater amounts of protein to speed up post-exercise protein synthesis (see Chapter 10 for details).[72] Middle-aged and older people who wish to retain vitality should start now and continue to build and defend their muscle mass through life.

Customize the Plan

Each elderly person faces different degrees and types of physical limitations. Therefore, each should exercise in his or her own way. Modest exercise, such as a 10-minute walk a day, a flexibility routine, or resistance training (even while seated) provides progressive benefits.[73] Even obese elders who take up such exercising benefit impressively.[74] Great achievements are possible, improvements are inevitable, and it's never too late to benefit.

start now! Ready to make a change? If you are an older person, or if you care for an older person, devise a sensible exercise plan and track your activity in Diet & Wellness Plus in MindTap for one week. At the end of that week, look at your total physical activity and decide if a higher activity level is desirable and achievable for the following week.

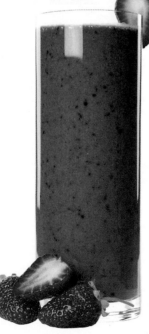

Olvina/Shutterstock.com

supplemental nutrient-fortified formulas in liquid, pudding, cookie, or other forms between meals can supply needed energy, protein, and other nutrients.

KEY POINT

- Protein DRI values remain about the same through adult life, but physical conditions change and may affect both the amounts of protein needed and its sources.

Carbohydrates and Fiber

Ample whole-grain breads, cereals, rice, and pasta provide the steady supply of carbohydrate that the brain demands for optimal functioning. The fiber in these foods takes on extra importance in aging to prevent constipation, a common complaint among older adults and nursing home residents in particular.

> For fiber sources and tips for increasing intakes, see Figure 4–16, p. 133.

Fruit and vegetables supply soluble fibers and other food components to help ward off chronic diseases. With aging, however, come problems of transportation, limited cooking facilities, and chewing disabilities that limit some elderly people's intakes of fresh fruit and vegetables. For these people, a blender can yield a refreshing, nutritious drink from frozen or fresh fruit and vegetables, a banana, and some milk or yogurt. In truth, most older adults, even those without limitations, fail to obtain the recommended 25 or so grams of fiber each day (14 grams per 1,000 calories).[75] When low fiber intakes combine with low fluid intakes, inadequate exercise, and many medications, constipation becomes inevitable.

KEY POINT

- Adequate fiber can help older adults to avoid constipation.

Fats and Arthritis

Older adults must attend to fat intakes for several reasons. Consuming enough of the essential fatty acids and limiting intakes of saturated and *trans* fats remain priorities for disease prevention in aging.

Osteoarthritis The common type of **arthritis**, osteoarthritis, often causes loss of mobility as people age. Normally, the ends of healthy bones are protected by small sacs of fluid that act as joint lubricants. With arthritis, the sacs erode, cartilage and bone ends disintegrate, joints become malformed, and moving becomes painful. In overweight people, loss of body weight often brings relief, particularly in the knees; physical activities such as walking, bicycling, and swimming can reduce arthritis pain in most joints and improve physical function, mental health, and quality of life.[76]

Rheumatoid Arthritis Rheumatoid arthritis arises from an immune system malfunction: the immune system mistakenly attacks the bone coverings as if they were foreign tissue. The lining around the joints becomes swollen and inflamed, and as a result, joints become painful to move. Some evidence suggests a role for the omega-3 fatty acid EPA in treatment of rheumatoid arthritis (but not of osteoarthritis).[77]

Many ineffective or unproven "cures" are sold for arthritis relief. Research is mixed on whether the popular dietary supplements chondroitin sulfate and glucosamine, both components of cartilage, provide relief.[78]

Gout A form of inflammatory arthritis known as gout affects millions of U.S. adults, and its prevalence increases with age. An increased incidence of gout has been observed with "triggers" such as insulin resistance, overweight, and a "Western-style" diet high in meats, sweets, and fats. Adherence to a diet known for its other health benefits, the DASH diet, is associated with a lower risk of gout.[79] (The DASH diet plan is in Appendix E.)

KEY POINT

- Arthritis causes pain and immobility, and older people with arthritis often fall for quack cures.

Vitamin Needs

Vitamin needs change as people age. Among factors affecting these needs are changes in absorption, metabolism, and excretion of vitamins.

Vitamin A Vitamin A stands alone among the vitamins in that its absorption appears to increase with aging. For this reason, some researchers have proposed lowering the vitamin A requirement for aged populations. Others resist this proposal because foods containing vitamin A and its precursor beta-carotene confer health benefits and because many of these foods, notably green leafy vegetables, are frequently lacking in the diet.

Vitamin D Changes with aging can interfere with vitamin D metabolism, so the DRI for vitamin D is slightly higher for older people (DRI lists are at the back of the book, pp. A and B). In aging, these factors combine to reduce blood vitamin D concentrations:

- Intakes decrease with lower intake of fortified milk.
- Sunlight exposure decreases as more time is spent indoors.
- Synthesis in the skin declines fourfold.
- Activation by the kidneys diminishes.

Supplements may help normalize blood vitamin D and may prevent some number of falls in elderly people. Anyone with osteoporosis should follow medical advice.

Vitamin B_{12} By age 60, reduced stomach acid production can reduce the ability to absorb vitamin B_{12} from food, making deficiency likely. Stomach acid-reducing medications, frequently prescribed for older people, worsen the problem and may raise the risk of vitamin B_{12} deficiency by as much as 80 percent.[80] Many elderly people suffer marginal deficiencies, but most of these cases go unrecognized and untreated because vitamin B_{12} tests are rarely performed. Elderly people often choose less meat and milk, rich suppliers

arthritis a usually painful inflammation of joints caused by many conditions, including infections, metabolic disturbances, or injury; usually results in altered joint structure and loss of function.

of vitamin B_{12}, so dietary insufficiency may also contribute to these deficiencies. Synthetic vitamin B_{12} is reliably absorbed and injections are available. Much misery can be averted by testing for and reversing deficiencies of vitamin B_{12} in elderly people.

Diet and Vision   Losses of vision in the elderly correlates with loss of life that cannot be explained by other risk factors. Dark green, leafy vegetables, which are rich in certain carotenoid phytochemicals, may protect the eyes from one cause of blindness: macular degeneration.[§] Carotenoid and other nutrient supplements are unproven for eye protection, although some physicians may prescribe them in hopes of slowing the advance of macular degeneration.

By age 75, half of all U.S. adults have developed **cataracts**.[81] A cataract is a clouding of the lens that impairs vision and leads to blindness. Only 5 percent of people younger than 50 years have cataracts; afterward, the percentage jumps to between 20 and 30 percent. The lens of the eye is easily oxidized. Some studies suggest that a diet high in *foods* that provide ample antioxidants—carotenoids, vitamin C, and vitamin E— may reduce the risk of early onset and progression of cataracts.[82] High-dose vitamin C or E supplements, conversely, may increase some people's cataract risks.[83]

KEY POINTS

- Vitamin A absorption increases with aging.
- Elderly people are vulnerable to deficiencies of vitamin D and vitamin B_{12}.

Water and the Minerals

Dehydration is a major risk for older adults. Total body water decreases with age, so even mild stresses, such as a hot day or a fever, can quickly dehydrate the tissues. The thirst mechanism may diminish, and even healthy older people may go for long periods without drinking. The kidneys also lose efficiency in recapturing water before it is lost as urine. Dehydration then leads to problems such as constipation, bladder problems, and mental confusion that is easily mistaken for **senile dementia**. This effect may occur with a water loss of as little as 2 percent of body weight. In a person with asthma, dehydration thickens mucus in the lungs, blocking airways and leading to pneumonia. In a bedridden person, dehydration can lead to **pressure ulcers**. To prevent dehydration, older adults should consume sufficient fluid each day. The beverage recommendations for adults 51 years and older suggest that women consume 9 cups of fluid each day; for men, recommendations increase to 13 cups.

Fluid choices, strategically made, can improve the nutrition status of an elderly person. For example, an underweight person with diminished appetite and weight loss may be tempted by a smoothie of bananas, frozen strawberries or other frozen fruit, milk or soy milk, and a touch of chocolate syrup or powdered sugar. Hearty, soft-cooked meat and vegetable soups, milk-based seafood or vegetable bisque, puddings, and commercial liquid meal replacers all provide fluid along with calories, protein, and other nutrients essential for health. In contrast, an overweight elderly person needs tempting low- or no-calorie beverages: plain or sparkling water with lemon or lime, broth-based soups, artificially sweetened tea or coffee, and low-sodium vegetable juices.

Iron   Iron status generally improves in later life, especially in women after menstruation ceases and in those who take iron supplements, eat red meat regularly, and include vitamin C–rich fruit in their daily diet. When iron-deficiency anemia does occur, diminished appetite with low food intake is often the cause. Aside from diet, other factors make iron deficiency likely in older people:

- Chronic blood loss from ulcers or hemorrhoids.
- Poor iron absorption due to reduced stomach acid secretion.
- Antacid use, which interferes with iron absorption.
- Use of medicines that cause blood loss, including anticoagulants, aspirin, and arthritis medicines.

cataract (CAT-uh-ract) clouding of the lens of the eye that can lead to blindness. Cataracts can be caused by injury, viral infection, toxic substances, genetic disorders, and possibly some nutrient deficiencies or imbalances.

senile dementia the loss of brain function beyond the normal loss of physical adeptness and memory that occurs with aging.

pressure ulcers damage to the skin and underlying tissues as a result of unrelieved compression and poor circulation to the area; also called *bed sores*.

[§]The carotenoids are lutein and zeaxanthin, which help to form pigments of the macula of the eye.

Chapter 14 Child, Teen, and Older Adult

Older people take more medicines than others, and drug and nutrient interactions are common.

Zinc Zinc deficiencies, common in older people, are known to impair immune function and may increase the likelihood of infectious diseases, such as pneumonia. Zinc deficiency can also depress the appetite and blunt the sense of taste, thereby reducing food intakes and worsening zinc status. Many medications interfere with the body's absorption or use of zinc, and an older adult's medicine load can worsen zinc deficiency.

Multinutrient Supplements Overall, elderly people often benefit from a single balanced low-dose vitamin and mineral supplement. Older people taking such supplements suffer fewer sicknesses caused by infection. A summary of the effects of aging on nutrient needs appears in Table 14–15.

Table 14–15
Summary of Nutrient Concerns in Aging

Nutrient	Effects of Aging	Comment
Energy	Need decreases.	Physical activity moderates the decline.
Fiber	Low intakes make constipation likely; beneficial for controlling weight and reducing the risk of heart disease and type 2 diabetes.	Inadequate water intakes and physical activity, along with some medications, compound risks of constipation.
Protein	Needs may stay the same or slightly increase; intake often decreases.	Low-fat milk and other high-quality protein foods are appropriate; high-fiber legumes provide protein and other nutrients.
Vitamin A	Absorption increases.	Supplements normally not needed.
Vitamin D	Increased likelihood of inadequate intake; synthesis in skin tissue declines.	Daily moderate exposure to sunlight may be of benefit.
Vitamin B_{12}	Malabsorption of some forms.	Foods fortified with synthetic vitamin B_{12} or a supplement may be of benefit in addition to a balanced diet.
Water	Lack of thirst and increased urine output make dehydration likely.	Mild dehydration is a common cause of confusion.
Iron	In women, status improves after menopause; deficiencies linked to chronic blood losses and low stomach acid output.	Stomach acid is required for absorption; antacid or other medicine use may aggravate iron deficiency; vitamin C and meat enhance absorption.
Zinc	Intakes are often inadequate and absorption may be poor, but needs may also increase.	Medications interfere with absorption; deficiency may depress appetite and sense of taste.
Calcium	Intakes may be low; osteoporosis becomes common.	Lactose intolerance commonly limits milk intake; calcium-rich substitutes or supplements are needed (consider supplements that include vitamin D).
Potassium	Increased intake might decrease the risk of high blood pressure.	Include fruit, vegetables, and low-fat or fat-free milk and yogurt in the diet.
Sodium	Decreasing intake might lower the risk of high blood pressure.	Choose and prepare foods with little to no added salt; consider herbs or salt substitutes to add flavor to foods.
Fat	Increased risk of cardiovascular disease.	Look for foods low in saturated fats, *trans* fats, and cholesterol, and make most fats polyunsaturated or monounsaturated.

Table 14–16

What to Expect in Aging

Changes with Age You Probably Can Slow or Prevent

By exercising, eating an adequate diet, reducing stress, and planning ahead, you may be able to slow or prevent:

✓ Wrinkling of skin due to sun damage
✓ Some forms of mental confusion
✓ Elevated blood pressure
✓ Accelerated resting heart rate
✓ Reduced lung capacity and oxygen uptake
✓ Increased body fatness
✓ Elevated blood cholesterol
✓ Slowed energy metabolism
✓ Decreased maximum work rate
✓ Loss of sexual functioning
✓ Loss of joint flexibility
✓ Diminished oral health: loss of teeth, gum disease
✓ Bone loss
✓ Digestive problems, constipation

Changes with Age You Probably Must Accept

These changes are probably beyond your control:

✓ Graying hair
✓ Balding
✓ Some drying and wrinkling of skin
✓ Impairment of near vision
✓ Some loss of hearing
✓ Reduced taste and smell sensitivity
✓ Reduced touch sensitivity
✓ Slowed reactions (reflexes)
✓ Slowed mental function
✓ Diminished visual memory
✓ Menopause (women)
✓ Loss of fertility (men)
✓ Loss of joint elasticity

KEY POINT

■ Aging alters vitamin and mineral needs; some rise, while others decline.

Can Diet Choices Lengthen Life?

Although people cannot alter the year of their birth, they can probably alter the length and quality of their lives. Lifestyle choices make a difference.

Lifestyle Factors   Have you ever noticed that some older adults seem younger than their chronological ages? Research on this observation has focused on health habits of older people and has identified three major factors related to nutrition:

■ Abstinence from, or moderation in, alcohol use.

■ Regular nutritious meals.

■ Weight control.

Three additional factors are recognized: regular adequate sleep, abstinence from smoking, and regular physical activity. The physical health of those who engage in all six positive health practices may be comparable to that of people 30 years younger who engage in few or none. Some changes of aging, such as graying hair and reduced senses of smell, taste, and eyesight are inescapable, but others may yield to individual life choices (see Table 14–16).

Energy Restriction   Evidence that diet might influence the life span emerged decades ago when researchers starved young rats, feeding them diets extremely low in energy. The starved rats stopped growing, while a group of control rats ate and grew normally. Many of the starved rats died young from malnutrition. The survivors, although permanently deformed from their ordeal, remained alive far beyond the normal life span for such animals and developed diseases of aging much later than normal. Since then, this result has been repeated in many species (see Table 14–17).

With moderate energy restriction, animals also retain youthfulness longer and develop fewer disease risk factors such as high blood pressure, glucose intolerance, and immune system impairments.[84] In monkeys, moderate calorie restriction generally prolongs life and reduces the incidence of diabetes, cancer, and cardiovascular disease.[85] No one can say conclusively whether any of these findings might also apply to human beings.[86]

On the negative side, severely energy-restricted mice are more susceptible to acute infections.[87] Also, although energy restriction may improve chronic disease risks, it stunts growth and may damage some systems to benefit others. Moreover, without supplements, calorie-restricted diets lack needed nutrients. Scientists are

---

Table 14–17

Effects of Energy Restriction on Life Span

Differences in maximum life span are observed between animals eating normally and those whose energy intakes are restricted.

	Normal Diet	Energy Restricted
Rats	33 months	47 months
Spiders	100 days	139 days
Single-celled animals (protozoa)	13 days	25 days

---

hoping to discover drugs that mimic the benefits of calorie restriction while minimizing risks.[88] For now, however, any supplement or treatment claiming to prolong human life is a hoax.

KEY POINT

- In rats and other species, food energy deprivation lengthens the lives of individuals.

Aging, Immunity, and Inflammation

A free-radical theory blames chronic inflammation for physical deterioration in aging. As people age, the body's internal antioxidant enzymes diminish and the immune system loses function. When illness strikes, the immune system becomes overstimulated but less able to cope with the challenge. The result is chronic inflammation, with increasing frailty and illness.[89]

Most chronic diseases—such as atherosclerosis, Alzheimer's disease, and rheumatoid arthritis—involve inflammation. Therefore, inflammation is believed to be a partly harmful process; yet at the same time it plays a critical role in the destruction of invading organisms and repair of damaged tissues. The longest-lived people, the theory states, have an optimal balance between inflammatory and anti-inflammatory influences.

These lines of research have promoted a storm of worthless and sometimes hazardous "life-extending" pills, supplements, and treatments, such as DHEA, testosterone, and growth hormone. Better to spend money on legumes, fresh fruit, and vegetables, along with a good pair of walking shoes.

KEY POINT

- Claims for life extension through antioxidants or other supplements are unsubstantiated.

Can Diet Affect the Course of Alzheimer's Disease?

The cause of Alzheimer's disease (AD), the most prevalent form of senile dementia, is unknown, but genetic inheritance clearly contributes. The devastation of AD occurs when areas of the brain that coordinate memory and cognition become littered with clumps of abnormal protein fragments and tangles of nerve tissue that damage or kill brain cells.** Soon, memory fails and reasoning powers diminish, followed by loss of communication skills; loss of physical capabilities; onset of anxiety, delusions, depression, anger, inappropriate behavior, and sleep disturbance; and eventually loss of life itself. Once the destruction begins, the outlook for its reversal is bleak.

Healthy eating patterns, including the nutrient-rich Mediterranean diet, have been associated with slowed mental declines in aging.[90] The Mediterranean diet includes seafood, and seafood raises blood omega-3 fatty acids. Among people with mild AD, those with higher blood omega-3 fatty acids may experience slower cognitive decline than others, possibly because of a modulating effect on gene expression.[91] The mineral zinc, once viewed as a hoped-for nutrition link with AD, has been dismissed as such—dietary zinc content and blood values seem unrelated to the condition, although the actions of enzymes that rely on these minerals are impaired.[92]

In addition to AD, other forms of dementia are common among the elderly; Figure 14–10 presents some controllable risk factors associated with them. Once AD has set in, preventing excessive weight loss becomes a primary concern. Depression and forgetfulness can lead to skipped meals and poor food choices. Caregivers can help by providing well-liked, well-balanced, and well-tolerated meals and snacks served in a cheerful, peaceful atmosphere with companions to spur interest in eating.

**The protein fragments are called *beta-amyloid*.

Figure 14–10

Controlling Dementia Risk Factors

Dementia is common among elderly people and often unpreventable, but some factors associated with its development can be controlled.

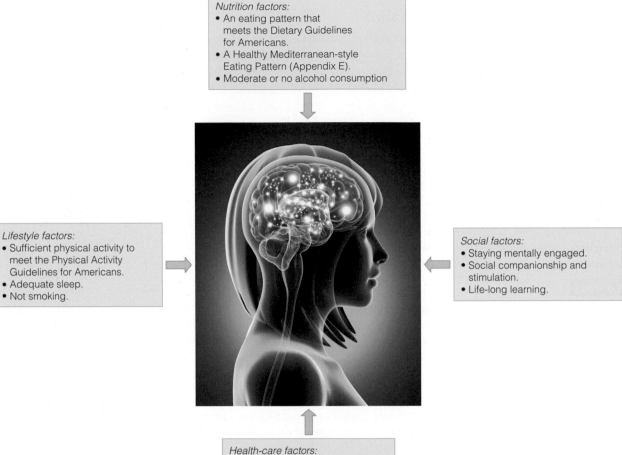

Nutrition factors:
- An eating pattern that meets the Dietary Guidelines for Americans.
- A Healthy Mediterranean-style Eating Pattern (Appendix E).
- Moderate or no alcohol consumption

Lifestyle factors:
- Sufficient physical activity to meet the Physical Activity Guidelines for Americans.
- Adequate sleep.
- Not smoking.

Social factors:
- Staying mentally engaged.
- Social companionship and stimulation.
- Life-long learning.

Health-care factors:
- All medical tests on schedule.
- Effective treatment of diabetes, cardiovascular diseases, or hypertension.
- Correction of hearing or vision loss.

iStock.com/pixologicstudio

Sources: Adapted from P. B. Gorelick and coauthors, Defining optimal brain health in adults: A presidential advisory from the American Heart Association/American Stroke Association, Stroke (2017), epub ahead of print, doi.org/10.1161/STR.0000000000000148; B. Sabayan and F. Sorond, Reducing risk of dementia in older age, Journal of the American Medical Association 317 (2017): 2028.

KEY POINTS

- Alzheimer's disease causes some degree of brain deterioration in many people older than age 65.
- Nutrition care gains importance as Alzheimer's disease progresses.

Food Choices of Older Adults

Most older people are independent, socially sophisticated, mentally lucid, fully participating members of society who report being happy and healthy. Many have cut down on intakes of saturated fats and are eating slightly more vegetables and whole-grain breads, although few meet the recommended intakes of these foods. Older people who eat a wide variety of foods are better nourished and enjoy a better quality of life than those who subsist on a monotonous diet. Grocers assist the elderly by prominently displaying good-tasting, low-fat, nutritious foods in easy-to-open, single-serving packages with labels that are easy to read.

Obstacles to Adequacy   Many factors affect the food choices and eating habits of older people, including whether they live alone or with others, at home or in an institution. Men living alone, for example, are likely to consume poorer-quality diets than those living with spouses.

Two other factors stand out: increasing use of multiple medications and abuse of alcohol.[93] People older than age 65 consume about a fourth of all the medications, both prescription and over-the-counter (OTC), sold in the United States. Although these medications enable people with health problems to live longer and more comfortably, they also pose a threat to nutrition status because they may interfere with nutrients, depress the appetite, or alter taste perception (see Controversy 14, p. 562).

The incidence of alcoholism, alcohol abuse, or problem drinking among the elderly in the United States is estimated at between 2 and 10 percent. Loneliness, isolation, and depression accompany overuse of alcohol and lessen nutrient intakes. Table 14–18 provides an easily remembered means of identifying those who might be at risk for malnutrition.

Programs that Help   Several federal programs can provide help for older people. Social Security provides income to retired people older than age 62 who paid into the system during their working years. The Supplemental Nutrition Assistance Program (SNAP), formerly called the Food Stamp Program, assists the very poor by supplementing their monthly food budgets. The Administration on Aging coordinates services governed by the Older Americans Act, including the provision of nutritious meals in a social congregate setting, education and shopping assistance, counseling and referral to other needed services, and transportation to necessary appointments. For the homebound, Meals on Wheels volunteers deliver meals to the door. Nutritionists are

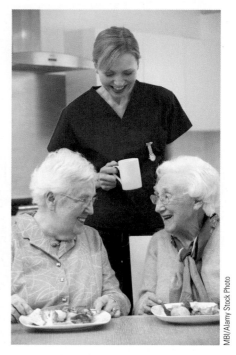

Shared meals can be the high point of the day.

MBI/Alamy Stock Photo

Table 14–18

Predictors of Malnutrition in the Elderly

Here is a quick and easy-to-remember list of factors that increase the likelihood of malnutrition in the elderly. The first letters spell the word *DETERMINE*.

To Determine:	Ask:
Disease	▪ Do you have an illness or condition that changes the types or amounts of foods you eat?
Eating poorly	▪ Do you eat fewer than two meals a day? Do you eat fruit, vegetables, and milk products daily?
Tooth loss or mouth pain	▪ Is it difficult or painful to eat?
Economic hardship	▪ Do you have enough money to buy the food you need?
Reduced social contact	▪ Do you eat alone most of the time?
Multiple medications	▪ Do you take three or more different prescribed or OTC medications daily?
Involuntary weight loss or gain	▪ Have you lost or gained 10 pounds or more in the last 6 months?
Needs assistance	▪ Are you physically able to shop, cook, and feed yourself?
Elderly person	▪ Are you older than 80?

wise not to focus solely on nutrient and food intakes of the elderly because enjoyment and social interactions may be as important as food itself.

Many older people, even able-bodied ones with financial resources, find themselves unable to perform all the needed cooking, cleaning, and shopping tasks. For anyone living alone, and particularly for those of advanced age, it is important to work through the problems that food preparation presents. This chapter's Food Feature presents some ideas.

KEY POINTS

- Food choices of the elderly are affected by aging, altered health status, and changed life circumstances.
- Federal programs can help provide nourishment, transportation, and social interactions.

FOOD FEATURE

Single Survival and Nutrition on the Run

LO 14.5 Describe the challenges associated with regularly eating alone.

A single person of any age, whether a busy student in a college dormitory, an elderly person in a retirement apartment, or a professional in an efficiency suite, faces challenges in obtaining nourishing meals. People without access to kitchens and freezers find storing foods problematic, so they often eat out. Following is a collection of ideas gathered from single people who have devised ways to nourish themselves despite obstacles.

Is Eating in Restaurants a Wise Choice?

Restaurant foods are convenient, but can such foods meet nutrient needs or

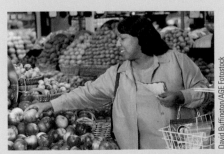

Shopping for and preparing nutritious foods for one person takes some special know-how.

David Buffington/AGE Fotostock

support health as well as homemade foods? The answer is "perhaps," but making it so takes some effort. A few chefs and restaurant owners are concerned with the nutritional health of their patrons, but more often chefs strive only to please the palate. Restaurant foods are often overly endowed with calories, fat, saturated fat, sugar, and salt but often lack fiber, folate, or calcium. Vegetables and fruit may be in short supply, and a single meat or pasta portion may exceed an entire day's recommended intake. To improve restaurant meals, follow these suggestions:

- Restrict your portions to sizes that do not exceed your energy needs.
- Ask that excess portions be placed in take-out containers at the start of the meal.
- Ask for extra vegetables, fruit, or salad.
- Request whole-grain breads and pasta (more restaurants now supply these, and others may do so with repeated requests).

- Make judicious choices of foods that stay within intake guidelines for solid fats, added sugars, and salt.

The Food Feature of Chapter 5 offered specific suggestions for ordering fast food and other foods with an eye to keeping fat intakes within bounds, and Chapter 8 listed foods high in sodium. Table 14–19 provides tips for single survival in the grocery store and at home.

Managing Loneliness

Loneliness affects many people, young and old alike, and can negatively influence overall health. For nutrition's sake, among many reasons, it is important to attend to loneliness, and mealtimes provide an opportunity to do so. People who are living alone must learn to connect food with socializing. Invite guests and make enough food so that you can enjoy the leftovers later on. If you know of a friend or acquaintance who frequently eats alone, you can bet that person would love to join you for a meal now and then.

Table 14–19

Smart Shopping and Creative Cooking

Smart Shopper Tips

- Make a list to reduce impulse buying; buy on sale, and use coupons for needed items.
- Watch sizes: gallons of milk may be cheaper than pints per ounce, but the savings are lost if the milk sours. Dry milk and small shelf-stable milk boxes often make sense.
- Bulk staple foods, such as dry milk, oatmeal, ready-to-eat cereals, or rice are cheapest, but they must be stored properly (see Chapter 15 for hints to avoid food waste).
- If freezer space allows, buy whole chickens or "family pack" meats at bargain prices. Divide into single servings, wrap well, mark the date, freeze, and use as needed.
- Ask grocers to break open large packages of fresh foods; buy only the amount you can use up. More expensive but convenient small bags of cut and washed fresh vegetables may be an option.
- Frozen vegetables in large resealable bags are more economical than small boxes.

- Freeze a loaf of whole-grain bread; defrost or toast as needed.
- Eggs keep for weeks in the refrigerator. After their sell-by date, hard-boil and refrigerate them for handy protein servings that last a week longer.
- Buy several tomatoes, pears, and other fresh fruits in various stages of ripeness: a ripe one to eat right away, a nearly ripe one to eat soon after, and a green one to ripen in a few days.
- Buy ready-to-heat and eat foods from the grocery store delicatessen section—these cost less than similar foods from restaurants. Choose nutrient-dense items; skip stuffing, macaroni and cheese, meat loaf and gravy, vegetables in sauce, mayonnaise-dressed mixed salads, and fried foods.
- Buy a ready-roasted chicken; use the main pieces for several dinners; simmer the remainder with herbs and vegetables in a broth for soup.

Creative Kitchen Tricks

- Divide a head of cauliflower or broccoli into thirds. Cook one-third right away; marinate one-third in Italian salad dressing to use later in a salad; toss the remainder into a casserole, soup, or stew, or eat it raw with dip for a crunchy snack.
- Stir-fry ready-to-use blends of cabbage, snow peas, and onions; bags of slaw-cut vegetables; or raw vegetables for a delicious dinner. Add Asian seasonings and leftover chicken or seafood. Bonus: one pan to wash.
- Microwavable bags of brown rice cost more but provide a whole-grain food for those less able to cook.

- Treat leftovers with respect. Nothing beats a plate of delicious leftovers for speed and convenience—plate, reheat in the microwave, and eat.
- Use nutritious frozen dinners judiciously (caution: these can be very high in solid fats, added sugars, and salt—read Nutrition Facts panels). Round out the meal with a salad, a whole-grain roll, and a glass of fat-free milk.

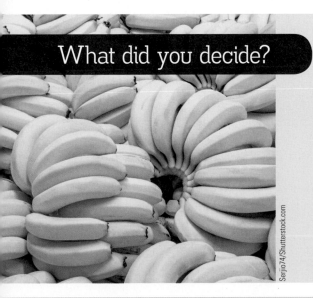

What did you decide?

Do you need **special information** to properly nourish children, or are they like "little adults" in their needs?

Do you suspect that symptoms you feel may be caused by a **food allergy**?

Are **teenagers** old enough to decide for themselves what to eat?

Can good nutrition help you live **better and longer**?

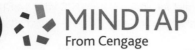

Self Check

1. (LO 14.1) Children often fail to consume adequate amounts of _____.
   a. dairy
   b. meats
   c. vegetables
   d. sugar-sweetened beverages

2. (LO 14.1) A healthy child's normal appetite control system
   a. cannot be trusted to provide the right level of calories for growth.
   b. can be short-circuited by a constant stream of foods high in added sugars, saturated fat, and refined grains.
   c. holds the child's appetite constant, without much fluctuation from day to day.
   d. none of the above.

3. (LO 14.1) On a pound-for-pound basis, a 5-year-old's need for vitamin A is about double the need of an adult man.
   T   F

4. (LO 14.1) Which of the following can contribute to choking in children?
   a. peanut butter eaten by the spoonful
   b. hot dogs and tough meat
   c. grapes and hard candy
   d. all of the above.

5. (LO 14.1) Lead toxicity in young children
   a. is no longer a problem in the United States.
   b. is especially likely in a child whose diet lacks calcium, iron, or zinc.
   c. arises primarily from ingesting of foods packed in metal cans.
   d. all of the above.

6. (LO 14.1) Research to date supports the idea that food allergies or intolerances are common causes of hyperactivity in children.
   T   F

7. (LO 14.1) A child who ate cream of broccoli soup and became ill now feels ill whenever it is served. The child most likely has a _____.
   a. food allergy
   b. food intolerance
   c. food aversion
   d. food antibody

8. (LO 14.2) Which of the following is most commonly deficient in adolescents?
   a. folate
   b. zinc
   c. iron
   d. vitamin D

9. (LO 14.2) Which of the following may worsen the symptoms associated with PMS?
   a. exercise
   b. caffeine
   c. vitamin D
   d. all of the above.

10. (LO 14.2) Which of the following is *not* associated with peak bone mass?
    a. physical activity
    b. scholastic achievement
    c. vitamin D status
    d. calcium intake

11. (LO 14.3) Physical changes of aging that can affect nutrition include _____.
    a. reduced stomach acid
    b. increased saliva output
    c. tooth loss and gum disease
    d. a and c

12. (LO 14.3) In research, which of the following is associated with a longer life span in many species?
    a. energy restriction
    b. superoxide dismutase
    c. omega-3 fatty acids
    d. none of the above.

13. (LO 14.4) Nutrition does not seem to play a role in the causation of osteoarthritis.
    T   F

14. (LO 14.4) Vitamin A absorption decreases with age.
    T   F

15. (LO 14.4) Antioxidant supplements have been shown to slow down the progression of Alzheimer's disease.
    T   F

16. (LO 14.4) A person planning a nutritious diet for an elderly person should pay particular attention to providing enough _____.
    a. vitamin A
    b. vitamin B$_{12}$
    c. iron
    d. b and c

17. (LO 14.4) The word DETERMINE is an acronym used in assessing an elderly person's _____.
    a. risk of malnutrition
    b. bone integrity
    c. degree of independence
    d. all of the above.

18. (LO 14.5) Single elderly people who routinely eat alone most often prefer isolation and should be left to themselves.
    T   F

19. (LO 14.6) Nutrient–drug interactions are common in people who:
    a. take a medicine for a long time or take multiple medications.
    b. drink alcohol.
    c. are poorly nourished to begin with.
    d. all of the above.

Answers to these Self Check questions are in Appendix G.

Nutrient–Drug Interactions: Who Should Be Concerned?

LO 14.6   Summarize the concerns surrounding nutrient–drug interactions.

A 45-year-old Chicago business executive attempts to give up smoking with the help of nicotine gum. She replaces smoking breaks with beverage breaks, drinking frequent servings of tomato juice, coffee, and colas. She is discouraged when her stomach becomes upset and her craving for tobacco continues unabated, despite the nicotine gum. Problem: nutrient–drug interaction.

A 14-year-old girl develops frequent and prolonged respiratory infections. Over the past 6 months, she has suffered constant fatigue despite adequate sleep, has had trouble completing school assignments, and has given up playing volleyball because she runs out of energy on the court. During the same 6 months, she has been taking antacid pills several times a day because she heard this was a sure way to lose weight. Her pediatrician has diagnosed iron–deficiency anemia. Problem: nutrient–drug interaction.

A 30-year-old schoolteacher who benefits from antidepressant medication attends a faculty wine and cheese party. After sampling the cheese with a glass or two of red wine, his face becomes flushed. His behavior prompts others to drive him home. In the early morning hours, he awakens with severe dizziness, a migraine headache, vomiting, and trembling. An ambulance delivers him to an emergency room where a physician takes swift action to save his life. Problem: nutrient–drug interaction.

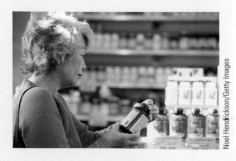

The Potential for Harm

People sometimes think that medical drugs do only good, not harm. As the opening stories illustrate, however, both prescription and OTC medicines can have unintended consequences, among which are significant interactions with nutrition.[1]*

Figure C14–1 shows that drugs can interact with foods, nutrients, and herbs in a number of ways. Each may affect the absorption, action, metabolism, or excretion of the others.

Some drugs are known to interact with specific nutrients (see Table C14–1). In addition, alcohol is infamous for its interactions with nutrients, and the more

*Reference notes are in Appendix F.

alcohol ingested, the more likely that a significant nutrient interaction will occur (see Controversy 3, p. 95).

Factors that Make Interactions Likely

Significant interactions do not occur every time a person takes a drug. The potential for interactions is greatest in those who take medicines for a long time, who take multiple drugs, who drink alcohol daily, or who are poorly nourished to begin with. The great majority of people age of 65 and older receive at least one prescription medication, and 40 percent take five or more drugs at a time.[2] The risk of an adverse effect rises substantially among older people taking five or more daily

Figure C14–1

How Foods, Drugs, and Herbs Can Interact

The arrows show that foods, drugs, and herbs can interfere with each other's absorption, actions, metabolism, or excretion.

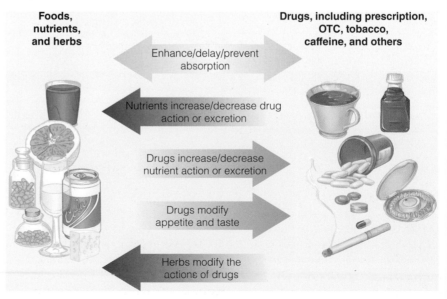

Foods, nutrients, and herbs

Drugs, including prescription, OTC, tobacco, caffeine, and others

Enhance/delay/prevent absorption

Nutrients increase/decrease drug action or excretion

Drugs increase/decrease nutrient action or excretion

Drugs modify appetite and taste

Herbs modify the actions of drugs

Selected Nutrient–Drug Interactions

Drugs	Effects on Nutrient Absorption	Effects on Nutrient Excretion	Effects on Nutrient Metabolism
Acid controllers	Reduce iron, folate, and vitamin B_{12} absorption		
Antacids (aluminum containing)	Reduce iron, folate, and vitamin B_{12} absorption	Accelerate calcium and phosphorus excretion	May accelerate destruction of thiamin
Antibiotics (long-term usage)	Reduce absorption of fats, amino acids, folate, fat-soluble vitamins, vitamin B_{12}, calcium, copper, iron, other minerals	Accelerate excretion of folate, niacin, potassium, riboflavin, and vitamin C	Destroy vitamin K–producing bacteria and reduce vitamin K production
Antidepressants (monoamine oxidase inhibitors, MAOI)			Slow breakdown of tyramine, producing dangerous blood pressure spikes and other symptoms on consuming tyramine-rich foods (Table C14–2, p. 564) or alcoholic beverages (sherry, vermouth, red wines, some beers)
Aspirin (large doses, long-term usage)	Reduces folate absorption and blood concentration	Accelerates excretion of thiamin, vitamin C, and vitamin K; causes iron and potassium losses through gastric blood loss	
Caffeine		Accelerates excretion of small amounts of calcium and magnesium	Stimulates release of fatty acids into the blood
Diabetes drug (metformin, long-term use)	Reduces vitamin B_{12} absorption and blood concentration		
Cholesterol-lowering "statin" drugs (Zocor, Lipitor)			Grapefruit juice slows drug metabolism, causing buildup of high drug levels. Potentially life-threatening muscle toxicity can result.
Diuretics		Raise blood calcium and zinc; lower blood folate, phosphorus, electrolytes, vitamin B_{12}; increase excretion of calcium, water-soluble nutrients	Interfere with storage of zinc
Laxatives (effects vary with type)	Reduce absorption of many nutrients	Accelerate excretion of all unabsorbed nutrients	
Oral contraceptives	Reduce absorption of folate, may improve absorption of calcium	Cause sodium retention	Raise blood vitamin A, vitamin D, copper, and iron; may lower blood beta-carotene, riboflavin, vitamin B_{12}, and vitamin C; may elevate requirements for riboflavin and vitamin B_6; alter blood lipids

medications, and it compounds further when herbs and other supplements are added to the mix.

The details of nutrient–drug interactions are many and far more extensive than can be presented here. These discussions are intended to raise awareness of the most common ones and offer a preventive strategy.

Absorption of Drugs and Nutrients

The business executive described earlier felt the effects of chemical incompatibility. Acids from the tomato juice, coffee, and colas she drank before chewing the nicotine gum kept the nicotine from being absorbed into the bloodstream

through the lining of her mouth as intended, and so did not quell her craving. Instead, it traveled to her stomach and caused nausea.†

---

† These items also interfere with the action of nicotine gum: beer; coffee; condiments (ketchup, mustard, and soy sauce); juices (apple, grape, orange, and pineapple); and lemon-lime soda.

Similarly, dairy products or calcium-fortified juices interfere with the absorption of certain antibiotics. Drug label instructions, such as "Take on an empty stomach" or "Do not combine with dairy products," help avert most such interactions.

Certain drugs can also interfere with the small intestine's absorption of minerals. This interaction explains the experience of the tired 14-year-old. Her overuse of antacids neutralized her stomach's normal acidity, on which iron absorption depends. The medicine bound tightly to the iron molecules, forming an insoluble, unabsorbable complex. Her iron stores already bordered on deficiency, as iron stores for young girls typically do, so her misuse of antacids pushed her over the edge into iron-deficiency anemia.

Chronic laxative use can also lead to malnutrition. Laxatives can carry nutrients through the intestines so rapidly that vitamins in the tract have no time to be absorbed. Mineral oil, a laxative the body cannot absorb, can rob a person of important fat-soluble vitamins and potentially beneficial phytochemicals by dissolving them and carrying them out in the feces.

Metabolic Interactions

The teacher who landed in the emergency room was taking an antidepressant medicine, one of the monoamine oxidase inhibitors (MAOI). At the party, he suffered a dangerous chemical interaction between the medicine and the compound tyramine in his cheese and wine. Tyramine is produced during the fermenting process in cheese and wine manufacturing. Table C14–2 lists some foods high in tyramine.

The MAOI medication works by depressing the activity of enzymes that destroy the brain neurotransmitter dopamine. With less enzyme activity, more dopamine is left, and depression lifts. As a side effect, the drug also depresses enzymes in the liver that destroy tyramine. Ordinarily, the man's liver would have quickly destroyed the tyramine from the cheese and wine, but due to the MAOI medication, tyramine built up and caused the potentially fatal reaction.

Table C14–2

Some Foods High in Tyramine

- Aged cheeses
- Aged meats
- Alcoholic beverages (beer, wine)
- Anchovies
- Caviar
- Fava beans
- Fermented foods (sauerkraut, sausages)
- Feta cheese
- Lima beans
- Mushrooms
- Pickled fish or meat
- Prepared soy foods (miso, tempeh, tofu)
- Smoked fish or meat
- Soy sauce
- Yeast extract (Marmite); yeast supplements

Note: The tyramine content of foods depends on storage conditions and processing; thus, the amounts in similar products can vary substantially.

Other culprits affecting drug metabolism include food and spice phytochemicals and popular herbal supplements.[3] A chemical constituent of grapefruit juice suppresses an enzyme responsible for breaking down many kinds of medical drugs. With less drug breakdown, doses build up to toxic levels in the body. A person who drinks either grapefruit or cranberry juice and also takes the blood-thinning drug warfarin may exhibit delayed blood clotting with dangerously prolonged bleeding times.

Caffeine and Tobacco

People in every society use caffeine in some form for its well-known "wake-up" effect. Caffeine is a true stimulant drug. Like all stimulants, it increases the respiratory rate, heart rate, and secretion of stress and other hormones. Caffeine also raises the blood pressure, an effect that lasts for hours after consumption.

Caffeine's interactions with foods and nutrients are subtle but may be significant because caffeine is ubiquitous in foods and beverages—see Figure C14–2. Chocolate bars, colas, and other foods favored by children contain caffeine, and children are most sensitive to its effects. Many popular cold and headache remedies also offer about a cup of coffee's worth of caffeine per dose because, in addition to being a mild pain reliever in its own right, this amount of caffeine remedies the caffeine-withdrawal headache that no other pain reliever can touch.[4] The 2015 Dietary Guidelines for Americans committee has concluded that excessive intakes of caffeine

(>400 milligrams per day for adults) can lead to caffeine toxicity and fatal cardiovascular events.[5] Deaths from pure powdered caffeine, sold as a "dietary supplement" but actually a powerful stimulant drug, have triggered Food and Drug Administration (FDA) warnings to manufacturers and other actions. A single teaspoon of the powder delivers the caffeine of more than 30 cups of coffee.

Caffeine is also a diuretic (which causes water loss from the body). However, when taken in moderation, caffeinated beverages can contribute to daily fluid intakes without impairing the body's water balance (see Chapter 8 for details).

Regarding moderate caffeine intakes, research is limited, but it mostly refutes any causative links between daily caffeine and cancer, cardiovascular disease, or birth defects. In fact, observational research suggests that consuming caffeine or coffee, including decaffeinated coffee, may reduce the risk of type 2 diabetes.[6] Such correlations cannot establish cause, however. It may be that people who choose coffee over sugar-sweetened soft drinks take in fewer calories and weigh less, and that it is these factors that reduce diabetes risk. Much more research is needed to clarify these associations.

As for cigarettes and other tobacco products, they are delivery systems for the drug nicotine. Tobacco's dangers are well known, and most are beyond the scope of nutrition. Smoking does depress hunger and, as a result, sometimes reduces body fatness; it also accelerates the breakdown of vitamin C, upping requirements.

These foods and beverages all contain caffeine, but few, if any, of their labels state how much. A product's manufacturer may offer caffeine information on its website.

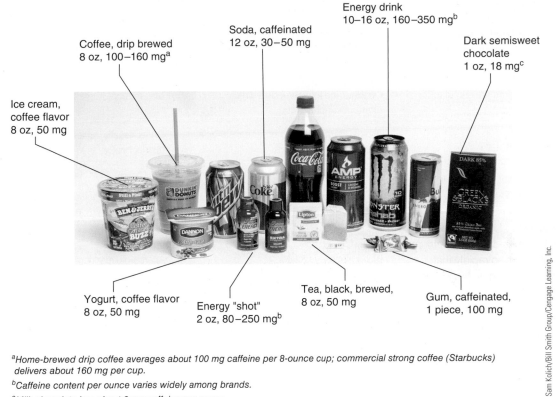

Coffee, drip brewed
8 oz, 100–160 mg[a]

Soda, caffeinated
12 oz, 30–50 mg

Energy drink
10–16 oz, 160–350 mg[b]

Dark semisweet chocolate
1 oz, 18 mg[c]

Ice cream, coffee flavor
8 oz, 50 mg

Yogurt, coffee flavor
8 oz, 50 mg

Energy "shot"
2 oz, 80–250 mg[b]

Tea, black, brewed,
8 oz, 50 mg

Gum, caffeinated,
1 piece, 100 mg

[a]Home-brewed drip coffee averages about 100 mg caffeine per 8-ounce cup; commercial strong coffee (Starbucks) delivers about 160 mg per cup.

[b]Caffeine content per ounce varies widely among brands.

[c]Milk chocolate has about 6 mg caffeine per ounce.

© Sam Kolich/Bill Smith Group/Cengage Learning, Inc.

Herbal Remedies, Alcohol, Other Drugs

Herbs can also interact with drugs, sometimes dangerously (see Table C14–3, p. 566). For example, people may take ginkgo biloba hoping to improve memory (evidence disproves this effect), but they may instead experience increased bleeding (ginkgo opposes blood clotting). When combined with other blood-thinning medications, such as aspirin or vitamin E, ginkgo biloba is associated with dangerous hemorrhaging.[7]

People who drink alcohol take note: alcohol interacts with a wide range of medications, including cardiovascular agents, central nervous system agents, and metabolic agents, causing symptoms ranging from nausea and headaches to loss of coordination, internal bleeding, heart problems, and breathing difficulties.[8] When taken with diuretics, alcohol can cause dehydration; when taken with sedatives such as sleeping pills or pain relievers, alcohol can suppress brain areas that maintain breathing, heart rate, and other life-sustaining functions. Always check with the prescribing physician about whether a medication may interact with alcohol.

Compounds in marijuana produce an enhanced enjoyment of eating, especially of sweets. Proposed medical uses of marijuana include relieving certain types of chronic pain, increasing food intake among patients with failing appetites and weight loss (in HIV/AIDS and other wasting diseases), and quelling nausea and vomiting caused by cancer and its treatments.[9] It also may produce significant adverse effects such as addiction (particularly in adolescents), panic attacks, disorientation, confusion, increased heart rate, and lung problems.[10]

Many other drugs of abuse cause loss of appetite, weight loss, and malnutrition among people who abuse them heavily. The stronger the craving for the drug, the less a drug abuser wants nutritious food. Rats given unlimited access to cocaine will choose the drug over food until they die of starvation. Drug abusers face multiple nutrition problems, and an important aspect of addiction recovery is their identification and correction.

Herb and Drug Interactions

Herb	Drug	Interaction
Bilberry, dong quai, feverfew, garlic, ginger, ginkgo biloba, ginseng, meadowsweet, St. John's wort, turmeric, willow	Warfarin, coumadin (anticlotting drugs, "blood thinners"); aspirin, ibuprofen, and other nonsteroidal anti-inflammatory drugs	Prolonged bleeding time; danger of hemorrhage
Black tea, St. John's wort, saw palmetto	Iron supplement; antianxiety drug	Tannins in herbs inhibit iron absorption; St. John's wort speeds clearance of many drugs.
Borage, evening primrose oil	Anticonvulsants	Seizures
Echinacea (possible immunostimulant)	Cyclosporine and corticosteroids (immunosuppressants)	May reduce drug effectiveness
Feverfew	Aspirin, ibuprofen, and other nonsteroidal anti-inflammatory drugs	Drugs negate the effect of the herb for headaches
Garlic supplements	Protease inhibitors (HIV-AIDS[a]) drug	Decreased blood concentrations of the drug
Ginseng	Estrogens, corticosteroids	Enhanced hormonal response
Ginseng, hawthorn, kyushin, licorice, plantain, St. John's wort, uzara root	Digoxin (cardiac antiarrhythmic drug derived from the herb foxglove)	Interference with drug action and monitoring
Ginseng, karela	Blood glucose regulators	Altered blood glucose level
Kelp (iodine source)	Synthroid or other thyroid hormone replacers	Interference with drug action
Licorice	Corticosteroids (oral and topical)	Overreaction to drug (potentiation)
Panax ginseng	Antidepressants	Overexcitability, mania
St. John's wort	Cyclosporine (immunosuppressant); anti-retroviral drugs (HIV/AIDS[a] drugs); warfarin (reduces blood clotting); MAOIs (used to treat depression)[a]	Increased enzymatic destruction of many drugs; decreased drug effectiveness; increased organ transplant rejection; reduced anticoagulant effect. Potentiation, with serotonin syndrome (mild): sweating, chills, blood pressure spike, abnormal heartbeat, seizures
Valerian	Barbiturates (sedatives)	Enhanced sedation

Note: A valuable free resource for reliable online information about herbs is offered by the Memorial Sloan-Kettering Cancer Center at www.mskcc.org/aboutherbs.

[a]MAOI stands for monoamine oxidase inhibitors.

Sources: M. Z. Liu and coauthors, Pharmacogenomics and herb-drug interactions: Merge of future and tradition, Evidence-Based Complementary and Alternative Medicine (2015), epub, doi:10.1155/2015/321091; B. Ge, Z. Zhang, and Z. Zuo, Updates on the clinical evidenced herb–warfarin interactions, Evidence-Based Complementary and Alternative Medicine (2014), epub, doi:10.1155/2014/9573.

Personal Strategy

In conclusion, when you need to take a medicine, do so wisely. Ask your physician, pharmacist, or other health-care provider for specific instructions about the doses, times, and how to take the medication—for example, with meals or on an empty stomach. If you notice new symptoms or if a drug seems not to be working well, consult your physician.

In general, strive to live life with less chemical assistance. If you are sleepy, try a 15-minute nap or 15 minutes of stretching exercises instead of a 15-minute coffee break. The coffee will stimulate your nerves for an hour, but the alternatives can refresh your attitude for the rest of the day. If you suffer constipation, try getting enough exercise, fiber, and water for a few days. Chances are that a laxative will be unnecessary. Given adequate nutrition, rest, exercise, and hygiene, your body's ability to fine tune itself may surprise you.

Critical Thinking

1. List all of the foods and drinks that you consume in one day that contain caffeine. Calculate your total caffeine intake. Do you think this intake is appropriate for you? Why or why not?

2. Choose three nutrient–drug interactions that are of concern to you. Create a chart that lists each interaction and states how the interaction affects absorption, excretion, and metabolism.

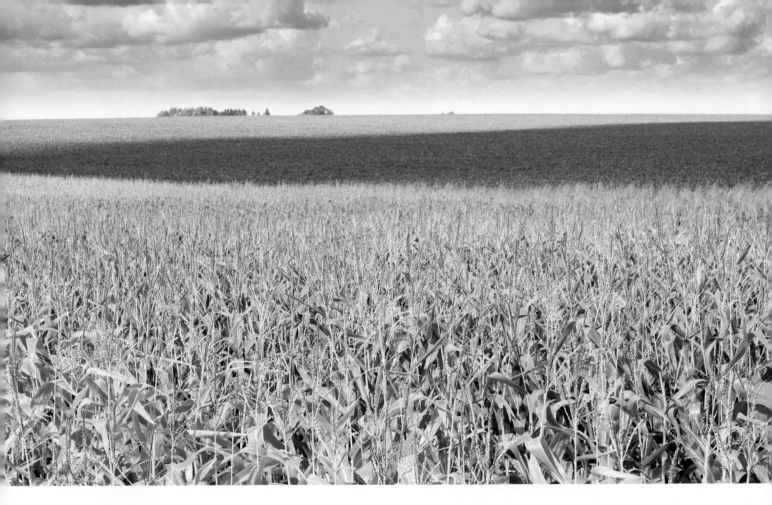

15 Hunger and the Future of Food

Learning Objectives

After completing this chapter, you should be able to accomplish the following:

LO 15.1   Describe food insecurity in the United States.

LO 15.2   Describe the severity and extent of poverty and starvation in the developing world.

LO 15.3   Describe how extreme poverty affects nutrition status in adults and children.

LO 15.4   Describe the world food supply and the factors that affect it.

LO 15.5   Outline the steps that governments, private enterprises, and individuals can take to ensure a sustainable food supply.

LO 15.6   Describe low-input agriculture and its importance to future food production.

What do you think?

With our abundant food supply, is anyone in the United States **hungry**?

Can **one person** make a difference to the world's problems?

Will the earth yield **enough food** to feed human populations in the future?

Is a meal's **monetary price** its only cost?

I n the United States today, over 6 million households live with **very low food security**—one or more members of these households, many of them children, repeatedly have little or nothing to eat because of a lack of money (Table 15–1 defines terms).[1]* Another 15.6 million food-insecure households have food, but not the food they need. Food insecurity often leads to **hunger**—not the healthy appetite triggered by anticipation of a hearty meal but the pain, illness, or weakness caused by prolonged food deprivation.

Worldwide, hunger problems are much more severe. At least 815 million people living in the poorest developing nations suffer chronic food insufficiency, hunger, and severe malnutrition, while their neighbors are food secure or even overfed.[2] Today, many a nation is facing a **food crisis** in which already meager food supplies have dwindled further, and rates of malnutrition have risen sharply.

The tragedy described on these pages may seem at first to be beyond the influence of the ordinary person. What possible difference can one person make? As it turns out, quite a bit. Students in particular play a powerful role in bringing about change. Students everywhere are helping to change governments, support education, improve human predicaments, and solve environmental problems. Students offer major services to communities through soup kitchens, home repair programs, and childhood education. The young people of today are the world's single best hope for a better tomorrow.

U.S. Food Insecurity

LO 15.1   Describe food insecurity in the United States.

In the United States, poverty and low food security exist side by side with affluence and the **high food security** enjoyed by most U.S. citizens. Survey questions (offered in Table 15–2) help determine the existence and degree of food insecurity in the United States. Figure 15–1 (p. 570) depicts trends in food insecurity over recent decades.

Food Poverty in the United States

In developed countries, hunger results primarily from **food poverty**.[3] People go without nourishing meals not because there is no food nearby to purchase but because they lack sufficient money to pay both for the food they need and for other necessities, such as clothing, housing, medicines, and utilities. More than 12 percent of the population of the United States, including 18 percent of U.S. children, lives in poverty.[4] The likelihood of food poverty increases with problems such as abuse of alcohol and other drugs, mental or physical illness, lack of awareness of or access to available food programs, and reluctance to accept what some perceive as "government handouts" or charity.

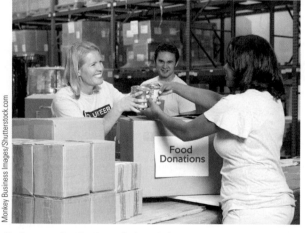

Each person's efforts can help to bring about needed change.

hunger physical discomfort, illness, weakness, or pain beyond a mild uneasy sensation arising from a prolonged involuntary lack of food; a consequence of food insecurity.

food crisis a steep decline in food availability with a proportional rise in hunger and malnutrition at the local, national, or global level.

food poverty hunger occurring when enough food exists in an area but some of the people cannot obtain it because they lack money, are being deprived for political reasons, live in a country at war, or suffer from other problems such as underemployment, unemployment, or lack of transportation.

Limited Nutritious Food Intakes   To stretch meager food supplies, adults may skip meals or cut their portions. When desperate, they may be forced to break social rules—begging from strangers, stealing from markets, consuming pet foods, or even scavenging through garbage cans. In the latter case, the foods they find may be spoiled or contaminated and inflict dangerous foodborne illnesses that compound the harm to health from borderline malnutrition. Children in such families sometimes go hungry for entire days until the adults can obtain food.

Significant numbers of U.S. children in families with low food security consume enough calories each day but from a steady diet of inexpensive, low-nutrient foods, such as white bread, fats, sugary punches, chips, and snack cakes, with few of the fruit, vegetables, milk products, and other nutritious foods children need to be healthy. The more severe their circumstances, the more likely children are to be in poor or fair health, and the greater their likelihood of hospitalization.

*Reference notes are in Appendix F.

Table 15–1

U.S. Food Security Terms

Food security exists on a continuum. Food security status is assessed in the context of specially designed questions (see Table 15–2, below).

Term	Definition	Example
Food Security		
▪ **High food security**	No reported indications of food access problems or limitations.	A family that has a full refrigerator and pantry, without shortages.
▪ **Marginal food security**	One or two reported indications of problems—typically of anxiety over food sufficiency or shortage of food in the house. Little or no indication of changes in diets or food intake.	A parent who worries that the food purchased will not last until the next paycheck.
Food Insecurity		
▪ **Low food security**	Reports of reduced quality, variety, or desirability of diet. Little or no indication of reduced food intake.	A family whose diet centers on inexpensive, low-nutrient foods such as refined grains, processed meats, sweets, and fats.
▪ **Very low food security**	Reports of multiple indications of disrupted eating patterns and reduced food intake.	A family in which one or more members have gone to bed hungry, have lost weight, or have not eaten for a whole day because they did not have enough food.

Source: United States Department of Agriculture, Economic Research Service, Definitions of food security, available at http://www.ers.usda.gov/topics/food-nutrition -assistance/food-security-in-the-us/definitions-of-food-security.aspx.

Table 15–2

Food Security Questions for U.S. Households

Questions such as these help identify households that have trouble meeting their basic food needs. Households reporting two or fewer of these conditions are classified as *food secure*; those with more than two are *food insecure* (for scoring details, visit the website listed in the source note).

1. "We worried whether our food would run out before we got money to buy more." Was that often, sometimes, or never true for you in the last 12 months?

2. "The food that we bought just didn't last and we didn't have money to get more." Was that often, sometimes, or never true for you in the last 12 months?

3. "We couldn't afford to eat balanced meals." Was that often, sometimes, or never true for you in the last 12 months?

4. In the last 12 months, did you or other adults in the household ever cut the size of your meals or skip meals because there wasn't enough money for food? (Yes/No)

5. (If yes to question 4) How often did this happen—almost every month, some months but not every month, or in only 1 or 2 months?

6. In the last 12 months, did you ever eat less than you felt you should because there wasn't enough money for food? (Yes/No)

7. In the last 12 months, were you ever hungry, but didn't eat, because there wasn't enough money for food? (Yes/No)

8. In the last 12 months, did you lose weight because there wasn't enough money for food? (Yes/No)

9. In the last 12 months, did you or other adults in your household ever not eat for a whole day because there wasn't enough money for food? (Yes/No)

10. (If yes to question 9) How often did this happen—almost every month, some months but not every month, or in only 1 or 2 months?

Source: A. Coleman-Jensen, M. P. Rabbitt, C. A. Gregory, A. Singh, USDA Economic Research Service, Household Food Security in the United States in 2016, (2017), Economic Research Report 237, available at www.ers.usda.gov/publications/pub-details/?pubid=84972.

Figure 15–1

Trends in Prevalence Rates of Food Insecurity and Very Low Food Security in U.S. Households, 1995–2016

Food insecurity has declined somewhat over the past decade, but still affects millions of people.

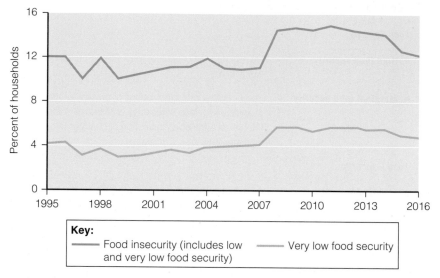

Key:
—— Food insecurity (includes low and very low food security)   —— Very low food security

Note: Prevalence rates for 1996 and 1997 were adjusted for the estimated effects of differences in data collection screening protocols used in those years.

Source: USDA Economic Research Service, using data from Current Population Survey Food Security Supplement.

Poverty and Obesity Food insecurity and obesity often exist side by side—sometimes within the same household or even in the same person.[5] With obesity comes an increased risk of developing chronic diseases, such as diabetes and hypertension, while poverty worsens the outlook for controlling those diseases.

KEY POINTS

- As poverty in the United States increases, food insecurity does, too.
- Children living in food-insecure households often lack the food they need.
- People with low food security may suffer obesity alongside hunger in the same community, family, or person.

What U.S. Food Programs Address Low Food Security?

An extensive network of food assistance programs delivers life-giving food daily to tens of millions of U.S. citizens living in poverty (see Table 15–3). As of 2017, one of every four Americans was receiving food assistance of some kind, at a total cost of over $100 billion per year.[6] Figure 15–2 shows the distribution of this cost across the programs.

Nationwide Efforts The centerpiece U.S. food program for low-income people is the Supplemental Nutrition Assistance Program (SNAP),† administered by the United States Department of Agriculture (USDA).† It provides assistance to tens of millions of citizens, about half of them children, but these benefits may not meet the entire cost of a health-promoting diet for all family members.[7] Eligible households receive electronic debit transfer cards that they use like cash to purchase food and food-bearing plants and seeds but not tobacco, cleaning items, alcohol, or other nonfood items. To help stretch consumer food dollars and SNAP credits, the USDA provides guidance on planning thrifty meals, together with daily menus and recipes.

†SNAP was formerly known as the Food Stamp Program.

Table 15–3

U.S. Federal and State Food Assistance Programs

This is a sampling of national and state programs aimed at reducing hunger in the United States.

- Commodity Supplemental Food Program
- Child and Adult Care Food Program
- Emergency Food Assistance Program
- Food Distribution Program on Indian Reservations
- National School Lunch and Breakfast Programs (see Chapter 14)
- Special Supplemental Nutrition Program for Women, Infants, and Children (WIC; see Chapter 13)
- Supplemental Nutrition Assistance Program (SNAP), formerly called the Food Stamp Program

Community Efforts To *relieve* hunger when government programs fall short, concerned citizens in many communities work through local agencies and religious organizations to help deliver food to hungry people. National **food recovery** programs, such as Feeding America, coordinate the efforts of **food banks**, **food pantries**, **emergency kitchens**, and homeless shelters that provide food to tens of millions of people a year.‡

To *eradicate* hunger, a community must do much more than provide immediate food relief to its citizens. It must also root out the underlying causes of hunger by:

- identifying and concentrating on communities most affected.
- committing to ending racial and gender discrimination and disparities, which create and worsen poverty.
- strengthening and implementing U.S. programs that aim to address hunger and poverty.
- supporting policies that protect lower-wage workers and enable them to become financially secure.

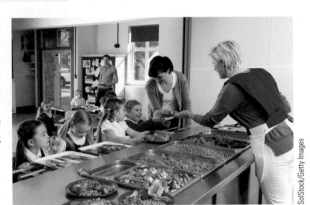

School breakfasts and lunches provide low-income children with nourishment at little or no cost.

Figure 15–2

Percentages of Expenditures for U.S. Food Programs (Rounded Values)

The Supplemental Nutrition Assistance Program (SNAP) accounts for almost three-quarters of U.S. food assistance expenditures. (Values are rounded.)

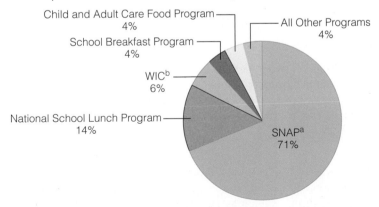

- Child and Adult Care Food Program 4%
- School Breakfast Program 4%
- WIC[b] 6%
- National School Lunch Program 14%
- All Other Programs 4%
- SNAP[a] 71%

[a]SNAP = Supplemental Nutrition Assistance Program.
[b]WIC = Special Supplemental Nutrition Program for Women, Infants, and Children.

Source: V. Olivera, U.S. Department of Agriculture, Economic Research Service, The food assistance landscape: FY 2016 annual report (EIB-169), March 2017, available at www.ers.usda.gov/webdocs/publications/82994 /eib169_summary.pdf?v=42823.

food recovery collecting wholesome surplus food for distribution to low-income people who are hungry.

food banks facilities that collect and distribute food donations to authorized organizations feeding the hungry.

food pantries community food collection programs that provide groceries to be prepared and eaten at home.

emergency kitchens programs that provide prepared meals to be eaten on-site; often called *soup kitchens*.

‡For information about food pantries, food banks, and other agencies in your community, call the National Hunger Hotline: (800) GLEAN-IT.

With these actions and others like them, some predictions foresee an end to global and U.S. food insecurity by the year 2030.[8] To rephrase a well-known adage: If you give a man a fish, he will eat for a day. If you teach him to fish so that he can buy his own gear and bait, he will eat for a lifetime and help to feed you, too.

KEY POINTS

- Government programs help relieve poverty and hunger for many people.
- Communities help to build food security by eliminating the forces that cause or worsen poverty.

World Poverty and Hunger

LO 15.2 Describe the severity and extent of poverty and starvation in the developing world.

In the developing world, poverty and hunger are intense. Figure 15–3 offers a glimpse into the daily struggles to survive in such conditions. Figure 15–4 identifies nations of the world that suffer most from insufficiency. The primary problem is still food poverty, and in the hardest hit areas, the poverty is extreme.

The Staggering Statistics   Grasping the severity of poverty in the developing world can be difficult, but some statistics may help. One-fifth of the world's people have no land and no possessions *at all*. They survive on less than one U.S. dollar a day, they lack water that is safe to drink, and they cannot read or write.[9] The world's "poorest poor" spend about 80 percent of all they earn on food, but still they are hungry and malnourished. The average U.S. house cat eats twice as much protein every day as one of these people, and the yearly outlay for keeping that cat is greater than that person's annual income.

Women and Children   The world's poorest people are usually women and children. Many societies around the world undervalue females, providing girls with poorer diets, less or no education, and fewer opportunities than boys. Malnourished girls become malnourished mothers who give birth to low-birthweight infants—so the cycle of hunger, malnutrition, and poverty continues. Worldwide, three-fourths of those who die each year from starvation and related illnesses are children.[10] Those who survive simply cannot work hard enough to rise out of poverty. Most would have no borrowing power even if credit were available, and they lack the money needed to build even small businesses and incomes.

Figure 15–3

Images of World Poverty

Unclean water and poor sanitation spread parasites and infectious diseases that claim many lives, particularly among the young. To help feed the family, every pair of hands is needed, even children's.

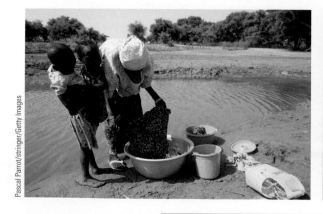
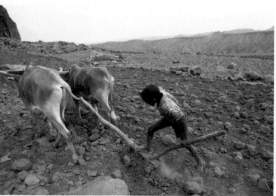

Figure 15–4

World Hunger Hot Spots

Hunger is most prevalent in the developing world.

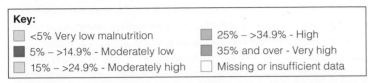

Key:
- <5% Very low malnutrition
- 5% – >14.9% - Moderately low
- 15% – >24.9% - Moderately high
- 25% – >34.9% - High
- 35% and over - Very high
- Missing or insufficient data

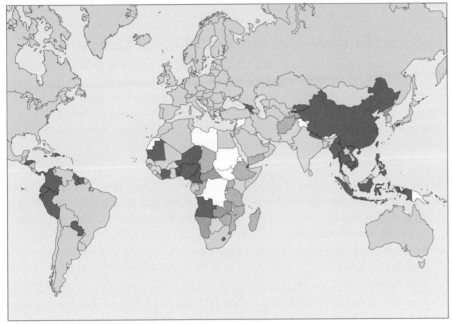

Source: Food and Agriculture Organization of the United Nations, The State of Food Insecurity in the World 2015, *available at http://www.fao.org/hunger/en/.*

An irony of poverty is that it drives people, even those without sufficient food, to bear more children. An impoverished family depends on its children to farm the land, haul water, and care for the adults in their old age. Malnutrition and disease kill many young children.[11] Therefore, parents often bear extra children to ensure that some will survive to adulthood.

Famine The most visible form of hunger is **famine**, an extreme food crisis in which multitudes of people in an area starve and die. The natural causes of famine—droughts, floods, and pests—occur, of course, but they take second place behind political and social causes.[12] For people of marginal existence, a sudden increase in food prices, a drop in workers' incomes, a change in government policy, or outbreak of war can suddenly leave millions hungry. The World Food Programme of the United Nations responds to food emergencies around the globe.

Intractable hunger and poverty remain enormous challenges to the world. In parts of Africa and the Middle East, killer famines recur whenever human conflicts converge with droughts in countries that have little food in reserve even in a peaceful year.[13] Racial, ethnic, and religious hatred along with monetary greed often underlies the food deprivation of whole groups of people. Farmers become warriors and agricultural fields become battlegrounds while citizens starve. Food becomes a weapon when warring factions repel international famine relief in hopes of starving their opponents before they themselves succumb.

KEY POINTS

- Natural causes, along with political and social causes, contribute to hunger and poverty in many developing countries.
- Women and children are generally the world's poorest poor.

famine widespread and extreme scarcity of food that causes starvation and death in a large portion of the population in an area.

The Malnutrition of Extreme Poverty

LO 15.3 Describe how extreme poverty affects nutrition status in adults and children.

In the world's most impoverished areas, persistent hunger inevitably leads to malnutrition. Multitudes of adults suffer day to day from the effects of malnutrition, but medical personnel often fail to properly diagnose these conditions. Most often, adults with malnutrition feel vaguely ill; they lose fat, muscle, and strength—they are thin and getting thinner. Their energy and enthusiasm are sapped away. With unrelenting food shortages, observable nutrient deficiency diseases develop.

Hidden Hunger—Vitamin and Mineral Deficiencies

Almost 2 billion people worldwide who consume sufficient calories still lack the variety and quality of foods needed to provide sufficient vitamins and minerals—they suffer the hidden hunger of deficiencies.[14] Nutrient deficiency diseases emerge as body systems begin to fail. Iron, iodine, vitamin A, and zinc are most commonly lacking, and the results can be severe—learning disabilities, mental retardation, impaired immunity, blindness, incapacity to work, and premature death.

The scope of nutrient deficiencies among adults and children is almost impossible to imagine:

- 40 percent of women in the developing world suffer poor health and debilitating fatigue from iron deficiency.[15] More than 50,000 women a year die during childbirth due to severe anemia.
- 18 million newborns every year have irreversible mental retardation (cretinism) from iodine deficiency.
- Half a million or more children (younger than age 5) become permanently blind from severe vitamin A deficiency.[16] Over 100 million more have marginally poor status that reduces their resistance to infections, such as measles.
- 25 percent of the world's population suffers from zinc deficiency that contributes to growth failure, diarrhea, and pneumonia.

These conditions are devastating not only to individuals but also to entire nations. When people suffer from mental retardation, blindness, infections, and early death due to malnutrition, national economies decline as productivity ceases and health-care costs soar.

KEY POINTS

- Malnutrition in adults most often appears as general thinness and loss of muscle.
- Vitamin and mineral deficiencies cause much misery worldwide.

Two Faces of Childhood Malnutrition

In contrast to malnourished adults, young impoverished and malnourished children often exhibit specific, more readily identifiable conditions. The form malnutrition takes in a hungry child depends partly on the nature of the food shortage that caused it. The most perilous condition, **severe acute malnutrition (SAM)**, occurs when food suddenly becomes unavailable, as in drought or war. Less immediately deadly but still damaging to health is **chronic malnutrition**, the unrelenting chronic food deprivation that occurs in areas where food supplies are chronically scanty and food quality is poor. Table 15–4 compares key features of SAM with those of chronic malnutrition.

SAM About 10 percent of the world's children suffer from SAM, often diagnosed by their degree of **wasting**. In the form of SAM called **marasmus**, lean and fat tissues have wasted away, burned off to provide energy to stay alive. Children with marasmus weigh too little for their height, and their upper arm circumferences measure smaller

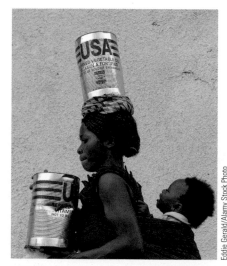

Donated food may temporarily ease hunger for some, but it is usually sporadic and insufficient to prevent nutrient deficiencies or support growth.

Eddie Gerald/Alamy Stock Photo

severe acute malnutrition (SAM) life-threatening malnutrition caused by recent severe food restriction; characterized in children by underweight for height (wasting).

chronic malnutrition malnutrition caused by long-term food deprivation; characterized in children by short height for age (stunting).

wasting in malnutrition, thinness for height, indicating recent rapid weight loss or failure to gain, often from severe acute malnutrition.

marasmus (ma-RAZ-mus) severe malnutrition characterized by poor growth, dramatic weight loss, loss of body fat and muscle, and apathy. From the Greek word meaning "dying away."

Table 15–4

Characteristics of Severe Acute Malnutrition (SAM) and Chronic Malnutrition

	Severe Acute Malnutrition	Chronic Malnutrition
FOOD DEPRIVATION	Current or recent lack of food	Long term lack of food quantity or quality
PHYSICAL FEATURES	Rapid weight loss Wasting (marasmus: underweight for height; small upper-arm circumference) Edema (kwashiorkor)	Stunting (short for age)

Note: Vitamin and mineral deficiencies are common in both types of malnutrition.

than normal (see Figure 15–5).[17] Loose skin on the buttocks and thighs often sags down, so that these children look as if they are wearing baggy pants. They often feel cold and are obviously ill. Sadly, such children are described as just "skin and bones."

Some starving children face this threat to life by engaging in as little activity as possible—not even crying for food. Others cry inconsolably. All of the muscles, including the heart muscle, are weak and deteriorating. Enzymes are in short supply, and the GI tract lining deteriorates. Consequently, what little food is eaten often cannot be absorbed.

A less common form of SAM is **kwashiorkor**. Its distinguishing feature is edema, a fluid shift out of the blood and into the tissues that causes swelling.[18] Loss of hair color is also common, and telltale patchy and scaly skin develops, often with sores that fail to heal. In a dangerous combination condition—**marasmic kwashiorkor**—muscles waste, but the wasting may not be apparent because the child's face, limbs, and abdomen are swollen with edema. Historically, kwashiorkor was attributed to too little protein in the diet, but today researchers recognize that the meager diets of starving children do not differ much—they all lack protein and many other nutrients.

Each year, 3.1 million children, as many as 6 children *every minute*, die as a result of poor nutrition. Most of them do not starve to death—they die from the diarrhea and dehydration that accompany infections.

Chronic Malnutrition A much greater number of children worldwide live with chronic malnutrition. They subsist on diluted cereal drinks that supply scant energy and even less protein; such food allows them to survive but not to thrive. Intestinal parasites drain nourishment away, too.[19] Growth ceases because they chronically lack the nutrients required to grow normally—they develop **stunting**, and it is often irreversible.[20] They may appear normal because their bodies are normally proportioned, but these stunted children may be no larger at age 4 than at 2, and they often suffer the miseries of malnutrition: frequent infections and diarrhea, and vitamin and mineral deficiencies. Severe malnutrition during these years irreversibly impairs brain development and learning ability, and greatly diminishes future prospects for escaping from poverty.

KEY POINTS

- Malnutrition in adults is widespread but is often overlooked; severe observable deficiency diseases develop as body systems fail.
- Many of the world's children suffer from wasting due to severe acute malnutrition, the deadliest form of malnutrition.
- Many more children's growth is stunted because they chronically lack the nutrients needed to grow normally.

Figure 15–5

Arm Circumference

Measuring a child's mid-upper-arm circumference helps to assess the severity of SAM.

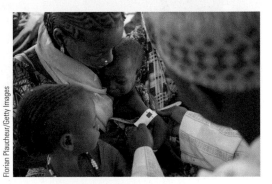

Florian Plaucheur/Getty Images

kwashiorkor (kwash-ee-OR-core, kwash-ee-or-CORE) severe malnutrition characterized by failure to grow and develop, edema, changes in the pigmentation of hair and skin, fatty liver, anemia, and apathy.

marasmic kwashiorkor a particularly lethal form of severe acute malnutrition, in which a child's dangerously reduced lean body tissue is masked by edema, making the condition hard to detect.

stunting low height for age, indicating limited growth in children due to chronic malnutrition.

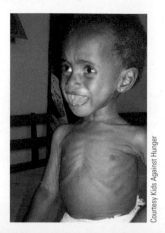
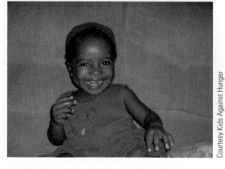
Figure 15–6

A Medical Nutrition Therapy Rescue

This 2-year-old girl was suffering from severe acute malnutrition. After a few weeks of medical nutrition therapy, she gained substantial weight and health along with a new appetite for living.

oral rehydration therapy (ORT) oral fluid replacement for children with severe diarrhea caused by infectious disease. A simple recipe for ORT: ½ L boiled water, 4 tsp sugar, ½ tsp salt.

ready-to-use therapeutic food (RUTF) highly caloric food products offering carbohydrate, lipid, protein, and micronutrients in a soft-textured paste used to promote rapid weight gain in malnourished people, particularly children.

world food supply the quantity of food, including stores from previous harvests, available to the world's people at a given time.

Medical Nutrition Therapy

Loss of appetite and impaired food assimilation interfere with attempts to provide nourishment to a malnourished child. To restore metabolic balance and promote physical growth, mental development, and recovery from illnesses, malnourished children need specially formulated fluids and foods. SAM often demands hospitalization, intensive nursing care, gradual nutrient reintroduction, and medication.

Children dehydrated from diarrhea need immediate rehydration. With severe fluid and mineral losses, blood pressure drops and the heartbeat weakens. The right fluid, given quickly by knowledgeable providers, can help raise the blood pressure and strengthen the heartbeat, thereby averting death. Health-care workers save millions of lives each year by reversing dehydration with **oral rehydration therapy (ORT)**. In addition, such children need adequate sanitation and a safe water supply to prevent infectious diseases.

Once medically stable, malnourished children benefit from **ready-to-use therapeutic food (RUTF)**, specially formulated food products intended to promote rapid reversal of weight loss and nutrient deficiencies.[21] Manufacturers blend smooth pastes of oil and sugars with ground peanuts, powdered milk, or other protein sources and seal premeasured single doses in sterilized pouches. RUTF are ready to eat: they need not be mixed with water (a plus in areas with unclean water sources) or prepared in any way, and the pouches resist bacterial contamination. Importantly, RUTF can be safely stored for 3 to 4 months without refrigeration, a rare luxury in many impoverished areas.

Cost is the downside of commercial RUTF products: they are expensive to buy and ship to impoverished areas. A child may need to receive daily RUTF for up to 3 months for a full recovery with a low risk of relapse.[22] To lower the cost, RUTF pastes can often be made on site from affordable local ingredients, increasing its availability to children suffering from severe malnutrition (see Figure 15–6).[23]

KEY POINTS

- Oral rehydration therapy and ready-to-use therapeutic foods, if properly administered, can save the lives of starving children.
- Commercial RUTF products are costly, but similar foods made from local ingredients cost less.

The Future Food Supply and the Environment

LO 15.4 Describe the world food supply and the factors that affect it.

Banishing hunger for all of the world's people poses two major challenges. The first is to provide enough food to meet the needs of the earth's expanding population without destroying the natural resources needed to continue producing food. The second challenge is to ensure that all people have access to enough nutritious food to live active, healthy lives.

By all accounts, today's total **world food supply** can abundantly feed the entire current population.[24] For future supplies to remain ample, the world must cope with forces that threaten the production and distribution of its food.

Threats to the Food Supply

Many forces compound to threaten world food production and distribution, both today and in coming decades. The following list names just some of them.

- *Hunger, poverty, and population growth.* Every 60 seconds, 109 people die in the world, but in that same 60 seconds 255 are born to replace them.[25] Every year, the earth gains another 76,854,987 new residents to feed, most of them born in impoverished areas. By 2050, a billion additional tons of grain will be needed to feed the world's population, but such an increase may not be possible beyond the earth's human **carrying capacity**.

- *Loss of food-producing land.* Food-producing land is becoming saltier, eroding, and being paved over. The world's deserts are expanding.

- *Fossil fuel use.* Fossil fuel use underlies much world economic growth, with associated pollution of air, soil, and water.

- *Atmosphere and global climate change.* That climate change is occurring is no longer a serious academic debate.[26] The National Academies of Science conclude that "there is a strong, credible body of evidence, based on multiple lines of research, documenting that Earth is warming. Strong evidence also indicates that recent warming is largely caused by human activities, especially the release of **greenhouse gases** through the burning of fossil fuels."

  Society's slow response to heed these warnings has jeopardized human life and livelihoods.[27] The associated heat waves, droughts, fires, storms, and floods thwart farmers and destroy crops, particularly in the poorest areas of the world. Arid deserts are projected to expand by 200 million acres in coming years in sub-Saharan Africa alone. As ocean heat builds up, ocean food chains are likely to fail.

- *Ozone loss from the outer atmosphere.* The outer atmosphere's protective ozone layer continues to grow thinner, permitting more harmful radiation from the sun to penetrate. As radiation contributes to the earth's temperature rise, polar ice caps are melting, causing global sea-level rise and threatening the world's coastlines. Radiation may also directly damage important crops.

- *Fresh water shortages.* Growing food requires great quantities of fresh water. The earth's fresh water supply is unevenly distributed, and too much of it is wasted, polluted, and unsustainably managed. Over a billion people lack access to drinkable clean water today. If climate change continues on its current trajectory, almost half the world's population may be living in areas of high **water stress** just 20 years from now and water scarcity may displace many millions of people from their homelands.[28] Figure 15-7 illustrates this threat.

- *Increased flooding.* Crop-damaging localized heavy storms are becoming more frequent and severe, causing flash floods that erode vast acreages of topsoil from parched land.

- *Ocean pollution, warming, and acidification.* Ocean pollution of many kinds is killing fish in large "dead zones" that expand as excessive algal growth depletes dissolved oxygen in the water. Ocean water acidity increases as it dissolves excess carbon dioxide from fossil fuel emissions, threatening the acid-base balance and other environmental conditions critical to sea life.[29]

The global problems just described are all related, and, often, so are their solutions. To think positively, this means that any initiative people take to address one problem will help solve many others.

KEY POINTS

- The world's current food supply is sufficient, but distribution remains a problem.
- Future food security is currently threatened by many forces.

Figure 15–7

Desertification

As groundwater is used up, deserts spread.

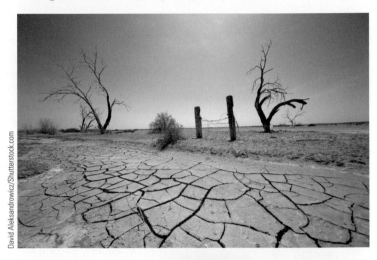

David Aleksandrowicz/Shutterstock.com

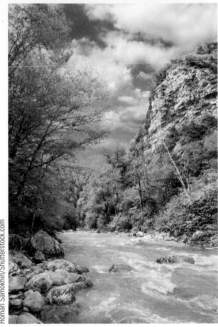

Roman Samokhin/Shutterstock.com

Pure rivers, lakes, and streams represent irreplaceable water resources.

carrying capacity the total number of living organisms that a given environment can support without deteriorating in quality.

greenhouse gases gases that contribute to global climate change by absorbing the sun's infrared radiation and trapping heat; examples of greenhouse gases are carbon dioxide and methane.

water stress the pressure placed on water resources by human activities such as municipal water supplies, industries, power plants, and agricultural irrigation.

Fisheries and Food Waste

Many other aspects of food production and sustainability are worth investigating. This section presents just two more: the changing world supply of fish and seafood and the huge quantities of food that are wasted after production.

Wild Fisheries and Aquaculture People around the world love seafood and demand is rising, but overfishing in past decades has caused the near collapse of some species.[30] Today, more than 60 percent of the world's food fish stocks are fully exploited or overexploited, meaning that harvests cannot expand, despite increasing efforts to catch more. The fish stocks are too small. International efforts to protect important food fish species include seasonal quotas, "no fishing zones" in breeding and recovery areas, and rules against illegal harvesting. Some species have returned from the brink of extinction, but rebuilding wild oceanic fish stocks to a **sustainable** level will require worldwide cooperation.

Wild fish shortages and large profits have spurred the rapid growth of **aquaculture** businesses, which now provide more than half of the world's food fish and shellfish. Some aquaculture "fish farms" consist of vast net cages that enclose fish in ocean inlets or freshwater lakes, where natural water flow refreshes the cages, as shown in Figure 15–8. Other types house fish in artificial ponds positioned inland close to coastlines. Natural water is diverted through the ponds, bringing in clean water and washing wastes into streams, lakes, or oceans. Farther inland, pond water is continuously filtered and cleansed. All farmed fish must be fed chow that contains fish, such as sardines, harvested from wild stocks, diverting them from direct human use and from larger wild fish species, such as cod, that depend on them. As for consumer safety and nutrition, the 2015 Dietary Guidelines for Americans committee concluded that consumers can freely choose between wild and farm-raised tuna and salmon because their

---

> **Figure 15–8**
>
> **Aquaculture**

An open net cage houses fish in an ocean or a lake, where natural flow refreshes the cages.

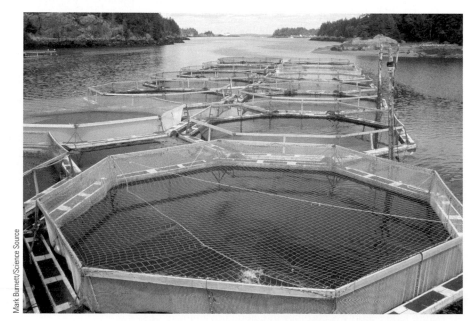

Mark Burnett/Science Source

sustainable able to continue indefinitely; the use of resources in ways that maintain both natural resources and human life into the future; the use of natural resources at a pace that allows the earth to replace them and does not cause pollution to accumulate.

aquaculture the farming of aquatic organisms for food, generally fish, mollusks, or crustaceans, that involves such activities as feeding immature organisms, providing habitat, protecting them from predators, harvesting them, and selling or consuming them.

levels of contamination and nutrients are similar.[31] In general, smaller species are less contaminated and more sustainable.[§]

Food Loss and Waste In a hungry world, 1.3 billion tons of nourishing food, one-third of total annual production, are lost to spoilage, pests, or waste each year, squandering not just the food but the resources spent to produce, package, and transport it.[32] More than 25 percent of all the fresh water used each year is spent producing food that is ultimately wasted. Similarly, about 300 million barrels of oil are spent to fuel the production of that wasted food. If this waste goes on unchecked, food production will have to increase by an estimated 70 percent by the year 2050 to feed the predicted world population. This is unlikely to be achievable (see the Controversy).[33]

The scope of U.S. food waste is enormous (see Figure 15–9). Discarded food constitutes the single greatest component of municipal waste—even greater than yard waste or plastics.[34] As food waste decomposes, it releases both methane and carbon dioxide, greenhouse gases that contribute to climate change.

The old proverb "Waste not, want not" seems to apply: preventing even half of the current food waste could provide food for huge numbers of people without using a single additional acre of farmland, drop of water, or barrel of oil. In less developed areas of the world, safer storage, better transportation, and more effective packaging are needed to keep food wholesome for human consumption. In this country, better food planning, purchasing, and use by food service industries and consumers are needed to put food where it belongs: on the plates of hungry people. Figure 15–10 illustrates food recovery methods for food industries, and Table 15–5 (p. 580) provides a guide for individuals who want to cut food waste and save substantial money.

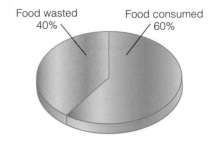

Figure 15–9

U.S. Food Waste—Calories Per Capita

About 40 percent of the food produced in the United States each year is wasted. For each person, daily food waste amounts to 1,400 calories worth of food, easily enough to cover the energy needs of a hungry child.

Food wasted 40%   Food consumed 60%

KEY POINTS

- Unsustainable harvesting threatens the world's wild fish stocks.
- Aquaculture provides a substantial portion of the world's seafood.
- Food loss and waste pose challenges, and reducing them would expand the food supply without additional production inputs.

Figure 15–10

Food Recovery Hierarchy

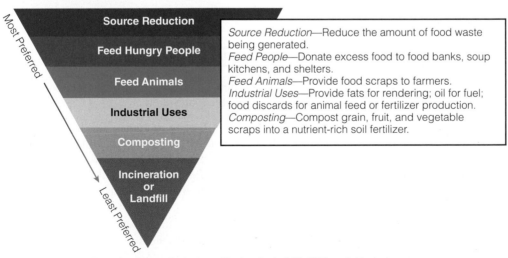

FOOD RECOVERY HIERARCHY

Most Preferred

Source Reduction
Feed Hungry People
Feed Animals
Industrial Uses
Composting
Incineration or Landfill

Least Preferred

Source Reduction—Reduce the amount of food waste being generated.
Feed People—Donate excess food to food banks, soup kitchens, and shelters.
Feed Animals—Provide food scraps to farmers.
Industrial Uses—Provide fats for rendering; oil for fuel; food discards for animal feed or fertilizer production.
Composting—Compost grain, fruit, and vegetable scraps into a nutrient-rich soil fertilizer.

Source: Environmental Protection Agency, Generators of food waste, April 26, 2012, available at www.epa.gov.

[§]For a guide to sustainable species by state, visit www.seafoodwatch.org/seafood-recommendations/consumer-guides.

The Future Food Supply and the Environment

579

Table 15–5

How to Reduce Waste and Stretch Food Dollars

Eating well on a budget can pose a challenge, but reducing waste is a good first step. For daily menus and recipes for healthy, thrifty meals, visit the USDA Center for Nutrition Policy and Promotion: www.cnpp.usda.gov.

Plan Ahead

- Plan your menus, write grocery lists, and shop only for foods on your list to avoid expensive "impulse" buying.
- Center meals on whole grains, legumes, and vegetables; use smaller quantities of meat, poultry, fish, or eggs.
- Cook large quantities when time and money allow; freeze portions for convenient later meals.
- Check for sales, and use coupons for products you need; plan meals to take advantage of sale items.

Shop Smart

- Do not shop when hungry.
- Select whole foods instead of convenience foods (raw whole potatoes instead of refrigerated prepared mashed potatoes, for example).
- Try store brands.
- Buy fresh produce in season; buy canned or frozen items at other times.
- Buy large bags of frozen items or dry goods; use as needed and store the remainder.
- Buy cereals to cook, such as oatmeal instead of ready-to-eat breakfast cereals.
- Buy fat-free dry milk; mix and refrigerate quantities needed for a day or two. Buy fresh milk by the gallon or half gallon only if you can use it up before it spoils.
- Buy less red meat. Use inexpensive cuts, such as beef chuck and pork shoulder roasts; cook with liquid long enough to make the meat tender, and add ample vegetables and grains to the meal.
- Buy whole chickens instead of pieces; ask a butcher to show you how to cut them up.
- Frequent discount stores instead of grocery stores for non-food items such as toilet paper and detergent.

Reduce Waste

- Change your thinking from "what do I want to eat" to "what do I have available to eat." You paid for the food you have on hand, so use it up.
- Buy only the amount of fresh food that you will eat before it spoils. The FDA website offers a refrigerator and freezer storage chart to estimate how long fresh foods will last (see www.fda.gov/downloads/food/foodborneillnesscontaminants/ucm109315.pdf).
- Peel away the tough outer layers from stems of asparagus and broccoli; slice and cook the tender stems or add raw to salads.
- Scrub, but don't peel, potatoes before cooking—the skins add color, texture, and nutrients to the dish.
- Before buying food in bulk, plan how to store it properly. If it spoils before use, you'll throw away your savings.
- If your "bargain" bulk food is more than you can use but is still fresh, donate it to your local food bank or homeless shelter. (It won't save you money, but it will provide a wealth of satisfaction.)
- If space permits, compost fruit and vegetable scraps to feed shrubs and other outdoor plants.

How Can People Help?

LO 15.5 Outline the steps that governments, private enterprises, and individuals can take to ensure a sustainable food supply.

Today, the keys to solving the world's poverty, hunger, and environmental problems are within the reach of both poor and rich nations—if they muster the will to employ them. In this country, the federal government, the states, local communities, big businesses and small companies, educators, and all individuals, including dietitian nutritionists and food service managers, have many opportunities to drive the effort forward.

Government Action

Government policies can change to promote sustainability:

- The 2015 Dietary Guidelines for Americans committee focused on sustainability as an essential element of food security for the U.S. population.[35]
- The U.S. government is currently devoting record amounts of tax dollars to subsidizing conservation programs for agricultural lands.

- Local and state governments are banning plastic bags and straws and setting goals for 100 percent renewable energy use, among other initiatives.

However, more can be done.

Private and Community Enterprises

Businesses can help to change the nation's ways; some already have—AT&T, Prudential, and Kraft General Foods are major supporters of anti-hunger programs. Restaurants and other food facilities are planning for less food waste and participating in gleaning efforts by giving their fresh leftover foods to community distribution centers. Food producers are increasingly choosing sustainable methods to meet a growing demand for products produced with integrity.

Educators and Students

Educators, including nutrition educators, have a crucial role to play. The nation and world look to scientists to solve problems and innovate for the future, so a solid science curriculum is critical for students at every level of education. While still learning, students can share the knowledge they gain with families, friends, and communities and take action in their communities and beyond.

Food and Nutrition Professionals

Registered dietitian nutritionists, dietetic technicians, and food service managers can make careful, conservative choices in procurement, reuse, recycling, energy use, water use, leadership, and capital improvements both in business and in their personal lives. In addition, the Academy of Nutrition and Dietetics urges its members to work for policy changes in private and government food assistance programs, to intensify education about hunger and sustainability, and to be advocates on the local, state, and national levels to help end hunger in the United States.[36]

Individuals

All individuals can become involved in these large trends. Many small decisions each day add up to large impacts on the environment. The quote of Figure 15–11 means that everyone on earth must make sustainable choices. The Consumer's Guide sums up some of these decisions and actions.

Conclusion

No part of the world is safely insulated against future food shortages. Developed countries may be the last to feel the effects, but they will ultimately go as the world goes. To limit the threat will require no less than a major shift in how the world uses its resources. This chapter's Controversy highlights one part of that larger effort: new approaches to continued food abundance through advanced low-input agriculture.

KEY POINT

- Government, business, educators, and individuals have opportunities to promote wise resource use at home and around the world.

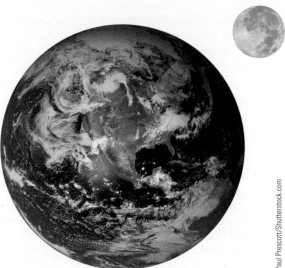

Figure 15–11

Sustainable Choices Help Protect the Planet

"For every person in the world to reach present U.S. levels of consumption with existing technology would require four more planet Earths."

—E. O. Wilson, 2002

Paul Prescott/Shutterstock.com

"We do not inherit the earth from our ancestors, we borrow it from our children."

Ascribed to Chief Seattle, a 19th-century Native American leader

A CONSUMER'S GUIDE TO . . .

Making "Green" Choices (Without Getting "Greenwashed")

Concerned consumers want to shop responsibly. How can they know whether label claims about environmental benefits are truthful? Like the word *natural* on food labels, appealing *green* claims, such as *eco-friendly*, have no legal meaning but may give a false impression that using the product could have far-reaching environmental benefits. Such labels amount to "greenwashing," the shallow use of vague terms or catchy symbols to feign environmental concern and hook unsuspecting consumers.[1]*

Honest manufacturers of "green" products make a sincere effort to mitigate environmental harms from their goods. They make specific, valid claims that are easy to spot: "Made with 60 percent recycled material," for example. Such labels may also provide a website or phone number for more information. All products exert impacts on the environment, however—even the "greenest" ones.

Less Buying, More Doing

As it turns out, the most beneficial choices for the environment often involve less buying and more doing, a trade many consumers are reluctant to make. Viewed from a broader perspective, simple green lifestyle actions such as the following are not purely altruistic—they benefit your health and your budget as well as your planet:

- Ride a bike to work or classes instead of joining a gym to save time and money.

- Shop "carless," to save money on gasoline—use public transportation, bicycle, or walk; carpool when buying bulky items.

- Reduce food waste (review Table 15–5, p. 580).

- Carry clean reusable grocery sacks when biking or driving. Even clean plastic sacks from the store can be

*Reference notes are in Appendix F.

reused, and recycled when they wear out.

- Use fewer electric gadgets. Mix batters, chop vegetables, and open cans by hand.

- Eat more foods from plants, fewer from animals.

Choosing Wisely

- Choose sustainable fish species (for a printable guide, visit http://www.seafoodwatch.org.)

- Choose minimally packaged items; buy bulk items or those with reusable or recyclable packaging. Packaging uses resources to produce, is bulky to store and handle, and adds substantially to the cost of goods.

- Choose reusable pans, dishes, cups, and utensils, and cloth napkins and kitchen towels rather than disposable ones to save cash and reduce trash.

- Buy reusable plastic food storage containers instead of aluminum foil, plastic wraps, or plastic storage bags. The containers quickly pay for themselves in money *not* spent on disposables.

- Choose coffee and other imported food products labeled "Fair Trade," available at many stores. *Fair Trade* indicates that businesses work toward food security, fair wages for workers, and conservation of natural resources.

- Plant a vegetable or herb garden, or join a community garden. Gardening provides physical activity and food, too. Just a few pots of herbs, lettuces, and radishes planted in a sunny spot can provide you with a tasty salad from time to time.

- Shop at farmers' markets and roadside stands for foods grown close to home. Locally grown foods require less transportation, packaging, and refrigeration than shipped foods.

- Try picking produce at local farms—it's fun, it's exercise, and it saves money, too.

Bigger Ideas

- Join organizations of like-minded people who work to make things better. You'll enjoy meeting new people and making a difference.

- Buy efficient appliances. ENERGY STAR (see Figure 15–12) appliances rank in the top 25 percent for energy efficiency. These products save money on utility bills year after year, and their use has reduced impacts on the climate.

- Consider buying an electric car for your next vehicle. Rebates and savings on gas can make them affordable as well as sustainable.

Figure 15–12

ENERGY STAR

By choosing ENERGY STAR–certified products, a typical household can save almost $400 per year in energy costs. ENERGY STAR–certified new homes are designed and built to standards that deliver energy savings of about 30 percent compared with other new homes. Read more at www.energystar.gov/.

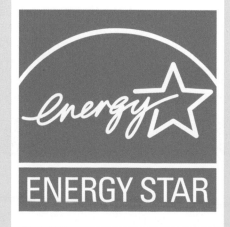

- Buy from ENERGY STAR–certified manufacturers. They effectively prevent substantial greenhouse gases from entering the air.[2†]

- Insulate your home to save energy and money.

- Consider using solar power, especially to heat water; check with local utilities for reimbursement grants.

- *Reduce.* Save the most money, time, and resources by consuming less. Buy less stuff. Even recycling costs energy.

- *Reuse.* If an item is necessary, go for durable, not disposable.

[†]*Find ENERGY STAR–certified partners at www.epa.gov.*

- *Recycle.* When the last drop of usefulness seems gone, put items into the recycling stream so they can be remade into new useful things.[‡]

Moving Ahead

Beyond daily choices, people can make the greatest impact by teaching others and by volunteering with like-minded people in their communities—in local cleanup efforts, in tree-planting projects, and in community gardens. Local food pantries and gleaners also welcome volunteers. If you take action today, you'll soon see the benefits of a "less buying and more doing" lifestyle begin to emerge.

[‡]*To help to find out where to recycle common items in your own community, try this website: www.earth911.com.*

Review Questions[§]

1. A consumer choosing a product that says "green" or "eco-friendly" on the label can be assured that it is safe for the environment.   T   F

2. Foods from plants require fewer resources to produce and are generally less expensive to buy than foods from animals.   T   F

3. Adopting some green lifestyle habits can
   a. save money and benefit personal fitness.
   b. reduce household trash.
   c. help preserve the environment.
   d. all of the above.

[§]*Answers to Consumer's Guide review questions are in Appendix G.*

What did you decide?

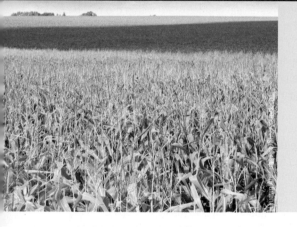

With our abundant food supply, is anyone in the United States **hungry**?

Can **one person** make a difference to the world's problems?

Will the earth yield **enough food** to feed human populations in the future?

Is a meal's **monetary price** its only cost?

What's online?

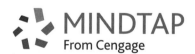
MINDTAP
From Cengage

Visit www.Cengage.com to access MindTap, a complete digital course that includes Diet & Wellness Plus, interactive quizzes, videos, and more.

Self Check

1. (LO 15.1) Which of the following is a symptom of food insecurity?
   a. You worry about gaining weight but cannot afford "diet" foods.
   b. You cannot always afford to purchase the quality or variety of nutritious foods needed for balanced meals.
   c. You shop daily to get the best prices and use coupons to stretch your budget.
   d. You buy fresh rather than frozen foods to save money.

2. (LO 15.1) Which of these items can be purchased with electronic debit transfer cards from the Supplemental Nutrition Assistance Program?
   a. hot dogs
   b. cigarettes
   c. dishwashing liquid
   d. red wine

3. (LO 15.1) The primary cause of hunger in the United States is
   a. living in food deserts.
   b. a lack of food aid.
   c. a lack of nutrition knowledge.
   d. food poverty.

4. (LO 15.2) Today, famine is most often a result of _____.
   a. global food shortage
   b. drought
   c. social causes such as war
   d. flood

5. (LO 15.2) The world's "poorest poor" spend about 80 percent of their income on food.
   T F

6. (LO 15.2) Worldwide, _____ of those who die each year from starvation and related illnesses are children.
   a. three-fourths
   b. one-third
   c. one-fourth
   d. none of the above.

7. (LO 15.2) Poverty and hunger drive people to bear more children.
   T F

8. (LO 15.3) The malnutrition of poverty inflicts all of the following except _____.
   a. learning disabilities
   b. mental retardation
   c. deafness
   d. blindness

9. (LO 15.3) Most children who die of malnutrition starve to death.
   T F

10. (LO 15.3) A particularly perilous form of malnutrition, which occurs when food suddenly becomes unavailable, such as in drought or war, is called _____.
    a. severe acute malnutrition (SAM)
    b. chronic malnutrition (CM)
    c. vitamin deficiency malnutrition (VDM)
    d. pericardial abdominal malnutrition (PAM)

11. (LO 15.4) To save a starving child who has a weak heart-beat and low blood pressure, a necessary first step is to quickly administer _____.
    a. protein supplements
    b. vitamin A supplements
    c. oral rehydration therapy (ORT)
    d. ready-to-use therapeutic food (RUTF)

12. (LO 15.4) Which of the following is a threat to the future food supply?
    a. fossil fuel use
    b. water shortages
    c. ocean pollution
    d. all of the above.

13. (LO 15.4) What percentage of its food supply does the United States waste each year?
    a. 20 percent
    b. 30 percent
    c. 40 percent
    d. 50 percent

14. (LO 15.4) Reducing food waste is a great way to save money.
    T F

15. (LO 15.5) Today, the keys to solving the world's poverty, hunger, and environmental problems are within the reach of both poor and rich nations.
    T F

16. (LO 15.5) Only the federal government and large corporations have the resources necessary to make an impact in the fight against poverty, hunger, and environmental degradation.
    T F

17. (LO 15.6) A vegetarian diet requires just one-third of the energy needed to produce the average meat-containing diet.
    T F

18. (LO 15.6) The scientific discipline that uses ecological theory to study, design, manage, and evaluate productive agricultural systems to conserve critical resources is known as _____.
    a. integrated pest management
    b. sustainability
    c. agroecology
    d. none of the above

Answers to these Self Check questions are in Appendix G.

How Can We Feed Ourselves Sustainably?

LO 15.6 Describe low-input agriculture and its importance to future food production.

If predictions hold true, the world's farmers will soon face greater pressure than ever before to feed a burgeoning world population. To produce this food will require more land, water, and energy, and it must be accomplished while conserving the resources that make growing crops and animals possible into the future. What is needed is nothing short of a second **green revolution**, except that this one must be doubly green: increasing the productivity of available land while protecting or restoring the environment.[1]* In addition, people today are urged to adopt a **sustainable diet**, to ensure that resources are conserved as people are fed.

Costs of Current Food Production Methods

Producing food costs the earth dearly. The environmental impacts of agriculture and the food industry take many forms, including water use and pollution, greenhouse gas emissions, and resource overuse. Table C15–1 offers definitions of terms relevant to these concepts. Important, but beyond the scope of this discussion, are the costs in terms of human health and other problems associated with farm work, such as overexposure to pesticides.

Impacts on Land and Water

To produce food, first, we clear land—prairie, wetland, or forest—replacing native ecosystems with crops or food animals. Crops pull nutrients from the soil. With each harvest, some of those nutrients are removed, so manufactured fertilizers are applied to replace them. Some of the nitrogen in this fertilizer flies

*Reference notes are in Appendix F.

off as gas, contributing to greenhouse gas emissions.

With rain or irrigation, fertilizer from fields and manure from grazing lands and feed lots run off into waterways, causing algae overgrowth. The algae die and decompose, forming ocean **dead zones** where whole areas are depleted of oxygen. Some plowed soil runs off, too, clouding the water and burying aquatic plants and animals. To protect crops, herbicides and pesticides are applied. These poisons also kill native plants, native insects, and animals that eat those plants and insects. Meanwhile, with continued chemical use, weeds and pests grow resistant to their effects.

Finally, we irrigate, a practice that adds salts to the soil—the water evaporates, but the salts do not. As soils become salty, plant growth fails. Irrigation also depletes the local fresh water supply over time because much of the water taken from surface or underground supplies evaporates or runs off. This process, carried to an extreme, dries up whole rivers and lakes and lowers the water tables of entire regions.

Soil Depletion

The soil can also be depleted by other agricultural practices, particularly indiscriminate land clearing (deforestation) and overuse by cattle (overgrazing). Traditional farming methods that turn over all topsoil each season expose vast areas to the forces of wind and water. Exposed topsoil blows away on the wind (see Figure C15–1) or washes into the sea, leaving unfertile areas behind.

Unsustainable agriculture has already destroyed many once-fertile regions where civilizations formerly flourished. The dry, salty deserts of North Africa were once plowed and irrigated wheat fields, the breadbasket of the

Vast areas under the plow are exposed to erosion, and those that must be irrigated will, over time, become salty and unusable.

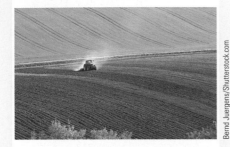

Bernd Juergens/Shutterstock.com

Roman Empire. Today's mistreatment of soil and water is causing destruction on an unprecedented scale.

Loss of Species

Agriculture also weakens its own underpinnings when it fails to conserve species diversity. By the year 2050, some 40,000 plant species that exist today may go extinct. The United Nations Food and Agriculture Organization attributes many of the losses to modern farming practices, as well as to human population growth.

Global eating habits are growing more uniform, a trend that contributes to species loss. As people everywhere eat the same limited array of foods, demand for local, genetically diverse, native plants is insufficient to make them financially worth preserving. Yet, in the future, as the climate warms, those very plants may be needed for food. A wild species of corn that grows in a dry climate, for example, might contain just the genetic information necessary to help make the domestic corn crop resistant to drought. For this and other reasons, protecting biodiversity is a critical human need.

Fuel Use and Energy Sources

Energy and fertilizers from fossil fuels have spurred unprecedented gains in agricultural output, but scientists now recognize that, with limited fossil fuel resources, such gains are not sustainable into the future. Fossil fuel use itself also threatens the future of food production by contributing to pollution and global climate change.

Biofuels made from renewable corn and soybeans were once hailed as safer alternatives to fossil fuels, but these also carry high environmental costs. Strong world demand for corn or soybean ethanol triggers the conversion of wild native habitats into corn and soybean fields, diverts resources away from growing food crops needed to feed hungry local populations, and adds to greenhouse gas emissions. Other plants, such as native grasses and even genetically engineered algae, appear to be more promising than food crops for biofuel production.[2] Other potential energy sources, such as wind and solar energy, are now surpassing fossil fuels in producing economic benefits.

Hidden Costs of Food Production

To produce the roughly 300 calories of food energy available in a can of corn, more than 6,000 calories of fuel (including those needed for the can and transportation) are used; add 2,000 more calories of fuel to that if the corn comes frozen. Food production represents a quarter of U.S. fossil energy consumption, mainly for fertilizers, pesticides, and irrigation.

Clearly, food imposes an additional cost on the environment—a constellation of inputs not simple to grasp—and not reflected in the price tag. These "hidden" costs must be accounted for, so that our food systems can adapt to changing conditions with workable plans to feed future populations.

The Burden of Livestock

Raising livestock takes an enormous toll on land and energy resources. Like plant crops, herds of livestock occupy land that once maintained itself in a natural state. Converted land suffers losses of native plants and animals, soil erosion, water depletion, and desert formation.

U.S. Meat Production

When animals are raised in concentrated areas such as cattle feedlots or giant hog "farms," huge masses of manure produced in these overcrowded, factory-style farms leach into local soils and water supplies, and pollute them. In an effort to control this source of pollution, the U.S. Environmental Protection Agency (EPA) offers incentives to livestock farmers who agree to clean up their wastes and allow their operations to be overseen to prevent pollution.

In addition, animals in such feedlots must be fed, and grain is grown for them on other land (Figure C15–2 compares the grain amounts required to produce various foods). That grain may require fertilizers, herbicides, pesticides, and irrigation, too. In the United States, one-fifth of all cropland is used to produce feed for livestock—more land than is used to produce grain for people.

World Trends in Meat Consumption

The world is demanding more meat and dairy products, putting pressure on ecological systems.[3] In 1999, for example, meat and milk consumption in East Asia was a little over 100 pounds per person per year; by 2030, yearly consumption will have risen to almost 170 pounds per person. This trend has been underestimated in long-term projections of the world's demand for food and energy.

The Future Starts Now

For each of the problems just described, solutions are being devised, and their use is growing worldwide.[4] Around the world, ideas for sustainable food production are emerging from the field of **agroecology**. This scientific discipline applies ecological theory to develop agricultural systems that balance ecological soundness, economic viability, and social justice.

The crop yields from farms that employ agroecological practices often compare favorably with those from farms using methods of the green revolution. The first of these practices, **low-input agriculture**,

Figure C15–2

Pounds of Grain Needed to Produce One Pound of Bread and One Pound of Animal Weight Gain[a]

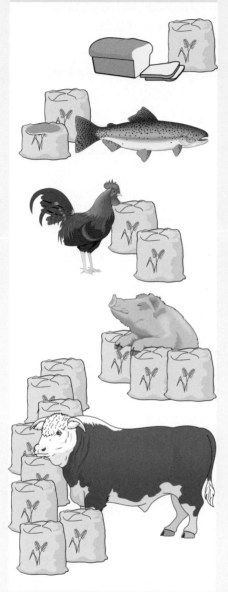

[a]Estimates of grain intakes for beef vary from less than 2.5 to more than 10 pounds of grain depending upon how long the animal is allowed to graze and how long it spends in a feedlot.

emphasizes strategic use of natural processes wherever possible, reducing the need for chemically intensive methods.

Another innovation, urban vertical farming, attacks the problem from another angle. They use the vertical space in old warehouses and other structures for growing edible crops in a highly controlled environment (see Figure C15–3).

Figure C15–3

Innovative Indoor Farming

Vertical farms make use of air space instead of acreage. Farming this way requires 95 percent less water than conventional farms, uses no pesticides, and generates no polluting runoff.

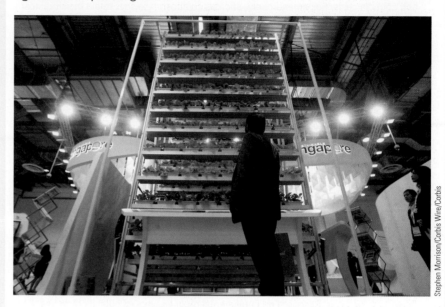

Stephen Morrison/Corbis Wire/Corbis

Low-Input and Precision Agriculture

Farmers may use low-input agriculture, adopting **integrated pest management (IPM)** strategies, such as rotating crops and introducing natural predators to control pests, rather than depending on pesticides alone. Many low-input techniques are not really new—they would be familiar to our great-grandparents. Many farmers today are rediscovering the benefits of old techniques while also taking advantage of newer technologies, such as precision agriculture, that their predecessors could not have imagined.

The term *precision agriculture* means what it sounds like: farmers adjust soil and crop management to target the precise needs of various areas of the farm. *Global positioning satellite (GPS)* units in the sky beam data about a field to GPS receiving devices on equipment here on earth. Farmers use the information to target, within a meter's accuracy, land areas that need treatments. The potential dollar and environmental savings in terms of water, fertilizers, and

pesticides are enormous. The initial cost of the equipment, however, is high.

Soil Conservation

The U.S. Conservation Reserve Program provides federal assistance to farmers and ranchers who wish to improve their conservation of soil, water, and related natural resources on environmentally sensitive lands. It encourages farmers to plant native grasses, food plants for wildlife, or trees instead of cash crops on highly erodible cropland, wetlands, or other environmentally sensitive acreage. It also encourages conservative techniques such as shallow tilling and the planting of grassy strips to control the flow of water off fields, reducing erosion, and protecting local water quality.

Other programs offer incentives for improving air quality or water quality or for purchasing sensitive lands for conservation. Private foundations or other groups may get help in funding such programs from local, state, or federal agencies.

Twelve Steps for the Future of Food

1. *Employ agroforestry.* Trees planted in and around farms reduce soil erosion by providing a natural barrier against strong winds and rainfall, and their roots stabilize and nourish soils.

2. *Improve soil management.* Alternating crop species allows soil to rest, restores nutrients, and controls pests. Soil amendments, such as compost, help soils retain moisture near plant roots.

3. *Increase crop diversity.* Growing many crop varieties helps control pests and diseases and reduces reliance on single varieties, increasing domestic food security.

4. *Increase livestock diversity.* Genetic diversity in food animals strengthens disease resistance. Lesser-known livestock such as North American bison are often hardier and produce richer milk than typical dairy livestock.

5. *Improve food production from existing livestock.* Feeding grass rather than corn or soybeans to animals cuts the demand for feedstuffs and helps relieve pressure on global human food supplies.

6. *Support "Meatless Mondays."* Forgoing meat on one day a week reduces environmental impacts. This practice is also widely associated with lower risks of chronic disease in people.

7. *Use smarter irrigation.* Installing water sensors or micro-irrigation technology and planning water-efficient gardens or farms using specific crops and locations can conserve crucial water supplies.

8. *Use integrated farming systems.* Integrated farming systems, such as permaculture, improve soil fertility and agricultural productivity by using natural resources as efficiently as possible. Research on implementation of techniques such as recycling wastewater and planting groups of plants that use the same resources in related ways is expanding rapidly across the United States.

9. *Use organic and agroecological farming.* Organic and agroecological farming methods are designed to build soil quality and promote plant and animal health in harmony with local ecosystems.

10. *Support small-scale farmers.* Small farms often specialize in growing fruit and vegetables for local human consumption, whereas large farms often focus on corn and soybeans for industrial uses.

11. *Reevaluate ethanol as fuel.* Encouraging clean energy alternatives to crop-based biofuels will increase the amount of food available for consumption.

12. *Support agricultural research.* Government support for agricultural research and its applications can help address issues such as hunger, malnutrition, and poverty.

Source: Adapted from Worldwatch Institute, 12 innovations to combat drought, improve food security, and stabilize food prices, August 2, 2012, available at www.worldwatch.org/12-innovations-combat-drought-improve-food-security-and-stabilize-food-prices.

The Potential of Genetic Engineering

Many farmers worldwide report both financial and conservation benefits from planting genetically engineered crops (see Controversy 12, p. 477).Growing herbicide-resistant crops, for example, requires less tilling of the soil to reduce weed growth, reducing soil loss from wind and water erosion. Pesticide-resistant crops demand less use of both petroleum-based pesticides and the fuel to run the equipment to apply them. Salt-resistant crops can grow in salty areas where conventional crops wither. If approached carefully, genetic engineering promises economically feasible, environmentally conservative options for agricultural lands. Table C15–2 provides other approaches to food sustainability. In the struggle to secure global food and energy for the future, no resource can be overlooked or wasted.

Roles of Consumers

Conscientious consumers can reduce pollution and the use of resources through the choices they make. Some new, fresh ways of thinking about how to obtain foods, and which foods to choose, can enliven the diet and enrich daily life.

Keeping Local Profits Local

Farmers selling their broccoli, carrots, and apples at city farmers' markets and roadside stands often net a higher profit than when selling to wholesalers. In addition, families who buy homegrown produce tend to eat greater quantities and varieties of fruit and vegetables, and the health benefits of this practice are well known. Through a **farm share**, consumers can buy weekly shares of a local farmer's crops, harvested in season and picked up while fresh.

Good for You, Good for the Planet

An often overlooked point: food choices that benefit the environment also benefit human health.[5] A sustainable diet is higher than the typical U.S. diet in legumes, whole grains, nuts, seeds, fruit, and vegetables and lower in red meats and highly processed foods. The same kind of diet also reduces risks of chronic diseases.

Overall, a vegetarian diet requires just a third of the energy needed to produce the average meat-based diet. Among meats, a lower-input option is livestock raised on the open range; these animals eat grass and plants not directly edible by people. Most of our beef is grain-fed, however, and the average energy requirement to produce it is high.

All in all, our choices as a nation add up to a measurable "ecological footprint"—the productive land and water required to supply all of the resources individuals consume and to absorb all of the wastes generated using prevailing practices. The footprint of each individual is four times larger in an industrialized country than in a developing one (see Figure C15–4). To help size up your own ecological footprint, take the quiz in Table C15–3, p. 590.

Conclusion

The problems of providing food for future generations are global in scope, yet the actions of individual people lie at the heart of their solutions. Do what you can to tread lightly on the earth. Celebrate changes that are possible today by making them permanent and reap the benefits of increased health and well-being. Do the same with changes that become possible tomorrow—and every day thereafter.

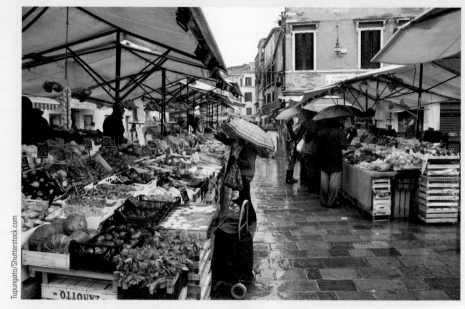

Tupungato/Shutterstock.com

Farmers' markets and farm share arrangements provide fresh foods from local growers.

Figure C15–4
Ecological Footprints

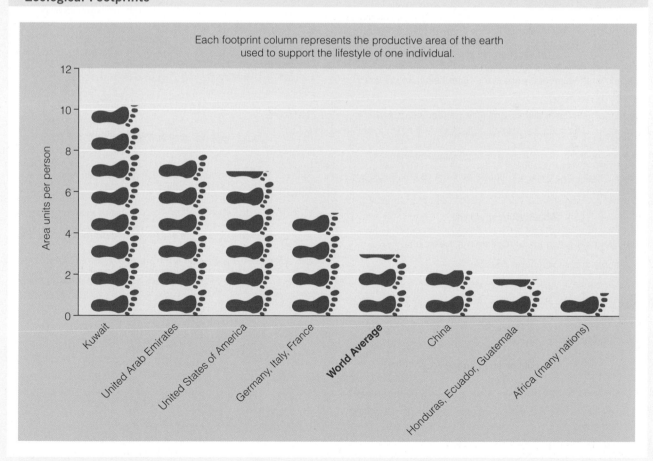

Each footprint column represents the productive area of the earth used to support the lifestyle of one individual.

Area units per person (y-axis, 0 to 12)

Categories: Kuwait, United Arab Emirates, United States of America, Germany, Italy, France, **World Average**, China, Honduras, Ecuador, Guatemala, Africa (many nations)

Source: Data from Global Footprint Network, Footprint by country, 2014, available at www.footprintnetwork.org/index.php.

This quiz can help you evaluate your impact on the earth. The higher you score, the smaller your "footprint."

At home, do you

1. Recycle everything you can: newspapers, cans, glass bottles and jars, scrap metal, used oil, etc.?
2. Use cold water in the washer whenever possible?
3. Turn off the tap while you scrub your hands or brush your teeth?
4. Stop using appliances (such as electric can openers) to do things you can do by hand?
5. Reuse grocery bags to line your wastebasket? Reuse or recycle bread bags, butter tubs, shipping boxes, etc.?
6. Store food in reusable containers rather than plastic wrap, disposable bags and containers, or aluminum foil?

In the yard, do you

7. Pull weeds instead of using herbicides?
8. Fertilize with manure and compost, rather than with chemical fertilizers?
9. Compost your leaves and yard debris, rather than burning them?
10. Return extra plastic and rubber pots to the plant nursery?

On vacation, do you

11. Turn down the heat and turn off the water heater before you leave?
12. Carry reusable cups, dishes, and flatware (and use them)?
13. Dispose of trash appropriately (never litter)?
14. Buy no souvenirs made from wild or endangered animals?
15. Stay on roads and trails, and not trample dunes and fragile undergrowth?

About your car, do you

16. Keep your car tuned up for maximum fuel efficiency?
17. Use public transit whenever possible?
18. Ride your bike or walk whenever possible?
19. Plan to replace your car with a more fuel-efficient model when you can?
20. Recycle your engine oil?

At school or work, do you

21. Recycle used paper?
22. Send electronic text messages, and use scrap paper for writing lists and notes?
23. Print or copy on both sides of the paper?
24. Reuse envelopes and file folders?
25. Use the stairs instead of the elevator whenever you can?

When buying, do you

26. Buy as little plastic and foam packaging as possible?
27. Buy permanent, rather than disposable, products?
28. Buy paper rather than plastic, if you must buy disposable products?
29. Buy fresh produce grown locally?
30. Buy in bulk to avoid unnecessary packaging?

In other areas, do you

31. Volunteer your time to conservation projects?
32. Encourage your family, friends, and neighbors to save resources, too?
33. Write letters to support conservation issues?

Scoring

First, give yourself 4 points for answering this quiz: ____

Then, give yourself 1 point each for all the habits you know people should adopt. This is to give you credit for your awareness, even if you haven't acted on it yet (total possible points = 33): ____

Finally, give yourself 2 more points for each habit you have adopted—or honestly would if you could (total possible points = 66): ____

Total score:

1 to 25: You are a beginner in stewardship of the earth. Try to improve.

26 to 50: You are on your way and doing better than many consumers.

51 to 75: Good. Pat yourself on the back, and keep on improving.

76 or more: Excellent. You are a shining example for others to follow.

Source: Adapted from Conservation Action Checklist, produced by the Washington Park Zoo, Portland, Oregon, and available from Conservation International, 1015 18th St. N.W., Suite 1000, Washington, D.C. 20036: 1-800-406-2306 (website: www.conservation.org). Call or write for copies of the original or for more information.

Appendix Contents

Chemical Structures: Carbohydrates, Lipids, and Amino Acids

The chapters of this book use simplified ball-and-stick models to illustrate the structures of molecules. This appendix provides a bit more detail about the chemical notations associated with carbohrates, lipids, amino acids, and peptides. Note that the four main types of atoms found in molecules of energy nutrients are hydrogen (H), oxygen (O), nitrogen (N), and carbon (C). Each atom has a characteristic number of bonds that it can form with other atoms:

$$H- \qquad -O- \qquad -N- \qquad -C-$$

$$1 \qquad\qquad 2 \qquad\qquad 3 \qquad\qquad 4$$

You can count the number of bonds for each atom in the molecule (ethyl alcohol) below: each H has one bond, O has two, and each C has four:

$$H-\overset{\displaystyle H}{\underset{\displaystyle H}{C}}-\overset{\displaystyle H}{\underset{\displaystyle H}{C}}-O-H$$

Carbohydrates

Chapter 4 described the classes of carbohydrates and demonstrated that monosaccharides can join together to form disaccharides and larger polysaccharides. Here are some of these carbohydrate structures, starting with glucose.

GLUCOSE

The chemical notation on the left shows all of the bonds of a glucose molecule; the center and right notations show common abbreviations, with fewer illustrated bonds and hydrogen atoms.

Glucose

Glucose

Glucose

DISACCHARIDES

When two monosaccharides are joined together, they form a disaccharide. The abbreviated chemical notations of the three disaccharides are shown below.

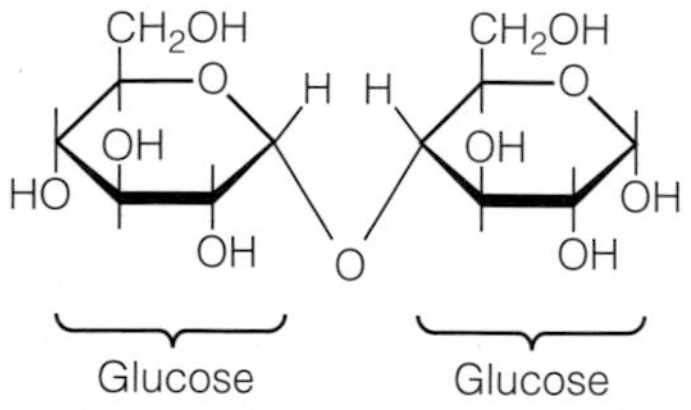

Maltose

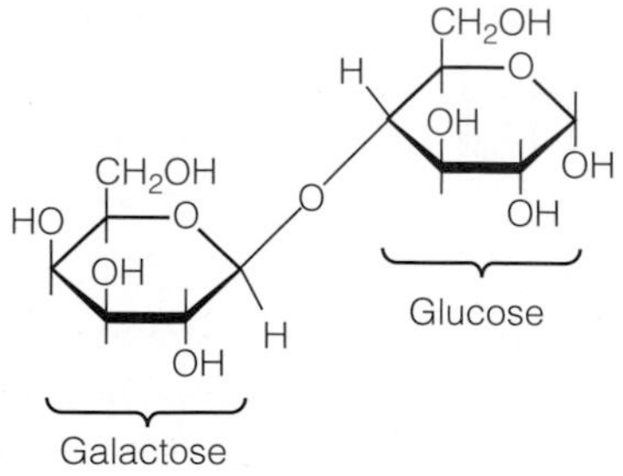

Lactose (alpha form)

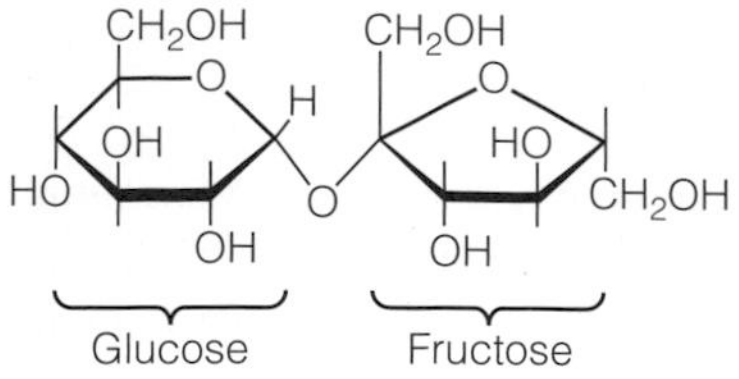

Sucrose

STARCHES

Starch, glycogen, and cellulose are all long chains of glucose molecules linked together. Some starch is branched, but the structure below is an unbranched starch.

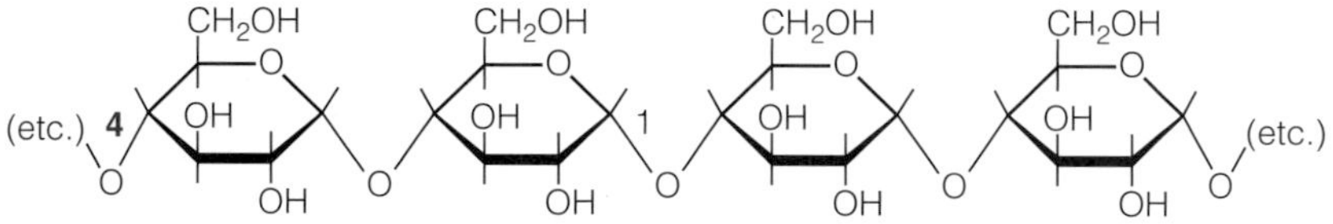

Amylose (unbranched starch)

Lipids

Chapter 5 notes that triglycerides are made up of three fatty acids attached to a glycerol molecule, forming the common fats in food and in the body. Below is a sampling of fatty acids; many others exist.

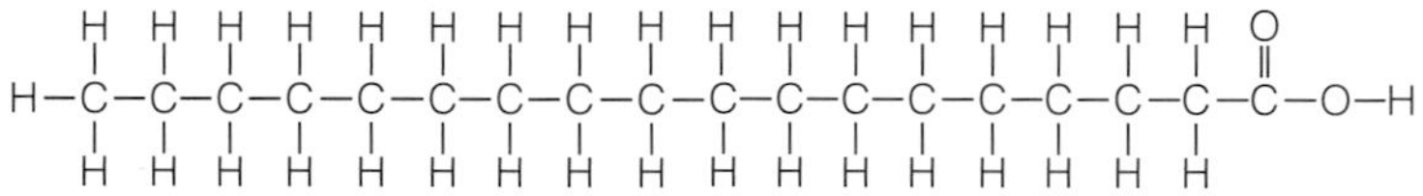

Stearic acid, an 18-carbon saturated fatty acid

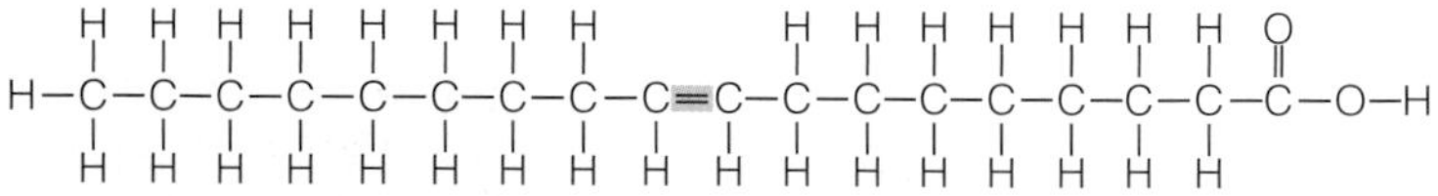

Oleic acid, an 18-carbon monounsaturated fatty acid

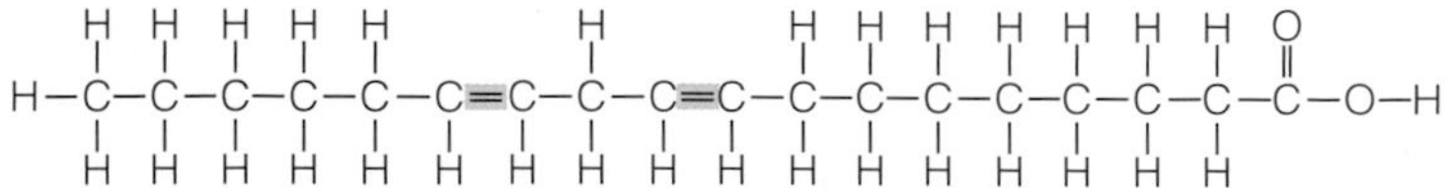

Linoleic acid, an 18-carbon polyunsaturated fatty acid

Appendix A Chemical Structures: Carbohydrates, Lipids, and Amino Acids

Fatty acids join with a glycerol molecule to make a triglyceride. Glycerol is shown below.

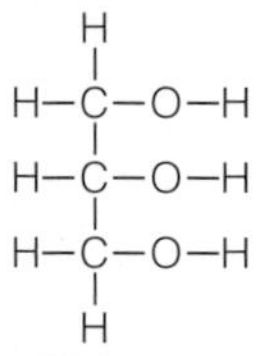

$$H-\overset{\overset{\displaystyle H}{|}}{\underset{\underset{\displaystyle H}{|}}{C}}-O-H$$

Glycerol

Most triglycerides contain a mixture of more than one type of fatty acid. The simplified notation used below makes it easy to pick out points of unsaturation (double bonds) in the fatty acid structures. Note that the top fatty acid is saturated, the one below it is monounsaturated, and the third is polyunsaturated. This notation makes it appear that all fatty acids are straight-line structures, but in real fats, points of unsaturation add kinks and bends, an effect illustrated in Figure 5–4 (p. 149).

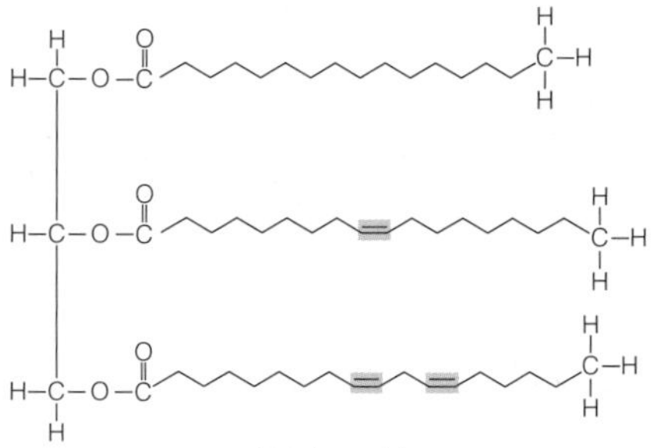

Triglyceride

A cholesterol molecule, one of the sterols, differs greatly in structure and function from the triglycerides; a molecule of cholesterol is depicted below.

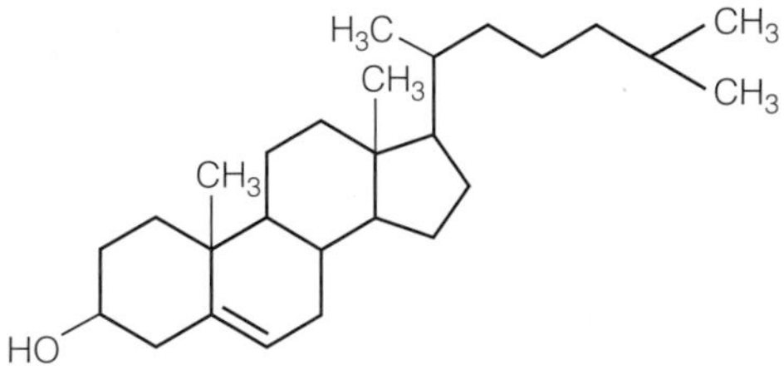

Cholesterol

Amino Acids

Proteins are formed from amino acids, as Chapter 6 made clear. All amino acids have a central carbon with an amino group (NH$_2$), an acid group (COOH), a hydrogen (H), and a side group attached. The side group structure (shown as a blank box) varies among amino acids.

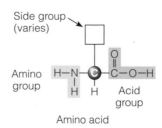

Side group (varies)

Amino group

Acid group

Amino acid

These are just a few of the amino acids (side group structures are shown in boxes to ease comparison):

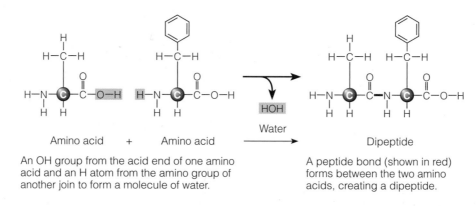

| Glycine | Alanine | Aspartic acid | Phenylalanine |

Making dipeptides, tripeptides, and polypeptides requires joining amino acids together with peptide bonds to make a chain.

Amino acid   +   Amino acid

An OH group from the acid end of one amino acid and an H atom from the amino group of another join to form a molecule of water.

Water

Dipeptide

A peptide bond (shown in red) forms between the two amino acids, creating a dipeptide.

World Health Organization Guidelines

The World Health Organization (WHO) is the source of nutrition guidance for many of the world's populations. These nutrient intake recommendations set the basis for country-specific dietary guidance, and they are listed in Table B–1.

TABLE B–1 World Health Organization Nutrient Intake Guidelines

The WHO has assessed the relationships between diet and the development of chronic diseases. Its recommendations include these:

- Energy: sufficient to support growth, physical activity, and a healthy body weight (BMI between 18.5 and 24.9) and to avoid weight gain greater than 11 lb (5 kg) during adult life
- Total fat: 15% to 35% of total energy
- Saturated fatty acids: <10% of total energy
- Polyunsaturated fatty acids: 6% to 11% of total energy
- Omega-6 polyunsaturated fatty acids: 2.5% to 9% of total energy
- Omega-3 polyunsaturated fatty acids: 0.5% to 2% of total energy
- *Trans*-fatty acids: <1% of total energy
- Total carbohydrate: 55% to 75% of total energy
- Sugars: <10% of total energy (< 5% of total energy would provide additional health benefits)
- Protein: 10% to 15% of total energy
- Cholesterol: <300 mg/day
- Salt (sodium): <5 g salt/day (<2 g sodium/day), appropriately iodized
- Fruit and vegetables: ≥400 g/day (about 1 lb)
- Total dietary fiber: >25 g/day from foods
- Physical activity: 1 hour of moderate-intensity activity, such as walking, on most days of the week

Source: Compiled from tables available at www.who.int/publications/guidelines/nutrition/en/index.html and www.who.int/nutrition/publications/guidelines/sugars_intake/en/.

M athematical problems have been worked out for you as examples at appropriate places in the text. This appendix aims to help with the use of the metric system and with those problems not fully explained elsewhere.

Conversion Factors

Conversion factors are useful mathematical tools in everyday calculations, like the ones encountered in the study of nutrition. A conversion factor is a fraction in which the numerator (top) and the denominator (bottom) express the same quantity in different units. For example, 2.2 pounds (lb) and 1 kilogram (kg) are equivalent; they express the same weight. The conversion factor used to change pounds to kilograms or vice versa is:

$$\frac{2.2 \text{ lb}}{1 \text{ kg}} \quad \text{or} \quad \frac{1 \text{ kg}}{2.2 \text{ lb}}$$

Because both factors equal 1, measurements can be multiplied by the factor without changing the value of the measurement. Thus, the units can be changed.

The correct factor to use in a problem is the one with the unit you are seeking in the numerator (top) of the fraction. Following are some examples of problems commonly encountered in nutrition study; they illustrate the usefulness of conversion factors.

EXAMPLE 1

Convert the weight of 130 pounds to kilograms:

1. Choose the conversion factor in which the unit you are seeking is on top:

$$\frac{1 \text{ kg}}{2.2 \text{ lb}}$$

2. Multiply 130 pounds by the factor:

$$130 \text{ lb} \times \frac{1 \text{ kg}}{2.2 \text{ lb}} = \frac{130 \text{ kg}}{2.2}$$

$$= 59 \text{ kg (rounded off to the nearest whole number)}$$

EXAMPLE 2

How many grams (g) of saturated fat are contained in a 3-ounce (oz) hamburger?

1. Appendix A shows that a 4-ounce hamburger contains 7 grams of saturated fat. You are seeking grams of saturated fat; therefore, the conversion factor is:

$$\frac{7 \text{ g saturated fat}}{4 \text{ oz hamburger}}$$

2. Multiply 3 ounces of hamburger by the conversion factor:

$$3 \text{ oz hamburger} \times \frac{7 \text{ g saturated fat}}{4 \text{ oz hamburger}} = \frac{3 \times 7}{4} = \frac{21}{4}$$

$$= 5 \text{ g saturated fat (rounded off to the nearest whole number)}$$

Energy Units

1 calorie* (cal) = 4.2 kilojoules

1 millijoule (MJ) = 240 cal

1 kilojoule (kJ) = 0.24 cal

1 gram (g) carbohydrate = 4 cal = 17 kJ

1 g fat = 9 cal = 37 kJ

1 g protein = 4 cal = 17 kJ

1 g alcohol = 7 cal = 29 kJ

Nutrient Unit Conversions

Sodium

To convert milligrams of sodium to grams of salt:

$$\text{mg sodium} \div 400 = \text{g of salt}$$

The reverse is also true:

$$\text{g salt} \times 400 = \text{mg sodium}$$

Folate

To convert micrograms (μg) of synthetic folate in supplements and enriched foods to Dietary Folate Equivalents (μg DFE):

$$\mu\text{g synthetic folate} \times 1.7 = \mu\text{g DFE}$$

For naturally occurring folate, assign each microgram of folate a value of 1 μg DFE:

$$\mu\text{g folate} = \mu\text{g DFE}$$

EXAMPLE 3

Consider a pregnant woman who takes a supplement and eats a bowl of fortified cornflakes, 2 slices of fortified bread, and a cup of fortified pasta:

1. From the supplement and fortified foods, she obtains synthetic folate:

Supplement	100 μg folate
Fortified cornflakes	100 μg folate
Fortified bread	40 μg folate
Fortified pasta	60 μg folate
	300 μg folate

2. To calculate the DFE, multiply the amount of synthetic folate by 1.7:

$$300\ \mu\text{g} \times 1.7 = 510\ \mu\text{g DFE}$$

3. Now add the naturally occurring folate from the other foods in her diet—in this example, another 90 μg of folate.

$$510\ \mu\text{g DFE} + 90\ \mu\text{g} = 600\ \mu\text{g DFE}$$

Notice that if we had not converted synthetic folate from supplements and fortified foods to DFE, then this woman's

---

Throughout this book and in the appendixes, the term calorie is used to mean kilocalorie. Thus, when converting calories to kilojoules, do not enlarge the calorie values—they are kilocalorie values.

intake would appear to fall short of the 600 μg recommendation for pregnancy (300 μg + 90 μg = 390 μg). But as this example shows, her intake does meet the recommendation.

Vitamin A

Equivalencies for vitamin A:

1 μg RAE = 1 μg retinol

= 12 μg beta-carotene

= 24 μg other vitamin A carotenoids

1 international unit (IU) = 0.3 μg retinol

= 3.6 μg beta-carotene

= 7.2 μg other vitamin A carotenoids

To convert older retinol equivalents (RE) values to micrograms retinal activity equivalents (RAE):

1 μg RE retinol = 1 μg RAE retinol

6 μg RE beta-carotene = 12 μg RAE beta-carotene

12 μg RE other vitamin A carotenoids = 24 μg RAE other vitamin A carotenoids

International Units (IU)

To convert IU to:

- μg vitamin D: divide by 40 or multiply by 0.025.
- 1 IU natural vitamin E = 0.67 mg alpha-tocopherol.
- 1 IU synthetic vitamin E = 0.45 mg alpha-tocopherol.
- vitamin A, see above.

Percentages

A percentage is a comparison between a number of items (perhaps your intake of energy) and a standard number (perhaps the number of calories recommended for your age and gender—your energy DRI). The standard number is the number you divide by. The answer you get after the division must be multiplied by 100 to be stated as a percentage (percent means "per 100").

EXAMPLE 4

What percentage of the DRI recommendation for energy is your energy intake?

1. Find your energy DRI value on the inside front cover. We'll use 2,368 calories to demonstrate.

2. Total your energy intake for a day—for example, 1,200 calories.

3. Divide your calorie intake by the DRI value:

$$1{,}200\ \text{cal (your intake)} \div 2{,}368\ \text{cal (DRI)} = 0.507$$

4. Multiply your answer by 100 to state it as a percentage:

$$0.507 \times 100 = 50.7 = 51\% \text{ (rounded off to the nearest whole number)}$$

In some problems in nutrition, the percentage may be more than 100. For example, suppose your daily intake of vitamin A is 3,200 and your DRI is 900 μg. Your intake as a percentage of the DRI is more than 100 percent (i.e., you consume more than 100 percent of your recommendation for vitamin A). The following calculations show your vitamin A intake as a percentage of the DRI value:

$$3,200 \div 900 = 3.6 \text{ (rounded)}$$
$$3.6 \times 100 = 360\% \text{ of DRI}$$

EXAMPLE 5

Food labels express nutrients and energy contents of foods as percentages of the Daily Values. If a serving of a food contains 200 milligrams of calcium, for example, what percentage of the calcium Daily Value does the food provide?

1. Find the calcium Daily Value on the inside back cover, page Y.

2. Divide the milligrams of calcium in the food by the Daily Value standard:

$$\frac{200}{1,300} = 0.15 \text{ (rounded)}$$

3. Multiply by 100:

$$0.15 \times 100 = 15\% \text{ of the Daily Value}$$

EXAMPLE 6

This example demonstrates how to calculate the percentage of fat in a day's meals:

1. Recall the general formula for finding percentages of calories from a nutrient:

(one nutrient's calories $\div$ total calories) $\times$ 100 = the percentage of calories from that nutrient

2. Say a day's meals provide 1,754 calories and 54 grams of fat. First, convert fat grams to fat calories:

54 g $\times$ 9 cal per g = 486 cal from fat

3. Then apply the general formula for finding percentage of calories from fat:

(fat calories $\div$ total calories) $\times$ 100 = percentage of calories from fat
$$(486 \div 1,754) \times 100 = 27.7 \text{ (28\%, rounded)}$$

Weights and Measures

Length

1 inch (in.) = 2.54 centimeters (cm)
1 foot (ft) = 30.48 cm
1 meter (m) = 39.37 in

Temperature

Steam	100°C	212°F	Steam
Body temperature	37°C	98.6°F	Body temperature
Ice	0°C	32°F	Ice
	Celsius[†]		Fahrenheit

- To find degrees Fahrenheit (°F) when you know degrees Celsius (°C), multiply by 9/5 and then add 32.
- To find degrees Celsius (°C) when you know degrees Fahrenheit (°F), subtract 32 and then multiply by 5/9.

Volume

Used to measure fluids or pourable dry substances such as cereal.

1 milliliter (ml) = $\frac{1}{5}$ teaspoon or 0.034 fluid ounce or $\frac{1}{1,000}$ liter
1 deciliter (dL) = $\frac{1}{10}$ liter
1 teaspoon (tsp or t) = 5 ml or about 5 grams (weight) salt
1 tablespoon (tbs or T) = 3 tsp or 15 ml
1 ounce, fluid (fl oz) = 2 tbs or 30 ml
1 cup (c) = 8 fl oz or 16 tbs or 250 ml
1 quart (qt) = 32 fl oz or 4 c or 0.95 liter
1 liter (L) = 1.06 qt or 1,000 ml
1 gallon (gal) = 16 c or 4 qt or 128 fl oz or 3.79 L

Weight

1 microgram (μg or mcg) = $\frac{1}{1,000}$ milligram
1 milligram (mg) = 1,000 mcg or $\frac{1}{1,000}$ gram
1 gram (g) = 1,000 mg or $\frac{1}{1,000}$ kilogram
1 ounce, weight (oz) = about 28 g or $\frac{1}{16}$ pound
1 pound (lb) = 16 oz (wt) or about 454 g
1 kilogram (kg) = 1,000 g or 2.2 lb

Food Lists for Diabetes and Weight Management

C hapter 2 introduces meal planning principles, and this appendix displays and explains the Food Lists from *Choose Your Foods: Food Lists for Diabetes* and *Choose Your Foods: Food Lists for Weight Management*. These lists can help people with diabetes to manage their blood glucose levels by controlling the amount and kinds of carbohydrates they consume. The lists can also help in planning diets for weight management by controlling calorie intake.

The Food Lists

The Food Lists sort foods by their proportions of carbohydrate, fat, and protein. These lists also fall into groups that reflect the dominant energy nutrient (Table D–1, p. D-2). For example, the Carbohydrates include these Food Lists:

- Starch
- Fruits
- Milk
- Nonstarchy Vegetables
- Sweets, Desserts, and Other Carbohydrates

Any food on a list can be traded for any other food on the same list without significantly affecting the intake of energy nutrients or total calories. The term *choice* is used throughout the lists to describe a certain quantity of food within a group of similar foods.

Serving Sizes

The serving sizes have been carefully adjusted and defined so that a serving of any food on a given list provides roughly the same amount of carbohydrate, fat, and protein—and therefore total energy. For example, a person may select 17 small grapes or ½ large grapefruit as one fruit serving, and either would provide roughly 15 grams of carbohydrate and 60 calories. A whole grapefruit, however, would count as 2 fruit servings.

To apply the system successfully, users must become familiar with the specified serving sizes. A convenient way to remember the serving sizes and energy values is to keep in mind a typical item from each list (review Table D–1).

The Foods on the Lists

Foods do not always appear on the Food Lists where you might first expect to find them. They are grouped according to their energy-nutrient contents rather than by their source, their outward appearance, or their vitamin and mineral contents. For example, cheeses are found among the meats on the Protein lists (not Milk and Milk Substitutes) because, like meats, cheeses contribute energy from protein and fat but provide negligible carbohydrate. For similar reasons, starchy vegetables such as corn, green peas, and potatoes are found on the Starch list with breads and cereals, not with the vegetables. Diet planners learn to view mixtures of foods, such as casseroles and soups, as combinations of foods from different lists.

Controlling Energy, Fat, and Sodium

The Food Lists help people control their energy intakes by paying close attention to serving sizes. Also, people wanting to lose weight can limit foods from the Sweets, Desserts, and Other Carbohydrates and Fats lists, and they might choose to avoid the Alcohol list altogether. The Free Foods list provide low-calorie choices.

The lists alert consumers to foods that are unexpectedly high in fat. For example, the Starch list specifies which grain products contain added fat (such as biscuits) by marking them with a symbol to indicate extra fat (the symbols are explained in the table keys). In addition, foods on the Milk and Milk Substitutes and Protein lists are separated into categories based on their fat contents (review Table D–1). The Protein list also includes plant-based proteins, which tend to be rich in fiber. Notice that many of these foods (p. D-9) bear the symbol for "good source of fiber."

People wanting to control the sodium in their diets can begin by eliminating any foods bearing the "high in sodium" symbol. In most cases, the symbol identifies foods that, in one serving, provide 480 milligrams or more of sodium. Foods on the Combination Foods and Fast Foods lists that bear the symbol provide more than 600 milligrams of sodium. Take time to explore the Food Lists (Tables D–2 through D–12). Doing so can provide a new focus on the energy-yielding nutrients that everyday foods provide.

TABLE D–1 The Food Lists

This table shows the amounts of nutrients and energy in one choice from each list.

Food Lists	Typical Item/Serving Size	Carbohydrate (g)	Protein (g)	Fat (g)	Energy[a] (cal)
Carbohydrates					
Starch[b]	1 slice bread	15	3	1	80
Fruits	1 small apple	15	—	—	60
Milk and milk substitutes					
Fat-free, low-fat (1%)	1 c fat-free milk	12	8	0–3	100
Reduced-fat (2%)	1 c reduced-fat milk	12	8	5	120
Whole	1 c whole milk	12	8	8	160
Nonstarchy vegetables	½ c cooked carrots	5	2	—	25
Sweets, desserts, and other carbohydrates	5 vanilla wafers	15	varies	varies	varies
Proteins					
Lean	1 oz chicken (no skin)	—	7	2	45
Medium-fat	1 oz ground beef	—	7	5	75
High-fat	1 oz pork sausage	—	7	8	100
Plant-based	½ c tofu	varies	7	varies	varies
Fats	1 tsp olive oil		—	5	45
Alcohol	12 fl oz beer	varies	—	—	100

[a]The energy value for each food list represents an approximate average for the group and does not reflect the precise number of grams of carbohydrate, protein, and fat. For example, a slice of bread contains 15 grams of carbohydrate (60 calories), 3 grams of protein (12 calories), and 1 gram of fat (9 calories)—rounded to 80 calories for ease in calculating. A ½ cup of nonstarchy vegetables contains 5 grams of carbohydrate (20 calories) and 2 grams of protein (8 calories), which has been rounded down to 25 calories.

[b]The Starch list includes cereals, grains and pasta, breads, crackers and snacks, starchy vegetables (such as corn, green peas, and potatoes), and legumes (dried beans, peas, and lentils).

Appendix D Food Lists for Diabetes and Weight Management

The Starch list includes breads, cereals, grains (including pasta and rice), starchy vegetables, crackers and snacks, and legumes (beans, peas, and lentils).
1 starch choice = 15 grams carbohydrate, 3 grams protein, 1 gram fat, and 80 calories.
Note: In general, one starch choice is ½ cup of cooked cereal, grain, or starchy vegetable; ⅓ cup of cooked rice or pasta; 1 ounce of bread product, such as 1 slice of bread; ¾ to 1 ounce of most snack foods.

Food	Serving Size	Food	Serving Size
Bread		**Starchy Vegetables** (continued)	
Bagel	¼ large bagel (1 oz)	Cassava or dasheen	⅓ cup
! Biscuit	1 (2½ in. across)	Corn	½ cup
Breads, loaf-type		on cob	4- to 4½-in. piece (½ large)
white, whole-grain, French, Italian, pumpernickel,	1 slice (1 oz)	✓ Hominy	¾ cup
rye, sourdough, unfrosted raisin or cinnamon		✓ Mixed vegetables with corn or peas	1 cup
✓ reduced-calorie, light	2 slices (1½ oz)	Marinara, pasta, or spaghetti sauce	½ cup
Breads, flat-type (flatbreads)		✓ Parsnips	½ cup
chapati	1 oz	✓ Peas, green	½ cup
ciabatta	1 oz	Plantain	⅓ cup
naan	3¼-in. square (1 oz)	Potato	
pita (6 in. across)	½ pita	baked with skin	¼ large (3 oz)
roti	1 oz	boiled, all kinds	½ cup or ½ medium (3 oz)
✓ sandwich flat buns, whole-wheat	1 bun (1½ oz)	! mashed, with milk and fat	½ cup
! taco shell	2 (each 5 in. across)	French-fried (oven-baked)ᶜ	1 cup (2 oz)
tortilla, corn	1 small (6 in. across)	✓ Pumpkin puree, canned, no sugar added	¾ cup
tortilla, flour (white or whole-wheat)	1 small (6 in. across) or ⅓ large	✓ Squash, winter (acorn, butternut)	1 cup
	(10 in. across)	✓ Succotash	½ cup
Cornbread	1¾-in. cube (1½ oz)	Yam or sweet potato, plain	½ cup (3½ oz)
English muffin	½ muffin	**Crackers and Snacks**	
Hot dog bun or hamburger bun	½ bun (¾ oz)	Crackers	
Pancake	1 (4 in. across, ¼ in. thick)	animal	8
Roll, plain	1 small (1 oz)	✓ crispbread	2–5 pieces (¾ oz)
! Stuffing, bread	⅓ cup	graham, 2½-in. square	3
Waffle	1 (4-in. square or 4 in. across)	nut and rice	10
Cereals		oyster	20
✓ Bran cereal (twigs, buds, or flakes)	½ cup	! round, butter-type	6
Cooked cereals (oats, oatmeal)	½ cup	saltine-type	6
Granola cereal	¼ cup	! sandwich-style, cheese or peanut	3
Grits, cooked	½ cup	butter filling	
Muesli	¼ cup	whole-wheat, baked	5 regular 1½-in. squares or
Puffed cereal	1½ cups		10 thins (¾ oz)
Shredded wheat, plain	½ cup	Granola or snack bar	1 (¾ oz)
Sugar-coated cereal	½ cup	Matzoh, all shapes and sizes	¾ oz
Unsweetened, ready-to-eat cereal	¾ cup	Melba toast	4 (2 in. by 4 in.)
Grainsᵃ		Popcorn	
Barley	⅓ cup	✓ no fat added	3 cups
Bran, dry		!! with butter added	3 cups
✓ oat	¼ cup	Pretzels	¾ oz
✓ wheat	½ cup	Rice cakes	2 (4 in. across)
✓ Bulgur	½ cup	Snack chips	
Couscous	⅓ cup	baked (potato, pita)	~8 (¾ oz)
Kasha	½ cup	!! regular (tortilla, potato)	~13 (1 oz)
Millet	⅓ cup	**Beans, Peas, and Lentils**ᵈ	
Pasta, white or whole-wheat	⅓ cup	The choices on this list count as 1 starch + 1 lean protein.	
Polenta	⅓ cup	✓ Baked beans, canned	⅓ cup
Quinoa, all colors	⅓ cup	✓ Beans (black, garbanzo, kidney, lima,	½ cup
Rice, all colors and types	⅓ cup	navy, pinto, white), cooked or canned,	
Tabbouleh (tabouli), prepared	½ cup	drained and rinsed	
Wheat germ, dry	3 tbs	✓ Lentils (any color), cooked	½ cup
Wild rice	½ cup	✓ Peas (black-eyed and split), cooked or canned,	½ cup
Starchy Vegetablesᵇ		drained and rinsed	
Breadfruit	¼ cup	Ⓢ ✓ Refried beans, canned	½ cup

ᵃ*Serving sizes are for cooked grains unless otherwise noted.* ᵇ*Serving sizes are for cooked vegetables.* ᶜ*Restaurant-style French fries are on the Fast Foods list.* ᵈ*Also found on the Protein list.*

Key:

✓ = Good source of fiber: 3 g/serving

! = Extra fat: +5 g/serving

!! = Extra fat: +10 g/serving

Ⓢ = High in sodium: ≥480 mg/serving

Appendix D Food Lists for Diabetes and Weight Management

TABLE D–3 Fruits

Fruit[a]

The Fruits list includes fresh, frozen, canned, and dried fruits and fruit juices.

1 fruit choice = 15 grams carbohydrate, 0 grams protein, 0 grams fat, and 60 calories.

Note: In general, one fruit choice is ½ cup of canned or frozen fruit or unsweetened fruit juice; 1 small fresh fruit (¾ to 1 cup); 2 tablespoons of dried fruit.

Food	Serving Size
Apple, unpeeled	1 small (4 oz)
Apples, dried	4 rings
Applesauce, unsweetened	½ cup
Apricots	
canned	½ cup
dried	8 halves
fresh	4 (5½ oz total)
Banana	1 extra-small, ~4 in. long (4 oz)
✓ Blackberries	1 cup
Blueberries	¾ cup
Cantaloupe	1 cup diced
Cherries	
sweet, canned	½ cup
sweet, fresh	12 (3½ oz)
Dates	3 small (deglet noor) or 1 large (medjool)
Dried fruits (blueberries, cherries, cranberries, mixed fruit, raisins)	2 tbs
Figs	
dried	3 small
✓ fresh	1½ large or 2 medium (3½ oz)
Fruit cocktail	½ cup
Grapefruit	
fresh	½ large (5½ oz)
sections, canned	¾ cup
Grapes	17 small (3 oz)
✓ Guava	2 small (2½ oz total)
Honeydew melon	1 cup diced
Kiwi	½ cup sliced
Loquat	¾ cup cubed
Mandarin oranges, canned	¾ cup
Mango	½ small (5½ oz) or ½ cup
Nectarine	1 medium (5½ oz)
✓ Orange	1 medium (6½ oz)
Papaya	½ (8 oz) or 1 cup cubed
Peaches	
canned	½ cup
fresh	1 medium (6 oz)
Pears	
canned	½ cup
✓ fresh	½ large (4 oz)
Pineapple	
canned	½ cup
fresh	¾ cup
Plantain, extra-ripe (black), raw	¼ (2¼ oz)
Plums	
canned	½ cup
dried (prunes)	3
fresh	2 small (5 oz total)
Pomegranate seeds (arils)	½ cup
✓ Raspberries	1 cup
✓ Strawberries	1¼ cup whole
Tangerine	1 large (6 oz)
Watermelon	1¼ cups diced
Fruit Juice	
Apple juice/cider	½ cup
Fruit juice blends, 100% juice	⅓ cup
Grape juice	⅓ cup
Grapefruit juice	½ cup
Orange juice	½ cup
Pineapple juice	½ cup
Pomegranate juice	½ cup
Prune juice	⅓ cup

[a]The weights listed include skin, core, seeds, and rind.

Key:
✓ = Good source of fiber: >3 g/serving

The Milk and Milk Substitutes list groups milks and yogurts based on the amount of fat they contain.

1 fat-free (skim) or low-fat (1%) milk = 12 grams carbohydrate, 8 grams protein, 0–3 grams fat, and 100 calories.

1 reduced-fat milk choice = 12 grams carbohydrate, 8 grams protein, 5 grams fat, and 120 calories.

1 whole milk choice = 12 grams carbohydrate, 8 grams protein, 8 grams fat, and 160 calories.

1 carbohydrate choice adds 15 grams carbohydrate and about 70 calories.

1 fat choice adds 5 grams fat and 45 calories.

Note: Cheeses are on the Protein list because they are rich in protein and have very little carbohydrate. Butter, cream, coffee creamers, almond milk, and unsweetened coconut milk lack protein and so are listed with the Fats. Ice cream and frozen yogurt are on the Sweets, Desserts, and Other Carbohydrates list.

Food	Serving Size	Choices per Serving
Milk and Yogurts		
Fat-free (skim) or low-fat (1%)		
milk, buttermilk, acidophilus milk, lactose-free milk	1 cup	1 fat-free milk
evaporated milk	½ cup	1 fat-free milk
yogurt, plain or Greek; may be sweetened with artificial sweetener	⅔ cup (6 oz)	1 fat-free milk
chocolate milk	1 cup	1 fat-free milk + 1 carbohydrate
Reduced-fat (2%)		
milk, acidophilus milk, kefir, lactose-free milk	1 cup	1 reduced-fat milk
yogurt, plain	⅔ cup (6 oz)	1 reduced-fat milk
Whole		
milk, buttermilk, goat's milk	1 cup	1 whole milk
evaporated milk	½ cup	1 whole milk
yogurt, plain	1 cup (8 oz)	1 whole milk
chocolate milk	1 cup	1 whole milk + 1 carbohydrate
Other Milk Foods and Milk Substitutes		
Eggnog		
fat-free	⅓ cup	1 carbohydrate
low-fat	⅓ cup	1 carbohydrate + ½ fat
whole milk	⅓ cup	1 carbohydrate + 1 fat
Rice drink		
plain, fat-free	1 cup	1 carbohydrate
flavored, low-fat	1 cup	2 carbohydrates
Soy milk		
light or low-fat, plain	1 cup	½ carbohydrate + ½ fat
regular, plain	1 cup	½ carbohydrate + 1 fat
Yogurt with fruit, low-fat	⅔ cup (6 oz)	1 fat-free milk + 1 carbohydrate

TABLE **D–5** Nonstarchy Vegetables

The Nonstarchy Vegetables list includes vegetables that contain small amounts of carbohydrates and few calories; starchy vegetables that contain higher amounts of carbohydrate and calories are found on the Starch list. Salad greens (like arugula, chicory, endive, escarole, lettuce, radicchio, romaine, and watercress) are on the Free Foods list.

1 nonstarchy vegetable choice = 5 grams carbohydrate, 2 grams protein, 0 grams fat, and 25 calories.

Note: In general, one nonstarchy vegetable choice is ½ cup of cooked vegetables or vegetable juice or 1 cup of raw vegetables. Count 3 cups of raw vegetables or 1½ cups of cooked nonstarchy vegetables as one carbohydrate choice.

Amaranth leaves (Chinese spinach)	Hearts of palm
Artichoke	✓ Jicama
Artichoke hearts (no oil)	Kale
Asparagus	Kohlrabi
Baby corn	Leeks
Bamboo shoots	Mixed vegetables (without starchy vegetables, legumes,
Bean sprouts (alfalfa, mung, soybean)	or pasta)
Beans (green, wax, Italian, yard-long)	Mushrooms, all kinds, fresh
Beets	Okra
Broccoli	Onions
Broccoli slaw, packaged, no dressing	Pea pods
✓ Brussels sprouts	Peppers (all varieties)
Cabbage (green, red, bok choy, Chinese)	Radishes
✓ Carrots	Rutabaga
Cauliflower	⑤ Sauerkraut, drained and rinsed
Celery	Spinach
Chayote	Squash, summer varieties (yellow, pattypan, crookneck, zucchini)
Coleslaw, packaged, no dressing	Sugar snap peas
Cucumber	Swiss chard
Daikon	Tomato
Eggplant	Tomatoes, canned
Fennel	⑤ Tomato sauce (unsweetened)
Gourds (bitter, bottle, luffa, bitter melon)	Tomato/vegetable juice
Green onions or scallions	Turnips
Greens (collard, dandelion, mustard, purslane, turnip)	Water chestnuts

Key:
✓ = Good source of fiber: >3 g/serving
⑤ = High in sodium: ≥480 mg/serving

TABLE **D–6** Sweets, Desserts, and Other Carbohydrates

The Sweets, Desserts, and Other Carbohydrates list contains foods with added sugars, added fats, or both, and their total calories vary accordingly.

1 carbohydrate choice = 15 grams carbohydrate and about 70 calories.
1 fat choice = 5 grams fat and 45 calories.

Food	Serving Size	Choices per Serving
Beverages, Soda, and Sports Drinks		
Cranberry juice cocktail	½ cup	1 carbohydrate
Fruit drink or lemonade	1 cup (8 oz)	2 carbohydrates
Hot chocolate, regular	1 envelope (2 tbs or ¾ oz) added to 8 oz water	1 carbohydrate
Soft drink (soda), regular	1 can (12 oz)	2½ carbohydrates
Sports drink (fluid replacement type)	1 cup (8 oz)	1 carbohydrate
Brownies, Cake, Cookies, Gelatin, Pie, and Pudding		
Biscotti	1 oz	1 carbohydrate + 1 fat
Brownie, small, unfrosted	1½-in. square, ⅞-in. high (~1 oz)	1 carbohydrate + 1 fat
Cake		
angel food, unfrosted	¹⁄₁₂ of cake (~2 oz)	2 carbohydrates
frosted	2-in. square (~2 oz)	2 carbohydrates + 1 fat
unfrosted	2-in. square (~1 oz)	1 carbohydrate + 1 fat
Cookies		
100-calorie pack	1 oz	1 carbohydrate + ½ fat
chocolate chip cookies	2, 2¼ in. across	1 carbohydrate + 2 fats
gingersnaps	3 small, 1½ in. across	1 carbohydrate
large cookie	1, 6 in. across (~3 oz)	4 carbohydrates + 3 fats
sandwich cookies with crème filling	2 small (~⅔ oz)	1 carbohydrate + 1 fat
sugar-free cookies	1 large or 3 small (¾ to 1 oz)	1 carbohydrate + 1–2 fats
vanilla wafer	5	1 carbohydrate + 1 fat
Cupcake, frosted	1 small (~1¾ oz)	2 carbohydrates + 1–1½ fats
Flan	½ cup	2½ carbohydrates + 1 fat

TABLE D-6 Sweets, Desserts, and Other Carbohydrates (*continued*)

Food	Serving Size	Choices per Serving
Brownies, Cake, Cookies, Gelatin, Pie, and Pudding (continued)		
Fruit cobbler	½ cup (3½ oz)	3 carbohydrates + 1 fat
Gelatin, regular	½ cup	1 carbohydrate
Pie		
commercially prepared fruit, 2 crusts	⅙ of 8-in. pie	3 carbohydrates + 2 fats
pumpkin or custard	⅛ of 8-in. pie	1½ carbohydrates + 1½ fats
Pudding		
regular (made with reduced-fat milk)	½ cup	2 carbohydrates
sugar-free or sugar- and fat-free (made with fat-free milk)	½ cup	1 carbohydrate
Candy, Spreads, Sweets, Sweeteners, Syrups, and Toppings		
Blended sweeteners (mixtures of artificial sweeteners and sugar)	1½ tbs	1 carbohydrate
Candy		
chocolate, dark or milk type	1 oz	1 carbohydrate + 2 fats
chocolate "kisses"	5 pieces	1 carbohydrate + 1 fat
hard	3 pieces	1 carbohydrate
Coffee creamer, nondairy type		
powdered, flavored	4 tsp	½ carbohydrate + ½ fat
liquid, flavored	2 tbs	1 carbohydrate
Fruit snacks, chewy (pureed fruit concentrate)	1 roll (¾ oz)	1 carbohydrate
Fruit spreads, 100% fruit	1½ tbs	1 carbohydrate
Honey	1 tbs	1 carbohydrate
Jam or jelly, regular	1 tbs	1 carbohydrate
Sugar	1 tbs	1 carbohydrate
Syrup		
chocolate	2 tbs	2 carbohydrates
light (pancake-type)	2 tbs	1 carbohydrate
regular (pancake-type)	1 tbs	1 carbohydrate
Condiments and Sauces		
Barbecue sauce	3 tbs	1 carbohydrate
Cranberry sauce, jellied	¼ cup	1½ carbohydrates
[S] Curry sauce	1 oz	1 carbohydrate + 1 fat
[S] Gravy, canned or bottled	½ cup	½ carbohydrate + ½ fat
Hoisin sauce	1 tbs	½ carbohydrate
Marinade	1 tbs	½ carbohydrate
Plum sauce	1 tbs	½ carbohydrate
Salad dressing, fat-free, cream-based	3 tbs	1 carbohydrate
Sweet-and-sour sauce	3 tbs	1 carbohydrate
Doughnuts, Muffins, Pastries, and Sweet Breads		
Banana nut bread	1-in. slice (2 oz)	2 carbohydrates + 1 fat
Doughnut		
cake, plain	1 medium (1½ oz)	1½ carbohydrates + 2 fats
hole	2 (1 oz)	1 carbohydrate + 1 fat
yeast-type, glazed	1, 3¾ in. across (2 oz)	2 carbohydrates + 2 fats
Muffin		
regular	1 (4 oz)	4 carbohydrates + 2½ fats
lower-fat	1 (4 oz)	4 carbohydrates + ½ fat
Scone	1 (4 oz)	4 carbohydrates + 3 fats
Sweet roll or Danish	1 (2½ oz)	2½ carbohydrates + 2 fats
Frozen Bars, Frozen Desserts, Frozen Yogurt, and Ice Cream		
Frozen pops	1	½ carbohydrate
Fruit juice bars, frozen, 100% juice	1 (3 oz)	1 carbohydrate
Ice cream		
fat-free	½ cup	1½ carbohydrates
light	½ cup	1 carbohydrate + 1 fat
no-sugar-added	½ cup	1 carbohydrate + 1 fat
regular	½ cup	1 carbohydrate + 2 fats
Sherbet, sorbet	½ cup	2 carbohydrates
Yogurt, frozen		
fat-free	⅓ cup	1 carbohydrate
regular	½ cup	1 carbohydrate + 0–1 fat
Greek, lower-fat or fat-free	½ cup	1½ carbohydrates

Key:
[S] = High in sodium: ≥480 mg/serving

TABLE D–7 Protein

The Protein list groups foods based on the amount of fat they contain.
1 lean protein choice = 0 grams carbohydrate, 7 grams protein, 2 grams fat, and 45 calories.
1 medium-fat protein choice = 0 grams carbohydrate, 7 grams protein, 5 grams fat, and 75 calories.
1 high-fat protein choice = 0 grams carbohydrate, 7 grams protein, 8 grams fat, and 100 calories.

Food	Serving Size	Food	Serving Size
Lean Protein		**Medium-Fat Protein**	
Beef: ground (90% or higher lean/10% or lower fat); select or choice grades trimmed of fat, such as roast (chuck, round, rump, sirloin), steak (cubed, flank, porterhouse, T-bone), tenderloin	1 oz	Beef trimmed of visible fat: ground beef (85% or lower lean/15% or higher fat), corned beef, meatloaf, prime cuts of beef (rib roast), short ribs, tongue	1 oz
⑤ Beef jerky	½ oz	Cheeses with 4–7 g fat/oz: feta, mozzarella, pasteurized processed cheese spread, reduced-fat cheeses	1 oz
Cheeses with ≥3 g fat/oz	1 oz	Cheese, ricotta (regular or part-skim)	¼ cup (2 oz)
Curd-style cheeses: cottage-type (all kinds); ricotta (fat-free or light)	¼ cup (2 oz)	Egg	1
Egg substitutes, plain	¼ cup	Fish: any fried	1 oz
Egg whites	2	Lamb: ground, rib roast	1 oz
Fish		Pork: cutlet, ground, shoulder roast	1 oz
fresh or frozen, such as catfish, cod, flounder, haddock, halibut, orange roughy, tilapia, trout	1 oz	Poultry with skin: chicken, dove, pheasant, turkey, wild duck, or goose; fried chicken	1 oz
salmon, fresh or canned	1 oz	⑤ Sausage with 4–7 g fat/oz	1 oz
sardines, canned	2 small	**High-Fat Protein**	
tuna, fresh or canned in water or oil and drained	1 oz	These foods are high in saturated fat, cholesterol, and calories and may raise blood cholesterol levels if eaten on a regular basis. Try to eat 3 or fewer choices from this group per week.	
⑤ smoked: herring or salmon (lox)	1 oz	Bacon, pork	2 slices (1 oz each before cooking)
Game: buffalo, ostrich, rabbit, venison	1 oz		
⑤ Hot dog[a] with ≤3 g fat/oz	1 (1¾ oz)	⑤ Bacon, turkey	3 slices (½ oz each before cooking)
Lamb: chop, leg, or roast	1 oz		
Organ meats: heart, kidney, liver[b]	1 oz	Cheese, regular: American, blue-veined, brie, cheddar, hard goat, Monterey jack, Parmesan, queso, and Swiss	1 oz
Oysters, fresh or frozen	6 medium		
Pork, lean		! Hot dog: beef, pork, or combination	1 (10 per 1 lb-sized package)
⑤ Canadian bacon	1 oz		
⑤ ham	1 oz	Hot dog: turkey or chicken	1 (10 per 1 lb-sized package)
rib or loin chop/roast, tenderloin	1 oz		
Poultry, without skin: chicken; Cornish hen; domestic duck or goose (well-drained of fat); turkey; lean ground turkey or chicken	1 oz	Pork: sausage, spareribs	1 oz
⑤ Processed sandwich meats with ≤3 g fat/oz: chipped beef, thin-sliced deli meats, turkey ham, turkey pastrami	1 oz	⑤ Processed sandwich meats with ≥8 g fat/oz: bologna, hard salami, pastrami	1 oz
⑤ Sausage with ≤3 g fat/oz	1 oz	⑤ Sausage with ≥8 g fat/oz: bratwurst, chorizo, Italian, knockwurst, Polish, smoked, summer	1 oz
Shellfish: clams, crab, imitation shellfish, lobster, scallops, shrimp	1 oz		
Veal: cutlet (no breading), loin chop, roast	1 oz		

[a]May contain carbohydrate.

[b]May be high in cholesterol.

Key:
! = Extra fat

⑤ = High in sodium: ≥480 mg/serving (based on the sodium content of a typical 3-oz serving of meat, unless 1 oz or 2 oz is the normal serving size)

TABLE D-7 Protein (*continued*)

Plant-Based Protein

Beans, peas, and lentils are also on the Starch list; nut butters in small amounts are on the Fats list. Because carbohydrate content varies among plant-based proteins, read food labels.

1 plant-based protein choice = variable grams carbohydrate, 7 grams protein, variable grams fat, and variable calories.

Food	Serving Size	Choices per Serving
"Bacon" strips, soy-based	2 (½ oz)	1 lean protein
✓ Baked beans, canned	⅓ cup	1 starch + 1 lean protein
✓ Beans (black, garbanzo, kidney, lima, navy, pinto, white), cooked or canned, drained and rinsed	½ cup	1 starch + 1 lean protein
"Beef" or "sausage" crumbles, meatless	1 oz	1 lean protein
"Chicken" nuggets, soy-based	2 (1½ oz)	½ carbohydrate + 1 medium-fat protein
✓ Edamame, shelled	½ cup	½ carbohydrate + 1 lean protein
Falafel (spiced chickpea and wheat patties)	3 patties (~2 in. across)	1 carbohydrate + 1 high-fat protein
Hot dog, meatless, soy-based	1 hot dog (1½ oz)	1 lean protein
✓ Hummus	⅓ cup	1 carbohydrate + 1 medium-fat protein
✓ Lentils, any color, cooked or canned, drained and rinsed	½ cup	1 starch + 1 lean protein
Meatless burger, soy-based	3 oz	½ carbohydrate + 2 lean proteins
✓ Meatless burger, vegetable- and starch-based	1 patty (~2½ oz)	½ carbohydrate + 1 lean protein
Meatless deli slices	1 oz	1 lean protein
Mycoprotein ("chicken" tenders or crumbles), meatless	2 oz	½ carbohydrate + 1 lean protein
Nut spreads: almond butter, cashew butter, peanut butter, soy nut butter	1 tbs	1 high-fat protein
✓ Peas (black-eyed and split peas), cooked or canned, drained and rinsed	½ cup	1 starch + 1 lean protein
✓ [S] Refried beans, canned	½ cup	1 starch + 1 lean protein
"Sausage" breakfast-type patties, meatless	1 (1½ oz)	1 medium-fat protein
Soy nuts, unsalted	¾ oz	½ carbohydrate + 1 medium-fat protein
Tempeh, plain, unflavored	¼ cup (1½ oz)	1 medium-fat protein
Tofu	½ cup (4 oz)	1 medium-fat protein
Tofu, light	½ cup (4 oz)	1 lean protein

Key:
✓ = Good source of fiber: >3 g/serving   [S] = High in sodium: ≥480 mg/serving

TABLE D-8 Fats

Fats and oils have mixtures of unsaturated (polyunsaturated and monounsaturated) and saturated fats. Foods on the Fats list are grouped together based on the major type of fat they contain.

1 fat choice = 0 grams carbohydrate, 0 grams protein, 5 grams fat, and 45 calories.

Note: In general, one fat choice is 1 teaspoon of oil or solid fat or 1 tablespoon of salad dressing.

When used in large amounts, bacon and nut butters are counted as high-fat protein choices (see Protein list). Fat-free salad dressings are on the Sweets, Desserts, and Other Carbohydrates list. Fat-free products such as margarines, salad dressings, mayonnaise, sour cream, and cream cheese are on the Free Foods list.

Food	Serving Size
Unsaturated Fats—Monounsaturated Fats	
Almond milk (unsweetened)	1 cup
Avocado, medium	2 tbs (1 oz)
Nut butters (*trans* fat-free): almond butter, cashew butter, peanut butter (smooth or crunchy)	1½ tsp
Nuts	
almonds	6 nuts
Brazil	2 nuts
cashews	6 nuts
filberts (hazelnuts)	5 nuts
macadamia	3 nuts
mixed (50% peanuts)	6 nuts
peanuts	10 nuts
pecans	4 halves
pistachios	16 nuts
Oil: canola, olive, peanut	1 tsp
Olives	
black (ripe)	8
green, stuffed	10 large
Spread, plant stanol ester-type	
light	1 tbs
regular	2 tsp

Food	Serving Size
Unsaturated Fats—Polyunsaturated Fats	
Margarine	
lower-fat spread (30%–50% vegetable oil, *trans* fat–free)	1 tbs
stick, tub, or squeeze (*trans* fat–free)	1 tsp
Mayonnaise	
reduced-fat	1 tbs
regular	1 tsp
Mayonnaise-style salad dressing	
reduced-fat	1 tbs
regular	2 tsp
Nuts	
pignolia (pine nuts)	1 tbs
walnuts, English	4 halves
Oil: corn, cottonseed, flaxseed, grapeseed, safflower, soybean, sunflower	1 tsp
Salad dressing	
reduced-fat[a]	2 tbs
regular	1 tbs
Seeds	
flaxseed, ground	1½ tbs
pumpkin, sesame, sunflower	1 tbs
Tahini or sesame paste	2 tsp

[a]*May contain carbohydrate.*

(*continued*)

TABLE D–8 Fats (continued)

Food	Serving Size	Food	Serving Size
Saturated Fats		**Saturated Fats** (continued)	
Bacon, cooked, regular or turkey	1 slice	Cream	
Butter		half-and-half	2 tbs
reduced-fat	1 tbs	heavy	1 tbs
stick	1 tsp	light	1½ tbs
whipped	2 tsp	whipped	2 tbs
Butter blends made with oil		Cream cheese	
reduced-fat or light	1 tbs	reduced-fat	1½ tbs (¾ oz)
regular	1½ tsp	regular	1 tbs (½ oz)
Chitterlings, boiled	2 tbs (½ oz)	Lard	1 tsp
Coconut, sweetened, shredded	2 tbs	Oil: coconut, palm, palm kernel	1 tsp
Coconut milk, canned, thick		Salt pork	¼ oz
light	⅓ cup	Shortening, solid	1 tsp
regular	1½ tbs	Sour cream	
Coconut milk beverage (thin), unsweetened	1 cup	reduced-fat or light	3 tbs
		regular	2 tbs

TABLE D–9 Free Foods

Most foods on the Free Foods list should be limited to 3 servings per day and eaten throughout the day. Eating all 3 servings at one time could raise blood glucose levels. Food and drink choices listed without a serving size can be eaten whenever you like.

1 free food choice = ≤5 grams carbohydrate and ≤20 calories.

Food	Serving Size	Food	Serving Size
Low-Carbohydrate Foods		**Condiments** (continued)	
Candy, hard (regular or sugar-free)	1 piece	Hot pepper sauce	
Fruits: cranberries or rhubarb, sweetened with sugar substitute	½ cup	Lemon juice	
Gelatin dessert, sugar-free, any flavor		Miso	1½ tsp
Gum, sugar-free		Mustard	
Jam or jelly, light or no-sugar-added	2 tsp	honey	1 tbs
Salad greens (such as arugula, chicory, endive, escarole, leaf or iceberg lettuce, purslane, romaine, radicchio, spinach, watercress)		brown, Dijon, horseradish-flavored, wasabi-flavored, or yellow	
		Parmesan cheese, grated	1 tbs
Sugar substitutes (artificial sweeteners)		Pickle relish (dill or sweet)	1 tbs
Syrup, sugar-free	2 tbs	Pickles	
Vegetables: any **raw** nonstarchy vegetables (such as broccoli, cabbage, carrots, cucumber, tomato)	½ cup	⑤ dill	1½ medium
		sweet, bread and butter	2 slices
Vegetables: any **cooked** nonstarchy vegetables (such as carrots, cauliflower, green beans)	¼ cup	sweet, gherkin	¾ oz
		Pimento	
Reduced-Fat or Fat-Free Foods		Salsa	¼ cup
Cream cheese, fat-free	1 tbs (½ oz)	⑤ Soy sauce, light or regular	1 tbs
Coffee creamers, nondairy		Sweet-and-sour sauce	2 tsp
liquid, flavored	1½ tsp	Taco sauce	1 tbs
liquid, sugar-free, flavored	4 tsp	Vinegar	
powdered, flavored	1 tsp	Worcestershire sauce	
powdered, sugar-free, flavored	2 tsp	Yogurt, any type	2 tbs
Margarine spread		**Drinks/Mixes**	
fat-free	1 tbs	⑤ Bouillon, broth, consommé	
reduced-fat	1 tsp	Bouillon or broth, low-sodium	
Mayonnaise		Carbonated or mineral water	
fat-free	1 tbs	Club soda	
reduced-fat	1 tsp	Cocoa powder, unsweetened	1 tbs
Mayonnaise-style salad dressing		Coffee, unsweetened or with sugar substitute	
fat-free	1 tbs	Diet soft drinks, sugar-free	
reduced-fat	2 tsp	Drink mixes (powder or liquid drops), sugar-free	
Salad dressing		Tea, unsweetened or with sugar substitute	
fat-free	1 tbs	Tonic water, sugar-free	
fat-free, Italian	2 tbs	Water	
Sour cream, fat-free or reduced-fat	1 tbs	Water, flavored, sugar-free	
Whipped topping		**Seasonings**	
light or fat-free	2 tbs	Flavoring extracts (for example, vanilla, almond, or peppermint)	
regular	1 tbs	Garlic, fresh or powder	
Condiments		Herbs, fresh or dried	
Barbecue sauce	2 tsp	Kelp	
Catsup (ketchup)	1 tbs	Nonstick cooking spray	
Chili sauce, sweet, tomato-type	2 tsp	Spices	
Horseradish		Wine, used in cooking	

Key:

⑤ = High in sodium: ≥480 mg/serving

Appendix D Food Lists for Diabetes and Weight Management

TABLE D–10 Combination Foods

Many foods are eaten in various combinations, such as casseroles. Because "combination" foods do not fit into any one choice list, this list of choices provides some typical combination foods.
1 carbohydrate choice = 15 grams carbohydrate and about 70 calories.

Food	Serving Size	Choices per Serving
Entrees		
S Casserole-type entrees (tuna noodle, lasagna, spaghetti with meatballs, chili with beans, macaroni and cheese)	1 cup (8 oz)	2 carbohydrates + 2 medium-fat proteins
S Stews (beef/other meats and vegetables)	1 cup (8 oz)	1 carbohydrate + 1 medium-fat protein + 0–3 fats
Frozen Meals/Entrees		
S ✓ Burrito (beef and bean)	1 (5 oz)	3 carbohydrates + 1 lean protein + 2 fats
Dinner-type healthy meal (includes dessert and is usually <400 cal)	~9–12 oz	2–3 carbohydrates + 1–2 lean proteins + 1 fat
"Healthy"-type entree (usually <300 cal)	~7–10 oz	2 carbohydrates + 2 lean proteins
Pizza		
S cheese/vegetarian, thin crust	¼ of a 12-in. pizza (4½–5 oz)	2 carbohydrates + 2 medium-fat proteins
S meat topping, thin crust	¼ of a 12-in. pizza (5 oz)	2 carbohydrates + 2 medium-fat proteins + 1½ fats
S cheese/vegetarian or meat topping, rising crust	⅙ of a 12-in. pizza (4 oz)	2½ carbohydrates + 2 medium-fat proteins
S Pocket sandwich	1 sandwich (4½ oz)	3 carbohydrates + 1 lean protein + 1–2 fats
S Pot pie	1 (7 oz)	3 carbohydrates + 1 medium-fat protein + 3 fats
Salads (Deli-Style)		
Coleslaw	½ cup	1 carbohydrate + 1½ fats
Macaroni/pasta salad	½ cup	2 carbohydrates + 3 fats
S Potato salad	½ cup	1½–2 carbohydrates + 1–2 fats
Tuna salad or chicken salad	½ cup (3½ oz)	½ carbohydrate + 2 lean proteins + 1 fat
Soups		
S ✓ Bean, lentil, or split pea soup	1 cup (8 oz)	1½ carbohydrates + 1 lean protein
S Chowder (made with milk)	1 cup (8 oz)	1 carbohydrate + 1 lean protein + 1½ fats
S Cream soup (made with water)	1 cup (8 oz)	1 carbohydrate + 1 fat
S Miso soup	1 cup (8 oz)	½ carbohydrate + 1 lean protein
S Ramen noodle soup	1 cup (8 oz)	2 carbohydrates + 2 fats
Rice soup/porridge (congee)	1 cup (8 oz)	1 carbohydrate
S Tomato soup (made with water), borscht	1 cup (8 oz)	1 carbohydrate
S Vegetable beef, chicken, noodle, or other broth-type soup (including "healthy"-type soups, such as those lower in sodium and/or fat)	1 cup (8 oz)	1 carbohydrate + 1 lean protein

Key:
✓ = Good source of fiber: >3 g/serving
S = High in sodium: ⩾600 mg/serving for main dishes/meals and ⩾480 mg/serving for side dishes

TABLE D–11 Fast Foods

The choices in the Fast Foods list are not specific fast-food meals or items but are estimates based on popular foods. Ask the restaurant or check its website for nutrition information about your favorite fast foods.
1 carbohydrate choice = 15 grams carbohydrate and about 70 calories.

Food	Serving Size	Choices per Serving
Main Dishes/Entrees		
Chicken		
S breast, breaded and fried[a]	1 (~7 oz)	1 carbohydrate + 6 medium-fat proteins
breast, meat only[b]	1	4 lean proteins
drumstick, breaded and fried[a]	1 (~2½ oz)	½ carbohydrate + 2 medium-fat proteins
drumstick, meat only[b]	1	1 lean protein + ½ fat
S nuggets or tenders	6 (~3½ oz)	1 carbohydrate + 2 medium-fat proteins + 1 fat
S thigh, breaded and fried[a]	1 (~5 oz)	1 carbohydrate + 3 medium-fat proteins + 2 fats
thigh, meat only[b]	1	2 lean proteins + ½ fat
wing, breaded and fried[a]	1 wing (~2 oz)	½ carbohydrate + 2 medium-fat proteins
wing, meat only[b]	1 wing	1 lean protein
S ✓ Main dish salad (grilled chicken-type, no dressing or croutons)	1 salad (~11½ oz)	1 carbohydrate + 4 lean proteins

[a]*Definition and weight refer to food **with** bone, skin, and breading.*
[b]*Definition refers to food **without** bone, skin, and breading.*

(continued)

TABLE D–11 Fast Foods (*continued*)

Food	Serving Size	Choices per Serving
Pizza		
🅢 cheese, pepperoni, or sausage, regular or thick crust	⅛ of a 14-in. pizza (~4 oz)	2½ carbohydrates + 1 high-fat protein + 1 fat
🅢 cheese, pepperoni, or sausage, thin crust	⅛ of a 14-in. pizza (~2¾ oz)	1½ carbohydrates + 1 high-fat protein + 1 fat
🅢 cheese, meat, and vegetable, regular crust	⅛ of a 14-in. pizza (~5 oz)	2½ carbohydrates + 2 high-fat proteins
Asian		
🅢 Beef/chicken/shrimp with vegetables in sauce	1 cup (~6 oz)	1 carbohydrate + 2 lean proteins + 1 fat
Egg roll, meat	1 egg roll (~3 oz)	1½ carbohydrates + 1 lean protein + 1½ fats
Fried rice, meatless	1 cup	2½ carbohydrates + 2 fats
Fortune cookie	1	½ carbohydrate
🅢 Hot-and-sour soup	1 cup	½ carbohydrate + ½ fat
🅢 Meat with sweet sauce	1 cup (~6 oz)	3½ carbohydrates + 3 medium-fat proteins + 3 fats
🅢 Noodles and vegetables in sauce (chow mein, lo mein)	1 cup	2 carbohydrates + 2 fats
Mexican		
🅢 ✓ Burrito with beans and cheese	1 small (~6 oz)	3½ carbohydrates + 1 medium-fat protein + 1 fat
🅢 Nachos with cheese	1 small order (~8)	2½ carbohydrates + 1 high-fat protein + 2 fats
🅢 Quesadilla, cheese only	1 small order (~5 oz)	2½ carbohydrates + 3 high-fat proteins
Taco, crisp, with meat and cheese	1 small (~3 oz)	1 carbohydrate + 1 medium-fat protein + ½ fat
🅢 ✓ Taco salad with chicken and tortilla bowl	1 salad (1 lb including bowl)	3½ carbohydrates + 4 medium-fat proteins + 3 fats
🅢 Tostada with beans and cheese	1 small (~5 oz)	2 carbohydrates + 1 high-fat protein
Sandwiches		
Breakfast sandwiches		
🅢 breakfast burrito with sausage, egg, cheese	1 (~4 oz)	1½ carbohydrates + 2 high-fat proteins
🅢 egg, cheese, meat on an English muffin	1	2 carbohydrates + 3 medium-fat proteins + ½ fat
🅢 egg, cheese, meat on a biscuit	1	2 carbohydrates + 3 medium-fat proteins + 2 fats
🅢 sausage biscuit sandwich	1	2 carbohydrates + 1 high-fat protein + 4 fats
Chicken sandwiches		
🅢 grilled with bun, lettuce, tomatoes, spread	1 (~7½ oz)	3 carbohydrates + 4 lean proteins
🅢 crispy, with bun, lettuce, tomatoes, spread	1 (~6 oz)	3 carbohydrates + 2 lean proteins + 3½ fats
Fish sandwich with tartar sauce and cheese	1 (5 oz)	2½ carbohydrates + 2 medium-fat proteins + 1½ fats
Hamburger		
regular with bun and condiments (catsup, mustard, onion, pickle)	1 (~3½ oz)	2 carbohydrates + 1 medium-fat protein + 1 fat
🅢 4 oz meat with cheese, bun, and condiments (catsup, mustard, onion, pickle)	1 (~8½ oz)	3 carbohydrates + 4 medium-fat proteins + 2½ fats
Hot dog with bun, plain	1 (~3½ oz)	1½ carbohydrates + 1 high-fat protein + 2 fats
Submarine sandwich (no cheese or sauce)		
🅢 <6 g fat	1 6-in. sub	3 carbohydrates + 2 lean proteins
🅢 regular	1 6-in. sub	3 carbohydrates + 2 lean proteins + 1 fat
🅢 Wrap, grilled chicken, vegetables, cheese, and spread	1 small (~4–5 oz)	2 carbohydrates + 2 lean proteins + 1½ fats
Sides/Appetizers		
🅢 ! French fries	1 small order (~3½ oz)	2½ carbohydrates + 2 fats
	1 medium order (~5 oz)	3½ carbohydrates + 3 fats
	1 large order (~6 oz)	4½ carbohydrates + 4 fats
🅢 Hash browns	1 cup/medium order (~5 oz)	3 carbohydrates + 6 fats
🅢 Onion rings	1 serving (8–9 rings, ~4 oz)	3½ carbohydrates + 4 fats
Salad, side (no dressing, croutons, or cheese)	1 small	1 nonstarchy vegetable
Beverages and Desserts		
Coffee, latte (fat-free milk)	1 small (~12 oz)	1 fat-free milk
Coffee, mocha (fat-free milk, no whipped cream)	1 small (~12 oz)	1 fat-free milk + 1 carbohydrate
Milkshake, any flavor	1 small (~12 oz)	5½ carbohydrates + 3 fats
	1 medium (~16 oz)	7 carbohydrates + 4 fats
	1 large (~22 oz)	10 carbohydrates + 5 fats
Soft-serve ice cream cone	1 small	2 carbohydrates + ½ fat

Key:
✓ = Good source of fiber: >3 g/serving
! = Extra fat
🅢 = High in sodium: ≥600 mg/serving for main dishes/meals and ≥480 mg/serving for side dishes

TABLE D-12 Alcohol

NOTE: For those who choose to drink alcohol, guidelines suggest limiting alcohol intake to 1 drink or less per day for women and 2 drinks or less per day for men. To reduce the risk of low blood glucose (hypoglycemia), especially when taking insulin or a diabetes pill that increases insulin, alcohol should always be consumed with food, not alone. Although alcohol, by itself, does not directly affect blood glucose, be aware of the carbohydrate (for example, in mixed drinks, beer, and wine) that may raise blood glucose.

1 alcohol equivalent (½ oz ethanol) = 100 calories. 1 carbohydrate choice = 15 g carb and about 70 calories.

Alcoholic Beverage[a]	Serving Size	Choices per Serving
Beer		
light (<4.5% abv)	12 fl oz	1 alcohol equivalent + ½ carbohydrate
regular (~5% abv)	12 fl oz	1 alcohol equivalent + 1 carbohydrate
dark (>5.7% abv)	12 fl oz	1 alcohol equivalent + 1–1½ carbohydrates
Distilled spirits (80 or 86 proof): vodka, rum, gin, whiskey, tequila	1½ fl oz	1 alcohol equivalent
Liqueur, coffee (53 proof)	1 fl oz	½ alcohol equivalent + 1 carbohydrate
Sake	1 fl oz	½ alcohol equivalent
Wine		
champagne/sparkling	5 fl oz	1 alcohol equivalent
dessert (sherry)	3½ fl oz	1 alcohol equivalent + 1 carbohydrate
dry, red or white (10% abv)	5 fl oz	1 alcohol equivalent

[a] "% abv" refers to the percentage of alcohol by volume.

The Food Lists are the basis of a meal planning system designed by a committee of the American Diabetes Association and the Academy of Nutrition and Dietetics. While originally designed for people with diabetes and others who must follow special diets, the Food Lists are based on principles of good nutrition that apply to everyone. © 2014 by the American Diabetes Association and the Academy of Nutrition and Dietetics.

Appendix E Eating Patterns to Meet the Dietary Guidelines for Americans

This appendix presents several eating patterns that meet the ideals of the Dietary Guidelines for Americans. First, Table E–1 lists the USDA Healthy U.S.-Style Eating Pattern in full. Next, Tables E–2 and E–3 present the Dietary Approaches to Stop Hypertension, or DASH, Eating Plan. Although it was originally developed to fight high blood pressure, the DASH plan has proved useful for cutting people's risks of many diseases while meeting nutrient needs superbly.

A Healthy Vegetarian adaptation of the Healthy U.S.-Style Pattern, offered in Table E–4, demonstrates the flexibility of the patterns. This table provides guidance for vegetarians and shows how to meet nutrient needs without meat.

A Healthy Mediterranean-Style food intake pattern can also meet the goals of the Dietary Guidelines for Americans. Table E–5 presents the Healthy Mediterranean-Style eating pattern, and Table E–6 compares it with the Healthy U.S.-Style and Healthy Vegetarian patterns. Figure E–1 illustrates a Mediterranean food pyramid, and Table E–7 provides tips for choosing healthy Mediterranean-style meals. Two cautions are in order, however: First, Mediterranean-style fat sources, such as olives, olive oil, and nuts, although more healthful than saturated fat sources, are high in calories and contribute to weight gain when overconsumed. Second, beware of meals served in Greek, Italian, or other "Mediterranean" restaurants in this country. They often center on generous portions of meats, cheeses, and other foods rich in saturated fats that appeal to the Western palate, and are not in keeping with a Healthy Mediterranean pattern.

TABLE E–1 USDA Healthy U.S.-Style Eating Patterns

Recommended daily intake amounts; weekly amounts for vegetable and protein foods subgroups.

Energy Level of Pattern[a,b]	1,000	1,200	1,400	1,600	1,800	2,000	2,200	2,400	2,600	2,800	3,000	3,200
Food Group[c]												
Fruits	1 c	1 c	1½ c	1½ c	1½ c	2 c	2 c	2 c	2 c	2½ c	2½ c	2½ c
Vegetables[d]	1 c	1½ c	1½ c	2 c	2½ c	2½ c	3 c	3 c	3½ c	3½ c	4 c	4 c
Dark green vegetables (c/wk)	½	1	1	1½	1½	1½	2	2	2½	2½	2½	2½
Red/orange vegetables (c/wk)	2½	3	3	4	5½	5½	6	6	7	7	7½	7½
Dry beans and peas (c/wk)	½	½	½	1	1½	1½	2	2	2½	2½	3	3
Starchy vegetables (c/wk)	2	3½	3½	4	5	5	6	6	7	7	8	8
Other vegetables (c/wk)	1½	2½	2½	3½	4	4	5	5	5½	5½	7	7
Grains[e]	3 oz-eq	4 oz-eq	5 oz-eq	5 oz-eq	6 oz-eq	6 oz-eq	7 oz-eq	8 oz-eq	9 oz-eq	10 oz-eq	10 oz-eq	10 oz-eq
Whole grains	1½ oz-eq	2 oz-eq	2½ oz-eq	3 oz-eq	3 oz-eq	3 oz-eq	3½ oz-eq	4 oz-eq	4½ oz-eq	5 oz-eq	5 oz-eq	5 oz-eq
Other grains	1½ oz-eq	2 oz-eq	2½ oz-eq	2 oz-eq	3 oz-eq	3 oz-eq	3½ oz-eq	4 oz-eq	4½ oz-eq	5 oz-eq	5 oz-eq	5 oz-eq
Protein Foods[d]	2 oz-eq	3 oz-eq	4 oz-eq	5 oz-eq	5 oz-eq	5½ oz-eq	6 oz-eq	6½ oz-eq	6½ oz-eq	7 oz-eq	7 oz-eq	7 oz-eq
Meat, poultry, eggs (oz/wk)	10	14	19	23	23	26	28	31	31	33	33	33
Seafood (oz/wk)	3	4	6	8	8	8	9	10	10	10	10	10
Nuts seeds, soy (oz/wk)	2	2	3	4	4	5	5	5	5	6	6	6
Dairy	2 c	2.5 c	2.5 c	3 c	3 c	3 c	3 c	3 c	3 c	3 c	3 c	3 c
Oils	15 g	17 g	17 g	22 g	24 g	27 g	29 g	31 g	34 g	36 g	44 g	51g
Limit on Calories for Other Uses, calories (% of calories)[e]	150 (15%)	100 (8%)	110 (8%)	130 (8%)	170 (9%)	270 (14%)	280 (13%)	350 (15%)	380 (15%)	400 (14%)	470 (16%)	610 (19%)

[a]Food group amounts shown in cup (c) or ounce equivalents (oz-eq). Oils, solid fats, and added sugars are shown in grams (g).

[b]Eating patterns at 1,000, 1,200, and 1,400 calories meet the nutritional needs of children ages 2 to 8 years. Patterns from 1,600 to 3,200 calories meet the nutritional needs of children ages 9 years and older and adults. If a child ages 4 to 8 years needs more calories and, therefore, is following a pattern at 1,600 calories or more, the recommended amount from the dairy group can be 2½ cups per day. Children ages 9 years and older and adults should not use the 1,000, 1,200, or 1,400 calorie patterns.

[c]Quantity equivalents for each food group are:

- Grains, 1 ounce equivalent is: ½ cup cooked rice, pasta, or cooked cereal; 1 ounce dry pasta or rice; 1 slice bread; 1 small muffin (1 oz); 1 cup ready-to-eat cereal flakes.
- Fruits and Vegetables, 1 cup equivalent is: 1 cup raw or cooked fruit or vegetable, 1 cup fruit or vegetable juice, 2 cups leafy salad greens.
- Protein Foods, 1 ounce equivalent is: 1 ounce lean meat, poultry, or fish; 1 egg; ¼ cup cooked dry beans or tofu; 1 tbs peanut butter; ½ ounce nuts or seeds.
- Dairy, 1 cup equivalent is: 1 cup milk or yogurt, 1½ ounces natural cheese such as Cheddar cheese or 2 ounces of processed cheese.

[d]Vegetable and protein foods subgroup amounts are shown in this table as weekly amounts because it would be difficult for consumers to select foods from all subgroups daily.

[e]Whole-grain subgroup amounts shown in this table are minimums. More whole grains up to all of the grains recommended may be selected, with offsetting decreases in the amounts of enriched refined grains.

Source: U.S. Department of Health and Human Services and U.S. Department of Agriculture, 2015–2020 Dietary Guidelines for Americans, *8th edition (2015),* available at http://health.gov/dietaryguidelines/2015/guidelines/.

TABLE E–2 DASH Eating Plan—Number of Daily Food Servings by Calorie Level

Food Group	1,200 Calories	1,400 Calories	1,600 Calories	1,800 Calories	2,000 Calories	2,600 Calories	3,100 Calories
Grains[a]	4–5	5–6	6	6	6–8	10–11	12–13
Vegetables	3–4	3–4	3–4	4–5	4–5	5–6	6
Fruits	3–4	4	4	4–5	4–5	5–6	6
Fat-free or low-fat dairy products[b]	2–3	2–3	2–3	2–3	2–3	3	3–4
Lean meats, poultry, and fish	3 or less	3–4 or less	3–4 or less	6 or less	6 or less	6 or less	6–9
Nuts, seeds, and legumes	3 per week	3 per week	3–4 per week	4 per week	4–5 per week	1	1
Fats and oils[c]	1	1	2	2–3	2–3	3	4
Sweets and added sugars	3 or less per week	3 or less per week	3 or less per week	5 or less per week	5 or less per week	≤2	≤2
Maximum sodium limit[d]	2,300 mg/day	2,300 mg/day	2,300 mg/day	2,300 mg/day	2,300 mg/day	2,300 mg/day	2,300 mg/day

[a]Whole grains are recommended for most grain servings as a good source of fiber and nutrients.

[b]For lactose intolerance, try either lactase enzyme pills with dairy products, lactose-free or lactose-reduced milk, or soy milk fortified with vitamin D and calcium. Other milk-like products may lack protein.

[c]Fat content changes the serving amount for fats and oils. For example, 1 tbs regular salad dressing = one serving; 1 tbs low-fat dressing = one-half serving; 1 tbs fat-free dressing = zero servings.

[d]The DASH eating plan has a sodium limit of either 2,300 mg or 1,500 mg per day.

Source: National Heart, Lung, and Blood Institute; National Institutes of Health; U.S. Department of Health and Human Services, 2018, available at www.nhlbi.nih.gov /health-topics/dash-eating-plan.

Food Group	Serving Sizes	Examples and Notes	Significance of Each Food Group to the DASH Eating Plan
Grains[a]	1 slice bread 1 oz dry cereal[b] ½ cup cooked rice, pasta, or cereal[b]	Whole-wheat bread and rolls, whole-wheat pasta, English muffin, pita bread, bagel, cereals, grits, oatmeal, brown rice, unsalted pretzels and popcorn	Major sources of energy and fiber
Vegetables	1 cup raw leafy vegetable ½ cup cut-up raw or cooked vegetable ½ cup vegetable juice	Broccoli, carrots, collards, green beans, green peas, kale, lima beans, potatoes, spinach, squash, sweet potatoes, tomatoes	Rich sources of potassium, magnesium, and fiber
Fruits	1 medium fruit ¼ cup dried fruit ½ cup fresh, frozen, or canned fruit ½ cup fruit juice	Apples, apricots, bananas, dates, grapes, oranges, grapefruit, grapefruit juice, mangoes, melons, peaches, pineapples, raisins, strawberries, tangerines	Important sources of potassium, magnesium, and fiber
Fat-free or low-fat dairy products[c]	1 cup milk or yogurt 1½ oz cheese	Fat-free milk or buttermilk; fat-free, low-fat, or reduced fat cheese; fat-free/low-fat regular or frozen yogurt	Major sources of calcium and protein
Lean meats, poultry, and fish	1 oz cooked meats, poultry, or fish 1 egg	Select only lean; trim away visible fats; broil, roast, or poach; remove skin from poultry	Rich sources of protein and magnesium
Nuts, seeds, and legumes	⅓ cup or 1½ oz nuts 2 tbs peanut butter 2 tbs or ½ oz seeds ½ cup cooked legumes (dried beans, peas)	Almonds, filberts, mixed nuts, peanuts, walnuts, sunflower seeds, peanut butter, kidney beans, lentils, split peas	Rich sources of energy, magnesium, protein, and fiber
Fats and oils[d]	1 tsp soft margarine 1 tsp vegetable oil 1 tbs mayonnaise 2 tbs salad dressing	Soft margarine, vegetable oil (canola, corn, olive, safflower), low-fat mayonnaise, light salad dressing	The DASH study had 27% of calories as fat, including fat in or added to foods
Sweets and added sugars	1 tbs sugar 1 tbs jelly or jam ½ cup sorbet, gelatin dessert 1 cup lemonade	Fruit-flavored gelatin, fruit punch, hard candy, jelly, maple syrup, sorbet and ices, sugar	Sweets should be low in fat

[a]Whole grains are recommended for most grain servings as a good source of fiber and nutrients.

[b]Serving sizes vary between ½ cup and 1¼ cups, depending on cereal type. Check the product's Nutrition Facts label.

[c]For lactose intolerance, try either lactase enzyme pills with dairy products, lactose-free or lactose-reduced milk, or soy milk fortified with vitamin D and calcium. Other milk-like products may lack protein.

[d]Fat content changes the serving amount for fats and oils. For example, 1 tbs regular salad dressing = one serving; 1 tbs low-fat dressing = one-half serving; 1 tbs fat-free dressing = zero servings.

Source: National Heart, Lung, and Blood Institute; National Institutes of Health; U.S. Department of Health and Human Services, 2018, available at www.nhlbi.nih.gov/health-topics/dash-eating-plan.

TABLE E-4 Healthy Vegetarian Eating Patterns

Vegans can use this pattern by replacing all dairy choices with fortified soy beverages (soymilk) or other fortified plant-based dairy substitutes.

Calorie Level of Pattern[a]	1,000	1,200	1,400	1,600	1,800	2,000	2,200	2,400	2,600	2,800	3,000	3,200
Food Group[b]	Daily Amount[c] of Food from Each Group (vegetable and protein foods subgroup amounts are per week)											
Vegetables	1 c-eq	1½ c-eq	1½ c-eq	2 c-eq	2½ c-eq	2½ c-eq	3 c-eq	3 c-eq	3½ c-eq	3½ c-eq	4 c-eq	4 c-eq
Dark-green vegetables (c-eq/wk)	½	1	1	1½	1½	1½	2	2	2½	2½	2½	2½
Red and orange vegetables (c-eq/wk)	2½	3	3	4	5½	5½	6	6	7	7	7½	7½
Legumes (beans and peas) (c-eq/wk)[d]	½	½	½	1	1½	1½	2	2	2½	2½	3	3
Starchy vegetables (c-eq/wk)	2	3½	3½	4	5	5	6	6	7	7	8	8
Other vegetables (c-eq/wk)	1½	2½	2½	3½	4	4	5	5	5½	5½	7	7
Fruits	1 c-eq	1 c-eq	1½ c-eq	1½ c-eq	1½ c-eq	2 c-eq	2 c-eq	2 c-eq	2 c-eq	2½ c-eq	2½ c-eq	2½ c-eq
Grains	3 oz-eq	4 oz-eq	5 oz-eq	5½ oz-eq	6½ oz-eq	6½ oz-eq	7½ oz-eq	8½ oz-eq	9½ oz-eq	10½ oz-eq	10½ oz-eq	10½ oz-eq
Whole grains[e] (oz-eq/day)	1½	2	2½	3	3½	3½	4	4½	5	5½	5½	5½
Refined grains (oz-eq/day)	1½	2	2½	2½	3	3	3½	4	4½	5	5	5
Dairy	2 c-eq	2.5 c-eq	2.5 c-eq	3 c-eq	3 c-eq	3 c-eq	3 c-eq	3 c-eq	3 c-eq	3 c-eq	3 c-eq	3 c-eq
Protein Foods	1 oz-eq	1½ oz-eq	2 oz-eq	2½ oz-eq	3 oz-eq	3½ oz-eq	3½ oz-eq	4 oz-eq	4½ oz-eq	5 oz-eq	5½ oz-eq	6 oz-eq
Eggs (oz-eq/wk)	2	3	3	3	3	3	3	3	3	4	4	4
Legumes (beans and peas) (oz-eq/wk)[d]	1	2	4	4	6	6	6	8	9	10	11	12
Soy products (oz-eq/wk)	2	3	4	6	6	8	8	9	10	11	12	13
Nuts and seeds (oz-eq/wk)	2	2	3	5	6	7	7	8	9	10	12	13
Oils	15 g	17 g	17 g	22 g	24 g	27 g	29 g	31 g	34 g	36 g	44 g	51 g
Limit on Calories for Other Uses, calories (% of calories)	190 (19%)	170 (14%)	190 (14%)	180 (11%)	190 (11%)	290 (15%)	330 (15%)	390 (16%)	390 (15%)	400 (14%)	440 (15%)	550 (17%)

[a,b,c,e]See Table E–1 notes.

[d]About half of total legumes are shown as vegetables, in cup-eq, and half as protein foods, in oz-eq. Total legumes in the Patterns, in cup-eq, is the amount in the vegetable group plus the amount in protein foods group (in oz-eq) divided by 4.

TABLE E-5 Healthy Mediterranean-Style Eating Patterns

Calorie Level of Pattern[a]	1,000	1,200	1,400	1,600	1,800	2,000	2,200	2,400	2,600	2,800	3,000	3,200
Food Group[b]	Daily Amount[c] of Food from Each Group (vegetable and protein foods subgroup amounts are per week)											
Vegetables	1 c-eq	1½ c-eq	1½ c-eq	2 c-eq	2½ c-eq	2½ c-eq	3 c-eq	3 c-eq	3½ c-eq	3½ c-eq	4 c-eq	4 c-eq
Dark-green vegetables (c-eq/wk)	½	1	1	1½	1½	1½	2	2	2½	2½	2½	2½
Red and orange vegetables (c-eq/wk)	2½	3	3	4	5½	5½	6	6	7	7	7½	7½
Legumes (beans and peas) (c-eq/wk)	½	½	½	1	1½	1½	2	2	2½	2½	3	3
Starchy vegetables (c-eq/wk)	2	3½	3½	4	5	5	6	6	7	7	8	8
Other vegetables (c-eq/wk)	1½	2½	2½	3½	4	4	5	5	5½	5½	7	7
Fruits	1 c-eq	1 c-eq	1½ c-eq	2 c-eq	2 c-eq	2½ c-eq	2½ c-eq	2½ c-eq	2½ c-eq	3 c-eq	3 c-eq	3 c-eq
Grains	3 oz-eq	4 oz-eq	5 oz-eq	5 oz-eq	6 oz-eq	6 oz-eq	7 oz-eq	8 oz-eq	9 oz-eq	10 oz-eq	10 oz-eq	10 oz-eq
Whole grains[d] (oz-eq/day)	1½	2	2½	3	3	3	3½	4	4½	5	5	5
Refined grains (oz-eq/day)	1½	2	2½	2	3	3	3½	4	4½	5	5	5
Dairy	2 c-eq	2½ c-eq	2½ c-eq	2 c-eq	2 c-eq	2 c-eq	2 c-eq	2½ c-eq	2½ c-eq	2½ c-eq	2½ c-eq	2½ c-eq
Protein Foods	2 oz-eq	3 oz-eq	4 oz-eq	5½ oz-eq	6 oz-eq	6½ oz-eq	7 oz-eq	7½ oz-eq	7½ oz-eq	8 oz-eq	8 oz-eq	8 oz-eq
Seafood (oz-eq/wk)[e]	3	4	6	11	15	15	16	16	17	17	17	17
Meats, poultry, eggs (oz-eq/wk)	10	14	19	23	23	26	28	31	31	33	33	33
Nuts, seeds, soy products (oz-eq/wk)	2	2	3	4	4	5	5	5	5	6	6	6
Oils	15 g	17 g	17 g	22 g	24 g	27 g	29 g	31 g	34 g	36 g	44 g	51 g
Limit on Calories for Other Uses, calories (% of calories)	150 (15%)	100 (8%)	110 (8%)	140 (9%)	160 (9%)	260 (13%)	270 (12%)	300 (13%)	330 (13%)	350 (13%)	430 (14%)	570 (18%)

[a,b,c,d]See Table E–1, notes a through d.

[e]The U.S. Food and Drug Administration (FDA) and the U.S. Environmental Protection Agency (EPA) provide joint guidance regarding seafood consumption for women who are pregnant or breastfeeding and young children. For more information, see the FDA or EPA websites www.FDA.gov/fishadvice; www.EPA.gov/fishadvice.

TABLE E–6 Three USDA Eating Patterns Compared

Three USDA Eating Patterns (Healthy U.S.-Style, Healthy Vegetarian, and Healthy Mediterranean-Style) are recognized as useful for meeting the ideals of the Dietary Guidelines for Americans. The following columns compare them at the 2,000-calorie level.

Food Group	Healthy U.S.-Style Pattern	Healthy Vegetarian Pattern	Healthy Mediterranean Pattern
Fruit	2 c per day	2 c per day	2½ c per day
Vegetables	2½ c per day	2½ c per day	2½ c per day
Legumes	1½ c per wk	3 c per wk	1½ c per wk
Whole Grains	3 oz-eq per day	3 oz-eq per day	3 oz-eq per day
Dairy	3 c per day	3 c per day	2 c per day
Protein Foods	5½ oz-eq per day	3½ oz-eq per day	6½ oz-eq per day
Meat	12½ oz-eq/wk	–	12½ oz-eq/wk
Poultry	10½ oz-eq/wk	–	10½ oz-eq/wk
Seafood	8 oz-eq/wk	–	15 oz-eq/wk
Eggs	3 oz-eq/wk	3 oz-eq/wk	3 oz-eq/wk
Nuts/seeds	4 oz-eq/wk	7 oz-eq/wk	4 oz-eq/wk
Processed soy	½ oz-eq/wk	8 oz-eq/wk	½ oz-eq/wk
Oils	27 g per day	27 g per day	27 g per day

Source: U.S. Department of Agriculture and U.S. Department of Health and Human Services, Scientific Report of the 2015 Dietary Guidelines Advisory Committee, *2015, D-1: 125, available at www.health.gov.*

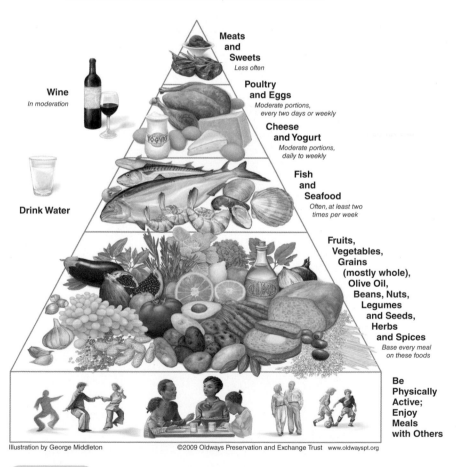

Mediterranean Diet Pyramid
A contemporary approach to delicious, healthy eating

Meats and Sweets
Less often

Wine
In moderation

Poultry and Eggs
Moderate portions, every two days or weekly

Cheese and Yogurt
Moderate portions, daily to weekly

Drink Water

Fish and Seafood
Often, at least two times per week

Fruits, Vegetables, Grains (mostly whole), Olive Oil, Beans, Nuts, Legumes and Seeds, Herbs and Spices
Base every meal on these foods

Be Physically Active; Enjoy Meals with Others

Illustration by George Middleton   ©2009 Oldways Preservation and Exchange Trust   www.oldwayspt.org

TABLE E–1 A Mediterranean Diet Pyramid

TABLE E-7 Ideas for Healthy Mediterranean-Style Meals

As a general rule, fill half your plate with vegetables, a fourth with whole grains, and a quarter with protein foods. Eat fish or seafood 1–2 times a week, and choose baked, steamed, grilled, or poached preparations over fried. One day a week, substitute vegetable proteins for all meats.

Choose this	Instead of this
Breakfast	
Whole fruit pieces; cut fruit or fruit salad without added sugar	Fruit juice; fruit salad with sugars or marshmallows
Low-sugar whole-grain granola (no hydrogenated oils) with nuts and dried fruit; oatmeal (including instant oatmeal) with apples, cinnamon, or a teaspoon of berry or other fruit jam	Commercial high-sugar granola with hydrogenated oils; refined, sugar-sweetened, ready-to-eat cereal
Mediterranean protein foods (peanut butter, hummus, egg, yogurt); turkey, chicken, or soy breakfast sausages	Sausage, bacon, breakfast steak
100% whole-grain toasted bread slice, bagel, or English muffin with hummus, mashed avocado, or nut butter	Refined white toast with butter and jelly
Omelet with sautéed onions, mushrooms, broccoli, or leftover vegetables, or cooked or smoked salmon with a sprinkle of hard cheese, salsa, or olive tapenade	Omelet with sausage or ham and cheese
Smoothies with milk or fortified soy milk, frozen overripe bananas, and berries (a handful of spinach or other greens blends well and adds a fresh flavor and nutrients)	High-sugar commercial smoothies; milkshakes with ice cream, chocolate syrup
Plain yogurt or Greek yogurt with fresh fruit, homemade granola, or a teaspoon of fruit jam or syrup	Commercial sugar-sweetened yogurt
Lunch	
Creative salads with a variety of ingredients: nuts, beans, fish, hard cheese sprinkles, olives, or berries and other fruit	Repetitive, boring lettuce and tomato salads
Canned tuna, sardines, or mackerel (olive oil or water packed) mixed with hummus, lemon juice, and seasonings; add chopped apple or dried cranberries for sweetness	Canned fish salads made with regular mayonnaise and sugar-sweetened pickle relish
Whole-grain crackers, wraps, or breads	Refined flour crackers, wraps, or breads
Whole-grain wheat flour or corn tortillas for burritos, wraps, and quesadillas	Refined flour tortillas
Tapenades, avocado, or hummus spread on sandwiches	Mayonnaise for sandwiches (or choose a mayonnaise made with olive oil)
Broth-based vegetable soups (preferably low-sodium) with whole-grain pasta	Cream-based soups with refined starches
Vegetarian pizza with tomatoes, olives, spinach, artichokes, or other vegetables on whole-grain crust	Sausage, pepperoni, or hamburger pizza on refined flour crust
Supper	
Whole-grain pasta or fortified "extra protein" pasta (½ to 1 c for most adults), with beans or seafood and tomato sauce, garlic, onions, artichokes, frozen peas, or other vegetables to fill in the plate	Refined flour pasta with cream, butter, and cheese sauces
Turkey burgers (made with ground turkey breast and oatmeal); chicken or turkey Italian sausage; serve burgers or sausages with wilted spinach and sliced tomatoes on a whole-grain bun	Ground beef burgers; pork Italian sausage; refined white buns
Prepared salsa for topping potatoes, beans, veggie burgers, rice, or eggs	Creamy, cheesy sauces
Poultry or seafood; limited lean red meat	Frequent use of fatty beef, lamb, or pork

Source: Many of these ideas and more can be found at http://oldwayspt.org/.

Chapter 1

1. M. Sotos-Prieto and coauthors, Association of changes in diet quality with total and cause-specific mortality, *New England Journal of Medicine* 377 (2017): 143–153; Position of the Academy of Nutrition and Dietetics: Total diet approach to healthy eating, *Journal of the Academy of Nutrition and Dietetics* 113 (2013): 307–317 (reaffirmed 2016).
2. U.S. Department of Health and Human Services, *Healthy People 2020* (Washington, D.C.: U.S. Government Printing Office, 2010), available at www.healthypeople.gov.
3. National Center for Health Statistics, *Overview of Midcourse Progress and Health Disparities in Healthy People 2020 Midcourse Review* (Hyattsville, MD: U.S. Government Printing Office, 2016), available at www.cdc.gov/nchs/healthy_people/hp2020/hp2020_midcourse_review.htm; Healthy People 2020, Leading Health Indicators: Nutrition, Physical Activity, and Obesity, May 2014, available at www.healthypeople.gov/sites/default/files/HP2020_LHI_Nut_PhysActiv.pdf.
4. J. B. Kohn, Is dietary fiber considered an essential nutrient? *Journal of the Academy of Nutrition and Dietetics* 116 (2016): 360.
5. P. C. Konturek and coauthors, Malnutrition in hospitals: It was, is now, and must not remain a problem, *Medical Science Monitor* (2015), epub available at doi: 10.12659/MSM.894238.
6. Centers for Disease Control and Prevention, Adults meeting fruit and vegetable intake recommendations—United States, 2013, *Morbidity and Mortality Weekly Report* 64 (2015): 709–713.
7. C. A. Monteiro and coauthors, Ultra-processed products are becoming dominant in the global food system, *Obesity Reviews* 14 (2013): 21–28.
8. T. Fiolet and coauthors, Consumption of ultra-processed foods and cancer risk: Results from NutriNet-Santé prospective cohort, *BMJ* (2018), epub, doi: 10.1136/bmj.k322; E. M. Steele and coauthors, Ultra-processed foods and added sugars in the US diet: Evidence from a nationally representative cross-sectional study, *BMJ Open* (2016), epub, doi: 10.1136/bmjopen-2015-009892.
9. Position of the American Dietetic Association: Functional foods, *Journal of the American Dietetic Association* 113 (2013): 1096–1103 (reaffirmed 2016).
10. Position of the Academy of Nutrition and Dietetics: Total diet approach to healthy eating, 2013 (reaffirmed 2016).
11. S. L. Connor, Think globally, practice locally: Culturally competent dietetics, *Journal of the Academy of Nutrition and Dietetics* 115 (2015): S55.

12. A. Afshin and coauthors, The prospective impact of food pricing on improving dietary consumption: A systematic review and meta-analysis, *PLoS One* (2017), epub available at doi: 10.1371/journal.pone.0172277; L. Hebden and coauthors, You are what you choose to eat: Factors influencing young adults' food selection behaviour, *Journal of Human Nutrition and Dietetics* (2015), epub, doi: 10.1111/jhn.12312.
13. J. A. Wolfson and S. N. Bleich, Is cooking at home associated with better diet quality or weight-loss intention? *Public Health Nutrition* 18 (2015): 1397–1406.
14. A. Afshin and coauthors, The prospective impact of food pricing on improving dietary consumption, 2017; K. Ball and coauthors, Influence of price discounts and skill-building strategies on purchase and consumption of healthy food and beverages: Outcomes of the Supermarket Healthy Eating for Life randomized controlled trial, *American Journal of Clinical Nutrition* 101 (2015): 1055–1064.
15. E. Robinson and coauthors, What everyone else is eating: A systematic review and meta-analysis of the effect of informational eating norms on eating behavior, *Journal of the Academy of Nutrition and Dietetics* 114 (2014): 414–429.
16. International Food Information Council Foundation, 2017 Food and Health Survey: "A Healthy Perspective: Understanding American Food Values" (May 2017), available at www.foodinsight.org/2017-food-and-health-survey.
17. B. Liebman, Stacking the deck? How industry funding can influence science and create confusion, *Nutrition Action* (March 2017): 3–5; B. Liebman, What's the catch? Why the latest study is rarely the final answer, *Nutrition Action Health Letter* (April 2014): 1, 3.
18. S. B. Soumerai and coauthors, How do you know which health care effectiveness research you can trust? A guide to study design for the perplexed, *Preventing Chronic Disease* 2 (2015), epub, doi: http://dx.doi.org/10.5888/pcd12.150187.
19. M. C. Nisbet and D. Fahy, The need for knowledge-based journalism in politicized science debates, *Annals of the American Academy of Political and Social Science* (2015): 223–234.
20. National Center for Health Statistics, National Health and Nutrition Examination Survey (NHANES), *What We Eat in America*, available at www.cdc.gov/nchs/nhanes/wweia.htm.
21. Practice paper of the Academy of Nutrition and Dietetics, Selecting nutrient-dense foods for good health, *Journal of the Academy of Nutrition and Dietetics* 116 (2016): 1473–1479.

22. J. Di Noia, Defining powerhouse fruits and vegetables: A nutrient density approach, *Preventing Chronic Disease* 11 (2014), epub, doi: http://dx.doi.org/10.5888/pcd11.130390.
23. U.S. Department of Health and Human Services and U.S. Department of Agriculture, *2015–2020 Dietary Guidelines for Americans*, 8th edition (2015), available at health.gov/dietaryguidelines/2015/guidelines.

Controversy 1

1. Practice Paper of the Academy of Nutrition and Dietetics: Social media and the dietetics practitioner: Opportunities, challenges and best practices, *Journal of the Academy of Nutrition and Dietetics* 116 (2016): 1825–1835.
2. L. McKeever and coauthors, Demystifying the search button: A comprehensive PubMed search strategy for performing an exhaustive literature review, *Journal of Parenteral and Enteral Nutrition* 39 (2015): 622–635.
3. D. M. Eisenberg and J. D. Burgess, Nutrition education in an era of global obesity and diabetes: Thinking outside the box, *Academic Medicine* 90 (2015): 854–860.
4. Academy of Nutrition and Dietetics, Definition of terms list (2017), available at eatrightpro.org/~/media/eatrightpro%20files/practice/scope%20standards%20of%20practice/academydefinitionoftermslist.ashx; from Position of the Academy of Nutrition and Dietetics, Dietitians of Canada, and the American College of Sports Medicine: Nutrition and athletic performance, *Journal of the Academy of Nutrition and Dietetics* 116 (2016): 501–528.
5. D. Rogers and coauthors, Distinctions in entry-level Registered Dietetic Nutritionist, and Nutrition and Dietetics Technicians, Registered, practice: Further results from the 2015 Commission on Dietetic Registration entry-level dietetics practice audit, *Journal of the Academy of Nutrition and Dietetics* 116 (2016): 1685–1696.

Chapter 2

1. Standing Committee on the Scientific Evaluation of Dietary Reference Intakes, Food and Nutrition Board, Institute of Medicine, *Dietary Reference Intakes: Applications in Dietary Assessment* (Washington, D.C.: National Academies Press, 2000), pp. 5–7.
2. U.S. Department of Agriculture and U.S. Department of Health and Human Services, *Scientific Report of the 2015 Dietary Guidelines Advisory Committee* (2015), C:15, available at https://health.gov/dietaryguidelines/2015-scientific-report/.

3. Food and Drug Administration, Food labeling: Revision of the nutrition and supplement facts labels (Docket No. FDA–2012–N–1210), *Federal Register* 79 (2014): 11880–11987.

4. U.S. Department of Health and Human Services and U.S. Department of Agriculture, *Dietary Guidelines for Americans 2015–2020*, 8th edition (2015), available at health.gov/dietaryguidelines /2015/guidelines.

5. M. M. Wilson, J. Reedy, and S. M. Krebs-Smith, American diet quality: Where it is, where it is heading, and what it could be, *Journal of the Academy of Nutrition and Dietetics* 116 (2016): 302–310.

6. 2018 Physical Activity Guidelines Advisory Committee, *2018 Physical Activity Guidelines Advisory Committee Scientific Report* (Washington, DC: U.S. Department of Health and Human Services, 2018), available at https://health.gov /paguidelines/second-edition/report/pdf/PAG _Advisory_Committee_Report.pdf.

7. E. M. Steele and coauthors, Ultra-processed foods and added sugars in the US diet: Evidence from a nationally representative cross-sectional study, *BMJ Open* (2016), epub, doi: 10.1136 /bmjopen-2015-009892; M. Poti and coauthors, Is the degree of food processing and convenience linked with the nutritional quality of foods purchased by US households?, *American Journal of Clinical Nutrition* 101 (2015): 1251–1262.

8. U.S. Department of Agriculture and U.S. Department of Health and Human Services, *Scientific Report of the 2015 Dietary Guidelines Advisory Committee* (2015): E-5:4; S. J. Nielsen and coauthors, Calories consumed from alcoholic beverages by U.S. adults, 2007–2010 (*NCHS Data Brief* 110) (Hyattsville, MD: National Center for Health Statistics, November 2012), available at www.cdc.gov/nchs/data/databriefs/db110.htm.

9. USDA, ChooseMyPlate.gov, updated April 2017.

10. Food and Drug Administration, Changes to the Nutrition Facts label, 2017, available at www.fda.gov/Food/GuidanceRegulation /GuidanceDocumentsRegulatoryInformation /LabelingNutrition/ucm385663.htm#dates.

11. S. S. Sanjari, S. Jahn, and Y. Boztug, Dual-process theory and consumer response to front-of-package nutrition label formats, *Nutrition Reviews* 75 (2018): 871–882; M. S. Edge and coauthors, The impact of variation in a fact-based front-of-package nutrition labeling system on consumer comprehension, *Journal of the Academy of Nutrition and Dietetics* 114 (2014): 843–854.

12. Grocery Manufacturers Association, Facts Up Front front-of-pack labeling initiative, 2017, available at www.gmaonline.org/issues-policy /health-nutrition/facts-up-front-front-of-pack -labeling-initiative.

Consumer's Guide 2

1. D. Benton, Portion size: What we know and what we need to know, *Critical Reviews in Food Science and Nutrition* 55 (2015): 988–1004.

2. A. Tiwari and coauthors, Cooking at home: A strategy to comply with U.S. Dietary Guidelines at no extra cost, *American Journal of Preventive Medicine* 52 (2017): 616–624.

Controversy 2

1. B. Shitt-Hale and coauthors, The beneficial effects of berries on cognition, motor behavior and neuronal function in ageing, *British Journal of Nutrition* 114 (2015): 1542–1549.

2. X. Jiang and coauthors, Increased consumption of fruit and vegetables is related to a reduced risk of cognitive impairment and dementia: Meta-analysis, *Frontiers in Aging Neuroscience* (2017), epub, doi: 10.3389/fnagi.2017.00018.

3. J. L. Bowtell and coauthors, Enhanced task-related brain activation and resting perfusion in healthy older adults after chronic blueberry supplementation, *Applied Physiology, Nutrition, and Metabolism* 42 (2017): 773–779.

4. A. L. Macready and coauthors, Flavonoid-rich fruit and vegetables improve microvascular reactivity and inflammatory status in men at risk of cardiovascular disease—FLAVURS: A randomized controlled trial, *American Journal of Clinical Nutrition* 99 (2014): 479–489.

5. G. Annuzzi and coauthors, Diets naturally rich in polyphenols improve fasting and post-prandial dyslipidemia and reduce oxidative stress: A randomized controlled trial, *American Journal of Clinical Nutrition* 99 (2014): 463–471.

6. D. A. Steinhaus and coauthors, Chocolate intake and incidence of heart failure: Findings from the Cohort of Swedish Men, *American Heart Journal* 183 (2017): 18–23; S. Kwok and coauthors, Habitual chocolate consumption and risk of cardiovascular disease among health men and women, *Heart* 101 (2015): 1279–1287; C. Matsumoto and coauthors, Chocolate consumption and risk of diabetes mellitus in the Physicians' Health Study, *American Journal of Clinical Nutrition* 101 (2015): 362–367; D. Esser and coauthors, Dark chocolate consumption improves leukocyte adhesion factors and vascular function in overweight men, *FASEB Journal* 28 (2014): 1466–1473.

7. D. M. Delman and coauthors, Effects of flaxseed lignan secoisolariciresinol diglucosideon preneoplastic biomarkers of cancer progression in a model of simultaneous breast and ovarian cancer development, *Nutrition and Cancer* 67 (2015): 857–864; S. H. Sawant and S. L. Bodhankar, Flax lignan concentrate reverses alterations in blood pressure, left ventricular functions, lipid profile and antioxidant status in DOCA-salt induced renal hypertension in rats, *Renal Failure* 38 (2016): 411–423.

8. A. Sorice and coauthors, Differential response of two human breast cancer cell lines to the phenolic extract from flaxseed oil, *Molecules* (2016), epub, doi:10.3390/molecules21030319.

9. J. K. Mason and L. U. Thompson, Flaxseed and its lignan and oil components: Can they play a role in reducing the risk of and improving the treatment of breast cancer? *Applied Physiology, Nutrition, and Metabolism* 39 (2014): 663–678.

10. M. Atkin, D. Laight, and M. H. Cummings, The effects of garlic extract upon endothelial function, vascular inflammation, oxidative stress and insulin resistance in adults with type 2 diabetes at high cardiovascular risk: A pilot double blind randomized placebo controlled trial, *Journal of Diabetes and Its Complications* 30 (2016): 723–727.

11. Y. X. Zhang and coauthors, Trends in overweight and obesity among rural children and adolescents from 1985 to 2014 in Shandong, China, *European Journal of Preventive Cardiology* 23 (2016): 1314–1320; P. Gordon-Larsen, H. Wang, and B. M. Popkin, Overweight dynamics in Chinese children and adults, *Obesity Reviews* 15 (2014): 37–48.

12. Z. Yan and coauthors, Association between consumption of soy and risk of cardiovascular disease: A meta-analysis of observational studies, *European Journal of Preventive Cardiology* 24 (2017): 735–747.

13. T. Chalvon-Demersay and coauthors, A systematic review of the effects of plant compared with animal protein sources on features of metabolic syndrome, *Journal of Nutrition* 147 (2017): 281–292; H. Gylling and coauthors, Plant sterols and plant stanols in the management of dyslipidaemia and prevention of cardiovascular disease, *Atherosclerosis* 232 (2014): 346–360.

14. G. L. Arellano-Martinez and coauthors, Soya protein stimulates bile acid excretion by the liver and intestine through direct and indirect pathways influenced by the presence of dietary cholesterol, *British Journal of Nutrition* 111 (2014): 2059–2066.

15. X. Guo and coauthors, Long-term soy consumption and tumor tissue MicroRNA and gene expression in triple-negative breast cancer, *Cancer* 15 (2016): 2544–2551; M. Messina, Soy foods, isoflavones, and the health of postmenopausal women, *American Journal of Clinical Nutrition* 100 (2014): 423S–430S.

16. M. Chen and coauthors, Association between soy isoflavone intake and breast cancer risk for pre- and post-menopausal women: A meta-analysis of epidemiological studies, *PLoS One* 9 (2014), epub, doi:10.1371/journal. pone.0089288.

17. A. Uifalean and coauthors, Soy isoflavones and breast cancer cell lines: Molecular mechanisms and future perspectives, *Molecules* (2016), epub, doi:10.3390/molecules21010013.

18. L. H. Kushi and coauthors, American Cancer Society guidelines on nutrition and physical activity for cancer prevention: Reducing the risk of cancer with healthy food choices and physical activity, *CA: A Cancer Journal for Clinicians* 62 (2012): 30–67.

19. L. G. Zhao and coauthors, Green tea consumption and cause-specific mortality: Results from two prospective cohort studies in China, *Journal of Epidemiology* 27 (2017): 36–41.

20. G. Myers and coauthors, Tea and flavonoid intake predict osteoporotic fracture risk in elderly Australian women: A prospective study, *American Journal of Clinical Nutrition* 102 (2015): 958–965.

21. W. E. Ek and coauthors, Tea and *coffee consumption in relation to DNA methylation in four European cohorts, Human Molecular Genetics* (2017), epub, doi: 10.1093/hmg/ddx194.

F

22. Zhao and coauthors, Green tea consumption and cause-specific mortality, 2017.

23. J. Yarmolinsky, G. Gon, and P. Edwards, Effect of tea on blood pressure for secondary prevention of cardiovascular disease: A systematic review and meta-analysis of randomized controlled trials, *Nutrition Reviews* 73 (2015): 236–246; S. Khalesi and coauthors, Green tea catechins and blood pressure: A systematic review and meta-analysis of randomised controlled trials, *European Journal of Nutrition* 53 (2014): 1299–1311.

24. C. S. Yang and H. Wang, Cancer preventive activities of tea catechins, *Molecules* (2016), epub, doi:10.3390/molecules21121679.

25. W. Dekant and coauthors, Safety assessment of green tea based beverages and dried green tea extracts as nutritional supplements, *Toxicology Letter* (2017), epub, doi: 10.1016/j.toxlet.2017.06.008.

26. I. Fernandes and coauthors, Wine flavonoids in health and disease prevention, *Molecules* (2017), epub, doi:10.3390/molecules22020292.

27. K. Palluf and coauthors, Resveratrol and lifespan in model organisms, *Current Medicinal Chemistry* 23 (2016): 4639–4680.

28. M. Fernandez and coauthors, Yogurt and cardiometabolic diseases: A critical review of potential mechanisms, *Advances in Nutrition* 8 (2017): 812–829; R. Pei and coauthors, Evidence for the effects of yogurt on gut health and obesity, *Critical Reviews in Food Science and Nutrition* 57 (2017): 1569–1583.

29. T. Bohn, Dietary factors affecting polyphenol bioavailability, *Nutrition Reviews* 72 (2014): 429–452.

30. A. Soare and coauthors, Multiple dietary supplements do not affect metabolic and cardiovascular health, *Aging* 6 (2014): 149–157.

31. S. F. Nabavi and coauthors, Cranberry for urinary tract infection: From bench to bedside, *Current Topics in Medicinal Chemistry* 17 (2017): 331–339.

Chapter 3

1. R. Søberg and coauthors, Fgf21 is a sugar-induced hormone associated with sweet intake and preference in humans, *Cell Metabolism* 25 (2017): 1045–1053; J. A. Mennella, N. K. Bobowski, and D. R. Reed, The development of sweet taste: From biology to hedonics, *Reviews in Endocrine and Metabolic Disorders* 17 (2016): 171–178.

2. R. Shamir and S. M. Donovan, Introduction to the Second Global Summit on the Health Effects of Yogurt, *Nutrition Reviews* 73 (2015): 1–3; A. Kuwahara, Contributions of colonic short-chain fatty acid receptors in energy homeostasis, *Frontiers in Endocrinology* 5 (2014), epub, doi: 10.3389/fendo.2014.00144.

3. K. Tuohy and D. Del Rio, eds., *Diet-microbe interactions in the gut* (San Diego, CA: Academic Press, 2014).

4. S. V. Lynch and O. Pedersen, The human intestinal microbiome in health and disease, *New England Journal of Medicine* 375 (2016): 2369–2379; D. S. Spasova and C. D. Surh, Blowing on embers: Commensal microbiota and our immune system, *Frontiers in Immunology* 5 (2014): 1–20.

5. J. Bienenstock, W. Kunze, and P. Forsythe, Microbiota and the gut-brain axis, *Nutrition Reviews* 73 (2015): 28–31; D. S. Spasova and C. D. Surh, Blowing on embers: Commensal microbiota and our immune system, *Frontiers in Immunology* 5 (2014), epub, doi: 10.3389/fimmu.2014.00318.

6. M. Fernandez and coauthors, Yogurt and cardiometabolic diseases: A critical review of potential mechanisms, *Advances in Nutrition* 8 (2017): 812–829; C. M. Ferreira and coauthors, The central role of the gut microbiota in chronic inflammatory diseases, *Journal of Immunology Research* (2014), epub, doi: 10.1155/2014/689492; Y. J. Lee and K. S. Park, Irritable bowel syndrome: Emerging paradigm in pathophysiology, *World Journal of Gastroenterology* 20 (2014): 2456–2469; H. Zeng, D. L. Lazarova, and M. Bordonaro, Mechanisms linking dietary fiber, gut microbiota and colon cancer prevention, *World Journal of Gastrointestinal Oncology* 6 (2014): 41–51; I. Moreno-Indias and coauthors, Impact of the gut microbiota on the development of obesity and type 2 diabetes mellitus, *Frontiers in Microbiology* 5 (2014), epub, doi: 10.3389/fmicb.2014.00190.

7. A. E. Mikolajczyk and coauthors, Assessment of tandem measurements of pH and total gut transit time in healthy volunteers, *Clinical and Translational Gastroenterology* (2015), epub, doi: 10.1038/ctg.2015.22.

8. L. Wei and coauthors, Acid suppression medications and bacterial gastroenteritis: A population-based cohort study, *British Journal of Pharmacology* (2017), epub, doi: 10.1111.bcp.13205.

9. S. Jain and S. Dhingra, Pathology of esophageal cancer and Barrett's esophagus, *Annals of Cardiothoracic Surgery* 6 (2017): 99–109.

10. A. F. Peery and coauthors, Risk factors for hemorrhoids on screening colonoscopy, *PLoS One* (2015), epub, doi:10.1371/journal.pone.0139100.

11. A. C. Ford, B. E. Lacy, and N. J. Talley, Irritable bowel syndrome, *New England Journal of Medicine* (2017): 2566–2578; Y. J. Lee and K. S. Park, Irritable bowel syndrome: Emerging paradigm in pathophysiology, *World Journal of Gastroenterology* 20 (2014): 2456–2469.

12. 12 M. Simrén and coauthors, Management of the multiple symptoms of irritable bowel syndrome, *Lancet Gastroenterology and Hepatology* 2 (2017): 112–122.

Controversy 3

1. Centers for Disease Control and Prevention, Alcohol and public health, Data and maps, 2017, available at www.cdc.gov/alcohol/data-stats.htm; M. Stahre and coauthors, Contribution of excessive alcohol consumption to deaths and years of potential life lost in the United States, *Preventing Chronic Disease* 11 (2014), doi: http://dx.doi.org/10.5888/pcd11.130293.

2. Centers for Disease Control and Prevention, Binge drinking (2017), Fact Sheet, available at www.cdc.gov/alcohol/fact-sheets/binge-drinking.htm.

3. Centers for Disease Control and Prevention, Binge drinking, 2017.

4. *Dietary Guidelines for Americans 2010*, reaffirmed in 2015, www.dietaryguidelines.gov.

5. B. F. Grant and coauthors, Prevalence of 12-month alcohol use, high-risk drinking, and DSM-IV alcohol use disorder in the United States, 2001–2002 to 2012–2013: Results from the National Epidemiologic Survey on Alcohol and Related Conditions, *JAMA Psychiatry* 74 (2017): 911–923.

6. K. L. Hess and coauthors, Binge drinking and risky sexual behavior among HIV-negative and unknown HIV status men who have sex with men, 20 US cities, *Alcohol and Drug Dependence* 147 (2015): 46–52; X. Zhang and coauthors, Changes in density of on-premises alcohol outlets and impact on violent crime, Atlanta, Georgia, 1997–2007, *Preventing Chronic Disease* 12 (2015), available at www.cdc.gov/pcd/issues/2015/14_0317.htm.

7. A. Voskoboinik and coauthors, Alcohol and atrial fibrillation: A sobering review, *Journal of the American College of Cardiology* 68 (2016): 2567–2576.

8. J. H. O'Keefe and coauthors, Alcohol and cardiovascular health: The dose makes the poison . . . or the remedy, *Mayo Clinic Proceedings* 89 (2014): 382–393.

9. M. V. Holmes and coauthors, Association between alcohol and cardiovascular disease: Mendelian randomisation analysis based on individual participant data, *British Medical Journal* 349 (2014), epub, doi: 10.1136/bmj.g4164.

10. O'Keefe and coauthors, Alcohol and cardiovascular health, 2014.

11. L. C. Del Gobbo and coauthors, Contribution of major lifestyle risk factors for incident heart failure in older adults: The Cardiovascular Health Study, *JACC: Heart Failure* 3 (2015): 520–528; [Refuting evidence] A. Gonçalves and coauthors, Relationship between alcohol consumption and cardiac structure and function in the elderly, *Epidemiology* (2015), epub, doi: 10.1161/circimaging.114.002846.

12. I. Fernandes and coauthors, Wine flavonoids in health and disease prevention, *Molecules* (2017), epub, doi: 10.3390/molecules22020292.

13. N. K. LoConte and coauthors, Alcohol and Cancer: A statement of the American Society of Clinical Oncology, *Journal of Clinical Oncology* 36 (2018): 83–93; World Cancer Research Fund/American Institute for Cancer Research, *Diet, Nutrition, Physical Activity, and Breast Cancer*, Continuous Update Project Report, 2017, available at www.aicr.org/continuous-update-project/reports/breast-cancer-report-2017.pdf; K. D. Shield, I. Soerjomataram, and J. Rehm, Alcohol use and breast cancer: A critical review, *Alcohol, Clinical and Experimental Research* 40 (2016): 1166–1181; H. Yen and coauthors, Alcohol intake and risk of nonmelanoma skin cancer:

A systematic review and dose-response meta-analysis, *British Journal of Dermatology* 177 (2017): 696–707.

14. A. Russo and coauthors, CYP4F2 repression and a modified alpha-tocopherol (vitamin E) metabolism are two independent consequences of ethanol toxicity in human hepatocytes, *Toxicology in Vitro* 40 (2017): 124–133; O. Ogunsakin and coauthors, Chronic ethanol exposure effects on vitamin D levels among subjects with alcohol use disorder, *Environmental Health Insights* 10 (2016): 191–199; V. S. Subramanian, P. Srinivasan, and H. M. Said, Uptake of ascorbic acid by pancreatic acinar cells is negatively impacted by chronic alcohol exposure, *American Journal of Physiology–Cell Physiology* 311 (2016): C129–C135.

15. B. F. Palmer and D. J. Clegg, Electrolyte disturbances in patients with chronic alcohol-use disorder, *New England Journal of Medicine* 377 (2017): 1368–1377.

16. L. C. Vedder and coauthors, Interactions between chronic ethanol consumption and thiamine deficiency on neural plasticity, spatial memory, and cognitive flexibility, *Alcoholism, Clinical and Experimental Research* 39 (2015): 2143–2153.

Chapter 4

1. M. M. Adeva-Andany and coauthors, Glycogen metabolism in humans, *BBA (Biochimica et Biophysica Acta) Clinical* (2016), epub, doi: 10.1016/j.bbacli.2016.02.001.

2. Position of the Academy of Nutrition and Dietetics: Health implications of dietary fiber, *Journal of the Academy of Nutrition and Dietetics* 115 (2015): 1861–1870; G. Tang and coauthors, Meta-analysis of the association between whole grain intake and coronary heart disease risk, *American Journal of Cardiology* 115 (2015): 625–629; P. Vitaglione and coauthors, Whole-grain wheat consumption reduces inflammation in a randomized controlled trial on overweight and obese subjects with unhealthy dietary and lifestyle behaviors: Role of polyphenols bound to cereal dietary fiber, *American Journal of Clinical Nutrition* 101 (2015): 251–261.

3. J. W. McRorie, Evidence-based approach to fiber supplements and clinically meaningful health benefits, Part I, *Nutrition Today* 50 (2015): 82–89; J. W. McRorie, Evidence-based approach to fiber supplements and clinically meaningful health benefits, Part II, *Nutrition Today* 50 (2015): 90–97.

4. J. M. Pickard and coauthors, Gut microbiota: Role in pathogen colonization, immune responses, and inflammatory disease, *Immunology Reviews* 279 (2017): 70–89; H. Zeng, D. L. Lazarova, and M. Bordonaro, Mechanisms linking dietary fiber, gut microbiota and colon cancer prevention, *World Journal of Gastrointestinal Oncology* 6 (2014): 41–51.

5. R. Mica and coauthors, Etiologic effects and optimal intakes of foods and nutrients for risk of cardiovascular diseases and diabetes: Systematic reviews and meta-analyses from the Nutrition and Chronic Diseases Expert Group (NutriCoDE), *PLoS ONE* (2017), epub, doi.org/10.1371/journal.pone; Position of the Academy of Nutrition and Dietetics: Health implications of dietary fiber, 2015.

6. A. Whitehead and coauthors, Cholesterol-lowering effects of oat β-glucan: A meta-analysis of randomized controlled trials, *American Journal of Clinical Nutrition* 100 (2014): 114–121.

7. C. J. Rebello, C. E. O'Neil, and F. L. Greenway, Dietary fiber and satiety: The effects of oats on satiety, *Nutrition Reviews* 74 (2016): 131–147.

8. G. Marion and coauthors, Effects of ready-to-eat-cereals on key nutritional and health outcomes: A systematic review, *PLoS One* (2016), epub, doi: 10.1371/journal.pone.0164931.

9. S. M. Vanegas and coauthors, Substituting whole grains for refined grains in a 6-wk randomized trial has a modest effect on gut microbiota and immune and inflammatory markers of healthy adults, *American Journal of Clinical Nutrition* 105 (2017): 635–650.

10. M. Rezapour, A. Ali, and N. Stollman, Diverticular disease: An update on pathogenesis and management, *Gut and Liver* (2017), epub, doi.org/10.5009/gnl16552.

11. Centers for Disease Control and Prevention, Colon Cancer Statistics, 2017, available at www.cdc.gov/cancer/colorectal/statistics/index.htm.

12. World Cancer Research Fund and the American Institute for Cancer Research, Continuous Update Project report: Diet, nutrition, physical activity and colorectal cancer, 2017, available at wcrf.org/colorectal-cancer-2017; B. Moen and coauthors, Effect of dietary fibers on cecal microbiota and intestinal tumorigenesis in azoxymethane treated a/j min/+ mice, *PLoS ONE* (2016), epub, doi: 10.1371/ journal.pone.0155402; S. L. Navarro and coauthors, The interaction between dietary fiber and fat and risk of colorectal cancer in the women's health initiative, *Nutrients* (2016), epub, doi: 10.3390/nu8120779.

13. Pickard and coauthors, Gut microbiota, 2017; Zeng, Lazarova, and Bordonaro, Mechanisms linking dietary fiber, gut microbiota and colon cancer prevention, 2014.

14. A. L. Carreiro and coauthors, The macronutrients, appetite, and energy intake, *Annual Review of Nutrition* 36 (2016): 73–103; C. S. Byrne and coauthors, The role of short chain fatty acids in appetite regulation and energy homeostasis, *International Journal of Obesity* 39 (2015): 1331–1338.

15. M. K. Hoy and J. D. Goldman, Fiber intake of the U.S. population: What we eat in America, NHANES 2009–2010 (Food Surveys Research Group Dietary Data Brief 12), September 2014, available at www.ars.usda.gov/SP2UserFiles/Place/80400530/pdf/DBrief/12_fiber_intake_0910.pdf.

16. A. M. Albertson and coauthors, Whole grain consumption trends and associations with body weight measures in the United States: Results from the cross sectional National Health and Nutrition Examination Survey 2001–2012, *Nutrition Journal* (2016), epub, doi: 10.1186/s12937-016-0126-4.

17. H. Wu and coauthors, Whole grain intake and mortality: Two large prospective studies in U.S. men and women, *JAMA Internal Medicine* 175 (2015): 373–384.

18. M. J. Keenan and coauthors, Role of resistant starch in improving gut health, adiposity, and insulin resistance, *Advances in Nutrition* 6 (2015): 198–205.

19. National Institutes of Health, Genetics Home Reference, Lactose intolerance (2017), available at https://ghr.nlm.nih.gov/condition/lactose-intolerance#statistics.

20. D. A. Saviano, Lactose digestion from yogurt: Mechanism and relevance, *American Journal of Clinical Nutrition* 99 (2014): 1251S–1255S.

21. S. J. Koppel and R. H. Swerdlow, Neuroketotherapeutics: A modern review of a century-old therapy, *Neurochemistry International* (2017), epub ahead of print, doi: 10.1016/j.neuint.2017.05.019; E. H. Kossoff and coauthors, Diet redux: Outcomes from reattempting dietary therapy for epilepsy, *Journal of Child Neurology* 31 (2016): 1052–1056; A. Lin and coauthors, Complications during ketogenic diet initiation: Prevalence, treatment, and influence on seizure outcomes, *Pediatric Neurology* 68 (2017): 35–39; P. J. Simm and coauthors, The effect of the ketogenic diet on the developing skeleton, *Epilepsy Research* 136 (2017): 62–66.

22. Standing Committee on the Scientific Evaluation of *Dietary Reference Intakes*, *Dietary Reference Intakes for Energy, Carbohydrate, Fiber, Fat, Fatty Acids, Cholesterol, Protein, and Amino Acids* (National Academies Press: Washington, D.C., 2002/2005), pp. 265–338.

23. R. Rosset, A. Surowska, and L. Tappy, Pathogenesis of cardiovascular and metabolic diseases: Are fructose-containing sugars more involved than other dietary calories?, *Current Hypertension Reports* (2016), epub, doi: 10.1007/s11906-016-0652-7.

24. H. Meng and coauthors, Effect of macronutrients and fiber on postprandial glycemic responses and meal glycemic index and glycemic load value determinations, *American Journal of Clinical Nutrition* 105 (2017): 842–853.

25. N. R. Matthan and coauthors, Estimating the reliability of glycemic index values and potential sources of methodological and biological variability, *American Journal of Clinical Nutrition* 104 (2016): 1004–1013; D. Zevi and coauthors, Personalized nutrition by prediction of glycemic responses, *Cell* 163 (2015): 1079–1094.

26. S. Sieri and V. Krogh, Dietary glycemic index, glycemic load and cancer: An overview of the literature, *Nutrition, Metabolism, and Cardiac Diseases* 27 (2017): 18–31; R. de la Iglasia and coauthors, Review of dietary strategies implicated in the prevention and treatment of metabolic syndrome, *International Journal of Molecular Sciences* (2016), epub, doi: 10.3390/ijms17111877.

27. A. B. Evert and coauthors, Nutrition therapy recommendations for management of adults with diabetes, *Diabetes Care* 37 (2014): S120–S143.

28. F. M. Sacks and coauthors, Effects of high vs low glycemic index of dietary carbohydrate on cardiovascular disease risk, *Journal of the American Medical Association* 312 (2014): 2531–2541.

29. M. J. Franz and coauthors, Academy of Nutrition and Dietetics Nutrition practice guideline for type 1 and type 2 diabetes in adults: Systematic review of evidence for medical nutrition therapy effectiveness and recommendations for integration into the nutrition care process, *Journal of the Academy of Nutrition and Dietetics* 117 (2017): 1659–1679.

30. A. E. Thompson, Hypoglycemia, *Journal of the American Medical Association* 313 (2015): 1284.

31. A. C. Godswill, Sugar alcohols: Chemistry, production, health concerns and nutritional importance of mannitol, sorbitol, xylitol, and erythritol, *International Journal of Advanced Academic Research* 3 (2017), epub, available at www.ijaar.org/articles/Volume3-Number2/Sciences-Technology-Engineering/ijaar-ste-v3n2-feb17-p2.pdf.

Consumer's Guide 4

1. U.S. Department of Health and Human Services and U.S. Department of Agriculture, 2015–2020 *Dietary Guidelines for Americans*, 8th edition (2015), available at health.gov/dietaryguidelines/2015/guidelines.

Controversy 4

1. World Health Organization, Guideline: *Sugars intake for adults and children* (Geneva: World Health Organization, 2015), available at http://who.int/nutrition/publications/guidelines/sugars_intake/en/; U.S. Department of Health and Human Services and U.S. Department of Agriculture, 2015–2020 *Dietary Guidelines for Americans*, 8th edition (2015), available at http://health.gov/dietaryguidelines/2015/guidelines/.

2. U. Ladabaum and coauthors, Obesity, abdominal obesity, physical activity, and caloric intake in U.S. adults: 1988–2010, *American Journal of Medicine* 127 (2014): 717–727.

3. U.S. Department of Health and Human Services and U.S. Department of Agriculture, 2015–2020 Dietary Guidelines for Americans, 8th edition (2015), available at http://health.gov/dietaryguidelines/2015/guidelines/.

4. S. A. Bowman and coauthors, *Food patterns equivalents intakes by Americans: What we eat in America*, NHANES 2003–2004 and 2013–2014, *Food Surveys Research Group Dietary Data Brief* 17, (2017), available at www.ars.usda.gov./ARSUserFiles/80400530/pdf/DBrief/17_Food_Patterns_Equivalents_0304_1314.pdf.

5. M. Luger and coauthors, Sugar-sweetened beverages and weight gain in children and adults: A systematic review from 2013 to 2015 and a comparison with previous studies, *Obesity Facts* 10 (2017): 647–693; K. L. Stanhope, Sugar consumption, metabolic disease and obesity: The state of the controversy, *Critical Reviews in Clinical Laboratory Sciences* (2015), epub, doi: 10.3109/10408363.2015.1084990.

6. N. I. Toufel-Shone and coauthors, Demographic characteristics and food choices of participants in the Special Diabetes Program for American Indians Diabetes Prevention Demonstration Project, *Ethnicity and Health* 20 (2014): 327–340.

7. A. Kolderup and B. Svihus, Fructose metabolism and relation to atherosclerosis, type 2 diabetes, and obesity, *Journal of Nutrition and Metabolism* (2015), epub, doi: 10.1155/2015/823081.

8. K. L. Stanhope, Sugar consumption, metabolic disease and obesity, 2015.

9. U.S. Department of Agriculture, *2015–2020 Dietary Guidelines for Americans*, 2015.

10. M. B. Vos and coauthors, Added sugars and cardiovascular disease risk in children: A scientific statement from the American Heart Association, *Circulation* 135 (2017): e1017–31034.

11. A. H. Malik and coauthors, Impact of sugar-sweetened beverages on blood pressure, *American Journal of Cardiology* 113 (2014): 1574–1580; K. P. Kell and coauthors, Added sugars in the diet are positively associated with diastolic blood pressure and triglycerides in children, *American Journal of Clinical Nutrition* 100 (2014): 46–52.

12. M. Siervo and coauthors, Sugar consumption and global prevalence of obesity and hypertension: An ecological analysis, *Public Health Nutrition* 17 (2014): 587–596; L. A. Te Morenga and coauthors, Dietary sugars and cardiometabolic risk: Systematic review and meta-analyses of randomized controlled trials of the effects on blood pressure and lipids, *American Journal of Clinical Nutrition* 100 (2014): 65–79.

13. K. P. Kell and coauthors, Added sugars in the diet are positively associated with diastolic blood pressure and triglycerides in children, *American Journal of Clinical Nutrition* 100 (2014): 46–52.

14. M. B. Vos and coauthors, Added sugars and cardiovascular disease risk in children: A scientific statement from the American Heart Association, 2017.

15. V. S. Malik and F. B. Hu, Fructose and cardiometabolic health: What the evidence from sugar-sweetened beverages tells us, *Journal of the American College of Cardiology* 66 (2015): 1615–1614.

16. G. A. Bray and B. M. Popkin, Dietary sugar and body weight: Have we reached a crisis in the epidemic of obesity and diabetes? *Diabetes Care* 37 (2014): 950–956.

17. M. Dehghan and coauthors, Associations of fats and carbohydrate intake with cardiovascular disease and mortality in 18 countries from five continents (PURE): a prospective cohort study, *Lancet* 390 (2017): 2050–2062; K. L. Stanhope, Sugar consumption, metabolic disease and obesity, 2015.

18. D. Zanchi and coauthors, The impact of gut hormones on the neural circuit of appetite and satiety: A systematic review, *Neuroscience and Biobehavioral Reviews* 80 (2017): 457–475.

19. A. Kolderup and B. Svihus, Fructose metabolism and relation to atherosclerosis, type 2 diabetes, and obesity, *Journal of Nutrition and Metabolism* (2015), epub, doi.org/10.1155/2015/823081.

20. J. Lowndes and coauthors, The effect of normally consumed amounts of sucrose or high fructose corn syrup on lipid profiles, body composition, and related parameters in overweight/obese subjects, *Nutrients* 6 (2014): 1128–1144.

21. Kolderup and Svihus, Fructose metabolism and relation to atherosclerosis, type 2 diabetes, and obesity, 2015.

22. J. Ma and coauthors, Sugar-sweetened beverage, diet soda, and fatty liver disease in the Framingham Heart Study cohorts, *Journal of Hepatology* 63 (2015): 462–469; R. Jin and M. B. Vos, Fructose and liver function--is this behind nonalcoholic liver disease? *Current Opinion in Clinical Nutrition and Metabolic Care* 18 (2015): 490–495.

23. J. M. Schwartz and coauthors, Effects of dietary fructose restriction on liver fat, de novo lipogenesis, and insulin kinetics in children with obesity, *Gastroenterology* 153 (2017): 743–752; J. M. Schwartz and coauthors, Effect of a high-fructose weight-maintaining diet on lipogenesis and liver fat, *Journal of Clinical Endocrinology and Metabolism* 100 (2015): 2434–2442.

24. M. Vos and coauthors, Added sugars and cardiovascular disease risk in children: A scientific statement from the American Heart Association, *Circulation* 135 (2017): e1017–e1034; J-M. Schwarz, M. Clearfield, and K. Mulligan, Conversion of sugar to fat: Is hepatic de novo lipogenesis leading to metabolic syndrome and associated chronic diseases? *Journal of the American Osteopathic Association* 117 (2017): 520–527; R. Kelishadi, M. Mansourian, and M. Heidari-Beni, Association of fructose consumption and components of metabolic syndrome in human studies: A systematic review and meta-analysis, *Nutrition* 30 (2014): 503–510.

25. K. Stanhope and coauthors, A dose-response study of consuming high fructose corn syrup-sweetened beverages on lipid/lipoprotein risk factors for cardiovascular disease in young adults, *American Journal of Clinical Nutrition* 101 (2015): 1144–1154; A. K. Lee and coauthors, Consumption of less than 10% of total energy from added sugars is associated with increasing HDL in females during adolescence: A longitudinal analysis, *Journal of the American Heart Association* 3 (2014), doi:10.1161/JAHA.113.000615.

26. U.S. Department of Health and Human Services and U.S. Department of Agriculture, *2015–2020 Dietary Guidelines for Americans*, 8th edition (2015), available at http://health.gov/dietaryguidelines/2015/guidelines/.

27. E. M. Steele and coauthors, Ultra-processed foods and added sugars in the US diet: Evidence from a nationally representative cross-sectional study, *BMJ Open* (2016), epub, doi:10.1136/bmjopen-2015-009892.

28. P. M. Wise and coauthors, Reduced dietary intake of simple sugars alters perceived sweet taste

intensity but not perceived pleasantness, *American Journal of Clinical Nutrition* 103 (2016): 50–60.

Chapter 5

1. A. Rodriguez and coauthors, Revisiting the adipocyte: A model for integration of cytokine signaling and the regulation of energy metabolism, *American Journal of Physiology: Endocrinology and Metabolism* (2015), epub, doi: 10.1152/ajpendo.00297.2015.

2. S. Kaviani and J. A. Cooper, Appetite responses to high-fat meals or diets or varying fatty acid composition: A comprehensive review, *European Journal of Clinical Investigation* 71 (2017): 1154–1165; N. V. DiPatrizio and D. Piomelli, Intestinal lipid derived signals that sense dietary fat, *Journal of Clinical Investigation* 125 (2015): 891–898.

3. A. L. Carreiro and coauthors, The macronutrients, appetite, and energy intake, *Annual Review of Nutrition* 36 (2016): 73–103.

4. A. Romano and coauthors, High dietary fat intake influences the activation of specific hindbrain and hypothalamic nuclei by the satiety factor oleoylethanolamide, *Physiology and Behavior* 136 (2014): 55–62; F. A. Duca, Y. Sakar, and M. Covasasa, The modulatory role of high fat feeding on gastrointestinal signals in obesity, *Journal of Nutritional Biochemistry* 24 (2013): 1663–1677.

5. L. Eyres and coauthors, Coconut oil consumption and cardiovascular risk factors in humans, *Nutrition Reviews* 74 (2016): 267–280;Position of the Academy of Nutrition and Dietetics: Dietary fatty acids for healthy adults, *Journal of the Academy of Nutrition and Dietetics* 114 (2014): 136–153.

6. D. S. Mackay and coauthors, Lathosterol-to-cholesterol ratio in serum predicts cholesterol-lowering response to plant sterol consumption in a dual-center, randomized single-blind placebo-controlled trial, *American Journal of Clinical Nutrition* 101 (2015): 432–439; D. A. Taha and coauthors, Lipid-lowering activity of natural and semi-synthetic sterols and stanols, *Journal of Pharmacy and Pharmaceutical Sciences* 18 (2015): 344–367.

7. Centers for Disease Control and Prevention, National Center for Health Statistics, Fast Stats (2017), available at www.cdc.gov/nchs/fastats/deaths.htm.

8. D. Mozaffarian and coauthors, Heart disease and stroke statistics-2016 update: A report from the American Heart Association, *Circulation* 133 (2016): e38–e360.

9. USDA, *What we eat In America*, NHANES 2013-2014, available at www.ars.usda.gov/nea/bhnrc/fsrg.

10. R. Mateo-Gallego and coauthors, Adherence to a Mediterranean diet is associated with the presence and extension of atherosclerotic plaques in middle-aged asymptomatic adults: The Aragon Workers' Health Study, *Journal of Clinical Lipidology* 11 (2017): 1372–1382; M. A. Martinez and M. Bes-Rastrollo, Dietary patterns, Mediterranean diet, and cardiovascular disease, *Current Opinion in Lipidology* 25 (2014): 20–26; I. R. Estruch and coauthors, Primary prevention of cardiovascular disease with a Mediterranean diet, *New England Journal of Medicine* 368 (2013): 1279–1290.

11. M. Guasch-Ferré and coauthors, Nut consumption and risk of cardiovascular disease, *Journal of the American College of Cardiology* 70 (2017): 2519–2532; M. Garcia and coauthors, The effect of the traditional Mediterranean-style diet on metabolic risk factors: A meta-analysis, *Nutrients* (2016), epub, doi: 10.3390/nu8030168; M. L. Bertoia and coauthors, Mediterranean and Dietary Approaches to Stop Hypertension dietary patterns and risk of sudden cardiac death in postmenopausal women, *American Journal of Clinical Nutrition* 99 (2014): 344–351; E. Ros and coauthors, Mediterranean diet and cardiovascular health: Teachings of the PREDIMED study, *Advances in Nutrition* 5 (2014): 330S–336S; H. Gardener and coauthors, Mediterranean diet and carotid atherosclerosis in the Northern Manhattan Study, *Atherosclerosis* 234 (2014): 303–310.

12. S. Dash and coauthors, New insights into the regulation of chylomicron production, *Annual Review of Nutrition* 35 (2015): 265–294.

13. D. Saleheen and coauthors, Association of HDL cholesterol efflux capacity with incident coronary heart disease events: A prospective case-control study, *Lancet. Diabetes and Endocrinology* 3 (2015): 507–513.

14. D. Mozaffarian and coauthors, Heart disease and stroke statistics-2016 update, 2016.

15. R. H. Eckel and coauthors, 2013 AHA/ ACC Guideline on Lifestyle Management to Reduce Cardiovascular Risk: A report of the American College of Cardiology/American Heart Association Task Force on Practice Guidelines, *Journal of the American College of Cardiology* 63 (2014): 2960–2984; D. J. McNamara, Dietary cholesterol, heart disease risk and cognitive dissonance, *Proceedings of the Nutrition Society* 73 (2014): 161–166.

16. R. C. Cristall and coauthors, Impact of egg consumption on cardiovascular risk factors in individuals with type 2 diabetes and at risk for developing diabetes: A systematic review of randomized nutritional intervention studies, *Canadian Journal of Diabetes* 41 (2017): 453–463; J. Diez-Espino and coauthors, Egg consumption and cardiovascular disease according to diabetic status: The PREDIMED study, *Clinical Nutrition* 36 (2017): 1015–1021; D. Mozaffarian, Dietary and policy priorities for cardiovascular disease, diabetes, and obesity: A comprehensive review, *Circulation* 133 (2016): 187–225.

17. U.S. Department of Agriculture and U.S. Department of Health and Human Services, Scientific Report of the 2015 Dietary Guidelines Advisory Committee (2015), p. 52.

18. E. J. Benjamin and coauthors, Heart disease and stroke statistics—2018 update: A report from the American Heart Association, *Circulation* (2018), epub ahead of print, doi: 10.1161/CIR.0000000000000558.

19. E. A. Dennis and P. C. Norris, Eicosanoid storm in infection and inflammation, *Nature Reviews: Immunology* 15 (2015): 511–523.

20. H. Ohnishi and Y. Saito, Eicosapentaenoic acid (EPA) reduces cardiovascular events: Relationship with the EPA/arachidonic acid ratio, *Journal of Atherosclerosis and Thrombosis* 20 (2013): 861–877.

21. Mozaffarian, Dietary and policy priorities for cardiovascular disease, diabetes, and obesity: A comprehensive review, 2016; T. A. Mori, Conference on "Dietary Strategies for the Management of Cardiovascular Risk," Dietary n-3 PUFA and CVD: A review of the evidence, *Proceedings of the Nutrition Society* 73 (2014): 57–64; K. Takada and coauthors, Effects of eicosapentaenoic acid on platelet function in patients taking long-term aspirin following coronary stent implantation, *International Heart Journal* 55 (2014): 228–233; M. van Bilsen and A. Planavila, Fatty acids and cardiac disease: Fuel carrying a message, *Acta Physiologica* 211 (2014): 476–490.

22. J. Veenstra and coauthors, Genome-wide interaction study of omega-3 PUFAS and other fatty acids on inflammatory biomarkers of cardiovascular health in the Framingham heart study, *Nutrients* (2017), epub, doi: 10.3390/nu9080900.

23. W. Lian and coauthors, Fish intake and the risk of brain tumor: A meta-analysis with systematic review, *Journal of Nutrition* (2017), epub, doi: 10.1186/s12937-016-0223-4; M. T. Dinwiddie and coauthors, Omega-3 fatty acid consumption and prostate cancer: A review of exposure measures and results of epidemiological studies, *Journal of the American College of Nutrition* 35 (2016): 452–468.

24. M. Hennebelle and coauthors, Omega-3 polyunsaturated fatty acids and chronic stress-induced modulations of glutamatergic neurotransmission in the hippocampus, *Nutrition Reviews* 72 (2014): 99–112; J. V. Pottala and coauthors, Higher RBC EPA + DHA corresponds with larger total brain and hippocampal volumes: WHIMS–MRI study, *Neurology* 82 (2014): 435–442.

25. U.S. Department of Agriculture and U.S. Department of Health and Human Services, Scientific Report of the 2015 Dietary Guidelines Advisory Committee (2015), p. 31.

26. A. S. Abdelhamid and coauthors, Omega-3 fatty acids for the primary and secondary prevention of cardiovascular disease, *Cochrane Database of Systematic Reviews*, (2018), epub, doi: 10.1002/14651858.CD003177.pub3; E. M. Balk and coauthors, Omega-3 fatty acids and cardiovascular disease: An updated systematic review, AHRQ Publication No. 16-E002-EF, (2016), available at www.ncbi.nlm.nih.gov/books/NBK384547/; D. S. Siscovick and coauthors, Omega-3 polyunsaturated fatty acid (fish oil) supplementation and the prevention of clinical cardiovascular disease: A science advisory from the American Heart Association, *Circulation* 135 (2017): e867–e884.

27. F. M. Sacks and coauthors, Dietary fats and cardiovascular disease: A Presidential

Advisory from the American Heart Association, *Circulation* 136 (2017), epub, doi: 10.1161/CIR.0000000000000510; L. Haibo and coauthors, Plasma *trans*-fatty acids levels and mortality: A cohort study based on 1999–2000 National Health and Nutrition Examination Survey (NHANES), *Lipids in Health and Disease* (2017), epub, doi: 10.1186/s12944-017-0567-6; D. Mozaffarian, Dietary and policy priorities for cardiovascular disease, diabetes, and obesity: A comprehensive review, *Circulation* 133 (2016): 187–225; K. Gebauer and coauthors, Vaccenic acid and *trans*-fatty acid isomers from partially hydrogenated oil both adversely affect LDL cholesterol: A double-blind, randomized controlled trial, *American Journal of Clinical Nutrition* 102 (2015): 1339–1346; R. Ganguly and G. N. Pierce, The toxicity of dietary *trans* fats, *Food and Chemical Toxicology* 78 (2015): 170–176.

28. Q. Yang and coauthors, Plasma *trans*-fatty acid concentrations continue to be associated with serum lipid and lipoprotein concentrations among us adults after reductions in *trans*-fatty acid intake, *Journal of Nutrition* 147 (2017: 896–907.

29. U.S. Food and Drug Administration, Final Determination Regarding Partially Hydrogenated Oils (Removing *Trans* Fat), June 2018, available at www.fda.gov/food/ingredientspackaginglabeling/foodadditivesingredients/ucm449162.htm.

30. A. A. Kadhum and M. N. Shamma, Edible lipids modification processes: A review, *Critical Reviews in Food Science and Nutrition* 57 (2017): 48–58; F. Mohamedshah and J. Ruff, IFT addresses sodium, sugars, and fats for DGAC, *Food Technology*, May 2014, available at www.ift.org.

31. USDA Nutrient Data Laboratory, Release 27.

32. S. Bulotta and coauthors, Beneficial effects of the olive oil phenolic components oleuropein and hydroxytyrosol: Focus on protection against cardiovascular and metabolic diseases, *Journal of Translational Medicine* 12 (2014), doi: 10.1186/ s12967-014-0219-9.

33. H. N. Luu and coauthors, Prospective evaluation of the association of nut/peanut consumption with total and cause-specific mortality, *JAMA Internal Medicine* 175 (2015): 755–766; A. Afshin and coauthors, Consumption of nuts and legumes and risk of incident ischemic heart disease, stroke, and diabetes: A systematic review and meta-analysis, *American Journal of Clinical Nutrition* 100 (2014): 278–288.

Consumer's Guide 5

1. M. R. Simões and coauthors, Chronic mercury exposure impairs the sympathovagal control of the rat heart, *Clinical and Experimental Pharmacology and Physiology* 43 (2016): 1038–1045.

2. Food and Drug Administration and Environmental Protection Agency, Eating fish: What pregnant women and parents should know, 2017, available at www.fda.gov/Food/ResourcesForYou/Consumers/ucm393070.htm.

3. Food and Drug Administration and Environmental Protection Agency, Eating fish: What pregnant women and parents should know, 2017.

4. H. Jiang and coauthors, Comparative study of the nutritional composition and toxic elements of farmed and wild *Chanodichthys mongolicus*, *Chinese Journal of Oceanology and Limnology* 35 (2017): 737–744.

Controversy 5

1. F. M. Sacks and coauthors, Dietary fats and cardiovascular disease: A presidential advisory from the American Heart Association, *Circulation* 130 (2017): e1–e23; D. Mozaffarian, Dietary and policy priorities for cardiovascular disease, diabetes, and obesity: A comprehensive review, *Circulation* 133 (2016): 187–225.

2. Keys, *Seven Countries: A multivariate analysis of death and coronary heart disease* (Cambridge, Mass.: Harvard University Press, 1980).

3. U.S. Department of Agriculture and U.S. Department of Health and Human Services, Scientific Report of the 2015 Dietary Guidelines Advisory Committee, 2015, D-6:11, available at www.health.gov.

4. M. A. Briggs, K. S. Petersen, and P. M. Kris-Etherton, Saturated fatty acids and cardiovascular disease: replacements for saturated fat to reduce cardiovascular risk, *Healthcare* (2017), epub, 10.3390/healthcare5020029; M. R. Flock, J. A. Fleming, and P. M. Kris-Etherton, Macro-nutrient replacement options for saturated fat: Effects on cardiovascular health, *Current Opinion in Lipidology* 25 (2014): 67–74.

5. F. M. Sacks and coauthors, Dietary fats and cardiovascular disease: A presidential advisory from the American Heart Association, *Circulation* 136 (2017): e1–e23; D. D. Wang and F. B. Hu, Dietary fat and Risk of cardiovascular disease: Recent controversies and advances, *Annual Review of Nutrition* 37 (2017): 423–446; P. M. Clifton and J. B. Keogh, A systematic review of the effect of dietary saturated and polyunsaturated fat on heart disease, *Nutrition, Metabolism and Cardiovascular Diseases* 27 (2017): 1060–1080; U.S. Department of Agriculture and U.S. Department of Health and Human Services, *Scientific report of the 2015 Dietary Guidelines Advisory Committee*, 2015, D-6:15, available at www.health.gov.

6. R. J. de Souza and coauthors, Intake of saturated and *trans* unsaturated fatty acids and risk of all cause mortality, cardiovascular disease, and type 2 diabetes: Systematic review and meta-analysis of observational studies, *British Medical Journal* (2015), epub, doi: 101136/bmj.h3978.

7. M. Dehghan and coauthors, Associations of fats and carbohydrate intake with cardiovascular disease and mortality in 18 countries from five continents (PURE): A prospective cohort study, *Lancet* (2017), epub ahead of print, doi: 10.1016/S0140-6736(17)32252-3.

8. U.S. Department of Agriculture and U.S. Department of Health and Human Services, *Scientific report of the 2015 Dietary Guidelines Advisory Committee*, 2015, A:3–5, available at www.health.gov.

9. Sacks and coauthors, Dietary fats and cardiovascular disease: A presidential advisory

from the American Heart Association, 2017; A. M. Fretts and coauthors, Plasma phospholipid saturated fatty acids and incident atrial fibrillation: The Cardiovascular Health Study, *Journal of the American Heart Association* (2014), epub, doi:10l1161/JAHA.114.000889; Flock, Fleming, and Kris-Etherton, Macro-nutrient replacement options for saturated fat, 2014.

10. R. H. Eckel and coauthors, 2013 AHA/ACC guideline on lifestyle management to reduce cardiovascular risk: A report of the American College of Cardiology/American Heart Association Task Force on Practice Guidelines, *Circulation* 129 (2014): S76–S99.

11. J. A. Nettleton, P. Legrand, and R. P. Mensink, ISSFAL 2014 debate: Is it time to update saturated fat recommendations? *Annals of Nutrition and Metabolism* (2015), epub, doi:10.1159/000371585; G. Michas, R. Micha, and A. Zampelas, Dietary fats and cardiovascular disease: Putting together the pieces of a complicated puzzle, *Atherosclerosis* 234 (2014): 320–328; G. D. Lawrence, Dietary fats and health: Dietary recommendations in the context of scientific evidence, *Advances in Nutrition* 4 (2013): 294–302.

12. M. Weech and coauthors, Replacement of dietary saturated fat with unsaturated fats increases numbers of circulating endothelial progenitor cells and decreases numbers of microparticles: findings from the randomized, controlled Dietary Intervention and VAScular function (DIVAS) study, *American Journal of Clinical Nutrition* 107 (2018): 876–882; U. Ravnskov and coauthors, The questionable benefits of exchanging saturated fat with polyunsaturated fat, *Mayo Clinic Proceedings* 89 (2014): 451–453.

13. R. P. Mensink, Effects of saturated fatty acids on serum lipids and lipoproteins: A systematic review and regression analysis (Geneva: World Health Organization, 2016), available at http://apps.who.int/iris/bitstream/handle/10665/246104/9789241565349-eng.pdf;jsessionid=F70A75589E5F53565F613DAA9231DD9B?sequence=1; G. Zong and coauthors, Intake of individual saturated fatty acids and risk of coronary heart disease in U.S. men and women: Two prospective longitudinal cohort studies, *BMJ* (2016), epub, doi.org/10.1136/bmj.i5796; J. Praagman and coauthors, The association between dietary saturated fatty acids and ischemic heart disease depends on the type and source of fatty acid in the European Prospective Investigation into Cancer and Nutrition-Netherlands cohort, *American Journal of Clinical Nutrition* 103 (2016): 356–365.

14. B. Walsh, Eat butter: Scientists labeled fat the enemy: Why they were wrong, *Time*, June 23, 2014; M. Bittman, Butter is back, *New York Times*, March 26, 2014, p. A-23.

15. R. Chowdhury and coauthors, Association of dietary, circulating, and supplement fatty acids with coronary risk, *Annals of Internal Medicine* 160 (2014): 398–407.

16. Comments and response, *Annals of Internal Medicine* 161 (2014): 453–459; M. Katan, as interviewed in B. Liebman, Fat under fire: New findings or shaky science? *Nutrition Action Healthletter*, May 2014, pp. 3–7; D. Kromhout and coauthors, The confusion about dietary fatty acids recommendations for CHD prevention, *British Journal of Nutrition* 106 (2011): 627–632.

17. U.S. Department of Agriculture and U.S. Department of Health and Human Services, *Scientific report of the 2015 Dietary Guidelines Advisory Committee*, 2015, D-6:16, available at www.health.gov.

18. G. Zong and coauthors, Intake of individual saturated fatty acids and risk of coronary heart disease in US men and women: Two prospective longitudinal cohort studies, *British Medical Journal* 355 (2016), doi: 10.1136/bmj.i5796.

19. M. Weech and coauthors, Replacement of dietary saturated fat with unsaturated fats increases numbers of circulating endothelial progenitor cells and decreases numbers of microparticles (2018); Y. Wang and coauthors, Saturated palmitic acid induces myocardial inflammatory injuries through direct binding to TLR4 accessory protein MD2, *Nature Communications* (2017), epub, doi:10.1038/ncomms13997.

20. N. G. Puaschitz and coauthors, Dietary intake of saturated fat is not associated with risk of coronary events or mortality in patients with established coronary artery disease, *Journal of Nutrition* 145 (2015): 299–305.

21. J. Praagman and coauthors, The association between dietary saturated fatty acids and ischemic heart disease depends on the type and source of fatty acid in the European Prospective Investigation into Cancer and Nutrition–Netherlands cohort, *American Journal of Clinical Nutrition* 103 (2016): 356–365.

22. D. D. Wang and F. B. Hu, Dietary fat and risk of cardiovascular disease: recent controversies andadvances, *Annual Review of Nutrition* 37 (2017), epub ahead of print, doi.org/10.1146/annurev-nutr-071816-064607.

23. W. Shen and M. K. McIntosh, Nutrient regulation: Conjugated linoleic acid's inflammatory and browning properties in adipose tissue, *Annual Review of Nutrition* 36 (2016): 183–210.

24. R. M. Kolahdouz and coauthors, Ruminant *trans*-fatty acids and risk of breast cancer: A systematic review and meta-analysis of observational studies, abstract, *Minerva Endocrinology* 42 (2017): 385–396; A. R. Rahbar and coauthors, Effect of conjugated linoleic acid as a supplement or enrichment in foods on blood glucose and waist circumference in humans: A meta-analysis, *Endocrine, Metabolic & Immune Disorders-Drug Targets* 17 (2017): 5–18.

25. Y. Wang and coauthors, Saturated palmitic acid induces myocardial inflammatory injuries through direct binding to TLR4 accessory protein MD2, 2017; T. Moguchi and coauthors, Excessive intake of *trans* fatty acid accelerates atherosclerosis through promoting inflammation and oxidative stress in a mouse model of hyperlipidemia, *Journal of Cardiology* 70 (2017): 121–127.

26. Haring and coauthors, Healthy dietary interventions and lipoprotein (a) plasma levels: Results from the Omni Heart Trial, *PLOS ONE* (2014), epub, doi: 10.1371/journal.pone.0114859.

27. F. M. Sacks and coauthors, Dietary fats and cardiovascular disease: A Presidential Advisory from the American Heart Association, *Circulation* 136 (2017), epub, doi: 10.1161/CIR.0000000000000510; R. Micha and coauthors, Etiologic effects and optimal intakes of foods and nutrients for risk of cardiovascular diseases and diabetes: Systematic reviews and meta-analyses from the nutrition and chronic diseases expert group (NutriCoDE), *PLoS One* (2017), epub, doi: 10.1371/journal.pone.0175149; R. J. de Souza and coauthors, Intake of saturated and *trans* unsaturated fatty acids and risk of all cause mortality, cardiovascular disease, and type 2 diabetes: Systematic review and meta-analysis of observational studies, *British Medical Journal* (2015), epub, doi: 101136/bmj.h3978.

28. D. Mozaffarian, Dietary and policy priorities for cardiovascular disease, diabetes, and obesity: A comprehensive review, *Circulation* 133 (2016): 187–225; J. A. Dias and coauthors, A high quality diet is associated with reduced systemic inflammation in middle-aged individuals, *Atherosclerosis* 238 (2015): 38–44.

29. U.S. Department of Health and Human Services and U.S. Department of Agriculture, 2015–2020 *Dietary Guidelines for Americans*, 8th edition (2015), available at health.gov/dietaryguidelines/2015/guidelines/.

30. V. Miller and coauthors, Fruit, vegetable, and legume intake and cardiovascular disease and deaths in 18 countries (PURE): A prospective cohort study, *Lancet* (2017), epub ahead of print, doi: 10.1016/S0140-6736(17)32253-5; N. Veronese and coauthors, Fried potato consumption is associated with elevated mortality: An 8-y longitudinal cohort study, *American Journal of Clinical Nutrition* 106 (2017): 162–167.

Chapter 6

1. Standing Committee on the Scientific Evaluation of Dietary Reference Intakes, Food and Nutrition Board, Institute of Medicine, *Dietary Reference Intakes for energy, carbohydrate, fiber, fat, fatty acids, cholesterol, protein, and amino acids* (Washington, D.C.: National Academies Press, 2002/2005), pp. 589–768.

2. M. A. Bender, Sickle cell disease, in M.P Adam and coeditors, GeneReviews [Internet] (University of Washington: Seattle, 2017), available at www.ncbi.nlm.nih.gov/books/NBK1377/.

3. N. M. Sales, P. B. Pelegrini, and M. C. Goersch, Nutrigenomics: Definitions and advances of this new science, *Journal of Nutrition and Metabolism* (2014): epub, doi: 10.1155/2014/202759.

4. E. Arentson-Lantz and coauthors, Protein: A nutrient in focus, *Applied Physiology, Nutrition, and Metabolism* 40 (2015): 755–761; N. R. Rodriguez and S. L. Miller, Effective translation of current dietary guidance: Understanding and communication the concepts of minimal and optimal levels of dietary protein, *American Journal of Clinical Nutrition* 101 (2015): 1353S–1358S; M. Rafii and coauthors, Dietary protein requirement of female adults >65 years determined by the indicator amino acid oxidation technique is higher than current recommendations, *Journal of Nutrition* 145 (2015): 18–24; A. N. Pedersen and T. Cederholm, Health effects of protein intake in healthy elderly populations: A systematic literature review, *Food and Nutrition Research* 58 (2014): epub, doi:10.3402/fnr.v58.23364.

5. V. Melina, W. Craig, and S. Levin, Position of the Academy of Nutrition and Dietetics: Vegetarian diets, *Journal of the Academy of Nutrition and Dietetics* 116 (2016): 1970–1980.

6. Centers for Disease Control and Prevention, Diet/Nutrition, Fast Facts, June 2014, available at www.cdc.gov/nchs/fastats/diet.htm.

7. A. L. Carreiro and coauthors, The macronutrients, appetite, and energy intake, *Annual Review of Nutrition* 36 (2016): 73–103; C. D. Morrison and T. Laeger, Protein-dependent regulation of feeding and metabolism, *Trends in Endocrinology and Metabolism* 26 (2015): 256–262.

8. A. Etemadi and coauthors, Mortality from different causes associated with meat, heme iron, nitrates, and nitrites in the NIH-AARP Diet and Health Study: Population based cohort study, *British Medical Journal* (2017) epub, doi.org/10.1136/bmj.j1957; P. Hernández-Alonso and coauthors, High dietary protein intake is associated with an increased body weight and total death risk, *Clinical Nutrition* 35 (2016): 496–505.

9. A. Kamper and S. Strandgaard, Long-term effects of high-protein diets on renal function, *Annual Review of Nutrition* 37 (2017): 347–369; M. Cuenca-Sánchez, D. Navas-Carrillo, and E. Orenes-Piñero, Controversies surrounding high-protein diet intake: Satiating effect and kidney and bone health, *Advances in Nutrition* 6 (2015): 260–266.

10. M. Kitada and coauthors, A low-protein diet exerts a beneficial effect on diabetic status and prevents diabetic nephropathy in Wistar fatty rats, an animal model of type 2 diabetes and obesity, *Nutrition and Metabolism (London)* (2018), epub, doi: 10.1186/s12986-018-0255-1. eCollection 2018; D. H. Pesta and V. T. Samuel, A high-protein diet for reducing body fat: Mechanisms and possible caveats, *Nutrition and Metabolism* 11 (2014), epub, doi: 10.1186/1743-7075-11-53.

11. K. Kalantar-Zadeh and D. Foque, Nutritional management of chronic kidney disease, *New England Journal of Medicine* 377 (2017): 1765–1776; M. Snelson, R. E. Clarke, and M. T. Coughlan, Stirring the pot: Can dietary modification alleviate the burden of CKD? *Nutrients* (2017), epub, doi: 10.3390/nu9030265.

12. V. Bouvard, Carcinogenicity of consumption of red and processed meat, *Lancet Oncology* (2015): 1599–1600; P. J. Tárraga López, J. S. Albero, and J. A. Rodríguez-Montes, Primary and secondary prevention of colorectal cancer, *Clinical Medicine Insights: Gastroenterology* 14 (2014): 33–46.

13. U.S. Preventive Services Task Force, Screening for celiac disease: U.S. Preventive Services Task Force recommendation statement, *Journal of the American Medical Association* 317 (2017): 1252–1257.

14. A Fasano and coauthors, Nonceliac gluten sensitivity, *Gastroenterology* 148 (2015): 1195–1204; L. Eli, L. Roncoroni, and M. T. Bardella, Non-celiac gluten sensitivity: Time for sifting the grain, *World Journal of Gastroenterology* 21 (2015): 8221–8226; M. M. Leonard and B. Vasagar, US perspective on gluten-related diseases, *Clinical and Experimental Gastroenterology* 7 (2014), epub, doi:10.2147/CEG.S54567.

15. J. Molina-Infante and A. Carroccio, Suspected nonceliac gluten sensitivity confirmed in few patients after gluten challenge in double-blind, placebo-controlled trials, *Clinical Gastroenterology and Hepatology* 15 (2017): 339–348; M. Uhde and coauthors, Intestinal cell damage and systemic immune activation in individuals reporting sensitivity to wheat in the absence of coeliac disease, *Gut* 65 (2016): 1930–1937.

16. N. J. Talley and M. M. Walker, Celiac disease and nonceliac gluten or wheat sensitivity: The risks and benefits of diagnosis, *JAMA Internal Medicine* 177 (2017): 615–616; E. Lionetti and coauthors, Celiac disease from a global perspective, *Best Practice and Research: Clinical Gastroenterology* 29 (2015): 365–379.

Consumer's Guide 6

1. C. D. Morrison and T. Laeger, Protein-dependent regulation of feeding and metabolism, *Trends in Endocrinology and Metabolism* 26 (2015): 256–262.

2. D. H. Pesta and V. T Samuel, A high-protein diet for reducing body fat: Mechanisms and possible caveats, *Nutrition & Metabolism* (2014), epub, doi: 10.1186/1743-7075-11-53.

3. C. C. Chi and coauthors, Interventions for prevention of herpes simplex labialis (cold sores on the lips), *Cochrane Database of Systematic Reviews* 8 (2015): CD010095.

4. H. Y. Guo and coauthors, Hyper-homocysteinemia independently causes and promotes atherosclerosis in LDL receptor-deficient mice, *Journal of Geriatric Cardiology* 11 (2014): 74–78; R. H. Mendes and coauthors, Moderate hyper-homocysteinemia provokes dysfunction of cardiovascular autonomic system and liver oxidative stress in rats, *Autonomic Neuroscience: Basic and Clinical* 180 (2014): 43–47.

5. K. Kalantar-Zadeh and D. Foque, Nutritional management of chronic kidney disease, *New England Journal of Medicine* 377 (2017): 1765–1776; L. Wandrag and coauthors, Impact of supplementation with amino acids or their metabolites on muscle wasting in patients with critical illness or other muscle wasting illness: A systematic review, *Journal of Human Nutrition and Dietetics* 28 (2015): 313–330.

6. Standing Committee on the Scientific Evaluation of Dietary Reference Intakes, Food and Nutrition Board, Institute of Medicine, *Dietary Reference Intakes for Energy, carbohydrate, fiber, fat, fatty acids, cholesterol, protein, and amino acids* (Washington, D.C.: National Academies Press, 2002/2005), pp. 589–768.

Controversy 6

1. A. Etemadi and coauthors, Mortality from different causes associated with meat, heme iron, nitrates, and nitrites in the NIH-AARP Diet and Health Study: Population based cohort study, *British Medical Journal* (2017) epub, doi. org/10.1136/bmj.j1957; M. J. Orlich and G. E. Frasier, Vegetarian diets in the Adventist Health Study 2: A review of initial published findings, *American Journal of Clinical Nutrition* 100 (2014): 353S–358S.

2. L. E. O'Connor, J. E. Kim, and W. W. Campbell, Total red meat intake of ≥0.5 servings/d does not negatively influence cardiovascular disease risk factors: A systemically searched meta-analysis of randomized controlled trials, American Journal of Clinical Nutrition 105 (2017): 57–59.

3. V. Melina, W. Craig, and S. Levin, Position of the Academy of Nutrition and Dietetics: Vegetarian diets, *Journal of the Academy of Nutrition and Dietetics* 116 (2016): 1970–1980.

4. X. Wang and coauthors, Fruit and vegetable consumption and mortality from all causes, cardiovascular disease, and cancer: Systematic review and dose-response meta-analysis of prospective cohort studies, *British Medical Journal* 349 (2014), epub, doi:10.1136/bmj.g4490.

5. O. Oyebode and coauthors, Fruit and vegetable consumption and all-cause, cancer and CVD mortality: Analysis of Health Survey for England data, *Journal of Epidemiology and Community Health* 68 (2014): 856–862.

6. P. N. Singh and coauthors, Global epidemiology of obesity, vegetarian dietary patterns, and noncommunicable disease in Asian Indians, *American Journal of Clinical Nutrition* 100 (2014): 359S–364S.

7. Y. Yokoyama, S. M. Levin, and N. D. Barnard, Association between plant-based diets and plasma lipids: a systematic review and meta-analysis, *Nutrition Reviews* 75 (2017): 683–698; Z. H. Jian and coauthors, Vegetarian diet and cholesterol and TAG levels by gender, *Public Health Nutrition* 18 (2015): 721–726; F. Wang and coauthors, Effects of vegetarian diets on blood lipids: A systematic review and meta-analysis of randomized controlled trials, *Journal of the American Heart Association* (2015), epub, doi: 10.1161/JAHA.115.002408.

8. A. Satija and coauthors, Healthful and unhealthful plant-based diets and the risk of coronary heart disease in U.S. adults, *Journal of the American College of Cardiology* (2017), epub, doi: 10.1016/j.jacc.2017.05.047.

9. D. Demeyer and coauthors, Mechanisms linking colorectal cancer to the consumption of (processed) red meat: A review, *Food Science and Nutrition* 56 (2016): 2747–2766; World Health Organization, International Agency for Research on Cancer, IARC Monographs evaluate consumption of red meat and processed meat, 2015, www.iarc.fr/en/media-centre/iarcnews/pdf/Monographs-Q&A_Vol114.pdf; M. J. Orlich and coauthors, Vegetarian dietary patterns and the risk of colorectal cancers, *JAMA Internal Medicine* 175 (2015): 767–776.

10. T. J. Key and coauthors, Cancer in British vegetarians: Updated analyses of 4998 incident cancers in a cohort of 32,491 meat eaters, 8,612 fish eaters, 18,298 vegetarians, and 2,246 vegans, *American Journal of Clinical Nutrition* 100 (2014): 378S–385S.

11. A. Etemadi and coauthors, Mortality from different causes associated with meat, heme iron, nitrates, and nitrites in the NIH-AARP Diet and Health Study: Population based cohort study, 2017.

12. U. Hammerling and coauthors, Consumption of red/processed meat and colorectal carcinoma: Possible mechanisms underlying the significant association, *Critical Reviews in Food Science and Nutrition* 56 (2016): 614–634.

13. G. B. Piccoli and coauthors, Vegan-vegetarian diets in pregnancy: Danger or panacea? A systematic narrative review, *BJOG* 122 (2015): 623–633.

14. B. Allès and coauthors, Comparison of socio-demographic and nutritional characteristics between self-reported vegetarians, vegans, and meat-eaters from the Nutrinet-Santé study, *Nutrients* (2017), epub, doi: 10.3390/nu9091023; R. Pawlak, S. E. Lester, and T. Babatunde, The prevalence of cobalamin deficiency among vegetarians assessed by serum vitamin B12: A review of literature, *European Journal of Clinical Nutrition* 68 (2014): 541–548.

15. C. Kocaoglu and coauthors, Cerebral atrophy in a vitamin B12-deficient infant of a vegetarian mother, *Journal of Health, Population, and Nutrition* 32 (2014): 367–371.

16. G. J. Lee and coauthors, Consumption of non-cow's milk beverages and serum vitamin D levels in early childhood, *Canadian Medical Association Journal* 186 (2014): 1287–1293; N. F. Krebs and coauthors, Meat consumption is associated with less stunting among toddlers in four diverse low-income settings, *Food and Nutrition Bulletin* 32 (2011): 185–191; M. Van Winckel and coauthors, Clinical practice: Vegetarian infant and child nutrition, *European Journal of Pediatrics* 170 (2011): 1489–1494.

17. R. S. Gibson, A. M. Heath, and E. A. Szymlek-Gay, Is iron and zinc nutrition a concern for vegetarian infants and young children in industrialized nations? *American Journal of Clinical Nutrition* 100 (2014): 459S–468S.

18. P. D. Genaro and coauthors, Dietary protein intake in elderly women: Association with muscle and bone mass, *Nutrition in Clinical Practice* 30 (2015): 283–289.

19. K. L. Tucker, Vegetarian diets and bone status, *American Journal of Clinical Nutrition* 100 (2014): 329S–335S.

Chapter 7

1. N. Kono and H. Arai, Intracellular transport of fat-soluble vitamins A and E, *Traffic* 16 (2015): 19–34.

2. A. S. Green and A. J. Fascetti, Meeting the vitamin A requirement: The Efficacy and importance of β-carotene in animal species, *Scientific World Journal* (2016), epub, doi: 10.1155/2016/7393620.

3. S. A. Tanumihardjo and coauthors, Biomarkers of nutrition for development (BOND)—vitamin A review, *The Journal of Nutrition* 146 (2016): 1816S–1848S; G. Bakdash and coauthors, Retinoic acid primes human dendritic cells to induce gut-homing, IL-10-producing regulatory T cells, *Mucosal Immunology* 8 (2015): 265–278; C. Rochette-Egly, Retinoic acid signaling and mouse embryonic stem cell differentiation: Cross talk between genomic and non-genomic effects of RA, *Biochemica et Biophysica acta* 1851 (2015): 66–75.

4. J. T. Busada and C. B. Geyer, The role of retinoic acid (RA) in spermatogonial differentiation, *Biology of Reproduction* 94 (2016): 1–10; T. J. Cunningham and G. Duester, Mechanisms of retinoic acid signaling and its roles in organ and limb development, *Nature Reviews Molecular Cell Biology* 16 (2015): 110–123.

5. A. Imdad and coauthors, Vitamin A supplementation for preventing morbidity and mortality in children from six months to five years of age, *Cochrane Database Systematic Reviews* (2017), epub, doi: 10.1002/14651858.CD008524.pub3; A. Parafita-Fernandez and coauthors, Acquired night blindness due to bad eating patterns, *European Journal of Clinical Nutrition* 69 (2015): 752–754.

6. A. Sommer, Preventing blindness and saving lives: The centenary of vitamin A, *Journal of the American Medical Association Ophthalmology* 132 (2014): 115–117.

7. K. Feroze and E. Kaufman, Xerophthalmia, *StatPearls* (2017): Bookshelf ID: NBK431094 PMID: 28613746.

8. T. J. Cunningham and G. Duester, Mechanisms of retinoic acid signaling and its roles in organ and limb development, 2015.

9. L. M. Fettig and coauthors, Cross talk between progesterone receptors and retinoic acid receptors in regulation of cytokeratin 5-positive breast cancer cells, *Oncogene* 36 (2017): 6074–6084; A. Roy and coauthors, Multiple roles of RARRES1 in prostate cancer: Autophagy induction and angiogenesis inhibition, *PLos One* (2017), epub, doi: 10.1371/journal.pone.0180344; X. Xu and coauthors, KDM3B shows tumor-suppressive activity and transcriptionally regulates HOXA1 through retinoic acid response elements in acute myeloid leukemia, *Leukemia & Lymphoma* 25 (2017): 1–10.

10. M. R. Bono and coauthors, Retinoic acid as a modulator or T cell immunity, *Nutrients* (2016), doi: 10.3390/nu8060349.

11. A. C. Palmer and coauthors, Maternal vitamin A supplementation increases natural antibody concentrations of preadolescent offspring in rural Nepal, *Nutrition* 31 (2015): 813–819; S. A. van de Pavert and coauthors, Maternal retinoids control type 3 innate lymphoid cells and set the offspring immunity, *Nature* 508 (2014): 123–127.

12. World Health Organization, Measles fact sheet, January 2017, available at www.who.int/mediacentre/factsheets/fs286/en.

13. M. A. Metzler and L. L. Sandell, Enzymatic metabolism of vitamin A in developing vertebrate embryos, *Nutrients* (2016), epub, doi: 10.3390/nu8120812.

14. A. C. Green, T. J. Martin, and L. E. Purton, The role of vitamin A and retinoic acid receptor signaling in post-natal maintenance of bone, *The Journal of Steroid Biochemistry and Molecular Biology* 155 (2016): 135–146.

15. S. Pinkaew and coauthors, Triple-fortified rice containing vitamin A reduced marginal vitamin A deficiency and increased vitamin A liver stores in school-aged Thai children, *The Journal of Nutrition* 144 (2014): 519–524.

16. CDC, Measles (*Rubeola*), in The Yellow Book 2018: Health Information for International Travelers' Health (2017), available at www.cdc.gov.

17. National Institutes of Health Office of Dietary Supplements, Vitamin A fact sheet for health professionals (2016), available at ods.od.nih.gov.

18. S. Khalil and coauthors, Retinoids: A journey from the molecular structures and mechanisms of action to clinical uses in dermatology and adverse effects, *The Journal of Dermatological Treatment* (2017): 1–13.

19. B. Gopinath and coauthors, Intake of key micronutrients and food groups in patients with late-stage age-related macular degeneration compared with age-sex-matched controls, *The British Journal of Ophthalmology* 101 (2017): 1027–1031; K. J. Meyers and coauthors, Joint associations of diet, lifestyle, and genes with age-related macular degeneration, *Ophthalmology* 122 (2015): 2286–2294.

20. J. R. Evans and J. G. Lawrenson, Antioxidant vitamin and mineral supplements for slowing the progression of age-related macular degeneration, *Cochrane Database of Systematic Reviews* (2017), epub, doi: 10.1002/14651858; F. Corvi and coauthors, Pilot evaluation of short-term changes in macular pigment and retinal sensitivity in different phenotypes of early age-related macular degeneration after carotenoid supplementation, *The British Journal of Ophthalmology* 101 (2017): 770–773; B. Eisenhauer and coauthors, Lutein and zeaxanthin-food sources, bioavailability and dietary variety in age-related macular degeneration protection, *Nutrients* (2017), epub, doi: 10.3390/nu9020120; A. Gorusupudi, K. Nelson, and P. S. Bernstein, The age-related eye disease 2 study: Micronutrients in the treatment of macular degeneration, *Advances in Nutrition* 8 (2017): 40–53; C. J. Chiu and coauthors, The relationship of

major American dietary patterns to age-related macular degeneration, *American Journal of Ophthalmology* 158 (2014): 118–127.

21. K. Pezdirc and coauthors, Consuming high-carotenoid fruit and vegetables influences skin yellowness and plasma carotenoids in young women: A single-blind randomized crossover trial, *Journal of the Academy of Nutrition and Dietetics* 116 (2016): 1257–1265.

22. R. L. Schleicher and coauthors, The vitamin D status of the U.S. population from 1988 to 2010 using standardized serum concentrations of 25-hydroxyvitamin D shows recent modest increases, *The American Journal of Clinical Nutrition* 104 (2016): 454–461.

23. E. Wintermeyer and coauthors, Crucial role of vitamin D in the musculoskeletal system, *Nutrients* 8 (2016): 319; G. Carmeliet, V. Dermauw, and R. Bouillon, Vitamin D signaling in calcium and bone homeostasis: a delicate balance, *Best Practice & Research Clinical Endocrinology & Metabolism* 29 (2015): 621–631.

24. C. M. Weaver and coauthors, Calcium plus vitamin D supplementation and risk of fractures: An updated meta-analysis from the National Osteoporosis Foundation, *Osteoporosis International* 27 (2016): 367–376; P. R. Ebeling, Vitamin D and bone health: Epidemiologic studies, *BoneKEy Reports* 3 (2014), epub, doi:10.1038/bonekey.2014.6; P. Lips, E. Gielen, and N. M. van Schoor, Vitamin D supplements with or without calcium to prevent fractures, *BoneKEy Reports* (2014), epub, doi:10.1038/bonekey.2014.7.

25. N. Trehan and coauthors, Vitamin D deficiency, supplementation, and cardiovascular health, *Critical Pathways in Cardiology* 16 (2017): 109–118; D. D. Binkle, Extraskeletal actions of vitamin D, *Annals of the New York Academy of Sciences* 1376 (2016): 29–52; A. R. Martineau and coauthors, Vitamin D supplementation to prevent acute respiratory tract infections: Systematic review and meta-analysis of individual participant data, *The British Medical Journal* 356 (2017): i6583; E. T. Jacobs and coauthors, Vitamin D and colorectal, breast, and prostate cancers: A review of the epidemiological evidence, *Journal of Cancer* 7 (2016): 232–240; S. L. McDonnell and coauthors, Serum 25-hydroxyvitamin D concentrations ≥40 ng/ml are associated with >65% lower cancer risk: Pooled analysis of randomized trial and prospective cohort study, *PLoS One* 11 (2016): e0152441; D. B. Matchar and coauthors, Vitamin D levels and the risk of cognitive decline in Chinese elderly people: The Chinese Longitudinal Healthy Longevity Survey, *The Journals of Gerontology. Series A, Biological Sciences and Medical Sciences* 71 (2016): 1363–1368; J. Wang and coauthors, Meta-analysis of the association between vitamin D and autoimmune thyroid disease, *Nutrients* 7 (2015): 2485–2498; L. E. Mokry and coauthors, Vitamin D and risk of multiple sclerosis: A Mendelian randomization study, *PLoS Medicine* 12 (2015): e1001866, K. Amrein and coauthors, Effect of high-dose vitamin D3 on hospital length of stay in

Appendix F Chapter 7 Notes

critically ill patients with vitamin D deficiency: The VITdAL-ICU randomized clinical trial, *Journal of the American Medical Association* 312 (2014): 1520–1530; D. Dutta and coauthors, Vitamin-D supplementation in prediabetes reduced progression to type 2 diabetes and was associated with decreased insulin resistance and systemic inflammation: An open label randomized prospective study from Eastern India, *Diabetes Research and Clinical Practice* 103 (2014): e18–e23; N. J. Groves, J. J. McGrath, and T. H. Burne, Vitamin D as a neurosteroid affecting the developing and adult brain, *Annual Review of Nutrition* 34 (2014): 117–141.

26. C. D'Amore and coauthors, Vitamin D deficiency and clinical outcome in patients with chronic heart failure: A review, *Nutrition, Metabolism, and Cardiovascular Diseases* 27 (2017): 837–849; R. Scragg and coauthors, Effect of monthly high-dose vitamin D supplementation on cardiovascular disease in the Vitamin D Assessment Study: A randomized clinical trial, *JAMA Cardiology* 2 (2017): 608–616; J. Lappe and coauthors, Effect of vitamin D and calcium supplementation on cancer-incidence in older women: A randomized clinical trial, *Journal of the American Medical Association* 317 (2017): 1234–1243; A. M. Goodwill and C. Szoeke, A systematic review and meta-analysis of the effect of low vitamin D on cognition, *Journal of the American Geriatrics Association* (2017): doi: 10.1111/jgs.15012; W. Dankers and coauthors, Vitamin D in autoimmunity: Molecular mechanisms and therapeutic potential, *Frontiers in Immunology* 7 (2016): 697; C. Mathieu, Vitamin D and diabetes: where do we stand?, *Diabetes Research and Clinical Practice* 108 (2015): 201–209; K. de Haan and coauthors, Vitamin D deficiency as a risk factor for infection, sepsis and mortality in the critically ill: Systematic review and meta-analysis, *Critical Care* 18 (2014): 660.

27. A. L. Creo and coauthors, Nutritional rickets around the world: An update, *Paediatrics and International Child Health* 37 (2017): 84–98; R. Singleton and coauthors, Rickets and vitamin D deficiency in Alaska native children, *Journal of Pediatric Endocrinology and Metabolism* 28 (2015): 815–823.

28. T. R. Hill and T. J. Aspray, The role of vitamin D in maintaining bone health in older people, *Therapeutic Advances in Musculoskeletal Disease* 9 (2017): 89–95; K. Shikino, M. Ikusaka, and T. Yamashita, Vitamin D-deficient osteomalacia due to excessive self-restrictions for atopic dermatitis, *BMJ Case Reports* (2014), doi: 10.1136/bcr-2014-204558.

29. J. Zhao and coauthors, Association between calcium or vitamin D supplementation and fracture incidence in community-dwelling older adults: A systematic review and meta-analysis, *Journal of the American Medical Association* 318 (2017): 2466–2482; N. M. Van Schoor, M. W. Heymans, and P. Lips, Vitamin D status in relation to physical performance, falls and fractures in the Longitudinal Aging Study Amsterdam: A reanalysis of previous findings using standardized serum 25-hydroxyvitamin D values, *The Journal of Steroid Biochemistry and Molecular Biology* 177 (2017): 255–260; T. R. Hill and T. J. Aspray, The role of vitamin D in maintaining bone health in older people, 2017; H. Macdonald and T. J. Aspray, Vitamin D supplements and bone mineral density, *Lancet* 383 (2014): 1292; H. A. Bischoff-Ferrari and coauthors, Monthly high-dose vitamin D treatment for the prevention of functional decline: A randomized clinical trial, *Journal of the American Medical Association Internal Medicine* 176 (2016): 175–183.

30. S. Savastano and coauthors, Low vitamin D status and obesity: Role of nutritionist, *Reviews in Endocrine and Metabolic Disorders* 18 (2017): 215–225; P. Prasad and A. Kochhar, Interplay of vitamin D and metabolic syndrome: A review, *Diabetes & Metabolic Syndrome: Clinical Research & Reviews* 10 (2016): 105–112; M. Pereira-Santos and coauthors, Obesity and vitamin D deficiency: A systematic review and meta-analysis, *Obesity Reviews* 16 (2015): 341–349; Y. Yao and coauthors, A meta-analysis of the relationship between vitamin D deficiency and obesity, *International Journal of Clinical and Experimental Medicine* 8 (2015): 14977–14984.

31. S. Barja-Fernandez and coauthors, 25-Hydroxyvitamin D levels of children are inversely related to adiposity assessed by body mass index, *Journal of Physiology and Biochemistry* 74 (2017): 111–118; C. E. Moore and Y. Liu, Low serum 25-hydroxyvitamin D concentrations are associated with total adiposity of children in the United States: National Health and Nutrition Examination Survey 2005 to 2006, *Nutrition Research* 36 (2016): 72–79.

32. C. Himbert and coauthors, A systematic review of the interrelation between diet- and surgery-induced weight loss and vitamin D status, *Nutrition Review* 38 (2017): 13–26; P. K. Pannu, Y. Zhao, and M. J. Soares, Reductions in body weight and percent fat mass increase the vitamin D status of obese subjects: A systematic review and metaregression analysis, *Nutrition Research* 36 (2016): 201–213; A. Gangloff and coauthors, Changes in circulating vitamin D levels with loss of adipose tissue, *Current Opinion in Clinical Nutrition and Metabolic Care* 19 (2016): 464–470.

33. C. F. Dix, J. L. Barcley, and O. R. L. Wright, The role of vitamin D in adipogenesis, *Nutrition Reviews* 76 (2018): 47–59; S. Savastano and coauthors, Low vitamin D status and obesity: role of nutritionist, 2017; J. E. Heller and coauthors, Relation between vitamin D status and body composition in collegiate athletes, *International Journal of Sport Nutrition and Exercise Metabolism* 25 (2015): 128–135; L. K. Pourshahidi, Vitamin D and obesity: Current perspectives and future directions, *The Proceedings of the Nutrition Society* 74 (2015): 115–124; C. Cipriani and coauthors, Vitamin D and its relationship with obesity and muscle, *International Journal of Endocrinology* (2014), epub, doi: 10.1155/2014/841248

34. M. S. Razzaque, Can adverse effects of excessive vitamin D supplementation occur without developing hypervitaminosis D?, *Journal of Steroid Biochemistry and Molecular Biology* (2017), epub ahead of print, doi: 10.1016/j.jsbmb.2017.07.006; R. L. Shea and J. D. Berg, Self-administration of vitamin D supplements in the general public may be associated with high 25-hydroxyvitamin D concentrations, *Annals of Clinical Biochemistry* 54 (2017): 355–361; G. Conti and coauthors, Vitamin D intoxication in two brothers: Be careful with dietary supplements, *Journal of Pediatric Endocrinology and Metabolism* 27 (2014): 763–767.

35. S. Schramm and coauthors, Impact of season and different vitamin D thresholds on prevalence of vitamin D deficiency in epidemiological cohorts—a note of caution, *Endocrine* 56 (2017): 658–666; M. A. Serdar and coauthors, Analysis of changes in parathyroid hormone and 25 (OH) vitamin D levels with respect to age, gender, and season: A data mining study, *Journal of Medical Biochemistry* 36 (2017): 73–83; G. Olerod and coauthors, The variation in free 25-hydroxy vitamin D and vitamin D-binding protein with season and vitamin D status, *Endocrine Connections* 6 (2017): 111–120; I. Ohlund and coauthors, Increased vitamin D intake differentiated according to skin color is needed to meet requirements in young Swedish children during winter: A double-blind randomized clinical trial, *The American Journal of Clinical Nutrition* 106 (2017): 105–112; C. M. O'Neill and coauthors, Seasonal changes in vitamin D-effective UVB availability in Europe and associations with population serum 25-hydroxyvitamin D, *Nutrients* 8 (2016), epub, doi: 10.3390/nu8090533.

36. Committee on Dietary Reference Intakes, Dietary Reference Intakes for Calcium and Vitamin D, p. 6.; U.S. Department of Health and Human Services and U.S. Department of Agriculture, Dietary Guidelines for Americans 2015–2020, available at www.health.gov.

37. D. Ferrari, G. Lombardi, and G. Banfi, Concerning the vitamin D reference range: Pre-analytical and analytical variability of vitamin D measurement, *Biochemia Medica* 27 (2017), epub, doi: 10.11613/BM.2017.030501; M. Kiely, A. Hemmingway, and K. M. O'Callaghan, Vitamin D in pregnancy: Current perspectives and future directions, *Therapeutic Advances in Musculoskeletal Disease* 9 (2017): 145–154; P. J. Veugelers, T. M. Pham, and J. P. Ekwaru, Optimal vitamin D supplementation doses that minimize the risk for both low and high serum 25-hydroxyvitamin D concentrations in the general public, *Nutrients* (2015), epub, doi: 10.3390/nu7125527

38. J. B. Kohn, Are mushrooms a significant source of vitamin D?, *Journal of the Academy of Nutrition and Dietetics* 116 (2016): 1520; K. D. Cashman and coauthors, Effect of ultraviolet light-exposed mushrooms on vitamin D status: Liquid chromatography-tandem mass spectrometry reanalysis of biobanked sera from

a randomized controlled trial and a systematic review plus meta-analysis, *The Journal of Nutrition* 146 (2016): 565–575; P. K. Kamweru and E. L. Tindibale, Vitamin D and vitamin D from ultraviolet-irradiated mushrooms (Review), *International Journal of Medicinal Mushrooms* 18 (2016): 205–214.

39. J. X. Chen and coauthors, δ- and γ-tocopherols inhibit phIP/DSS-induced colon carcinogenesis by protection against early cellular and DNA damages, *Molecular Carcinogenesis* 56 (2017): 172–183; A. J. Burbank and coauthors, Gamma tocopherol-enriched supplement reduces a sputum eosinophilia and endotoxin-induced sputum neutrophilia in volunteers with asthma, *The Journal of Allergy and Clinical Immunology* (2017): epub ahead of print, doi: 10.1016/j.jaci.2017.06.029.

40. S. Budhathoki and coauthors, Plasma 25-hydroxyvitamin D concentration and subsequent risk of total and site specific cancers in Japanese population: Large case-cohort study within Japan Public Health Center-based Prospective Study cohort, *BMJ* (2018), epub, doi: 10.1136/bmj.k671; I. Korovila and coauthors, Proteostasis, oxidative stress and aging, *Redox Biology* 13 (2017): 550–567; J. C. Jha and coauthors, The emerging role of NADPH oxidase NOX5 in vascular disease, *Clinical Science* 131 (2017): 981–990; M. Höll and coauthors, ROS signaling by NADPH oxidase 5 modulates the proliferation and survival of prostate carcinoma cells, *Molecular Carcinogenesis* 55 (2016): 27–39; J. C. Jha and coauthors, Genetic targeting or pharmacologic inhibition of NADPH oxidase Nox4 provides renoprotection in long-term diabetic nephropathy, *Journal of the American Society of Nephrology* 25 (2014): 1237–1254.

41. Q. Jiang, Natural forms of vitamin E: metabolism, antioxidant, and anti-inflammatory activities and their role in disease prevention and therapy, *Free Radical Biology and Medicine* 72 (2014): 76–90.

42. J. Cook-Mills and coauthors, Interaction of vitamin E isoforms on asthma and allergic airway disease, *Thorax* 71 (2016): 954–956; P. Ambrogini and coauthors, α-tocopherol and hippocampal neural plasticity in physiological and pathological conditions, *International Journal of Molecular Science* 17 (2016): doi: 10.3390/ijms17122107; A. W. Ashor and coauthors, Effect of vitamin C and vitamin E supplementation on endothelial function: A systematic review and meta-analysis of randomized controlled trials, *British Journal of Nutrition* 113 (2015): 1182–1194.

43. S. Khanna and coauthors, Excessive alpha-tocopherol exacerbates microglial activation and brain injury caused by acute ischemic stroke, *FASEB Journal: Official Publication of the Federation of American Societies for Experimental Biology* 29 (2015): 828–836; C. K. Desai and coauthors, The role of vitamin supplementation in the prevention of cardiovascular disease events, *Clinical Cardiology* 37 (2014): 576–581.

44. G. Bjelakovic, D. Nikolova, and C. Gluud, Antioxidant supplements and mortality, *Current Opinion in Clinical Nutrition and Metabolic Care* 17 (2014): 40–44.

45. A. J. Curtis and coauthors, Vitamin E supplementation and mortality in healthy people: A meta-analysis of randomized controlled trials, *Cardiovascular Drugs and Therapy* 28 (2014): 563–573; S. Jiang and coauthors, Meta-analysis: Low-dose intake of vitamin E combined with other vitamins or minerals may decrease all-cause mortality, *Journal of Nutritional Science and Vitaminology* 60 (2014): 194–205. G. Y. Lai and coauthors, Effects of alpha-tocopherol and beta-carotene supplementation on liver cancer incidence and chronic liver disease mortality in the ATBC study, *British Journal of Cancer* 111 (2014): 2220–2223; J. Virtamo and coauthors, Effects of alpha-tocopherol and beta-carotene supplementation on cancer incidence and mortality: 18-year postintervention follow-up of the Alpha-tocopherol, Beta-carotene Cancer Prevention Study, *International Journal of Cancer* 135 (2014): 178–185.

46. Committee on Dietary Reference Intakes, Dietary Reference Intakes for Calcium and Vitamin D, p. 6.; U.S. Department of Health and Human Services and U.S. Department of Agriculture, Dietary Guidelines for Americans 2015–2020, available at www.health.gov.

47. E. M. Hawes and A. J. Viera, Anticoagulation: managing adverse events in patients receiving anticoagulation and perioperative care, *FP Essentials* 422 (2014): 31–39.

48. J. K. Villa and coauthors, Effect of vitamin K in bone metabolism and vascular calcification: A review of mechanisms of action and evidences, *Critical Reviews in Food Science and Nutrition* (2016): epub ahead of print, doi: 10.1080/10408398.2016.1211616; A. Urano and coauthors, Vitamin K deficiency evaluated by serum levels of undercarboxylated osteocalcin in patients with anorexia nervosa with bone loss, *Clinical Nutrition* 34 (2015): 443–448.

49. G. Hao and coauthors, Vitamin K intake and the risk of fractures: A meta-analysis, *Medicine* 96 (2017): e6725; T. E. Finnes and coauthors, A combination of low serum concentrations of vitamins K1 and D is associated with increased risk of hip fractures in elderly Norwegians: A NOREPOS study, *Osteoporosis International* 27 (2016): 1645–1652; A. C. Torbergsen and coauthors, Vitamin K1 and 25(OH)D are independently and synergistically associated with a risk for hip fracture in an elderly population: A case control study, *Clinical Nutrition* 34 (2015): 101–106.

50. Z. B. Huang and coauthors, Does vitamin K2 play a role in the prevention and treatment of osteoporosis for postmenopausal women: A meta-analysis of randomized controlled trials, *Osteoporosis International* 26 (2015): 1175–1186; M. S. Hamidi and A. M. Cheung, Vitamin K and musculoskeletal health in postmenopausal women, *Molecular Nutrition and Food Research* 58 (2014): 1647–1657.

51. J. C. Phillippi and coauthors, Prevention of vitamin K deficiency bleeding, *Journal of Midwifery & Women's Health* (2016): doi: 10.1111/jmwh.12470; R. Schulte and coauthors, Rise in late onset vitamin K deficiency bleeding in young infants because of omission or refusal of prophylaxis at birth, *Pediatric Neurology* 50 (2014): 564–568.

52. J. Loyal and coauthors, Refusal of vitamin K by parents of newborns: A survey of the better outcomes through research for newborns network, *Academic Pediatrics* 17 (2017): 368–373; L. H. Marcewicz and coauthors, Parental refusal of vitamin K and neonatal preventive services: A need for surveillance, *Maternal and Child Health Journal* 21 (2017): 1079–1084; R. Schulte and coauthors, Rise in late onset vitamin K deficiency bleeding in young infants because of omission or refusal of prophylaxis at birth, 2014.

53. G. Akolkar and coauthors, Vitamin C mitigates oxidative/nitrosative stress and inflammation in Doxorubicin-induced cardiomyopathy, *American Journal of Physiology Heart and Circulatory Physiology* (2017): doi: 10.1152/ajpheart.00253.2017; A. Ludke and coauthors, Time course of changes in oxidative stress and stress-induced proteins in cardiomyocytes exposed to doxorubicin and prevention by vitamin C, *PLoS One* 12 (2017), epub, doi.org/10.1371/journal.pone.0179452.

54. R. F. Mendes-da-Silva and coauthors, Prooxidant versus antioxidant brain action of ascorbic acid in well-nourished and malnourished rats as a function of dose: A cortical spreading depression and malondialdehyde analysis, *Neuropharmacology* 86 (2014): 155–160; A. Chakraborthy and coauthors, Antioxidant and pro-oxidant activity of vitamin C in oral environment, *Indian Journal of Dental Research* 25 (2014): 499–504.

55. S. S. Gropper and J. L. Smith, Vitamin C (Ascorbic Acid), in Advanced *nutrition and human metabolism* (Cengage Learning: Boston, 2018), pp. 303–312.

56. G. M. Allan and B. Arroll, Prevention and treatment of the common cold: Making sense of the evidence, *Canadian Medical Association Journal* 186 (2014): 190–199.

57. H. Hemilä, Vitamin C and infections, *Nutrients* 9 (2017), epub, doi: 10.3390/nu9040339.

58. R. A. Wijkmans and K. Talsma, Modern scurvy, *Journal of Surgical Case Reports* (2016), https://doi.org/10.1093/jscr/rjv168; M. Levavasseur and coauthors, Severe scurvy: An underestimated disease, *European Journal of Clinical Nutrition* 69 (2015): 1076–1077; J. Ong and R. Randhawa, Scurvy in an alcoholic patient treated with intravenous vitamins, *BMJ Case Reports* (2014), epub, doi: 10.1136/bcr-2013-009479.

59. S. Yaich and coauthors, Secondary oxalosis due to excess vitamin C intake: A cause of graft loss in a renal transplant recipient, *Saudi Journal of Kidney Disease and Transplantation* 25 (2014): 113–116; X. Tang and J. C. Lieske, Acute and chronic kidney injury in nephrolithiasis,

Current Opinion in Nephrology and Hypertension 23 (2014): 385–390.

60. A. Sanvisens and coauthors, Long-term mortality of patients with alcohol-related Wernicke-Korsakoff syndrome, *Alcohol and Alcoholism* 52 (2017): 466–471.

61. T. Udhayabanu and coauthors, Riboflavin responsive mitochondrial dysfunction in neurodegenerative diseases, *Journal of Clinical Medicine* (2017), epub, doi: 10.3390/jcm6050052; Y. P. Wang and coauthors, Riboflavin supplementation improves energy metabolism in mice exposed to acute hypoxia, *Physiological Research* 63 (2014): 341–350.

62. S. K. Luthe and R. Sato, Alcoholic pellagra as a course of altered mental status in the emergency department, *The Journal of Emergency Medicine* (2017), epub, doi: 10.1016/j.jemermed.2017.05.008; N. Terada and coauthors, Wernicke encephalopathy and pellagra in an alcoholic and malnourished patient, *BMJ Case Reports* (2015), epub, doi: 10.1136/bcr-2015-209412; A. A. Badawy, Pellagra and alcoholism: A biochemical perspective, *Alcohol and Alcoholism* 49 (2014): 238–250.

63. G. Matapandeu, S. H. Dunn, and P. Pagels, An outbreak of pellagra in the Kasese catchment area, Dowa, Malawi, *The American Journal of Tropical Medicine and Hygiene* 96 (2017): 1244–1247.

64. R. L. Dunbar and H. Goel, Niacin alternatives for dyslipidemia: Fool's gold or gold mine? Part 1: Alternative niacin regimens, *Current Atherosclerosis Reports* 18 (2016): 11.

65. C. Minto and coauthors, Definition of a tolerable upper intake level of niacin: A systematic review and meta-analysis of the dose-dependent effects of nicotinamide and nicotinic acid supplementation, *Nutrition Reviews* (2017), epub ahead of print, doi: 10.1093/nutrit/nux011; S. Schandelmaier and coauthors, Niacin for primary and secondary prevention of cardiovascular events, *The Cochrane Database of Systematic Reviews* 6 (2017), epub, doi: 10.1002/14651858.CD009744.pub2.

66. S. Schandelmaier and coauthors, Niacin for primary and secondary prevention of cardiovascular events, 2017; A. R. Last, J. D. Ference, and E. R. Menzel, Hyperlipidemia: Drugs for cardiovascular risk reduction in adults, *American Family Physician* 95 (2017): 78–87; W. E. Boden, M. S. Sidhu, and P. P. Toth, The therapeutic role of niacin in dyslipidemia management, *Journal of Cardiovascular Pharmacology and Therapeutics* 19 (2014): 141–158.

67. R. B. Goldberg and coauthors, Effects of extended-release niacin added to simvastatin/ezetimibe on glucose and insulin values in AIM-HIGH, *The American Journal of Medicine* 129 (2016): e13–e22; R. Haynes and K. Rahimi, Niacin: Old habits die hard, *Heart* 102 (2016): 170–171; T. J. Anderson and coauthors, Safety profile of extended-release niacin in the AIM-HIGH trial, *The New England Journal of Medicine* 371 (2014): 288–290.

68. R. Haynes and K. Rahimi, Niacin: Old habits die hard, 2016.

69. M. McGee, S. Bainbridge, and B. Fontaine-Bisson, A crucial role for maternal dietary methyl donor intake in epigenetic programming and fetal growth outcomes, *Nutrition Reviews* 76 (2018): 469–478; M. Hiraoka and Y. Kagawa, Genetic polymorphisms and folate status, *Congenital Anomalies* 57 (2017): 142–149.

70. M. Matejcic and coauthors, Biomarkers of folate and vitamin B12 and breast cancer risk: Report from the EPIC cohort, *International Journal of Cancer* 140 (2017): 1246–1259; C. D. Cantarella and coauthors, Folate deficiency as predisposing factor for childhood leukaemia: A review of the literature, *Genes & Nutrition* 12 (2017): 14; S. J. Kim and coauthors, Plasma folate, vitamin B-6, and vitamin B-12 and breast cancer risk in BRCA1- and BRCA2-mutation carriers: A prospective study, *The American Journal of Clinical Nutrition* 104 (2016): 671–677; Y. Peng, B. Dong, and Z. Wang, Serum folate concentrations and all-cause, cardiovascular disease and cancer mortality: A cohort study based on 1999–2010 National Health and Nutrition Examination Survey (NHANES), *International Journal of Cardiology* 219 (2016): 136–142; R. Wang and coauthors, Folate intake, serum folate levels, and prostate cancer risk: A meta-analysis of prospective studies, *BMC Public Health* 14 (2014): 1326.

71. A. S. Parnell and A. Correa, Analyses of trends in prevalence of congenital heart defects and folic acid supplementation, *Journal of Thoracic Disease* 9 (2017): 495–500; A. Xu and coauthors, A meta-analysis of the relationship between maternal folic acid supplementation and the risk of congenital heart defects, *International Heart Journal* 57 (2016): 725–728; A. E. Czeizel, A. Vereczkey, and I. Szabo, Folic acid in pregnant women associated with reduced prevalence of severe congenital heart defects in their children: A national population-based case-control study, *European Journal of Obstetrics, Gynecology, and Reproductive Biology* 193 (2015): 34–39.

72. M. Viswanathan and coauthors, Folic acid supplementation for the prevention of neural tube defects: An updated evidence report and systematic review for the U.S. Preventive Services Task Force, *Journal of the American Medical Association* 317 (2017): 190–203.

73. J. Williams and coauthors, Updated estimates of neural tube defect prevented by mandatory folic acid fortification—United States, 1995–2011, *Centers for Disease Control and Prevention Morbidity and Mortality Weekly Report* 64 (2015): 1–5; K. S. Crider and coauthors, Population red blood cell folate concentrations for prevention of neural tube defects: Bayesian model, *British Medical Journal* 349 (2014), epub, doi: 10.1136/bmj.g4554.

74. H. N. Moussa and coauthors, Folic acid supplementation: What is new? Fetal, obstetric, long-term benefits and risks, *Future Science Open Access* 2 (2016), epub, doi: 10.4155/fsoa-2015-0015.

75. A. M. Orozco and coauthors, Characteristics of U.S. adults with usual daily folic acid intake above the tolerable upper intake level: National Health and Nutrition Examination Survey, 2003–2010, *Nutrients* 8 (2016): 195.

76. R. H. Bahous and coauthors, High dietary folate in pregnant mice leads to pseudo-MTHFR deficiency and altered methyl metabolism, with embryonic growth delay and short-term memory impairment in offspring, *Human Molecular Genetics* 26 (2017): 888–900; K. E. Christensen and coauthors, Moderate folic acid supplementation and MTHFD1-synthetase deficiency in mice, a model for the R653Q variant, result in embryonic defects and abnormal placental development, *American Journal of Clinical Nutrition* 104 (2016): 1459–1469; A. N. Mudryi and coauthors, Folate intakes from diet and supplements may place certain Canadians at risk for folic acid toxicity, *British Journal of Nutrition* 116 (2106): 1236–1245.

77. U.S. Preventive Services Task Force, Folic Acid Supplementation for the prevention of neural tube defects: Recommendation statement, (2017), available at www.uspreventiveservicestaskforce.org/Page/Document/RecommendationStatementFinal/folic-acid-for-the-prevention-of-neural-tube-defects-preventive-medication; Scientific Report of the 2015 Dietary Guidelines Advisory Committee (2015): available at www.health.gov.

78. H. N. Moussa and coauthors, Folic acid supplementation: what is new? Fetal, obstetric, long-term benefits and risks, 2016.

79. C. Hui and coauthors, Associations between Alzheimer's Disease and blood homocysteine, vitamin B12, and folate: A case-control study, *Current Alzheimer Research* 12 (2015): 88–94.

80. A. Brito and coauthors, The human serum metabolome of vitamin B-12 deficiency and repletion, and associations with neurological function in elderly adults, *Journal of Nutrition* 147 (2017): 1839–1849; E. J. de Koning and coauthors, Effects of two-year vitamin B_{12} and folic acid supplementation on depressive symptoms and quality of life in older adults with elevated homocysteine concentrations: Additional results from the B-PROOF study, an RCT, *Nutrients* (2016), epub, doi: 10.3390/nu8110748; O. I. Okereke and coauthors, Effect of long-term supplementation with folic acid and B vitamins on risk of depression in older women, *The British Journal of Psychiatry* 206 (2015): 324–331.

81. F. Franceschi and coauthors, Role of *Helicobacter pylori* infection on nutrition and metabolism, *World Journal of Gastroenterology* 20 (2014): 12809–12817.

82. V. R. Aroda and coauthors, Long-term metformin use and vitamin B_{12} deficiency in the Diabetes Prevention Program Outcomes study, *The Journal of Clinical Endocrinology & Metabolism* 101 (2016): 1754–1761; M. A. Ahmed, G. Muntingh, and P. Rheeder, Vitamin B_{12} deficiency in metformin-treated type-2 diabetes patients, prevalence and association with peripheral neuropathy, *BioMed Central*

Pharmacology & Toxicology 17 (2016), epub, doi: 10.1186/s40360-016-0088-3; D. Kang and coauthors, Higher prevalence of metformin-induced vitamin B12 deficiency in sulfonylurea combination compared with insulin combination in patients with type 2 diabetes: A cross-sectional study, *PLoS One* 9 (2014), epub, doi: 10.1371/journal.pone.0109878.

83. J. Y. Huang and coauthors, Dietary intake of one-carbon metabolism-related nutrients and pancreatic cancer risk: The Singapore Chinese Health Study, *Cancer Epidemiology Biomarkers & Prevention* 25 (2016): 417–424; X. Wu and coauthors, The role of genetic polymorphisms as related to one-carbon metabolism, vitamin B_6, and gene-nutrient interactions in maintaining genomic stability and cell viability in Chinese breast cancer patients, *International Journal of Molecular Sciences* 17 (2016), epub, doi: 10.3390/ijms17071003; D. C. Muller and coauthors, Circulating concentrations of vitamin B_6 and kidney cancer prognosis: A prospective case-cohort study, *PLoS One* 10 (2015), epub, doi: 10.1371/journal.pone.0140677; H. Dong and coauthors, Efficacy of supplementation with B vitamins for stroke prevention: A network meta-analysis of randomized controlled trials, *PLoS One* (2015), epub, doi: 10.1371/journal.pone.0137533.

84. D. M. Mock, Biotin: From nutrition to therapeutics, *Journal of Nutrition* 147 (2017): 1487–1492; K. Dakshinamurti and coauthors, Microarray analysis of pancreatic gene expression during biotin repletion in biotin-deficient rats, *Canadian Journal of Physiology and Pharmacology* 93 (2015): 1103–1110; C. A. Perry and coauthors, Pregnancy and lactation alter biomarkers of biotin metabolism in women consuming a controlled diet, *The Journal of Nutrition* 144 (2014): 1977–1984.

85. H. T. Rajarethnem and coauthors, Combined supplementation of choline and docosahexaenoic acid during pregnancy enhances neurodevelopment of fetal hippocampus, *Neurology Research International* (2017), epub, doi 10.1155/2017/8748706; J. H. King and coauthors, Maternal choline supplementation alters fetal growth patterns in a mouse model of placental insufficiency, *Nutrients* 9 (2017): 765, doi:10.3390/nu9070765; Y. Wang and coauthors, Maternal dietary intake of choline in mice regulates development of the cerebral cortex in the offspring, *FASEB Journal* 30 (2016): 1566–1578; B. J. Strupp and coauthors, Maternal choline supplementation: A potential prenatal treatment for Down syndrome and Alzheimer's disease, *Current Alzheimer Research* 13 (2016): 97–106.

86. T. C. Wallace and V. L. Fulgoni, Assessment of total choline intakes in the United States, *Journal of the American College of Nutrition* 35 (2016): 108–112; T. C. Wallace and V. L. Fulgoni, Usual choline intakes are associated with egg and protein food consumption in the United States, *Nutrients* (2017), epub, doi: 10.3390/nu9080839.

87. B. J. Strupp and coauthors, Maternal choline supplementation: A potential prenatal

treatment for Down syndrome and Alzheimer's disease, 2016; X. Jiang, A. A. West, and M. A. Caudill, Maternal choline supplementation: A nutritional approach for improving offspring health?, *Trends in Endocrinology & Metabolism* 25 (2014): 263–273.

88. "M. Jessri, W. Y. Lou, and M. R. L'Abbe, The 2015 Dietary Guidelines for Americans is associated with a more nutrient-dense diet and a lower risk of obesity, The American Journal of Clinical Nutrition 104 (2016): 1378–1392; M. D. Hingle, J. Kandiah, and A. Maggi, Practice paper of the Academy of Nutrition and Dietetics: selecting nutrient-dense foods for good health, Journal of the Academy of Nutrition and Dietetics 116 (2016): 1473–1479."

Controversy 7

1. National Institutes of Health Office of Dietary Supplements, Multivitamin/mineral supplements (2017), available at https://ods.od.nih.gov/factsheets/MVMS-HealthProfessional/.

2. National Institutes of Health Office of Dietary Supplements, Multivitamin/mineral supplements, 2017.

3. Rao N. Rao and coauthors, An increase in dietary supplement exposures reported to US poison control centers, *Journal of Medical Toxicology* 13 (2017): 227–237.

4. A. A. Yates and coauthors, Bioactive nutrients: Time for tolerable upper intake levels to address safety, *Regulatory Toxicology and Pharmacology* 84 (2017): 94–101; A. J. Geller and coauthors, Emergency department visits for adverse events related to dietary supplements, *New England Journal of Medicine* 373 (2015): 1531–1540.

5. V. Navarro and coauthors, Liver injury from herbal and dietary supplements, *Hepatology* 65 (2017): 363–373; A. M. Abe, D. J. Hein, and P. J. Gregory, Regulatory alerts for dietary supplements in Canada and the United States, 2005-13, *American Journal of Health-System Pharmacology* 72 (2015): 966–971.

6. ConsumerLab.com, Product review: Multivitamin and multimineral supplements review, 2014, available at www.consumerlab.com.

7. P. Gusev and coauthors, Over-the-counter prenatal multivitamin/mineral products: Chemical analysis for the dietary supplement ingredient database, *Journal of the Federation of American Societies for Experimental Biology* 28 (2014): 809.3.

8. D. D. Bickle, Extraskeletal actions of vitamin D, *Annals of the New York Academy of Sciences*, 1376 (2016): 29–52; J. A. Baron and coauthors, A trial of calcium and vitamin D for the prevention of colorectal adenomas, *New England Journal of Medicine* 373 (2015): 1519–1530.

9. U.S. Preventive Services Task Force, Vitamin supplementation to prevent cancer and CVD: Preventive medication, February 2014, Final Update September 2016, available at www.uspreventiveservicestaskforce.org/Page/Document/UpdateSummaryFinal/vitamin-supplementation-to-prevent-cancer-and-cvd-counseling.

10. P. Lance and coauthors, Colorectal adenomas in participants of the SELECT random-

ized trial of selenium and vitamin e for prostate cancer prevention, *Cancer Prevention Research* 10 (2017): 45–54; B. A. Vučković and coauthors, Vitamin supplementation on the risk of venous thrombosis: Results from the MEGA case-control study, *American Journal of Clinical Nutrition* 101 (2015): 606–612.

11. U.S. Preventive Services Task Force, Vitamin supplementation to prevent cancer and CVD: Preventive medication, February 2014, Final Update September 2016.

12. L. Schwingshackl and coauthors, Dietary supplements and risk of cause-specific death, cardiovascular disease, and cancer: A systematic review and meta-analysis of primary prevention trials, *Advances in Nutrition* 8 (2017): 27–39; U.S. Preventive Services Task Force, Vitamin supplementation to prevent cancer and CVD: Preventive medication, February 2014, Final Update September 2016.

13. S. Rautiainen, and coauthors, Effect of baseline nutritional status on long-term multivitamin use and cardiovascular disease risk: A secondary analysis of the Physicians' Health Study II Randomized Clinical Trial, *JAMA Cardiology* 2 (2017): 617–625; N. G. Zaorsky and coauthors, Men's health supplement use and outcomes in men receiving definitive intensity-modulated radiation therapy for localized prostate cancer, *American Journal of Clinical Nutrition* 104 (2016): 1582–1593.

Chapter 8

1. U.S. Department of Health and Human Services and U.S. Department of Agriculture, *2015–2020 Dietary Guidelines for Americans*, 8th edition (2015), available at http://health.gov/dietaryguidelines/2015/guidelines/.

2. J. D. Adams and coauthors, Dehydration Impairs Cycling Performance, Independently of Thirst: A Blinded Study, *Medicine and Science in Sports and Exercise* 50 (2018): 1697–1703; S. N. Cheuvront and R. W. Kenefick, Dehydration: Physiology, assessment, and performance effects, *Comprehensive Physiology* 4 (2014): 257–285.

3. A. Rosinger and K. Herrick, Daily water intake among U.S. men and women, 2009–2012, *CDC Data Brief* 242 (2016), available at www.cdc.gov/nchs/products/databriefs/db242.htm.

4. Daily water intake among U.S. men and women, 2009–2012, *NCHS DataBrief* 242, April 2016.

5. World Health Organization, Drinking-water: Fact sheet, July 2017, available at www.who.int/mediacentre/factsheets/fs391/en/.

6. U.S. Environmental Protection Agency, Basic Information about lead in drinking water, 2018, available at www.epa.gov/ground-water-and-drinking-water/basic-information-about-lead-drinking-water#reducehome.

7. K. M. Benedict and coauthors, Surveillance for waterborne disease outbreaks associated with drinking water—the United States, 2013–2014, *Morbidity and Mortality Weekly Report* 66 (2017): 1216–1225; M. Hanna-Attisha and coauthors, Elevated blood lead levels in children associated with the Flint drinking water crisis:

A spatial analysis of risk and public health response, *American Journal of Public Health* 106 (2016): 283–290.

8. Flint Water Advisory Task Force Final Report, March 2016, available at www.michigan.gov/documents/snyder/FWATF_FINAL_REPORT_21March2016_517805_7.pdf.

9. Natural Resources Defense Council, The truth about tap: Lots of people think drinking bottled water is safer. Is it? January 2016, available at www.nrdc.org/stories/truth-about-tap.

10. U.S. Food and Drug Administration, FDA regulates the safety of bottled water beverages including flavored water and nutrient-added water beverages, Food Facts, 2014, available at www.fda.gov/food/foodborneillnesscontaminants/buystoreservesafefood/ucm046894.htm.

11. U.S. Department of Agriculture and U.S. Department of Health and Human Services, Scientific report of the 2015 Dietary Guidelines Advisory Committee, 2015, D-6: 8–15, available at www.health.gov; S. Agarwal and coauthors, Comparison of prevalence of inadequate nutrient intake based on body weight status of adults in the United States: An analysis of NHANES 2001–2008, *Journal of the American College of Nutrition* 7 (2015): 1–9; C. E. O'Neil and coauthors, Ethnic disparities among food sources of energy and nutrients of public health concern and nutrients to limit in adults in the United State: NHANES 2003–2006, *Food and Nutrition Research* 58 (2014): 15784.

12. I. Mosialou and coauthors, MC4R-dependent suppression of appetite by bone-derived lipocalin 2, *Nature* 543 (2017): 385–390.

13. S. L. Lennon and coauthors, 2015 evidence analysis library evidence-based nutrition practice guideline for the management of hypertension in adults, *Journal of the Academy of Nutrition and Dietetics* 117 (2017): 1445–1458; P. A. James and coauthors, 2014 evidence-based guideline for the management of high blood pressure in adults: Report from the panel members appointed to the eighth Joint National Committee (JNC 8), *Journal of the American Medical Association* 311 (2014): 507–520.

14. L. Moore-Schiltz and coauthors, Dietary intake of calcium and magnesium and the metabolic syndrome in the National Health and Nutrition Examination (NHANES) 2001–2010 data, *British Journal of Nutrition* 114 (2015): 924–935; Y. Park and J. Kim, Association of dietary vitamin D and calcium with genetic polymorphisms in colorectal neoplasia, *Journal of Cancer Prevention* 20 (2015): 97–105.

15. J. A. Beto, The role of calcium in aging, *Clinical Nutrition Research* 4 (2015): 1–8.

16. 16 D. Goltzman and coauthors, Approach to hypercalcemia, Endotext (2016), NCBI Bookshelf available at www.ncbi.nlm.nih.gov/books/NBK279129/.

17. S. Astbury and coauthors, Nutrient availability, the microbiome, and intestinal transport during pregnancy, *Applied Physiology, Nutrition, and Metabolism* 40 (2015): 1100–1106.

18. A. Fang and coauthors, Habitual dietary calcium intakes and calcium metabolism in healthy adults Chinese: A systematic review and meta-analysis, *Asia Pacific Journal of Clinical Nutrition* 25 (2016): 776–784.

19. J. Gao and coauthors, Age-related regional deterioration patterns and changes in nanoscale characterizations of trabeculae in the femoral head, *Experimental Gerontology* 62C (2015): 63–72; R. D. Jackson and W. J. Mysiw, Insights into the epidemiology of postmenopausal osteoporosis: The Women's Health Initiative, *Seminars in Reproductive Medicine* 32 (2014): 454–462.

20. R. Zhao, Z. Xu, and M. Zhao, Antiresorptive agents increase the effects of exercise on preventing postmenopausal bone loss in women: A meta-analysis, *PLoS One* 10 (2015): e0116729.

21. C. M. Weaver and coauthors, The National Osteoporosis Foundation's position statement on peak bone mass development and lifestyle factors: A systematic review and implementation recommendations, *Osteoporosis International* 27 (2016): 1281–1386.

22. U.S. Department of Health and Human Services and U.S. Department of Agriculture, *2015–2020 Dietary Guidelines for Americans*, 8th edition (2015), available at http://health.gov/dietaryguidelines/2015/guidelines/.

23. J. Uribarri and M. S. Calvo, Dietary phosphorus intake and health, *American Journal of Clinical Nutrition* 99 (2014): 247–248.

24. A. R. Chang and C. Anderson, Dietary phosphorus intake and the kidney, *Annual Review of Nutrition* 37 (2017): 321–346; R. Nicoll, J. M. Howard, and M. Y. Henein, A review of the effect of diet on cardiovascular calcification, *International Journal of Molecular Sciences* 16 (2015): 8861–8883.

25. P. L. Lutsey and coauthors, Serum magnesium, phosphorus, and calcium are associated with risk of incident heart failure: The Atherosclerosis Risk in Communities (ARIC) study, *American Journal of Clinical Nutrition* 100 (2014): 756–764; D. Kolte and coauthors, Role of magnesium in cardiovascular diseases, *Cardiology in Review* 22 (2014): 182–192.

26. S. L. Lennon and coauthors, 2015 Evidence Analysis Library evidence-based nutrition practice guideline for the management of hypertension in adults, 2017; H. Han and coauthors, Dose-response relationship between dietary magnesium intake, serum magnesium concentration and risk of hypertension: A systematic review and meta-analysis of prospective cohort studies, *Nutrition Journal* (2017), epub, doi: 10.1186/s12937-017-0247-4; X. Fang and coauthors, Dietary magnesium intake and the risk of cardiovascular disease, type 2 diabetes, and all-cause mortality: A dose-response meta-analysis of prospective cohort studies, *BMC Medicine* (2016), epub, doi: 10.1186/s12916-016-0742-z.

27. M. J. Hannon and J. G. Verbalis, Sodium homeostasis and bone, *Current Opinion in Nephrology and Hypertension* 23 (2014): 370–376.

28. S. L. Jackson and coauthors, Prevalence of excess sodium intake in the United States—NHANES, 2009–2012, *Morbidity and Mortality Weekly Report* 64 (2016): 1393–1397.

29. S. Selvaraj and coauthors, Association of estimated sodium intake with adverse cardiac structure and function, *Journal of the American College of Cardiology* 70 (2017): 715–724;U.S. Department of Agriculture and U.S. Department of Health and Human Services, Scientific report of the 2015 Dietary Guidelines Advisory Committee, 2015, D-6:4, available at www.health.gov; M. D. Ritchey and coauthors, Million hearts: Prevalence of leading cardiovascular disease risk factors—United States, 2005–2012, *Morbidity and Mortality Weekly Report* 63 (2014): 462–467.

30. 30 S. J. Taler, Initial treatment of hypertension, *New England Journal of Medicine* 378 (2018): 636–644; S. L. Lennon and coauthors, 2015 evidence analysis library evidence-based nutrition practice guideline for the management of hypertension in adults, 2017; R. H. Eckel and coauthors, 2013 AHA/ACC Guideline on Lifestyle Management to Reduce Cardiovascular Risk, *Circulation* 129 (2014): S76–S99.

31. U.S. Department of Agriculture and U.S. Department of Health and Human Services, Scientific report of the 2015 Dietary Guidelines Advisory Committee, 2015, D-6:5, available at www.health.gov.

32. N. R. C. Campbell and coauthors, 2016 Dietary Salt Fact Sheet and Call to Action: The World Hypertension League, International Society of Hypertension, and the International Council of Cardiovascular Prevention and Rehabilitation, *Journal of Clinical Hypertension* 18 (2016): 1082–1085.

33. S. Selvaraj and coauthors, Association of Estimated sodium intake with adverse cardiac structure and function, *Journal of the American College of Cardiology* 70 (2017): 715–724.

34. W. B. Farquhar and coauthors, Dietary sodium and health: More than just blood pressure, *Journal of the American College of Cardiology* 65 (2015): 1042–1050.

35. J. D. Williamson and coauthors, Intensive vs. standard blood pressure control and cardiovascular disease outcomes in adults aged ≥75 years: A randomized clinical trial, *Journal of the American Medical Association* 315 (2016): 2673–2682; A. A. Razmaria, Chronic kidney disease, *Journal of the American Medical Association* 315 (2016): 2248.

36. L. Pilic, C. R. Pedlar, and Y. Mavrommatis, Salt-sensitive hypertension: Mechanisms and effects of dietary and other lifestyle factors, *Nutrition Reviews* (2016): 645–658.

37. Y. Wang and coauthors, Genetic variants in renalase and blood pressure responses to dietary salt and potassium interventions: A family-based association study, *Kidney and Blood Pressure Research* 39 (2014): 497–506.

38. R. S. Sebastian and coauthors, Sandwiches are major contributors of sodium in the diets of American adults: Results from *What We*

Eat in America, National Health and Nutrition Examination Survey 2009–2010, *Journal of the Academy of Nutrition and Dietetics* 115 (2015): 272–277; U.S. Department of Agriculture and U.S. Department of Health and Human Services, *Scientific report of the 2015 Dietary Guidelines Advisory Committee*, 2015, D-1:39, 43–44, available at www.health.gov.

39. M. E. Cogswell and coauthors, Modeled changes in U.S. sodium intake from reducing sodium concentration of commercially processed and prepared foods to meet voluntary standards established in North American: NHANES, *American Journal of Clinical Nutrition* 106 (2017): 530–540.

40. J. M. Poti and coauthors, Sodium reduction in U.S. households' packaged food and beverage purchases, 2000 to 2014, *JAMA Internal Medicine* 177 (2017): 986-994.

41. S. P. Jurascheck and coauthors, Effects of sodium reduction and the DASH diet in relation to baseline blood pressure, *Journal of the American College of Cardiology* 70 (2017): 2841–2848; U.S. Department of Agriculture and U.S. Department of Health and Human Services, *Scientific report of the 2015 Dietary Guidelines Advisory Committee*, 2015, D-2:9–11, available at www.health.gov; M. Siervo and coauthors, Effects of the Dietary Approach to Stop Hypertension (DASH) diet on cardiovascular risk factors: A systematic review and meta-analysis, *British Journal of Nutrition* 113 (2015): 1–15.

42. Q. Li and coauthors, Enjoyment of spicy flavor enhances central salty-taste perception and reduces salt intake and blood pressure, *Hypertension* 70 (2017): 1291–1299; A. M. Janssen and coauthors, Reduced-sodium lunches are well-accepted by uninformed consumers over a 3-week period and result in decreased daily dietary sodium intakes: A randomized controlled trial, *Journal of the Academy of Nutrition and Dietetics* 115 (2015): 16141625.

43. R. H. Sterns, Disorders of plasma sodium: Causes, consequences, and correction, *New England Journal of Medicine* 372 (2015): 55–65.

44. J. Stamler and coauthors, Relation of dietary sodium (salt) to blood pressure and its possible modulation by other dietary factors, *Hypertension* (2018), epub ahead of print, doi: 10.1161/hypertensionaha.117.09928; U.S. Department of Health and Human Services and U.S. Department of Agriculture, *2015–2020 Dietary Guidelines for Americans*, 8th edition (2015), available at http://health.gov/dietaryguidelines/2015/guidelines/.

45. M. P. Vanderpump, Epidemiology of iodine deficiency, *Minerva Medica* 108 (2017): 116–123.

46. E. N. Pearce and coauthors, Consequences of iodine deficiency and excess in pregnant women: An overview of current knowns and unknowns, *American Journal of Clinical Nutrition* 104 (2016): 918S–923S.

47. Z. Abebe, E. Gebeye, and A. Tariku, Poor dietary diversity, wealth status and use of un-iodized salt are associated with goiter among school children: A cross-sectional study in Ethiopia, *BMC Public Health* (2017), epub, doi: 10.1186/s12889-016-3914-z.

48. A. D. Gernand and coauthors, Micronutrient deficiencies in pregnancy worldwide: Health effects and prevention, *Nature Reviews Endocrinology* 12 (2016): 274–289.

49. W. Chen and coauthors, Associations between iodine intake, thyroid volume, and goiter rate in school-aged Chinese children from areas with high iodine drinking water concentrations, *American Journal of Clinical Nutrition* 105 (2017): 228–233.

50. A. L. Carriquiry and coauthors, Variation in the iodine concentrations of foods: Considerations for dietary assessment, *American Journal of Clinical Nutrition* 104 (2016): 877S–887S.

51. H. Padmanabhan, M. J. Brookes, and T. Iqubal, Iron and colorectal cancer: Evidence from in vitro and animal studies, *Nutrition Reviews* 73 (2015): 308–317; H. Aljwaid and coauthors, Non-transferrin-bound iron is associated with biomarkers of oxidative stress, inflammation, and endothelial dysfunction in type 2 diabetes, *Journal of Diabetes Complications* 29 (2015): 943–949.

52. A. L. Fisher and E. Nemeth, Iron homeostasis during pregnancy, *American Journal of Clinical Nutrition* 106 (2017): 1567S–1574S; C. Cao and K. O. O'Brien, Pregnancy and iron homeostasis: An update, *Nutrition Reviews* 71 (2013): 35–51; A. A. Khalafallah and A. E. Dennis, Iron deficiency anaemia in pregnancy and postpartum: Pathophysiology and effect of oral versus intravenous iron therapy, *Journal of Pregnancy* (2012): 630519, doi:10.1155/2012/630519.

53. S. R. Pasricha, K. McHugh, H. Drakesmith, Regulation of hepcidin by erythropoiesis: The story so far, *Annual Review of Nutrition* 36 (2017): 417–434.

54. L. E. Murray-Kolb and coauthors, Consumption of iron-biofortified beans positively affects cognitive performance in 18- to 27-year old Rwandan female college students in an 18-week randomized controlled efficacy trial, *Journal of Nutrition* 147 (2017): 2109–2117; J. P. Wirth and coauthors, Predictors of anemia in women of reproductive age: Biomarkers Reflecting Inflammation and Nutritional Determinants of Anemia (BRINDA) Project, *American Journal of Clinical Nutrition* 106 (2017): 416S–427S.

55. R. A. Lumish and coauthors, Gestational iron deficiency is associated with pica behaviors in adolescents, *Journal of Nutrition* 144 (2014): 1533–1539.

56. M. S. Low and coauthors, Daily iron supplementation for improving anaemia, iron status and health in menstruating women, *Cochrane Database of Systematic Reviews* (2016), epub, doi: 10.1002/14651858.CD009747.pub2.

57. P. M. Gupta and coauthors, Iron status of toddlers, nonpregnant females, and pregnant females in the United States, *American Journal of Clinical Nutrition* 106 (2017): 1640S–1646S.

58. World Health Organization, Micronutrients: Iron deficiency anaemia, www.who.int/nutrition/topics/ida/en, January 2017.

59. H. Padmanabhan, M. J. Brookes, and T. Iqbal, Iron and colorectal cancer: Evidence from in vitro and animal studies, *Nutrition Reviews* 73 (2015): 308–317.

60. P. C. Adams, Epidemiology and diagnostic testing for hemochromatosis and iron overload, *International Journal of Laboratory Hematology* 37 (2015): 25–30; E. Gammella and coauthors, Iron-induced damage in cardiomyopathy: Oxidative-dependent and independent mechanisms, *Oxidative Medicine and Cellular Longevity* 2015 (2015): 230182.

61. M. L. Maia and coauthors, Invariant natural killer T cells are reduced in hereditary hemochromatosis patients, *Journal of Clinical Immunology* 35 (2015): 68–74.

62. F. Wang and coauthors, Zinc might prevent heat-induced hepatic injury by activating the Nrf2-antioxidant in mice, *Biological Trace Element Research* 165 (2015): 86–95; P. I. Oteiza, Zinc and the modulation of redox homeostasis, *Free Radical Biology and Medicine* 53 (2012): 1748–1759.

63. D. C. Hamm, E. R. Bondra, and M. M. Harrison, Transcriptional activation is a conserved feature of the early embryonic factor Zelda that requires a cluster of four zinc fingers for DNA binding and a low-complexity activation domain, *Journal of Biological Chemistry* 290 (2014): 3508–3518; S. D. Gower-Winter and C. W. Levenson, Zinc in the central nervous system: From molecules to behavior, *Biofactors* 38 (2012): 186–193.

64. M. Maares and H. Haase, Zinc and immunity: An essential interrelation, *Archives of Biochemistry and Biophysics* 611 (2016): 58–65.

65. S. C. Liberato, G. Singh, and K. Mulholland, Zinc supplementation in young children: A review of the literature focusing on diarrhoea prevention and treatment, *Clinical Nutrition* 34 (2015): 181–188.

66. Liberato and coauthors, Zinc supplementation in young children, 2015; E. Mayo-Wilson and coauthors, Zinc supplementation for preventing mortality, morbidity, and growth failure in children aged 6 months to 12 years of age, *Cochrane Database of Systematic Reviews* (2014), doi:10.1002/14651858.CD009384.pub2.

67. R. R. Das and M. Singh, Oral zinc for the common cold, *Journal of the American Medical Association* 311 (2014): 1440–1441.

68. B. Farmer, Nutritional adequacy of plant-based diets for weight management: Observations from the NHANES, *American Journal of Clinical Nutrition* 100 (2014): 365S–368S; M. Foster and coauthors, Effect of vegetarian diets on zinc status: A systematic review and meta-analysis of studies in humans, *Journal of the Science of Food and Agriculture* 93 (2013): 2362–2371.

69. A. H. Rose and P. R. Hoffmann, Selenoproteins and cardiovascular stress, *Thrombosis and Haemostasis* 113 (2015): 494–504; Z. Zhang, J. Zhang, and J. Xiao, Selenoproteins and selenium status in bone physiology and pathology, *Biochemica et Biophysica Acta* 1840 (2014): 3246–3256.

70. K. E. Geillinger and coauthors, Hepatic metabolite profiles in mice with a suboptimal selenium status, *Journal of Nutritional Biochemistry* 25 (2014): 914–922.

71. F. Brigo and coauthors, Selenium supplementation for primary prevention of cardiovascular disease: Proof of no effectiveness, *Nutrition, Metabolism, and Cardiovascular Diseases* 24 (2014): e2–e3.

72. K. S. Prabhu and X. G. Lei, Selenium, *Advanced Nutrition* 15 (2016): 415–417; N. Babaknejad and coauthors, The relationship between selenium levels and breast cancer: A systematic review and meta-analysis, *Biological Trace Element Research* 159 (2014): 1–7.

73. M. Vinceti and coauthors, Selenium for preventing cancer, *Cochrane Database of Systematic Reviews* 3 (2014): CD005195; S. A. Kenfield and coauthors, Selenium supplementation and prostate cancer mortality, *Journal of the National Cancer Institute* 107 (2014): 360.

74. P. Agarwal, S. Sharma, and U. S. Agarwal, Selenium toxicity: A rare diagnosis, *Indian Journal of Dermatology, Venereology and Leprology* 82 (2016): 690–693.

75. E. J. Joy and coauthors, Soil type influences crop mineral composition in Malawi, *Science of the Total Environment* 505 (2015): 587–595.

76. J. P. Brown and coauthors, The dynamic behavior of the early dental caries lesion in caries-active adults and implications, *Community Dentistry and Oral Epidemiology* (2015), doi:10.1111/cdoe.

77. D. M. Proctor and coauthors, Assessment of the mode of action for hexavalent chromium-induced lung cancer following inhalation exposures, *Toxicology* 325 (2014): 160–179.

78. National Institutes of Health, Chromium: Dietary supplement fact sheet, March 2018, available at https://ods.od.nih.gov/factsheets /Chromium-HealthProfessional/; N. J. Hoffman and coauthors, Chromium enhances insulin responsiveness via AMPK, *Journal of Nutritional Biochemistry* 25 (2014): 565–572.

79. S. Zlatic and coauthors, Molecular basis of neurodegeneration and neurodevelopmental defects in Menkes disease, *Neurobiology of Disease* (2015), doi:10.1016/j.nbd.2014.12.024; O. Bandmann, K. H. Weiss, and S. G. Kaler, Wilson's disease and other neurological copper disorders, *Lancet Neurology* 14 (2015): 103–113.

Consumer's Guide 8

1. A. Qaseem and coauthors, Dietary and pharmacologic management to prevent recurrent nephrolithiasis in adults: A clinical practice guideline from the American College of Physicians, *Annals of Internal Medicine* 161 (2014): 659–667.

2. K. L. Stanhope, Sugar consumption, metabolic disease and obesity: The state of the controversy, *Critical Reviews in Clinical Laboratory Sciences* (2015), epub, doi: 10.3109/10408363.2015.1084990; M. Siervo and coauthors, Sugar consumption and global prevalence of obesity and hypertension:

An ecological analysis, *Public Health Nutrition* 17 (2014): 587–596.

3. B. M. Popkin and C. Hawkes, Sweetening of the global diet, particularly beverages: Patterns, trends, and policy responses, *Lancet. Diabetes and Endocrinology* 4 (2016): 174–186; Q. Yang and coauthors, Added sugar intake and cardiovascular diseases mortality among U.S. adults, *Journal of the American Medical Association Internal Medicine* 174 (2014): 516–524.

Controversy 8

1. National Osteoporosis Foundation, www.nof .org, January 2017.

2. C. M. Weaver and coauthors, The National Osteoporosis Foundation's position statement on peak bone mass development and lifestyle factors: A systematic review and implementation recommendations, *Osteoporosis International* 27 (2016): 1281–1386.

3. A. Bachelot and coauthors, Poor compliance to hormone therapy and decreased bone mineral density in women with premature ovarian insufficiency, *PLoS One* (2016), epub, doi: 10.1371/ journal.pone.0164638; N. Kurtoglu-Aksoy and coauthors, Implications of premature ovarian failure on bone turnover markers and bone mineral density, *Clinical and Experimental Obstetrics and Gynecology* 41 (2014): 149–153.

4. T. Willson and coauthors, The clinical epidemiology of male osteoporosis: A review of the recent literature, *Clinical Epidemiology* 7 (2015): 65–76; A. D. Manthripragada and coauthors, Fracture incidence in a large cohort of men age 30 years and older with osteoporosis, *Osteoporosis International* 26 (2015): 1619–1627.

5. N. Lucif and coauthors, Association between plasma testosterone level and bone mineral density in healthy elderly men, *Journal of the American Geriatrics Society* 62 (2014): 981–982; L. Modekilde, P. Vestergaard, and L. Rejnmark, The pathogenesis, treatment and prevention of osteoporosis in men, *Drugs* 73 (2013): 15–29.

6. E. Nieschlag, Current topics in testosterone replacement of hypogonadal men, *Best Practice and Research: Clinical Endocrinology and Metabolism* 29 (2015): 77–90.

7. P. Zhang and coauthors, Visceral adiposity is negatively associated with bone density and muscle attenuation, *American Journal of Clinical Nutrition* 101 (2015): 337–343; P. Y. Liu and coauthors, New insight into fat, muscle and bone relationship in women: Determining the threshold at which body fat assumes negative relationship with bone mineral density, *International Journal of Preventive Medicine* 5 (2014): 1452–1463.

8. J. Xu and coauthors, Effects of exercise on bone status in female subjects, from young girls to postmenopausal women: An overview of systematic reviews and meta-analyses, *Sports Medicine* 46 (2016): 1165–1182; J. M. Lappe and coauthors, The longitudinal effects of physical activity and dietary calcium on bone mass accrual across stages of pubertal development, *Journal of Bone and Mineral Research* 30 (2015): 156–164.

9. K. G. Avin and coauthors, Biomechanical aspects of the muscle-bone interaction, *Current Osteoporosis Reports* 13 (2015): 1–8.

10. A. A. Shanb and E. F. Youssef, The impact of adding weight-bearing exercise versus nonweight bearing programs to the medical treatment of elderly patients with osteoporosis, *Journal of Family and Community Medicine* 21 (2014): 176–181; M. Behringer and coauthors, Effects of weight-bearing activities on bone mineral content and density in children and adolescents: A meta-analysis, *Journal of Bone and Mineral Research* 29 (2014): 467–478.

11. R. I. Ray and coauthors, Predictors of poor clinical outcome following hip fracture in middle aged-patients, *Injury* (2014), doi: 10.1016 /j.injury.2014.11.005.

12. G. W. Gaddini and coauthors, Twelve months of voluntary heavy alcohol consumption in male rhesus macaques suppresses intracortical bone remodeling, *Bone* 71 (2015): 227–236; D. B. Maurel and coauthors, Alcohol and bone: Review of dose effects and mechanisms, *Osteoporosis International* 23 (2012): 1–16.

13. C. M. Weaver and coauthors, The National Osteoporosis Foundation's position statement on peak bone mass development and lifestyle factors: A systematic review and implementation recommendations, 2016.

14. T. T. Fung and coauthors, Soda consumption and risk of hip fractures in postmenopausal women in the Nurses' Health Study, *American Journal of Clinical Nutrition* 100 (2014): 953–958.

15. M. Halfon, O. Phan, and D. Teta, Vitamin D: A review on its effects on muscle strength, the risk of fall, and frailty, *BioMed Research International* (2015), epub, doi. org/10.1155/2015/953241; V. A. Moyer and the U.S. Preventive Services Task Force, Vitamin D and calcium supplementation to prevent fractures in adults: U.S. Preventive Services Task Force recommendation statement, *Annals of Internal Medicine* 158 (2013): 691–696.

16. J. P. Bonjour, The dietary protein, IGF-I, skeletal health axis, *Hormone Molecular Biology and Clinical Investigation* 28 (2016): 39–53; P. D. Genaro and coauthors, Dietary protein intake in elderly women: Association with muscle and bone mass, *Nutrition in Clinical Practice* 30 (2015): 283–289.

17. T. Hu and coauthors, Protein intake and lumbar bone density: The multi-ethnic study of atherosclerosis (MESA), *British Journal of Nutrition* 112 (2014): 1384–1392.

18. K. L. Tucker, Vegetarian diets and bone status, *American Journal of Clinical Nutrition* 100 (2014): 329S–335S; A. R. Mangels, Bone nutrients for vegetarians, *American Journal of Clinical Nutrition* 100 (2014): 469S–475S.

19. G. Hao and coauthors, Vitamin K intake and the risk of fractures: A meta-analysis, *Medicine* (Baltimore) 96 (2017), epub, doi: 10.1097/MD.0000000000006725.

20. T. S. Orchard and coauthors, Magnesium intake, bone mineral density, and fractures:

Results from the Women's Health Initiative Observational Study, *American Journal of Clinical Nutrition* 99 (2014): 926–933.

21. M. S. LeBoff and coauthors, VITAL-Bone Health: Rationale and design of two ancillary studies evaluating the effects of vitamin D and/or omega-3 fatty acid supplements on incident fractures and bone health outcomes in the Vitamin D and OmegA-3 Trial, *Contemporary Clinical Trials* (2015), doi: 10.1016/j.cct.2015.01.007; T. S. Orchard and coauthors, A systematic review of omega-3 fatty acids and osteoporosis, *British Journal of Nutrition* 107 (2012): S253–S260.

22. North American Menopause Society, 2017 hormone therapy position statement, *Journal of the North American Menopause Society* 24 (2017): 728–753; R. D. Langer, The evidence base for HRT: What can we believe? *Climacteric* 20 (2017): 91–96; R. A. Lobo and coauthors, Back to the future: Hormone replacement therapy as part of a prevention strategy for women at the onset of menopause, *Atherosclerosis* 254 (2016): 282–290.

23. J. Hess and J. Slavin, Snacking for a cause: Nutritional insufficiencies and excesses of U.S. children: A critical review of food consumption patterns and macronutrient and micronutrient intake of U.S. children, *Nutrients* 6 (2014): 4750–4759.

24. S. D. Crockett and coauthors, Calcium and vitamin D supplementation and increased risk of serrated polyps: Results from a randomised clinical trial, *Gut* (2018), epub ahead of print, doi: 10.1136.gutjnl-2017-315242; N. C. Harvey and coauthors, The role of calcium supplementation in healthy musculoskeletal aging: An expert consensus meeting of the European Society for Clinical and Economic Aspects of Osteoporosis, Osteoarthritis and Musculoskeletal Diseases (ESCEO) and the International Foundation for Osteoporosis (IOF), *Osteoporosis International* (2017): 447–462; J. J. B. Anderson and coauthors, Calcium intake from diet and supplements and the risk of coronary artery calcification and its progression among older adults: 10-year follow-up of the Multi-Ethnic Study of Atherosclerosis (MESA), *Journal of the American Heart Association* 5 (2016): e003815; J. R. Lewis and coauthors, The effects of calcium supplementation on verified coronary heart disease hospitalization and death in postmenopausal women: A collaborative meta-analysis of randomized controlled trials, *Journal of Bone and Mineral Research* 30 (2015): 165–175; C. S. Shin and K. M. Kim, The risks and benefits of calcium supplementation, *Endocrinology and Metabolism* 30 (2015): 27–34; D. Challoumas and coauthors, Effects of combined vitamin D-calcium supplements on the cardiovascular system: Should we be cautious? *Atherosclerosis* 238 (2015): 388–398.

25. J. Zhao and coauthors, Association between calcium or vitamin D supplementation and fracture incidence in community-dwelling older adults: A systematic review and meta-analysis, *Journal of the American Medical Association* 318 (2017): 2466–2482; V. A. Moyer and the U.S. Preventive Services Task Force, Vitamin D and calcium supplementation to prevent fractures in adults, 2013.

26. S. L. Lennon and coauthors, 2015 evidence analysis library evidence-based nutrition practice guideline for the management of hypertension in adults, *Journal of the Academy of Nutrition and Dietetics* 117 (2017): 1445–1458.

27. U.S. Department of Agriculture and U.S. Department of Health and Human Services, Scientific Report of the 2015 Dietary Guidelines Advisory Committee, 2015, D-1:18, available at www.health.gov.

Chapter 9

1. C. M. Hales and coauthors, Prevalence of obesity among adults and youth: United States, 2015–2016, *NCHS Data Brief* 288 (2017), available at www.cdc.gov/nchs/products/databriefs/db288.htm; National Center for Health Statistics, *Health, United States, 2015: With Special Feature on Racial and Ethnic Health Disparities*, Report No.: 2016-1232, (Hyattsville, MD: 2016).

2. The GBD 2015 Obesity Collaborators, Health effects of overweight and obesity in 195 countries over 25 years, *New England Journal of Medicine* 377 (2017): 13–27; World Health Organization, Obesity and overweight fact sheet, June 2016, available at www.who.int/mediacentre/factsheets/fs311/en.

3. W. Dietz, Current epidemiology of obesity in the United States, in *The Current State of Obesity Solutions in the United States* (Washington, D.C.: National Academies Press, 2014), pp. 5–14.

4. Global BMI Mortality Collaboration, Body-mass index and all cause mortality: Individual-participant-data meta-analysis of 239 prospective studies in four continents, *Lancet* 388 (2017): 776–786; C. D. Fryar and C. L. Ogden, Prevalence of underweight among adults aged 20 and over: United States, 1960–1962 through 2011–2012, NCHS Health E-Stats, updated September 2014, available at www.cdc.gov/nchs/data/hestat/underweight_adult_11_12/underweight_adult_11_12.htm.

5. Centers for Disease Control and Prevention, Obesity is common, serious and costly, Obesity and Overweight Facts, updated September 2017, available at www.cdc.gov/chronicdisease/overview/index.htm.

6. Global BMI Mortality Collaboration, Body-mass index and all cause mortality: Individual-participant-data meta-analysis of 239 prospective studies in four continents, 2017; A. V. Patel, J. S. Hildebrand, and S. M. Gapstur, Body mass index and all-cause mortality in a large prospective cohort of white and black U.S. adults, *PLoS One* 9 (2014), epub, doi: 10.1371/journal.pone.0109153.

7. L. A. Smith and coauthors, Translating mechanism-based strategies to break the obesity-cancer link: A narrative review, *Journal of the Academy of Nutrition and Dietetics* 118 (2018): 652–657; The GBD 2015 Obesity Collaborators, Health effects of overweight and obesity in 195 countries over 25 years, 2017; M. Bastien and coauthors, Overview of epidemiology and contribution of obesity to cardiovascular disease, *Progress in Cardiovascular Diseases* 56 (2014): 369–381; V. G. Gilby and T. A. Ajith, Role of adipokines and peroxisome proliferator-activated receptors in nonalcoholic fatty liver disease, *World Journal of Hepatology* 6 (2014): 570–579.

8. D. N. Lorenzo and V. Bennett, Cell-autonomous adiposity through increased cell surface GLUT4 due to ankyrin-B deficiency, Proceedings of the National Academy of Sciences of the United States of America 114 (2017): 12743–12748; N. Sattar and J. M. R. Gill, Type 2 diabetes as a disease of ectopic fat? *BMC Medicine* 12 (2014), epub, doi: 10.1186/s12916-014-0123-4.

9. A. Rodríguez and coauthors, Revisiting the adipocyte: A model for integration of cytokine signaling and the regulation of energy metabolism, *American Journal of Physiology: Endocrinology and Metabolism* (2015), epub, doi: 10.1152/ajpendo.00297.2015; H. J. Yoo and K. M. Choi, Adipokines as a novel link between obesity and atherosclerosis, *World Journal of Diabetes* 5 (2014): 357–363.

10. J. I. Mechanick, D. L. Hurley, and W. T. Garvey, Adiposity-based chronic disease as a new diagnostic term: The American Association of Clinical Endocrinologists and American College of Endocrinology Position statement, *Endocrine Practice* 23 (2017): 372–378.

11. J. J. Lee and coauthors, Association of changes in abdominal fat quantity and quality with incident cardiovascular disease risk factors, *Journal of the American College of Cardiology* 68 (2016): 1509–1521; Bastien and coauthors, Overview of epidemiology and contribution of obesity to cardiovascular disease, 2014; J. R. Cerhan and coauthors, A pooled analysis of waist circumference and mortality in 650,000 adults, *Mayo Clinic Proceedings* 89 (2014): 335–345.

12. S. Sharma and coauthors, Normal-weight central obesity and mortality risk in older adults with coronary artery disease, *Mayo Clinic Proceedings* 91 (2016): 343–351; K. R. Sahakyan and coauthors, Normal-weight central obesity: Implications for total and cardiovascular mortality, *Annals of Internal Medicine* 163 (2015): 827–835; A. Steffen and coauthors, General and abdominal obesity and risk of esophageal and gastric adenocarcinoma in the European Prospective Investigation into Cancer and Nutrition, *International Journal of Cancer* 137 (2015): 646–657.

13. D. Mozaffarian and coauthors, Heart disease and stroke statistics—2015 update: A report from the American Heart Association, *Circulation* 131 (2015): e29–322.

14. Lee and coauthors, Association of changes in abdominal fat quantity and quality with incident cardiovascular disease risk factors, 2016.

15. G. Traversy and J. P. Chaput, Alcohol consumption and obesity: An update, *Current Obesity Reports* 4 (2015): 122–130; A. Philipsen and coauthors, Associations of objectively

measured physical activity and abdominal fat distribution, *Medicine and Science in Sports and Exercise* 47 (2015): 983–989.

16. American College of Cardiology/American Heart Association Task Force on Practice Guidelines and the Obesity Society, Executive summary: Guidelines for the management of overweight and obesity in adults, *Obesity* 22 (2014): S5–S39.

17. G. H. Goossens, The metabolic phenotype in obesity: Fat mass, body fat distribution, and adipose tissue function, *Obesity Facts* 10 (2017): 207–215; P. D. Loprinzi and E. Frith, Cardiometabolic healthy obesity paradigm and all-cause mortality risk, *European Journal of Internal Medicine* 43 (2017): 42–45.

18. S. W. Flint and coauthors, Obesity discrimination in the recruitment process: "You're Not Hired!" *Frontiers of Psychology* 7 (2016): 657; J. Locher and D. Allison, Fat tax: Weight penalties for women in academia throughout their lifetimes, *Association for Women in Science Magazine* (Spring 2016): 38–39.

19. E. Manzato and coauthors, Risk factors for weight gain: A longitudinal study in non-weight loss treatment-seeking overweight adults, *Eating and Weight Disorders* 20 (2015): 371–378; A. R. Sutin and A. Terracciano, Perceived weight discrimination and obesity, *PLoS One* (2014), epub, doi: 10.1371/journal. pone.0070048; G. M. Coelho, Prevention of eating disorders in female athletes, *Journal of Sports Medicine* (2014), epub, doi: 10.2147/ OAJSM.S36528.

20. H. Banack and coauthors, Is BMI a valid measure of obesity in postmenopausal women? *Menopause* 25 (2017): 307–313; N. Stefan, F. Schick, and H. U. Häring, Causes, characteristics, and consequences of metabolically unhealthy normal weight in humans, *Cell Metabolism* 26 (2017): 292–300; P. B. Maffetone, I. Rivera-Dominguez, and P. B. Laursen, Overfat adults and children in developed countries: The public health importance of identifying excess body fat, *Frontiers of Public Health* (2017), epub, doi: 10.3389/fpubh.2017.00190.

21. D. Gallagher and coauthors, Changes in skeletal muscle and organ size after a weight-loss intervention in overweight and obese type 2 diabetic patients, *American Journal of Clinical Nutrition* 105 (2017): 78–84.

22. O. A. Massadi and coauthors, What is the real relevance of endogenous ghrelin? *Peptides* 70 (2015): 1–6.

23. G. D. M. Potter and coauthors, Longer sleep is associated with lower BMI and favorable metabolic profiles in UK adults: Findings from the National Diet and Nutrition Survey, *PLoS One* (2017), epub, doi: 10.1371/journal. pone.0182195; J. L. Broussard and coauthors, Elevated ghrelin predicts food intake during experimental sleep restriction, *Obesity* (Silver Spring) 24 (2016): 132–138; H. K. Al Khatib and coauthors, The effects of partial sleep deprivation on energy balance: A systematic review and meta-analysis, *European Journal of Clinical Nutrition* (2016): doi: 10.1038/ejcn.2016.201; H.

S. Dashti and coauthors, Habitual sleep duration is associated with BMI and macronutrient intake and may be modified by CLOCK genetic variants, *American Journal of Clinical Nutrition* 101 (2015): 135–143.

24. L. Sominsky and S. J. Spencer, Eating behavior and stress: A pathway to obesity, *Frontiers in Psychology* 5 (2014), epub, doi: 10.3389/fpsyg.2014.00434.

25. M. A. Deluca, Habituation of the responsiveness of mesolimbic and mesocortical dopamine transmission to taste stimuli, *Frontiers in Integrative Neuroscience* 8 (2014), epub, doi: 10.3389/fnint.2014.00021.

26. I. Momken and coauthors, A new leptin-mediated mechanism for stimulating fatty acid oxidation: A pivotal role for sarcolemmal FAT/CD36, *Biochemical Journal* 474 (2017): 149–162; M. B. Allison and M. G. Myers Jr., Connecting leptin signaling to biological function, *Journal of Endocrinology* 223 (2014), epub, doi: 10.1530/JOE-14-0404; C. Sobrino Crespo and coauthors, Peptides and food intake, *Frontiers in Endocrinology* 5 (2014), epub, doi: 10.3389/fendo.2014.00058R.

27. H. K. Park and R. S. Ahima, Physiology of leptin: Energy homeostasis, neuroendocrine function and metabolism, *Metabolism* 64 (2015): 24–34; A. B. Crujeiras and coauthors, Leptin resistance in obesity: An epigenetic landscape, *Life Sciences* 140 (2015): 57–63.

28. C. D. Morrison and T. Laeger, Protein-dependent regulation of feeding and metabolism, *Trends in Endocrinology and Metabolism* 26 (2015): 256–262.

29. B. Burton-Freeman and coauthors, Ratios of soluble and insoluble dietary fibers on satiety and energy intake in overweight pre- and postmenopausal women, *Nutrition and Healthy Aging* 4 (2017): 157–168.

30. T. S. Bruna and coauthors, A systematic review and meta-analysis of the prebiotics and synbiotics effects on glycaemia, insulin concentrations and lipid parameters in adult patients with overweight or obesity, *Clinical Nutrition* 34 (2015): 845–858.

31. E. Ferrannini, M. Rosenbaum, and R. O. Leibel, The threshold shift paradigm of obesity: Evidence from surgically induced weight loss, *American Journal of Clinical Nutrition* 100 (2014): 996–1002.

32. S. Kajimura and M. Saito, A new era in brown adipose tissue biology: Molecular control of brown fat development and energy homeostasis, *Annual Review of Physiology* 76 (2014): 225–249.

33. I. Shimizu and coauthors, Vascular rarefaction mediates whitening of brown fat in obesity, *Journal of Clinical Investigation* 124 (2014): 2099–2112.

34. A. Vargas-Castillo and coauthors, Understanding the biology of thermogenic fat: Is browning a new approach to the treatment of obesity? *Archives of Medical Research* 48 (2017): 401–413; P. Lee and coauthors, Irisin and FGF21 are cold-induced endocrine activators of

brown fat function in humans, *Cell Metabolism* 19 (2014): 302–309; Y. Oiq and coauthors, Eosinophils and type 2 cytokine signaling in macrophages orchestrate development of functional beige fat, *Cell* 157 (2014): 1292–1308.

35. F. B. Seganfredo and coauthors, Weight-loss interventions and gut microbiota changes in overweight and obese patients: A systematic review, *Obesity Reviews* 10 (2017): 832–851; M. E. Dumas and coauthors, Microbial-host cometabolites are prodromal markers predicting phenotypic heterogeneity in behavior, obesity, and impaired glucose tolerance, *Cell Reports* 20 (2017): 136–148; C. Graham, A. Mullen, and K. Whelan, Obesity and the gastrointestinal microbiota: A review of associations and mechanisms, *Nutrition Reviews* 73 (2015): 376–385.

36. R. C. Schugar and coauthors, The TMAO-producing enzyme flavin-containing monooxygenase 3 regulates obesity and the beiging of white adipose tissue, *Cell Reports* 19 (2017): 2451–2461.

37. M. K. Hamilton and H. E. Raybould, Bugs, guts and brains, and the regulation of food intake and body weight, *International Journal of Obesity* 6 (2016): S8–S14; Graham, Mullen, and Whelan, Obesity and the gastrointestinal microbiota: A review of associations and mechanisms, 2015.

38. D. K. Dahiya and coauthors, Gut microbiota modulation and its relationship with obesity using prebiotic fibers and probiotics: A review, *Frontiers in Microbiology* (2017), epub, doi: 10.3389/fmicb.2017.00563.

39. A. E. Locke and coauthors, Genetic studies of body mass index yield new insights for obesity biology, *Nature* 518 (2015): 197–206; D. Shungin and coauthors, New genetic loci link adipose and insulin biology to body fat distribution, *Nature* 518 (2015): 187–196."

40. D. N. Lorenzo and V. Bennett, Cell-autonomous adiposity through increased cell surface GLUT4 due to ankyrin-B deficiency, Proceedings of the National Academy of Sciences of the United States of America 114 (2017): 12743–12748.

41. B. de Lauzon-Guillain and coauthors, Mediation and modification of genetic susceptibility to obesity by eating behaviors, *American Journal of Clinical Nutrition* 106 (2017): 996–1004.

42. I. C. de Macedo, I. S. de Freitas, and I. L. da Silva Torres The influence of palatable diets in reward system activation: A mini review, *Advances in Pharmacological Sciences* (2016), epub, doi: 10.1155/2016/7238679; T. South and coauthors, Rats eat a cafeteria-style diet to excess but eat smaller amounts and less frequently when tested with chow, *PLoS One* 9 (2014), epub, doi: 10.1371/journal. pone.0093506.

43. A. C. Reichelt, M. J. Morris, and R. R. Westbrook, Cafeteria diet impairs expression of sensory-specific satiety and stimulus-outcome learning, *Frontiers in Psychology* 5 (2014), epub, doi: 10.3389/fpsyg.2014.00852.

44. B. Wansink and J. Kim, Bad popcorn in big buckets: Portion size can influence intakes as much as taste, *Journal of Nutrition Education and Behavior* 37 (2005): 242–245.

45. B. Wansink, K. van Ittersum, and C. R. Payne, Larger bowl size increases the amount of cereal children request, consume, and waste, *Journal of Pediatrics* 164 (2014): 323–326.

46. A. Carter and coauthors, The neurobiology of "food addiction" and its implications for obesity treatment and policy, *Annual Review of Nutrition* 36 (2016): 105–128.

47. G. Wang and coauthors, Brain dopamine and obesity, *Lancet* 357 (2001): 354–357.

48. de Macedo, de Freitas, and da Silva Torres The influence of palatable diets in reward system activation: A mini review, 2016.

49. A. Sfera and coauthors, The obesity-impulsivity axis: Potential metabolic interventions in chronic psychiatric patients, *Frontiers in Psychiatry* (2017), epub, doi: 10.3389/fpsyt.2017.00020; A. Michaud and coauthors, Overlapping neural endophenotypes in addiction and obesity, *Frontiers in Endocrinology* (2017), epub, doi: 10.3389/fendo.2017.00127.

50. A. Garfinkel-Castro and coauthors, Obesity and the built environment at different urban scales: Examining the literature, *Nutrition Reviews* 75, Supplement 1 (2017): 51–61.

51. D. W. Barnett and coauthors, Built environmental correlates of older adults' total physical activity and walking: A systematic review and meta-analysis, *International Journal of Behavior, Nutrition, and Physical Activity* (2017), epub, doi: 10.1186/s12966-017-0558-z.

52. A. Feathers and coauthors, Food environments are relevant to recruitment and adherence in dietary modification trials, *Nutrition Research* 35 (2015): 480–488; C. Larson and coauthors, Development of a community-sensitive strategy to increase availability of fresh fruits and vegetables in Nashville's urban food deserts, *Preventing Chronic Disease* 10 (2014), epub, doi: 10.5888/pcd10.130008; N. M. Wedick and coauthors, Access to healthy food stores modifies effect of a dietary intervention, *American Journal of Preventive Medicine* (2014), epub, doi: 10.1016/j.amepre.2014.08.020.

53. T. Dubowitz and coauthors, Healthy food access for urban food desert residents: Examination of the food environment, food purchasing practices, diet and BMI, *Public Health Nutrition* 18 (2015): 2220–2230.

54. D. McDermot, B. Igoe, and M. Stahre, Assessment of healthy food availability in Washington state—Questioning the food desert paradigm, *Journal of Nutrition Education and Behavior* 49 (2017): 130–136.

55. 55 Institute of Medicine, Committee on Accelerating Progress in Obesity Prevention, *Accelerating progress in obesity prevention: Solving the weight of the nation* (Washington, D.C.: National Academies Press, 2012), available at www.nap.edu.

56. J. Cawley, D. Dragone, and S. Von Hinke Kessler Scholder, The demand for cigarettes as derived from the demand for weight loss: A theoretical and empirical investigation, *Health Economics* 25 (2015): 8–23.

57. S. M. Raefsky and M. P. Mattson, Adaptive responses of neuronal mitochondria to bioenergetic challenges: Roles in neuroplasticity and disease resistance, *Free Radicals In Biology and Medicine* 102 (2017): 203–216; T. Murphy, G. P. Dias, and S. Thuret, Effects of diet on brain plasticity in animal and human studies: Mind the gap, *Neural Plasticity* (2014), epub, doi: 10.1155/2014/563160; C. Baumeier and coauthors, Caloric restriction and intermittent fasting alter hepatic lipid droplet proteome and diacylglycerol species and prevent diabetes in NZO mice, *Biochimica et Biophysica Acta* 1851 (2015): 566–576; N. Makino and coauthors, Calorie restriction increases telomerase activity, enhances autophagy, and improves diastolic dysfunction in diabetic rat hearts, *Molecular and Cellular Biochemistry* 403 (2015): 1–11; S. E. Olivo-Marston and coauthors, Effects of calorie restriction and diet-induced obesity on murine colon carcinogenesis, growth and inflammatory factors, and microRNA expression, *PLoS One* (2014), epub, doi: 10.1371/journal.pone.0094765; R. J. Colman and coauthors, Caloric restriction reduces age-related and all-cause mortality in rhesus monkeys, *Nature Communications* (2014), epub, doi: 10.1038/ncomms4557; M. P. Mattson, Interventions that improve body and brain bioenergetics for Parkinson's disease risk reduction and therapy, *Journal of Parkinson's Disease* 4 (2014): 1–13; V. D. Longo and M. P. Mattson, Fasting: Molecular mechanisms and clinical applications, *Cell Metabolism* 19 (2014): 181–192.

58. R. E. Patterson and D. D. Sears, Metabolic effects of intermittent fasting, *Annual Review of Nutrition* 37 (2017): 371–393.

59. M. Harvie and A. Howell, Potential benefits and harms of intermittent energy restriction and intermittent fasting amongst obese, overweight and normal weight subjects—A narrative review of human and animal evidence, *Behavioral Sciences* (2017), epub, doi: 103390/bs7010004.

60. J. F. Trepanowski, C. M. Kroeger, and Adrienne Barnosky, Effect of alternate-day fasting on weight loss, weight maintenance, and cardioprotection among metabolically healthy obese adults, *JAMA Internal Medicine* 177 (2017): 930–938.

61. Position of the Academy of Nutrition and Dietetics: Interventions for the treatment of overweight and obesity in adults, *Journal of the Academy of Nutrition and Dietetics* 116 (2016): 129–147.

62. U.S. Department of Agriculture and U.S. Department of Health and Human Services, Scientific report of the 2015 Dietary Guidelines Advisory Committee, 2015, D-2:66, available at www.health.gov; D. J. Johns and coauthors, Diet or exercise interventions vs. combined behavioral weight management programs: A systematic review and meta-analysis of direct comparisons, *Journal of the Academy of Nutrition and Dietetics* 114 (2014): 1557–1568.

63. Position of the Academy of Nutrition and Dietetics: Interventions for the treatment of overweight and obesity in adults, 2016.

64. Position of the Academy of Nutrition and Dietetics: Interventions for the treatment of overweight and obesity in adults, *Journal of the Academy of Nutrition and Dietetics* 116 (2016): 129–147; American College of Cardiology/American Heart Association Task Force on Practice Guidelines and the Obesity Society, Executive summary: Guidelines (2013) for the management of overweight and obesity in adults, 2014.

65. M. Jessri, W. Y. Lou, and M. R. L'Abbé, The 2015 Dietary Guidelines for Americans is associated with a more nutrient-dense diet and a lower risk of obesity, *American Journal of Clinical Nutrition* 104 (2016): 1378–1392; U.S. Department of Agriculture and U.S. Department of Health and Human Services, Scientific report of the 2015 Dietary Guidelines Advisory Committee, 2015, D-2:43, available at www.health.gov; N. D. Barnard, S. M. Levin, and Y. Yokoyama, A systematic review and meta-analysis of changes in body weight in clinical trials of vegetarian diets, *Journal of the Academy of Nutrition and Dietetics* 115 (2015): 954–969; J. D. Smith and coauthors, Changes in intake of protein foods, carbohydrate amount and quality, and long-term weight change: Results from 3 prospective cohorts, *American Journal of Clinical Nutrition* 101 (2015): 1216–1224.

66. J. Dhillon, S. Y. Tan, and R. D. Mattes, Almond consumption during energy restriction lowers truncal fat and blood pressure in compliant overweight or obese adults, *Journal of Nutrition* 146 (2016): 2513–2519; C. L. Jackson and F. B. Hu, Long-term associations of nut consumption with body weight and obesity, *American Journal of Clinical Nutrition* 100 (2014): 408S–411S.

67. A. A. Aragon and coauthors, International society of sports nutrition position stand: Diets and body composition, *Journal of the International Society of Sports Nutrition* 14 (2017), epub, doi: 10.1186/s12970-017-0174-y.

68. H. Stewart and R. M. Morrison, New regulations will inform consumers about calories in restaurant foods, Amber Waves, 2015, available at www.ers.usda.gov/amber-waves.aspx; U.S. Food and Drug Administration, How many calories? Look at the menu, Consumer Health Information, November 2014, available at www.fda.gov/consumer.

69. M. H. Alhussain, I. A. Macdonald, and M. A. Taylor, Irregular meal-pattern effects on energy expenditure, metabolism, and appetite regulation: A randomized controlled trial in healthy normal-weight women, American College of Clinical Nutrition 104 (2016): 21–32."

70. S. Kucukgoncu, M. Midura, and C. Tek, Optimal management of night eating syndrome: Challenges and solutions, *Neuropsychiatric Disease and Treatment* 11 (2015): 751–760.

71. M. H. Rouhani and coauthors, Associations between dietary energy density and obesity: A systematic review and meta-analysis of observational studies, *Nutrition* 32 (2016): 1037–1047.

72. R. Estruch and coauthors, Effect of a high-fat Mediterranean diet on bodyweight and waist circumference: A prespecified secondary outcomes analysis of the PREDIMED randomised controlled trial, *Lancet Diabetes and Endocrinology* 4 (2016): 666–676; M. Garcia and coauthors, The effect of the traditional Mediterranean-style diet on metabolic risk factors: A meta-analysis, *Nutrients* (2016), epub, doi: 10.3390/nu8030168.

73. C. E. O'Neil, V. L. Fulgoni, and T. A. Nicklas, Tree Nut consumption is associated with better adiposity measures and cardiovascular and metabolic syndrome health risk factors in U.S. Adults: NHANES 2005–2010, *Nutrition Journal* (2015), epub, doi: 10.1186/s12937-015-0052-x.

74. M. B. Azad and coauthors, Nonnutritive sweeteners and cardiometabolic health: A systematic review and meta-analysis of randomized controlled trials and prospective cohort studies, *Canadian Medical Association Journal* 189 (2017): E929–E939; Position of the Academy of Nutrition and Dietetics: Interventions for the treatment of overweight and obesity in adults, 2016; L. B. Sørensen and coauthors, Sucrose compared with artificial sweeteners: A clinical intervention study of effects on energy intake, appetite, and energy expenditure after 10 wk of supplementation in overweight subjects, *American Journal of Clinical Nutrition* 100 (2014): 36–45; R. Muckelbauer and coauthors, Association between water consumption and body weight outcomes: A systematic review, *American Journal of Clinical Nutrition* 98 (2013): 282–299; D. F. Tate and coauthors, Replacing caloric beverages with water or diet beverages for weight loss in adults: Main results of the Choose Healthy Options Consciously Everyday (CHOICE) randomized clinical trial, *American Journal of Clinical Nutrition* 95 (2012): 555–563.

75. X. Bian and coauthors, The artificial sweetener acesulfame potassium affects the gut microbiome and body weight gain in CD-1 mice, *PLoS One* (2017), epub, doi: 10.1371/journal.pone.0178426; J. Suez and coauthors, Artificial sweeteners induce glucose intolerance by altering the gut microbiota, *Nature* 514 (2014): 181–186.

76. M. Fantino and coauthors, Beverages containing low energy sweeteners do not differ from water in their effects on appetite, energy intake and food choices in healthy, non-obese French adults, *Appetite* 125 (2018): 557–565; A. D. Mooradian, M. Smith, and M. Tokuda, The role of artificial and natural sweeteners in reducing the consumption of table sugar: A narrative review, *Clinical Nutrition ESPEN* (2017), epub, doi: 10.1016/j.clnesp.2017.01.004; C. W. Chia and coauthors, Chronic low-calorie sweetener use and risk of abdominal obesity among older adults: A cohort study, *PLoS One* (2016), epub, doi: 10.1371/journal.pone.0167241; S. P. Fowler, Low-calorie sweetener use and energy balance: Results from experimental studies in animals, and large-scale prospective studies in humans, *Physiology and Behavior* 164 (2016): 517–523.

77. J. A. Douglas and coauthors, Acute exercise and appetite-regulating hormones in overweight and obese individuals: A meta-analysis, *Journal of Obesity* (2016), epub, doi: 10.1155/2016/2643625; K. Deighton and D. J. Stensel, Creating an acute energy deficit without stimulating compensatory increases in appetite: Is there an optimal exercise protocol? *Proceedings of the Nutrition Society* 73 (2014): 352–358.

78. J. Zibellini and coauthors, Does diet-induced weight loss lead to bone loss in overweight or obese adults? A systematic review and meta-analysis of clinical trials, *Journal of Bone and Mineral Research* 30 (2015): 168–178.

79. 2018 Physical Activity Guidelines Advisory Committee, *2018 Physical Activity Guidelines Advisory Committee Scientific Report* (Washington, DC: U.S. Department of Health and Human Services, 2018); National Academies of Sciences, Engineering, and Medicine, The challenge of treating obesity and overweight: Proceedings of a workshop, (2017), epub, doi: https://doi.org/10.17226/24855; B. Kleist and coauthors, Moderate walking enhances the effects of an energy-restricted diet on fat mass loss and serum insulin in overweight and obese adults in a 12-week randomized controlled trial, *Journal of Nutrition* 147 (2017): 1875–1884.

80. T. Baranowski, Are active video games useful to combat obesity? (editorial) *American Journal of Clinical Nutrition* 101 (2015): 1107–1108; A. Gribbon and coauthors, Active video games and energy balance in male adolescents: A randomized crossover trial, *American Journal of Clinical Nutrition* 101 (2015): 1126–1134.

81. U.S. Food and Drug Administration, Beware of products promising miracle weight loss, Consumer Health Information, 2015, available at www.fda.gov/consumer.

82. S. H. Chang and coauthors, Effectiveness and risks of bariatric surgery: An updated systematic review and meta-analysis, 2003–2012, *JAMA Surgery* 19 (2014): 275–287.

83. T. D. Adams and coauthors, Weight and metabolic outcomes 12 years after gastric bypass, *New England Journal of Medicine* 377 (2017): 1143–1165; M. L. Maciejewski and coauthors, Bariatric surgery and long-term durability of weight loss, *JAMA Surgery* (2016): doi:10.1001/jamasurg.2016.2317.

84. S. S. Dagan and coauthors, Nutritional recommendations for adult bariatric surgery patients: Clinical practice, *Advances in Nutrition* 8 (2017): 382–394.

85. J. Hoffstedt and coauthors, Long-term protective changes in adipose tissue after gastric bypass, *Diabetes Care* 40 (2017): 77–84; D. Arterburn and D. McCulloch, Bariatric surgery for type 2 diabetes getting closer to the long-term goal, *JAMA Surgery* 150 (2015): 931–940; L. Sjöström and coauthors, Association of bariatric surgery with long-term remission of type 2 diabetes and with microvascular and macrovascular complications, *Journal of the American Medical Association* 311 (2014): 2297–2304; C. S. Kwok and coauthors, Bariatric surgery and its impact on cardiovascular disease and mortality: A systematic review and meta-analysis, *International Journal of Cardiology* 173 (2014): 20–28; P. R. Schauer and coauthors, Bariatric surgery versus intensive medical therapy for diabetes—3-year outcomes, *New England Journal of Medicine* 370 (2014): 2002–2013; B. M. Wolfe and S. H. Belle, Long-term risks and benefits of bariatric surgery: A research challenge, *Journal of the American Medical Association* 312 (2014): 1792–1793; D. S. Casagrande and coauthors, Incidence of cancer following bariatric surgery: Systematic review and meta-analysis, *Obesity Surgery* 24 (2014): 1499–1509.

86. V. Tremaroli and coauthors, Roux-en-Y gastric bypass and vertical banded gastroplasty induce long-term changes on the human gut microbiome contributing to fat mass regulation, *Cancer Bioenergetics* 22 (2015): 228–238; A. P. Liou and coauthors, Conserved shifts in the gut microbiota due to gastric bypass reduce host weight and adiposity, *Science Translational Medicine* (2014), epub, doi: 10.1126/scitranslmed.3005687; L. C. Kong and coauthors, Gut microbiota after gastric bypass in human obesity: Increased richness and associations of bacterial genera with adipose tissue genes, *American Journal of Clinical Nutrition* 98 (2013): 16–24.

87. U.S. Food and Drug Administration, Medical Devices that Treat Obesity: What to Know, Consumer Health Information, June 2018, available at www.fda.gov/ForConsumers/ConsumerUpdates.

88. P. G. de Moura-Grec and coauthors, Impact of bariatric surgery on oral health conditions: 6-months cohort study, *International Dental Journal* 64 (2014): 144–149.

89. K. Dogan and coauthors, Long-term nutritional status in patients following Roux-en-Y gastric bypass surgery, *Clinical Nutrition* 37 (2018): 612–617; R. A. Guerreiro and R. Ribeiro, Ophthalmic complications of bariatric surgery, *Obesity Surgery* 25 (2015): 165–173; C. Karefylakis and coauthors, Vitamin D status 10 years after primary gastric bypass: Gravely high prevalence of hypovitaminosis D and raised PTH levels, *Obesity Surgery* 24 (2014): 343–348; A. A. Al Hassany, Night blindness due to vitamin A deficiency associated with copper deficiency myelopathy secondary to bowel bypass surgery, *BMJ Case Reports* (2014) epub, doi: 10.1136/bcr-2013-202478.

90. J. Parrott and coauthors, American Society for Metabolic and Bariatric Surgery

Integrated health nutritional guidelines for the surgical weight loss patient 2016 update: Micronutrients, *Surgery for Obesity and Related Disorders* 13 (2017): 727–741.

91. U.S. Food and Drug Administration, Liquid-filled intragastric balloon systems: Letter to healthcare providers-potential risks, 2017, available at https://www.fda.gov/MedicalDevices/Safety/LetterstoHealthCareProviders/ucm609597.htm.

92. R. Abdullah and coauthors, Risk assessment of plant food supplements and other herbal products containing aristolochic acids using the margin of exposure (MOE) approach, *Food Additives and Contaminants: Part A* 34 (2017): 135–144.

93. P. S. MacLean and coauthors, NIH working group report: Innovative research to improve maintenance of weight loss, *Obesity* 23 (2015): 7–15.

94. G. M. Mackie, D. Samocha-Bonet, and C. S. Tam, Does weight cycling promote obesity and metabolic risk factors? *Obesity Research and Clinical Practice* 11 (2017): 131–139; S. E. Schofield and coauthors, Metabolic dysfunction following weight-cycling in male mice, *International Journal of Obesity* (London) 41 (2017): 402–411.

95. J. P. Montani, Y. Schutz, and A. G. Dulloo, Dieting and weight cycling as risk factors for cardiometabolic diseases: Who is really at risk? *Obesity Reviews* 16 (2015): 7–18.

96. E. Burgess and coauthors, Behavioural treatment strategies improve adherence to lifestyle intervention programmes in adults with obesity: A systematic review and meta-analysis, *Clinical Obesity* 7 (2017) 105–114.

Consumer's Guide 9

1. Market Data Enterprises, The U.S. Weight Loss & Diet Control Market (2017), available at www.marketresearch.com.

2. C. D. Gardner and coauthors, Effect of low-fat vs low-carbohydrate diet on 12-month weight loss in overweight adults and the association with genotype pattern or insulin secretion: The DIETFITS randomized clinical trial, *Journal of the American Medical Association* 319 (2018): 667–679.

3. J. Schwarz, M. Clearfield, and K. Mulligan, Conversion of sugar to fat: Is hepatic de novo lipogenesis leading to metabolic syndrome and associated chronic diseases? *Journal of the American Osteopathic Association* 117 (2017): 520–527.

4. A. L. Carreiro and coauthors, The macronutrients, appetite, and energy intake, *Annual Review of Nutrition* 36 (2016): 73–103; H. J. Leidy and coauthors, The role of protein in weight loss and maintenance, *American Journal of Clinical Nutrition* 101 (2015): 1320S–1329S; A. Astrup, A. Raben, and N. Gieker, The role of higher protein diets in weight control and obesity-related comorbidities, *International Journal of Obesity* 39 (2015): 721–726; E. A. Martens and M. S. Westerterp-Plantenga, Protein diets, body weight loss and weight mainte-

nance, *Current Opinion in Clinical Nutrition and Metabolic Care* 17 (2014): 75–79; D. H. Pesta and V. T. Samuel, A high-protein diet for reducing body fat: Mechanisms and possible caveats, *Nutrition and Metabolism* 11 (2014), epub, doi: 10.1186/1743- 7075-11–53.

5. A. A. Aragon and coauthors, International society of sports nutrition position stand: Diets and body composition, *Journal of the International Society of Sports Nutrition* 14 (2017), epub, doi: 10.1186/s12970-017-0174-y; D. L. Layman and coauthors, Defining meal requirements for protein to optimize metabolic roles of amino acids, *American Journal of Clinical Nutrition* 101 (2015): 1330S–1338S; A. J. Hector and coauthors, Whey protein supplementation preserves postprandial myofibrillar protein synthesis during short-term energy restriction in overweight and obese adults, *Journal of Nutrition* (2015), epub, doi: 10.3945/jn.114.200832.

6. Leidy and coauthors, The role of protein in weight loss and maintenance, 2015.

7. J. D. Smith and coauthors, Changes in intake of protein foods, carbohydrate amount and quality, and long-term weight change: Results from 3 prospective cohorts, *American Journal of Clinical Nutrition* 101 (2015): 1216–1224.

8. A. Kamper and S. Strandgaard, Long-term effects of high-protein diets on renal function, *Annual Review of Nutrition* 37 (2017): 347–369.

Controversy 9

1. National Institute of Mental Health, Eating disorders among children, available at www.nimh.nih.gov/health/statistics/prevalence/eating-disorders-among-children.shtml; K. Campbell and R. Peebles, Eating disorders in children and adolescents: State of the art review, *Pediatrics* 134 (2014): 582–592.

2. B. Herpertz-Dahlmann and coauthors, Eating disorder symptoms do not just disappear: The implications of adolescent eating-disordered behaviour for body weight and mental health in young adulthood, *European Child and Adolescent Psychiatry* 24 (2015): 675–684.

3. S. A. McLean, S. J. Paxton, and E. H. Wertheim, The role of media literacy in body dissatisfaction and disordered eating: A systematic review, *Body Image* 19 (2016): 9–23; L. P. MacNeill and L. A. Best, Perceived current and ideal body size in female undergraduates, *Eating Behaviors* 18 (2015): 71–75; L. Das, R. Mohan, and T. Makaya, The bid to lose weight: Impact of social media on weight perceptions, weight control and diabetes, *Current Diabetes Reviews* 10 (2014): 291–297.

4. E. Stice, Interactive and mediational etiologic models of eating disorder onset: Evidence from prospective studies, *Annual Review of Clinical Psychology* 12 (2016): 359–381; K. M. Pike, H. W. Hoek, and P. E. Dunne, Cultural trends and eating disorders, *Current Opinion in Psychiatry* 27 (2014): 436–442.

5. J. Mingoia and coauthors, The relationship between social networking site use and the internalization of a thin ideal in females: A meta-analytic review, *Frontiers in Psychology* (2017), epub, doi: 10.3389/fpsyg.2017.01351; A. Dakanalis and coauthors, The developmental effects of media-ideal internalization and self-objectification processes on adolescents' negative body-feelings, dietary restraint, and binge eating, *European Child and Adolescent Psychiatry* 24 (2015): 997–1010; A. G. Mabe, K. J. Forney, and P. K. Keel, Do you "like" my photo? Facebook use maintains eating disorder risk, *International Journal of Eating Disorders* 47 (2014): 516–523.

6. R. L. Carl, M. D. Johnson, and T. J. Martin, Promotion of healthy weight-control practices in young athletes, *Pediatrics* (2017), epub, doi: 10.1542/peds.2017-1871.

7. D. Neumark-Sztainer and M. E. Eisenberg, Body image concerns, muscle-enhancing behaviors, and eating disorders in males, *Journal of the American Medical Association* 312 (2014): 2156–2157.

8. A. K. W. Kelly and S. Hect, The female athlete triad, *Pediatrics* 138 (2016), epub, doi: 10.1542/peds.2016-0922.

9. M. T. Barrack and coauthors, Higher incidence of bone stress injuries with increasing female athlete triad–related risk factors: A prospective multisite study of exercising girls and women, *American Journal of Sports Medicine* 42 (2014): 949–958.

10. Carl, Johnson, and Martin, Promotion of healthy weight-control practices in young athletes, 2017.

11. American Psychiatric Association, *Diagnostic and statistical manual of mental disorders,* 5th edition (Washington, D.C.: APA, 2013), pre-publication, available at www.dsm5.org/ProposedRevision/Pages/FeedingandEatingDisorders.aspx.

12. M. M. Fichter and coauthors, Long-term outcome of anorexia nervosa: Results from a large clinical longitudinal study, *International Journal of Eating Disorders* 50 (2017): 1018–1030.

13. L. M. de Barse and coauthors, Does maternal history of eating disorders predict mothers' feeding practices and preschoolers' emotional eating? *Appetite* 85 (2015): 1–7.

14. M. M. Fichter and N. Quadflieg, Mortality in eating disorders-results of a large prospective clinical longitudinal study, *International Journal of Eating Disorders* 49 (2016): 391–401; A. Keshaviah and coauthors, Re-examining premature mortality in anorexia nervosa: A meta-analysis redux, *Comprehensive Psychiatry* 55 (2014): 1773–1784; G. Di Cola and coauthors, Cardiovascular disorders in anorexia nervosa and potential therapeutic targets, *Internal and Emergency Medicine* 9 (2014): 717–721.

15. C. M. Grilo, Psychological and behavioral treatments for binge-eating disorder, *Journal of Clinical Psychiatry* 78, Supplement 1 (2017): 20–24.

16. M. Kells and S. Kelly-Weeder, Nasogastric tube feeding for individuals with anorexia nervosa: An integrative review, *Journal of the American Psychiatric Nurses Association* 22 (2016): 449–468.

17. S. S. Khalsa and coauthors, What happens after treatment? A systematic review of relapse, remission, and recovery in anorexia nervosa, *Journal of Eating Disorders* (2017), epub, doi: 10.1186/s40337-017-0145-3.

18. APA, *Diagnostic and statistical manual of mental disorders*, 2013.

19. A. M Chao and coauthors, Binge eating and weight loss outcomes in individuals with type 2 diabetes: 4-year results from the Look AHEAD study, *Obesity* 25 (2017): 1830–1837; S. E. Racine and coauthors, Examining associations between negative urgency and key components of objective binge episodes, *International Journal of Eating Disorders* 41 (2015): 527–538.

20. R. D. Rienecke, Family-based treatment of eating disorders in adolescents: Current insights, *Adolescent Health, Medicine, and Therapeutics* 8 (2017): 69–79.

21. A. Raevuori and coauthors, Highly increased risk of type 2 diabetes in patients with binge eating disorder and bulimia nervosa, *International Journal of Eating Disorders* 48 (2015): 555–562.

22. A. Meule and A. N. Gearhardt, Food addiction in the light of DSM-5, *Nutrients* 6 (2014): 3653–3671; A. J. Flint and coauthors, Food-addiction scale measurement in 2 cohorts of middle-aged and older women, *American Journal of Clinical Nutrition* 99 (2014): 578–586.

23. A. Goracci and coauthors, Pharmacotherapy of binge-eating disorder: A review, *Journal of Addiction Medicine* 9 (2015): 1–19; M. E. Bocarsly and coauthors, GS 455534 selectively suppresses binge eating of palatable food and attenuates dopamine release in the accumbens of sugar-bingeing rats, *Behavioral Pharmacology* 25 (2014): 147–157; N. A. Hadad and L. A. Knackstedt, Addicted to palatable foods: Comparing the neurobiology of bulimia nervosa to that of drug addiction, *Psychopharmacology* 231 (2014): 1897–1912.

24. N. H. Golden and coauthors, Preventing obesity and eating disorders in adolescents, *Pediatrics* 138 (2016): 114–123.

Chapter 10

1. 2018 Physical Activity Guidelines Advisory Committee, *2018 Physical Activity Guidelines Advisory Committee Scientific Report* (Washington, DC: U.S. Department of Health and Human Services, 2018); K. M. Diaz and coauthors, Patterns of sedentary behavior and mortality in U.S. middle-aged and older adults: A national cohort study, *Annals of Internal Medicine* 167 (2017): 465–475; American Heart Association, Sedentary behavior and cardiovascular morbidity and mortality: A science advisory from the American Heart Association, *Circulation* 134 (2016): e262–e279.

2. Centers for Disease Control and Prevention, Exercise or physical activity, 2017, available at www.cdc.gov/nchs/fastats/exercise.htm; Healthy People.gov, 2020 Topics and objectives, Physical activity, available at www.healthypeople .gov/2020/topics-objectives/topic/physical-activity.

3. B. Bond and coauthors, Exercise intensity and the protection from postprandial vascular dysfunction in adolescents, *Heart and Circulatory Physiology* (2015), epub, doi: 10.1152/ ajpheart.00074.2015; M. Catoire and S. Kersten, The search for exercise factors in humans, *FASEB Journal* 29 (2015): 1615–1628; R. Y. Aysano and coauthors, Acute effects of physical exercise in type 2 diabetes: A review, *World Journal of Diabetes* 15 (2014): 659–665; K. Iizuka, T. Machida, and M. Hirafuji, Skeletal muscle is an endocrine organ, *Journal of Pharmacological Sciences* 125 (2014): 125–131.

4. W. Fan and R. M. Evans, Exercise mimetics: Impact on health and performance, *Cell Metabolism* 25 (2017): 242–247; J. Giudice and J. M. Taylor, Muscle as a paracrine and endocrine organ, *Current Opinion in Pharmacology* 34 (2017): 49–55; J. O. Chen and coauthors, Irisin: A new molecular marker and target in metabolic disorder, *Lipids in Health and Disease* 14 (2015), epub, doi: 10.1186/1476-511X-14-2.

5. C. Handschin, Caloric restriction and exercise "mimetics": Ready for prime time? *Pharmacological Research* 103 (2016): 158–166.

6. 2018 Physical Activity Guidelines Advisory Committee. *2018 Physical Activity Guidelines Advisory Committee Scientific Report* (Washington, DC: U.S. Department of Health and Human Services, 2018).

7. M. McCarthy and coauthors, Breaking up sedentary time with seated upper body activity can regulate metabolic health in obese high risk adults: A randomised crossover trial, *Diabetes, Obesity, and Metabolism* 19 (2017): 1732–1739; E. Stamatakis and coauthors, Association of "weekend warrior" and other leisure time physical activity patterns with risks for all-cause, cardiovascular disease, and cancer mortality, *JAMA Internal Medicine* 177 (2017): 335–342; M. E. Armstrong and coauthors, Frequent physical activity may not reduce vascular disease risk as much as moderate activity: Large prospective study of UK women, *Circulation* 131 (2015): 721–729; U. Ekelund and coauthors, Physical activity and all-cause mortality across levels of overall and abdominal adiposity in European men and women: The European Prospective Investigation into Cancer and Nutrition Study (EPIC), *American Journal of Clinical Nutrition* 101 (2015): 613–621; C. Y. Wu and coauthors, The association of physical activity with all-cause, cardiovascular, and cancer mortality among older adults, *Preventive Medicine* 72(2015): 23–29.

8. 2018 Physical Activity Guidelines Advisory Committee, *2018 Physical Activity Guidelines Advisory Committee Scientific Report* (Washington, DC: U.S. Department of Health and Human Services, 2018).

9. F. Damas and coauthors, A review of resistance training-induced changes in skeletal muscle protein synthesis and their contribution to hypertrophy, *Sports Medicine* 45 (2015): 801–807; S. Phillips, Building an "optimal diet": Putting protein into practice, presented at the Academy of Nutrition and Dietetics' Food and Nutrition Conference and Expo, Atlanta, October 2014.

10. Y. Hellsten and M. Nyberg, Cardiovascular adaptations to exercise training, *Comprehensive Physiology* 6 (2015): 1–32; C. Y. Wu and coauthors, The association of physical activity with all-cause, cardiovascular, and cancer mortality among older adults, *Preventive Medicine* 72 (2015): 23–29.

11. S. Steib and coauthors, Dose-response relationship of neuromuscular training for injury prevention in youth athletes: A meta-analysis, *Frontiers in Physiology* (2017), epub, doi: 10.3389/fphys.2017.00920; M. S. Vavilala and coauthors, Early changes in cerebral autoregulation among youth hospitalized after sports-related traumatic brain injury, *Brain Injury* 32 (2017): 269–275; A. C. McKee and coauthors, The neuropathology of sport, *Acta Neuropathologica* 127 (2014): 29–51; J. Calatayud and coauthors, Exercise and ankle sprain injuries: A comprehensive review, *Physician and Sportsmedicine* 42 (2014): 88–93.

12. American College of Sports Medicine, *ACSM's Guidelines for Exercise Testing and Prescription*, 9th ed. (Philadelphia: Lippincott, Williams, and Wilkins, 2014).

13. J. S. Baker, M. C. McCormick, and R. A. Robergs, Interaction among skeletal muscle metabolic energy systems during intense exercise, *Journal of Nutrition and Metabolism* (2010), epub, doi: 10.1155/2010/905612.

14. S. Kuzmiak-Glancy and W. T. Willis, Skeletal muscle fuel selection occurs at the mitochondrial level, *Journal of Experimental Biology* 217 (2014): 1993–2003.

15. Position of the Academy of Nutrition and Dietetics, Dietitians of Canada, and the American College of Sports Medicine: Nutrition and athletic performance, *Journal of the Academy of Nutrition and Dietetics* 116 (2016): 501–528.

16. D. Ndahimana and coauthors, Accuracy of dietary reference intake predictive equation for estimated energy requirements in female tennis athletes and non-athlete college students: Comparison with the doubly labeled water method, *Nutrition Research and Practice* 11 (2017): 51–56.

17. Position of the Academy of Nutrition and Dietetics, Dietitians of Canada, and the American College of Sports Medicine: Nutrition and athletic performance, 2016.

18. C. Cabral-Santos and coauthors, Physiological acute response to high-intensity intermittent and moderate-intensity continuous 5 km running performance: Implications for training prescription, *Journal of Human Kinetics* 56 (2017): 127–137; B. K. Greer and coauthors,

EPOC comparison between isocaloric bouts of steady-state aerobic, intermittent aerobic, and resistance training, *Research Quarterly for Exercise and Sport* (2015): 190–195.

19. K. Karstoft and coauthors, The effects of interval- vs. continuous exercise on excess post-exercise oxygen consumption and substrate oxidation rates in subjects with type 2 diabetes, *Metabolism* 65 (2016): 1316–1325; I. Larsen and coauthors, High- and moderate-intensity aerobic exercise and excess post-exercise oxygen consumption in men with metabolic syndrome, *Scandinavian Journal of Medicine & Science in Sports* 24 (2014): e174–e179.

20. B. Murray and C. Rosenbloom, Fundamentals of glycogen metabolism for coaches and athletes, *Nutrition Reviews* 76 (2018): 243–259; J. Bergstrom and coauthors, Diet, muscle glycogen and physical performance, *Acta Physiologica Scandanavica* 71 (1967): 140–150.

21. K. J. Stuempfle and coauthors, Race diet of finishers and non-finishers in a 100 mile (161 km) mountain footrace, *Journal of the American College of Nutrition* 30 (2011): 529–535.

22. R. J. S. Costa and coauthors, Systematic review: Exercise-induced gastrointestinal syndrome—implications for health and intestinal disease, *Alimentary Pharmacology & Therapeutics* 46 (2017): 246–265; R. J. S. Costa and coauthors, The impact of gastrointestinal symptoms and dermatological injuries on nutritional intake and hydration status during ultramarathon events, *Sports Medicine* (2016), epub, doi: 10.1186/s40798-015-0041-9.

23. M. Cole and coauthors, The effects of acute carbohydrate and caffeine feeding strategies on cycling efficiency, *Journal of Sports Sciences* 36 (2018): 817–823.

24. K. A. Pollak and coauthors, Exogenously applied muscle metabolites synergistically evoke sensations of muscle fatigue and pain in human subjects, *Experimental Physiology* 99 (2014): 368–380.

25. P. Proia and coauthors, Lactate as a metabolite and a regulator in the central nervous system, *International Journal of Molecular Sciences* (2016), epub, doi: 10.3390/ijms17091450.

26. M. M. Hall and coauthors, Lactate: Friend or foe, *PM and R: The Journal of Injury, Function, and Rehabilitation* 8 (2016): S8–S15; J. F. Moxnes and Ø. Sandbakk, The kinetics of lactate production and removal during whole-body exercise, *Theoretical Biology and Medical Modeling* 9 (2012), epub, doi: 10.1186/1742-4682-9-7.

27. K. D. Gejl and coauthors, Muscle glycogen content modifies SR Ca2+ release rate in elite endurance athletes, *Medicine and Science in Sports and Exercise* 46 (2014): 496–505.

28. M. B. Reid, Redox interventions to increase exercise performance, *Journal of Physiology* 594 (2016): 5125–5133.

29. S. G. Impey and coauthors, Fuel for the work required: A practical approach to amalgamating train-low paradigms for endurance athletes, *Physiological Reports* (2016), epub, doi: 10.14814/phy2.12803.

30. M. Pöchmüller and coauthors, A systematic review and meta-analysis of carbohydrate benefits associated with randomized controlled competition-based performance trials, *Journal of the International Society of Sports Medicine* (2016), epub, doi: 10.1186/s12970-016-0139-6; C. Williams and I. Rollo, Carbohydrate nutrition and team sport performance, *Sports Medicine* 45 (2016): S13–S22.

31. E. Prado de Oliveira, R. C. Burnini, and A. Jeukendrup, Gastrointestinal complaints during exercise: Prevalence, etiology, and nutritional recommendations, *Sports Medicine* 44 (2014): S79–S85.

32. A. F. Alghannam and coauthors, Influence of post-exercise carbohydrate-protein ingestion on muscle glycogen metabolism in recovery and subsequent running exercise, *International Journal of Sport Nutrition and Exercise Metabolism* 26 (2016): 572–580.

33. L. L. Spriet, New insights into the interaction of carbohydrate and fat metabolism during exercise, *Sports Medicine* 44 (2014): S87–S96.

34. C. K. Chang, K. Borer, and P. J. Lin, Low-carbohydrate-high-fat diet: Can it help exercise performance? *Journal of Human Kinetics* 56 (2017): 81–92; E. R. Helms and coauthors, High-protein, low-fat, short-term diet results in less stress and fatigue than moderate-protein moderate-fat diet during weight loss in male weightlifters: A pilot study, *International Journal of Sport Nutrition and Exercise Metabolism* 25 (2015): 163–170.

35. Position of the Academy of Nutrition and Dietetics, Dietitians of Canada, and the American College of Sports Medicine: Nutrition and athletic performance, *Journal of the Academy of Nutrition and Dietetics* 116 (2016): 501–528.

36. M. Martorell and coauthors, Docosahexaenoic acid supplementation promotes erythrocyte antioxidant defense and reduces protein nitrosative damage in male athletes, *Lipids* 50 (2015): 131–148; F. M. DiLorenzo, C. J. Drager, and J. W. Rankin, Docosahexaenoic acid affects markers of inflammation and muscle damage after eccentric exercise, *Journal of Strength and Conditioning Research* 28 (2014): 2768–2774.

37. D. M. Camera and coauthors, Selective modulation of microRNA expression with protein ingestion following concurrent resistance and endurance exercise in human skeletal muscle, *Frontiers in Physiology* (2016), epub, doi: 10.3389/fphys.2016.00087.

38. W. J. Smiles and coauthors, Modulation of autophagy signaling with resistance exercise and protein ingestion following short-term energy deficit, *American Journal of Physiology–Regulatory, Integrative and Comparative Physiology* (2015), epub, doi: 10.1152/ajpregu.00413.2014.

39. W. K. Mitchell and coauthors, Human skeletal muscle protein metabolism responses to amino acid nutrition, *Advances in Nutrition* 7 (2016): 828S–838S; D. M. Camera and coauthors, Protein ingestion increases myofibrillar

protein synthesis after concurrent exercise, *Medicine and Science in Sports and Exercise* 47 (2015): 82–91; D. K. Layman and coauthors, Defining meal requirements for protein to optimize metabolic roles of amino acids, *American Journal of Clinical Nutrition* 101 (2015): 1330S–1338S.

40. I. Kim, N. E. P. Deutz, and R. R. Wolfe, Update on maximal anabolic response to dietary protein, *Clinical Nutrition* 37 (2018): 411–418; C. M. Kersick and coauthors, International Society of Sports Nutrition position stand: Nutrient timing, *Journal of the International Society of Sports Nutrition* (2017), epub, doi: 10.1186/s12970-0189-4.

41. E. Simmons, J. D. Fluckey, and S. E. Riechman, Cumulative muscle protein synthesis and protein intake requirements, *Annual Review of Nutrition* 36 (2016): 17–43; D. J. Beale, Evidence inconclusive—comment on article by Schoenfeld et al., *Journal of the International Society of Sports Nutrition* (2016), epub, doi: 10.1186/s12970-016-0148-5B; J. Schoenfeld, A. A. Aragon, and J. W. Krieger, The effect of protein timing on muscle strength and hypertrophy: A meta-analysis, *Journal of the International Society of Sports Nutrition* (2013), epub, doi: 10.1186/1550-2783-10-53.

42. C. J. Mitchell and coauthors, Acute post-exercise myofibrillar protein synthesis is not correlated with resistance training-induced muscle hypertrophy in young men, *PLoS One* 9 (2014), epub, doi: 10.1371/journal.pone.0089431.

43. P. T. Reidy and coauthors, Protein supplementation does not affect myogenic adaptations to resistance training, *Medicine and Science in Sports and Exercise* 49 (2017): 1197–1208; T. M. McLellan, S. M. Pasiakos, and H. R. Lieberman, Effects of protein in combination with carbohydrate supplements on acute or repeat endurance exercise performance: A systematic review, *Sports Medicine* 44 (2014): 535–550.

44. Simmons, Fluckey, and Riechman, Cumulative muscle protein synthesis and protein intake requirements, 2016.

45. Reidy and coauthors, Protein supplementation does not affect myogenic adaptations to resistance training, 2017.

46. Position of the Academy of Nutrition and Dietetics, Dietitians of Canada, and the American College of Sports Medicine: Nutrition and athletic performance, *Journal of the Academy of Nutrition and Dietetics* 116 (2016): 501–528; N. R. Rodriguez and S. L. Miller, Effective translation of current dietary guidance: Understanding and communicating the concepts of minimal and optimal levels of dietary protein, *American Journal of Clinical Nutrition* 101 (2015): 1353S–1358S.

47. I. Alaunyte, V. Stojceska, and A. Plunkett, Iron and the female athlete: A review of dietary treatment methods for improving iron status and exercise performance, *Journal of the International Society of Sports Nutrition* (2015), epub, doi: 10.1186/s12970-015-0099-2; Y. H. Chiu

Appendix F Chapter 10 Notes

and coauthors, Early changes of the anemia phenomenon in male 100-km ultramarathoners, *Journal of the Chinese Medical Association* 78 (2015): 108–113.

48. R. B. Parks, S. J. Hetzel, and M. A. Brooks, Iron deficiency and anemia among collegiate athletes: A retrospective chart review, *Medicine and Science in Sports and Exercise* 49 (2017): 1711–1715; W. Kong, G. Gao, and Y. Chang, Hepcidin and sports anemia, *Cell and Bioscience* 4 (2014), epub, doi: 10.1186/2045-3701-4-19.

49. A. Coates, M. Mountjoy, and J. Burr, Incidence of iron deficiency and iron deficient anemia in elite runners and triathletes, *Clinical Journal of Sports Medicine* 27 (2017): 493–498; D. M. DellaValle and J. D. Haas, Iron supplementation improves energetic efficiency in iron-depleted female rowers, *Medicine and Science in Sports and Exercise* 46 (2014): 1204–1215; S. Pasricha and coauthors, Iron supplementation benefits physical performance in women of reproductive age: A systematic review and meta-analysis, *Journal of Nutrition* 144 (2014): 906–914.

50. A. N. Peiris, S. Jaroudi, and R. Noor, Heat stroke, *Journal of the American Medical Association* 318 (2018): 2503; Executive summary of National Athletic Trainers' Association position statement on exertional heat illnesses, 2014, available at www.nata.org/sites/default/files/Heat-Illness-Executive-Summary.pdf.

51. Position of the Academy of Nutrition and Dietetics, Dietitians of Canada, and the American College of Sports Medicine: Nutrition and athletic performance, *Journal of the Academy of Nutrition and Dietetics* 116 (2016): 501–528.

52. J. D. Adams and coauthors, Dehydration Impairs Cycling Performance, Independently of Thirst: A Blinded Study, *Medicine and Science in Sports and Exercise* 50 (2018): 1697–1703.

53. E. L. Earhart and coauthors, Effects of oral sodium supplementation on indices of thermoregulation in trained, endurance athletes, *Journal of Sports Science and Medicine* 14 (2015): 172–178.

54. E. R. Parr and coauthors, Alcohol ingestion impairs maximal post-exercise rates of myofibrillar protein synthesis following a single bout of concurrent training, *PLoS One* 9 (2014), epub, doi: 10.1371/journal.pone.0088384.

55. M. J. Cramer and coauthors, Postexercise glycogen recovery and exercise performance is not significantly different between fast food and sport supplements, *Journal of the International Society of Sports Medicine* 25 (2015): 448–455.

56. Kersick and coauthors, International Society of Sports Nutrition position stand: Nutrient timing, 2017.

57. B. Besbrow and coauthors, Comparing the rehydration potential of different milk-based drinks to a carbohydrate-electrolyte beverage, *Applied Physiology and Nutrition Metabolism* 39 (2014): 1366–1372.

Controversy 10

1. M. Comassi and coauthors, Acute effects of different degrees of ultra-endurance exercise on systemic inflammatory responses, *Internal Medicine Journal* 45 (2015): 74–79.

2. M. B. Reid, Redox interventions to increase exercise performance, *Journal of Physiology* 594 (2016): 5125–5133; C. L. Draeger and coauthors, Controversies of antioxidant vitamins supplementation in exercise: Ergogenic or ergolytic effects in humans? *Journal of the International Society of Sports Nutrition* 11 (2014), epub, doi: 10.1186/1550-2783-11-4; T. D. Scribbans and coauthors, Resveratrol supplementation does not augment performance adaptations or fibre-type-specific responses to high-intensity interval training in humans, *Applied Physiology, Nutrition, and Metabolism* 39 (2014): 1305–1313.

3. R. C. Leonardo-Mendonça and coauthors, Redox status and antioxidant response in professional cyclists during training, *European Journal of Sport Science* 14 (2014): 830–838; S. K. Powers and coauthors, Exercise-induced improvements in myocardial antioxidant capacity: The antioxidant players and cardio-protection, *Free Radical Research* 48 (2014): 43–51; G. Sharifi, A. B. Najafabadi, and F. E. Ghashghaei, Oxidative stress and total antioxidant capacity in handball players, *Advances in Biomedical Research* 3 (2014), epub, doi: 10.4103/2277-9175.139538.

4. L. L. Petiz and coauthors, Vitamin A oral supplementation induces oxidative stress and suppresses IL-10 and HSP70 in skeletal muscle of trained rats, *Nutrients* (2017), epub, doi: 10.3390/nu9040353; G. Paulsen and coauthors, Vitamins C and E supplementation alters protein signaling after a strength training session, but not muscle growth during 10 weeks of training, *Journal of Physiology* 592 (2014): 5391–5408.

5. S. Porcelli and coauthors, Aerobic fitness affects the exercise performance responses to nitrate supplementation, *Medicine and Science in Sports and Exercise* 47 (2015): 1643–1651; R. K. Boorsma, J. Whitfield, and L. L. Spriet, Beetroot juice supplementation does not improve performance of elite 1500-m runners, *Medicine and Science in Sports and Exercise* 46 (2014): 2326–2334; W. T. Clements, S. R. Lee, and R. J. Bloomer, Nitrate ingestion: A review of the health and physical performance effects, *Nutrients* 6 (2014): 5224–5264.

6. M. B. Reid, Redox interventions to increase exercise performance, *Journal of Physiology* 594 (2016): 5125–5133.

7. A. M. Jones, Influence of dietary nitrate on the physiological determinants of exercise performance: A critical review, *Applied Physiology in Nutrition and Metabolism* 39 (2014): 1019–1028.

8. J. Nyakayiru and coauthors, Beetroot juice supplementation improves high-intensity intermittent type exercise performance in trained soccer players, *Nutrients* (2017), epub, doi: 10.3390/nu9030314.

9. L. J. Wylie and coauthors, Influence of beetroot juice supplementation on intermittent exercise performance, *European Journal of Applied Physiology* 116 (2016): 416–425.

10. G. L. Kent and coauthors, Dietary nitrate supplementation does not improve cycling time-trial performance in the heat, *Journal of Sports Sciences* 36 (2018): 1204–1211; S. Porcelli and coauthors, Aerobic fitness affects the exercise performance responses to nitrate supplementation, *Medicine and Science in Sports and Exercise* 47 (2015): 1643–1651; Boorsma, Whitfield, and Spriet, Beetroot juice supplementation does not improve performance of elite 1500-m runners, 2014.

11. A. L. Friis and coauthors, Dietary beetroot juice – effects on physical performance in COPD patients: A randomized controlled crossover trial, *International Journal of Chronic Obstructive Pulmonary Disease* (2017), epub, doi: 10.2147/COPD.S135752.

12. L. Nybäck and coauthors, Physiological and performance effects of nitrate supplementation during roller-skiing in normoxia and normobaric hypoxia, *Nitric Oxide* 70 (2017): 1–8.

13. G. M. K. Rossetti and coauthors, Dietary nitrate supplementation increases acute mountain sickness severity and sense of effort during hypoxic exercise, *Journal of Applied Physiology* 123 (2017): 983–992.

14. B. H. Jacobson and coauthors, Effect of energy drink consumption on power and velocity of selected sport performance activities, *Journal of Strength and Conditioning Research* (2017), epub ahead of print, doi: 10.1519/JSC.0000000000002026; L. Arcoverde and coauthors, Effect of caffeine ingestion on anaerobic capacity quantified by different methods, *PLoS One* (2017), epub, doi: 10.1371/journal.pone.0179457; R. S. Cruz and coauthors, Caffeine affects time to exhaustion and substrate oxidation during cycling at maximal lactate steady state, *Nutrients* 7 (2015): 5254–5264; S. M. An, J. S. Park, and S. H. Kim, Effect of energy drink dose on exercise capacity, heart rate recovery and heart rate variability after high-intensity exercise, *Journal of Exercise Nutrition and Biochemistry* 18 (2014): 31–39.

15. M. Cole and coauthors, The effects of acute carbohydrate and caffeine feeding strategies on cycling efficiency, *Journal of Sports Sciences* (2017), epub ahead of print, doi: 10.1080/02640414.2017.1343956.

16. J. L. Temple and coauthors, The safety of ingested caffeine: A comprehensive review, *Frontiers in Psychiatry* (2017), epub, doi: 10.3389/fpsyt.2017.00080; G. Mohney, Teen's caffeine-related death highlights the dangers of the common stimulant, *ABC News*, May 16, 2017, available at abcnews.go.com/Health/teens-caffeine-related-death-highlights-dangers-common-stimulant/story?id=47437035.

17. K. Novakova and coauthors, Effect of L-carnitine supplementation on the body carnitine pool, skeletal muscle energy metabolism and physical performance in male vegetarians,

European Journal of Nutrition (2015), epub ahead of print, doi: 10.1007/s00394-015-0838-9.
18. L. W. Judge and coauthors, Creatine usage and education of track and field throwers at NCAA Division I universities, *Journal of Strength and Conditioning Research* (2014), epub ahead of print, doi: 10.1519/JSC.0000000000000818.
19. C. L. Camic and coauthors, The effects of polyethylene glycosylated creatine supplementation on anaerobic performance measure and body composition, *Journal of Strength and Conditioning Research* 28 (2014): 825–833; M. C. Devries and S. M. Phillips, Creatine supplementation during resistance training in older adults—A meta-analysis, *Medicine and Science in Sports and Exercise* 46 (2014): 1194–1203.
20. Devries and Phillips, Creatine supplementation during resistance training in older adults, 2014; Judge and coauthors, Creatine usage and education of track and field throwers at NCAA Division I universities, 2014.
21. L. M. Burke, Practical considerations for bicarbonate loading and sports performance, *Nestlé Nutrition Institute Workshop Series* 75 (2013): 15–26.
22. P. M. Bellinger, β-alanine supplementation for athletic performance: An update, *Journal of Strength and Conditioning Research* 28 (2014): 1751–1770; R. M. Hobson and coauthors, Effects of β-alanine supplementation on exercise performance: A meta-analysis, *Amino Acids* 43 (2012): 25–37; A. E. Smith and coauthors, Exercise-induced oxidative stress: The effects of β-alanine supplementation in women, *Amino Acids* 43 (2012): 77–90; A. E. Smith-Ryan and coauthors, High-velocity intermittent running: Effects of beta-alanine supplementation, *Journal of Strength and Conditioning Research* 26 (2012): 2798–2805.
23. P. M. Bellinger and C. L. Minahan, Performance effects of acute β-alanine induced paresthesia in competitive cyclists, *European Journal of Sport Science* 30 (2015): 1–8.
24. P. T. Reidy and B. B. Rasmussen, Role of ingested amino acids and protein in the promotion of resistance exercise-induced muscle protein anabolism, *Journal of Nutrition* 146 (2016): 155–183.
25. N. Babault and coauthors, Pea proteins oral supplementation promotes muscle thickness gains during resistance training: A double-blind, randomized, placebo-controlled clinical trial vs. whey protein, *Journal of the International Society of Sports Nutrition* 12 (2015), epub, doi: 10.1186/s12970-014-0064-5.
26. S. M. Pasiakos, T. M. McLellan, and H. R. Lieberman, The effects of protein supplements on muscle mass, strength, and aerobic and anaerobic power in healthy adults: A systematic review, *Sports Medicine* 45 (2015): 111–131.
27. P. A. Cohen, J. C. Travis, and B. J. Venhuis, A synthetic stimulant never tested in humans, 1,3-dimethylbutylamine (DMBA) is identified in multiple dietary supplements, *Drug Testing and Analysis* 7 (2015): 83–87.
28. M. E. Arensberg and coauthors, Summit on Human Performance and Dietary Supplements summary report, Nutrition Today 49 (2014): 7–15.

Chapter 11

1. E. J. Benjamin and coauthors, Heart disease and stroke statistics—2017 update: A report from the American Heart Association, *Circulation* 135 (2017): e146–e603.
2. Benjamin and coauthors, Heart disease and stroke statistics—2017, 2017.
3. Benjamin and coauthors, Heart disease and stroke statistics--2017, 2017.
4. S. M. Alfonso and coauthors, The impact of dietary fatty acids on macrophage cholesterol homeostasis, *Journal of Nutritional Biochemistry* 25 (2014): 95–103; B. Messner and D. Bernhard, Smoking and cardiovascular disease: Mechanisms of endothelial dysfunction and early atherogenesis, *Arteriosclerosis, Thrombosis, and Vascular Biology* 34 (2014): 509–515.
5. Benjamin and coauthors, Heart disease and stroke statistics—2017 update, 2017.
6. American Heart Association, Menopause and heart disease, updated June 23, 2017, available at www.heart.org/HEARTORG/Conditions/More/MyHeartandStrokeNews/Menopause-and-Heart-Disease_UCM_448432_Article.jsp.
7. A. V. Khera and coauthors, Genetic risk, adherence to a healthy lifestyle, and coronary disease, *New England Journal of Medicine* 375 (2016): 2349–2358.
8. Benjamin and coauthors, Heart disease and stroke statistics—2017, 2017.
9. P. A. James and coauthors, 2014 Evidence-based guidelines for the management of high blood pressure in adults: Report from the panel members appointed to the Eighth Joint National Committee (JNC8), *Journal of the American Medical Association* 311 (2014): 507–520.
10. Benjamin and coauthors, Heart disease and stroke statistics—2017, 2017; R. V. Same and coauthors, Relationship between sedentary behavior and cardiovascular risk, *Current Cardiology Reports* 18 (2016): 6.
11. C. Tudor-Locke and coauthors, Step-based physical activity metrics and cardiometabolic risk: NHANES 2005–2006, *Medicine and Science in Sports and Exercise* 49 (2017): 283–291; G. N. Healy and coauthors, Replacing sitting time with standing or stepping: Associations with cardio-metabolic risk biomarkers, *European Heart Journal* 36 (2015): 2643–2649.
12. A. Rao, V. Pandya, and A. Whaley-Connell, Obesity and insulin resistance in resistant hypertension: Implications for the kidney, *Advances in Chronic Kidney Disease* 22 (2015): 211–217.
13. Benjamin and coauthors, Heart disease and stroke statistics—2017 update, 2017.
14. H. O'Keefe and coauthors, Alcohol and cardiovascular health: The dose makes the poison . . . or the remedy, *Mayo Clinic Proceedings* 89 (2014): 382–393.
15. C. S. Ceron and coauthors, Vascular oxidative stress: A key factor in the development of hypertension associated with ethanol consumption, *Current Hypertension Reviews* 10 (2014): 213–222.
16. R. C. Hoogeveen and coauthors, Small dense low-density lipoprotein cholesterol concentrations predict risk for coronary heart disease: The Atherosclerosis Risk in Communities (ARIC) study, *Arteriosclerosis, Thrombosis, and Vascular Biology* 34 (2014): 1069–1077; N. B. Allen and coauthors, Blood pressure trajectories in early adulthood and subclinical atherosclerosis in middle age, *Journal of the American Medical Association* 311 (2014): 490–497.
17. A. Ramirez and P. P. Hu, Low high-density lipoprotein and risk of myocardial infarction, *Clinical Medicine Insights: Cardiology* 9 (2015): 113–117; H. K. Siddiqi, D. Kiss, and D. Rader, HDL-cholesterol and cardiovascular disease: Rethinking our approach, *Current Opinion in Cardiology* 30 (2015): 536–542.
18. A. Tenenbaum, R. Klempfner, and E. Z. Fisman, Hypertriglyceridemia: A too long unfairly neglected major cardiovascular risk factor, *Cardiovascular Diabetology* 13 (2014): 159.
19. F. M. Sacks and coauthors, Dietary fats and cardiovascular disease: A Presidential Advisory from the American Heart Association, *Circulation* 136 (2017): e1–e23; R. Micha and coauthors, Etiologic effects and optimal intakes of foods and nutrients for risk of cardiovascular diseases and diabetes: Systematic reviews and meta-analyses from the Nutrition and Chronic Diseases Expert Group (NutriCoDE), *PLoS One*, 2017, https://doi.org/10.1371/journal.pone.0175149.
20. Sacks and coauthors, Dietary fats and cardiovascular disease, 2017; Benjamin and coauthors, Heart disease and stroke statistics—2017 update, 2017; A. M. Freeman and coauthors, Trending cardiovascular nutrition controversies, *Journal of the American College of Cardiology* 69 (2017): 1172–1187; U.S. Department of Health and Human Services and U.S. Department of Agriculture, *2015–2020 Dietary Guidelines for Americans*, 8th ed. (2015), available at http://health.gov/dietaryguidelines/2015/guidelines/; R. H. Eckel and coauthors, 2013 AHA/ACC guideline on lifestyle management to reduce cardiovascular risk: A report of the American College of Cardiology/American Heart Association Task Force on Practice Guidelines, *Circulation* 129 (2014): S76–S99.
21. D. Mozzaffarian, Dietary and policy priorities for cardiovascular disease, diabetes, and obesity, *Circulation* 133 (2016): 187–225.
22. Benjamin and coauthors, Heart disease and stroke statistics—2017 update, 2017.
23. M. Al Rifai and coauthors, The association of nonalcoholic fatty liver disease, obesity, and metabolic syndrome with systemic inflammation and subclinical atherosclerosis: The Multi-Ethnic Study of Atherosclerosis (MESA), *Atherosclerosis* 239 (2015): 629–633; F. Bonomini, L. F. Rodella, and R. Rezzani, Metabolic syndrome, aging,

and involvement of oxidative stress, *Aging and Disease* 10 (2015): 109–120.

24. Benjamin and coauthors, Heart disease and stroke statistics—2017 update, 2017.

25. G. N. Healy and coauthors, Replacing sitting time with standing or stepping: Associations with cardio-metabolic risk biomarkers, *European Heart Journal* 36 (2015): 2643–2649; M. Hamer, E. Stamatakis, and A. Steptoe, Effects of substituting sedentary time with physical activity on metabolic risk, *Medicine and Science in Sports and Exercise* 46 (2014): 1946–1950.

26. Benjamin and coauthors, Heart disease and stroke statistics—2017 update, 2017.

27. Y. Huang and coauthors, Prehypertension and the risk of stroke: A meta-analysis, *Neurology* 82 (2014): 1153–1161.

28. D. C. Goff and coauthors, 2013 ACC/AHA guidelines on the assessment of cardiovascular risk: A report of the American College of Cardiology/American Heart Association Task Force on Practice Guidelines, *Circulation* 129 (2014): S49–S73; Eckel and coauthors, 2013 AHA/ACC guideline on lifestyle management to reduce cardiovascular risk, 2014; N. J. Stone and coauthors, ACC/AHA guideline on the treatment of blood cholesterol to reduce atherosclerotic cardiovascular risk in adults: A report of the American College of Cardiology/American Heart Association Task Force on Practice Guidelines, *Circulation* 129 (2014): S1–S45.

29. R. Micha and coauthors, Association between dietary factors and mortality from heart disease, stroke, and type 2 diabetes in the United States, *Journal of the American Medical Association* 317 (2017): 912–924.

30. S. N. Adebamowo and coauthors, Association between intakes of magnesium, potassium, and calcium and risk of stroke: 2 cohorts of US women and updated meta-analyses, *American Journal of Clinical Nutrition* 101 (2015): 1269–1277; H. M. Noh and coauthors, Association between high blood pressure and intakes of sodium and potassium among Korean adults: Korean National Health and Nutrition Examination Survey, 2007–2012, *Journal of the Academy of Nutrition and Dietetics* 115 (2015): 1950–1957; A. Binia and coauthors, Daily potassium intake and sodium-to-potassium ratio in the reduction of blood pressure: A meta-analysis of randomized controlled trials, *Journal of Hypertension* 33 (2015): 1509–1520.

31. O. Oyebode and coauthors, Fruit and vegetable consumption and all-cause, cancer, and CVD mortality: Analysis of Health Survey for England data, *Journal of Epidemiology and Community Health* 68 (2014): 856–862; X. Wang and coauthors, Fruit and vegetable consumption and mortality from all causes, cardiovascular disease and cancer: Systematic review and dose-response meta-analysis of prospective cohort studies, *BMJ* (2014), doi: 10.1136/bmj.g4490; E. Garcia-Fernandez and coauthors, Mediterranean diet and cardiodiabesity: A review, *Nutrients* 6 (2014): 3474–3500.

32. Sacks and coauthors, Dietary fats and cardiovascular disease, 2017.

33. Sacks and coauthors, Dietary fats and cardiovascular disease, 2017.

34. J. Jiang and coauthors, Effect of marine-derived n-3 polyunsaturated fatty acids on major eicosanoids: A systematic review and meta-analysis from 18 randomized controlled trials, *PLoS One* 25 (2016): e0147351; O. A. Khawaja J. M. Gaziano, and L. Djoussé, N-3 fatty acids for the prevention of cardiovascular disease, *Current Atherosclerosis Reports* 16 (2014): 450–457.

35. M. Poreba and coauthors, Treatment with high-dose n-3 PUFAs has no effect on platelet function, coagulation, metabolic status or inflammation in patients with atherosclerosis and type 2 diabetes, *Cardiovascular Diabetology* (2017), epub, doi: 10.1186/s12933-017-0523-9; M. Lagarde and coauthors, In vitro and in vivo bimodal effects of docosahexaenoic acid supplements on redox status and platelet function, *Prostaglandins, Leukotrienes and Essential Fatty Acids* (2016), epub ahead of print, doi: 10.1016/j.plefa.2016.03.008.

36. A. Hernaez and coauthors, Mediterranean diet improves high-density lipoprotein function in high-cardiovascular-risk individuals, *Circulation* 135 (2017): 633–643; D. P. Redlinger and coauthors, How effective are current dietary guidelines for cardiovascular disease prevention in healthy middle-aged and older men and women? A randomized controlled trial, *American Journal of Clinical Nutrition* 101 (2015): 922–930.

37. Eckel and coauthors, 2013 AHA/ACC guideline on lifestyle management to reduce cardiovascular risk, 2014.

38. Centers for Disease Control and Prevention, *Diabetes: Working to reverse the US epidemic, at a glance, 2016,* www.cdc.gov/chronicdisease/resources/publications/aag/diabetes.htm.

39. E. Selvin and coauthors, Identifying trends in undiagnosed diabetes in U.S. adults by using a confirmatory definition: A cross-sectional study, *Annals of Internal Medicine* 167 (2017): 769–776.

40. International Diabetes Foundation, *Diabetes Atlas,* 7th ed., 2015, www.diabetesatlas.org.

41. American Diabetes Association, Classification and diagnosis of diabetes, *Diabetes Care* 40 (2017): S11–S24.

42. A. Llewellyn and coauthors, Childhood obesity as a predictor of morbidity in adulthood: A systematic review and meta-analysis, *Obesity Reviews* 17 (2016): 56–67; B. Tobisch, L. Blatniczky, and L. Barkai, Cardiometabolic risk factors and insulin resistance in obese children and adolescents: Relation to puberty, *Pediatric Obesity* 10 (2015): 37–44.

43. American Diabetes Association, Classification and diagnosis of diabetes, 2017.

44. K. J. Basile and coauthors, Genetic susceptibility to type 2 diabetes and obesity: Follow-up findings from genome-wide association studies, *International Journal of Endocrinology* (2014), epub, doi:10.1155/2014/769671.

45. American Diabetes Association, Classification and diagnosis of diabetes, 2017.

46. Centers for Disease Control and Prevention, *Diabetes: Working to reverse the US epidemic, at a glance, 2016,* www.cdc.gov/chronicdisease/resources/publications/aag/diabetes.htm.

47. Centers for Disease Control and Prevention, Prediabetes, updated December 28, 2016, available at www.cdc.gov/diabetes/basics/prediabetes.html.

48. American Diabetes Association, Classification and diagnosis of diabetes, 2017.

49. American Diabetes Association, Lifestyle management, *Diabetes Care* 40 (2017): S33–S43.

50. S. Ding and coauthors, Adjustable gastric band surgery or medical management in patients with type 2 diabetes: A randomized clinical trial, *Journal of Clinical Endocrinology and Metabolism* 100 (2015): 2546–2556; L. Sjöström and coauthors, Association of bariatric surgery with long-term remission of type 2 diabetes and with microvascular and macrovascular complications, *Journal of the American Medical Association* 311 (2014): 2297–2304.

51. S. Fan and coauthors, Physical activity level and incident type 2 diabetes among Chinese adults, *Medicine and Science in Sports and Exercise* 47 (2015): 751–756; D. T. Lackland and J. H. Voeks, Metabolic syndrome and hypertension: Regular exercise as part of lifestyle management, *Current Hypertension Reports* 16 (2014): 492; C. P. Earnest and coauthors, Aerobic and strength training in concomitant metabolic syndrome and type 2 diabetes, *Medicine and Science in Sports and Exercise* 46 (2014): 1293–1201.

52. A.B. Evert and coauthors, Nutrition therapy recommendations for the management of adults with diabetes: A position statement from the American Diabetes Association, *Diabetes Care* 37 (2014): S120–S143.

53. Evert and coauthors, Nutrition therapy recommendations for the management of adults with diabetes, 2014.

54. Position of the Academy of Nutrition and Dietetics: The role of medical nutrition therapy and Registered Dietitian Nutritionists in the prevention and treatment of prediabetes and type 2 diabetes, *Journal of the Academy of Nutrition and Dietetics* 118 (2018): 343–353; Evert and coauthors, Nutrition therapy recommendations for the management of adults with diabetes, 2014.

55. E. M. Balk and coauthors, Combined diet and physical activity promotion programs to prevent type 2 diabetes among persons at increased risk: A systematic review for the Community Preventive Services Task Force, *Annals of Internal Medicine* 163 (2015): 437–451; K. C. Portero and coauthors, Therapeutic interventions to reduce the risk of progression from prediabetes to type 2 diabetes mellitus, *Therapeutics and Clinical Risk Management* 10 (2014): 173–188.

56. American Cancer Society, *Cancer Facts and Figures 2017* (Atlanta, GA: American Cancer Society, 2017), available at www.cancer.org/research/cancer-facts-statistics.html.

57. American Cancer Society, *Cancer Facts and Figures 2017*.

58. American Cancer Society, *Cancer Prevention and Early Detection Facts and Figures 2017–2018* (Atlanta, GA: American Cancer Society, 2017), available at www.cancer.org/content/dam/cancer-org/research/cancer-facts-and-statistics/cancer-prevention-and-early-detection-facts-and-figures/cancer-prevention-and-early-detection-facts-and-figures-2017.pdf; E. Theodoratou and coauthors, Nature, nurture, and cancer risks: Genetic and nutritional contributions to cancer, *Annual Review of Nutrition* 37 (2017): 293–320; T. Lohse and coauthors, Adherence to the cancer prevention recommendations of the World Cancer Research Fund/American Institute for Cancer Research and mortality: A census-linked cohort, *American Journal of Clinical Nutrition* 104 (2016): 678–685.

59. M. Arnold and coauthors, Duration of adulthood overweight, obesity, and cancer risk in the Women's Health Initiative: A longitudinal study from the United States, *PLoS Medicine* 13 (2016): e1002081; M. Song and E. Giovannucci, Preventable incidence and mortality of carcinoma associated with lifestyle factors among white adults in the United States, *JAMA Oncology* 2 (2016): 1154–1161; M. L. Neuhouser and coauthors, Overweight, obesity, and postmenopausal invasive breast cancer risk: A secondary analysis of the Women's Health Initiative Randomized Clinical Trials, *JAMA Oncology* 1 (2015): 611–621; Y. Chen, C. Yu, and Y. Li, Physical activity and risks of esophageal and gastric cancers: A meta-analysis, *PLoS One* 9 (2014): e88082; S. Ghosh and coauthors, Association of obesity and circulating adipose stromal cells among breast cancer survivors, *Molecular Biology Reports* 41 (2014): 2907–2916.

60. D. T. Fisher, M. M. Appenheimer, and S. S. Evans, The two faces of IL-6 in the tumor environment, *Seminars in Immunology* 26 (2014): 38–47.

61. G. Grosso and coauthors, Possible role of diet in cancer: Systematic review and multiple metaanalyses of dietary patterns, lifestyle factors, and cancer risk, *Nutrition Reviews* 75 (2017): 405–419; C. Sapienza and J. P. Issa, Diet, nutrition, and cancer epigenetics, *Annual Review of Nutrition* 36 (2016): 665–681; W. C. Willett, T. Key, and I. Romieu, Diet, obesity, and physical activity, in B. W. Stewart and C. P. Wild (eds.), *World Cancer Report* (Lyon, France: International Agency for Research on Cancer, 2014), pp. 124–133.

62. Willett, Key, and Romieu, Diet, obesity, and physical activity, 2014.

63. M. L. Neuhouser and coauthors, Overweight, obesity, and postmenopausal invasive breast cancer risk: A secondary analysis of the Women's Health Initiative Randomized Clinical Trials, *JAMA Oncology* 1 (2015): 611–621; S. Ghosh and coauthors, Association of obesity and circulating adipose stromal cells among breast cancer survivors, *Molecular Biology Reports* 41 (2014): 2907–2916.

64. C. Scoccianti and coauthors, European code against cancer 4th edition: Alcohol drinking and cancer, *Cancer Epidemiology* 39 (2015): S67–S74; C. D. Castro and J. A. Castro, Alcohol drinking and mammary cancer: Pathogenesis and potential dietary preventive alternatives, *World Journal of Clinical Oncology* 5 (2014): 713–729; J. Rehm and K. Shield, Alcohol consumption, in B. W. Stewart and C. P. Wild (eds.), *World Cancer Report* (Lyon, France: International Agency for Research on Cancer, 2014), pp. 96–104.

65. U. Hammerling and coauthors, Consumption of red/processed meat and colorectal carcinoma: Possible mechanisms underlying the significant association, *Critical Reviews in Food Science and Nutrition* 56 (2016): 614–634; D. Demeyer and coauthors, Mechanisms linking colorectal cancer to the consumption of (processed) red meat: A review, *Critical Reviews in Food Science and Nutrition* 56 (2016): 2747–2766; World Health Organization, International Agency for Research on Cancer, IARC Monographs evaluate consumption of red meat and processed meat, Press release no. 240, October 2015, available at www.iarc.fr/en/media-centre/pr/2015/pdfs/pr240_E.pdf; Z. Abid, A. J. Cross, and R. Sinha, Meat, dairy, and cancer, *American Journal of Clinical Nutrition* 100 (2014): 386S–393S.

66. Abid, Cross, and Rashmi, Meat, dairy, and cancer, 2014; Willett, Key, and Romieu, Diet, obesity, and physical activity, 2014.

67. Abid, Cross, and Rashmi, Meat, dairy, and cancer, 2014.

68. J. Hooda, A. Shah, and L. Zhang, Heme, an essential nutrient from dietary proteins, critically impacts diverse physiological and pathological processes, *Nutrients* 6 (2014): 1080–1102.

69. American Cancer Society, Cancer Facts and Figures 2017 (Atlanta, GA: American Cancer Society, 2017), available at www.cancer.org/content/dam/cancer-org/research/cancer-facts-and-statistics/annual-cancer-facts-and-figures/2017/cancer-facts-and-figures-2017.pdf.

70. A. T. Kunzmann and coauthors, Dietary fiber intake and risk of colorectal cancer and incident and recurrent adenoma in the Prostate, Lung, Colorectal, and Ovarian Cancer Screening trial, *American Journal of Clinical Nutrition* 102 (2015): 881–890; T. Norat and coauthors, Fruits and vegetables: Updating the epidemiologic evidence for WCRF/AICR lifestyle recommendations for cancer prevention, *Cancer Treatment and Research* 159 (2014): 35–50.

71. F. Turati and coauthors, Fruit and vegetables and cancer risk: A review of southern European studies, *British Journal of Nutrition* 113 (2015): S102–S110; Norat and coauthors, Fruits and vegetables: Updating the epidemiologic evidence for WCRF/AICR lifestyle recommendations for cancer prevention; O. Oyebode and coauthors, Fruit and vegetable consumption and all-cause, cancer, and CVD mortality:

Analysis of Health Survey for England data, *Journal Epidemiology and Community Health* 68 (2014): 856–862.

72. Sapienza and Issa, Diet, nutrition, and cancer epigenetics, 2016; S. M. Tortorella and coauthors, Dietary sulforaphane in cancer chemoprevention: The role of epigenetic regulation and HDAC inhibition, *Antioxidants and Redox Signaling* 22 (2015): 1382–1424; P. Gupta and coauthors, Phenethyl isothiocyanate: A comprehensive review of anti-cancer mechanisms, *Biochimica et Biophysica Acta* 1846 (2014): 405–424.

73. American Cancer Society, Cancer Facts and Figures 2017 (Atlanta, GA: American Cancer Society, 2017), available at www.cancer.org/content/dam/cancer-org/research/cancer-facts-and-statistics/annual-cancer-facts-and-figures/2017/cancer-facts-and-figures-2017.pdf.

74. Willett, Key, and Romieu, Diet, obesity, and physical activity, 2014.

75. S. Brandhorst and V.D. Longo, Fasting and caloric restriction in cancer prevention and treatment, *Recent Results in Cancer Research* 2017 (2016): 241–266; A. Cangemi and coauthors, Dietary restriction: Could it be considered as speed bump on tumor progression road? *Tumor Biology* 37 (2016): 7109–7118.

Consumer's Guide 11

1. National Institutes of Health, National Center for Complementary and Integrative Health, Complementary, alternative, or integrative health: What's in a name? updated June, 2016, available at https://nccih.nih.gov/health/integrative-health; E. F. Myers, Herbal/botanical medicine, *Nutrition Today* 50 (2015): 194–206.

2. G. Onder and R. Liperoti, Herbal medications, *Journal of the American Medical Association* 315 (2016): 1068.

3. Onder and Liperoti, Herbal medications, 2016.

4. A. J. Vickers and K. Linde, Acupuncture for chronic pain, *Journal of the American Medical Association* 311 (2014): 955–956.

5. K. P. Hill, Medical marijuana for treatment of chronic pain and other medical and psychiatric problems: A clinical review, *Journal of the American Medical Association* 313 (2015): 2474–2483; P. F. Whiting and coauthors, Cannabinoids for medical use: A systematic review and meta-analysis, *Journal of the American Medical Association* 313 (2015): 2456–2473.

6. J. Meiman, R. Thiboldeaux, and H. Anderson, Lead poisoning and anemia associated with the use Ayurvedic medications purchased on the internet—Wisconsin, 2015, *Morbidity and Mortality Weekly Report* 64 (2015): 883.

7. Onder and Liperoti, Herbal medications, 2016.

8. National Institutes of Health, National Center for Complementary and Integrative Health, Herbs at a glance, Ginkgo, updated September 2016, available at https://nccih.nih.gov/health/ginkgo/ataglance.htm.

Controversy 11

1. N. M. Lindor, S. N. Thibodeau, and W. Burke, Whole-genome sequencing in healthy people, *Mayo Clinic Proceedings* 92 (2017): 159–172S; McGrath and D. Ghersi, Building towards precision medicine: Empowering medical professionals for the next revolution, *BMC Medical Genomics* (2016), epub, doi: 10.1186/s12920-016-0183-8.

2. FDA allows marketing of first direct-to-consumer tests that provide genetic risk information for certain conditions, *FDA News Release*, 2017, available at www.fda.gov/NewsEvents/Newsroom/PressAnnouncements/ucm551185.htm.

3. M. Kohlmeier and coauthors, Guide and position of the International Society of Nutrigenetics/Nutrigenomics on personalized nutrition, *Journal of Nutrigenetics and Nutrigenomics* 9 (2016): 28–46; Position of the Academy of Nutrition and Dietetics: Nutritional genomics, *Journal of the Academy of Nutrition and Dietetics* 114 (2014): 299–319.

4. Position of the Academy of Nutrition and Dietetics: Nutritional genomics, 2014. 5. E. Callaway, Epigenomics starts to make its mark, *Nature* 509 (2014): 33; C. Lavebratt, M. Almgren, and T. J. Eström, Epigenetic regulation in obesity, *International Journal of Obesity* 36 (2012): 757–765.

5. A. P. Feinberg, The key role of epigenetics in human disease prevention and mitigation, *New England Journal of Medicine* 378 (2018): 1323–1334; M. Lahti-Pulkkinen and coauthors, Intergenerational transmission of birth weight across 3 generations, American Journal of Epidemiology 187 (2018): 1165–1173.

6. S. M. Tortorella and coauthors, Dietary sulforaphane in cancer chemoprevention: The role of epigenetic regulation and HDAC inhibition, *Antioxidants and Redox Signaling* 22 (2015): 1382–1424.

7. J. I. Young, S. Züchner, and G. Wang, Regulation of the epigenome by vitamin C, *Annual Review of Nutrition* 35 (2015): 545–564.

8. R. H. Bahous and coauthors, High dietary folate in pregnant mice leads to pseudo-MTHFR deficiency and altered methyl metabolism, with embryonic growth delay and short-term memory impairment in offspring, *Human Molecular Genetics* 26 (2017): 888–900; K. E. Christensen and coauthors, Moderate folic acid supplementation and MTHFD1-synthetase deficiency in mice, a model for the R653Q variant, result in embryonic defects and abnormal placental development, *American Journal of Clinical Nutrition* 104 (2016): 1459–1469.

9. M. McGee, S. Bainbridge, and B. Fontaine-Bisson, A crucial role for maternal dietary methyl donor intake in epigenetic programming and fetal growth outcomes, *Nutrition Reviews* 76 (2018): 469–478; R. Dominguez-Salas and coauthors, Maternal nutrition at conception modulates DNA methylation of human metastable epialleles, *Nature Communications* (2014), epub, doi: 10.1038/ncomms4746; J. Zhang and coauthors, DNA methylation: The pivotal interaction between early-life nutrition and glucose metabolism in later life, *British Journal of Nutrition* 112 (2014): 1850–1857.

10. Federal Trade Commission, Direct-to-consumer genetic tests, 2014, available at www.consumer.ftc.gov/articles/0166-direct-consumer-genetic-tests.

11. M. Fox, What you're giving away in those home DNA tests, nbcnews.com, 2017, available at www.nbcnews.com/health/health-news/what-you-re-givingaway-those-home-dna-tests-n824776; R. Poinhos and coauthors, Psychological determinants of consumer acceptance of personalised nutrition in 9 European countries, *PLOS ONE* (2014), epub, doi: 10.1371/journal.pone.0110614.

12. T. Haeusermann and coauthors, Open sharing of genomic data: Who does it and why? *PLoS One* (2017), epub, doi: 10.1371/journal.pone.0177158.

13. Position of the Academy of Nutrition and Dietetics: Nutritional genomics, 2014.

14. D. E. Nielsen and coauthors, Diet and exercise changes following direct-to-consumer personal genomic testing, *BMC Medical Genomics* (2017), epub, doi: 10.1186/s12920-017-0258-1.

15. S. W. Gray and coauthors, Personal genomic testing for cancer risk: Results from the impact of personal genomics study, *Journal of Clinical Oncology* 35 (2017): 636–644.

16. D. Corella and coauthors, Effects of the Ser-326Cys polymorphism in the DNA repair OGG1 gene on cancer, cardiovascular, and all-cause mortality in the PREDIMED study: Modulation by diet, *Journal of the Academy of Nutrition and Dietetics* 118 (2018): 589–604.

Chapter 12

1. Position of the Academy of Nutrition and Dietetics: Food and water safety, *Journal of the Academy of Nutrition and Dietetics* 114 (2014): 1819–1829.

2. Centers for Disease Control and Prevention, Estimates of Foodborne Illness in the United States, 2017, available www.cdc.gov/foodborneburden/index.html.

3. U.S. Food and Drug Administration, Food Safety Modernization Act (FSMA), 2017, available at www.fda.gov/Food/GuidanceRegulation/FSMA/.

4. Centers for Disease Control and Prevention, Incidence and trends of infection with pathogens transmitted commonly through food—Food-borne Diseases Active Surveillance Network, 10 U.S. sites, 2006–2013, *Morbidity and Mortality Weekly Report* 63 (2014): 328–332.

5. Centers for Disease Control and Prevention, List of multistate foodborne outbreak investigations, 2015, available at www.cdc.gov/foodsafety/outbreaks/multistate-outbreaks/outbreaks-list.html.

6. L. Bottichio and coauthors, Outbreak of *Salmonella* Oslo infections linked to Persian cucumbers—United States, 2016, *Morbidity and Mortality Weekly Report* 65 (2017):1430–1433.

7. U.S. Food and Drug Administration, FDA investigating multistate outbreak of *E. coli* O157:H7 infections likely linked to romaine lettuce from Yuma growing region, May 2018, available at www.fda.gov/Food/RecallsOutbreaksEmergencies/Outbreaks/ucm604254.htm.

8. United States Department of Agriculture, Food product dating, 2016, available at www.fsis.usda.gov.

9. C. P. Gerba and coauthors, Bacterial occurrence in kitchen hand towels, *Food Protection Trends* 34 (2014): 312–317.

10. M. Cardinale and coauthors, Microbiome analysis and confocal microscopy of used kitchen sponges reveal massive colonization by *Acinetobacter, Moraxella* and *Chryseobacterium* species, *Scientific Reports* (2017), epub, doi: 10.1038/s41598-017-06055-9.

11. Cardinale and coauthors, Microbiome analysis and confocal microscopy of used kitchen sponges reveal massive colonization by *Acinetobacter, Moraxella* and *Chryseobacterium* species, 2017.

12. A. Lando and coauthors, U.S. Food and Drug Administration, *2016 FDA food safety survey*, available at www.fda.gov/downloads/Food/FoodScienceResearch/ConsumerBehaviorResearch/UCM529453.pdf.

13. Centers for Disease Control and Prevention, Foodborne illness, foodborne disease, 2014, available at www.cdc.gov/foodsafety/facts.html.

14. S. J. Chai and coauthors, *Salmonella enterica* serotype Enteritidis: Increasing incidence of domestically acquired infections, *Clinical Infectious Diseases* 54 (2012): S488–S497.

15. W. Wang, M. Li, and Y. Li, Intervention strategies for reducing *Vibrio Parahaemolyticus* in seafood: A review, *Journal of Food Science* 80 (2015): R10–R19.

16. C. M. Cossaboom and coauthors, *Brucella abortus* vaccine strain RB51 infection and exposures associated with raw milk consumption—Wise County, Texas, 2017, *Morbidity and Mortality Weekly Report* 67 (2018): 286; Centers for Disease Control and Prevention, Raw milk, (2016), available at www.cdc.gov/foodsafety/rawmilk/raw-milk-index.html.

17. U.S. Department of Agriculture and U.S. Department of Health and Human Services, *Scientific report of the 2015 Dietary Guidelines Advisory Committee, 2015*, A-4, available at www.health.gov.

18. Centers for Disease Control and Prevention, Multistate outbreak of Listeriosis linked to whole cantaloupes from Jensen farms, Colorado, August 2012, available at www.cdc.gov/listeria/outbreaks/cantaloupes-jensen-farms/082712/.

19. Centers for Disease Control and Prevention, Multistate outbreak of *E. coli* O157:H7 infections linked to romaine lettuce, April 2018, available at www.cdc.gov/ecoli/2018/o157h7-04-18/index.html; M. Berlanga and R. Guerrero, Living together in biofilms: The microbial cell factory and its biotechnological implications, *Microbial Cell Factories* (2015), epub, doi: 10.1186/s12934-016-0569-5; Position of the Academy of Nutrition and Dietetics: Food and water safety, 2014..

20. Centers for Disease Control and Prevention, Multistate outbreak of Shiga toxin–producing *Escherichia coli* O121 infections linked to raw clover sprouts, 2014, available at www.cdc.gov/ecoli/2014/0121-05-14/index.html.

21. L. H. Gould and coauthors, Outbreaks of disease associated with food imported into the United States, 1996–2014, *Emerging Infectious Diseases* (2017): 525–528.

22. U.S. Food and Drug Administration, *FDA Food Safety Modernization Act* (FSMA), 2018, available at www.fda.gov/Food/GuidanceRegulation/FSMA/default.htm.

23. U.S. Department of Agriculture, Agricultural Marketing Service, Country of origin labeling, 2014, available at www.ams.usda.gov/AMSv1.0/cool.

24. U.S. Department of Agriculture, Keeping "bag" lunches safe, 2013, available at www.fsis.usda.gov.

25. U.S. Food and Drug Administration, Food irradiation: What you need to know, 2014, available at www.fda.gov/Food/ResourcesForYou/Consumers/ucm261680.htm.

26. U.S. Food and Drug Administration, Kinetics of microbial inactivation for alternative food processing technologies—High pressure processing, 2014, available at www.fda.gov/Food/FoodScienceResearch/ucm100158.htm.

27. A. Valdés and coauthors, State of the art of antimicrobial edible coatings for food packaging applications, *Coatings* (2017), epub, doi: 10.3390/coatings7040056.

28. World Health Organization, *Antimicrobial resistance: Global Report on Surveillance* (Geneva: WHO, 2014), pp. 3–6; C. Nathan and O. Cars, Antibiotic resistance—Problems, progress, and prospects, *New England Journal of Medicine* 371 (2014): 1761–1763; Institute of Medicine, *Anti-microbial resistance: A problem without borders* (Washington, DC: National Academies Press, 2014).

29. FDA Annual Summary Report on Antimicrobials Sold or Distributed in 2015 for Use in Food-Producing Animals, available at www.fda.gov/AnimalVeterinary/NewsEvents/CVMUpdates/ucm534244.htm.

30. U.S. Food and Drug Administration, For consumers: Seven things pregnant women and parents need to know about arsenic in rice and rice cereal (2017), available at www.fda.gov/ForConsumers/ConsumerUpdates/ucm493677.htm.

31. S. Munera-Picazo and coauthors, Inorganic and total arsenic contents in rice-based foods for children with celiac disease, *Journal of Food Science* 79 (2014): T122–T128 .

32. F. Maqbool and coauthors, Immunotoxicity of mercury: Pathological and toxicological effects, *Journal of Environmental Science and Health, Part C Environmental Carcinogenesis and Ecotoxicology Reviews* 35 (2017): 29–46.

33. K. M. Rice and coauthors, Environmental mercury and its toxic effects, *Journal of Preventive Medicine and Public Health* 47 (2014): 74–83.

34. P. E. Drevnick and coauthors, Spatiotemporal patterns of mercury accumulation in lake sediments of western North America, *Science of the Total Environment* 568 (2016): 1157–1170; P. W. Drevnick, C. H. Lamborg, and M. J. Horgan, Increase in mercury in Pacific yellowfin tuna, *Environmental Toxicology* (2015), epub, doi: 10.1002/etc.2883.

35. K. Kindy, Food additives on the rise as FDA scrutiny wanes, *Washington Post*, August 17, 2015, available at www.washingtonpost.com/national/food-additives-on-the-rise-as-fda-scrutiny-wanes/2014/08/17/828e9bf8-1cb2-11e4-ab7b-696c295ddfd1_story.html

36. A. Etemadi and coauthors, Mortality from different causes associated with meat, heme iron, nitrates, and nitrites in the NIH-AARP Diet and Health Study: Population based cohort study, *British Medical Journal* (2017) epub, doi.org/10.1136/bmj.j1957.

37. J. Suez and coauthors, Artificial sweeteners induce glucose intolerance by altering the gut microbiota, *Nature* 514 (2014): 181–186.

38. J. L. Kuk and R. E. Brown, Aspartame intake is associated with greater glucose intolerance in individuals with obesity, *Applied Physiology, Nutrition, and Metabolism* 41 (2016): 796–798.

39. T. Sathyapain and coauthors, Aspartame sensitivity? A double blind randomised crossover study, *PLoS ONE* 10 (2015), epub, doi: 10.1371/ journal.pone.0116212; U.S. Department of Agriculture and U.S. Department of Health and Human Services, *Scientific report of the 2015 Dietary Guidelines Advisory Committee*, 2015, D-5:35–41, available at www.health.gov; American Cancer Institute, Aspartame, 2014, available at www.cancer.org/cancer/cancercauses/othercarcinogens/athome/aspartame; M. L. McCullough and coauthors, Artificially and sugar-sweetened carbonated beverage consumption is not associated with risk of lymphoid neoplasms in older men and women, *Journal of Nutrition* 144 (2014): 2041–2049.

40. A. Sharma, Monosodium glutamate-induced oxidative kidney damage and possible mechanisms: A mini-review, *Journal of Biomedical Science* 22 (2015), epub, doi: 10.1186/s12929-015-0192-5; M. Lee, MSG: Can an amino acid really be harmful? *Clinical Correlations* (2014), epub, available at www.clinicalcorrelations.org/?p=7655.

41. C. Philippat and coauthors, Prenatal exposure to nonpersistent endocrine disruptors and behavior in boys at 3 and 5 years, *Environmental Health Perspectives* (2017), epub, doi: 10.1289/EHP1314; D. Chen and coauthors, Bisphenol analogues other than BPA: Environmental occurrence, human exposure, and toxicity-a review, *Environmental Science and Technology* 50 (2016): 5438–5453; Y. Chen and coauthors, Exposure to the BPA-substitute Bisphenol S causes unique alterations of germline function, *PLoS Genetics* (2016), epub, doi: 10.1371/journal.pgen.1006223; B. Mole, Doubts grow over BPA replacement, *Science News*, April 4, 2015, p. 10; M. D. Mersha and coauthors, Effects of BPA and BPS exposure limited to early embryogenesis persist to impair non-associative learning in adults, *Behavior and Brain Function* (2015), epub, doi: 10.1186/s12993-015-0071-y; J. R. Rochester and A. L. Bolden, Bisphenol S and F: A systematic review and comparison of the hormonal activity of Bisphenol A substitutes, *Environmental Health Perspectives* 123 (2015): 643–650.

42. National Toxicology Program, Draft NTP research report on the CLARITY-BPA Core Study: A perinatal and chronic extended-dose-range study of bisphenol A in rats, (2018), available at https://ntp.niehs.nih.gov/ntp/about_ntp/rrprp/2018/april/rr09peerdraft.pdf.

43. U.S. Food and Drug Administration, Statement from Stephen Ostroff M.D., Deputy Commissioner for Foods and Veterinary Medicine, on National Toxicology Program draft report on Bisphenol A, (2018), available at www.fda.gov/NewsEvents/Newsroom/PressAnnouncements/ucm598100.htm.

Consumer's Guide 12

1. Organic Trade Association, Maturing U.S. organic sector sees steady growth of 6.4 percent in 2017, available at https://ota.com/news/press-releases/20201.

2. J. L. Wan-chen and coauthors, You taste what you see: Do organic labels bias taste perceptions? *Food Quality and Preference* 29 (2013): 33–39.

3. M. Barański and coauthors, Higher antioxidant and lower cadmium concentrations and lower incidence of pesticide residues in organically grown crops: A systematic literature review and meta-analysis, *British Journal of Nutrition* 112 (2014): 794–811.

4. C. L. Curl and coauthors, Estimating pesticide exposure from dietary intake and organic food choices: The Multi-ethnic Study of Atherosclerosis (MESA), *Environmental Health Perspectives* (2015), epub, doi: 10.1289/ ehp.1408197.

5. Environmental Working Group, Shoppers guide to pesticides in produce, 2015, available at www.ewg.org/foodnews/.

6. U.S. Department of Agriculture and U.S. Department of Health and Human Services, *Scientific report of the 2015 Dietary Guidelines Advisory Committee*, 2015, A-4, available at www.health.gov.

7. Barański and coauthors, Higher antioxidant and lower cadmium concentrations and lower incidence of pesticide residues in organically grown crops, 2014.

8. D. Średnicka-Tober and coauthors, Composition differences between organic and conventional meat: A systematic literature review and meta-analysis, *British Journal of Nutrition* 115 (2016): 994–1011.

9. C. Strassner and coauthors, How the organic food system supports sustainable diets and translates these into practice, *Frontiers in Nutrition* (2015), epub, doi: 10.3389/fnut.2015.00019.

10. T. Yang and coauthors, Effectiveness of commercial and homemade washing agents in removing pesticide residues on and in apples, *Journal of Agricultural and Food Chemistry* 65 (2017): 9744–9752.

Controversy 12

1. J. Lyon, Nobel laureates pick food fight with GMO foes, *Journal of the American Medical Association* 316 (2016): 1752–1753; S. Wunderlich and K. A. Gatto, Consumer perception of genetically modified organisms and sources of information, *Advances in Nutrition* 6 (2015): 842–851.

2. D. R. Schilling, Genetically engineered "spider goat" spins out elastic material superior to Kevlar, Industry Tap into News, May 2014, available at www.industrytap.com/genetically -engineered-spider-goat-spins-elastic-material -superior-kevlar/19392.

3. Hypoallergenic peanuts: Who cares and why? Accessed March 2015, epub available at www .ncat.edu/caes/agresearch/impacts/NCAT%20 -%20Ibrahim%20ph.pdf.

4. E. Waltz, USDA approves next-generation GM potato, *Nature Biotechnology* 33 (2015): 12–13.

5. E. Lief, Embrace of "Golden Rice" globally remains frustratingly slow, *American Council on Science and Health,* 2017, available at www.acsh .org/news/2017/05/18/embrace-golden-rice -globally-remains-frustratingly-slow-11297.

6. M. R. La Frano and coauthors, Bioavailability of iron, zinc, and provitamin A carotenoids in biofortified staple crops, *Nutrition Reviews* 72 (2014): 289–307.

7. H. Jin and coauthors, Engineering biofuel tolerance in non-native producing microorganisms, *Biotechnology Advances* 32 (2014): 541–548.

8. U.S Environmental Protection Agency, EPA can strengthen its oversight of herbicide resistance with better management controls, 2017, available at www.epa.gov/sites/production/files/2017-06 /documents/_epaoig_20170621-17-p-0278.pdf.

9. U.S. Food and Drug Administration, AquAdvantage salmon fact sheet, 2017, available at www.fda.gov/AnimalVeterinary /DevelopmentApprovalProcess/GeneticEngineering /GeneticallyEngineeredAnimals/ucm473238.htm.

10. Union of Concerned Scientists, Protect our food: A campaign to take the harm out of pharma and industrial crops, available at www .ucsusa.org/food_and_environment/genetic _engineering/protect-our-food.html.

11. M. V. DiLeo and coauthors, An assessment of the relative influences of genetic background, functional diversity at major regulatory genes, and transgenic constructs on the tomato fruit metabolome, *Plant Genome* 7 (2014), epub, doi: 10.3835/plantgenome2013.06.0021.

12. International Food Information Council Foundation, A guide to understanding modern agricultural biotechnology, 2013, available at www.foodinsight.org/sites/default/files/Undstg%20 Modern%20Ag%20Biotechnology.pdf.

13. J. Fernandez-Cornejo and coauthors, Genetically Engineered Crops in the United States (Economic Research Report 162) (Washington, D.C.: U.S. Department of Agriculture, 2014), pp. 24–26.

14. National Bioengineered Food Disclosure Standard: A Proposed Rule by the Agricultural Marketing Service, Federal Register, 05/04/2018, available at www.federalregister.gov/documents /2018/05/04/2018-09389/national-bioengineered -food-disclosure-standard.

Chapter 13

1. J. Abbasi, The paternal epigenome makes its mark, *Journal of the American Medical Association* 317 (2017): 2049–2051; L. Giahi and coauthors, Nutritional modifications in male infertility: A systematic review covering 2 decades, *Nutrition Reviews* 74 (2016): 118–130; T. K. Jensen and coauthors, Habitual alcohol consumption associated with reduced semen quality and changes in reproductive hormones: A cross-sectional study among 1221 young Danish men, *BMJ Open* 4 (2014): e005462.

2. R. F. Goldstein and coauthors, Association of gestational weight gain with maternal and infant outcomes, *Journal of the American Medical Association* 317 (2017): 2207–2225; E. Gresham and coauthors, Effects of dietary interventions on neonatal and infant outcomes: A systematic review and meta-analysis, *American Journal of Clinical Nutrition* 100 (2014): 1298–1321.

3. C. Berti and coauthors, Early-life nutritional exposures and lifelong health: Immediate and long-lasting impacts of probiotics, vitamin D, and breastfeeding, *Nutrition Reviews* 75 (2017): 83–97; D. Ley and coauthors, Early-life origin of intestinal inflammatory disorders, *Nutrition Reviews* 75 (2017): 175–187; J. G. O. Avila and coauthors, Impact of oxidative stress during pregnancy on fetal epigenetic patterns and early origin of vascular diseases, *Nutrition Reviews* 73 (2015): 12–21; T. L. Crume and coauthors, The long-term impact of intrauterine growth restriction in a diverse U.S. cohort of children; The EPOCH study, *Obesity (Silver Springs)* 22 (2014): 608–615.

4. A. M. W. Laerum and coauthors, Psychiatric disorders and general functioning in low birth weight adults: A longitudinal study, *Pediatrics* 139 (2017): e20162135; C. Xie and coauthors, Stunting at 5 years among SGA newborns, *Pediatrics* 137 (2016): e20152636; E. E. Ziegler, Nutrient needs for catch-up growth in low-birthweight infants, *Nestle Nutrition Institute Workshop Series* 81 (2015): 135–143; A. Lahat and coauthors, ADHD among young adults born at extremely low birth weight: The role of fluid intelligence in childhood, *Frontiers in Psychology* 19 (2014): 446.

5. S. L. Murphy and coauthors, Annual summary of vital statistics: 2013–2014, *Pediatrics* 139 (2017): e20163239.

6. Position of the Academy of Nutrition and Dietetics: Nutrition and lifestyle for a healthy pregnancy outcome, *Journal of the Academy of Nutrition and Dietetics* 114 (2014): 1099–1103.

7. Goldstein and coauthors, Association of gestational weight gain with maternal and infant outcomes, 2017; Position of the Academy of Nutrition and Dietetics: Obesity, reproduction and pregnancy outcomes, *Journal of the Academy of Nutrition and Dietetics* 116 (2016): 677–691.

8. Position of the Academy of Nutrition and Dietetics, Obesity, reproduction, and pregnancy outcomes, 2016; R. C. Ma and coauthors, Clinical management of pregnancy in the obese mother: Before conception, during pregnancy and post partum, *Lancet Diabetes and Endocrinology* 4 (2016): 1037–1049.

9. Position of the Academy of Nutrition and Dietetics, Obesity, reproduction, and pregnancy outcomes, 2016; J. Marchi and coauthors, Risks associated with obesity in pregnancy, for the mother and the baby: A systematic review of reviews, *Obesity Reviews* 16 (2015): 621–638.

10. 10 K. M. Godfrey and coauthors, Influence of maternal obesity on the long-term health of offspring, *Lancet Diabetes and Endocrinology* 5 (2017): 53–64; S. A. Leonard and coauthors, Trajectories of maternal weight from before pregnancy through postpartum and associations with childhood obesity, *American Journal of Clinical Nutrition* 106 (2017): 1295–1301.

11. Berti and coauthors, Early-life nutritional exposures and lifelong health: Immediate and long-lasting impacts of probiotics, vitamin D, and breastfeeding, 2017; Ley and coauthors, Early-life origin of intestinal inflammatory disorders, 2017; Avila and coauthors, Impact of oxidative stress during pregnancy on fetal epigenetic patterns and early origin of vascular diseases, 2015; J. Zheng and coauthors, DNA methylation: The pivotal interaction between early-life nutrition and glucose metabolism in later life, *British Journal of Nutrition* 112 (2014): 1850–1857.

12. C. G. Campbell and L. L. Kaiser, Practice Paper of the Academy of Nutrition and Dietetics: Nutrition and lifestyle for a healthy pregnancy outcome, 2014, available at www .eatrightpro.org.

13. V. Leventakou and coauthors, Fish intake during pregnancy, fetal growth, and gestational length in 19 European cohort studies, *American Journal of Clinical Nutrition* 99 (2014): 506–516; K. A. Mulder, D. J. King, and S. M. Innis, Omega-3 fatty acid deficiency in infants before birth identified using a randomized trial of maternal DHA supplementation in pregnancy, *PLoS One* 9 (2014): e83764.

14. P. M. Emmett, L. R. Jones, and J. Golding, Pregnancy diet and associated outcomes in the Avone Longitudinal Study of Parents and Children, *Nutrition Reviews* 73 (Suppl 3) (2015): 154–174.

15. Centers for Disease Control and Prevention, Birth defects COUNT, updated March 31, 2016, available at www.cdc.gov/ncbddd /birthdefectscount/data.html.

16. Centers for Disease Control and Prevention, Birth defects COUNT, 2016.

17. E. T. M. Leermakers and coauthors, Effects of choline on health across the life course: A systematic review, *Nutrition Reviews* 73 (2015): 500–522.

18. C. R. Peterson and D. Ayoub, Congenital rickets due to vitamin D deficiency in the mothers, *Clinical Nutrition* 34 (2015): 793–798.

19. M. K. Ozias and coauthors, Typical prenatal vitamin D supplement intake does not prevent decrease of plasma 25-hydroxyvitamin D at birth, *Journal of the American College of Nutrition* 33 (2014): 394–399.

20. A. L. Fisher and E. Nemeth, Iron homeostasis during pregnancy, *American Journal of Clinical Nutrition* 106 (2017): 1567S–1574S.

21. C. Cao and M. D. Fleming, The placenta: The forgotten essential organ of iron transport, *Nutrition Reviews* 74 (2016): 421–431.

22. Position of the Academy of Nutrition and Dietetics: Nutrition and lifestyle for a healthy pregnancy outcome, 2014.

23. D. G. Weismiller and K. M. Kolasa, Special concerns through an early pregnancy journey, *Nutrition Today* 51 (2016): 175–185; N. M. Nnam, Improving maternal nutrition for better pregnancy outcomes, *Proceedings of the Nutrition Society* 74 (2015): 454–459; L. Englund-Ögge and coauthors, Maternal dietary patterns and preterm delivery: Results from large prospective cohort study, *BMJ* 348 (2014): g1446; J. A. Grieger, L. E. Crzeskowiak, and V. L. Clifton, Preconception dietary patterns in human pregnancies are associated with preterm delivery, *Journal of Nutrition* 144 (2014): 1075–1080.

24. C. G. Campbell and L. L. Kaiser, Practice paper of the Academy of Nutrition and Dietetics: Nutrition and lifestyle for a healthy pregnancy outcome, July 2014, available at www.eatrightpro.org.

25. Women, Infants, and Children, WIC, Frequently asked questions about WIC, updated May 4, 2017, available at www.fns.usda.gov/wic/frequently-asked-questions-about-wic.

26. Goldstein and coauthors, Association of gestational weight gain with maternal and infant outcomes, 2017; N. P. Deputy, A. J. Sharma, and S. Y. Kim, Gestational weight gain—United States, 2012 and 2013, *Morbidity and Mortality Weekly Report* 64 (2015): 1215–1220; Position of the Academy of Nutrition and Dietetics: Nutrition and lifestyle for a healthy pregnancy outcome, 2014.

27. Position of the Academy of Nutrition and Dietetics: Obesity, reproduction, and pregnancy outcomes, 2016; Ma and coauthors, Clinical management of pregnancy in the obese mother: Before conception, during pregnancy and postpartum, 2016; A. B. Berenson and coauthors, Obesity risk knowledge, weight misperception, and diet and health-related attitudes among women intending to become pregnant, *Journal of the Academy of Nutrition and Dietetics* 116 (2016): 69–75; A. C. Flynn and coauthors, Dietary interventions in overweight and obese pregnant women: A systematic review of the content, delivery, and outcomes of randomized controlled trials, *Nutrition Reviews* 74 (2016): 312–328.

28. M. Z. Kapadia and coauthors, Weight loss instead of weight gain within the guidelines in obese women during pregnancy: A systematic review and meta-analyses of maternal and infant outcomes, *PLoS One* 10 (2015): e0132650.

29. M. Perales, R. Artal, and A. Lucia, Exercise during pregnancy, *Journal of the American Medical Association* 317 (2017): 1113–1114; M. Perales and coauthors, Maternal cardiac adaptations to a physical exercise program during pregnancy, *Medicine and Science in Sports and Exercise* 48 (2016): 896–906; S. E. Badon and coauthors, Leisure time physical activity and gestational diabetes mellitus in the Omega Study, *Medicine and Science in Sports and Exercise* 48 (2016): 1044–1052; Position of the Academy of Nutrition and Dietetics: Nutrition and Lifestyle for a healthy pregnancy outcome, 2014.

30. S. T. Harris and coauthors, Exercise during pregnancy and its association with gestational weight gain, *Maternal and Child Health Journal* 19 (2015): 528–537; R. Barakat and coauthors, A program of exercise throughout pregnancy: Is it safe to mother and newborn? *American Journal of Health Promotion* 29 (2014): 2–8.

31. U.S. Department of Health and Human Services, Office of Adolescent Health, Teen pregnancy and childbearing, 2016, available at www.hhs.gov/ash/oah/adolescent-development/reproductive-health-and-teen-pregnancy/teen-pregnancy-and-childbearing/index.html.

32. S. V. Dean and coauthors, Preconception care: Nutritional risks and interventions, *Reproductive Health* 11 (2014): S3.

33. J. L. Bottorff and coauthors, Tobacco and alcohol use in the context of adolescent pregnancy and postpartum: A scoping review of the literature, *Health and Social Care in the Community* 22 (2014): 561–574.

34. R. W. Corbett and K. M. Kolasa, Pica and weight gain in pregnancy, *Nutrition Today* 49 (2014): 101–108.

35. 35 G. Koren, S. Madjunkova, and C. Maltepe, The protective effects of nausea and vomiting of pregnancy against adverse fetal outcome—A systematic review, *Reproductive Toxicology* 47 (2014): 77–80.

36. A. Matthews and coauthors, Interventions for nausea and vomiting in early pregnancy, *Cochrane Database of Systemic Reviews* 3 (2014): CD007575.

37. Centers for Disease Control and Prevention, Reproductive Health: Tobacco use and pregnancy, updated September 29, 2017, available at www.cdc.gov/reproductivehealth/maternalinfanthealth/tobaccousepregnancy/index.htm; S. C. Curtin and T. J. Mathews, Smoking prevalence and cessation before and during pregnancy: Data from the birth certificate, 2014, *National Vital Statistics Reports* 65, February 10, 2016, Hyattsville, MD: National Center for Health Statistics. 2016.

38. S. Phelan, Smoking cessation in pregnancy, *Obstetrics and Gynecology Clinics of North America* 41 (2014): 255–266.

39. M. N. Kooijman and coauthors, Fetal smoke exposure and kidney outcomes in school-aged children, *American Journal of Kidney Diseases* 66 (2015): 412–420.

40. G. Banderali and coauthors, Short and long term health effects of parental tobacco smoking during pregnancy and lactation: A descriptive review, *Journal of Translational Medicine* 13 (2015): 327.

41. E. M. Hollams and coauthors, Persistent effects of maternal smoking during pregnancy on lung function and asthma in adolescents, *American Journal of Respiratory and Critical Care Medicine* 189 (2014): 401–407.

42. American Academy of Pediatrics, Task Force on Sudden Infant Death Syndrome, SIDS and other sleep-related infant deaths: Updated recommendations for a safe infant sleeping environment, *Pediatrics* 138 (2016): e20162938.

43. C. G. Campbell and L. L. Kaiser, Practice paper of the Academy of Nutrition and Dietetics: Nutrition and lifestyle for a healthy pregnancy outcome, July 2014, available at www.eatrightpro.org.

44. M. Neri and coauthors, Drugs of abuse in pregnancy, poor neonatal development, and future neurodegeneration. Is oxidative stress the culprit? *Current Pharmaceutical Design* 21 (2015): 1358–1368; A. M. Cressman and coauthors, Cocaine abuse during pregnancy, *Journal of Obstetrics and Gynaecology Canada* 36 (2014): 628–631.

45. United States Food and Drug Administration, Eating fish: What pregnant women and parents should know, updated October 19, 2017, available at www.fda.gov/Food/ResourcesForYou/Consumers/ucm393070.htm.

46. Centers for Disease Control and Prevention, People at risk—Pregnant women and newborns, updated June 29, 2017, available at www.cdc.gov/listeria/risk-groups/pregnant-women.html.

47. E. Pannia and coauthors, Role of maternal vitamins in programming health and chronic disease, *Nutrition Reviews* 74 (2016): 166–180.

48. The American College of Obstetricians and Gynecologists, Committee Opinion, Moderate caffeine consumption during pregnancy, reaffirmed 2016, available at www.acog.org/Resources-And-Publications/Committee-Opinions/Committee-on-Obstetric-Practice/Moderate-Caffeine-Consumption-During-Pregnancy.

49. L. W. Chen and coauthors, Maternal caffeine intake during pregnancy and risk of pregnancy loss: A categorical and dose-response meta-analysis of prospective studies, *Public Health Nutrition* 19 (2016): 1233–1244; J. Li and coauthors, A meta-analysis of risk of pregnancy loss and caffeine and coffee consumption during pregnancy, *International Journal of Gynaecology and Obstetrics* 130 (2015): 116–122; J. Rhee and coauthors, Maternal caffeine consumption during pregnancy and risk of low birth weight: A dose-response meta-analysis of observational studies, *PLoS One* 10 (2015): e0132334; D. C. Greenwood and coauthors, Caffeine intake during pregnancy and adverse birth outcomes: A systematic review and dose-response meta-analysis, *European Journal of Epidemiology* 29 (2014): 725–734; A. T. Hoyt and coauthors, Maternal caffeine consumption and small for

gestational age births: Results from a population-based case-control study, *Maternal and Child Health Journal* 18 (2014): 1540–1551.

50. Centers for Disease Control, Fetal alcohol spectrum disorders, updated June 6, 2017, available at www.cdc.gov/ncbddd/fasd/data.html; H. E. Hoyme and coauthors, Updated clinical guidelines for diagnosing fetal alcohol spectrum disorders, *Pediatrics* 138 (2016): e20154256.

51. Centers for Disease Control, Fetal alcohol spectrum disorders, updated June 6, 2017, available at www.cdc.gov/ncbddd/fasd/data.html.

52. Hoyme and coauthors, Updated clinical guidelines for diagnosing fetal alcohol spectrum disorders, 2016.

53. Position of the Academy of Nutrition and Dietetics, Obesity, reproduction, and pregnancy outcomes, 2016; A. Allalou and coauthors, A predictive metabolic signature for the transition from gestational diabetes to type 2 diabetes, *Diabetes* 65 (2016): 2529–2539; W. Bao and coauthors, Long-term risk of type 2 diabetes mellitus in relation to BMI and weight change among women with a history of gestational diabetes mellitus: A prospective cohort study, *Diabetologia* 58 (2015): 1212–1219.

54. American Diabetes Association, Classification and diagnosis of diabetes, *Diabetes Care* 40 (2017): S11–S24.

55. H. N. Moussa, S. E. Arian, and B. M. Sibai, Management of hypertension disorders in pregnancy, *Women's Health* 10 (2014): 385–404.

56. Moussa, Arian, and Sibai, Management of hypertension disorders in pregnancy, 2014.

57. J. A. Mennella, L. M. Daniels, and A. R. Reiter, Learning to like vegetables during breastfeeding: A randomized clinical trial of lactating mothers and infants, *American Journal of Clinical Nutrition* 106 (2017): 67–76; S. Nicklaus, The role of dietary experience in the development of eating behavior during the first years of life, *Nutrition and Metabolism* 70 (2017): 241–245.

58. Committee on Food Allergies: Global burden, causes, treatment, prevention, and public policy, in V. A. Stallings and M. P. Oria, eds., Food and Nutrition Board, Health and Medicine Division, National Academies of Sciences, Engineering, and Medicine, *Finding a Path to Safety in Food Allergy: Assessment of the Global Burden, Causes, Prevention, Management, and Public Policy* (Washington, D.C.: National Academies Press, 2016), available at www.nap.edu/23658.

59. C. G. Perrine and coauthors, Lactation and maternal cardio-metabolic health, *Annual Review of Nutrition* 36 (2016): 627–645; Position of the Academy of Nutrition and Dietetics, Obesity, reproduction, and pregnancy outcomes, 2016; N. Lòpez-Olmedo and coauthors, The associations of maternal weight change with breastfeeding, diet and physical activity during the postpartum period, *Maternal and Child Health Journal* 20 (2016): 270–280; M. P. Jarlenski and coauthors, Effects of breastfeeding

on postpartum weight loss among U.S. women, *Preventive Medicine* 69 (2014): 146–150.

60. A Zourladani and coauthors, The effect of physical exercise on postpartum fitness, hormone levels, and lipid levels: A randomized controlled trial in primiparous, lactating women, *Archives of Gynecology and Obstetrics* 291 (2015): 525–530; D. R. Evenson and coauthors, Summary of international guidelines for physical activity after pregnancy, *Obstetrical and Gynecological Survey* 69 (2014): 407–414.

61. Centers for Disease Control and Prevention, Health effects of Secondhand smoke, updated January 11, 2017, available at www.cdc.gov/tobacco/data_statistics/fact_sheets/secondhand_smoke/health_effects; J. D. Thacher and coauthors, Pre- and postnatal exposure to parental Smoking and allergic disease through adolescence, *Pediatrics* 134 (2014): 428–434.

62. Breastfeeding, in American Academy of Pediatrics, *Pediatric Nutrition*, 7th ed., ed. R. E. Kleinman (Elk Grove Village, Ill.: American Academy of Pediatrics, 2014), pp. 41–59.

63. Breastfeeding, in American Academy of Pediatrics, *Pediatric Nutrition*, 2014.

64. Formula feeding of term infants, in *Pediatric Nutrition*, 7th ed., ed. R. E. Kleinman (Elk Grove Village, IL: American Academy of Pediatrics, 2014), pp. 61–81.

65. Position of the Academy of Nutrition and Dietetics: Promoting and supporting breastfeeding, *Journal of the Academy of Nutrition and Dietetics* 115 (2015): 444–449; Breastfeeding, in American Academy of Pediatrics, *Pediatric Nutrition*, 2014.

66. Position of the Academy of Nutrition and Dietetics: Promoting and supporting breastfeeding, 2015; Breastfeeding, in American Academy of Pediatrics, *Pediatric Nutrition*, 2014.

67. American Academy of Pediatrics, *New Mother's Guide to Breastfeeding*, 3rd ed., ed. J. Y. Meek (New York, Bantam Books, 2017), pp. 64–94.

68. T. Jost and coauthors, Impact of human milk bacteria and oligosaccharides on neonatal gut microbiota establishment and gut health, *Nutrition Reviews* 73 (2015): 426–437.

69. Jost and coauthors, Impact of human milk bacteria and oligosaccharides on neonatal gut microbiota establishment and gut health, 2015; T. Smilowitz and coauthors, Breast milk oligosaccharides: Structure-function relationships in the neonate, *Annual Review of Nutrition* 34 (2014): 143–169.

70. J. T. Brenna and S. E. Carlson, Docosahexaenoic acid and human brain development: Evidence that a dietary supply is needed for optimal development, *Journal of Human Evolution* 77 (2014): 99–106.

71. S. M. Innis, Impact of maternal diet on human milk composition and neurological development of infants, *American Journal of Clinical Nutrition* 99 (2014): 734S–741S; Brenna and Carlson, Docosahexaenoic acid and human brain development: Evidence that a dietary supply is needed for optimal development, 2014.

72. U. Ramakrishnan and coauthors, Prenatal supplementation with DHA improves attention at 5 y or age: A randomized controlled trial, *American Journal of Clinical Nutrition* 104 (2016): 1075–1082; J. J. Qingqing and coauthors, Effect of n-3 PUFA supplementation on cognitive function throughout the life span from infancy to old age: A systematic review and meta-analysis of randomized controlled trials, *American Journal of Clinical Nutrition* 100 (2014): 1422–1436.

73. American Academy of Pediatrics, Fat-soluble vitamins, in *Pediatric Nutrition*, 7th ed., ed. R. E. Kleinman (Elk Grove Village, Ill.: American Academy of Pediatrics, 2014), pp. 495–515.

74. American Academy of Pediatrics, Breastfeeding, in *Pediatric Nutrition*, 7th ed., ed. R. E. Kleinman (Elk Grove Village, Ill.: American Academy of Pediatrics, 2014), pp. 41–59.

75. B. Lönnerdal, Human milk: Bioactive proteins/peptides and functional properties, *Nestle Nutrition Institute Workshop Series* 86 (2016): 97–107; M. A. Koch and coauthors, Maternal IgG and IgA antibodies dampen mucosal T helper cell responses in early life, *Cell* 165 (2016): 827–841; Jost and coauthors, Impact of human milk bacteria and oligosaccharides on neonatal gut microbiota establishment and gut health, 2015; Position of the Academy of Nutrition and Dietetics: Promoting and supporting breastfeeding, *Journal of the Academy of Nutrition and Dietetics* 115 (2015): 444–449; Smilowitz and coauthors, Breast milk oligosaccharides: Structure-function relationships in the neonate, 2014.

76. Jost and coauthors, Impact of human milk bacteria and oligosaccharides on neonatal gut microbiota establishment and gut health, 2015; B. M. Jakaitis and P. W. Denning, Human breast milk and the gastrointestinal innate immune system, *Clinics in Perinatology* 41 (2014): 423–435.

77. I. Tromp and coauthors, Breastfeeding and the risk of respiratory tract infections after infancy: The Generation R Study, *PLoS One* 12 (2017): e0172763; G. Bowatte and coauthors, Breastfeeding and childhood acute otitis media: A systematic review and meta-analysis, *Acta Paediatricsa* 104 (2015): 85–95.

78. K. Grimshaw and coauthors, Modifying the infant's diet to prevent food allergy, *Archives of Disease in Childhood* 102 (2017): 179–186; V. Bion and coauthors, Evaluating the efficacy of breastfeeding guidelines on long-term outcomes for allergic disease, *Allergy* 71 (2016): 661–670; C. J. Lodge and coauthors, Breastfeeding and asthma and allergies: A systematic review and meta-analysis, *Acta Paediatrica* 104 (2015): 38–53.

79. J. M. D. Thompson and coauthors, Duration of breastfeeding and risk of SIDS: An individual participant data meta-analysis, *Pediatrics* 140 (2017): e20171324; R. A. Danall and coauthors, American Academy of Pediatrics' Task Force on SIDS fully supports breastfeeding, *Breastfeeding Medicine* 9 (2014): 486–487.

80. P. Rzehak and coauthors, Infant feeding and growth trajectory patterns in childhood and body composition in young adulthood, *American Journal of Clinical Nutrition* 106 (2017): 568–580; W. Liang and coauthors, Breastfeeding reduces childhood obesity risks, *Childhood Obesity* 13 (2017): 197–204; A. Zamora-Kapoor and coauthors, Breastfeeding in infancy is associated with body mass index in adolescence: A retrospective cohort study comparing American Indians/Alaska Natives and Non-Hispanic whites, *Journal of the Academy of Nutrition and Dietetics* 117 (2017): 1049–1056; R. J. Hancox and coauthors, Association between breastfeeding and body mass index at age 6-7 years in an international survey, *Pediatric Obesity* 10 (2015): 283–287; C. M. Lefebvre and R. M. John, The effect of breastfeeding on childhood overweight and obesity: A systematic review of the literature, *Journal of the American Association of Nurse Practitioners* 26 (2014): 386–401.

81. Lefebvre and John, The effect of breastfeeding on childhood overweight and obesity: A systematic review of the literature, 2014.

82. S. Bar, R. Milanaik, and A. Adesman, Long-term neurodevelopmental benefits of breastfeeding, *Current Opinion in Pediatrics* 28 (2016): 559–566; S. Cai and coauthors, Infant feeding effects on early neurocognitive development in Asian children, *American Journal of Clinical Nutrition* 101 (2015): 326–336.

83. American Academy of Pediatrics, Formula feeding of term infants, in *Pediatric Nutrition*, 2014.

84. American Academy of Pediatrics, Formula feeding of term infants, in *Pediatric Nutrition*, 2014.

85. American Academy of Pediatrics, Formula feeding of term infants, in *Pediatric Nutrition*, 2014.

86. American Academy of Pediatrics, Complementary feeding, in *Pediatric Nutrition*, 7th ed., ed. R. E. Kleinman (Elk Grove Village, Ill.: American Academy of Pediatrics, 2014), pp. 123–139.

87. American Academy of Pediatrics, Complementary feeding, in *Pediatric Nutrition*, 2014.

88. R. Pérez-Escamilla, S. Segura-Pérez, and M. Lott, Feeding guidelines for infants and young toddlers, *Nutrition Today* 52 (2017): 223–231.

89. American Academy of Pediatrics, Complementary feeding, in *Pediatric Nutrition*, 2014.

90. M. B. Heyman and S. A. Abrams, Fruit juice in infants, children, and adolescents: Current recommendations, *Pediatrics* 139 (2017): e20170967.

91. Heyman and Abrams, Fruit juice in infants, children, and adolescents: Current recommendations, 2017.

92. P. J. Turner and D. E. Campbell, Implementing primary prevention for peanut allergy at a population level, *Journal of the American Medical Association* 317 (2017): 1111–1112; A. Togias and coauthors, Addendum guidelines for the prevention of peanut allergy in the United States: Report of the National Institute of Allergy and Infectious Deseases—sponsored expert panel, *Annals of Allergy, Asthma, and Immunology* 118 (2017): 166.e7–173.e7; G. Du Toit and coauthors, Randomized trial of peanut consumption in infants at risk for peanut allergy, *New England Journal of Medicine* 372 (2015): 803–813; D. M. Fleischer and coauthors, Consensus communication on early peanut introduction and the prevention of peanut allergy in high-risk infants, *Pediatrics* 136 (2015): 600–604.

Consumer's Guide 13

1. R. L. Dunn and coauthors, Engaging field-based professionals in a qualitative assessment of barriers and positive contributors to breastfeeding using the social ecological model, *Maternal and Child Health Journal* 19 (2015): 6–16; A. Brown, Maternal trait personality and breast- feeding duration: The importance of confidence and social support, *Journal of Advanced Nursing* 70 (2014): 587–598; A. S. Teich, J. Barnett, and K. Bonuck, Women's perceptions of breast-feeding barriers in early postpartum period: A qualitative analysis nested in two randomized controlled trials, *Breastfeeding Medicine* 9 (2014): 9–15.

2. J. M. Nelson, R. Li, and C. G. Perrine, Trends of U.S. hospitals distributing infant formula packs to breastfeeding mothers, 2007 to 2013, *Pediatrics* 135 (2015): 1051–1056.

3. Centers for Disease Control and Prevention, *Breastfeeding Report Card United States, 2016,* available at www.cdc.gov/breastfeeding/data/reportcard.htm.

4. U.S. Department of Health and Human Services, *Healthy People 2020,* available at www.healthypeople.gov.

Controversy 13

1. NCD Risk Factor Collaboration, Worldwide trends in body-mass index, underweight, overweight, and obesity from 1975 to 2016: A pooled analysis of 2416 population-based measurement studies in 128.9 million children, adolescents, and adults, *Lancet* (2017), epub ahead of print, doi: http://dx.doi.org/10.1016/S0140-6736(17)32129-3.

2. U.S. Preventive Services Task Force, Screening for obesity in children and adolescents: U.S. Preventive Services Task Force Recommendation Statement, *Journal of the American Medical Association* (2017): 2417–2426.

3. Y. Jo, The differences in characteristics among households with and without obese children: Findings from USDA's FoodAPS, EIB-179, April 2017, available at www.ers.usda.gov/webdocs/publications/85028/eib-179.pdf?v=42989; P. Dolton and M. Xiao, The intergenerational transmission of body mass index across countries, *Economics and Human Biology* 24 (2017): 140–152; M. Ng and coauthors, Global, regional, and national prevalence of overweight and obesity in children and adults during 1980–2013: A systematic analysis for the Global Burden of Disease Study 2013, *Lancet* (2014): 766–781; C. L. Ogden and coauthors, Prevalence of child and adult obesity in the United States, 2011–2012, *Journal of the American Medical Association* 311 (2014): 806–814.

4. Centers for Disease Control and Prevention, Prevalence of Childhood Obesity in the United States, 2011–2014 (2017), available at www.cdc.gov/obesity/data/childhood.html.

5. J. C. Jones-Smith and coauthors, Socioeconomic status and trajectory of overweight from birth to mid-childhood: The Early Childhood Longitudinal Study-Birth Cohort, *PLoS One* (2014), epub, doi: 10.1371/journal.pone.0100181.

6. M. Jones and coauthors, BMI health report cards: Parents' perceptions and reactions, *Health Promotion Practice* (2017), epub ahead of print, doi: 10.1177/1524839917749489; K. E. Rhee, R. McEachern, and E. Jelalian, Parent readiness to change differs for overweight child dietary and physical activity behaviors, *Journal of the Academy of Nutrition and Dietetics* (2014), epub, doi: 10.1016/j.jand.2014.04.029.

7. U.S. Preventive Services Task Force, Screening for obesity in children and adolescents: U.S. Preventive Services Task Force Recommendation Statement, 2017.

8. A. W. Harrist and coauthors, The social and emotional lives of overweight, obese, and severely obese children, *Child Development* 87 (2016): 1564–1580.

9. E. M. Throop and coauthors, Pass the popcorn: "Obesogenic" behaviors and stigma in children's movies, *Obesity* 22 (2014): 1694–1700.

10. Centers for Disease Control and Prevention, Healthy weight—It's not a diet, it's a lifestyle!: About BMI for Children and Teens, 2014, available at www.cdc.gov.

11. Mayo Clinic, Diseases and conditions: Type 2 diabetes in children: Definition, 2015, available at www.mayoclinic.org/diseases-conditions/type-2-diabetes-in-children/basics/definition/con-20030124-40k.

12. A. Umer and coauthors, Childhood obesity and adult cardiovascular disease risk factors: A systematic review with meta-analysis, *BMC Public Health* (2017), epub, doi: 10.1186/s12889-017-4691-z.

13. A. C. Skinner and coauthors, Cardiometabolic risks and severity of obesity in children and young adults, *New England Journal of Medicine* 373 (2015): 1307–1317.

14. T. W. Wang and coauthors, Tobacco product use among middle and high school students, United States, 2011–2017, *Morbidity and Mortality Weekly Report* 67 (2108): 629–633; W. L. Chan She Ping-Delfos and coauthors, Use of the Dietary Guideline Index to assess cardiometabolic risk in adolescents, *British Journal of Nutrition* 113 (2015): 1741–1752; Kids Health, Cholesterol and your child, 2015, available at kidshealth.org/parent/medical/heart/cholesterol.html.

15. S. L. Jackson and coauthors, Hypertension among youths—United States, 2001–2016, *Morbidity and Mortality Weekly Reports* 67 (2018): 758-762; L. Jing and coauthors, Ambulatory systolic blood pressure and obesity are

independently associated with left ventricular hypertrophic remodeling in children, *Journal of Cardiovascular Magnetic Resonance* (2017), epub, doi: 10.1186/s12968-017-0401-3.

16. M-J. Buscot and coauthors, BMI trajectories associated with resolution of elevated youth BMI and incident adult obesity, *Pediatrics* 141 (2018): e20172003.

17. N. H. Golden, M. Schneider, and C. Wood, Preventing obesity and eating disorders in adolescents, *American Academy of Pediatrics* 138 (2016): 114–123; B. Y. Rollins and coauthors, Maternal controlling feeding practices and girls' inhibitory control interact to predict changes in BMI and eating in the absence of hunger from 5 to 7 y, *American Journal of Clinical Nutrition* 99 (2014): 249–257.

18. American Academy of Pediatrics Policy Statement: Media and young minds, *Pediatrics* 138 (2016): 89–94; American Academy of Pediatrics, Media and children, 2015, available at www.aap.org.

19. E. J. Boyland and coauthors, Advertising as a cue to consume: A systematic review and meta-analysis of the effects of acute exposure to unhealthy food and nonalcoholic beverage advertising on intake in children and adults, *American Journal of Clinical Nutrition* 103 (2016): 519–533; M. R. Longacre and coauthors, Child-targeted TV advertising and preschoolers' consumption of high-sugar breakfast cereals, *Appetite* 108 (2016): 295–302.

20. M. M. Putnam, C. E. Cotto, and S. L. Calvert, Character apps for children's snacks: Effects of character awareness on snack selection and consumption patterns, *Games for Health Journal* (2018), epub, doi: 10.1089/g4h.2017.0097; American Psychological Association, The impact of food advertising on childhood obesity, 2017, available at www.apa.org/topics/kids-media /food.aspx.

21. W. C. Frazier III and J. L. Harris, Trends in television food advertising to young people: 2016 update, Rudd Brief, (2017), available at uconnruddcenter.org/files/TVAdTrends2017.pdf.

22. American Heart Association, Policy position statement on food advertising and marketing practices to children, 2015, available at www.heart.org/advocacy; World Health Organization, A framework for implementing the set of recommendations on the marketing of foods and non-alcoholic beverages to children, 2012, available at www.who.int.

23. M. Buscot and coauthors, BMI trajectories associated with resolution of elevated youth BMI and incident adult obesity, *Pediatrics* (2018), epub, doi: 10.1542/peds.2017-2003; A. H. Kristensen and coauthors, Reducing childhood obesity through U.S. federal policy: A microsimulation analysis, *American Journal of Preventive Medicine* 47 (2014): 604–612.

24. S. N. Bleich and coauthors, Interventions to prevent global childhood overweight and obesity: A systematic review, *Lancet Diabetes and Endocrinology* 6 (2018): 332–346; M. Hunsberger, Early feeding practices and family structure: Associations with overweight in children, *Proceedings of the Nutrition Society* 73 (2014): 132–136.

25. Mayo Clinic, Childhood obesity: Treatment and drugs, 2015, available at www.Mayoclinic .org.

26. H. Bergmeier, H. Skouteris, and M. Heatherington, Systematic research review of observational approaches used to evaluate mother–child mealtime interactions during preschool years, *American Journal of Clinical Nutrition* 101 (2015): 7–15.

27. J. Martin-Biggers and coauthors, Translating it into real life: A qualitative study of the cognitions, barriers, and supports for key obesogenic behaviors of parents of preschoolers, *BMC Public Health* 15 (2015): 189–203.

28. S. McGinty, T. K. Richmond, and N. K. Desai, Managing adolescent obesity and the role of bariatric surgery, *Current Opinion in Pediatrics* 27 (2015): 434–441; M. H. Zeller and coauthor, Severe obesity and comorbid condition impact on the weight-related quality of life of the adolescent patient, *Journal of Pediatrics* 166 (2015): 651–659.

29. A. S. Khalsa, Attainment of "5-2-1-0" obesity recommendations in preschool-aged children, *Preventive Medicine Reports* 8 (2017): 79–87.

30. U.S. Department of Agriculture and U.S. Department of Health and Human Services, Scientific report of the 2015 Dietary Guidelines Advisory Committee, 2015, D: 3–7, available at www.health.gov; R. B. Ervin and coauthors, Consumption of added sugar among U.S. children and adolescents, 2005–2008 (NCHS Data Brief 87), 2012.

31. J. A. Mitchell and coauthors, Physical activity and pediatric obesity: A quantile regression analysis, *Medicine and Science in Sports and Exercise* 49 (2017): 466–473; T. Skrede and coauthors, Moderate-to-vigorous physical activity, but not sedentary time, predicts changes in cardiometabolic risk factors in 10-y-old children: The Active Smarter Kids Study, *American Journal of Clinical Nutrition* 105 (2017): 1391–1398; I. Dias and coauthors, Effects of resistance training on obese adolescents, *Medicine and Science in Sports and Exercise* 47 (2015): 2636–2644.

32. P. T. Katzmarzyk and coauthors, An evolving scientific basis for the prevention and treatment of pediatric obesity, *International Journal of Obesity* 38 (2014): 887–905.

33. M. Miller and coauthors, Sleep duration and incidence of obesity in infants, children, and adolescents: A systematic review and meta-analysis of prospective studies, *Sleep* (2018), epub, doi: 10.1093/sleep/zsy018; A. Rangan and coauthors, Shorter sleep duration is associated with higher energy intake and an increase in BMI z-score in young children predisposed to overweight, *International Journal of Obesity* 42 (2017): 59–64; B. L. Jones, B. H. Fiese, and The STRONG Kids Team, Parent routines, child routines, and family demographics associated with obesity in parents and preschool-aged children, *Frontiers in Psychology* (2014), epub, doi: 10.3389/fpsyg.2014.00374.

34. E. N. Mullins and coauthors, Acute sleep restriction increases dietary intake in preschool-age children, *Journal of Sleep Research* 26 (2017): 48–54.

Chapter 14

1. E. C. Banfield and coauthors, Poor adherence to U.S. dietary guidelines for children and adolescents in the national health and nutrition examination survey population, *Journal of the Academy of Nutrition and Dietetics* 116 (2016): 21–27; Position of the Academy of Nutrition and Dietetics: Nutrition guidance for healthy children ages 2 to 11 years, *Journal of the Academy of Nutrition and Dietetics* 114 (2014): 1257–1276.

2. L. L. Birch and A. E. Doub, Learning to eat: Birth to age 2 y, *American Journal of Clinical Nutrition* 99 (2014): 723S–728S.

3. R. S. Gibson, A. M. Heath, and E. A. Szymlek-Gay, Is iron and zinc nutrition a concern for vegetarian infants and young children in industrialized countries? *American Journal of Clinical Nutrition* 100 (2014): 459S–468S.

4. Committee on Dietary Reference Intakes, *Dietary Reference Intakes for energy, carbohydrate, fiber, fat, fatty acids, cholesterol, protein, and amino acids* (Washington, D.C.: National Academies Press, 2005), Chapter 11.

5. Committee on Dietary Reference Intakes, *Dietary Reference Intakes for calcium and vitamin D* (Washington, D.C.: National Academies Press, 2011), pp. 5–35.

6. M. Nimesh and coauthors, An unsuspected pharmacological vitamin D toxicity in a child and its brief review of literature, *Toxicology International* 22 (2015): 167–169.

7. P. M. Gupta and coauthors, Iron status of toddlers, nonpregnant females, and pregnant females in the United States, *American Journal of Clinical Nutrition* 106 (2017): 1640S–1646S.

8. Banfield and coauthors, Poor adherence to U.S. dietary guidelines for children and adolescents in the national health and nutrition examination survey population, 2016.

9. K. J. Newens and J. Walton, A review of sugar consumption from nationally representative dietary surveys across the world, *Journal of Human Nutrition and Dietetics* 29 (2016): 225–240.

10. C. L. Brown and coauthors, Association of picky eating with weight status and dietary quality among low-income preschoolers, *Academic Pediatrics* (2017), epub ahead of print, doi: 10.1016/j.acap.2017.08.014.

11. A. Fildes and coauthors, Common genetic architecture underlying young children's food fussiness and liking for vegetables and fruit, *American Journal of Clinical Nutrition* 103 (2016): 1099–1104.

12. N. Zucker and coauthors, Psychological and psychosocial impairment in preschoolers with selective eating, *Pediatrics* 136 (2015): 574–575; S. Monnery-Patris and coauthors,

Smell differential reactivity, but not taste differential reactivity, is related to food neophobia in toddlers, *Appetite* 95 (2015): 303–309; V. Quick and coauthors, Relationships of neophobia and pickiness with dietary variety, dietary quality and diabetes management adherence in youth with type 1 diabetes, *European Journal of Clinical Nutrition* 68 (2014): 131–136.

13. J. A. Saltzman and coauthors, Predictors and outcomes of mealtime emotional climate in families with preschoolers, *Pediatric Psychology* 43 (2017): 195–206.

14. A. M. Ashman and coauthors, Maternal diet during early childhood, but not pregnancy, predicts diet quality and fruit and vegetable acceptance in offspring, *Maternal and Child Nutrition* 12 (2016): 579–590.

15. P. M. Gupta and coauthors, Iron, anemia, and iron deficiency anemia among young children in the United States, *Nutrients*, 2016, doi: 10.3390/nu8060330; J. R. Doom and M. K. Georgieff, Striking while the iron is hot: Understanding the biological and neurodevelopmental effects of iron deficiency to optimize intervention in early childhood, *Current Pediatric Reports* 2 (2014): 291–298.

16. B. B. Lanphear and coauthors, Prevention of childhood lead toxicity, *Pediatrics* (2016), epub, doi: 10.1542/peds.2016-1493; Centers for Disease Control and Prevention, Lead, available at www.cdc.gov/nceh/lead.

17. K. Dubanoski, Notes from the field: Lead poisoning in an infant associated with a metal bracelet—Connecticut, *Morbidity and Mortality Weekly Report* 66 (2016): 916.

18. World Health Organization, Lead poisoning and health (2017), available at www.who.int/mediacentre/factsheets/fs379/en/.

19. World Health Organization, Lead poisoning and health (2017), available at www.who.int/mediacentre/factsheets/fs379/en/.

20. KidsHealth, Lead poisoning (2015), available at kidshealth.org/parent/medical/brain/lead_poisoning.html.

21. B. P. Lanphear and Council on Environmental Health, American Academy of Pediatrics Policy Statement, Prevention of childhood lead toxicity, *Pediatrics* 138 (2016): 146–160.

22. Y. Wang, K. Wu, and W. Zhao, Blood zinc, calcium and lead levels in Chinese children aged 1–36 months, *International Journal of Clinical and Experimental Medicine* 8 (2015): 1424–1426; X. Ji and coauthors, Evaluation of blood zinc, calcium and blood lead levels among children aged 1–36 months, *Nutricion Hospitalaria* 30 (2014): 548–551; C. S. Sim and coauthors, Iron deficiency increases blood lead levels in boys and pre-menarche girls surveyed in NHANES 2010–2011, *Environmental Research* (2014), epub, doi: 10.1016/j.envres.2014.01.004.

23. Food Allergy Research & Education, About food allergies, 2015, available at www.foodallergy.org/about-food-allergies.

24. B. I. Nwaru and coauthors, Prevalence of common food allergies in Europe: A systematic review and meta-analysis, *Allergy* 69 (2014): 992–1007; S. H. Sicherer and coauthors, The natural history of egg allergy in an observational cohort, *Journal of Allergy and Clinical Immunology* 133 (2014): 492–499.

25. S. M. Jones and A. W. Burks, Food allergy, *New England Journal of Medicine* 377 (2017): 1168–1176.

26. R. Meyer and coauthors, A practical approach to vitamin and mineral supplementation in food allergic children, *Clinical and Translational Allergy* 5 (2015): 11.

27. S. C. Collins, Practice paper of the Academy of Nutrition and Dietetics: Role of the registered dietitian nutritionist in the diagnosis and management of food allergies, *Journal of the Academy of Nutrition and Dietetics* 116 (2016): 1621–1631.

28. R. G. Heine, Food allergy prevention and treatment by targeted nutrition, *Annals of Nutrition and Metabolism* 72 (2018): 33–45; Jones and Burks, Food allergy, 2017; D. M. H. Freeland and coauthors, Oral immunotherapy for food allergy, *Seminars in Immunology* (2017), epub ahead of print, doi: 10.1016/j.smim.2017.08.008; B. P. Vickery and coauthors, Early oral immunotherapy in peanut-allergic preschool children is safe and highly effective, *Journal of Allergy and Clinical Immunology* 139 (2016): 183–181.

29. V. A. Stallings and M. P. Oria, eds., National Academies of Sciences Engineering and Medicine Committee on Food Allergies: Global burden, causes, treatment, prevention, and public policy, (2017), epub available at www.nationalacademies.org/hmd/Activities/Nutrition/FoodAllergies.aspx.

30. Centers for Disease Control and Prevention, Attention-Deficit/Hyperactivity Disorder, Data and Statistics, (2017), available at www.cdc.gov/ncbddd/adhd/data.html.

31. J. T. Nigg and K. Holton, Restriction and elimination diets in ADHD treatment, *Child and Adolescent Psychiatric Clinics* 23 (2014): 937–953; E. Hawkey and J. T. Nigg, Omega-3 fatty acid and ADHD: Blood level analysis and meta-analytic extension of supplementation trials, *Clinical Psychology Review* 34 (2014): 496–505.

32. Centers for Disease Control and Prevention, Attention Deficit/Hyperactivity Disorder (ADHD), (2017), available at www.cdc.gov/ncbddd/adhd/facts.html.

33. National Institute of Dental and Craniofacial Research, Dental caries (tooth decay) in children (age 2 to 11), (2014), available at http://nidcr.nih.gov/DataStatistics/FindDataByTopic/DentalCaries/DentalCariesChildren2to11.htm.

34. S. Park and coauthors, Association of sugar-sweetened beverage intake during infancy with dental caries in 6-year olds, *Clinical Nutrition Research* 4 (2015): 9–17; A. Sheiham and W. P. T. James, A reappraisal of the quantitative relationship between sugar intake and dental caries: The need for new criteria for developing goals for sugar intake, *BMC Public Health* 14 (2014): 863.

35. U.S. Department of Agriculture and U.S. Department of Health and Human Services, Scientific Report of the 2015 Dietary Guidelines Advisory Committee (2015), C:15, available at health.gov/dietaryguidelines/2015-scientific-report/pdfs/scientific-report-of-the-2015-dietary-guidelines-advisory-committee.pdf.

36. J. D. Coulthard, L. Palla, and G. K. Pot, Breakfast consumption and nutrient intakes in 4-18-year olds: UK National Diet and Nutrition Survey Rolling Programme (2008–2012), *British Journal of Nutrition* 118 (2017): 280–290; S. S. Pineda Vargas and coauthors, Eating ready-to-eat cereal for breakfast is positively associated with daily nutrient intake, but not weight, in Mexican-American children and adolescents, *Nutrition Today* 51 (2016): 206–215.

37. C. N. Rasberry and coauthors, Health-related behaviors and academic achievement among high school students—United States, 2015, *Morbidity and Mortality Weekly Report* 66 (2017): 921–927.

38. F. Koohdani and coauthors, Midmorning snack programs have a beneficial effect on cognitive performance of students from high socioeconomic background, *Nutrition Today* 51 (2016): 310–315.

39. Position of the Academy of Nutrition and Dietetics, Society for Nutrition Education and Behavior, and School Nutrition Association: Comprehensive Nutrition Programs and Services in Schools, *Journal of the Academy of Nutrition and Dietetics* 118 (2018): 913–919; National School Lunch Program, 2016, available at www.fns.usda.gov/nslp/national-school-lunch-program-nslp.

40. K. L. Hubbard and coauthors, What's in children's backpacks? Foods brought from home, *Journal of the Academy of Nutrition and Dietetics* (2014), epub, doi: 10.1016/j.jand.2014.05.010; M. R. Longacre and coauthors, School food reduces household income disparities in adolescents' frequency of fruit and vegetable intake, *Preventive Medicine* 69 (2014): 202–207.

41. U.S. Department of Agriculture, Food and Nutrition Service, Nutrition standards in the National School Lunch and School Breakfast Programs: Final rule, *Federal Register* 77 (2012): 4088–4167.

42. M. A. Adams and coauthors, Location of school lunch salad bars and fruit and vegetable consumption in middle schools: A cross-sectional plate waste study, *Journal of the Academy of Nutrition and Dietetics* 116 (2016): 407–416.

43. American Academy of Pediatrics, Policy statement: Snacks, sweetened beverages, added sugars, and schools, *Pediatrics* 135 (2015): 575–583.

44. H. H. Laroche and coauthors, Healthy concessions: High school students' responses to healthy concession stand changes, *Journal of School Health* 87 (2017): 98–105; Centers for Disease Control and Prevention, Adolescent and school health: Competitive foods in schools,

2014, available at www.cdc.gov/healthyyouth /nutrition/standards.htm.

45. E. Hennessy and coauthors, State-level school competitive food and beverage laws are associated with children's weight status, *Journal of School Health* 84 (2014): 609–616.

46. E. C. Banfield and coauthors, Poor adherence to U.S. dietary guidelines for children and adolescents in the national health and nutrition examination survey population, 2016.

47. L. M. Lipsky and coauthors, Diet quality of US adolescents during the transition to adulthood: Changes and predictors, *American Journal of Clinical Nutrition* 105 (2017): 1424–1432; M. E. Harrison and coauthors, Systematic review of the effects of family meal frequency on psychosocial outcomes in youth, *Canadian Family Physician* 61 (2015): e96–e106.

48. Committee on Adolescent Healthy Care, Committee Opinion No. 714: Obesity in adolescents, *Obstetrics and Gynecology* 130 (2017): e127–e140.

49. J. L. Moss, B. Liu, and L. Zhu, Comparing percentages and ranks of adolescent weight-related outcomes among U.S. states: Implications for intervention development, *Preventive Medicine* 105 (2017): 109–115; B. S. Metcalf and coauthors, Exploring the adolescent fall in physical activity: A 10-yr cohort study (Early Bird 41), *Exercise and Science in Sports and Medicine* 47 (2015): 2084–2092.

50. C. M. Weaver and coauthors, The National Osteoporosis Foundation's position statement on peak bone mass development and lifestyle factors: A systematic review and implementation recommendations, *Osteoporosis International* 27 (2016): 1281–1386.

51. G. Miller and coauthors, Trends in beverage consumption among high school students—United States, 2007–2015, *Morbidity and Mortality Weekly Report* 66 (2017): 112–116.

52. M. Luger and coauthors, Sugar-sweetened beverages and weight gain in children and adults: A systematic review from 2013 to 2015 and a comparison with previous studies, *Obesity Facts* 10 (2017): 674–693; S. D. Poppitt, Beverage consumption: Are alcoholic and sugary drinks tipping the balance toward overweight and obesity? *Nutrients* 7 (2015): 6700–6715.

53. R. Katta and S. P. Desai, Diet and dermatology, *Journal of Clinical Aesthetic Dermatology* 7 (2014): 46–51.

54. L. M. Lipsky and coauthors, Diet quality of US adolescents during the transition to adulthood: Changes and predictors, *American Journal of Clinical Nutrition* 105 (2017): 1424–1432.

55. G. Miller and coauthors, Trends in beverage consumption among high school students—United States, 2007–2015, *Morbidity and Mortality Weekly Report* 66 (2017): 112–116; H. A. Hoertel, M. J. Will, and H. J. Leidy, A randomized crossover, pilot study examining the effects of a normal protein vs. high protein breakfast on food cravings and reward signals in overweight/obese "breakfast skipping," late-adolescent girls, *Nutrition Journal* (2014),

epub, doi: 101186/1475-2891-13-80; J. M. Poti, K. J. Duffey, and B. M. Popkin, The association of fast food consumption with poor dietary outcomes and obesity among children: Is it the fast food or the remainder of the diet? *American Journal of Clinical Nutrition* 99 (2014): 162–171.

56. J. M. Berge and coauthors, Family food preparation and its effects on adolescent dietary quality and eating patterns, *Journal of Adolescent Health* 59 (2016): 530–536.

57. Y. Li and coauthors, Impact of healthy lifestyle factors on life expectancies in the U.S. population, *Circulation* (2018), epub ahead of print, doi: 10.1161/CIRCULATIONAHA.117.032047; W. Rizza, N. Veronese, and L. Fontana, What are the roles of calorie restriction and diet quality in promoting healthy longevity? *Ageing Research Reviews* 13 (2014): 38–45.

58. E. Arias, M. Heron, J. Xu, United States Life Tables, 2013, National Vital Statistics Reports 66 (2017), epub, available at www.cdc.gov/nchs/ data/nvsr/nvsr66/nvsr66_03.pdf.

59. M. P. Rozing, T. B. L. Kirkwood, and R. G. J. Westendorp, Is there evidence for a limit to human lifespan? *Nature* 546 (2017): E11–E12; X. Dong, B. Milholland, and J. Vijg, Evidence for a limit to human lifespan, *Nature* 538 (2016): 257–259.

60. P. Liu and coauthors, Sarcopenia as a predictor of all-cause mortality among community-dwelling older people: A systematic review and meta-analysis, *Maturitas* 103 (2017): 16–22.

61. K. N. P. Starr and C. W. Bales, Excessive body weight in older adults: Concerns and recommendations, *Clinics in Geriatric Medicine* 31 (2015): 311–326.

62. Position of the Academy of Nutrition and Dietetics: Individualized nutrition approaches for older adults: Long-term care, post-acute care, and other settings, *Journal of the Academy of Nutrition and Dietetics* 118 (2018): 724–735; M. Hamer and G. O'Donovan, Sarcopenic obesity, weight loss and mortality: The English Longitudinal Study of Ageing, *American Journal of Clinical Nutrition* 106 (2017): 125–129.

63. P. JafariNasabian and coauthors, Osteosarcopenic obesity in women: Impact, prevalence, and management challenges, *International Journal of Women's Health* (2017), epub, doi: 10.2147/IJWH.S106107; D. T. Villareal and coauthors, Aerobic or resistance exercise, or both, in dieting obese older adults, *New England Journal of Medicine* 376 (2017): 1943–1955.

64. Federal Interagency Forum on Aging-Related Statistics, Older Americans 2016: Key indicators of well-being (Washington, DC: U.S. Government Printing Office, 2016), available at https://agingstats.gov/docs/LatestReport/Older -Americans-2016-Key-Indicators-of-WellBeing.pdf.

65. O. Theou and coauthors, Association between sedentary time and mortality across levels of frailty, *Canadian Medical Association Journal* 189 (2017): E1056–E1064; R. A. Fielding and coauthors, Dose of physical activity, physical functioning and disability risk in mobility-limited older adults: Results from the

LIFE study randomized trial, *PLoS One* (2017), epub, doi: 10.1371/journal.pone.0182155.

66. M. Steffl and coauthors, Relationship between sarcopenia and physical activity in older people: A systematic review and meta-analysis, *Clinical Interventions in Aging* 12 (2017): 835–845.

67. E. Arentson-Lantz and coauthors, Protein: A nutrient in focus, *Applied Physiology, Nutrition, and Metabolism* 40 (2015): 755–761; D. Paddon-Jones and coauthors, Protein and healthy aging, *American Journal of Clinical Nutrition* 101 (2015): 1339S–1345S; R. M. Daly and coauthors, Protein-enriched diet, with the use of lean red meat, combined with progressive resistance training enhances lean tissue mass and muscle strength and reduces circulating IL-6 concentrations in elderly women: A cluster randomized controlled trial, *American Journal of Clinical Nutrition* 99 (2014): 899–910; I. Kim and coauthors, Quantity of dietary protein intake, but not pattern of intake, affects net protein balance primarily through differences in protein synthesis in older adults, *American Journal of Physiology—Endocrinology and Metabolism* 308 (2014): E21–E28.

68. A. C. Tricco and coauthors, Comparisons of interventions for preventing falls in older adults: A systematic review and meta-analysis, *Journal of the American Medical Association* 318 (2017): 1687–1699; American College of Sports Medicine, Position stand: Exercise and physical activity for older adults, *Medicine and Science in Sports and Exercise* 41 (2009): 1510–1530.

69. Position of the Academy of Nutrition and Dietetics: Food and nutrition for older adults: Promoting health and wellness, *Journal of the Academy of Nutrition and Dietetics* 112 (2012): 1255–1277, reaffirmed 2016.

70. R. D. Pollock and coauthors, An investigation into the relationship between age and physiological function in highly active older adults, *Journal of Physiology* 593 (2015): 657–680.

71. W. K. Mitchell and coauthors, Human skeletal muscle protein metabolism responses to amino acid nutrition, *Advances in Nutrition* 7 (2016): 828S–838S.

72. D. R. Moore and coauthors, Protein ingestion to stimulate myofibrillar protein synthesis requires greater relative protein intakes in healthy older versus younger men, *Journals of Gerontology, Series A Biological Sciences and Medical Sciences* 70 (2015): 57–62.

73. S. A. Motalebi and coauthors, Effect of low-cost resistance training on lower-limb strength and balance in institutionalized seniors, *Experimental Aging Research* 44 (2018): 48–61; R. A. Fielding and coauthors, Dose of physical activity, physical functioning and disability risk in mobility-limited older adults: Results from the LIFE study randomized trial, *PLoS One* (2017), epub, doi: 10.1371/journal.pone.0182155.

74. S. B. Kritchevsky and coauthors, Exercise's effect on mobility disability in older adults with and without obesity: The LIFE study randomized clinical trial, *Obesity* 25 (2017): 1199–1205.

75. A. R. Mobley, Identifying practical solutions to meet America's fiber needs: Proceedings from the Food & Fiber Summit, *Nutrients* 6 (2014): 2540–2551; U.S. Department of Agriculture, *What we eat in America: Nutrient intakes from food by gender and age*, NHANES 2009–2010, available at www.ars.usda.gov /SP2UserFiles/Place/12355000/pdf/0910 /Table_1_NIN_GEN_09.pdf.

76. C. Reyes and coauthors, Association between overweight and obesity and risk of clinically diagnosed knee, hip, and hand osteoarthritis: A population-based cohort study, *Arthritis and Rheumatology* 68 (2016): 1869–1875; L. A. Zdziarski, J. G. Wasser, and H. K. Vincent, Chronic pain management in the obese patient: A focused review of key challenges and potential exercise solutions, *Journal of Pain Research* 8 (2015): 63–77; H. Bliddal, A. R. Leeds, and R. Christensen, Osteoarthritis, obesity and weight loss: Evidence, hypotheses and horizons—A scoping review, *Obesity Reviews* 15 (2014): 578–586.

77. M. Abdulrazaq and coauthors, Effect of omega-3 polyunsaturated fatty acids on arthritic pain: A systematic review, *Nutrition* 39-40 (2017): 57–66.

78. M. C. Hochberg and coauthors, Combined chondroitin sulfate and glucosamine for painful knee osteoarthritis: A multicentre, randomised, double-blind, non-inferiority trial versus celecoxib, *Annals of the Rheumatic Diseases* (2014), epub, doi: 10.1136/annrheumdis-2014-206792.

79. S. K. Rai and coauthors, The Dietary Approaches to Stop Hypertension (DASH) diet, Western diet, and risk of gout in men: Prospective cohort study, *British Medical Journal* 357 (2017), epub, doi: 10.1136/bmj.j1794.

80. M. L. Maes, D. R. Fixen, and S. A. Linnebur, Adverse effects of proton-pump inhibitor use in older adults: A review of the evidence, *Therapeutic Advances in Drug Safety* 8 (2017): 273–297.

81. National Eye Institute, Cataracts, www.nei .nih.gov/eyedata/cataract.

82. W. G. Christen and coauthors, Age-related cataract in men in the Selenium and Vitamin E Cancer Prevention Trial Eye Endpoints Study, *JAMA Ophthalmology* 133 (2015): 17–24; S. Rautiainen and coauthors, Total antioxidant capacity of the diet and risk of age-related cataract: A population-based prospective cohort of women, *JAMA Ophthalmology* 132 (2014): 247–252.

83. J. Zheng Selin and coauthors, High-dose supplements of vitamins C and E, low-dose multivitamins, and the risk of age-related cataract: A population-based prospective, *American Journal of Epidemiology* 177 (2013): 548–555.

84. C. Baumeier and coauthors, Caloric restriction and intermittent fasting alter hepatic lipid droplet proteome and diacylglycerol species and prevent diabetes in NZO mice, *Biochimica et Biophysica Acta* 1851 (2015): 566–576; N. Makino and coauthors, Calorie restriction increases telomerase activity, enhances autophagy, and improves diastolic dysfunction in diabetic rat hearts, *Molecular and Cellular Biochemistry* 403 (2015): 1–11; S. E. Olivo-Marston and coauthors, Effects of calorie restriction and diet-induced obesity on murine colon carcinogenesis, growth and inflammatory factors, and microRNA expression, *PLoS One* (2014), epub, doi: 10.1371/journal.pone.0094765.

85. J. A. Mattison and coauthors, Caloric restriction improves health and survival of rhesus monkeys, *Nature Communications* (2017), epub, doi: 10.1038/ncomms14063; R. J. Colman and coauthors, Caloric restriction reduces age-related and all-cause mortality in rhesus monkeys, *Nature Communications* (2014), epub, doi: 10.1038/ncomms4557.

86. J. C. Mathers, Impact of nutrition on the ageing process, *British Journal of Nutrition* 113 (2015): S18–S22; S. Steven and R. Taylor, Restoring normoglycaemia by use of a very low calorie diet in long- and short-duration Type 2 diabetes, *Diabetic Medicine* (2015), epub, doi: 10.1111/dme.12722; A. R. Barnosky and coauthors, Intermittent fasting vs. daily calorie restriction for type 2 diabetes prevention: A review of human findings, *Translational Research: The Journal of Laboratory and Clinical Medicine* 164 (2014): 302–311.

87. E. L. Goldberg and coauthors, Lifespan-extending caloric restriction or mTOR inhibition impair adaptive immunity of old mice by distinct mechanisms, *Aging Cell* 14 (2015): 130–138; D. Omodei and coauthors, Immune-metabolic profiling of anorexic patients reveals an anti-oxidant and anti-inflammatory phenotype, *Metabolism* 64 (2015): 396–405.

88. D. K. Ingram and G. S. Roth, Calorie restriction mimetics: Can you have your cake and eat it, too? *Ageing Research Reviews* 20 (2015): 46–62; J. H. Park and coauthors, Daumone fed late in life improves survival and reduces hepatic inflammation and fibrosis in mice, *Aging Cell* 13 (2014): 709–718; J. P. de Magalhães and coauthors, Genome-environment interactions that modulate aging: Powerful targets for drug discovery, *Pharmacological Reviews* 64 (2012): 88–101.

89. D. Monti and coauthors, Inflammaging and human longevity in the omics era, *Mechanisms of Ageing and Development* 165 (2017): 129–138.

90. P. B. Gorelick and coauthors, Defining optimal brain health in adults: A presidential advisory from the American Heart Association/American Stroke Association, *Stroke* (2017), epub ahead of print, doi.org/10.1161/ STR.0000000000000148; O. van de Rest and coauthors, Dietary patterns, cognitive decline, and dementia: A systematic review, *Advances in Nutrition* 6 (2015): 154–168; A. Smyth and coauthors, Healthy eating and reduced risk of cognitive decline: A cohort from 40 countries, *Neurology* 84 (2015): 2258–2265; L. Mosconi and coauthors, Mediterranean diet and magnetic resonance imaging-assessed brain atrophy in cognitively normal individuals at risk for Alzheimer's disease, *Journal of Prevention of Alzheimer's Disease* 1 (2014): 23–32.

91. M. Karimi and coauthors, DHA-rich n-3 fatty acid supplementation decreases DNA methylation in blood leukocytes: The OmegAD study, *American Journal of Clinical Nutrition* 106 (2017): 1157–1165.

92. G. P. Rodrigues and coauthors, Mineral status and superoxide dismutase enzyme activity in Alzheimer's disease, *Journal of Trace Elements in Medicine and Biology* 44 (2017): 83–87.

93. E. K. Kantor and coauthors, Trends in prescription drug use among adults in the United States from 1999-2012, *Journal of the American Medical Association* 314 (2015): 1818–1831.

Consumer's Guide 14

1. A. Ryu and T. H. Kim, Premenstrual syndrome: A mini review, *Maturitas* 82 (2015): 436–440; F. W. Tolossa and M. L. Bekele, Prevalence, impacts and medical managements of premenstrual syndrome among female students: Cross-sectional study in College of Health Sciences, Mekelle University, Mekelle, northern Ethiopia, *BMC Women's Health* 14 (2014): 52.

2. P. M. Tacani and coauthors, Characterization of symptoms and edema distribution in premenstrual syndrome, *International Journal of Women's Health* 7 (2015): 297–303; Tolossa and Bekele, Prevalence, impacts and medical managements of premenstrual syndrome among female students, 2014.

3. Ryu and Kim, Premenstrual syndrome: A mini review, 2015.

4. S. A. Elliott and coauthors, The influence of the menstrual cycle on energy balance and taste preference in Asian Chinese women, *European Journal of Nutrition* 54 (2015): 1323–1332.

5. E. R. Bertone-Johnson and coauthors, Plasma 25-hydroxyvitamin D and risk of premenstrual syndrome in a prospective cohort study, *BMC Women's Health* 14 (2014): 56.

6. F. Y. Azizieh, K. O. Alyahya, and K. Dingle, Association of self-reported symptoms with serum levels of vitamin D and multivariate cytokine profile in healthy women, *Journal of Inflammation Research* (2017), epub, doi: 10.2147/JIR.S127892.

7. M. Tartagni and coauthors, Vitamin D supplementation for premenstrual syndromerelated mood disorders in adolescents with severe hypovitaminosis D, *Journal of Pediatric and Adolescent Gynecology* 29 (2016): 357–361; Tolossa and Bekele, Prevalence, impacts and medical managements of premenstrual syndrome among female students, 2014; R. E. Anglin and coauthors, Vitamin D deficiency and depression in adults: Systematic review and meta-analysis, *British Journal of Psychiatry* 202 (2013): 100–107.

8. J. A. Shaffer and coauthors, Vitamin D supplementation for depressive symptoms: A systematic review and meta-analysis of randomized controlled trials, *Psychosomatic Medicine* 76 (2014): 190–196.

Controversy 14

1. J. H. Choi and C. M. Ko, Food and drug interactions, *Journal of Lifestyle Medicine* 7 (2017): 1–9.

2. C. J. Charlesworth and coauthors, Polypharmacy among adults aged 65 years and older in the United States: 1988–2010, *Journals Gerontology Series A: Biological Sciences and Medical Sciences* 70 (2015): 989–995; D. Gnjidic and coauthors, Polypharmacy cut-off and outcomes: Five or more medicines were used to identify community-dwelling older men at risk of different adverse outcomes, *Journal of Clinical Epidemiology* 65 (2012): 989–995.

3. Choi and Ko, Food and drug interactions, 2017.

4. V. T. Martin and B. Vij, Diet and headache: Part 1, *Headache* 56 (2016): 1543–1552.

5. U.S. Department of Agriculture and U.S. Department of Health and Human Services, *Scientific report of the 2015 Dietary Guidelines Advisory Committee,* 2015, D-5:32–35, available at www.health.gov.

6. G. Grosso and coauthors, Coffee, caffeine, and health outcomes: An umbrella review, *Annual Review of Nutrition* 37 (2017): 131–156; M. Ding and coauthors, Caffeinated and decaffeinated coffee consumption and risk of type 2 diabetes: A systematic review and a dose-response meta-analysis, *Diabetes Care* 37 (2014): 569–586.

7. U.S. Food and Drug Administration, Mixing medications and dietary supplements can endanger your health, Consumer Health Information, October 2014, available at www.fda.gov /consumer.

8. R. A. Breslow, C. Dong, and A. White, Prevalence of alcohol-interactive prescription medication use among current drinkers: United States, 1999–2010, *Alcoholism: Clinical and Experimental Research* 39 (2015): 371–379.

9. G. Lee and coauthors, Medical cannabis for neuropathic pain, *Current Pain and Headache Reports* (2018), epub, doi: 10.1007/s11916-018-0658-8; M. E. Gerich and coauthors, Medical marijuana for digestive disorders: High time to prescribe? *American Journal of Gastroenterology* 110 (2015): 208–214; P. J. Robson, Therapeutic potential of cannabinoid medicines, *Drug Testing and Analysis* 6 (2014): 24–30.

10. A. R. Turner and S. Agrawal, Marijuana (Treasure Island (FL): StatPearls Publishing, 2017), epub, available at www.ncbi.nlm.nih.gov /books/NBK430801/.

Chapter 15

1. A. Coleman-Jensen and coauthors, *Household food security in the United States in 2016, A repor summary from the Economic Research Service,* 2017, available at www.ers.usda.gov /webdocs/publications/84973/err237_summary .pdf?v=42979.

2. FAO, IFAD, UNICEF, WFP and WHO, *The state of food security and nutrition in the world 2017: Building resilience for peace and food security,* 2017, Rome, FAO, available at www.fao.org /state-of-food-security-nutrition/en/.

3. Position of the Academy of Nutrition and Dietetics: Food Insecurity in the United States, *Journal of the Academy of Nutrition and Dietetics* 117 (2017): 1991–2002.

4. J. L. Semega, K. R. Fontenot, and M. A. Kollar, U. S. Census Bureau, Income and poverty in the United States: 2016, (2017), Report Number: P60-259, available at www.census.gov/library /publications/2017/demo/p60-259.html.

5. D. C. Martins and coauthors, Assessment of food intake, obesity, and health risk among the homeless in Rhode Island, *Public Health Nursing* 32 (2015): 453–461; J. Kaur, M. M. Lamb, and C. L. Ogden, The association between food insecurity and obesity in children—The National Health and Nutrition Examination Survey, *Journal of the Academy of Nutrition and Dietetics* 115 (2015): 751–758.

6. K. Kassel, A. Melton, and R. M. Morrison, Selected charts from ag and food statistics: Charting the essentials, 2017, Economic Research Service Administrative Publication No. (AP-078), available at www.ers.usda.gov /publications/pub-details/?pubid=85462.

7. K. Mulik and L. Haynes-Maslow, The affordability of MyPlate: An analysis of SNAP benefits and the actual cost of eating according to the Dietary Guidelines, *Journal of Nutrition Education and Behavior* 49 (2017): 623–631.

8. M. D. Gamlin, *Ending U.S. hunger and poverty by focusing on communities where it's most likely,* Bread for the World Briefing Paper 31, March 2017, available at www.bread.org/library/ending -us-hunger-and-poverty-focusing-communities -where-its-most-likely.

9. Food and Agriculture Organization of the United Nations, International Fund for Agricultural Development, and World Food Programme, *The state of food insecurity in the world 2014,* 2014, p. 4.

10. Food and Agriculture Organization of the United Nations, International Fund for Agricultural Development, and World Food Programme, *The state of food insecurity in the world 2014,* 2014.

11. P. L. Tigga, J. Sen, and N. Mondal, Association of some socio-economic and socio-demographic variables with wasting among pre-school children of North Bengal, India, *Ethiopian Journal of Health Sciences* 25 (2015): 63–72.

12. E. Andresen and coauthors, Malnutrition and elevated mortality among refugees from South Sudan, *Morbidity and Mortality Weekly Report* 63 (2014): 700; N. Gupta, Conflict, children and malnutrition in CAR, *Borgen Magazine,* February 19, 2015, available at www .borgenmagazine.com/conflict-children -malnutrition-car/; K. Fahim, Malnutrition hits millions of children in Yemen, *New York Times,* December 18, 2014, available at www.nytimes .com/2014/12/19/world/middleeast/yemen -children-starve-as-government-weakens.html?r=0.

13. A. Seal and coauthors, A weak health response is increasing the risk of excess mortality as food crisis worsens in Somalia, *Conflict and Health* (2017), epub, doi: 10.1186/s13031-017-0114-0.

14. World Health Organization, Nutrition: Micronutrient deficiencies, (2018), available at www.who.int.

15. International Food Policy Research Institute, 2014 Global Hunger Index: The challenge of hidden hunger, available at www.ifpri.org.

16. C. Shekhar, Hidden hunger: Addressing micronutrient deficiencies using improved crop varieties, *Chemistry and Biology* 20 (2013): 1305–1306; World Health Organization, Global prevalence of vitamin A deficiency in populations at risk: 1995–2005 (Geneva: World Health Organization, 2009); Standing Committee on the Scientific Evaluation of Dietary Reference Intakes, Food and Nutrition Board, Institute of Medicine, Dietary Reference Intakes for vitamin A, Vitamin K, arsenic, boron, chromium, copper, iodine, iron, manganese, molybdenum, nickel, silicon, vanadium, and zinc (Washington, D.C.: National Academies Press, 2001), pp. 4-9–4-10.

17. P. J. Becker and coauthors, Consensus statement of the Academy of Nutrition and Dietetics/ American Society for Parenteral and Enteral Nutrition: Indicators recommended for the identification and documentation of pediatric malnutrition (undernutrition), *Journal of the Academy of Nutrition and Dietetics* 114 (2014): 1988–2000.

18. I. Trehan and M. J. Manary, Management of severe acute malnutrition in low-income and middle-income countries, *Archives of Disease in Childhood* 100 (2015): 283–287.

19. B. de Gier and coauthors, Helminth infections and micronutrients in school-age children: A systematic review and meta-analysis, *American Journal of Clinical Nutrition* 99 (2014): 1499–1509.

20. M. Wolde, Y. Berhan, and A. Chala, Determinants of underweight, stunting and wasting among schoolchildren, *BMC Public Health* (2015), epub, doi: 10.1186/s12889- 014-1337-2.

21. P. Bahwere and coauthors, Soya, maize, and sorghum-based ready-to-use therapeutic food with amino acid is as efficacious as the standard milk and peanut paste-based formulation for the treatment of severe acute malnutrition in children: A noninferiority individually randomized controlled efficacy clinical trial in Malawi, *American Journal of Clinical Nutrition* 106 (2017): 1100–1112.

22. I. Trehan and coauthors, Extending supplementary feeding for children younger than 5 years with moderate acute malnutrition leads to lower relapse rates, *Journal of Pediatric Gastroenterology and Nutrition* 60 (2015): 544–549.

23. Bahwere and coauthors, Soya, maize, and sorghum-based ready-to-use therapeutic food

with amino acid is as efficacious as the standard milk and peanut paste-based formulation for the treatment of severe acute malnutrition in children: A noninferiority individually randomized controlled efficacy clinical trial in Malawi, 2017.

24. Food and Agriculture Organization of the United Nations, World agriculture: Towards 2015/2030, 2015.

25. U.S. Census Bureau, World vital events per time unit: 2018, available at www.census.gov /popclock/.

26. A. J. McMichael, Globalization, climate change, and human health, *New England Journal of Medicine* 368 (2015): 1335–1343; National Academies of Science and the Royal Society, Climate change evidence and causes, 2014, available at http://nas-sites.org/americasclimate-choices/events/a-discussion-on-climate-change -evidence-and-causes.

27. T. Watts and coauthors, The *Lancet* Countdown on health and climate change: From 25 years of inaction to a global transformation for public health, *Lancet* 391 (2018): 581–630.

28. United Nations, International Decade for Action: Water for life 2005–2015, available at www.un.org/waterforlifedecade/scarcity.shtml.

29. National Oceanic and Atmospheric Administration, NOAA, USGS and partners predict third largest Gulf of Mexico summer "dead zone" ever, (2017), available at www.noaa .gov/media-release/noaa-usgs-and-partners -predict-third-largest-gulf-of-mexico-summer -dead-zone-ever; Pacific Marine Environmental Laboratory, National Oceanic and Atmospheric Administration, Ocean acidification: How will changes in ocean chemistry affect marine life?

(2017), available at www.pmel.noaa.gov /co2/story/Ocean+Acidification; K. Minogue, Climate change expected to expand majority of ocean dead zones, *Smithsonian Science News* 5 (2014), available at http://smithsonianscience .org/2014/11/climate-change-expected-expand-majority-ocean-dead-zones.

30. Food and Agricultural Organization of the United Nations, *The State of the world fisheries and aquaculture*, 2014, available at www.fao .org/3/a-i3720e.pdf.

31. U.S. Department of Agriculture and U.S. Department of Health and Human Services, *Scientific report of the 2015 Dietary Guidelines Advisory Committee*, 2015, D-5:17–20, available at www.health.gov.

32. D. Gunders with J. Bloom, *Wasted: How America is losing up to 40 percent of its food from farm to fork to landfill*, (2017), available at www .nrdc.org.

33. J. Bayala and coauthors, Editorial for the Thematic Series in Agriculture & Food Security: Climate-smart agricultural technologies in West Africa: Learning from the ground AR4D experiences, *Agriculture and Food Security* (2017), epub, doi.org/10.1186/s40066-017-0117-5.

34. Environmental Protection Agency, *Basic information about food waste*, April 26, 2014, available at www.epa.gov.

35. U.S. Department of Agriculture and U.S. Department of Health and Human Services, *Scientific report of the 2015 Dietary Guidelines Advisory Committee*, 2015.

36. C. Vogliano, A. Steiber, and K. Brown, Linking agriculture, nutrition, and health: The role of the Registered Dietitian Nutritionist, *Journal of the Academy of Nutrition and Dietetics* 115 (2015): 1710–1714.

37. Controversy 15

1. National Academies of Sciences, Engineering, and Medicine, Consensus Study Report Highlights: Science Breakthroughs to Advance Food and Agricultural Research by 2030 (July 2018), available at https://www.nap.edu/resource/25059 /ScienceBreakthroughs2030ReportBrief.pdf; Food and Agriculture Organization of the United Nations, *World agriculture: Towards 2015/2030*, Summary report, 2015, available at www.fao.org /docrep/004/y3557e/y3557e00.htm.

2. C. Brown and coauthors, Switchgrass biofuel production on reclaimed surface mines: I. Soil quality and dry matter yield, *BioEnergy Research* (2015), epub, doi: 10.1007/s12155-015-9658-2; B. Mole, Bacteria make plants into biofuel, *Science News*, July 12, 2014, p. 16.

3. World Health Organization, Global and regional food consumption patterns and trends: Availability and changes in consumption of animal products, April 2015, available at www .who.int/nutrition/topics/3_foodconsumption/en /index4.html.

4. U.S. Department of Agriculture and U.S. Department of Health and Human Services, *Scientific report of the 2015 Dietary Guidelines Advisory Committee*, 2015, D-5:9–16, available at www.health.gov.

5. K. Bälter and coauthors, Is a diet low in greenhouse gas emissions a nutritious diet? Analyses of self-selected diets in the LifeGene study, *Archives of Public Health* (2017), epub doi: 10.1186/s13690-017-0185-9; U.S. Department of Agriculture and U.S. Department of Health and Human Services, *Scientific report of the 2015 Dietary Guidelines Advisory Committee*, 2015; J. Sabaté and S. Soret, Sustainability of plant-based diets: Back to the future, *American Journal of Clinical Nutrition* 100 (2014): 476S–482S.

Answers to Chapter Questions
Answers to Consumer's Guide Review and Self-Check Questions

CHAPTER 1

Consumer's Guide Review

1. d
2. b
3. b

Self Check Questions

1. False. Heart disease and cancer are influenced by many factors with genetics and diet among them.
2. c
3. d
4. a
5. a
6. a
7. T
8. c
9. b
10. False. The choice of where, as well as what, to eat is often based more on taste and social considerations than on nutrition judgments.
11. b
12. a
13. T
14. F
15. b
16. a
17. d
18. False. In this nation, profiteers selling diplomas and certificates make it easy to obtain a bogus nutrition credential.

CHAPTER 2

Consumer's Guide Review

1. False. Restaurant portions are not held to standards and should not be used as a guide for choosing portion sizes.
2. T
3. False. Most consumers overestimate both the calories and fat in restaurant foods.

Self Check Questions

1. b
2. d
3. T

4. False. The DRI are estimates of the needs of healthy people only. Medical problems alter nutrient needs.
5. c
6. T
7. c
8. d
9. False. People who choose to eat no meats or products taken from animals can still use the USDA Food Patterns to make their diets adequate.
10. a
11. False. A properly planned diet should include healthy snacks as part of the total daily food intake, if so desired.
12. c
13. T
14. T
15. T
16. d
17. T
18. False. Although they are natural constituents of foods, phytochemicals have not been proven safe to consume in large amounts.

CHAPTER 3

Self Check Questions

1. a
2. False. Each gene is a blueprint that directs the production of one or more of the body's proteins, such as an enzyme.
3. c
4. a
5. b
6. T
7. c
8. d
9. False. Absorption of the majority of nutrients takes place across the specialized cells of the small intestine.
10. d
11. a
12. c
13. False. The kidneys straddle the cardiovascular system and filter the blood.
14. b

15. T
16. a
17. False. Alcohol is a natural toxin that can cause severe damage to the liver, brain, and other organs, and can be lethal in high enough doses.

CHAPTER 4

Consumer's Guide Review

1. b
2. b
3. a

Self Check Questions

1. b
2. a
3. T
4. T
5. c
6. T
7. b
8. a
9. False. Ketosis is the result of too little carbohydrate in the body tissues.
10. False. The liver's glycogen storage is limited to about 2,000 calories' worth.
11. False. Type 2 diabetes is most often prevented by successful weight-loss management.
12. c
13. T.
14. T.
15. d
16. T
17. T
18. a

CHAPTER 5

Consumer's Guide Review

1. False. Methylmercury is a highly toxic industrial pollutant concentrated in the flesh of certain species of fish, and it is unaffected by cooking.
2. False. Children and pregnant or lactating women should strictly follow recommendations set for them and choose fish species that are rich in omega-3 fatty acids *and* lower in mercury.
3. False. Cod provides little EPA and DHA.

Self Check Questions

1. c
2. False. In addition to providing abundant fuel, fat cushions tissues, serves as insulation, forms cell membranes, and serves as raw material, among other functions.
3. b
4. False. In general, vegetable and fish oils are excellent sources of polyunsaturated fats.
5. c

6. T
7. b
8. d
9. T
10. T
11. False. Chylomicrons are produced in small intestinal cells.
12. False. Consuming large amounts of saturated fatty acids elevates serum LDL cholesterol and thus *raises* the risk of heart disease and heart attack.
13. d
14. False. Fish, not supplements, is the recommended source of fish oil.
15. T
16. b
17. b
18. d
19. T
20. T
21. d

CHAPTER 6

Consumer's Guide Review

1. False. Evidence does not support taking protein supplements such as commercial shakes and energy bars to lose weight.
2. T
3. False. In high doses, tryptophan may cause nausea and skin disorders as unwanted side effects.

Self Check Questions

1. b
2. c
3. a
4. a
5. b
6. T
7. T
8. d
9. a
10. T
11. T
12. d
13. False. Excess protein in the diet may have adverse effects, such as worsening kidney disease.
14. a
15. a
16. T
17. d
18. T
19. c
20. False. Fried banana or vegetable chips are often high in calories and saturated fat, and are best reserved for an occasional treat.

CHAPTER 7

Consumer's Guide Review

1. T
2. T
3. False. Many kinds of food processing make nutritious foods more accessible and safer to consume.

Self Check Questions

1. b
2. c
3. T
4. a
5. d
6. False. Vitamin A supplements have no effect on acne.
7. T
8. d
9. a
10. c
11. T
12. c
13. b
14. a
15. False. No study to date has conclusively demonstrated that vitamin C can prevent colds or reduce their severity.
16. d
17. c
18. T
19. a
20. b
21. b
22. False. The FDA has little control over supplement sales.

CHAPTER 8

Consumer's Guide Review

1. a
2. d
3. d

Self Check Questions

1. d
2. False. Water intoxication occurs when too much plain water floods the body's fluids and disturbs their normal composition.
3. c
4. b
5. T
6. a
7. d
8. c
9. d
10. False. After about age 40, the bones typically begin to lose density.
11. T
12. c
13. b
14. a
15. False. Calcium is the most abundant mineral in the body.
16. False. The Academy of Nutrition and Dietetics, among others, recommends the consumption of fluoridated water.
17. False. Butter, cream, and cream cheese contain negligible calcium, being almost pure fat. Some vegetables, such as broccoli, are good sources of available calcium.
18. T
19. T
20. b

CHAPTER 9

Consumer's Guide Review

1. False. A diet book that addresses eicosanoids and adipokines may or may not present accurate nutrition science or effective diet advice.
2. False. Limiting calories is a key strategy for weight loss.
3. True.

Self Check Questions

1. d
2. T
3. b
4. False. The thermic effect of food is believed to have negligible effects on total energy expenditure.
5. False. The BMI are unsuitable for use with athletes and adults over age 65.
6. c
7. d
8. d
9. a
10. b
11. False. Genomic researchers have identified multiple genes likely to play roles in obesity development but have not so far identified a single genetic cause of common obesity.
12. T
13. d
14. a
15. T
16. T
17. b
18. False. Over-the-counter drugs for obesity most often present risk without benefit.
19. b
20. False. Disordered eating behaviors in early life set a pattern that likely continues into young adulthood.

CHAPTER 10

Consumer's Guide Review

1. a
2. a
3. b

Self Check Questions

1. b
2. c
3. False. Athletes who wish to excel in sports must develop muscle power, quick reaction time, agility, and resistance to muscle fatigue.
4. False. Muscle cells and tissues respond to a physical activity overload by altering the structures and metabolic equipment needed to perform the work.
5. c
6. c
7. a
8. T
9. T
10. a
11. d
12. T
13. a
14. False. Frequent nutritious between-meal snacks can provide extra calories to help maintain body weight.
15. T
16. d
17. a
18. b
19. d

CHAPTER 11

Consumer's Guide Review

1. T
2. False. The National Center for Complementary and Integrative Health (NCCIH) does not promote laetrile therapy.
3. T

Self Check Questions

1. False. Chronic diseases have risk factors that show correlations with disease development but are not distinct causes.
2. d
3. False. Atherosclerosis is an accumulation of lipids within the artery wall, but it also involves a complex response of the artery to tissue damage and inflammation.
4. T
5. False. Men do have more heart attacks than women, but CVD kills more women than any other cause of death.

6. a
7. c
8. T
9. T
10. c
11. False. For managing type 2 diabetes, regular physical activity can help by reducing excess body fat and increasing tissue sensitivity to insulin.
12. T
13. d
14. False. The DASH diet is designed for helping people with hypertension to control the disease.
15. d
16. False. Currently, for the best chance of consuming adequate nutrients and staying healthy, people should eat a well-planned diet of whole foods, as described in Chapter 2.

CHAPTER 12

Consumer's Guide Review

1. d
2. T
3. a

Self Check Questions

1. T
2. a
3. c
4. d
5. c
6. False. Today, the chance of getting a foodborne illness from eating produce is similar to the chance of becoming ill from eating meat, eggs, and seafood.
7. T
8. a
9. b
10. T
11. False. Nature has provided many plants used for food with natural poisons to fend off diseases, insects, and other predators.
12. False. The EPA and FDA warn of unacceptably high methylmercury levels in certain fish species and advise all pregnant women to eat fish species with lower methylmercury levels.
13. T
14. c
15. c
16. d
17. T
18. b
19. b
20. T

CHAPTER 13

Consumer's Guide Review

1. False. Despite convincing advertising, no commercial formula can fully match the benefits of human milk.
2. False. Only about 30 percent of infants are still breastfeeding at 1 year of age.
3. False. Lactation consultants are employed by hospitals to help new mothers establish healthy breastfeeding relationships with their newborns and to help ensure successful long-term breastfeeding.

Self Check Questions

1. c
2. T
3. b
4. d
5. d
6. T
7. b
8. False. The American Academy of Pediatrics urges all women to stop drinking as soon as they plan to become pregnant, and to abstain throughout the pregnancy.
9. a
10. T
11. d
12. T
13. a
14. a
15. d
16. d
17. False. There is no proof for the theory that "stuffing the baby" at bedtime will promote sleeping through the night.
18. T
19. False. In light of the developmental needs of one-year-olds, parents should discourage unacceptable behaviors, such as standing at the table or throwing food.
20. c

CHAPTER 14

Consumer's Guide Review

1. T
2. False. Ongoing research suggests that taking multivitamins, magnesium, manganese, or diuretics is *not* useful.
3. False. During the two weeks *before* menstruation, women may experience a natural, hormone-governed increase of appetite.

Self Check Questions

1. c
2. b
3. T
4. d
5. b
6. False. Research to date does not support the idea that food allergies or intolerances cause hyperactivity in children, but studies continue.
7. c
8. c
9. b
10. b
11. d
12. a
13. T
14. False. Vitamin A absorption appears to increase with aging.
15. False. To date, no proven benefits are available from herbs or other remedies.
16. b
17. a
18. False. Most single elderly people would love an invitation to join someone for a meal.
19. d

CHAPTER 15

Consumer's Guide Review

1. False. The terms *green* and *eco-friendly* are meaningless without scientific evidence to back them up.
2. T
3. d

Self Check Questions

1. b
2. a
3. d
4. c
5. T
6. a
7. T
8. c
9. False. Most children who die of malnutrition do not starve to death—they die because their health has been compromised by dehydration from infections that cause diarrhea.
10. a
11. c
12. d
13. c
14. T
15. T
16. False. The federal government, the states, local communities, big business and small companies, educators, and all individuals, including dietitians and food service managers, have many opportunities to make an impact in the fight against poverty, hunger, and environmental degradation.
17. T
18. c

Appendix H Physical Activity Levels and Energy Requirements

C hapter 9 described how to calculate ranges of the estimated energy requirement (EER) for an adult by using an equation that accounts for age and gender
alone. This appendix offers a way of establishing estimated calorie needs per day by
age, gender, and physical activity level, as endorsed by the *Dietary Guidelines for
Americans 2015*, and based on the equations of the Committee on Dietary Reference
Intakes.

Table H–1 describes activity levels for three groups of people: sedentary, moderately
active, and active. Once you have identified an activity level that approximates your
own, find your daily calorie need in Table H–2.

Table H–3 specifies the American College of Sports Medicine's Guidelines
for Physical Fitness. These guidelines are more demanding and also more specific
than USDA's Physical Activity Guidelines (see Chapter 10). Table H–4 offers a sample
workout program that meets or exceeds both sets of recommendations.

TABLE H–1 Sedentary, Moderately Active, and Active People

Sedentary	A lifestyle that includes only the light physical activity associated with typical day-to-day life.
Moderately active	A lifestyle that includes physical activity equivalent to walking about 1.5 to 3 miles per day at 3 to 4 miles per hour in addition to the light physical activity associated with typical day-to-day life.
Active	A lifestyle that includes physical activity equivalent to walking more than 3 miles per day at 3 to 4 miles per hour in addition to the light physical activity associated with typical day-to-day life.

*Source: U.S. Department of Agriculture and U.S. Department of Health and Human Services, Dietary
Guidelines for Americans 2010, (reaffirmed 2015) available at www.dietaryguidelines.gov.*

TABLE H–2 Estimated Calorie Needs per Day by Age, Gender, and Physical Activity Level (Detailed)

Estimated amounts of calories needed to maintain calorie balance for various gender and age groups at three different levels of physical activity.[a] The estimates are rounded to the nearest 200 calories. An individual's calorie needs may be higher or lower than these average estimates.

Age (years)	Male/ Sedentary	Male/ Moderately Active	Male/Active	Female[b]/ Sedentary	Female[b]/ Moderately Active	Female[b]/Active
2	1,000	1,000	1,000	1,000	1,000	1,000
3	1,200	1,400	1,400	1,000	1,200	1,400
4	1,200	1,400	1,600	1,200	1,400	1,400
5	1,200	1,400	1,600	1,200	1,400	1,600
6	1,400	1,600	1,800	1,200	1,400	1,600
7	1,400	1,600	1,800	1,200	1,600	1,800
8	1,400	1,600	2,000	1,400	1,600	1,800
9	1,600	1,800	2,000	1,400	1,600	1,800
10	1,600	1,800	2,200	1,400	1,800	2,000
11	1,800	2,000	2,200	1,600	1,800	2,000
12	1,800	2,200	2,400	1,600	2,000	2,200
13	2,000	2,200	2,600	1,600	2,000	2,200
14	2,000	2,400	2,800	1,800	2,000	2,400
15	2,200	2,600	3,000	1,800	2,000	2,400
16	2,400	2,800	3,200	1,800	2,000	2,400
17	2,400	2,800	3,200	1,800	2,000	2,400
18	2,400	2,800	3,200	1,800	2,000	2,400
19–20	2,600	2,800	3,000	2,000	2,200	2,400
21–25	2,400	2,800	3,000	2,000	2,200	2,400
26–30	2,400	2,600	3,000	1,800	2,000	2,400
31–35	2,400	2,600	3,000	1,800	2,000	2,200
36–40	2,400	2,600	2,800	1,800	2,000	2,200
41–45	2,200	2,600	2,800	1,800	2,000	2,200
46–50	2,200	2,400	2,800	1,800	2,000	2,200
51–55	2,200	2,400	2,800	1,600	1,800	2,200
56–60	2,200	2,400	2,600	1,600	1,800	2,200
61–65	2,000	2,400	2,600	1,600	1,800	2,000
66–70	2,000	2,200	2,600	1,600	1,800	2,000
71–75	2,000	2,200	2,600	1,600	1,800	2,000
76+	2,000	2,200	2,400	1,600	1,800	2,000

[a]Based on estimated energy requirements (EER) equations, using reference heights (average) and reference weights (healthy) for each age-gender group. For children and adolescents, reference height and weight vary. For adults, the reference man is 5 feet 10 inches tall and weighs 154 pounds. The reference woman is 5 feet 4 inches tall and weighs 126 pounds. EER equations are from the Institute of Medicine, Dietary Reference Intakes for Energy, Carbohydrate, Fiber, Fat, Fatty Acids, Cholesterol, Protein, and Amino Acids (Washington, D.C. National Academies Press, 2002).

[b]Estimates for females do not include women who are pregnant or breastfeeding.

Source: U.S. Department of Agriculture and U.S. Department of Health and Human Services, Dietary Guidelines for Americans 2010, (reaffirmed 2015) available at www.dietaryguidelines.gov.

TABLE H–3 American College of Sports Medicine's Guidelines for Physical Fitness

Type of Activity	Aerobic activity that uses large-muscle groups and can be maintained continuously	Resistance activity that is performed at a controlled speed and through a full range of motion	Stretching activity that uses the major muscle groups
Frequency	5 to 7 days per week	2 to 3 nonconsecutive days per week	2 to 7 days per week
Intensity	Moderate (equivalent to walking at a pace of 3 to 4 mph)[a]	Enough to enhance muscle strength and improve body composition	Enough to feel tightness or slight discomfort
Duration	At least 30 minutes per day	2 to 4 sets of 8 to 12 repetitions involving each major muscle group	2 to 4 repetitions of 15 to 30 seconds per muscle group
Examples	Running, cycling, dancing, swimming, inline skating, rowing, power walking, cross-country skiing, kickboxing, water aerobics, jumping rope; sports activities such as basketball, soccer, racquetball, tennis, volleyball	Pull-ups, push-ups, sit-ups, weightlifting, pilates	Yoga

[a]For those who prefer vigorous-intensity aerobic activity such as walking at a very brisk pace (>4.5 mph) or running (≥5 mph), a minimum of 20 minutes per day, 3 days per week is recommended.

TABLE H–4 A Sample Balanced Fitness Program

Monday	Tuesday	Wednesday	Thursday	Friday	Saturday or Sunday
5-min warm-up[a]	5-min warm-up[a]	5-min warm-up[a]	5-min warm-up[a]	5-min warm-up[a]	
Resistance training: chest, back, arms, and shoulders 15–45 min[b]	Resistance training: legs, core (abdomen/lower back) 15–45 min		Resistance training: chest, back, arms, and shoulders 15–45 min	Resistance training: legs, core (abdomen/lower back) 15–45 min	Active leisure pursuits: Sports, walking, hiking, biking, swimming
Moderate aerobic activity: 15–20 min	Moderate aerobic activity: 15–20 min	Moderate aerobic activity: 15–20 min	Moderate aerobic activity: 15–20 min	Moderate aerobic activity: 15–20 min	
Stretching: 5 min	Stretching: 5 min	Stretching: 5 min	Stretching: 5 min	Stretching: 5 min	

[a]The warm-up consists of a slower or less-intense version of the activity ahead and may count toward the week's total activity requirement if it is performed at moderate intensity.

[b]Lower-intensity exercise requires more time; higher-intensity exercise requires less time.

Source: Designed for Nutrition: Concepts and Controversies by P. Spencer Webb, MS, RDN, CSCS, Exercise/Human Performance Instructor, U.S. Military Special Operations Forces.

Glossary

A

A1C test a blood test for type 2 diabetes that measures the percentage of hemoglobin (a blood protein) with glucose attached to it. The test reflects blood glucose control over the previous few months. Also called *glycosylated hemoglobin test* or *HbA1C test* (*Hb* stands for *hemoglobin*).

absorb to take in, as nutrients are taken into the intestinal cells after digestion; the main function of the digestive tract with respect to nutrients.

Academy of Nutrition and Dietetics (AND) the professional organization of dietitians in the United States (formerly the American Dietetic Association). The Canadian equivalent is the Dietitians of Canada (DC), which operates similarly.

acceptable daily intake (ADI) the estimated amount of a sweetener that can be consumed daily over a person's lifetime without any adverse effects.

Acceptable Macronutrient Distribution Ranges (AMDR) values for carbohydrate, fat, and protein expressed as percentages of total daily caloric intake; ranges of intakes set for the energy-yielding nutrients that are sufficient to provide adequate total energy and nutrients while minimizing the risk of chronic diseases.

accredited approved; in the case of medical centers or universities, certified by an agency recognized by the U.S. Department of Education.

acetaldehyde (ass-et-AL-deh-hide) a substance to which ethanol is metabolized on its way to becoming harmless waste products that can be excreted.

acid-base balance equilibrium between acid and base concentrations to maintain a proper pH in the body fluids.

acidosis (acid-DOH-sis) the condition of excess acid in the blood, indicated by a below-normal pH (*osis* means "too much").

acid reducers prescription and over-the-counter drugs that reduce the acid output of the stomach; effective for treating severe, persistent forms of heartburn but not for neutralizing acid already present. Also called *acid controllers*.

acids compounds that release hydrogens in a watery solution.

acne chronic inflammation of the skin's follicles and oil-producing glands, which leads to an accumulation of oils inside the ducts that surround hairs; usually associated with the maturation of young adults.

acupuncture (AK-you-punk-chur) a technique that involves piercing the skin with long, thin needles at specific anatomical points to relieve pain or illness.

added sugars sugars and syrups added to a food for any purpose, such as to add sweetness or bulk or to aid in browning (baked goods). Also called *carbohydrate sweeteners*, they include concentrated fruit juice, glucose, fructose, high-fructose corn syrup, sucrose, and other sweet carbohydrates.

addiction a chronic, relapsing brain disease that is characterized by compulsive drug seeking and use, despite harmful consequences; addiction is classified as a brain disease because addictive drugs change the brain's structure and functioning.

additives substances that are added to foods but are not normally consumed by themselves as foods.

adequacy the dietary characteristic of providing all of the essential nutrients, fiber, and energy in amounts sufficient to maintain health and body weight.

Adequate Intakes (AI) nutrient intake goals for individuals set when scientific data are insufficient to allow establishment of an RDA value and assumed to be adequate for healthy people.

adipokines (AD-ih-poh-kynz) protein hormones made and released by adipose tissue (fat) cells.

adipose tissue the body's fat tissue, consisting of masses of fat-storing cells and blood vessels to nourish them.

adiposity-based chronic disease a clinical name used in diagnosing obesity. *Adiposity* refers to fat cells and tissues, identifying them as the source of the disease.

adolescence the period from the beginning of puberty until maturity.

a drink any alcoholic beverage that delivers 0.6 ounce of pure ethanol.

advertorials lengthy advertisements in newspapers and magazines that read like feature articles but are written for the purpose of touting the virtues of products and may or may not be accurate.

aerobic (air-ROH-bic) requiring oxygen.

aerobic activity physical activity that involves the body's large muscles working at light to moderate intensity for a sustained period of time. Brisk walking, running, swimming, and bicycling are examples. Also called *endurance activity*.

aflatoxin (af-lah-TOX-in) a toxin from a mold that grows on corn, grains, peanuts, and tree nuts stored in warm, humid conditions; a cause of liver cancer prevalent in tropical developing nations.

agave syrup a carbohydrate-rich sweetener made from a Mexican plant; a high fructose content gives some agave syrups a greater sweetening power per calorie than sucrose.

agility nimbleness; the ability to quickly change directions.

agroecology a scientific discipline that combines biological, physical, and social sciences with ecological theory to develop methods for producing food sustainably.

alcohol abuse see *problem drinking*.

alcoholism dependency on alcohol characterized by compulsive, uncontrollable drinking with negative effects on physical health, family relationships, and social health.

alcohol dehydrogenase (dee-high-DRAH-gen-ace) **(ADH)** an enzyme system that breaks down alcohol.

alcohol-related birth defects (ARBD) malformations in the skeletal and organ systems (heart, kidneys, eyes, ears) associated with prenatal alcohol exposure.

alcohol-related neurodevelopmental disorder (ARND) behavioral, cognitive, or central nervous system abnormalities associated with prenatal alcohol exposure.

alcohols chemical compounds that consist of a carbon atom or chain of carbons to which a hydroxyl (oxygen-hydrogen) group is attached. The alcohol of alcoholic beverages is ethanol, which has two carbon atoms.

alkalosis (al-kah-LOH-sis) the condition of excess base in the blood, indicated by an above-normal blood pH (*alka* means "base"; *osis* means "too much").

allergies immune reactions to foreign substances, such as components of foods. Also called *hypersensitivities* by researchers.

alpha-lactalbumin (lact-AL-byoo-min) the chief protein in human breast milk.

amine (a-MEEN) **group** the nitrogen-containing portion of an amino acid.

amino acid chelates (KEY-lates) compounds of minerals (such as calcium) combined with amino acids in a form that favors their absorption. A chelating agent is a molecule that binds to another molecule and can then either promote or prevent its movement from place to place (*chele* means "claw").

amino (a-MEEN-o) **acids** the building blocks of protein. Each has an amine group at one end, an acid group at the other, and a distinctive side chain.

amniotic (AM-nee-OTT-ic) **sac** the "bag of waters" in the uterus in which the fetus floats.

anabolic steroid hormones chemical messengers related to the male sex hormone testosterone that stimulate the building up of body tissues (*anabolic* means "promoting growth"; *sterol* refers to compounds chemically related to cholesterol).

anaerobic (AN-air-ROH-bic) not requiring oxygen.

anaphylactic (an-ah-feh-LACK-tick) **shock** a life-threatening whole-body allergic reaction to an offending substance.

androstenedione (AN-droh-STEEN-die-own) a precursor of testosterone that elevates both testosterone and estrogen in the blood of both males and females. Often called *andro*, it is sold with claims of producing increased muscle strength, but controlled studies disprove such claims.

anecdotal evidence information based on interesting and entertaining, but not scientific, personal stories.

anemia a blood condition in which red blood cells, the body's oxygen carriers, are inadequate or impaired and so cannot meet the oxygen demands of the body.

anencephaly (an-en-SEFF-ah-lee) an uncommon and always fatal neural tube defect in which the brain fails to form.

aneurysm (AN-you-rism) the ballooning out of an artery wall at a point that is weakened by deterioration.

anorexia nervosa an eating disorder characterized by extreme restriction of energy intake relative to requirements leading to a dangerously low body weight, and a disturbed perception of body weight and shape; seen (usually) in teenage girls and young women

(*anorexia* means "without appetite"; *nervos* means "of nervous origin").

Antabuse a drug that increases acetaldehyde, which produces such misery in combination with alcohol that a drinker will refrain from drinking after taking it. (Acetaldehyde is a product formed during alcohol metabolism.) The generic form is *disulfiram*.

antacids medications that react directly and immediately with the acid of the stomach, neutralizing it. Antacids are most suitable for treating occasional heartburn.

antibiotic-resistant bacteria bacterial strains that cause increasingly common and potentially fatal infectious diseases that do not respond to standard antibiotic therapy. An example is MRSA (pronounced MER-suh), a multidrug-resistant *Staphyloccocus aureus* bacterial strain.

antibodies (AN-te-bod-ees) large proteins of the blood, produced by the immune system in response to an invasion of the body by foreign substances (antigens). Antibodies combine with and inactivate the antigens.

anticarcinogens compounds in foods that act in any of several ways to oppose the formation of cancer.

antidiuretic (AN-tee-dye-you-RET-ick) **hormone** a hormone of the brain that signals the kidneys to conserve water in response to dehydration.

antigen a microbe or substance foreign to the body that elicits the formation of antibodies or an inflammation reaction from immune system cells. Food antigens are usually large proteins. Inflammation consists of local swelling and irritation and attracts white blood cells to the site.

antioxidant nutrients vitamins and minerals that oppose the effects of oxidants on human physical functions. The antioxidant vitamins are vitamin E, vitamin C, and beta-carotene. The mineral selenium also participates in antioxidant activities.

antioxidants (an-tee-OX-ih-dants) compounds that protect other compounds from damaging reactions involving oxygen by themselves reacting with oxygen (*anti* means "against"; *oxy* means "oxygen"). *Oxidation* is a potentially damaging effect of normal cell chemistry involving oxygen.

aorta (ay-OR-tuh) the large artery that conducts oxygenated blood away from the heart to the rest of the circulatory system.

appendicitis inflammation and/or infection of the appendix. (The appendix is a sac about 4 inches long, protruding from the large intestine. It may become infected if fragments of the intestinal contents become trapped within it.)

appetite the psychological desire to eat; a learned motivation and a positive sensation that accompanies the sight, smell, or thought of appealing foods.

appliance thermometer a thermometer that verifies the temperature of an appliance. An *oven thermometer* verifies that the oven is heating properly; a *refrigerator/freezer thermometer* tests for proper refrigerator temperature (<40°F, or <4°C) or freezer temperature (0°F, or −17°C).

aquaculture the farming of aquatic organisms for food, generally fish, mollusks, or crustaceans, that involves such activities as feeding immature organisms, providing habitat, protecting them from predators, harvesting them, and selling or consuming them.

arachidonic (ah-RACK-ih-DON-ik) **acid** an omega-6 fatty acid derived from linoleic acid.

arsenic a poisonous metallic element. In trace amounts, arsenic is believed to be an essential nutrient in some animal species. Arsenic is often added to insecticides and weed killers and, in tiny amounts, to certain animal drugs.

arteries blood vessels that carry blood containing fresh oxygen supplies from the heart to the tissues.

arthritis a usually painful inflammation of joints caused by many conditions, including infections, metabolic disturbances, or injury; usually results in altered joint structure and loss of function.

artificial fats zero-energy fat replacers that are chemically synthesized to mimic the sensory and cooking qualities of naturally occurring fats but that are totally or partially resistant to digestion.

ascorbic acid one of the active forms of vitamin C (the other is *dehydroascorbic* acid); an antioxidant nutrient.

-ase (ACE) a suffix meaning *enzyme*. Categories of digestive and other enzymes and individual enzyme names often contain this suffix.

atherogenic diet a diet that promotes atherosclerosis—that is, a diet that is high in saturated fats and *trans* fats and low in vegetables, fruit, and whole grains. *Atherogenic* means able to initiate or promote atherosclerosis

atherosclerosis (ath-er-oh-scler-OH-sis) the most common form of cardiovascular disease; characterized by plaque along the inner walls of the arteries (*scleros* means "hard"; *osis* means "too much"). The term *arteriosclerosis* is often used to mean the same thing.

athlete a competitor in any sport, exercise, or game requiring physical skill; for the purpose of this book, anyone who trains at a high level of physical exertion, with or without competition. From the Greek *athlein*, meaning "to contend for a prize."

atrophy (AT-tro-fee) reduction in size (e.g., of a muscle) because of disuse.

autoimmune disorder a disease in which the body develops antibodies against its own proteins and then proceeds to destroy cells containing these proteins. Examples are type 1 diabetes and lupus.

B

baby water ordinary bottled water treated with ozone to make it safe but not sterile.

balance the dietary characteristic of providing foods of a number of types in proportion to each other, such that foods rich in some nutrients do not crowd out the diet foods that are rich in other nutrients.

balance study a laboratory study in which a subject is fed a controlled diet and the intake and excretion of a nutrient are measured. Balance studies are valid only for nutrients such as calcium (chemical elements) that do not change while they are in the body.

basal metabolic rate (BMR) the rate at which the body uses energy to support its basal metabolism.

basal metabolism the sum total of all the involuntary activities that are necessary to sustain life, including circulation, respiration, temperature maintenance, hormone secretion, nerve activity, and new tissue synthesis, but excluding digestion and voluntary activities. Basal metabolism is the largest component of the average person's daily energy expenditure.

bases compounds that accept hydrogens from solutions.

beetroot the root portion of the ordinary beet plant; the root vegetable, beet. Beetroot extracts may be sold as ergogenic aids.

behavior modification alteration of behavior using methods based on the theory that actions can be controlled by manipulating the environmental factors that cue, or trigger, the actions.

beriberi (berry-berry) the thiamin-deficiency disease; characterized by loss of sensation in the hands and feet, muscular weakness, advancing paralysis, and abnormal heart action.

beta-carotene an orange pigment with antioxidant activity; a vitamin A precursor made by plants and stored in human fat tissue.

bicarbonate a common alkaline chemical; a secretion of the pancreas. (Sodium bicarbonate is baking soda.)

bile a cholesterol-containing digestive fluid made by the liver, stored in the gallbladder, and released into the small intestine when needed. It emulsifies fats and oils to ready them for enzymatic digestion.

binge drinking see *heavy episodic drinking*.

binge eating disorder an eating disorder whose criteria are similar to those of bulimia nervosa, excluding purging or other compensatory behaviors.

bioaccumulation the accumulation of a contaminant in the tissues of living things at higher and higher concentrations along the food chain.

bioactive having chemical or physical properties that affect the functions of the body tissues.

bioactive food components compounds in foods, either nutrients or phytochemicals, that alter physiological processes.

biofilm a layer of microbes mixed with a sticky, protective coating of proteins and carbohydrates exuded by certain bacteria.

biotechnology the science of manipulating biological systems or organisms to modify their products or components or create new products; biotechnology includes recombinant DNA technology and traditional and accelerated selective breeding techniques.

biotin (BY-o-tin) a B vitamin; a coenzyme necessary for fat synthesis and other metabolic reactions.

bladder the sac that holds urine until time for elimination.

blind experiment an experiment in which the subjects do not know whether they are members of the experimental group or the control group. In a *double-blind experiment*, neither the subjects nor the researchers know to which group the members belong until the end of the experiment.

blood the fluid of the cardiovascular system; composed of water, red and white blood cells, other formed particles, nutrients, oxygen, and other constituents.

body composition the proportions of muscle, bone, fat, and other tissue that make up a person's total body weight.

body fat distribution the pattern of fat deposition in various body areas.

body mass index (BMI) an indicator of health risk from obesity or underweight, calculated by dividing the weight of a person by the square of the person's height.

body system a group of related organs that work together to perform a function. Examples are the circulatory system, respiratory system, and nervous system.

bone density a measure of bone strength, the degree of mineralization of the bone matrix.

bone meal or **powdered bone** crushed or ground bone preparations intended to supply calcium to the diet. Calcium from bone is not well absorbed and is often contaminated with toxic materials such as arsenic, mercury, lead, and cadmium.

botanical pertaining to or made from plants; any drug, medicinal preparation, dietary supplement, or similar substance obtained from a plant.

bottled water drinking water sold in single-use or reusable bottles commonly ranging in size from five ounces to five gallons.

botulism an often fatal foodborne illness caused by the botulinum toxin, a toxin produced by the *Clostridium botulinum* bacterium, which grows without oxygen in nonacidic canned foods.

bovine spongiform encephalopathy (BOH-vine SPUNJ-ih-form en-SEH-fal-AH-path-ee) **(BSE)** an often fatal illness of the nerves and brain observed in cattle and wild game and in people who consume affected meats. Also called *mad cow disease*.

BPA (bisphenol A) a compound that hardens plastic and a component of epoxy resin. BPA can leach from some plastic containers into the foods and beverages contained inside.

bran the protective fibrous coating around a grain; the chief fiber constituent of a grain.

broccoli sprouts the sprouted seed of *Brassica italica*, or the common broccoli plant; believed to be a functional food by virtue of its high phytochemical content.

brown adipose tissue (BAT) a type of adipose tissue abundant in hibernating animals and human infants and recently identified in human adults. Abundant pigmented enzymes of energy metabolism give BAT a dark appearance under a microscope; the enzymes release heat from fuels without accomplishing other work. Also called *brown fat*.

brown bread bread containing ingredients such as molasses that lend a brown color; these breads may be made with any kind of flour, including white flour.

brown sugar white sugar with molasses added, 95% pure sucrose.

buffers molecules that can help keep the pH of a solution from changing by gathering or releasing H ions.

built environment the buildings, roads, utilities, homes, fixtures, parks, and all the other man-made entities that form the physical characteristics of a community.

bulimia (byoo-LEEM-ee-uh) **nervosa** recurring episodes of binge eating combined with a morbid fear of becoming fat; usually followed by self-induced vomiting, misuse of laxatives or diuretics, fasting, or excessive exercise.

C

caffeine a stimulant that can produce alertness and reduce reaction time when used in small doses but that causes headaches, trembling, an abnormally fast heart rate, and other undesirable effects in high doses.

caffeine water bottled water with caffeine added.

calcium compounds the simplest forms of purified calcium. They include calcium carbonate, citrate, gluconate, hydroxide, lactate, malate, and phosphate. These supplements vary in the amount of calcium they contain, so read the labels carefully. A 500-milligram tablet of calcium gluconate may provide only 45 milligrams of calcium, for example.

caloric effect the drop in cancer incidence seen whenever calorie intakes are restricted.

calorie control the dietary characteristic of controlling energy intake; a feature of a sound diet plan.

calories units of energy. In nutrition science, the unit used to measure the energy in foods is a kilocalorie (also called *kcalorie* or *Calorie*): it is the amount of heat energy necessary to raise the temperature of a kilogram (a liter) of water 1 degree Celsius. This book follows the common practice of using the lowercase term *calorie* (abbreviated *cal*) to mean the same thing.

cancer a group of diseases characterized by the uncontrolled growth and spread of abnormal cells.

capillaries minute, weblike blood vessels that connect arteries to veins and permit transfer of materials between blood and tissues.

carbohydrase (car-boh-HIGH-drace) any of a number of enzymes that break the chemical bonds of carbohydrates.

carbohydrates compounds composed of single or multiple sugars. The name means "carbon and water," and a chemical shorthand for carbohydrate is CHO, signifying carbon (C), hydrogen (H), and oxygen (O).

carbonated water water that contains carbon dioxide gas, either naturally occurring or added, that causes bubbles to form in it; also called bubbling or sparkling water. Seltzer, soda, and tonic waters are legally soft drinks and are not regulated as water.

carcinogen (car-SIN-oh-jen) a cancer-causing substance; asbestos and tobacco smoke are examples of carcinogens.

carcinogenesis the process of cancer development (*carcin* means "cancer"; *gen* means "gives rise to").

cardiac output the volume of blood discharged by the heart each minute.

cardiorespiratory endurance the ability of the heart, lungs, and metabolism to sustain large-muscle exercise of moderate to high intensity for prolonged periods.

cardiovascular disease (CVD) a general term describing diseases of the heart and/or blood vessels. Examples of CVD include hypertension, coronary heart disease, and stroke.

carnitine nonessential nutrient that functions in cellular activities.

carotenoids (CARE-oh-ten-oyds) members of a group of pigments in foods that range in color from light yellow to reddish orange and are chemical relatives of beta-carotene. Many have a degree of vitamin A activity in the body.

carrying capacity the total number of living organisms that a given environment can support without deteriorating in quality.

case study a study of a single individual. When in clinical settings, researchers can observe treatments and their apparent effects. To prove that a treatment has produced an effect requires simultaneous observation of an untreated similar subject (a *case control*).

catalyst a substance that speeds the rate of a chemical reaction without itself being permanently altered in the process. All enzymes are catalysts.

cataract (CAT-uh-ract) clouding of the lens of the eye that can lead to blindness. Cataracts can be caused by injury, viral infection, toxic substances, genetic disorders, and possibly some nutrient deficiencies or imbalances.

cathartic a strong laxative.

celiac (SEE-lee-ack) **disease** a disorder characterized by an abnormal immune response, weight loss, and intestinal inflammation on exposure to the dietary protein gluten; also called *gluten-sensitive enteropathy* or *celiac sprue*.

cell differentiation (dih-fer-en-she-AY-shun) the process by which immature cells are stimulated to mature and gain the ability to perform functions characteristic of their cell type.

cells the smallest units in which independent life can exist. All living things are single cells or organisms made of cells.

cellulite (CELL-yoo-light) a term popularly used to describe dimpled fat tissue on the thighs and buttocks; not recognized in science.

central obesity excess fat in the abdomen and around the trunk.

Certified Diabetes Educator (CDE) a health-care professional who has completed an intensive professional training program and examination to earn a certificate attesting to the attainment of knowledge and skill in educating people with diabetes to help them manage their disease through medical and lifestyle means.

certified lactation consultant a health-care provider, often a registered nurse or a registered dietitian nutritionist, with specialized training and certification in breast and infant anatomy and physiology who teaches the mechanics of breastfeeding to new mothers.

Certified Specialist in Sports Dietetics (CSSD) a Registered Dietitian Nutritionist with special credentials and expertise to deliver safe, effective, evidence-based nutrition assessments and guidance for health and performance to athletes and other physically active people.

cesarean (see-ZAIR-ee-un) **section** surgical childbirth, in which the infant is taken through an incision in the woman's abdomen.

chelating agents (KEY-late-ing) molecules that attract or bind with other molecules and are therefore useful in either preventing or promoting movement of substances from place to place.

chlorophyll the green pigment of plants that captures energy from sunlight for use in photosynthesis.

cholesterol (koh-LESS-ter-all) a member of the group of lipids known as sterols; a soft, waxy substance made in the body and also found in animal-derived foods.

choline (KOH-leen) a nutrient used to make the phospholipid lecithin and other molecules.

chromosomes structures of mostly coiled DNA and proteins, housed in the nucleus of every cell. The DNA carries the genes for making cellular proteins; the protein and other constituents influence the configuration and functioning of the DNA.

chronic diseases degenerative conditions or illnesses that progress slowly, are long in duration, and lack immediate cures. Chronic diseases limit functioning, productivity, and the quality and length of life. Examples include heart disease, cancer, and diabetes.

chronic hypertension in pregnant women, hypertension that is present and documented before pregnancy; in women whose prepregnancy blood pressure is unknown, the presence of sustained hypertension before 20 weeks of gestation.

chronic malnutrition malnutrition caused by long-term food deprivation; characterized in children by short height for age (stunting).

chylomicrons (KYE-low-MY-krons) lipoproteins formed when lipids from a meal cluster with carrier proteins in the cells of the intestinal lining. Chylomicrons transport food fats through the watery body fluids to the liver and other tissues.

chyme (KIME) the fluid resulting from the actions of the stomach upon a meal.

cirrhosis (seer-OH-sis) advanced liver disease, often associated with alcoholism, in which liver cells have died, hardened, turned an orange color, and permanently lost their function.

clone an individual created asexually from a single ancestor, such as a plant grown from a single stem cell; a group of genetically identical individuals descended from a single common ancestor, such as a colony of bacteria arising from a single bacterial cell; in genetics, a replica of a segment of DNA, such as a gene, produced by genetic engineering.

coconut sugar a granulated sugar composed of sucrose, glucose, and fructose; made by evaporating the sap of the flower buds of coconut palm trees.

coconut water the fluid inside a young green coconut; heavily marketed for its substantial potassium content, it also provides about 45 calories per cup and little or no fat.

coenzyme (co-EN-zime) a small molecule that works with an enzyme to promote the enzyme's activity. Many coenzymes have B vitamins as part of their structure (*co* means "with").

cognitive behavioral therapy psychological therapy aimed at changing undesirable behaviors by changing underlying thought processes contributing to these behaviors; in anorexia, a goal is to replace false beliefs about body weight, eating, and self-worth with health-promoting beliefs.

cognitive skills as taught in behavior therapy, changes to conscious thoughts with the goal of improving adherence to lifestyle modifications; examples are problem-solving skills and the correction of false negative thoughts, termed *cognitive restructuring*.

collagen (COLL-a-jen) the chief protein of most connective tissues, including scars, ligaments, and tendons, and the underlying matrix on which bones and teeth are built.

colon the large intestine.

colostrum (co-LAHS-trum) a milklike secretion from the breasts during the first day or so after delivery before milk appears; rich in protective factors.

competitive foods unregulated meals, including fast foods, that compete side by side with USDA-regulated school lunches.

complementary and alternative medicine (CAM) a group of diverse medical and health-care systems, practices, and products that are not considered to be a part of conventional medicine. Examples include acupuncture, biofeedback, chiropractic, faith healing, and many others.

complementary foods nutrient- and energy-containing solid or semisolid foods (or liquids) fed to infants in addition to breast milk or infant formula.

complementary proteins two or more proteins whose amino acid assortments complement each other in such a way that the essential amino acids missing from one are supplied by the other.

complex carbohydrates long chains of sugar units arranged to form starch or fiber; also called *polysaccharides*.

concentrated fruit juice sweetener a concentrated sugar syrup made from dehydrated, deflavored fruit juice, commonly grape juice; used to sweeten products that can then claim to be "all fruit."

conditionally essential amino acid an amino acid that is normally nonessential but must be supplied by the diet in special circumstances when the need for it exceeds the body's ability to produce it.

confectioner's sugar finely powdered sucrose, 99.9% pure.

constipation infrequent, difficult, bowel movements, generally fewer than three per week, often caused by diet, inactivity, dehydration, or medication.

control group a group of individuals who are similar in all possible respects to the group being treated in an experiment but who receive a sham treatment instead of the real one. Also called *control subjects*.

controlled clinical trial an experiment in which one group of subjects (the experimental group) receives a treatment and a comparable group (the control group) receives an imitation treatment and outcomes for the two are compared Ideally, neither subjects nor researchers know who receives the treatment and who gets the placebo (a double-blind study).

cornea (KOR-nee-uh) the transparent hard, outer covering of the front of the eye.

corn sweeteners corn syrup and sugar solutions derived from corn.

corn syrup a syrup, mostly glucose, partly maltose, produced by the action of enzymes on cornstarch. Includes corn syrup solids.

coronary heart disease a chronic, progressive disease characterized by obstructive blood flow in the coronary arteries; also called *coronary artery disease*. The coronary arteries are those that feed the heart muscle itself. See also *peripheral artery disease*.

correlation the simultaneous change of two factors, such as the increase of weight with increasing height (a *direct* or *positive* correlation) or the decrease of cancer incidence with increasing fiber intake (an *inverse* or *negative*

correlation). A correlation between two factors suggests that one may cause the other but does not rule out the possibility that both may be caused by chance or by a third factor.

cortex the outermost layer of something. The brain's cortex is the part of the brain where conscious thought takes place.

cortical bone the ivorylike outer bone layer that forms a shell surrounding trabecular bone and that comprises the shaft of a long bone.

country of origin label (COOL) the required label stating the country of origination of certain imported fish and shellfish, certain other perishable foods, certain nuts, peanuts, and ginseng. Meats and poultry are no longer subject to COOL labeling.

creatine a nitrogen-containing compound that combines with phosphate to form a high-energy compound stored in muscle. Some studies suggest that creatine enhances energy and stimulates muscle growth, but long-term studies are lacking; digestive side effects may occur.

cretinism (CREE-tin-ism) severe mental and physical retardation of an infant caused by the mother's iodine deficiency during pregnancy.

critical thinking the mental activity of rationally and skillfully analyzing, synthesizing, and evaluating information.

critical period a finite period during development in which certain events may occur that will have irreversible effects on later developmental stages. A critical period is usually a period of cell division in a body organ.

cross-contamination the contamination of food through exposure to utensils, hands, or other surfaces that were previously in contact with contaminated food.

cruciferous vegetables vegetables with cross-shaped blossoms, members of the cabbage family. Intakes of these vegetables are associated with low cancer rates in human populations. Examples are broccoli, brussels sprouts, cabbage, cauliflower, rutabagas, and turnips.

cuisines styles of cooking.

cultural competence having an awareness and acceptance of one's own and others' cultures and abilities, leading to effective interactions with all kinds of people.

D

Daily Values nutrient standards used on food labels and on grocery store and restaurant signs.

dead zones columns of oxygen-depleted ocean water in which marine life cannot survive; often caused by algae blooms that occur when agricultural fertilizers and waste runoff enter natural waterways.

dehydration loss of water. The symptoms progress rapidly, from thirst to weakness to exhaustion and delirium, and end in death.

denaturation the irreversible change in a protein's folded shape brought about by heat, acids, bases, alcohol, salts of heavy metals, or other agents.

dental caries decay of the teeth (*caries* means "rottenness"). Also called *cavities*.

dextrose, anhydrous dextrose forms of glucose.

DHEA (dehydroepiandrosterone) a hormone made in the adrenal glands that serves as a precursor to the male hormone testosterone; recently banned by the U.S. Food and Drug Administration (FDA) because it poses the risk of life-threatening diseases, including cancer. Falsely promoted to burn fat, build muscle, and slow aging.

diabetes (dye-uh-BEET-eez) metabolic diseases that impair a person's ability to regulate blood glucose.

dialysis (die-AL-ih-sis) a medical treatment for failing kidneys in which a person's blood is circulated through a machine that filters out toxins and wastes and returns cleansed blood to the body; more properly called *hemodialysis*, meaning "dialysis of the blood."

diarrhea frequent, watery bowel movements usually caused by diet, stress, or irritation of the colon. Severe, prolonged diarrhea robs the body of fluid and certain minerals, causing dehydration and imbalances that can be dangerous if left untreated.

diet the foods (including beverages) a person usually eats and drinks.

dietary antioxidants compounds typically found in plant foods that counteract the adverse effects of oxidation on living tissues. The major antioxidant vitamins are vitamin E, vitamin C, and beta-carotene. Many phytochemicals are also antioxidants.

dietary folate equivalent (DFE) a unit of measure expressing the amount of folate available to the body from naturally occurring sources. The measure mathematically equalizes the difference in absorption between less absorbable food folate (folic acid) and highly absorbable synthetic folate added to enriched foods and found in supplements.

dietary nitrate a compound composed of one nitrogen and three oxygen atoms, often concentrated in extracts of vegetables, particularly beetroot, celery, and spinach; nitrate releases oxygen as it undergoes chemical conversions in the body.

Dietary Reference Intakes (DRI) a set of five lists of values for measuring the nutrient intakes of healthy people in the United States and Canada. The lists are Estimated Average Requirements (EAR), Recommended Dietary Allowances (RDA), Adequate Intakes (AI), Tolerable Upper Intake Levels (UL), and Acceptable Macronutrient Distribution Ranges (AMDR).

dietary supplements pills, liquids, or powders that contain purified nutrients or other ingredients.

dietetic technician see *Nutrition and Dietetics Technician, Registered.*

dietitian a person trained in the science of nutrition and dietetics. See also *Registered Dietitian Nutritionist.*

digest to break molecules into smaller molecules; a main function of the digestive tract with respect to food.

digestive system the body system composed of organs that break down complex food particles into smaller, absorbable products. The *digestive tract* and *alimentary canal* are names for the tubular organs that extend from the mouth to the anus. The whole system, including the pancreas, liver, and gallbladder, is sometimes called the *gastrointestinal*, or GI, system.

dipeptides (dye-PEP-tides) protein fragments that are two amino acids long (*di* means "two").

diploma mill an organization that awards meaningless degrees without requiring students to meet educational standards. Diploma mills are not the same as diploma forgers (providing fake diplomas and certificates bearing the names of real, respected institutions). Although visually indistinguishable from authentic diplomas, forgeries can be unveiled by checking directly with the institution.

disaccharides pairs of single sugars linked together (*di* means "two").

distilled water water that has been vaporized and recondensed, leaving it free of dissolved minerals.

diuretic (dye-you-RET-ic) a compound, usually a medication, causing increased urinary water excretion; a "water pill."

diverticula (dye-ver-TIC-you-la) sacs or pouches that balloon out of the intestinal wall, caused by weakening of the muscle layers that encase the intestine. The painful inflammation of one or more of the diverticula is known as *diverticulitis.*

DNA an abbreviation for deoxyribonucleic (dee-OX-ee-RYE-bow-nu-CLAY-ick) acid, the thread-like molecule that encodes genetic information in its structure; DNA strands coil up densely to form the chromosomes.

dolomite a compound of minerals (calcium magnesium carbonate) found in limestone and marble. Dolomite is powdered and is sold as a calcium-magnesium supplement but may be contaminated with toxic minerals, is not well absorbed, and interacts adversely with absorption of other essential minerals.

dopamine (DOH-pah-meen) a neurotransmitter that facilitates many important functions in the brain, including cognition, pleasure, motivation, mood, sleep, and others.

drink see *a drink.*

drug any substance that, when taken into a living organism, modifies one or more of its functions.

dual-energy X-ray absorptiometry (absorp-tee-OM-eh-tree) a noninvasive method of determining total body fat, fat distribution, and bone density by passing two low-dose X-ray beams through the body. Also used in evaluation of osteoporosis. Abbreviated DEXA.

E

eating disorder a disturbance in eating behavior that jeopardizes a person's physical or psychological health.

eating pattern the combination of foods and beverages that constitute an individual's complete dietary intake over time; a person's usual diet.

eclampsia (eh-CLAMP-see-ah) a severe complication during pregnancy in which seizures occur.

edamame fresh green soybeans, a source of phytoestrogens.

edema (eh-DEEM-uh) swelling of body tissue caused by leakage of fluid from the blood vessels; seen in protein deficiency (among other conditions).

eicosanoids (eye-COSS-ah-noyds) biologically active compounds that regulate body functions.

electrolytes compounds that partly dissociate in water to form ions, such as the potassium ion (K^+) and the chloride ion (Cl^-).

elemental diets diets composed of purified ingredients of known chemical composition; intended to supply, to the greatest extent possible, all essential nutrients to people who cannot eat foods.

embolism the event in which an embolus lodges in an artery and suddenly cuts off the blood supply to a part of the body. See also *thrombosis.*

embolus (EM-boh-luss) a clot that travels through the circulatory system (*embol* means "to insert").

embryo (EM-bree-oh) the stage of human gestation from the third to the eighth week after conception.

emergency kitchens programs that provide prepared meals to be eaten on-site; often called *soup kitchens.*

emetic (em-ETT-ic) an agent that causes vomiting.

empty calories calories provided by added sugars and solid fats with few or no other nutrients. Other empty calorie sources include alcohol, and highly refined starches, such as corn starch or potato starch, often found in ultra-processed foods.

emulsification the process of mixing lipid with water by adding an emulsifier.

emulsifier (ee-MULL-sih-fire) a compound with both water-soluble and fat-soluble portions that mixes with both fat and water and permanently disperses the fat in the water, forming an emulsion.

emulsion a mixture of two liquids that do not usually mix, in which tiny particles of one liquid are held suspended in the other.

endemic common or prevalent in a particular area or group of people.

endosperm the bulk of the edible part of a grain, the starchy part.

energy the capacity to do work. The energy in food is chemical energy; it can be converted to mechanical, electrical, thermal, or other forms of energy in the body. Food energy is measured in calories.

energy availability the amount of food energy consumed in a day minus the energy expended in physical activity; measured in calories per kilogram of lean body mass.

energy density a measure of the energy provided by a food relative to its weight (calories per gram).

energy drinks and **energy shots** sugar-sweetened beverages in various concentrations with supposedly ergogenic ingredients, such as vitamins, amino acids, caffeine, guarana, carnitine, ginseng, and others. Regulations of these drinks by the FDA is lax, and they are often high in caffeine or other stimulants.

energy reservoir a system of high-energy compounds that hold, store, and release energy derived from the energy-yielding nutrients and transfer it to cell structures to fuel cellular activities.

energy-yielding nutrients the nutrients the body can use for energy: carbohydrate, fat (also called *lipids*), and protein. These also may supply building blocks for body structures.

enriched foods and **fortified foods** foods to which nutrients have been added. If the starting material is a whole, basic food such as milk or whole grain, the result may be highly nutritious. If the starting material is a concentrated form of sugar or fat, the result is less nutritious.

enriched, fortified refers to the addition of nutrients to a refined food product. As defined by U.S. law, these terms mean that specified levels of thiamin, riboflavin, niacin, folate, and iron have been added to refined grains and grain products. The terms *enriched* and *fortified* can refer to the addition of more nutrients than just these five; read the label.

enterotoxins poisons that act on mucous membranes, such as those of the digestive tract.

environmental tobacco smoke the combination of exhaled smoke (mainstream smoke) and smoke from lighted cigarettes, pipes, or cigars (sidestream smoke) that enters the air around smokers and may be inhaled by other people. Also called *second-hand smoke*.

enzymes (EN-zimes) working proteins that speed up specific chemical reactions, such as releasing energy from nutrient molecules, without themselves being altered in the process.

EPA, DHA eicosapentaenoic (EYE-cossa-PENTA-ee-NO-ick) acid, docosahexaenoic (DOE-cossa-HEXA-ee-NO-ick) acid; omega-3 fatty acids made from linolenic acid in the tissues of fish.

epidemiological studies studies of populations; often used in nutrition to search for correlations between dietary habits and disease incidence; a first step in seeking nutrition-related causes of diseases.

epigenetics (ep-ih-gen-EH-tics) the science of heritable changes in gene function that occur without changes in the DNA sequence.

epigenome (ep-ih-GEE-nohm) the proteins and other molecules associated with chromosomes that affect gene expression. The epigenome is modulated by bioactive food components and other factors in ways that can be inherited. *Epi* is a Greek prefix, meaning "above" or "on."

epinephrine (epp-ih-NEFF-rin) a hormone of the adrenal gland that counteracts anaphylactic shock by opening the airways and maintaining heartbeat and blood pressure.

epiphyseal (eh-PIFF-ih-seal) **plate** a thick, cartilage-like layer that forms new cells that are eventually calcified, lengthening the bone (*epiphysis* means "growing" in Greek).

epithelial (ep-ith-THEE-lee-ull) **tissue** the layers of the body that serve as selective barriers to environmental factors. Examples are the cornea, the skin, the respiratory tract lining, and the lining of the digestive tract.

ergogenic (ER-go-JEN-ic) **aids** products that supposedly enhance performance, although few actually do so; the term *ergogenic* implies "energy giving" (*ergo* means "work"; *genic* means "give rise to").

erythrocyte (eh-REETH-ro-sight) **hemolysis** (HEE-moh-LIE-sis, hee-MOLL-ih-sis) rupture of the red blood cells that can be caused by vitamin E deficiency (*erythro* means "red"; *cyte* means "cell"; *hemo* means "blood"; *lysis* means "breaking"). The anemia produced by the condition is *hemolytic* (HEE-moh-LIT-ick) *anemia*.

essential amino acids amino acids that either cannot be synthesized at all by the body or cannot be synthesized in amounts sufficient to meet physiological need.

essential fatty acids fatty acids that the body needs but cannot make and so must be obtained from the diet.

essential nutrients the nutrients the body cannot make for itself (or cannot make fast enough) from other raw materials; nutrients that must be obtained from food to prevent deficiencies.

Estimated Average Requirements (EAR) the average daily nutrient intake estimated to meet the requirement of half of the healthy individuals in a particular life stage and gender group.

Estimated Energy Requirement (EER) the average dietary energy intake predicted to maintain energy balance in a healthy adult of a certain age, gender, weight, height, and level of physical activity consistent with good health.

ethanol the alcohol of alcoholic beverages, often called simply "alcohol"; a drug.

ethnic foods foods associated with particular cultural subgroups within a population.

euphoria (you-FOR-ee-uh) a state of intense happiness induced by an extremely pleasurable experience or by a drug such as ethanol.

evaporated cane juice raw sugar from which impurities have been removed.

excess postexercise oxygen consumption (EPOC) a measure of increased metabolism (energy expenditure) that continues for minutes or hours after cessation of exercise.

exclusive breastfeeding an infant's consumption of human milk with no supplementation of any type (no water, no juice, no nonhuman milk, and no foods) except for vitamins, minerals, and medications.

exercise planned, structured, and repetitive bodily movement that promotes or maintains physical fitness.

experimental group the people or animals participating in an experiment who receive the treatment under investigation. Also called *experimental subjects*.

extracellular fluid fluid residing outside the cells that transports materials to and from the cells.

extra virgin olive oil minimally processed olive oil produced by mechanical means, such as pressing (not chemical extraction), to preserve phytochemicals, green color, and flavor from the original olives. The highest grade of olive oil.

extreme obesity clinically severe overweight, presenting very high risks to health; the condition of having a BMI of 40 or above; also called *morbid obesity*.

extrusion processing techniques that transform grains, legumes, and other foods into fine particles that are cooked, shaped, colored, flavored, and often puffed, producing snacks, breakfast cereals, and other products.

F

famine widespread and extreme scarcity of food that causes starvation and death in a large portion of the population in an area.

farm share an arrangement in which a farmer offers the public a "subscription" for an allotment of the farm's products throughout the season.

fast foods restaurant foods that are available within minutes after customers order them—traditionally, hamburgers, French fries, and milkshakes; more recently, salads and other vegetable dishes as well. These foods may or may not meet people's nutrient needs, depending on the selections provided and on the energy allowances and nutrient needs of the eaters.

fasting plasma glucose test a blood test that measures the current blood glucose concentration in a person who has not ingested caloric beverages for at least 8 hours; the test can detect both diabetes and prediabetes. *Plasma* is the fluid part of whole blood.

fat cells cells that specialize in the storage of fat and form the fat tissue. Fat cells also produce fat-metabolizing enzymes; they also produce hormones involved in appetite and energy balance.

fat replacers ingredients that replace some or all of the functions of fat and may or may not provide energy.

fats lipids that are solid at room temperature (70°F or 21°C).

fatty acids organic acids composed of carbon chains of various lengths. Each fatty acid has an acid end and hydrogens attached to all of the carbon atoms of the chain.

fatty liver an early stage of liver deterioration seen in several diseases, including nonalcoholic and alcoholic liver diseases, in which fat accumulates in the liver cells.

fatty streaks deposits of fat on the inner surfaces of arteries, an early stage in the formation of plaques.

FDA Food Safety Modernization Act (FSMA) a law enacted in 2016 to build a new system of domestic and international controls for the detection, prevention, and correction of microbial contamination of the U.S. food supply.

FDA Produce Safety Rule a set of science-based standards that minimize microbial hazards during commercial growing, harvesting, packing, and holding of fruit and vegetables intended for U.S. consumption.

feces waste material remaining after digestion and absorption are complete; eventually discharged from the body.

Fellow of the Academy of Nutrition and Dietetics (FAND) members of the academy who are recognized for their outstanding service and integrity in the dietetics profession.

female athlete triad a potentially fatal triad of medical problems seen in female athletes: low energy availability (with or without disordered eating), menstrual dysfunction, and low bone mineral density.

fermentation the anaerobic (without oxygen) breakdown of carbohydrates by microorganisms that releases small organic compounds along with carbon dioxide and energy.

fertility the capacity of a woman to produce a normal ovum periodically and of a man to produce normal sperm; the ability to reproduce.

fetal alcohol spectrum disorders (FASD) a spectrum of physical, behavioral, and cognitive disabilities caused by prenatal alcohol exposure.

fetal alcohol syndrome (FAS) the cluster of symptoms including brain damage, growth restriction, mental retardation, and facial abnormalities seen in an infant or child whose mother consumed alcohol during her pregnancy.

fetus (FEET-us) the stage of human gestation from eight weeks after conception until the birth of an infant.

fiber a collective term for various indigestible plant materials, many of which bear links with human health.

fibers the indigestible parts of plant foods, largely nonstarch polysaccharides that are not digested by human digestive enzymes, although some are digested by resident bacteria of the colon. Fibers include cellulose, hemicelluloses, pectins, gums, mucilages, and a few non-polysaccharides such as lignin.

fight-or-flight reaction the body's instinctive hormone- and nerve-mediated reaction to danger. Also known as the *stress response*.

fitness the characteristics that enable the body to perform physical activity; more broadly, the ability to meet routine physical demands with enough reserve energy to rise to physical challenges and withstand stress.

fitness water lightly flavored bottled water enhanced with vitamins, supposedly to enhance athletic performance.

flavonoids (FLAY-von-oyds) a common and widespread group of phytochemicals, with over 6,000 identified members; physiologic effects may include antioxidant, antiviral, anticancer, and other activities. Some flavonoids are yellow pigments in foods; *flavus* means "yellow."

flavored waters lightly flavored beverages with few or no calories, but often containing vitamins, minerals, herbs, or other unneeded substances. Not superior to plain water for athletic competition or training.

flaxseed small brown seed of the flax plant; used in baking, cereals, or other foods. Valued in nutrition as a source of fatty acids, lignans, and fiber.

flexibility the capacity of the joints to move through a full range of motion; the ability to bend and recover without injury.

fluid and electrolyte balance maintenance of the proper amounts and kinds of fluids and minerals in each compartment of the body.

fluid and electrolyte imbalance failure to maintain the proper amounts and kinds of fluids and minerals in every body compartment; a medical emergency.

fluorapatite (floor-APP-uh-tight) a crystal of bones and teeth, formed when fluoride displaces the "hydroxy" portion of hydroxyapatite. Fluorapatite resists being dissolved back into body fluid.

fluorosis (floor-OH-sis) discoloration of the teeth due to ingestion of too much fluoride during tooth development. *Skeletal fluorosis* is characterized by unusually dense but weak, fracture-prone, often malformed bones, caused by excess fluoride in bone crystals.

foam cells foamy-looking cells formed during plaque formation: they develop from white blood cells that, while clearing fat from plaques, become engorged with it.

folate (FOH-late) a B vitamin that acts as part of a coenzyme important in the manufacture of new cells. The form added to foods and supplements is *folic acid*.

food scientifically, materials, usually of plant or animal origin, that contain essential nutrients, such as carbohydrates, fats, proteins, vitamins, or minerals, and that are ingested and assimilated by an organism to produce energy, stimulate growth, and maintain life; socially, a more limited number of such materials defined as acceptable by a culture.

food aversion an intense dislike of a food, biological or psychological in nature, resulting from an illness or other negative experience associated with that food.

food banks facilities that collect and distribute food donations to authorized organizations feeding the hungry.

foodborne illness illness transmitted to human beings through food; caused by an infectious agent (*foodborne infection*) or a poisonous substance arising from microbial toxins, poisonous chemicals, or other harmful substances (*food intoxication*). Also commonly called *food poisoning*.

food contaminant any substance occurring in food by accident; any food constituent that is not normally present.

food crisis a steep decline in food availability with a proportional rise in hunger and malnutrition at the local, national, or global level.

food deserts low-income communities where many people do not own cars and live more than a mile from a supermarket or large grocery store (in rural areas, more than 10 miles).

food group plan a diet-planning tool that sorts foods into groups based on their nutrient content and then specifies that people should eat certain minimum numbers of servings of foods from each group.

food intolerance an adverse reaction to a food or food additive not involving an immune response.

food neophobia (NEE-oh-FOE-beeah) the fear of trying new foods, common among toddlers.

food pantries community food collection programs that provide groceries to be prepared and eaten at home.

food poverty hunger occurring when enough food exists in an area but some of the people cannot obtain it because they lack money, are being deprived for political reasons, live in a country at war, or suffer from other problems such as lack of transportation.

food recovery collecting wholesome surplus food for distribution to low-income people who are hungry.

foodways the sum of a culture's habits, customs, beliefs, and preferences concerning food.

fork thermometer a utensil combining a meat fork and an instant-read food thermometer.

fraud or **quackery** the promotion, for financial gain, of devices, treatments, services, plans, or products (including diets and supplements) claimed to improve health, well-being, or appearance without proof of safety or effectiveness. (The word *quackery* comes from the term *quacksalver*, meaning a person who quacks loudly about a miracle product—a lotion or a salve.)

free radicals atoms or molecules with one or more unpaired electrons that make the atom or molecule unstable and highly reactive.

fructose (FROOK-tose) a monosaccharide; sometimes known as fruit sugar (*fruct* means "fruit"; *ose* means "sugar").

fructose, galactose, glucose the monosaccharides important in nutrition.

fruitarian includes only raw or dried fruit, seeds, and nuts in the diet; nutrient deficiencies and dental caries are associated with such diets.

fufu a low-protein staple food that provides abundant starch energy to many of the world's people; fufu is made by pounding or grinding root vegetables or refined grains and cooking them to a smooth, semisolid consistency.

functional foods whole or modified foods that contain bioactive food components believed to provide health benefits, such as reduced disease risks, beyond the benefits that their nutrients confer. However, all nutritious foods can support health in some ways.

G

galactose (ga-LACK-tose) a monosaccharide; part of the disaccharide lactose (milk sugar).

gastric juice the digestive secretion of the stomach.

gastroesophageal (GAS-tro-eh-SOFF-ahjeel) **reflux disease (GERD)** severe and chronic splashing of stomach acid and enzymes into the esophagus, throat, mouth, or airway that causes injury to those organs. Untreated GERD may increase the risk of esophageal cancer; treatment may require surgery or management with medication.

gatekeepers with respect to nutrition, key people who control other people's access to foods and thereby affect their nutrition profoundly. Examples are a spouse who buys and cooks the food, a parent who feeds the children, and a caregiver in a day-care center.

gelatin a protein product of collagen breakdown. In foods, it confers structure, such as in gelatin desserts; in nutrition, it supplies low-quality protein that lacks many essential amino acids.

gene editing a method of genetic engineering that employs CRISPR technology to alter an organism by adding, removing, or substituting molecules within a single gene's DNA strand with great precision. The acronym *CRISPR* refers to a particular DNA sequence employed in the method.

generally recognized as safe (GRAS) list a list, established by the FDA, of food additives long in use and believed to be safe.

genes units of a cell's inheritance; sections of the larger genetic molecule DNA (deoxyribonucleic acid). Each gene directs the making of one or more of the body's proteins.

genetically modified organism (GMO) popular term referring to an organism produced by genetic engineering; the term *genetically engineered organism (GEO)* is more scientifically accurate.

genetic engineering the direct, intentional manipulation of the genetic material of living things in order to obtain some desirable inheritable trait not present in the original organism. Also called *biotechnology*.

genetic profile the result of an analysis of genetic material that identifies unique characteristics of a person's DNA for forensic or diagnostic purposes.

genistein (GEN-ih-steen) a phytoestrogen found primarily in soybeans that both mimics and blocks the action of estrogen in the body; a type of flavonoid.

genome (GEE-nome) the full complement of genetic information in the chromosomes of a cell. In human beings, the genome consists of about 35,000 genes and supporting materials.

genomics the study of all the genes in an organism and their interactions with environmental factors.

germ the nutrient-rich inner part of a grain.

gestation the period of about 40 weeks (three trimesters) from conception to birth; the term of a pregnancy.

gestational diabetes abnormal glucose tolerance appearing during pregnancy.

gestational hypertension high blood pressure that develops in the second half of pregnancy and usually resolves after childbirth.

ghrelin (GREL-in) a hormone released by the stomach that signals the brain's hypothalamus and other regions to stimulate eating.

glands body organs that produce and release needed compounds, such as sweat, saliva, and hormones.

glucagon (GLOO-cah-gon) a hormone from the pancreas that stimulates the liver to release glucose into the blood when necessary to raise its concentration.

glucose (GLOO-cose) a single sugar used in both plant and animal tissues for energy; sometimes known as blood sugar or *dextrose*.

glucose polymers compounds that supply glucose not as single molecules but linked in chains somewhat like starch. The objective is to attract less water from the body into the digestive tract.

gluten (GLOO-ten) a type of protein in certain grain foods that is toxic to the person with celiac disease.

glycemic index (GI) a ranking of foods according to their potential for raising blood glucose relative to a standard food such as glucose.

glycerol (GLISS-er-all) an organic compound, three carbons long, of interest here because it serves as the backbone for triglycerides.

glycogen (GLY-co-gen) a storage form of carbohydrate energy (glucose); a highly branched polysaccharide that is made and held in liver and muscle tissues as a storage form of glucose. Glycogen is not a significant food source of carbohydrate and is not counted as one of the complex carbohydrates in foods.

goiter (GOY-ter) enlargement of the thyroid gland due to an iodine deficiency is *goiter*; enlargement due to an iodine excess is *toxic goiter*.

grams (g) metric units of weight. About 28 grams equal an ounce. A *milligram* is one-thousandth of a gram. A *microgram* is one-millionth of a gram.

granulated sugar common table sugar, crystalline sucrose, 99.9% pure.

granules small grains. Starch granules are packages of starch molecules. Various plant species make starch granules of varying shapes.

greenhouse gases gases that contribute to global climate change by absorbing the sun's infrared radiation and trapping heat; examples of greenhouse gases are carbon dioxide and methane.

green revolution a series of advances in technology made in the last century that dramatically increased farm yields worldwide. The techniques rely heavily on chemical fertilizers and pesticides, along with large farm machinery.

groundwater water that comes from underground aquifers.

growth hormone a hormone (somatotropin) that promotes growth and that is produced naturally in the pituitary gland of the brain.

growth spurt the marked rapid gain in physical size usually evident around the onset of adolescence.

H

hangover a delayed, usually morning-after, reaction to drinking too much alcohol too fast the night before, characterized by a headache and sometimes nausea.

hard liquor a beverage that is made by distilling a product such as wine or beer, which arose from fermentation; one that contains a higher percentage of alcohol. Examples are brandy, gin, rum, vodka, and whiskey.

hard water water with high calcium and magnesium concentrations.

hazard a state of danger; referring to any circumstance in which harm is possible under normal conditions of use.

Hazard Analysis Critical Control Point (HACCP) plan a systematic plan to identify and correct potential microbial hazards in the manufacturing, distribution, and commercial use of food products. HACCP may be pronounced "HASS-ip."

health claims FDA-approved food label statements that link food constituents with disease or health-related conditions. Examples: "Soluble fiber from daily oatmeal in a diet low in saturated fat and trans fat may reduce the risk of heart disease" or "A diet low in total fat may reduce the risk of some cancers."

heart attack sudden, unexpected cessation of the heartbeat, respiration, and consciousness, usually caused by a clot lodging in a coronary artery (thrombosis). If not quickly reversed, this is followed by death. Also called *cardiac arrest* or *myocardial infarction* (*myo* means "muscle"; *infarction* means "block of blood supply").

heartburn a burning sensation in the chest (in the area of the heart) caused by backflow of stomach acid into the esophagus.

heat cramps painful cramps of the abdomen, arms, or legs, often occurring hours after exercise; associated with inadequate intake of fluid or electrolytes or heavy sweating.

heat stroke an acute and life-threatening reaction to heat buildup in the body.

heavy drinking drinking five or more drinks on each of five or more days per month.

heavy episodic drinking engaging in heavy consumption of alcohol over a short time period, with the intention of becoming intoxicated; for a man: drinking five or more drinks; or for a woman: drinking four or more drinks on at least one occasion within a 30-day period. Also called *binge drinking*.

heavy metal any of a number of mineral ions such as mercury and lead, so called because they are of relatively high atomic weight; many heavy metals are poisonous.

heme (HEEM) the iron-containing portion of the hemoglobin and myoglobin molecules.

hemoglobin (HEEM-oh-globe-in) the oxygen-carrying protein of the blood; found in the red blood cells (*hemo* means "blood"; *globin* means "spherical protein").

hemolytic-uremic (HEEM-oh-LIT-ic you-REEM-ick) **syndrome** a severe result of infection with Shiga toxin-producing *E. coli*, characterized by abnormal blood clotting with kidney failure, damage to the central nervous system and other organs, and death, especially among children.

hemorrhage (HEM-orr-age) uncontrolled bleeding.

hemorrhoids (HEM-or-oids) swollen, hardened (varicose) veins in the rectum, usually caused by pressure resulting from constipation.

hepcidin (HEP-sid-in) a hormone secreted by the liver in response to elevated blood iron. Hepcidin reduces iron's absorption from the intestine and its release from storage.

herbal medicine the use of herbs and herbal preparations to prevent or cure diseases or to relieve symptoms.

hernia a protrusion of an organ or part of an organ through the wall of the body chamber that normally contains the organ. An example is a *hiatal* (high-AY-tal) *hernia*, in which part of the stomach protrudes up through the diaphragm into the chest cavity, which contains the esophagus, heart, and lungs.

hiccups spasms of both the vocal cords and the diaphragm, causing periodic, audible, short, inhaled coughs. These can result from irritation of the diaphragm, indigestion, or other causes. Hiccups usually resolve in a few minutes but can have serious effects if prolonged. Breathing into a paper bag (inhaling carbon dioxide) or dissolving a teaspoon of sugar in the mouth may stop them.

high-carbohydrate energy drinks flavored commercial beverages used to restore muscle glycogen after exercise or as pregame beverages.

high-carbohydrate gels semisolid, easy-to-swallow supplements of concentrated carbohydrate, commonly with potassium and sodium added; not a fluid source.

high-density lipoproteins (HDL) lipoproteins that return cholesterol from the tissues to the liver for dismantling and disposal; contain a large proportion of protein.

high food security no reported indications of food access problems or limitations.

high-fructose corn syrup (HFCS) a commercial sweetener used in many foods, including soft drinks, made by adding enzymes to cornstarch to convert some glucose to sweet-tasting fructose. Composed almost entirely of the monosaccharides fructose and glucose, its sweetness and caloric value are similar to sucrose.

high-quality proteins dietary proteins containing all the essential amino acids in relatively the same amounts that human beings require. They may also contain nonessential amino acids.

high-risk pregnancy a pregnancy characterized by risk factors that make it likely the birth will be complicated by premature delivery, difficult birth, retarded growth, birth defects, and early infant death. A *low-risk pregnancy* has none of these factors.

histamine a substance that participates in causing inflammation; produced by cells of the immune system as part of a local immune reaction to an antigen.

histones (HISS-tones) proteins that lend structural support to the chromosome structure and that help activate or silence gene expression.

homogenization a process by which milk fat is evenly dispersed within fluid milk; under high pressure, milk is passed through tiny nozzles to reduce the size of fat droplets and reduce their tendency to cluster and float to the top as cream.

honey a concentrated solution composed primarily of glucose and fructose, produced by enzymatic digestion of the sucrose in nectar by bees.

hormones chemicals that are secreted by glands into the blood in response to conditions in the body that require regulation. These chemicals serve as messengers, acting on other organs to maintain constant conditions.

hourly sweat rate the amount of weight lost plus fluid consumed during exercise per hour.

hunger (1) a consequence of food insecurity; physical discomfort, illness, weakness, or pain beyond a mild uneasy sensation arising from a prolonged involuntary lack of food.

hunger (2) the physiological need to eat, experienced as a drive for obtaining food; an unpleasant sensation that demands relief.

husk the outer, inedible part of a grain.

hydrochloric acid a strong, corrosive acid of hydrogen and chloride atoms, produced by the stomach to assist in digestion.

hydrogenation (high-dro-gen-AY-shun) the process of adding hydrogen to unsaturated fatty acids to make fat more solid and resistant to the chemical change of oxidation.

hydrolyzed (HIGH-druh-lyzed) **protein** a commercial protein ingredient made by way of hydrolysis, a type of chemical reaction that splits molecules into smaller fragments and attaches water components to make the split possible. *Hydro* = water, *lysis* = to cleave.

hydroxyapatite (hi-DROX-ee-APP-uh-tight) the chief crystal of bone and teeth, formed from calcium and phosphorus.

hyperactivity (in children) a syndrome characterized by inattention, impulsiveness, and excess motor activity; usually diagnosed before age 7, lasts 6 months or more, and usually does not entail mental illness or mental retardation. Properly called *attention-deficit/ hyperactivity disorder (ADHD)*.

hypertension higher than normal blood pressure.

hypertrophy (high-PURR-tro-fee) an increase in size (e.g., of a muscle) in response to use.

hypoglycemia (HIGH-poh-gly-SEE-mee-ah) an abnormally low blood glucose concentration, often accompanied by symptoms such as anxiety, rapid heartbeat, and sweating.

hyponatremia (HIGH-poh-nah-TREE-mee-ah) an abnormally low concentration of sodium in the blood.

hypothalamus (high-poh-THAL-uh-mus) a part of the brain that senses a variety of conditions in the body, such as temperature, glucose content, salt content, and others. It signals other parts of the brain or body to adjust those conditions when necessary.

hypothermia a below-normal body temperature.

I

immune system a large system of tissues and organs that defend the body against microbes or foreign materials that have penetrated the skin or body linings.

immunity protection from or resistance to a disease or infection by the development of antibodies and by the actions of cells and tissues in response to a threat.

implantation the stage of development, during the first two weeks after conception, in which the fertilized egg (fertilized ovum or zygote) embeds itself in the wall of the uterus and begins to develop.

inborn error of metabolism a genetic variation present from birth that may result in disease.

incidental additives substances that can get into food not through intentional introduction but as a result of contact with the food during growing, processing, packaging, storing, or some other stage before the food is consumed. Also called *accidental* or *indirect additives*.

infectious diseases diseases that are caused by bacteria, viruses, parasites, and other microbes and that can be transmitted from one person to another through air, water, or food; by contact; or through vector organisms such as mosquitoes and fleas.

inflammation (in-flam-MAY-shun) an immune response to cellular injury that produces an increase in white blood cells, redness, heat, pain, and swelling. Chronic inflammation accompanies many diseases.

infomercials feature-length television commercials that follow the format of regular programs but are intended to convince viewers to buy products and not to educate or entertain them.

initiation an event, probably occurring in a cell's genetic material, caused by radiation or by a chemical carcinogen, that gives rise to cancer.

inositol (in-OSS-ih-tall) a nonessential nutrient found in cell membranes.

insoluble fibers the tough, fibrous structures of fruit, vegetables, and grains; indigestible food components that do not dissolve in water.

instant-read thermometer a thermometer that, when inserted into food, measures its temperature within seconds; designed to test temperature of food at intervals.

insulin a hormone secreted by the pancreas in response to a high blood glucose concentration. It assists cells in drawing glucose from the blood.

insulin resistance a condition in which a normal or high concentration of circulating insulin produces a subnormal glucose-uptake response in muscle, liver, and adipose tissues; thought to be a metabolic consequence of obesity.

integrated pest management (IPM) management of pests using a combination of natural and biological controls and minimal or no application of pesticides.

intensity in exercise, the degree of effort required to perform a given physical activity.

intermittent fasting a pattern of consuming no or little food energy during 14 or more hours in a 24-hour day, interspersed with days of normal eating. Alternate-day fasts involve fasting every other day; other regimens call for fasting on two or three days per week. Modified fasts allow consumption of 20 to 25 percent of a person's energy need on fasting days.

intervention studies studies of populations in which observation is accompanied by experimental manipulation of some population members—for example, a study in which half of the subjects (the *experimental subjects*) follow diet advice to reduce fat intakes, while the other half (the *control subjects*) do not, and both groups' heart health is monitored.

intestine the body's long, tubular organ of digestion and the site of nutrient absorption.

intoxication a condition of diminished mental and physical ability, hyperexcitability, or stupor induced by intake of alcohol or other drug; a state of physical harm caused by a toxin; poisoning.

intracellular fluid fluid residing inside the cells that provides the medium for cellular reactions.

intrinsic factor a factor made by the stomach that is necessary for absorption of vitamin B_{12}.

invert sugar a mixture of glucose and fructose formed by the splitting of sucrose in an industrial process. Sold only in liquid form and sweeter than sucrose, invert sugar forms during certain cooking procedures and works to prevent crystallization of sucrose in soft candies and sweets.

ions (EYE-ons) electrically charged particles, such as sodium (positively charged) or chloride (negatively charged).

iron deficiency the condition of having depleted iron stores, which, at the extreme, causes iron-deficiency anemia.

iron-deficiency anemia a form of anemia caused by a lack of iron and characterized by red blood cell shrinkage and color loss. Accompanying symptoms are weakness, apathy, headaches, pallor, intolerance to cold, and inability to pay attention. (For other anemias, see the index.)

iron overload the state of having more iron in the body than it needs or can handle, usually arising from a hereditary defect. Also called *hemochromatosis*.

irradiation the application of ionizing radiation to foods to reduce insect infestation or microbial contamination or to slow the ripening or sprouting process. Also called *cold pasteurization*.

irritable bowel syndrome (IBS) intermittent disturbance of bowel function, especially diarrhea or alternating diarrhea and constipation, often with abdominal cramping or bloating; managed with diet, physical activity, or relief from psychological stress. The cause is uncertain, but inflammation is often involved, and a role for altered intestinal microbiota is suspected. IBS does not permanently harm the intestines or lead to serious diseases.

IU (international units) a measure of fat-soluble vitamin activity sometimes used in food composition tables and on supplement labels.

J

jaundice (JAWN-dis) yellowing of the skin due to spillover of the bile pigment bilirubin (bill-ee-ROO-bin) from the liver into the general circulation.

K

kefir (KEE-fur) a liquid form of yogurt, based on milk, probiotic microorganisms, and flavorings.

keratin (KERR-uh-tin) the normal protein of hair and nails.

keratinization accumulation of keratin in a tissue; a sign of vitamin A deficiency.

ketone (kee-tone) **bodies** acidic, water-soluble compounds that arise during the breakdown of fat when carbohydrate is not available. Also called by the broader term *ketones*, although some of these compounds vary chemically.

ketosis (kee-TOE-sis) an undesirably high concentration of ketone bodies, such as acetone, in the blood or urine.

kidneys a pair of organs that filter wastes from the blood, make urine, and release it to the bladder for excretion from the body.

kwashiorkor (kwash-ee-OR-core, kwash-ee-or-CORE) severe malnutrition characterized by failure to grow and develop, edema, changes in the pigmentation of hair and skin, fatty liver, anemia, and apathy.

L

laboratory studies studies that are performed under tightly controlled conditions and are designed to pinpoint causes and effects. Such studies often use animals as subjects.

lactase the intestinal enzyme that splits the disaccharide lactose to monosaccharides during digestion.

lactate an energy-yielding compound produced during the breakdown of glucose in anaerobic metabolism; with training, muscles gain efficiency in using lactate as fuel.

lactation production and secretion of breast milk for the purpose of nourishing an infant.

lactoferrin (lack-toe-FERR-in) a factor in breast milk that binds iron and keeps it from supporting the growth of the infant's intestinal bacteria.

lacto-ovo vegetarian includes dairy products, eggs, vegetables, grains, legumes, fruit, and nuts; excludes flesh and seafood.

lactose a disaccharide composed of glucose and galactose; sometimes known as milk sugar (*lact* means "milk"; *ose* means "sugar").

lactose intolerance impaired ability to digest lactose due to reduced amounts of the enzyme lactase.

lactose, maltose, sucrose the disaccharides important in nutrition.

lacto-vegetarian includes dairy products, vegetables, grains, legumes, fruit, and nuts; excludes flesh, seafood, and eggs; (*lacto* means "milk.").

lapses periods of returning to old habits.

large intestine the portion of the intestine that completes the absorption process.

lean body mass the weight of the body's lean tissues; body weight, minus fat tissue.

learning disability a condition resulting in an altered ability to learn basic cognitive skills such as reading, writing, and mathematics.

leavened (LEV-end) literally, "lightened" by yeast cells, which digest some carbohydrate components of the dough and leave behind bubbles of gas that make the bread rise.

lecithin (LESS-ih-thin) a phospholipid manufactured by the liver and also found in many foods; a major constituent of cell membranes.

legumes (leg-GOOMS, LEG-yooms) plants of the bean, pea, and lentil family that have roots with nodules containing special bacteria. These bacteria can trap nitrogen from the air in the soil and convert it into a form that becomes part of the plant's seeds. The seeds are rich in protein compared with those of most other plant foods.

leptin an appetite-suppressing hormone produced in the fat cells that conveys information about body fatness to the brain; believed to be involved in the maintenance of body composition (*leptos* means "slender").

leucine one of the essential amino acids; it is of current research interest for its role in stimulating muscle protein synthesis.

levulose an older name for fructose.

license to practice permission under state or federal law, granted on meeting specified criteria, to use a certain title (such as *dietitian*) and to offer certain services. Licensed dietitians may use the initials LD after their names.

life expectancy the average number of years lived by people in a given society.

life span the maximum number of years of life attainable by a member of a species.

lignans phytochemicals present mostly in seeds, particularly flaxseed, that are converted to phytoestrogens by intestinal bacteria and are under study as possible anticancer agents.

limiting amino acid an essential amino acid that is present in dietary protein in an insufficient amount, thereby limiting the body's ability to build protein.

linoleic (lin-oh-LAY-ic) **acid** an essential polyunsaturated fatty acid of the omega-6 family.

linolenic (lin-oh-LEN-ic) **acid** an essential polyunsaturated fatty acid of the omega-3 family. The full name of linolenic acid is *alpha-linolenic acid*.

lipase (LYE-pace) any of a number of enzymes that break the chemical bonds of fats (lipids).

lipid (LIP-id) a family of organic (carbon-containing) compounds soluble in organic solvents but not in water. Lipids include triglycerides (fats and oils), phospholipids, and sterols.

lipoic (lip-OH-ic) **acid** a nonessential nutrient.

lipoproteins (LYE-poh-PRO-teens, LIH-poh-PRO-teens) clusters of lipids associated with protein, which serve as transport vehicles for lipids in blood and lymph. The major lipoproteins include chylomicrons, VLDL, LDL, and HDL.

listeriosis a serious foodborne infection that can cause severe brain infection or death in a fetus or a newborn; caused by the bacterium *Listeria monocytogenes*, which is found in soil and water.

liver a large, lobed organ that lies just under the ribs. It filters the blood, removes and processes nutrients, manufactures materials for export to other parts of the body, and destroys toxins or stores them to keep them out of the circulatory system.

longevity long duration of life.

low birthweight a birthweight of less than 5½ pounds (2,500 grams); used as a predictor of probable health problems in the newborn and as a probable indicator of poor nutrition status of the mother before and/or during pregnancy. Low-birthweight infants may be born prematurely, or, if born at full term may be small for gestational age because they suffered growth failure in the uterus.

low-density lipoproteins (LDL) lipoproteins that transport lipids from the liver to other tissues such as muscle and fat; contain a large proportion of cholesterol.

low food security reports of reduced quality, variety, or desirability of diet. Little or no indication of reduced food intake.

low-input agriculture agriculture practiced on a small scale using individualized approaches that vary with local conditions so as to minimize technological, fuel, and chemical inputs.

lutein (LOO-teen) a plant pigment of yellow hue; a phytochemical believed to play roles in eye functioning and health.

lycopene (LYE-koh-peen) a pigment responsible for the red color of tomatoes and other red-hued vegetables; a phytochemical that may act as an antioxidant in the body.

lymph (LIMF) the fluid that moves from the bloodstream into tissue spaces and then travels in its own vessels, which eventually drain back into the bloodstream.

lymphocytes (LIM-foh-sites) white blood cells that participate in the immune response.

M

macrobiotic diet a vegan diet composed chiefly of whole grains, beans, and certain vegetables; taken to extremes, macrobiotic diets can compromise nutrient status.

macronutrients another name for the energy-yielding nutrients: carbohydrate, fat, and protein.

macular degeneration a common, progressive loss of function of the part of the retina that is most crucial to focused vision. This degeneration often leads to blindness.

major minerals essential mineral nutrients required in the adult diet in amounts greater than 100 milligrams per day. Also called *macrominerals*.

malnutrition any condition caused by excess or deficient food energy or nutrient intake or by an imbalance of nutrients.

Nutrient or energy deficiencies are forms of undernutrition; nutrient or energy excesses are forms of overnutrition.

maltose a disaccharide composed of two glucose units; sometimes known as malt sugar.

malt syrup a sweetener made from sprouted barley.

maple syrup a concentrated solution of sucrose derived from the sap of the sugar maple tree. This sugar was once common but is now usually replaced by sucrose and artificial maple flavoring.

marasmic kwashiorkor a particularly lethal form of severe acute malnutrition, in which a child's dangerously reduced lean body tissue is masked by edema, making the condition harder to detect.

marasmus (ma-RAZ-mus) severe malnutrition characterized by poor growth, dramatic weight loss, loss of body fat and muscle, and apathy. From the Greek word meaning "dying away."

marginal food security one or two reported indications of problems—typically of anxiety over food sufficiency or shortage of food in the house. Little or no indication of changes in diets or food intake.

margin of safety in reference to food additives, a zone between the concentration normally used and that at which a hazard exists. For common table salt, for example, the margin of safety is one-fifth (five times the amount normally used would be hazardous).

medical foods foods specially manufactured for use by people with medical disorders and administered on the advice of a physician.

medical nutrition therapy nutrition services used in the treatment of injury, illness, or other conditions; includes assessment of nutrition status and dietary intake and corrective applications of diet, counseling, and other nutrition services.

meta-analysis a computer-driven statistical summary of evidence gathered from multiple previous studies.

metabolic syndrome a combination of characteristic factors—high fasting blood glucose or insulin resistance, central obesity, hypertension, low blood HDL cholesterol, and elevated blood triglycerides—that greatly increase a person's risk of developing CVD. Also called *insulin resistance syndrome*.

metabolic water water generated in the tissues during the chemical breakdown of the energy-yielding nutrients in foods.

metabolism the sum of all physical and chemical changes taking place in living cells; includes all reactions by which the body obtains and spends the energy from food.

metastasis (meh-TASS-ta-sis) the migration of cancer cells from the original site to invade other sites in the body. (The cancer is said to be metastasizing.)

methyl (METH-il) **groups** molecular fragments consisting of one carbon and three hydrogen atoms that, among their many roles, can alter gene expression when attached by enzymes to strands of DNA.

methylmercury any toxic compound of mercury to which a characteristic chemical structure, a methyl group, has been added, usually by bacteria in aquatic sediments. Methylmercury is readily absorbed from the intestine and causes nerve damage in people.

microbes bacteria, viruses, fungi, or other organisms invisible to the naked eye, some of which cause diseases. Also called *microorganisms*.

microbiome the collective genes of a specific bacterial sample; for example, the particular array of genes in the bacterial species present in an individual's fecal sample.

microbiota any collection of microbes; for example, all of the bacteria, fungi, and viruses present in the human digestive tract.

micronutrients nutrients required in very small amounts: the vitamins and minerals.

microvilli (MY-croh-VILL-ee, MY-croh-VILL-eye) tiny, hairlike projections on each cell of every villus that greatly expand the surface area available to trap nutrient particles and absorb them into the cells (*singular*: microvillus).

milk anemia iron-deficiency anemia caused by drinking so much milk that iron-rich foods are displaced from the diet.

minerals naturally occurring, inorganic, homogeneous substances; chemical elements.

mineral water water from a spring or well that typically contains at least 250 parts per million (ppm) of naturally occurring minerals. Minerals give water a distinctive flavor. Many mineral waters are high in sodium.

miso fermented soybean paste used in Japanese cooking. Soy products are considered to be functional foods.

myokines (MY-oh-kynz) signaling proteins secreted by working skeletal muscles that contribute to widespread beneficial effects of exercise on body systems (*myo* = muscle).

moderate drinking drinking no more than one drink per day (for a woman) or no more than two drinks per day (for a man) and behaving normally while drinking.

moderation the dietary characteristic of providing constituents within set limits, not to excess.

modified atmosphere packaging (MAP) a technique used to extend the shelf life of perishable foods; the food is packaged in a

gas-impermeable container from which air is removed or to which an oxygen-free gas mixture, such as carbon dioxide and nitrogen, is added to deprive microbes of oxygen.

molasses a thick brown syrup left over from the refining of sucrose from sugar cane. The major micronutrient in molasses is iron, a contaminant from the machinery used in processing it.

monoglycerides (mon-oh-GLISS-er-ides) products of the digestion of lipids; a monoglyceride is a glycerol molecule with one fatty acid attached (*mono* means "one"; *glyceride* means "a compound of glycerol").

monosaccharides (mon-oh-SACK-ah-rides) single sugar units (*mono* means "one"; *saccharide* means "sugar unit").

monounsaturated fats triglycerides in which most of the fatty acids have one point of unsaturation (are monounsaturated).

monounsaturated fatty acid a fatty acid containing one point of unsaturation.

MSG symptom complex the acute, temporary, and self-limiting reactions, including burning sensations or flushing of the skin with pain and headache, experienced by sensitive people upon ingesting large doses of MSG.

mucus (MYOO-cus) a slippery coating of the digestive tract lining (and other body linings) that protects the cells from exposure to digestive juices (and other destructive agents). The adjective form is *mucous* (same pronunciation). The digestive tract lining is a *mucous membrane*.

multigrain a term used on food labels to indicate a food made with more than one kind of grain. Not an indicator of a whole-grain food.

muscle endurance the ability of a muscle to contract repeatedly within a given time without becoming exhausted. This muscle characteristic develops with increasing repetition rather than increasing workload and is associated with cardiorespiratory endurance.

muscle fatigue diminished force and power of muscle contractions despite consistent or increasing conscious effort to perform a physical activity.

muscle power the efficiency of a muscle contraction, measured by force and time.

muscle strength the ability of muscles to overcome physical resistance. This muscle characteristic develops with increasing workload rather than repetition and is associated with muscle size.

mutation a permanent, heritable change in an organism's DNA.

myoglobin (MYE-oh-globe-in) the oxygen-holding protein of the muscles (*myo* means "muscle").

N

National Health and Nutrition Examination Surveys (NHANES) a program of studies designed to assess the health and nutritional status of adults and children in the United States by way of interviews and physical examinations.

natural foods a term that has no legal definition but is often used to imply wholesomeness.

naturally occurring sugars sugars that are not added to a food but are present as its original constituents, such as the sugars of fruit or milk.

nectars concentrated juice and pulp of peach, pear, or other fruit.

nephrons (NEFF-rons) the working units of the kidneys, consisting of intermeshed blood vessels and tubules.

neural tube the embryonic tissue that later forms the brain and spinal cord.

neural tube defects (NTD) a group of abnormalities of the brain and spinal cord apparent at birth and caused by interruption of the normal early development of the neural tube.

neurotoxins poisons that act on the cells of the nervous system.

neurotransmitters chemicals that are released at the end of a nerve cell when a nerve impulse arrives there. They diffuse across the gap to the next cell and alter the membrane of that second cell to either inhibit or excite it.

niacin a B vitamin needed in energy metabolism. Niacin can be eaten preformed or made in the body from tryptophan, one of the amino acids. Other forms of niacin are *nicotinic acid*, *niacinamide*, and *nicotinamide*.

niacin equivalents (NE) the amount of niacin present in food, including the niacin that can theoretically be made from its precursor tryptophan that is present in the food.

night blindness slow recovery of vision after exposure to flashes of bright light at night; an early symptom of vitamin A deficiency.

night eating syndrome a disturbance in the daily eating rhythm associated with obesity, characterized by eating more than half of the daily calories after 7 p.m., awakening frequently at night to eat, and overconsuming calories.

nitrogen balance the amount of nitrogen consumed compared with the amount excreted in a given time period.

non-celiac gluten sensitivity a poorly defined collection of digestive symptoms that improves with elimination of gluten from the diet.

nonheme iron dietary iron not associated with hemoglobin; the iron of plants and other sources.

nonnutritive sweeteners sweet-tasting synthetic or natural food additives that offer sweet flavor but with negligible or no calories per serving; also called *artificial sweeteners*, *intense sweeteners*, *noncaloric sweeteners*, and *very low-calorie sweeteners*.

norepinephrine (NOR-EP-ih-NEFF-rin) a compound related to epinephrine that helps elicit the stress response.

nori a type of seaweed popular in Asian, particularly Japanese, cooking.

nucleotide (NU-klee-oh-tied) one of the subunits of which DNA and RNA are composed.

nutraceutical a term that has no legal or scientific meaning but that is sometimes used to refer to foods, nutrients, or dietary supplements believed to have medicinal effects. Often used to sell unnecessary or unproven supplements.

nutrient claims FDA-approved food label statements that describe the nutrient levels in food. Examples: "fat free" or "less sodium."

nutrient density a measure of nutrients provided per calorie of food. A *nutrient-dense food* provides needed nutrients with relatively few calories.

nutrients components of food that are indispensable to the body's functioning. They provide energy, serve as building material, help maintain or repair body parts, and support growth. The nutrients include water, carbohydrate, fat, protein, vitamins, and minerals.

nutrition the study of the nutrients in foods and in the body; sometimes also the study of human behaviors related to food.

Nutrition and Dietetics Technician, Registered (NDTR) a dietetics professional who has completed an academic degree from an accredited college or university and an approved dietetic technician program. This professional has also passed a national examination and maintains registration through continuing professional education.

nutritional equivalents the portion sizes of various foods needed to deliver similar amounts of any of the nutrients that characterize a particular food group.

nutritional genomics the science of how food components, such as nutrients, interact with the body's genetic material.

nutritionally enhanced beverages flavored beverages that contain any of a number of nutrients, including some carbohydrate, along with protein, vitamins, minerals, herbs, or other unneeded substances. Such "enhanced waters" may not contain useful amounts of carbohydrate or electrolytes to support athletic competition or training.

Nutrition Facts on a food label, the panel of nutrition information required to appear on almost every packaged food. Grocers may also provide the information for fresh produce, meats, poultry, and seafood.

nutritionist someone who studies or advises others on nutrition, and who may or may not have an academic degree in the nutrition. In states with responsible legislation, the term applies only to people who have master of science (MS) or doctor of philosophy (PhD) degrees from properly accredited institutions.

O

obesity excess body fatness associated with increased risks of mortality and chronic diseases; a body mass index of 30 or higher.

oils lipids that are liquid at room temperature (70°F or 21°C).

olestra a noncaloric artificial fat made from sucrose and fatty acids; formerly called *sucrose polyester*. A trade name is *Olean*.

omega-3 fatty acid a polyunsaturated fatty acid with its endmost double bond three carbons from the end of the carbon chain. Linolenic acid is an example.

omega-6 fatty acid a polyunsaturated fatty acid with its endmost double bond six carbons from the end of the carbon chain. Linoleic acid is an example.

omnivorous people who eat foods of both plant and animal origin, including animal flesh.

100% whole grain see *whole grain*.

oral rehydration therapy (ORT) oral fluid replacement for children with severe diarrhea caused by infectious disease. A simple recipe for ORT: ½ L boiled water, 4 tsp sugar, ½ tsp salt.

organic carbon containing. Four of the six classes of nutrients are organic: carbohydrate, fat, protein, and vitamins. Organic compounds include only those made by living things and do not include compounds such as carbon dioxide, diamonds, and a few carbon salts.

organic foods to be labeled organic, foods must meet strict USDA production regulations; in chemistry, however, all foods are made mostly of organic (carbon-containing) compounds.

organic gardens gardens grown with techniques of *sustainable agriculture*, such as using fertilizers made from composts (decayed organic materials) and introducing predatory insects to control pests, in ways that have minimal impact on soil, water, and air quality.

organosulfur compounds a large group of phytochemicals containing the mineral sulfur.

Organosulfur phytochemicals are responsible for the pungent flavors and aromas of foods belonging to the onion, leek, chive, shallot, and garlic family and are thought to stimulate cancer defenses in the body.

organs discrete structural units made of tissues that perform specific jobs. Examples are the heart, liver, and brain.

osteomalacia (OS-tee-o-mal-AY-shuh) the adult expression of vitamin D–deficiency disease, characterized by an overabundance of unmineralized bone protein (*osteo* means "bone"; *mal* means "bad"). Symptoms include bending of the spine and bowing of the legs.

osteopenia (OS-tee-oh-PEE-nee-ah) a condition of low bone mass that often progresses to osteoporosis.

osteoporosis (OSS-tee-oh-pore-OH-sis) a reduction of the bone mass of older people in which the bones become porous and fragile (*osteo* means "bones"; *poros* means "porous") ; also known as *adult bone loss*.

outbreak two or more cases of a disease arising from an identical organism acquired from a common food source within a limited time frame. Government agencies track and investigate outbreaks of foodborne illnesses, but tens of millions of individual cases go unreported each year.

outcrossing the unintended breeding of a domestic crop with a related wild species.

oven-safe thermometer a thermometer designed to remain in the food to give constant readings during cooking.

overload an extra physical demand placed on the body; an increase in the frequency, duration, or intensity of an activity. A principle of training is that for a body system to improve, it must be worked at frequencies, durations, or intensities that increase by increments.

overweight body weight above a healthy weight; BMI 25 to 29.9.

ovo-vegetarian includes eggs, vegetables, grains, legumes, fruit, and nuts, and excludes flesh, seafood, and milk products; *ovo* means "egg").

ovum the egg, produced by the mother, that unites with a sperm from the father to produce a new individual.

oxidants compounds (such as oxygen itself) that oxidize other compounds. Compounds that prevent oxidation are called *antioxidants*, whereas those that promote it are called *prooxidants* (*anti* means "against"; *pro* means "for").

oxidation interaction of a compound with oxygen; in this case, a damaging effect by a chemically reactive form of oxygen.

oxidative stress a theory of disease causation involving cell and tissue damage that arises when free radical reactions exceed the capacity of antioxidants to quench them.

oyster shell a product made from the powdered shells of oysters that is sold as a calcium supplement but is not well absorbed by the digestive system.

P

palmitic acid a 16-carbon saturated fatty acid found in tropical palm oil, among other foods. Palmitic acid intake is associated with atrial fibrillation, a dangerous form of irregular heartbeat.

pancreas a gland that produces the hormones insulin and glucagon, which regulate blood glucose concentrations. It also produces digestive enzymes, which it releases through a duct into the small intestine.

pancreatic juice fluid secreted by the pancreas that contains both enzymes to digest carbohydrates, fats, and proteins and sodium bicarbonate, an acid-neutralizing agent.

pantothenic (PAN-to-THEN-ic) **acid** a B vitamin and part of a critical coenzyme needed in energy metabolism, among other roles.

partial vegetarian a term sometimes used to mean an eating style that includes seafood, poultry, eggs, dairy products, vegetables, grains, legumes, fruit, and nuts; excludes or strictly limits certain meats, such as red meats. Also called *flexitarian*.

pasteurization the treatment of milk, juices, or eggs with heat sufficient to kill certain pathogenic (disease-causing) microbes commonly transmitted through these foods; not a sterilization process. Pasteurized products retain bacteria that cause spoilage.

pathogens bacteria, viruses, fungi, and other microbes capable of causing illness. *Pathogenic* is the adjective form.

PCBs (polychlorinated biphenyls) stable oily synthetic chemicals, once used in hundreds of U.S. industrial operations, that persist today in underwater sediments and contaminate fish and shellfish. Now banned from use in the U.S, PCBs circulate globally from areas where they are still in use. PCBs cause cancer, nervous system damage, immune dysfunction, and a number of other serious health effects.

peak bone mass the highest bone density attained by an individual; developed during the first three decades of life.

pellagra (pell-AY-gra) the niacin-deficiency disease (*pellis* means "skin"; *agra* means "rough"). Symptoms include the "4 Ds": diarrhea, dermatitis, dementia, and, ultimately, death.

peptide bond a bond that connects one amino acid with another, forming a link in a protein chain. A peptide is a strand of amino acids.

performance nutrition an area of nutrition science that pertains to maximizing physical performance in athletes, firefighters, military personnel, and others who must perform at high levels of physical ability. Also called *sports nutrition*.

peripheral artery disease any disease or disorder that affects the peripheral arteries, those that carry blood to the body's organs other than the heart. See also *coronary artery disease*.

peristalsis (per-ri-STALL-sis) the wavelike muscular squeezing of the esophagus, stomach, and small intestine that pushes their contents along.

pernicious (per-NISH-us) anemia a vitamin B_{12}–deficiency disease, caused by lack of intrinsic factor and characterized by large, immature red blood cells and damage to the nervous system (*pernicious* means "highly injurious or destructive").

persistent of a stubborn or enduring nature; with respect to food contaminants, the quality of remaining unaltered and unexcreted in plant foods or in the bodies of animals and human beings.

pesticides chemicals used to control insects, diseases, weeds, fungi, and other pests on crops and around animals. Used broadly, the term includes *herbicides* (to kill weeds), *insecticides* (to kill insects), and *fungicides* (to kill fungi).

pH a measure of acidity on a point scale. A solution with a pH of 1 is a strong acid; a solution with a pH of 7 is neutral; a solution with a pH of 14 is a strong base.

phenylketonuria (PKU) an inborn error of metabolism that interferes with the body's handling of phenylalanine (from dietary protein) and, left untreated, results in serious harm to the brain and nervous system.

phospholipids (FOSS-foh-LIP-ids) one of the three main classes of dietary lipids. These lipids are similar to triglycerides, but each has a phosphorus-containing acid in place of one of the fatty acids. Phospholipids are present in all cell membranes.

photosynthesis the process by which green plants make carbohydrates from carbon dioxide and water using the green pigment chlorophyll to capture the sun's energy (*photo* means "light"; *synthesis* means "making").

physical activity bodily movement produced by muscle contractions that substantially increase energy expenditure.

phytates (FYE-tates) compounds present in plant foods (particularly whole grains) that bind iron and may prevent its absorption.

phytochemicals (FYE-toe-KEM-ih-cals) bioactive compounds in plant-derived foods (*phyto*, pronounced FYE-toe, means "plant").

phytoestrogens (FYE-toe-ESS-troh-gens) phytochemicals structurally similar to the female sex hormone estrogen. Phytoestrogens weakly mimic estrogen or modulate hormone activity in the human body.

pica (PIE-ka) a craving and intentional consumption of nonfood substances. Also known as *geophagia* (gee-oh-FAY-gee-uh) when referring to clay eating and *pagophagia* (pag-oh-FAY-gee-uh) when referring to ice craving (*geo* means "earth"; *pago* means "frost"; *phagia* means "to eat").

placebo a sham treatment often used in scientific studies; an inert, harmless medication. The *placebo effect* is the healing effect that the act of treatment, rather than the treatment itself, often has.

placenta (pla-SEN-tuh) the organ of pregnancy in which maternal blood and fetal blood circulate in close proximity and exchange nutrients and oxygen (flowing into the fetus) and wastes (picked up by the mother's blood).

plant pesticides substances produced within plant tissues that kill or repel attacking organisms.

plant sterols phytochemicals that resemble cholesterol in structure but that lower blood cholesterol, possibly by interfering with cholesterol absorption in the intestine. Plant sterols include sterol esters and stanol esters, formerly called *phytosterols*.

plaques (placks; *singular*, plaque) mounds of lipid material mixed with smooth muscle cells and calcium that develop in the artery walls in atherosclerosis (*placken* means "patch"). The same word is also used to describe the accumulation of a different kind of deposit on teeth, which promotes dental caries.

plasma the cell-free fluid part of blood and lymph.

platelets tiny cell-like fragments in the blood, important in blood clot formation (*platelet* means "little plate").

point of unsaturation a site in a molecule where the bonding is such that additional hydrogen atoms can easily be attached.

polypeptide (POL-ee-PEP-tide) a protein fragment of about 10 to 50 amino acids bonded together (*poly* means "many").

polysaccharides another term for complex carbohydrates; compounds composed of long strands of glucose units linked together (*poly* means "many"). Also called *complex carbohydrates*.

polyunsaturated fats triglycerides in which most of the fatty acids have two or more points of unsaturation (are polyunsaturated).

polyunsaturated fatty acid a fatty acid with two or more points of unsaturation.

pop-up thermometer a disposable timing device commonly used in turkeys. The center of the device contains a spring that "pops up" when food reaches the right temperature.

prebiotic a substance that may not be digestible by the host, such as fiber, but that serves as food for probiotic bacteria and thus promotes their growth.

precision medicine an emerging approach for disease prevention and treatment that takes into account individual variability in the genes, environment, and lifestyle for each person. Also called *personalized medicine*.

precursors compounds that serve as starting materials for other compounds. In nutrition, vitamin precursors are compounds that can be converted into active vitamins. Also called *provitamins*.

prediabetes a condition in which the blood glucose concentration is above normal, but not high enough to be diagnosed as diabetes; a major risk factor for diabetes and cardiovascular diseases.

preeclampsia (PRE-ee-CLAMP-see-ah) a potentially dangerous condition during pregnancy characterized by hypertension and protein in the urine.

pregame meal the meal consumed in the hours before prolonged or repeated athletic training or competition, typically designed to boost the glycogen stores of endurance athletes.

premenstrual syndrome (PMS) a cluster of symptoms that some women experience prior to and during menstruation. They include, among others, abdominal cramps, back pain, swelling, headache, painful breasts, and mood changes.

prenatal (pree-NAY-tal) before birth.

prenatal supplements nutrient supplements specifically designed to provide the nutrients needed during pregnancy—particularly folate, iron, and calcium—without excesses or unneeded constituents.

pressure ulcers damage to the skin and underlying tissues as a result of unrelieved compression and poor circulation to the area; also called *bed sores*.

prion a disease agent consisting of an unusually folded protein that disrupts normal cell functioning. Prions cannot be controlled or killed by cooking or disinfecting, and the disease they cause cannot be treated. Prevention is the only form of control.

probiotic a live microorganism that, when administered in adequate amounts, alters the bacterial colonies of the body in ways believed to confer a health benefit on the host.

problem drinking (alcohol abuse) drinking behavior that causes social, emotional, family, job-related, or other problems because of alcohol overuse; a step on the way to alcoholism.

processed foods foods subjected to any process, such as milling, alteration of texture, addition of additives, cooking, or others. Depending on the starting material and the process, a processed food may or may not be nutritious.

processed meats a general term for meat products preserved by smoking, curing, salting, or adding chemical preservatives—for example, ham, bacon, jerky, hot dogs (including chicken and turkey), luncheon meats, salami and other sausages, SPAM, and Vienna sausages.

promoters factors such as certain hormones that speed up cancer development.

proof the percentage of alcohol in a beverage; a term used on labels. Water is the main ingredient in alcoholic beverages; proof equals twice the percentage of alcohol.

prooxidant a compound that triggers reactions involving oxygen.

protease (PRO-tee-ace) any of a number of enzymes that break the chemical bonds of proteins.

proteins compounds composed of carbon, hydrogen, oxygen, and nitrogen and arranged as strands of amino acids. (Some amino acids also contain the element sulfur.)

protein-sparing action the action of carbohydrate and fat in providing energy that allows protein to be used for purposes it alone can serve.

protein turnover the continuous breakdown and synthesis of body proteins involving the recycling of amino acids.

public health nutritionist a dietitian or other person with an advanced degree in nutrition who specializes in public health nutrition.

purified water water that has been treated by distillation or other physical or chemical processes that remove dissolved solids. Because purified water contains no minerals or contaminants, it is useful for medical and research purposes.

pyloric (pye-LORE-ick) **valve** the flap of muscle tissues of the lower stomach that regulates the flow of partly digested food into the small intestine and prevents backflow. Also called *pyloric sphincter*.

R

raw sugar the first crop of crystals harvested during sugar processing. Raw sugar cannot be sold in the United States because it contains too much filth (dirt, insect fragments, and the like). Sugar sold as U.S. "raw sugar" is actually evaporated cane juice.

reaction time the interval between stimulation and response.

ready-to-use therapeutic food (RUTF) highly caloric food products offering carbohydrate, lipid, protein, and micronutrients in a soft-textured paste used to promote rapid weight gain in malnourished people, particularly children.

recombinant bovine somatotropin (so-mat-oh-TROPE-in) **(rbST)** growth hormone of cattle, which is produced for agricultural use by way of genetic engineering. A *recombinant* protein arises from genetically engineered DNA. Also called *bovine growth hormone (bGH)*.

recombinant DNA (rDNA) technology a technique of genetic modification whereby scientists directly manipulate the genes of living things; includes methods of removing genes, doubling genes, introducing foreign genes, and changing gene positions to influence the growth and development of organisms.

Recommended Dietary Allowances (RDA) nutrient intake goals for individuals; the average daily nutrient intake level that meets the needs of nearly all (97 to 98 percent) healthy people in a particular life stage and gender group.

recovery drinks flavored beverages that contain protein, carbohydrate, and often other nutrients; intended to support postexercise recovery of energy fuels and muscle tissue.

reference dose an estimate of the intake of a substance over a lifetime that is considered to be without appreciable health risk; for pesticides, the maximum amount of a residue permitted in a food. Formerly called *tolerance limit*.

refined refers to the process by which the coarse parts of food products are removed. For example, the refining of wheat into white enriched flour involves removing three of the four parts of the kernel—the chaff, the bran, and the germ—leaving only the endosperm, which is composed mainly of starch and a little protein.

refined grains grains and grain products from which the bran, germ, or other edible parts of whole grains have been removed; not a whole grain. Many refined grains are low in fiber and are enriched with vitamins, as required by U.S. regulations.

Registered Dietitian Nutritionist (RDN) food and nutrition experts who have earned at least a bachelor's degree from an accredited college or university with a program approved by the Academy of Nutrition and Dietetics. The dietitian must also serve in an approved internship or coordinated program, pass the registration examination, and maintain professional competency through continuing education. Many states also require licensing of practicing dietitians. Also called *registered dietitian (RD)*.

registration listing with a professional organization that requires specific course work, experience, and passing of an examination.

requirement the amount of a nutrient that will just prevent the development of specific deficiency signs; distinguished from the DRI value, which is a generous allowance with a margin of safety.

residues whatever remains; in the case of pesticides, those amounts that remain on or in foods when people buy and use them.

resistance training physical activity that develops muscle strength, power, endurance, and mass. Resistance can be provided by free weights, weight machines, other objects, or the person's own body weight. Also called *weight training*, *resistance exercise*, or *strength exercise*.

resistant starch the fraction of starch in a food that is digested slowly, or not at all, by human enzymes.

responsive feeding an interactive feeding process in which a young child signals hunger and satiety vocally, through facial expressions, and through motor actions; the caregiver recognizes these cues and responds promptly in an emotionally supportive and developmentally appropriate manner. In this way, the child experiences a predictable response to hunger and satiety signals that supports healthy eating behaviors.

resveratrol (rez-VER-ah-trol) a phytochemical of grapes under study for potential health benefits.

retina (RET-in-uh) the layer of light-sensitive nerve cells lining the back of the inside of the eye.

retinol one of the active forms of vitamin A made from beta-carotene in animal and human bodies; an antioxidant nutrient. Other active forms are *retinal* and *retinoic acid*.

retinol activity equivalents (RAE) a new measure of the vitamin A activity of beta-carotene and other vitamin A precursors that reflects the amount of retinol that the body will derive from a food containing vitamin A precursor compounds.

rhodopsin (roh-DOP-sin) the light-sensitive pigment of the cells in the retina; it contains vitamin A (*opsin* means "visual protein").

riboflavin (RIBE-o-flay-vin) a B vitamin active in the body's energy-releasing mechanisms.

rickets the vitamin D–deficiency disease in children; characterized by abnormal growth of bone and manifested in bowed legs or knock-knees, outward-bowed chest deformity (pigeon chest), and knobs on the ribs.

risk factors traits, conditions, or lifestyle habits that increase people's chances of developing diseases; factors known to be correlated with diseases but not proven to be causal.

RNA (ribonucleic acid) cellular nucleic acids that play key roles in the process and control of protein synthesis.

S

safety the practical certainty that injury will not result from the use of a product or substance.

salts compounds composed of charged particles (ions). An example is potassium chloride (K^+Cl^-).

sarcopenia (SAR-koh-PEE-nee-ah) age-related loss of skeletal muscle mass, muscle strength, and muscle function.

satiation (SAY-she-AY-shun) the perception of fullness that builds throughout a meal, eventually reaching the degree of fullness and satisfaction that halts eating. Satiation generally determines how much food is consumed at one sitting.

satiety (sah-TIE-eh-tee) the feeling of fullness or satisfaction that people experience after meals. Satiety generally determines the length of time between meals.

saturated fats triglycerides in which most of the fatty acids are saturated.

saturated fatty acid a fatty acid carrying the maximum possible number of hydrogen atoms (having no points of unsaturation). A saturated fat is a triglyceride with three saturated fatty acids.

screen time sedentary time spent using an electronic device, such as a television, computer, or video game player.

scurvy the vitamin C–deficiency disease.

selective breeding a technique of genetic modification whereby organisms are chosen for reproduction based on their desirability for human purposes, such as high growth rate, high food yield, or disease resistance, with the intention of retaining or enhancing these characteristics in their offspring.

self-efficacy a person's belief in his or her ability to succeed in an undertaking.

senile dementia the loss of brain function beyond the normal loss of physical adeptness and memory that occurs with aging.

serotonin (SER-oh-TONE-in) a compound related in structure to (and made from) the amino acid tryptophan, with the help of vitamin B_6. It serves as one of the brain's principal neurotransmitters.

set-point theory a theory stating that the body's regulatory controls tend to maintain a particular body weight (the set point) over time, counteracting efforts to lose weight by dieting.

severe acute malnutrition (SAM) life-threatening malnutrition caused by recent severe food restriction; characterized in children by underweight for height (wasting).

Shiga toxin any of a group of protein toxins produced as certain bacteria strains multiply; when absorbed Shiga toxins cause severe illness.

shortening a semisolid fat made from vegetable oil commonly used for frying foods, or in baked goods to achieve a "short," or flaky, texture.

side chain the unique chemical structure attached to the backbone of each amino acid that distinguishes one amino acid from another.

simple carbohydrates sugars, including both single sugar units and linked pairs of sugar units. The basic sugar unit is a molecule containing six carbon atoms, together with oxygen and hydrogen atoms.

single-use temperature indicator a disposable instant-read thermometer that changes color to indicate temperature. This type is often used in commercial food establishments to eliminate cross-contamination.

skinfold test measurement of the thickness of a fold of skin and subcutaneous fat on the back of the arm (over the triceps muscle), below the shoulder blade (subscapular), or in other places, using a caliper; also called *fatfold test*.

small intestine the 20-foot length of small-diameter intestine, below the stomach and above the large intestine, which is the major site of food digestion and nutrient absorption.

smoking point the temperature at which fat gives off an acrid blue gas.

SNP (snip) a type of genetic variation involving a single changed nucleotide. The letters SNP stand for *single nucleotide polymorphism*.

soft water water with a high sodium concentration.

solid fats fats that are high in saturated fatty acids and usually solid at room temperature. Solid fats are found naturally in most animal foods and tropical oils, and also arise when vegetable oils are hydrogenated.

soluble fibers food components that readily dissolve in water, become viscous, and often impart gummy or gel-like characteristics to foods. An example is pectin from fruit, which is used to thicken jellies.

solvent a substance that dissolves another and holds it in solution.

soy milk a milklike beverage made from soybeans, claimed to be a functional food. Soy drinks should be fortified with vitamin A, vitamin D, riboflavin, and calcium to approach the nutritional equivalency of milk.

Special Supplemental Nutrition Program for Women, Infants, and Children (WIC) a USDA program offering low-income pregnant and lactating women and those with infants or preschool children coupons redeemable for specific foods that supply the nutrients deemed most necessary for growth and development.

sphincter (SFINK-ter) a circular muscle surrounding, and able to constrict, a body opening.

spina bifida (SPY-na BIFF-ih-duh) one of the most common types of neural tube defects, in which gaps occur in the bones of the spine. Often the spinal cord bulges and protrudes through the gaps, resulting in a number of motor and other impairments.

sports drinks flavored beverages designed to help athletes replace fluids and electrolytes and to provide carbohydrate before, during, and after physical activity, particularly endurance activities.

spring water water originating from an underground spring or well. It may be bubbly (carbonated) or "flat" or "still," meaning not carbonated. Brand names that include words such as "Spring" and "Pure" do not ensure that the water comes from a spring.

staple foods foods used frequently or daily—for example, rice (in East and Southeast Asia) or potatoes (in Ireland). Many of these foods are sufficiently nutritious to provide a foundation for a healthful diet.

starch a plant polysaccharide composed of glucose. After cooking, starch is highly digestible by human beings; raw starch often resists digestion.

stearic acid an 18-carbon saturated fatty acid found in most animal fats. Its role in heart disease is under study.

stem cell an undifferentiated cell that can mature into any of a number of specialized cell types. A stem cell of bone marrow may mature into one of many kinds of blood cells, for example.

sterols (STEER-alls) one of the three main classes of dietary lipids. Sterols have a structure similar to that of cholesterol.

stomach a muscular, elastic, pouchlike organ of the digestive tract that grinds and churns swallowed food and mixes it with acid and enzymes, forming chyme.

stone-ground refers to a milling process using limestone to grind any grain, including refined grains, into flour.

stone-ground flour flour made by grinding kernels of grain between heavy wheels made of limestone, a kind of rock derived from the shells and bones of marine animals. As the stones scrape together, bits of the limestone mix with the flour, enriching it with calcium.

stroke the shutting off of the blood flow to a part of the brain by a thrombus, an embolus, or the bursting of a blood vessel; these events are termed *cerebral thrombosis*, *cerebral embolism*, and *cerebral hemorrhage*, respectively. (The *cerebrum* is part of the brain.)

stroke volume the volume of oxygenated blood ejected from the heart toward body tissues at each beat.

structural proteins non-enzyme proteins of cells, such as the proteins of the cell membrane and of its interior structures.

structure-function claims legal but largely unregulated statements permitted on labels of foods and dietary supplements, describing the effect of a substance on the structure or function of the body, but that omit references to diseases. Examples: "Supports immunity and digestive health" or "Builds strong bones."

stunting low height for age, indicating limited growth in children due to chronic malnutrition.

subclinical deficiency a nutrient deficiency that has no outward clinical symptoms. Also called *marginal deficiency*.

subcutaneous (sub-cue-TAY-nee-us) located beneath the skin.

subcutaneous fat fat stored directly under the skin (*sub* means "beneath"; *cutaneous* refers to the skin).

sucrose (SOO-crose) a disaccharide composed of glucose and fructose; sometimes known as table, beet, or cane sugar and, often, as simply *sugar*.

sugar alcohols sugarlike compounds in the chemical family *alcohol* derived from fruit or manufactured from sugar dextrose or other carbohydrates; sugar alcohols are absorbed more slowly than sugars, are metabolized differently, and do not elevate the risk of dental caries. Also called *polyols*.

sugars simple carbohydrates; that is, molecules of either single sugar units or pairs of those sugar units bonded together. By common usage, *sugar* most often refers to sucrose.

surface water water that comes from lakes, rivers, and reservoirs.

sushi a Japanese dish that consists of vinegar-flavored rice, seafood, and colorful vegetables, typically wrapped in seaweed. Some sushi contains raw fish; other sushi contains only cooked ingredients.

sustainable able to continue indefinitely; the use of resources in ways that maintain both natural resources and human life into the future; the use of natural resources at a pace that allows the earth to replace them and does not cause pollution to accumulate.

sustainable diet a diet with low environmental impact that contributes to food and nutrition security and to healthy life for present and future generations. Sustainable diets are protective and respectful of biodiversity and ecosystems; culturally acceptable; accessible; economically fair and affordable; and nutritionally adequate, safe, and healthy while optimizing natural and human resources.

T

tannins compounds in tea (especially black tea) and coffee that bind iron. Tannins also denature proteins.

textured vegetable protein processed soybean protein used in products formulated to look and taste like meat, fish, or poultry.

thermic effect of food the body's speeded-up metabolism in response to having eaten a meal; also called *diet-induced thermogenesis*.

thermogenesis the generation and release of body heat associated with the breakdown of body fuels. *Adaptive thermogenesis* describes adjustments in energy expenditure related to changes in environment such as cold and to physiological events such as underfeeding or trauma.

thiamin (THIGH-uh-min) a B vitamin involved in the body's use of fuels.

thrombosis the event in which a thrombus grows large enough to close off a blood vessel and gradually cuts off the blood supply to a part of the body. See also *embolism*.

thrombus a stationary blood clot in the circulatory system.

thyroxine (thigh-ROX-in) a principal peptide hormone of the thyroid gland that regulates the body's rate of energy use.

tissues groups of cells working together to perform specialized tasks. Examples are muscles, nerves, blood, and bone.

tocopherol (tuh-KOFF-er-all) a kind of alcohol. The active form of vitamin E is alpha-tocopherol.

tofu (TOE-foo) a curd made from soybeans that is rich in protein, often enriched with calcium, and variable in fat content; used in many Asian and vegetarian dishes in place of meat.

Tolerable Upper Intake Levels (UL) the highest average daily nutrient intake levels that are likely to pose no risk of toxicity to almost all healthy individuals of a particular life stage and gender group.

toxicity the ability of a substance to harm living organisms. All substances, even pure water or oxygen, can be toxic in high enough doses.

trabecular (tra-BECK-you-lar) **bone** the weblike structure composed of calcium-containing crystals inside a bone's solid outer shell. It provides strength and acts like a calcium storage bank.

trace minerals essential mineral nutrients required in the adult diet in amounts less than 100 milligrams per day. Also called *microminerals*.

training regular practice of an activity, which leads to physical adaptations of the body with improvement in flexibility, strength, and/or endurance.

trans **fats** fats that contain any number of unusual fatty acids—*trans*-fatty acids—formed during processing.

trans-**fatty acids** fatty acids with unusual shapes that can arise when hydrogens are added to the unsaturated fatty acids of polyunsaturated oils (a process known as *hydrogenation*).

transgenic organism an organism resulting from the growth of an embryonic, stem, or germ cell into which a new gene has been inserted.

triglycerides (try-GLISS-er-ides) one of the three main classes of dietary lipids and the chief form of fat in foods and in the human body. A triglyceride is made up of three units of fatty acids and one unit of glycerol (*fatty acids* and *glycerol* are defined later).

trimester a period representing one-third of the term of gestation. A trimester is about 13 to 14 weeks.

tripeptides (try-PEP-tides) protein fragments that are three amino acids long (*tri* means "three").

turbinado (ter-bih-NOD-oh) **sugar** raw sugar from which the filth has been washed; legal to sell in the United States.

type 1 diabetes the type of diabetes in which the pancreas produces no or very little insulin; often diagnosed in childhood, although some cases arise in adulthood. Formerly called *juvenile-onset* or *insulin-dependent diabetes*.

type 2 diabetes the type of diabetes in which the pancreas makes plenty of insulin but the body's cells resist insulin's action; often diagnosed in adulthood. Formerly called *adult-onset* or *non-insulin-dependent diabetes*.

U

ulcer an eroded spot in the topmost, and sometimes underlying, layers of cells that form a lining. Ulcers of the digestive tract commonly form in the esophagus, stomach, or upper small intestine.

ultra-high temperature a process of sterilizing food by exposing it for a short time to temperatures above those normally used in processing.

ultra-processed foods a term used to describe highly palatable food products of manufacturing made with industrial ingredients and additives, such as sugars, refined starches, fats, salt, imitation flavors and colors, with little or no whole food added. Examples: sugary refined breakfast cereals, candies, cookies, fried chicken nuggets, potato "tots," ready-to-heat meals, snack chips and cakes, and soft drinks.

umbilical (um-BIL-ih-cul) **cord** the ropelike structure through which the fetus's veins and arteries reach the placenta; the route of nourishment and oxygen into the fetus and the route of waste disposal from the fetus.

unbleached flour a beige-colored refined endosperm flour with texture and nutritive qualities that approximate those of regular white flour.

underweight body weight below a healthy weight; BMI below 18.5.

unsaturated fatty acid a fatty acid that lacks some hydrogen atoms and has one or more points of unsaturation. An unsaturated fat is a triglyceride that contains one or more unsaturated fatty acids.

urban legends stories, usually false, that may travel rapidly throughout the world via the Internet, gaining the appearance of validity solely on the basis of repetition.

urea (yoo-REE-uh) the principal nitrogen-excretion product of protein metabolism; generated mostly by removal of amine groups from unneeded amino acids or from amino acids being sacrificed for energy.

uterus (YOO-ter-us) the womb, the muscular organ within which the infant develops before birth.

V

variety the dietary characteristic of providing a wide selection of foods—the opposite of monotony.

vegan includes only food from plant sources: vegetables, grains, legumes, fruit, seeds, and nuts. Also called strict vegetarian.

vegetarian includes plant-based foods and eliminates some or all animal-derived foods.

vegetarians people who exclude from their diets animal flesh and possibly other animal products such as milk, cheese, and eggs.

veins blood vessels that carry blood, with the carbon dioxide it has collected, from the tissues back to the heart.

very-low-density lipoproteins (VLDL) lipoproteins that transport triglycerides and other lipids from the liver to various tissues in the body.

very low food security reports of multiple indications of disrupted eating patterns and reduced food intake.

villi (VILL-ee, VILL-eye) fingerlike projections of the sheets of cells lining the intestinal tract. The villi make the surface area much greater than it would otherwise be (*singular*: villus).

visceral fat fat stored within the abdominal cavity in association with the internal abdominal organs; also called *intra-abdominal fat* or *visceral adipose tissue*.

viscous (VISS-cuss) having a sticky, gummy, or gel-like consistency that flows relatively slowly.

vitamin B$_{12}$ a B vitamin that helps to convert folate to its active form and also helps maintain the sheath around nerve cells. The vitamin's scientific name, not often used, is *cyanocobalamin*.

vitamin B$_6$ a B vitamin needed in protein metabolism. Its three active forms are *pyridoxine*, *pyridoxal*, and *pyridoxamine*.

vitamins organic compounds that are vital to life and indispensable to body functions but that are needed only in minute amounts; essential, noncaloric nutrients.

vitamin water bottled water with a few vitamins added; does not replace vitamins from a balanced diet and may worsen overload in people receiving vitamins from enriched food, supplements, and other enriched products such as "energy" bars.

VO$_{2max}$ the maximum rate of oxygen consumption by an individual (measured at sea level).

voluntary activities intentional activities (such as walking, sitting, or running) conducted by voluntary muscles.

W

waist circumference a measurement of abdominal girth that indicates visceral fatness.

wasting the progressive, relentless loss of the body's tissues that accompanies certain diseases and shortens survival time; in malnutrition, thinness for height, indicating recent rapid weight loss or failure to gain, often from severe acute malnutrition.

water balance the balance between water intake and water excretion, which keeps the body's water content constant.

water intoxication a dangerous dilution of the body's fluids resulting from excessive ingestion of plain water. Symptoms are headache, muscular weakness, mental confusion, seizures, and coma; fatalities can occur.

water stress the pressure placed on water resources by human activities such as municipal water supplies, industries, power plants, and agricultural irrigation.

wean to gradually replace breast milk with infant formula or other foods.

weight cycling repeated rounds of weight loss and subsequent regain that may pose health risks; also called *yo-yo dieting*.

Wernicke-Korsakoff (VER-nik-ee KOR-sah-koff) **syndrome** a cluster of symptoms involving nerve damage arising from a deficiency of the vitamin thiamin in alcoholism. Characterized by mental confusion, disorientation, memory loss, jerky eye movements, and staggering gait.

wheat bread bread made with any wheat flour, including refined enriched white flour.

wheat flour any flour made from wheat, including refined white flour.

whey (way) the watery part of milk, a by-product of cheese production. Once discarded as waste, whey is now recognized as a high-quality protein source for human consumption.

white flour an endosperm flour that has been refined and bleached for maximum softness and whiteness.

white sugar granulated sucrose, produced by dissolving, concentrating, and recrystallizing raw sugar. Also called *table sugar*.

white wheat a wheat variety developed to be paler in color than common red wheat (most familiar flours are made from red wheat). White wheat is similar to red wheat in carbohydrate, protein, and other nutrients, but it lacks the dark and bitter, but potentially beneficial, phytochemicals of red wheat.

whole foods milk and milk products; meats and similar foods such as fish and poultry; vegetables, including dried beans and peas; fruit; and grains. These foods are generally considered to form the basis of a nutritious diet. Also called *basic foods*.

100% whole grain a label term for food in which the grain is entirely whole grain, with no added refined grains.

whole grains grains or foods made from them that contain all the parts and naturally occurring nutrients of the entire grain seed, except the inedible husk.

whole-wheat flour flour made from whole-wheat kernels; a whole-grain flour. Also called *graham flour*.

world food supply the quantity of food, including stores from previous harvests, available to the world's people at a given time.

World Health Organization (WHO) an agency of the United Nations charged with improving human health and preventing or controlling diseases in the world's people.

X

xerophthalmia (ZEER-ahf-THALL-me-uh) progressive hardening of the cornea of the eye in advanced vitamin A deficiency that can lead to blindness (*xero* means "dry"; *ophthalm* means "eye").

xerosis (zeer-OH-sis) drying of the cornea; a symptom of vitamin A deficiency.

Z

zygote (ZYE-goat) the product of the union of ovum and sperm; a fertilized ovum.

Index

Stand-alone page letters A–E refer to the tables beginning after the index. The page numbers preceded by A through H are appendix page numbers. Bold-faced page numbers indicate definitions. Terms are also defined in the glossary. Page numbers followed by *n* indicate footnotes, by *t* indicate tables, and by *f* indicate figures.

Fatty acids (continued)
  melting point/fat hardness, 150
  monounsaturated, 149, 149f, 150f
  physical activity, 375f
  polyunsaturated, 149, 149f, 150f
  saturated (See Saturated fatty acids)
  saturation of, 149
  unsaturated, 149
  where found?, 151
Fatty fish, 499
Fatty streaks, **408t**
Feasting and fasting, 339f
Feces, **79**
Federal assistance programs, 557, 570, 571f, 571t
Fellow of the Academy of Nutrition and Dietetics (FAND), **27t**
Female athlete triad, **358t,** 359, 359f
Fermentation, **109**
Fertility, **485**
Fetal alcohol effects (FAE), 501n
Fetal alcohol spectrum disorders (FASD), **501**
Fetal alcohol syndrome (FAS), **501,** 501f
Fetus, **485.** See also Pregnancy
Feverfew, 566t
Fewer, 54t
Fiber
  adulthood, 550
  aging, 553t
  binders, 115–116
  blood glucose control, 112–113
  bowel movements, 89
  bread, 118f
  calculation (estimating fiber intake), 115t
  can my diet have too much fiber?, 115
  cancer, 114, 428
  characteristics, sources, and health effects, 113f
  cholesterol, 112, 114f
  defined, **8, 109**
  digestion, 83t
  digestive tract cancers, 114
  digestive tract health, 113–114
  DRI, 111t
  early and middle childhood, 529, 529t
  fermentation, 122
  fruit, 133f
  grains, 133f
  heart disease, 112
  high-fiber diet/low-fiber diet, compared, 114f
  insoluble, 112
  nonpregnant, pregnant, lactating women, 489f
  protein foods, 133f

recommended intake, 111t
soluble, 111–112
stroke, 112
vegetables, 133f
weight management, 115
whole grains, 119, 119t
Fiber fermentation, 115, 122
Fiber intakes and excesses, 115–116
Fiber-rich foods, 111–115
Fiber supplements, 114
Fiber terms, 54t
Fight Bac!, 447f
Fight-or-flight reaction, **74**
Fish. See Seafood
Fish oil, 150f, 151, 416
Fitness, **366.** See also Physical activity
Fitness water, **280t**
Flavonoids, 61, **62t**
Flavor, 76
Flavored waters, **389t**
Flavoring agents, 468–471
Flaxseed, 62–63, **62t**
Flaxseed oil, 150f
Flexibility, **369**
Flexitarian, 212
Flooding, 577
Flour types, 116–117
Fluid and electrolyte balance, **194**–195, 196t, **281**–282
Fluorapatite, **303**
Fluoridated water, 303, 303f
Fluoride, 302–303
  deficiency, 303
  infant, 509f
  overview, 306t
  roles of, in body, 303
  sources, 303
  toxicity, 303
Fluorosis, **303,** 303f, 306t
FMSA. See Food Safety Modernization Act (FSMA)
Foam cells, **408t**
FODMAP, 90n
Folacin, 257t. See also Folate
Folate, 248–250
  adult male vs. 5-month-old infant, 507f
  alcohol, and, 102
  birth defects, 248–249, 249f
  bread, 118f
  deficiency, 248, 257t
  defined, **248**
  dietary folate equivalent (DFE), 250
  food sources, 249, 250, 261t
  nonpregnant, pregnant, lactating women, 489f
  pregnancy, 490–492
  recommended intakes, 249, 250

summary/review, 250, 257t
toxicity, 249, 257t
Folate deficiency, 248, 257t
Folate toxicity, 249, 257t
Folic acid, 249, 257t. See also Folate
Food
  aroma, 76
  canned, 244
  colorful, 225
  competitive, 542
  complementary, 512
  cultural and social meanings, 12
  defined, **2**
  ethnic food choices, 46f
  fast (See Fast foods)
  flavor, 76
  fried, 427
  glycemic index (GI), 129–130, 130t
  "green" choices, 582–583
  joys of eating, 38
  plant-derived, 5
  restaurants (See Restaurant food)
  safety (See Food safety)
  whole (See Whole foods)
Food additives, 466–472
  artificial sweeteners, 468–470, 470f
  examples, 467t
  flavoring agents, 468–471
  functions, 467t
  incidental additives, 471–472
  microwave packages, 472
  monosodium glutamate (MSG), 470–471
  nitrites, 468
  regulations, 466–468
  salt and sugar, 468
  sulfites, 468
Food allergies, 514, 537–539
Food allergy warning label, 538f
Food and activity diary, 354f
Food and Agriculture Organization (FAO), 442t
Food and Drug Administration (FDA), 442t
  areas of concern, 441
  folic acid, 249
  foodborne illness, 441
  genetically engineered salmon, 480
  MedWatch, 265n
  pure powdered caffeine, 564
  quackery, 23n
  refrigerator and freezer storage chart, 580t
  seafood, 164
  sodium, 290
Food antigens, 537
Food assistance programs, 494, 570–572
Food aversion, **539**

Food banks, **571**
Food choices, 9–13
  cultural and social meanings of food, 12–13
  ethnic foods, 46f
  factors to consider, 13
  glossary of food types, 9, 10t
  nutritious foods, 11–12
  why people choose foods?, 12–13
Food combinations and digestion, 82
Food composition databases, 259n, 383n
Food contaminant, **464**–465, 466t
Food crisis, **568**
Food deserts, **335**
Food Feature boxes
  behavior modification, 354–355
  calcium requirements, 307–309
  DASH diet (preventive medicine), 431–432
  defensive dining, 171–175
  finding carbohydrates in foods, 132–136
  how to choose foods to meet vitamin needs, 259–261
  how to get enough nutrients, 20–21
  mealtimes with infants, 516
  nutrient-dense/less-nutrient-dense foods, 56–58
  performance diet, 392–395
  protein intake, 207–210
  real-life challenges in food safety, 472–474
  singlehood, 558, 559t
Food group plan, **39.** See also USDA Eating Patterns
Food groups, 39–42. See also individual subentries
  fruit, 40f
  grains, 40f, 42
  milk and milk products, 41f
  protein foods, 41f, 42
  vegetables, 39, 40f
Food Information Hotline, 451n
Food insecurity, 569t. See also U.S. food insecurity
Food intake (hunger, appetite, satiety)
  definitions, 328
  did my stomach shrink?, 330–331
  factors affecting appetite, 329–330
  "go signals," 328–330
  leptin, 331, 331f
  overview, 329f
  satiation, 330
  satiety, 331
  "stop" signals, 330

Dietary Reference Intakes (DRI)

The Dietary Reference Intakes (DRI) include two sets of values that serve as goals for nutrient intake—Recommended Dietary Allowances (RDA) and Adequate Intakes (AI). The RDA reflect the average daily amount of a nutrient considered adequate to meet the needs of most healthy people. If there is insufficient evidence to determine an RDA, an AI is set. AI values are more tentative than RDA, but both may be used as goals for nutrient intakes. (Chapter 2 provides more details.)

In addition to the values that serve as goals for nutrient intakes (presented in the tables on these two pages), the DRI include a set of values called Tolerable Upper Intake Levels (UL). The UL represent the maximum amount of a nutrient that appears safe for most healthy people to consume on a regular basis. Turn the page for a listing of the UL for selected vitamins and minerals.

Estimated Energy Requirements (EER), Recommended Dietary Allowances (RDA), and Adequate Intakes (AI) for Water, Fiber, and the Energy Nutrients

Age (yr)	Reference BMI (kg/m²)	Reference Height cm (in)	Reference Weight kg (lb)	Water[a] AI (L/day)	Energy EER[b] (cal/day)	Carbohydrate RDA (g/day)	Total Fiber AI (g/day)	Total Fat AI (g/day)	Linoleic Acid[d] AI (g/day)	Linolenic Acid[d,c] AI (g/day)	Protein RDA (g/day)[d]	Protein RDA (g/kg/day)
Males												
0–0.5	—	62 (24)	6 (13)	0.7[e]	570	60	—	31	4.4	0.5	9.1	1.52
0.5–1	—	71 (28)	9 (20)	0.8[f]	743	95	—	30	4.6	0.5	11	1.20
1–3[g]	—	86 (34)	12 (27)	1.3	1046	130	19	—	7	0.7	13	1.05
4–8[g]	15.3	115 (45)	20 (44)	1.7	1742	130	25	—	10	0.9	19	0.95
9–13	17.2	144 (57)	36 (79)	2.4	2279	130	31	—	12	1.2	34	0.95
14–18	20.5	174 (68)	61 (134)	3.3	3152	130	38	—	16	1.6	52	0.85
19–30	22.5	177 (70)	70 (154)	3.7	3067[h]	130	38	—	17	1.6	56	0.80
31–50	22.5[i]	177 (70)[i]	70 (154)[i]	3.7	3067[h]	130	38	—	17	1.6	56	0.80
>50	22.5[i]	177 (70)[i]	70 (154)[i]	3.7	3067[h]	130	30	—	14	1.6	56	0.80
Females												
0–0.5	—	62 (24)	6 (13)	0.7[e]	520	60	—	31	4.4	0.5	9.1	1.52
0.5–1	—	71 (28)	9 (20)	0.8[f]	676	95	—	30	4.6	0.5	11	1.20
1–3[g]	—	86 (34)	12 (27)	1.3	992	130	19	—	7	0.7	13	1.05
4–8[g]	15.3	115 (45)	20 (44)	1.7	1642	130	25	—	10	0.9	19	0.95
9–13	17.4	144 (57)	37 (81)	2.1	2071	130	26	—	10	1.0	34	0.95
14–18	20.4	163 (64)	54 (119)	2.3	2368	130	26	—	11	1.1	46	0.85
19–30	21.5	163 (64)	57 (126)	2.7	2403[j]	130	25	—	12	1.1	46	0.80
31–50	21.5[i]	163 (64)[i]	57 (126)[i]	2.7	2403[j]	130	25	—	12	1.1	46	0.80
>50	21.5[i]	163 (64)[i]	57 (126)[i]	2.7	2403[j]	130	21	—	11	1.1	46	0.80
Pregnancy												
1st trimester				3.0	+0	175	28	—	13	1.4	46	0.80
2nd trimester				3.0	+340	175	28	—	13	1.4	71	1.10
3rd trimester				3.0	+452	175	28	—	13	1.4	71	1.10
Lactation												
1st 6 months				3.8	+330	210	29	—	13	1.3	71	1.30
2nd 6 months				3.8	+400	210	29	—	13	1.3	71	1.30

NOTE: For all nutrients, values for infants are AI. Dashes indicate that values have not been determined.

[a]The water AI includes drinking water, water in beverages, and water in foods; in general, drinking water and other beverages contribute about 70 to 80 percent, and foods, the remainder. Conversion factors: 1 L = 33.8 fluid oz; 1 L = 1.06 qt; 1 cup = 8 fluid oz.

[b]The EER represents the average dietary energy intake that will maintain energy balance in a healthy person of a given gender, age, weight, height, and physical activity level. The values listed are based on an "active" person at the reference height and weight and at the midpoint ages for each group until age 19. Chapter 9 and Appendix H provide equations and tables to determine estimated energy requirements.

[c]The linolenic acid referred to in this table and text is the omega-3 fatty acid known as alpha-linolenic acid.

[d]The values listed are based on reference body weights.

[e]Assumed to be from human milk.

[f]Assumed to be from human milk and complementary foods and beverages. This includes approximately 0.6 L (~2½ cups) as total fluid including formula, juices, and drinking water.

[g]For energy, the age groups for young children are 1–2 years and 3–8 years.

[h]For males, subtract 10 calories per day for each year of age above 19.

[i]Because weight need not change as adults age if activity is maintained, reference weights for adults 19 through 30 years are applied to all adult age groups.

[j]For females, subtract 7 calories per day for each year of age above 19.

SOURCE: Adapted from the Dietary Reference Intakes series, National Academies Press. Copyright 1997, 1998, 2000, 2001, 2002, 2004, 2005, 2011 by the National Academy of Sciences.

Recommended Dietary Allowances (RDA) and Adequate Intakes (AI) for Vitamins

Age (yr)	Thiamin RDA (mg/day)	Riboflavin RDA (mg/day)	Niacin RDA (mg/day)[a]	Biotin AI (µg/day)	Pantothenic acid AI (mg/day)	Vitamin B$_6$ RDA (mg/day)	Folate RDA (µg/day)[b]	Vitamin B$_{12}$ RDA (µg/day)	Choline AI (mg/day)	Vitamin C RDA (mg/day)	Vitamin A RDA (µg/day)[c]	Vitamin D RDA (IU/day)[d]	Vitamin E RDA (mg/day)[e]	Vitamin K AI (µg/day)
Infants														
0–0.5	0.2	0.3	2	5	1.7	0.1	65	0.4	125	40	400	400 (10 µg)	4	2.0
0.5–1	0.3	0.4	4	6	1.8	0.3	80	0.5	150	50	500	400 (10 µg)	5	2.5
Children														
1–3	0.5	0.5	6	8	2	0.5	150	0.9	200	15	300	600 (15 µg)	6	30
4–8	0.6	0.6	8	12	3	0.6	200	1.2	250	25	400	600 (15 µg)	7	55
Males														
9–13	0.9	0.9	12	20	4	1.0	300	1.8	375	45	600	600 (15 µg)	11	60
14–18	1.2	1.3	16	25	5	1.3	400	2.4	550	75	900	600 (15 µg)	15	75
19–30	1.2	1.3	16	30	5	1.3	400	2.4	550	90	900	600 (15 µg)	15	120
31–50	1.2	1.3	16	30	5	1.3	400	2.4	550	90	900	600 (15 µg)	15	120
51–70	1.2	1.3	16	30	5	1.7	400	2.4	550	90	900	600 (15 µg)	15	120
>70	1.2	1.3	16	30	5	1.7	400	2.4	550	90	900	800 (20 µg)	15	120
Females														
9–13	0.9	0.9	12	20	4	1.0	300	1.8	375	45	600	600 (15 µg)	11	60
14–18	1.0	1.0	14	25	5	1.2	400	2.4	400	65	700	600 (15 µg)	15	75
19–30	1.1	1.1	14	30	5	1.3	400	2.4	425	75	700	600 (15 µg)	15	90
31–50	1.1	1.1	14	30	5	1.3	400	2.4	425	75	700	600 (15 µg)	15	90
51–70	1.1	1.1	14	30	5	1.5	400	2.4	425	75	700	600 (15 µg)	15	90
>70	1.1	1.1	14	30	5	1.5	400	2.4	425	75	700	800 (20 µg)	15	90
Pregnancy														
≤18	1.4	1.4	18	30	6	1.9	600	2.6	450	80	750	600 (15 µg)	15	75
19–30	1.4	1.4	18	30	6	1.9	600	2.6	450	85	770	600 (15 µg)	15	90
31–50	1.4	1.4	18	30	6	1.9	600	2.6	450	85	770	600 (15 µg)	15	90
Lactation														
≤18	1.4	1.6	17	35	7	2.0	500	2.8	550	115	1200	600 (15 µg)	19	75
19–30	1.4	1.6	17	35	7	2.0	500	2.8	550	120	1300	600 (15 µg)	19	90
31–50	1.4	1.6	17	35	7	2.0	500	2.8	550	120	1300	600 (15 µg)	19	90

NOTE: For all nutrients, values for infants are AI. The table on page Y defines units of nutrient measure.

[a]Niacin recommendations are expressed as niacin equivalents (NE), except for recommendations for infants younger than 6 months, which are expressed as preformed niacin.

[b]Folate recommendations are expressed as dietary folate equivalents (DFE).

[c]Vitamin A recommendations are expressed as retinol activity equivalents (RAE).

[d]Vitamin D recommendations are expressed as cholecalciferol and assume an absence of adequate exposure to sunlight. Pregnant or lactating girls ages 14–18 also need 15 micrograms vitamin D per day.

[e]Vitamin E recommendations are expressed as α-tocopherol.

Recommended Dietary Allowances (RDA) and Adequate Intakes (AI) for Minerals

Age (yr)	Sodium AI (mg/day)	Chloride AI (mg/day)	Potassium AI (mg/day)	Calcium RDA (mg/day)	Phosphorus RDA (mg/day)	Magnesium RDA (mg/day)	Iron RDA (mg/day)	Zinc RDA (mg/day)	Iodine RDA (µg/day)	Selenium RDA (µg/day)	Copper RDA (µg/day)	Manganese AI (mg/day)	Fluoride AI (mg/day)	Chromium AI (µg/day)	Molybdenum RDA (µg/day)
Infants															
0–0.5	120	180	400	200	100	30	0.27	2	110	15	200	0.003	0.01	0.2	2
0.5–1	370	570	700	260	275	75	11	3	130	20	220	0.6	0.5	5.5	3
Children															
1–3	1000	1500	3000	700	460	80	7	3	90	20	340	1.2	0.7	11	17
4–8	1200	1900	3800	1000	500	130	10	5	90	30	440	1.5	1.0	15	22
Males															
9–13	1500	2300	4500	1300	1250	240	8	8	120	40	700	1.9	2	25	34
14–18	1500	2300	4700	1300	1250	410	11	11	150	55	890	2.2	3	35	43
19–30	1500	2300	4700	1000	700	400	8	11	150	55	900	2.3	4	35	45
31–50	1500	2300	4700	1000	700	420	8	11	150	55	900	2.3	4	35	45
51–70	1300	2000	4700	1000	700	420	8	11	150	55	900	2.3	4	30	45
>70	1200	1800	4700	1200	700	420	8	11	150	55	900	2.3	4	30	45
Females															
9–13	1500	2300	4500	1300	1250	240	8	8	120	40	700	1.6	2	21	34
14–18	1500	2300	4700	1300	1250	360	15	9	150	55	890	1.6	3	24	43
19–30	1500	2300	4700	1000	700	310	18	8	150	55	900	1.8	3	25	45
31–50	1500	2300	4700	1000	700	320	18	8	150	55	900	1.8	3	25	45
51–70	1300	2000	4700	1200	700	320	8	8	150	55	900	1.8	3	20	45
>70	1200	1800	4700	1200	700	320	8	8	150	55	900	1.8	3	20	45
Pregnancy															
≤18	1500	2300	4700	1300	1250	400	27	12	220	60	1000	2.0	3	29	50
19–30	1500	2300	4700	1000	700	350	27	11	220	60	1000	2.0	3	30	50
31–50	1500	2300	4700	1000	700	360	27	11	220	60	1000	2.0	3	30	50
Lactation															
≤18	1500	2300	5100	1300	1250	360	10	13	290	70	1300	2.6	3	44	50
19–30	1500	2300	5100	1000	700	310	9	12	290	70	1300	2.6	3	45	50
31–50	1500	2300	5100	1000	700	320	9	12	290	70	1300	2.6	3	45	50

NOTE: For all nutrients, values for infants are AI.

Tolerable Upper Intake Levels (UL) for Vitamins

Age (yr)	Niacin (mg/day)[a]	Vitamin B6 (mg/day)[b]	Folate (µg/day)[a]	Choline (mg/day)	Vitamin C (mg/day)	Vitamin A (µg/day)[b]	Vitamin D (IU/day)	Vitamin E (mg/day)[c]
INFANTS								
0–0.5	—	—	—	—	—	600	1000 (25 µg)	—
0.5–1	—	—	—	—	—	600	1500 (38 µg)	—
CHILDREN								
1–3	10	30	300	1000	400	600	2500 (63 µg)	200
4–8	15	40	400	1000	650	900	3000 (75 µg)	300
9–13	20	60	600	2000	1200	1700	4000 (100 µg)	600
ADOLESCENTS								
14–18	30	80	800	3000	1800	2800	4000 (100 µg)	800
ADULTS								
19–70	35	100	1000	3500	2000	3000	4000 (100 µg)	1000
>70	35	100	1000	3500	2000	3000	4000 (100 µg)	1000
PREGNANCY								
≤18	30	80	800	3000	1800	2800	4000 (100 µg)	800
19–50	35	100	1000	3500	2000	3000	4000 (100 µg)	1000
LACTATION								
≤18	30	80	800	3000	1800	2800	4000 (100 µg)	800
19–50	35	100	1000	3500	2000	3000	4000 (100 µg)	1000

[a]The UL for niacin and folate apply to synthetic forms obtained from supplements, fortified foods, or a combination of the two.

[b]The UL for vitamin A applies to the preformed vitamin only.

[c]The UL for vitamin E applies to any form of supplemental α-tocopherol, fortified foods, or a combination of the two.

Tolerable Upper Intake Levels (UL) for Minerals

Age (yr)	Sodium (mg/day)	Chloride (mg/day)	Calcium (mg/day)	Phosphorus (mg/day)	Magnesium (mg/day)[d]	Iron (mg/day)	Zinc (mg/day)	Iodine (µg/day)	Selenium (µg/day)	Copper (µg/day)	Manganese (mg/day)	Fluoride (mg/day)	Molybdenum (µg/day)	Boron (mg/day)	Nickel (mg/day)	Vanadium (mg/day)
INFANTS																
0–0.5	—	—	1000	—	—	40	4	—	45	—	—	0.7	—	—	—	—
0.5–1	—	—	1500	—	—	40	5	—	60	—	—	0.9	—	—	—	—
CHILDREN																
1–3	1500	2300	2500	3000	65	40	7	200	90	1000	2	1.3	300	3	0.2	—
4–8	1900	2900	2500	3000	110	40	12	300	150	3000	3	2.2	600	6	0.3	—
9–13	2200	3400	3000	4000	350	40	23	600	280	5000	6	10	1100	11	0.6	—
ADOLESCENTS																
14–18	2300	3600	3000	4000	350	45	34	900	400	8000	9	10	1700	17	1.0	—
ADULTS																
19–50	2300	3600	2500	4000	350	45	40	1100	400	10,000	11	10	2000	20	1.0	1.8
51–70	2300	3600	2000	4000	350	45	40	1100	400	10,000	11	10	2000	20	1.0	1.8
>70	2300	3600	2000	3000	350	45	40	1100	400	10,000	11	10	2000	20	1.0	1.8
PREGNANCY																
≤18	2300	3600	3000	3500	350	45	34	900	400	8000	9	10	1700	17	1.0	—
19–50	2300	3600	2500	3500	350	45	40	1100	400	10,000	11	10	2000	20	1.0	—
LACTATION																
≤18	2300	3600	3000	4000	350	45	34	900	400	8000	9	10	1700	17	1.0	—
19–50	2300	3600	2500	4000	350	45	40	1100	400	10,000	11	10	2000	20	1.0	—

[d]The UL for magnesium applies to synthetic forms obtained from supplements or drugs only.

NOTE: A UL was not established for vitamins and minerals not listed and for those age groups listed with a dash (—) because of a lack of data, not because these nutrients are safe to consume at any level of intake. All nutrients can have adverse effects when intakes are excessive.

SOURCE: Adapted from the Dietary Reference Intakes series, National Academies Press. Copyright 1997, 1998, 2000, 2001, 2002, 2005, 2011 by the National Academy of Sciences.

Daily Values (DV) for Food Labels

The Daily Values (DV) are standards developed by the Food and Drug Administration (FDA) for use on food labels. The values are based on 2000 kcalories a day for adults and children aged 4 years and older. The proposed DV values will replace the current ones on updated Nutrition Fact panels (see Chapter 2 for food label details).

Nutrient	Current	Proposed
Vitamins		
Biotin	300 µg	30 µg
Choline	550 mg	550 mg
Folate	400 µg	400 µg DFE
Niacin	20 mg	16 mg NE
Pantothenic acid	10 mg	5 mg
Riboflavin	1.7 mg	1.3 mg
Thiamin	1.5 mg	1.2 mg
Vitamin A	1500 µg (5000 IU)	900 µg RAE
Vitamin B$_6$	2 mg	1.7 mg
Vitamin B$_{12}$	6 µg	2.4 µg
Vitamin C	60 mg	90 mg
Vitamin D	10 µg (400 IU)	20 µg
Vitamin E (α-tocopherol)	20 mg (30 IU)	15 mg
Vitamin K	80 µg	120 µg
Minerals		
Calcium	1000 mg	1300 mg
Chloride	3400 mg	2300 mg
Chromium	120 µg	35 µg
Copper	2 mg	0.9 mg
Iodine	150 µg	150 µg
Iron	18 mg	18 mg
Magnesium	400 mg	420 mg
Manganese	2 mg	2.3 mg
Molybdenum	75 µg	45 µg
Phosphorus	1000 mg	1250 mg
Potassium	3500 mg	4700 mg
Selenium	70 µg	55 µg
Sodium	2400 mg	2300 mg
Zinc	15 mg	11 mg

SOURCE: *Food and Drug Administration,* Food Labeling: Revision of the Nutrition and Supplement Facts Labels, *https://s3.amazonaws.com/public-inspection.federalregister.gov/2016-11867.pdf (pp. 903–904).*

Food Component	Amount	Calculation Factors
Fat	78 g	35% of kcalories
Saturated fat	20 g	10% of kcalories
Cholesterol	300 mg	–
Carbohydrate (total)	275 g	55% of kcalories
Fiber	28 g	14 g per 1000 kcalories
Added sugars	50 g	–
Protein	50 g	10% of kcalories

SOURCE: *Food and Drug Administration,* Food Labeling: Revision of the Nutrition and Supplement Facts Labels, *https://s3.amazonaws.com/public-inspection.federalregister.gov/2016-11867.pdf (pp. 905–906).*

GLOSSARY
NUTRIENT MEASURES

kcal: kcalories; a unit by which energy is measured (Chapter 1 provides more details).

g: grams; a unit of weight equivalent to about 0.03 ounces.

mg: milligrams; one-thousandth of a gram.

µg: micrograms; one-millionth of a gram.

IU: international units; an old measure of vitamin activity determined by biological methods (as opposed to new measures that are determined by direct chemical analyses). Many fortified foods and supplements use IU on their labels. For those still using IU, the following factors can be used for conversions.

- For vitamin A, 1 IU = 0.3 µg retinol
- For vitamin D, 1 IU = 0.05 µg cholecalciferol
- For vitamin E, 1 IU = 0.67 mg α-tocopherol

mg NE: milligrams niacin equivalents; a measure of niacin activity (Chapter 10 provides more details).

- 1 NE = 1 mg niacin
  = 60 mg tryptophan (an amino acid)

µg DFE: micrograms dietary folate equivalents; a measure of folate activity (Chapter 10 provides more details).

- 1 µg DFE = 1 µg food folate
  = 0.6 µg folic acid from fortified food or as a supplement taken with food

µg RAE: micrograms retinol activity equivalents; a measure of vitamin A activity (Chapter 11 provides more details).

- 1 µg RAE = 1 µg retinol
  = 12 µg β-carotene
  = 24 µg other vitamin A carotenoids

mmol: millimoles; one-thousanth of a mole, the molecular weight of a substance. To convert mmol to mg, multiply by the atomic weight of the substance.

- For sodium, mmol × 23 = mg Na
- For chloride, mmol × 35.5 = mg Cl
- For sodium chloride, mmol × 58.5 = mg NaCl

Body Mass Index (BMI)

Find your height along the left-hand column and look across the row until you find the number that is closest to your weight. The number at the top of that column identifies your BMI. Chapter 9 describes how BMI correlates with disease risks and defines obesity. The area shaded in blue represents healthy weight ranges.

	Under-weight	Healthy Weight						Overweight					Obese										
	(<18.5)	(18.5–24.9)						(25–29.9)					(≥30)										
	18	19	20	21	22	23	24	25	26	27	28	29	30	31	32	33	34	35	36	37	38	39	40
Height	**Body weight (pounds)**																						
4'10"	86	91	96	100	105	110	115	119	124	129	134	138	143	148	153	158	162	167	172	177	181	186	191
4'11"	89	94	99	104	109	114	119	124	128	133	138	143	148	153	158	163	168	173	178	183	188	193	198
5'0"	92	97	102	107	112	118	123	128	133	138	143	148	153	158	163	168	174	179	184	189	194	199	204
5'1"	95	100	106	111	116	122	127	132	137	143	148	153	158	164	169	174	180	185	190	195	201	206	211
5'2"	98	104	109	115	120	126	131	136	142	147	153	158	164	169	175	180	186	191	196	202	207	213	218
5'3"	102	107	113	118	124	130	135	141	146	152	158	163	169	175	180	186	191	197	203	208	214	220	225
5'4"	105	110	116	122	128	134	140	145	151	157	163	169	174	180	186	192	197	204	209	215	221	227	232
5'5"	108	114	120	126	132	138	144	150	156	162	168	174	180	186	192	198	204	210	216	222	228	234	240
5'6"	112	118	124	130	136	142	148	155	161	167	173	179	186	192	198	204	210	216	223	229	235	241	247
5'7"	115	121	127	134	140	146	153	159	166	172	178	185	191	198	204	211	217	223	230	236	242	249	255
5'8"	118	125	131	138	144	151	158	164	171	177	184	190	197	203	210	216	223	230	236	243	249	256	262
5'9"	122	128	135	142	149	155	162	169	176	182	189	196	203	209	216	223	230	236	243	250	257	263	270
5'10"	126	132	139	146	153	160	167	174	181	188	195	202	209	216	222	229	236	243	250	257	264	271	278
5'11"	129	136	143	150	157	165	172	179	186	193	200	208	215	222	229	236	243	250	257	265	272	279	286
6'0"	132	140	147	154	162	169	177	184	191	199	206	213	221	228	235	242	250	258	265	272	279	287	294
6'1"	136	144	151	159	166	174	182	189	197	204	212	219	227	235	242	250	257	265	272	280	288	295	302
6'2"	141	148	155	163	171	179	186	194	202	210	218	225	233	241	249	256	264	272	280	287	295	303	311
6'3"	144	152	160	168	176	184	192	200	208	216	224	232	240	248	256	264	272	279	287	295	303	311	319
6'4"	148	156	164	172	180	189	197	205	213	221	230	238	246	254	263	271	279	287	295	304	312	320	328
6'5"	151	160	168	176	185	193	202	210	218	227	235	244	252	261	269	277	286	294	303	311	319	328	336
6'6"	155	164	172	181	190	198	207	216	224	233	241	250	259	267	276	284	293	302	310	319	328	336	345

Body Mass Index-for-Age Percentiles: Boys and Girls, Age 2 to 20

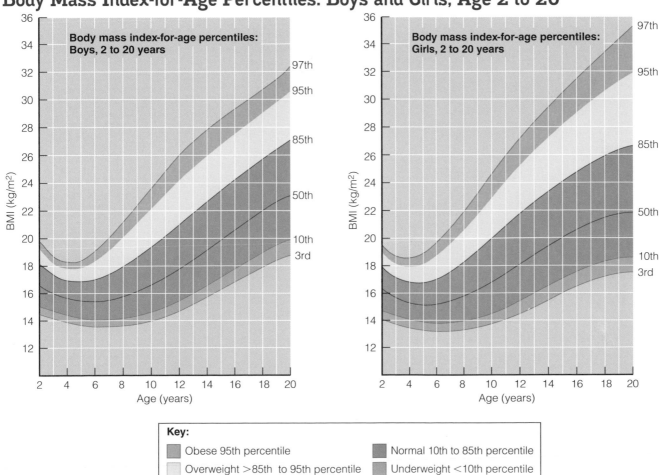

Key:

Obese 95th percentile

Overweight >85th to 95th percentile

Normal 10th to 85th percentile

Underweight <10th percentile

E

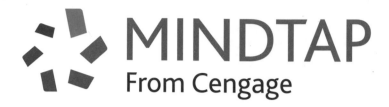

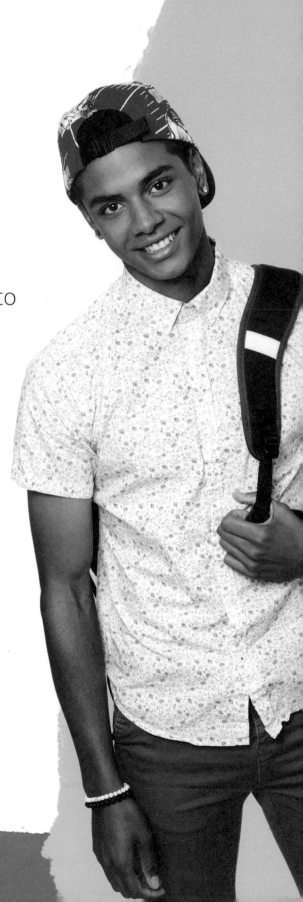